www.kanskionline.com
delivers CLINICAL OPHTHALMOLOGY: A SYSTEMATIC APPROACH 6th Edition online and more!

Thank you for purchasing
Clinical Ophthalmology: A Systematic Approach 6th Edition.
Your purchase entitles you to free online access to **www.kanskionline.com**

■ Fully searchable text
- Access by keyword, subject or index

■ Downloadable image library
- All 1800 images downloadable in PowerPoint format

■ Self-assessment questions
- Over 100 questions to test your knowledge

How to register

1. Scratch off the sticker on the right to reveal your unique PIN number

2. Connect to the internet and go to **www.kanskionline.com** for simple instructions on how to register – you'll need your PIN number and e-mail address to register

Important note: Your purchase of *Clinical Ophthalmology: A Systematic Approach*, Sixth Edition entitles you to access the website until the next edition is published, or until the current edition is no longer offered for sale by Elsevier, whichever occurs first. If the next edition is published less than a year after your purchase, you will be entitled to online access for 1 year from your date of purchase. Elsevier reserves the right to offer a suitable replacement product (such as a downloadable or CD-ROM-based electronic version) should online access to the website be discontinued.

Note
Book cannot be returned once panel is scratched off

Scratch off the sticker with care!

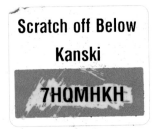

Scratch off Below

Kanski

7HQMHKH

Clinical Ophthalmology
A SYSTEMATIC APPROACH

Dedication

To the valiant Polish fighter pilots in the Battle of Britain.

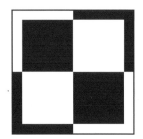

For Elsevier Butterworth-Heinemann:

Commissioning Editor: *Robert Edwards*

Development Editor: *Kim Benson*

Production Manager: *Frances Affleck*

Design: *Stewart Larking*

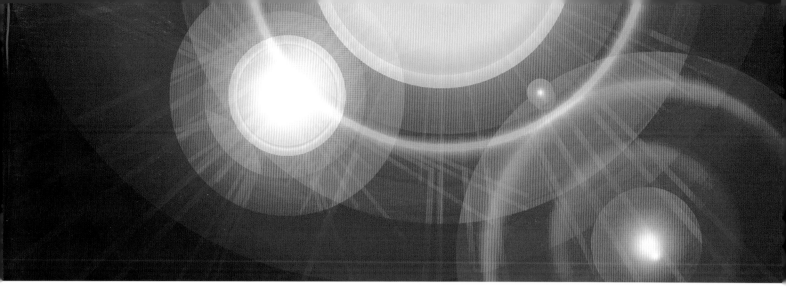

SIXTH EDITION

Clinical Ophthalmology

A SYSTEMATIC APPROACH

Jack J Kanski

MD, MS, FRCS, FRCOphth

Honorary Consultant Ophthalmic Surgeon
Prince Charles Eye Unit
King Edward VII Hospital
Windsor, UK

Photographers

Irina Gout MD, MScOphth, PhD
Kulwant Sehmi FRPS, ABIPP, AIMI
Anne Bolton BA, BIPP, DATEC

Artists

Terry R Tarrant
Phil Sidaway

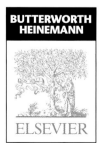

BUTTERWORTH
HEINEMANN

ELSEVIER

EDINBURGH LONDON NEW YORK OXFORD PHILADELPHIA ST LOUIS SYDNEY TORONTO 2007

BUTTERWORTH
HEINEMANN
ELSEVIER

First published 1984
Second edition 1989
Reprinted 1990 (twice), 1992, 1993
Third edition 1994
Reprinted 1995, 1996, 1997, 1998
Fourth edition 1999
Reprinted 2000, 2002
Fifth edition 2003
Reprinted 2003, 2006
Sixth edition 2007
Reprinted 2008

ISBN: 978-0-08-044969-2   Standard edition
ISBN: 978-0-08-045009-4   International edition

British Library Cataloguing in Publication Data
A catalogue record for this book is available from the British Library.

Library of Congress Cataloging in Publication Data
A catalog record for this book is available from the Library of Congress.

Note
Knowledge and best practice in this field are constantly changing. As new research and experience broaden our knowledge, changes in practice, treatment and drug therapy may become necessary or appropriate. Readers are advised to check the most current information provided (i) on procedures featured or (ii) by the manufacturer of each product to be administered, to verify the recommended dose or formula, the method and duration of administration, and contraindications. It is the responsibility of the practitioner, relying on their own experience and knowledge of the patient, to make diagnoses, to determine dosages and the best treatment for each individual patient, and to take all appropriate safety precautions. To the fullest extent of the law, neither the Publisher nor the Author assumes any liability for any injury and/or damage to persons or property arising out of or related to any use of the material contained in this book.

The Publisher

ELSEVIER
your source for books,
journals and multimedia
in the health sciences
www.elsevierhealth.com

Working together to grow
libraries in developing countries
www.elsevier.com | www.bookaid.org | www.sabre.org

ELSEVIER   BOOK AID International   Sabre Foundation

The publisher's policy is to use paper manufactured from sustainable forests

Printed in China

Contents

Preface to the sixth edition

Four years have elapsed since the publication of the fifth edition of *Clinical Ophthalmology*. Since then many advances have occurred in the speciality including the discovery of new disease processes as well as treatment modalities and diagnostic methods. This edition has therefore been completely revised and expanded to include much new material. The number of illustrations has been considerably increased so that the vast majority of clinical conditions are illustrated. The number of chapters has been increased from 20 to 24 with new chapters on examination, imaging techniques, congenital anomalies and drug-induced conditions. Emphasis is placed on understanding pathogenesis of disease processes and for the first time descriptions of histology have been included.

The aim of this book is not to replace the many excellent encyclopaedic multi-author texts and exhaustive bibliographies that are readily available in other publications but to provide the trainee with a systematic, concisely written, well-illustrated and easily assimilated single-volume text that provides basic knowledge and acts as a stepping-stone from which the reader can further expand his knowledge of ophthalmology.

JJK
Windsor 2007

Acknowledgements

I am greatly indebted to many colleagues and ophthalmic photographic departments for supplying images for this book. The source of each image is acknowledged in the legend. I would also thank my publishers, Caroline Makepeace in particular, for their support and encouragement over the years. I am very grateful to the following colleagues for reviewing the manuscript and providing many helpful suggestions:

PATHOLOGY
John Harry, FRCPath, FRCOphth
Honorary Consultant Ophthalmic Pathologist, Academic Unit of Ophthalmology, Birmingham and Midland Eye Centre, Birmingham, UK

ADNEXAL DISEASE
Andrew Pearson, MRCP, FRCOphth
Consultant Ophthalmic Surgeon, Prince Charles Eye Unit, Windsor, and Royal Berkshire Hospital, Reading, UK

STRABISMUS
John Sloper, D.Phil, FRCS, FRCOphth
Consultant Ophthalmic Surgeon, Moorfields Eye Hospital, London, UK

Ann McIntyre, DBO.T, BA (Hons)
Former Principal Orthoptist, Moorfields Eye Hospital, London, UK

EXTERNAL DISEASE
Stephen Tuft, MA, MChir, MD, FRCOphth
Consultant Ophthalmic Surgeon, Moorfields Eye Hospital, London, UK

UVEITIS AND SCLERITIS
Carlos Pavesio, MD, FRCOphth
Consultant Ophthalmic Surgeon, Moorfields Eye Hospital, London, UK

RETINAL DISEASE
Vaughan Tanner, BSc, FRCOphth
Consultant Ophthalmic Surgeon, Prince Charles Eye Unit, Windsor, and Royal Berkshire Hospital, Reading, UK

ONCOLOGY
Bertil Damato, PhD, FRCS, FRCOphth
Professor of Ophthalmology, Director Ocular Oncology Service, Royal Liverpool University Hospital, Liverpool, UK

NEUROIMAGING
Naomi Sibtain, MRCP, FRCR
Consultant Radiologist, St. Thomas' and King's College Hospitals, London, UK

CATARACT
Richard Packard, MD, FRCS, FRCOphth
Consultant Ophthalmic Surgeon, Prince Charles Eye Unit, Windsor, UK

PAEDIATRIC OPHTHALMOLOGY
Ken Nischal, FRCOphth
Consultant Ophthalmic Surgeon, Great Ormond Street Hospital for Children, London, UK

NEURO-OPHTHALMOLOGY
Ben Burton, MA, MRCP, FRCOphth
Fellow in Neuro-ophthalmology, King's College Hospital, London, UK

REFRACTIVE SURGERY
Paul Rosen, FRCOphth
Consultant Ophthalmic Surgeon, Oxford Eye Hospital, Oxford, UK

GLAUCOMA
John Salmon, MD, FRCS, FRCOphth
Consultant Ophthalmic Surgeon, Oxford Eye Hospital, Oxford, UK

OVERALL REVIEWER
Aasheet Desai, DOMS, FRCS(Ed)
Ophthalmic Surgeon, Prince Charles Eye Unit, Windsor, UK

IMPORTANT CONTRIBUTOR
Brad Bowling, FRCSEd (Ophth), FRCSOphth
Consultant Ophthalmic Surgeon, Buckinghamshire Hospitals NHS Trust, UK

CHAPTER 1

OCULAR EXAMINATION TECHNIQUES

SLIT-LAMP BIOMICROSCOPY OF THE ANTERIOR SEGMENT

The purpose of slit-lamp examination of the cornea and anterior segment is to determine the position, depth and size of any abnormalities (Fig. 1.1).

Direct illumination

Direct illumination with diffuse light is used to detect gross abnormalities:
a. A narrow obliquely directed slit-beam is used to visualize a cross-section of the cornea.
b. Further narrowing of the beam to a very thin optical section moved across the cornea can determine the depth of a lesion.
c. The height of the coaxial beam can be adjusted to measure the horizontal and vertical size of a lesion or associated epithelial defect.
d. The use of a red-free filter makes red objects appear black, thereby increasing contrast when observing vascular structures or rose bengal staining. A cobalt blue filter is normally used in conjunction with fluorescein.

Scleral scatter

Scleral scatter involves decentring the slit beam laterally so that the light is incident on the limbus with the microscope focused centrally. Light is then transmitted within the cornea by total internal reflection. A corneal stromal lesion will become illuminated because of forward light scatter. This technique is especially useful to detect subtle stromal haze, or cellular or lipid infiltration.

Retroillumination

Retroillumination uses reflected light from the iris or fundus after pupil dilation to illuminate the cornea. This allows the

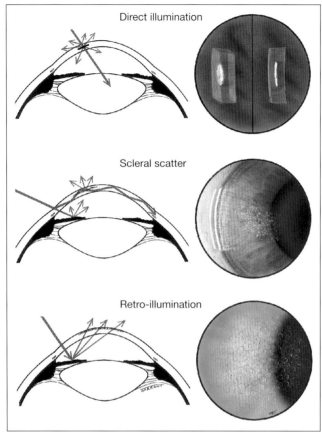

Fig. 1.1
Technique of slit-lamp biomicroscopy of the anterior segment

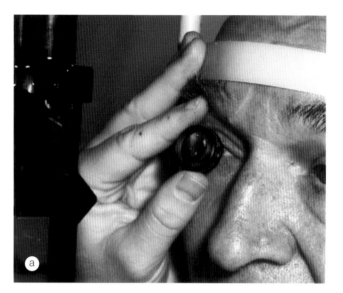

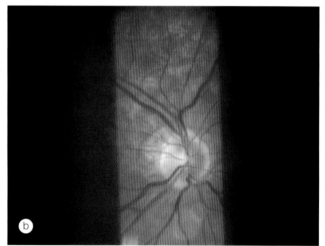

Fig. 1.2
(a) Indirect slit-lamp biomicroscopy; **(b)** fundus view (Courtesy of B Tompkins)

detection of fine epithelial and endothelial changes, such as epithelial cysts, keratic precipitates and small blood vessels.

Specular reflection

Specular reflection shows abnormalities of the endothelium such as reduced cell density and guttata. Pseudoguttata probably represent reversible endothelial cell oedema and inflammatory cells beneath the endothelial cell layer.

FUNDUS EXAMINATION

Slit-lamp biomicroscopy

Indirect ophthalmoscopy

Indirect ophthalmoscopy utilizes high power convex lenses designed to obtain a wide field of view of the fundus (Fig. 1.2); the image is vertically inverted and laterally reversed. The technique is as follows:

a. The slit beam is adjusted to a width about $\frac{1}{4}$ of its full round diameter.
b. The illumination is set at an angle coaxial with the slit-lamp viewing system.
c. The magnification and light intensity are adjusted to the lowest settings.
d. The light beam should be centred to pass directly through the patient's pupil.
e. The lens is held directly in front of the cornea just clearing the lashes so that the light beam passes through its centre.
f. The fundus is examined by moving the joystick and vertical adjustment mechanism of the slit-lamp whilst keeping the lens still.
g. Magnification is increased to show greater detail as necessary.
h. To view the peripheral retina the patient should be instructed to direct gaze accordingly.

Goldmann three-mirror examination

1. **Goldmann lens** consists of a central part and three mirrors set at different angles. Because the curvature of the contact surface of the lens is steeper than that of the cornea a viscous coupling substance with the same refractive index as the cornea is required to bridge the gap between the cornea and the goniolens. It is important to be familiar with each part of the lens as follows (Fig. 1.3):
   - The central part provides a 30° upright view of the posterior pole.
   - The equatorial mirror (largest and oblong shaped) enables visualization from 30° to the equator.
   - The peripheral mirror (intermediate in size and square shaped) enables visualization between the equator and the ora serrata.
   - The gonioscopy mirror (smallest and dome-shaped) may be used for visualizing the extreme periphery and pars plana. It is therefore apparent that the smaller the mirror the more peripheral the view obtained.

2. **Mirror positioning**
   - The mirror should be positioned opposite the area of the fundus to be examined; to examine the 12 o'clock position the mirror should be at 6 o'clock.
   - When viewing the vertical meridian, the image is upside down but not laterally reversed, as with indirect ophthalmoscopy, so that lesions located to the left of 12 o'clock in the retina will also appear in the mirror on the left-hand side (Fig. 1.4).
   - When viewing the horizontal meridian, the image is laterally reversed.

3. **Technique**
   a. The pupils are dilated.
   b. The locking screw is unlocked (Fig. 1.5a) to allow side tilting of the illumination column (Fig. 1.5b).
   c. Anaesthetic drops are instilled.
   d. Coupling fluid (high viscosity methylcellulose or equivalent) is inserted into the cup of the contact lens; it should be no more than half full.
   e. The patient is asked to look up; the inferior rim of the lens is inserted into the lower fornix (Fig. 1.6a) and pressed quickly against the cornea so that the coupling fluid has no time to escape (Fig. 1.6b).
   f. The illumination column should always be tilted except when viewing the 12 o'clock position in the fundus (i.e. with the mirror at 6 o'clock).
   g. When viewing horizontal meridians (i.e. 3 and 9 o'clock positions in the fundus) the column should be kept central.
   h. When viewing the vertical meridians (i.e. 6 and 12 o'clock positions) the column can be positioned left or right of centre (Fig. 1.7).
   i. When viewing oblique meridians (i.e. 1.30 and 7.30 o'clock) the column is kept right of centre, and vice versa when viewing the 10.30 and 4.30 o'clock positions.
   j. When viewing different positions of the peripheral retina the axis of the beam is rotated so that it is always at right angles to the mirror.
   k. To visualize the entire fundus the lens is rotated for 360°, using first the equatorial mirror and then the peripheral mirrors.

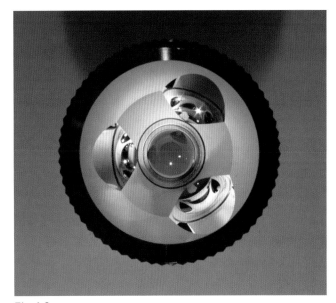

Fig. 1.3
Goldmann three-mirror lens

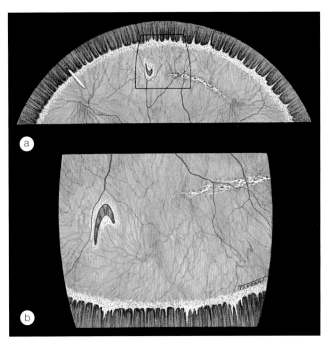

Fig. 1.4
(a) U-tear left of 12 o'clock and an island of lattice degeneration right of 12 o'clock; **(b)** the same lesions seen with the triple mirror positioned at 6 o'clock

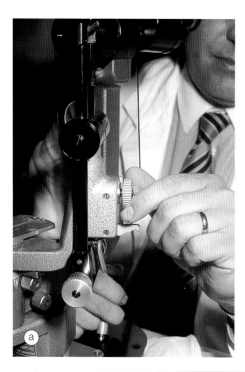 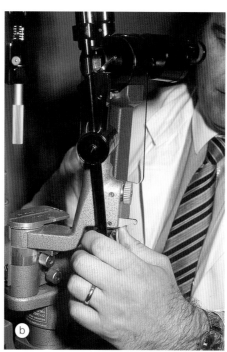

Fig. 1.5
Preparation of the slit-lamp for fundus examination. **(a)** Unlocking the screw; **(b)** tilting of the illumination column

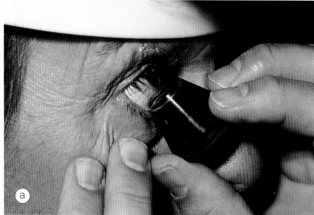

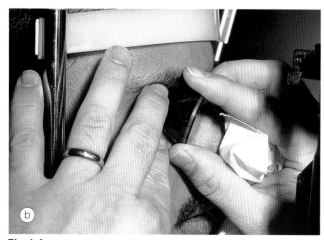

Fig. 1.6
(a) Insertion of the triple-mirror lens into the lower fornix with the patient looking up; **(b)** triple-mirror in position

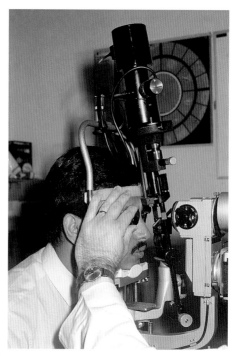

Fig. 1.7
Illumination column tilted and positioned right of centre to view the oblique meridians at 1.30 and 7.30 o'clock

l. To obtain a more peripheral view the lens is tilted to the opposite side asking the patient to move the eyes to the same side. For example, to obtain a more peripheral view of 12 o'clock (with mirrors at 6 o'clock) tilt the lens down and ask the patient to look up.

m. The vitreous cavity is examined with the central lens using both a horizontal and a vertical slit beam.

n. The posterior pole is examined.

Indirect ophthalmoscopy

Principles

Indirect ophthalmoscopy provides a stereoscopic view of the fundus. The light emitted from the instrument is transmitted to the fundus through a condensing lens, held at the focal point of the eye, which provides an inverted and laterally reversed image of the fundus (Fig. 1.8a). This image is viewed through a special viewing system in the ophthalmoscope. As the power of the condensing lens decreases, the working distance and the magnification are increased but the field of view is reduced, and vice versa.

Condensing lenses

The following condensing lenses of various powers and diameters are available for indirect ophthalmoscopy (Fig. 1.8b).

*   15D (magnifies ×4; field about 40°) is used for examination of the posterior pole.
*   20D (magnifies ×3; field about 45°) is the most commonly used for general examination of the fundus.
*   25D (magnifies ×2.5; field is about 50°).
*   30D (magnifies ×2; field is 60°) has a shorter working distance and is useful when examining patients with small pupils.
*   40D (magnifies ×1.5; field is about 65°) is used mainly to examine small children.
*   Panretinal 2.2 (magnifies ×3; field is about 55°).

Technique

a. Both pupils are dilated with 1% tropicamide and, if necessary, phenylephrine 10% so that they will not constrict when exposed to a bright light during examination.

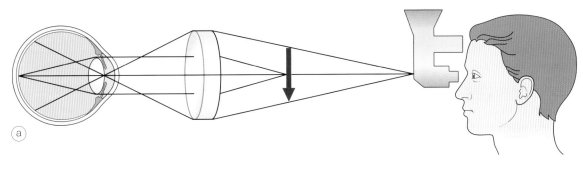

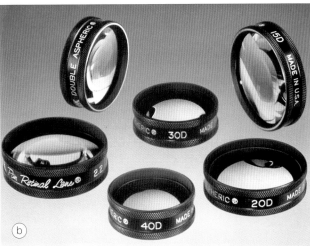

Fig. 1.8
(a) Principles of indirect ophthalmoscopy; **(b)** condensing lenses

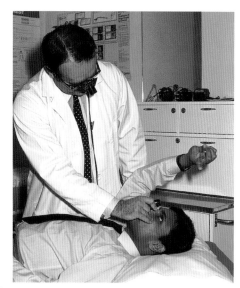

Fig. 1.9
Position of the patient during indirect ophthalmoscopy

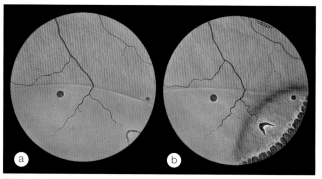

Fig. 1.10
Appearance of retinal breaks in detached retina. **(a)** Without scleral indentation; **(b)** with indentation

b. The patient should be in the supine position, with one pillow, on a bed (Fig. 1.9), reclining chair or couch, and not sitting upright in a chair.

c. The examination room is darkened.

d. The eyepieces are set at the correct interpupillary distance and the beam aligned so that it is located in the centre of the viewing frame.

e. The patient is instructed to keep both eyes open at all times.

f. The lens is taken into one hand with the flat surface facing the patient and throughout the examination is kept parallel to the patient's iris plane.

g. If necessary, the patient's eyelids are gently separated with the fingers.

h. In order to enable the patient to get used to the light he should be asked to look up so that the superior peripheral fundus is examined first.

i. The patient is asked to move the eyes and head into optimal positions for examination. For example, when examining the extreme retinal periphery, ask the patient to look away from you.

Scleral indentation

1. Purposes. Scleral indentation should be attempted only after the art of indirect ophthalmoscopy has been mastered. Its main function is to enhance visualization of the peripheral retina anterior to the equator (Fig. 1.10); it also permits a kinetic evaluation of the retina.

2. Technique

a. To view the ora serrata at 12 o'clock, the patient is asked to look down and the scleral indenter is applied to the outside of the upper eyelid at the margin of the tarsal plate (Fig. 1.11a).

b. With the indenter in place, the patient is asked to look up; at the same time the indenter is advanced into the anterior orbit parallel with the globe (Fig. 1.11b).

c. The examiner's eyes are aligned with the condensing lens and indenter.

d. Gentle pressure is exerted so that a mound is created (Fig. 1.11c) and then the indenter is moved to an adjacent part of the fundus.

NB The indenter should be kept tangential to the globe at all times, as perpendicular indentation will cause pain.

Fundus drawing

1. Technique. The image seen with the indirect ophthalmoscope is vertically inverted and laterally reversed. This phenomenon can be used to advantage when drawing the fundus if the top of the chart is placed towards the patient's feet (i.e. upside down). In this way the inverted position of the chart in relation to the patient's eye corresponds to the image of the fundus obtained by the observer. For example, a U-tear at 11 o'clock in the patient's right eye will correspond to the 11 o'clock position on the chart; the same applies to the area of lattice degeneration between 1 o'clock and 2 o'clock (Fig. 1.12a).

2. Colour code (Fig. 1.12b)

a. The boundaries of the RD are drawn by starting at the optic nerve and then extending to the periphery.

b. Detached retina is shaded blue and flat retina in red.

c. The course of retinal veins is indicated with blue. Retinal arterioles are not usually drawn unless they serve as a special guide to an important lesion.

d. Retinal breaks are drawn in red with blue outlines; the flat part of a retinal tear is also drawn in blue.

e. Thin retina is indicated by red hatchings outlined in blue; lattice degeneration is shown as blue hatchings outlined in blue; retinal pigment is black; retinal exudates yellow; and vitreous opacities green.

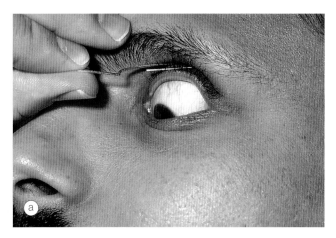

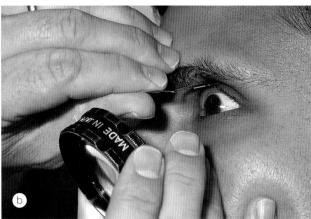

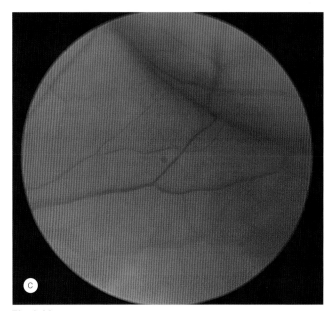

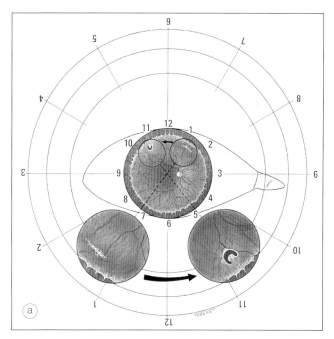

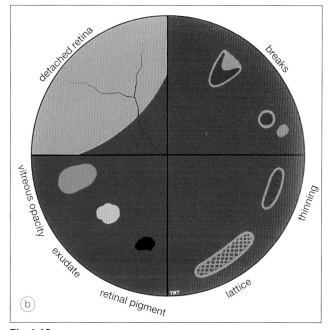

Fig. 1.11
Sclera indentation; **(a)** Insertion of indenter; **(b)** indentation;
(c) mound created by indentation
(Courtesy of N E Byer, from *The Peripheral Retina in Profile, a Stereoscopic
Atlas*, Criterion Press, Torrance, California, 1982 – fig. c)

Fig. 1.12
Technique of drawing retinal lesions. **(a)** Position of chart in
relation to the eye; **(b)** colour code for documenting retinal
lesions

TONOMETRY

Goldmann

Principles

Tonometry is the objective measurement of intraocular pressure (IOP), based most commonly on the force required to flatten the cornea, or the degree of corneal indentation produced by a fixed force. Goldmann applanation tonometry is based on the Imbert–Fick principle which states that for an ideal, dry, thin-walled sphere, the pressure inside the sphere (P) equals the force necessary to flatten its surface (F) divided by the area of flattening (A) (i.e. $P = F/A$). The IOP is proportional to the pressure applied to the globe (in practice the cornea) and the thickness of the walls of the globe (i.e. the thickness of the cornea, which is variable). The human eye is, however, not an ideal sphere – the cornea is rigid and resists flattening. Capillary attraction of the tear meniscus however, tends to pull the tonometer towards the cornea. Corneal rigidity and capillary attraction cancel each other when the flattened area has a diameter of 3.06mm, as in Goldmann tonometry (Fig. 1.13a). The Goldmann is a very accurate variable force tonometer consisting of a double prism (Fig. 1.13b).

Technique

a. The patient is positioned at the slit-lamp with the forehead firmly against the headrest.
b. Topical anaesthetic and fluorescein are instilled into the conjunctival sac.
c. With the cobalt blue filter and the brightest beam projected obliquely at the prism, the prism is centred in front of the apex of the cornea.
d. The dial is preset between 1 and 2 (i.e. between 10 and 20mmHg).
e. The prism is advanced until it just touches the apex of the cornea (Fig. 1.14a).
f. Viewing is switched to the ocular of the slit-lamp.
g. A pattern of two semicircles will be seen, one above and one below the horizontal midline which represent the fluorescein-stained tear film touching the upper and lower outer halves of the prism.
h. The dial on the tonometer is rotated to align the inner margins of the semicircles just touching (Fig. 1.14, right).
i. The reading on the dial, multiplied by ten, equals the IOP.

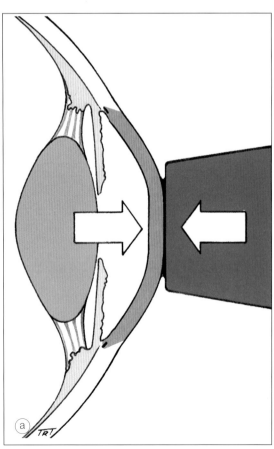

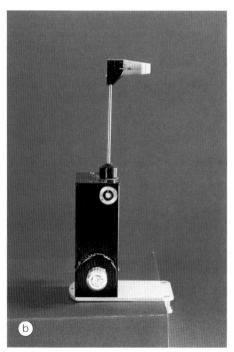

Fig. 1.13
Goldmann tonometry. **(a)** Physical principles; **(b)** tonometer (Courtesy of J Salmon – fig. b)

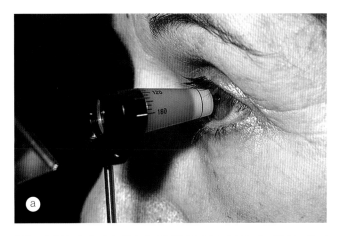

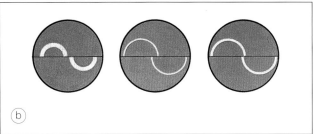

Fig. 1.14
Applanation tonometry. **(a)** Tonometer touching the cornea;
(b) fluorescein-stained semicircles during applanation tonometry

Potential errors

1. **Inappropriate fluorescein pattern** resulting from excessive fluorescein will make the semicircles too thick and the radius too small (Fig. 1.14, left), whereas insufficient fluorescein will make the semicircles too thin and the radius too large (Fig. 1.14, centre).
2. **Pressure on the globe** by the examiner or the patient squeezing the eyelids, and restricted extraocular muscles (e.g. thyroid myopathy), may result in an artificially high reading.
3. **Cornea oedema** may result in artificially low IOP by as much as 10mmHg compared with the true pressure.
4. **Corneal thickness.** Calculations of IOP assume that central corneal thickness is 520μm, with minimal normal variation from this value. If the cornea is thinner, underestimation of IOP may result, and if thicker an overestimation. Individuals with ocular hypertension tend to have corneas thicker than normal, whereas those with normal-tension glaucoma tend to have thinner corneas. Following refractive laser procedures the cornea is thinner and IOP is therefore underestimated, although in practice the difference is small. Tonometers are now available which take corneal thickness into account before a final reading is obtained.
5. **Incorrect calibration** of the tonometer can result in an incorrect reading. It is therefore important to check the calibration at regular intervals.

6. **Other factors** that may be associated with overestimation of IOP include a tight collar, which obstructs venous return and causes the IOP to rise, and anxiety.

Reducing the risk of cross-infection

The risk of transmission of infections such as adenovirus and human immunodeficiency virus (HIV) may be reduced by the following:
- Avoiding tonometry in individuals with overt infection.
- Using a disposable sleeve which covers the tip of the tonometer.
- Swabbing the tonometer tip thoroughly with an alcohol prep pad and allowing it to dry for approximately 10 minutes. This has been shown to be effective for HIV and other organisms, except hepatitis B and C and acanthamoeba.
- Wiping and then soaking the tonometer tip in a 3% solution of hydrogen peroxide for 5 minutes. This will disinfect a tip contaminated with hepatitis C. Since this solution is toxic to the corneal epithelium, extreme care must be taken to rinse the tip thoroughly before use.

Other tonometers

1. **Perkins** uses a Goldmann prism adapted to a small light source. It is hand-held and can therefore be used in bed-bound (Fig. 1.15a) or anaesthetized patients (Fig. 1.15b). Its use, however, requires considerable practice before reliable readings can be obtained.
2. **Tono-Pen** is a hand-held, self-contained, battery powered, portable, contact tonometer (Fig. 1.16). The probe tip contains a transducer that measures the applied force. A microprocessor analyses the force/time curve generated by the transducer during corneal indentation to calculate IOP. The instrument correlates well with Goldmann tonometry although it slightly overestimates a low IOP and underestimates a high IOP. Its main advantage involves the ability to measure IOP in eyes with distorted or oedematous corneas, as well as through a bandage contact lens.
3. **Non-contact tonometers** are based on the principle of applanation but, instead of using a prism, the central part of the cornea is flattened by a jet of air. The time required to sufficiently flatten the cornea relates directly to the level of IOP. The instrument is easy to use and does not require topical anaesthesia. It is therefore particularly useful for screening by non-ophthalmologists. Its main disadvantage is that it is accurate only within the low-to-middle range. The jet of air can startle the patient both with its apparent force and noise. A non-contact tonometer may be non-portable (Fig. 1.17a) or portable (Fig. 1.17b).
4. **Transpalpebral tonometers** are currently being developed. The Proview eye pressure monitor uses a psychophysiological test based on the entoptic phenomenon

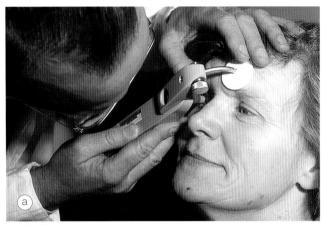
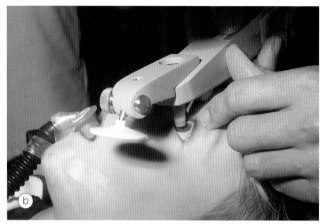

Fig. 1.15
Perkins tonometry; **(a)** In a bed-bound patient; **(b)** in an anaesthetized patient

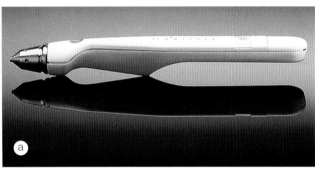

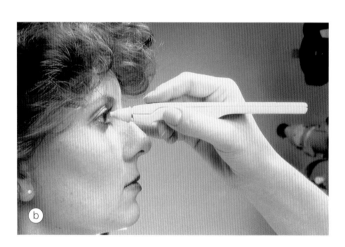

Fig. 1.16
(a) Tono-Pen; **(b)** Tono-Pen in use

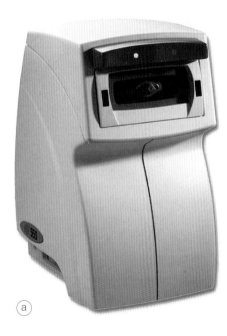
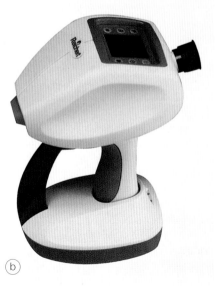

Fig. 1.17
Air-puff tonometers. **(a)** Non-portable; **(b)** portable

of pressure phosphenes to elevate IOP, and is designed for the patient to use at home.

GONIOSCOPY

Introduction

Purposes

The structures between the posterior corneal surface and the anterior surface of the iris constitutes the angle of the anterior chamber, the configuration of which is relevant to the pathogenesis of glaucoma. Contact between peripheral iris and cornea signifies a closed angle, which precludes aqueous access to the trabecular meshwork, whilst wide separation between the two signifies an open angle, implying that the obstruction to aqueous outflow lies in or beyond the trabecular meshwork. Gonioscopy involves the examination and analysis of the angle.

1. **Diagnostic** gonioscopy facilitates the identification of abnormal angle structures and estimation of the width of the chamber angle. It is particularly important in the management of eyes with narrow angles.
2. **Surgical** gonioscopy involves visualization of the angle during procedures such as laser trabeculoplasty and goniotomy.

Optical principles

The angle of the anterior chamber cannot be visualized directly through the intact cornea because light emitted from the angle undergoes total internal reflection at the anterior surface of the precorneal tear film. A goniolens eliminates total internal reflection by replacing the tear-film–air interface with a new tear-film–goniolens interface (Fig. 1.18).

1. **Indirect** goniolenses (goniomirrors) provide an image of the opposite angle and can be used only in conjunction with a slit-lamp.
2. **Direct** goniolenses (gonioprisms) provide a direct view of the angle. They do not require a slit-lamp and are used with the patient in the supine position.

Goniolenses

Goldmann

The Goldmann is an indirect goniolens with a contact surface diameter of approximately 12mm. It is relatively easy to master and affords an excellent view of the angle. It also stabilizes the globe and is therefore suitable for laser trabeculoplasty. The original Goldmann lens has three

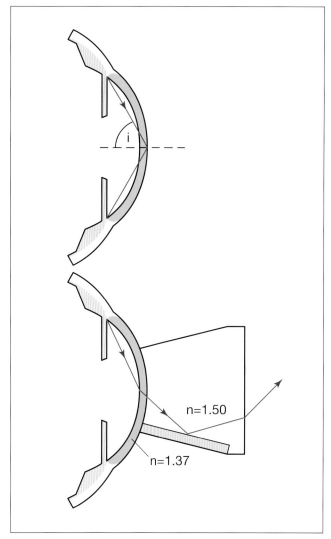

Fig. 1.18
Optical principles of gonioscopy; n = refractive index; i = angle of incidence

mirrors (see Fig. 1.3). Modifications with one mirror (Fig. 1.19a) and two mirrors with an antireflective coating have been designed for laser trabeculoplasty, enabling visualization of a wider circumference of the angle.

Zeiss

The Zeiss and the similar Posner and Sussman are indirect four-mirror goniolenses (Fig.1.19b). The contact surface of the lens has a diameter of 9mm and a curvature flatter than that of the cornea, negating the need for a coupling substance. Tears provide adequate contact material and lubrication for the lens. This permits quick and comfortable

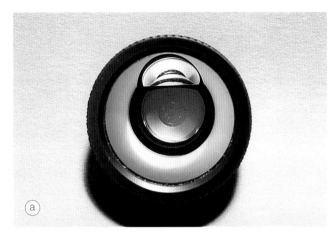

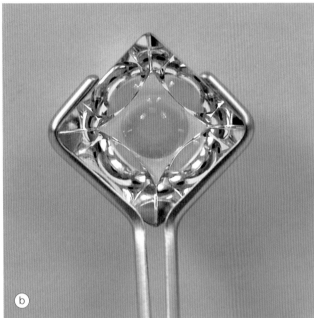

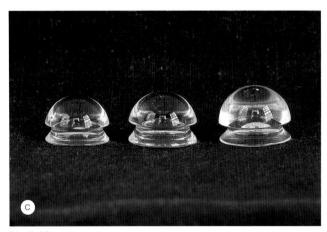

Fig. 1.19
Diagnostic goniolenses. **(a)** Goldmann single-mirror; **(b)** Zeiss four-mirror; **(c)** Koeppe

examination of the angle and importantly, does not interfere with subsequent examinations of the fundus. The four mirrors enable the entire circumference of the angle to be visualized with minimal rotation. This lens is useful for indentation gonioscopy (see below), but because it does not stabilize the globe, it cannot be used for laser trabeculoplasty.

Koeppe

The Koeppe is a dome-shaped direct diagnostic goniolens which comes in several sizes (Fig. 1.19c). It is easy to use and provides a panoramic view of the angle. It is therefore particularly useful for simultaneous comparison of one portion of the angle with another. Moreover, with the patient in the supine position the anterior chamber may become slightly deeper and the angle easier to visualize. When used in conjunction with a hand-held microscope, it offers great flexibility, allowing detailed inspection of the various subtleties of angle structures both by direct and retroillumination. It cannot be used in conjunction with a slit-lamp and therefore does not provide the same clarity, illumination and variable powers comparable with slit-lamp goniolenses.

Gonioscopic technique

Goldmann gonioscopy

The patient should be advised that the lens will touch the eye but not cause more than slight discomfort. The patient should also be requested to keep both eyes open at all times and not to move the head backwards when the lens is being inserted.

a. The preliminary steps are the same as already described for fundus examination.
b. The angle is visualized with the small dome-shaped gonioscopic mirror (if a three-mirror lens is being used).
c. Initially the mirror is placed at the 12 o'clock position to visualize the inferior angle and then rotated clockwise. The slit beam should be 2mm wide and when viewing different positions it is usually best to rotate the beam so that its axis is at right angles to the mirror.
d. When the view of the angle is obscured by a convex iris, it is possible to 'see over the hill' by asking the patient to look in the direction of the mirror.
e. When the plane of the iris is flat, the patient should be asked to look away from the mirror in order to obtain a view parallel to the iris with optimal image quality. This is particularly important when performing laser trabeculoplasty.

NB The image is laterally reversed with the mirror in the horizontal meridian and vertically.

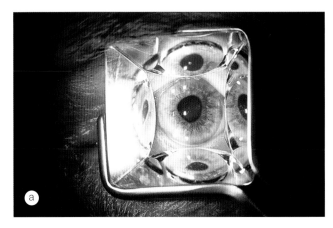
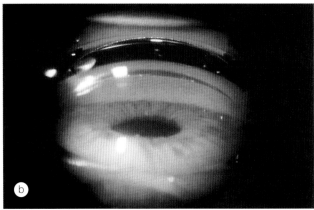
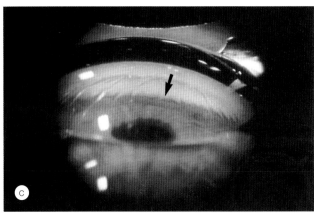

the centre of the cornea. Only gentle contact with the cornea is needed because excessive pressure will inadvertently distort angle structures.

c. Each quadrant of the angle is visualized with the opposite mirror (Fig. 1.20a).

d. Indentation gonioscopy may be performed by pressing posteriorly against the cornea. This will force aqueous into the angle of the anterior chamber, forcing the peripheral iris posteriorly.

- If the angle is closed by mere apposition between the iris and cornea (appositional closure – Fig. 1.20b), the angle will be forced open allowing visualization of the angle recess (Fig. 1.20c).
- If the angle is completely closed by adhesions between the peripheral iris and cornea (synechial closure) it will remain closed.
- If synechial closure is partial, part of the angle will open and a part will remain closed.

NB With practice, gentle indentation gonioscopy allows better visualization even of the normal angle. Goniolenses are a potential source of infection and should be disinfected in the same way as tonometer heads.

Identification of angle structures

Figure 1.21 shows the anatomy of angle structures.

1. **Schwalbe line** is the most anterior structure, appearing as an opaque line. Anatomically it demarcates the peripheral termination of Descemet membrane and the anterior limit of the trabeculum.
2. **The corneal wedge** is useful in locating an inconspicuous Schwalbe line as follows:
   a. Using a narrow slit beam, two linear reflections can be seen, one from the external surface of the cornea and its junction with the sclera, the other from the internal surface of the cornea.
   b. The two reflections meet at the apex of the corneal wedge which coincides with the Schwalbe line.

NB When performing laser trabeculoplasty a pigmented Schwalbe line should not be confused with the posterior pigmented trabeculum.

3. **The trabeculum** extends from the Schwalbe line to the scleral spur and has an average width of 600µm. Gonioscopically, it has a ground-glass appearance and appears to have depth. The anterior non-functional part lies adjacent to Schwalbe line and has a whitish colour. The posterior functional pigmented part lies adjacent to the scleral spur and has a greyish-blue translucent

Fig. 1.20
Indentation gonioscopy with a Zeiss lens. **(a)** Lens in place; **(b)** total angle closure prior to indentation; **(c)** following indentation the entire angle becomes visible (arrow) and the cornea develops folds (Courtesy of Wallace L M Alward, from *Color Atlas of Gonioscopy*, Wolfe, 1994 – figs b and c)

Zeiss gonioscopy

The preliminary steps are the same as for Goldmann gonioscopy but a coupling fluid is not required.
a. The patient is asked to look straight ahead.
b. Under slit-lamp visualization the lens is placed directly on

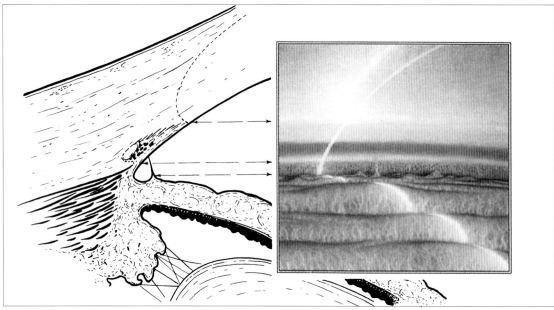

Fig. 1.21
Normal angle structures (Courtesy of Wallace L M Alward, from *Color Atlas of Gonioscopy*, Wolfe, 1994)

appearance. In laser trabeculoplasty burns are applied at the junction of the non-pigmented and pigmented trabeculum. Trabecular pigmentation is rare prior to puberty. In ageing eyes it involves the posterior trabeculum to a variable extent, most marked inferiorly and least in the horizontal meridian. Trabecular pigmentation is also most marked in brown eyes.

4. **Schlemm canal** may be identified in the non-pigmented angle as a slightly darker line deep to the posterior trabeculum. Blood can sometimes be seen in this canal if the goniolens compresses the episcleral veins such that the episcleral venous pressure exceeds the IOP.

5. **The scleral spur** is the most anterior projection of the sclera and the site of attachment of the longitudinal muscle of the ciliary body. Gonioscopically, the scleral spur is situated immediately posterior to the trabeculum and appears as a narrow, dense, often shiny, whitish band. It is a very important landmark because it has a relatively consistent appearance in different eyes.

NB In laser trabeculoplasty it is important to identify the scleral spur because the application of burns posterior to it will result in greater inflammation, with consequent increased risk of early post-laser rise in IOP and the formation of peripheral anterior synechiae.

6. **The ciliary body** stands out just behind the scleral spur as a pink to dull-brown to slate-grey band. Its width depends on the position of iris insertion and it tends to be narrower in hypermetropic eyes and wider in myopic eyes. The angle recess represents the posterior dipping of the iris as it inserts into the ciliary body.

7. **Iris processes** are small extensions of the anterior surface of the iris which insert at the level of the scleral spur and cover the ciliary body in varying extent. They are present in about one-third of normal eyes and are most prominent during childhood and in brown eyes. With increasing age they tend to wither and lose their continuity. Iris processes should not be confused with peripheral anterior synechiae which are broader and represent adhesions between the iris and angle structures. However, fine stellate peripheral anterior synechiae induced by inappropriate laser trabeculoplasty may easily be mistaken for iris processes.

8. **Blood vessels** running in a radial pattern at the base of the angle recess are often seen in normal eyes. Pathological blood vessels run randomly in various directions. As a general principle, any blood vessel that crosses the scleral spur onto the trabecular meshwork is abnormal.

Grading of angle width

Grading of angle width is performed to evaluate the functional status of the angle, the degree of closure and the risk of future closure. The following features should be noted and described in the superior and inferior halves of the angle

bearing in mind that most angles are narrowest superiorly:
- The shape and contour of the peripheral iris.
- The deepest structure seen.
- Amount of trabecular pigmentation.
- Presence of peripheral anterior synechiae.

The Shaffer system records the angle in degrees of arc subtended by two imaginary tangential lines drawn to the inner surface of the trabeculum and the anterior surface of the iris about one-third of the distance from its periphery. In practice, the angle is graded according to the visibility of various angle structures. The system assigns a numerical grade (4 to 0) to each angle with associated anatomical description, angle width in degrees and implied clinical interpretation (Fig. 1.22).

1. **Grade 4** (35–45°) is the widest angle characteristic of myopia in which the ciliary body can be visualized with ease; it is incapable of closure.
2. **Grade 3** (25–35°) is an open angle in which at least the scleral spur can be identified; it is also incapable of closure.
3. **Grade 2** (20°) is a moderately narrow angle in which only the trabeculum can be identified; angle closure is possible but unlikely.
4. **Grade 1** (10°) is a very narrow angle in which only Schwalbe line, and perhaps also the top of the trabeculum, can be identified; angle closure is not inevitable but the risk is high.
5. **Slit angle** is one in which there is no obvious iridocorneal contact but no angle structures can be identified; this angle has the greatest danger of imminent closure.
6. **Grade 0** (0°) is a closed angle due to iridocorneal contact and is recognized by the inability to identify the apex of the corneal wedge. Indentation gonioscopy with a Zeiss goniolens is necessary to differentiate 'appositional' from 'synechial' angle closure (see Fig. 1.20).

Pathological findings

It is important that gonioscopy is undertaken on all patients with glaucoma and glaucoma suspects. Failure to examine the filtration angle is one of the commonest causes of a missed diagnosis. Abnormal gonioscopic findings and their causes are as follows:

1. **Peripheral anterior synechiae**
   - Primary angle-closure glaucoma.
   - Anterior uveitis.
   - Iridocorneal endothelial (ICE) syndrome.
2. **Neovascularization**
   - Neovascular glaucoma.
   - Fuchs heterochromic cyclitis.
   - Chronic anterior uveitis.
3. **Hyperpigmentation**
   - Pigment dispersion syndrome.
   - Pseudophakic pigment dispersion.
   - Pseudoexfoliation syndrome.
   - Blunt ocular trauma.
   - Anterior uveitis.
   - Following acute angle-closure glaucoma.
   - Following YAG laser iridotomy.
   - Iris melanoma.
   - Iris pigment epithelial cysts.
   - Naevus of Ota.
   - After cataract surgery in uncontrolled diabetes.
4. **Trauma**
   - Angle recession.
   - Trabecular dialysis.
   - Cyclodialysis.
   - Foreign bodies.
5. **Blood in Schlemm canal**
   - Carotid-cavernous fistula and dural shunt.
   - Sturge–Weber syndrome.
   - Obstruction of the superior vena cava.

PSYCHOPHYSICAL TESTS

Visual acuity

Visual acuity (VA) is the easiest to perform and most important test of visual function. Spatial visual acuity is the ability to distinguish separate elements of a target and identify it as a whole. It is quantified by the minimum angle of separation (subtended at the nodal point of the eye) between two objects that allows them to be perceived as separate.

1. **Snellen** notation is described as the testing distance over the distance at which the letter would subtend 5 minutes of arc vertically. Thus at 6 metres a 6/6 letter subtends 5 minutes of arc, a 6/12 letter subtends 10 minutes and a 6/60 letter 50 minutes. The Snellen

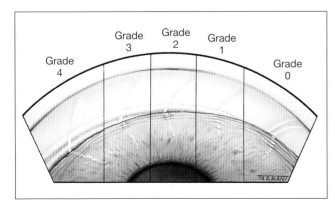

Fig. 1.22
Grading of angle width

fraction may also be expressed as a decimal (i.e. 6/6 = 1 and 6/12 = 0.5). Unfortunately, the Snellen chart (Fig. 1.23a) has many shortcomings. For example, the letters on the lower lines are more crowded than those towards the top, the spacing between each letter and each row bears no systematic relationship to the width or height of the letters and the small number of larger letters limits the chart's usefulness.

NB In patients with macular disease VA is frequently worse when the patient looks through a pin-hole.

2. **Bailey–Lovie** chart (Fig. 1.23b) is more accurate than the Snellen and is preferred in vision research. This records the minimum angle of resolution (MAR) which relates to the resolution required to resolve the elements of a letter. Thus 6/6 equates to a MAR of one minute of arc and 6/12 equates to two minutes. LogMAR is simply the log of the MAR. Each line of the chart comprises five letters and the spacing between each letter and each row is related to the width and height of the letters, respectively. The results are usually recorded in terms of a logMAR score with the notation 6/6 being equivalent to a logMAR of zero. As letter size changes by 0.1 logMAR units per row and there are five letters in each row, each letter can be assigned a score of 0.02. The final score takes account of every letter that has been read correctly read, thus avoiding the shortcomings of the Snellen chart.

Contrast sensitivity

1. **Principle.** Contrast sensitivity is a measure of the minimal amount of contrast required to distinguish a test object. The test is capable of detecting very early visual dysfunction, even when Snellen VA is normal.
2. **The Pelli–Robson** contrast sensitivity letter chart (Fig. 1.24) is viewed at 1 metre and consists of rows of letters of equal size but with decreasing contrast of 0.15 log units for every group of three letters.

Amsler grid

The grid charts evaluate the 20° of the visual field centred on fixation (Fig. 1.25) and is used mainly in screening and monitoring macular disease.

Charts

There are seven charts, each consisting of a 10cm square (Figs 1.26 and 1.27).

Chart 1 is the most commonly used. It comprises a high contrast white grid on a black background. The outer grid encloses 400 smaller 5mm squares. When viewed at about

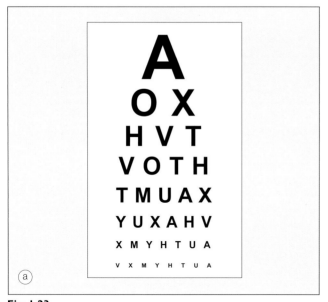

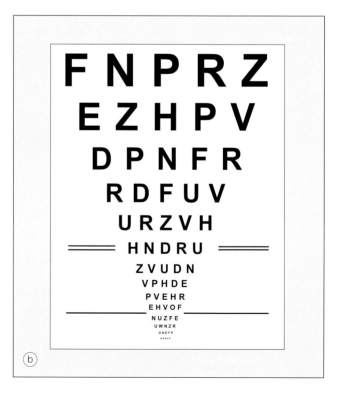

Fig. 1.23
Visual acuity charts. **(a)** Snellen; **(b)** Bailey–Lovie

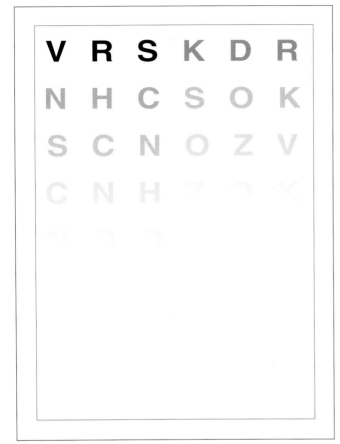

Fig. 1.24
Pelli–Robson contrast sensitivity letter chart

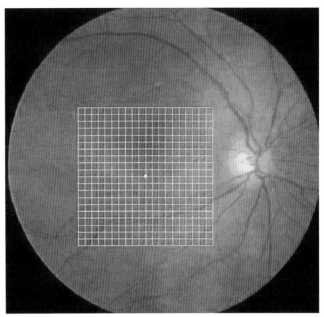

Fig. 1.25
Amsler grid superimposed onto the retina (Courtesy of A Franklin)

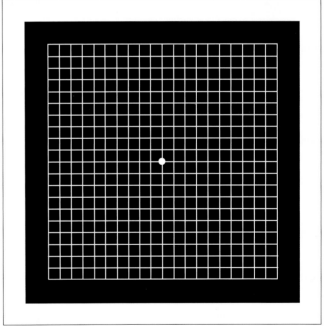

Fig. 1.26
Amsler grid chart 1 (Courtesy of A Franklin)

one-third of a metre, each small square subtends an angle of 1 degree.

Chart 2 is similar to chart 1 but has diagonal lines that aid fixation in patients unable to see the central spot as a result of a central scotoma.

Chart 3 is identical to chart 1 but has red squares. The red-on-black design aims to stimulate long wavelength foveal cones. It is used to detect colour scotomas and desaturation that may occur in toxic maculopathies, optic neuropathies and chiasmal lesions.

Chart 4 consisting only of random dots is used mainly to distinguish scotomas from metamorphopsia, as there is no form to be distorted.

Chart 5 consists of horizontal lines and is designed to detect metamorphopsia along specific meridians. It is of particular value in the evaluation of patients with reading difficulties.

Chart 6 is similar to chart 5 but has a white background and the central lines are closer together enabling more detailed evaluation.

Chart 7 exhibits a fine central grid, each square subtending an angle of half a degree and is therefore more sensitive.

Technique

a. Reading spectacles are worn, if appropriate, and one eye is covered.

b. The patient is asked to look directly at the central dot with the uncovered eye and report any distortion, blurred areas

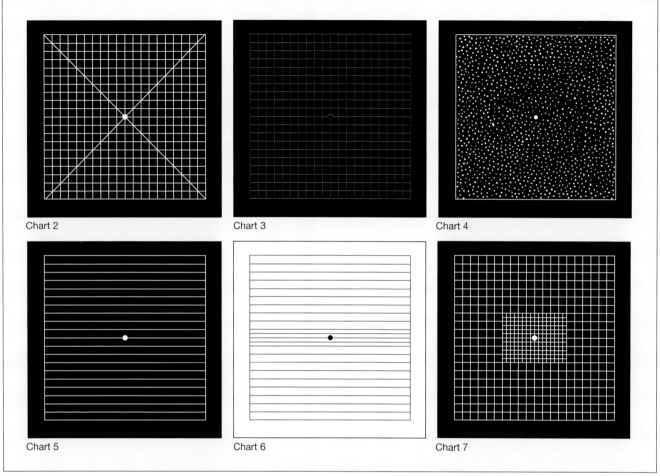

Fig. 1.27
Amsler grid charts 2–7 (Courtesy of A Franklin)

or blank spots anywhere on the grid. Patients with macular disease often report that the lines are wavy whereas those with optic neuropathy often remark that some of the lines are missing or faint but not distorted (Fig. 1.28).

c. The patient is asked if all four corners and all four sides of the square are visible. A missing corner or side (exterior scotoma) may have many causes such as glaucomatous field defects or retinitis pigmentosa.

Light brightness comparison test

This is essentially a test of optic nerve function which is usually normal in retinal disease, unless very advanced. It is performed as follows:

a. A light from an indirect ophthalmoscope is shone first into the normal eye and then the eye with suspected disease.

b. The patient is asked whether the light is symmetrically bright in both eyes.

c. In optic neuropathy the patient will report that the light is less bright in the affected eye.

d. The patient is asked to assign a relative value from 1 to 5 to the brightness of light in the diseased eye, as compared with the normal eye.

Photostress test

1. **Principles.** Photostress testing is a gross test of dark adaptation in which the visual pigments are bleached by light. This causes a temporary state of retinal insensitivity perceived by the patient as a scotoma. The recovery of vision is dependent on the ability of the photoreceptors to re-synthesize visual pigments. The test may be useful in detecting maculopathy when ophthalmoscopy is equivocal, as in mild cystoid macular oedema or central serous retinopathy; it may also differentiate visual loss caused by macular disease from that caused by an optic nerve lesion.

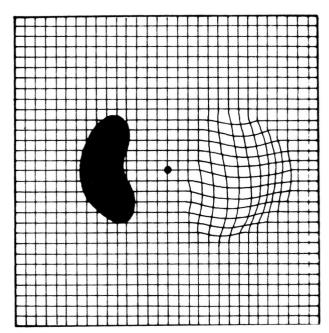

Fig. 1.28
Amsler recording showing wavy lines to indicate metamorphopsia and a scotoma

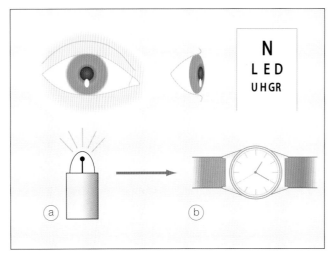

Fig. 1.29
Photostress test

2. Technique

a. The best corrected distance visual acuity is determined.

b. The patient fixates the light of a pen-torch or an indirect ophthalmoscope held about 3cm away for about 10 seconds (Fig. 1.29a).

c. The photostress recovery time (PSRT) is the time taken to read any three letters of the pre-test acuity line and is normally between 15 and 30 seconds (Fig. 1.29b).

d. The test is performed on the other, presumably normal, eye and the results are compared.

e. The PSRT is prolonged, relative to the normal eye, in macular disease (sometimes 50 seconds or more) but not in an optic neuropathy.

NB The pupillary reactions to light are usually normal in eyes with macular disease, although extensive retinal disease such as a retinal detachment or ischaemic central retinal vein occlusion may cause an afferent pupillary defect (APD). This is in contrast to optic neuropathy in which an APD occurs even in mild cases.

Dark adaptometry

1. Principle. Dark adaptation (DA) is the phenomenon by which the visual system (pupil, retina and occipital cortex) adapts to decreased illumination. This test is particularly useful in the investigation of patients complaining of night-blindness (nyctalopia). The retina is exposed to an intense light for a time sufficient to bleach 25% or more of the rhodopsin in the retina. Following this normal rods are insensitive to light and cones respond only to very bright stimuli. Subsequent recovery of light sensitivity can be monitored by placing the subject in the dark and periodically presenting spots of light of varying intensity in the visual field and asking the subject if they are perceived.

2. Technique of Goldmann–Weekes adaptometry

a. The subject is exposed to an intense light that bleaches the photoreceptors and then suddenly placed in the dark.

b. The threshold at which the subject just perceives the light is plotted.

c. The flashes are repeated at regular intervals; the sensitivity of the eye to light gradually increases.

3. The sensitivity curve is a plot of the light intensity of a minimally perceived spot versus time and is bipartite (Fig. 1.30).

a. *The cone branch* of the curve represents the initial 5–10 minutes of darkness during which cone sensitivity rapidly improves. The rod photoreceptors are also recovering during this time, but more slowly.

b. *The 'rod–cone' break* in normal subjects occurs after 7–10 minutes when cones achieve their maximum sensitivity, and the rods become perceptibly more sensitive than cones.

c. *The rod branch* of the curve is slower and represents the continuation of improvement of rod sensitivity. After 15–30 minutes, the fully dark-adapted rods allow the subject to perceive a spot of light over 100 times dimmer than would be possible with cones alone. If the flashes are focused onto the foveola (where rods are absent), only a rapid segment, corresponding to cone adaptation, is recorded.

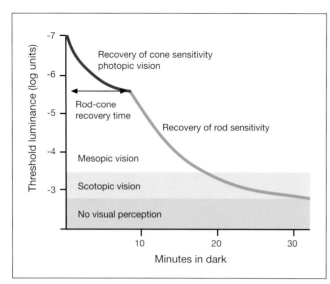

Fig. 1.30
Dark adaptation curve

Colour vision tests

Colour vision (CV) testing is sometimes useful in the clinical evaluation of hereditary fundus dystrophies, where impairment may be present prior to the development of visual acuity and visual field changes.

Principles

CV is a function of three populations of retinal cones each with its specific sensitivity: blue (tritan) at 414–424nm, green (deuteran) 522–539nm and red (protan) at 549–570nm. A normal person requires all these primary colours to match those within the spectrum. Any given cone pigment may be deficient (e.g. protanomaly – red weakness) or entirely absent (e.g. protanopia – red blindness). Trichromats possess all three types of cones (although not necessarily functioning perfectly) while absence of one or two types of cones renders an individual a dichromat or a monochromat respectively. Most individuals with congenital colour defects are anomalous trichromats and use abnormal proportions of the three primary colours to match those in the light spectrum. Those with red-green deficiency caused by abnormality of red-sensitive cones are protanomalous, those with abnormality of green-sensitive cones are deuteranomalous and those with blue-green deficiency caused by abnormality of blue-sensitive cones are tritanomalous.

NB Acquired macular disease tends to produce blue-yellow defects and optic nerve lesions red-green defects.

Colour vision tests

1. **Ishihara** test is used mainly to screen for congenital protan and deuteran defects. It consists of a test plate followed by 16 plates each with a matrix of dots arranged to show a central shape or number which the subject is asked to identify (Fig.1.31a). A colour deficient person will only be able to identify some of the figures. Inability to identify the test plate (provided visual acuity is sufficient) indicates malingering.
2. **Hardy–Rand–Rittler** is similar to Ishihara but more sensitive since it can detect all three congenital defects (Fig. 1.31b).
3. **City University** test consists of ten plates each containing a central colour and four peripheral colours (Fig. 1.31c). The subject selects one of the peripheral colours which most closely matches the central colour.
4. **Farnsworth–Munsell 100-hue** is the most sensitive for both congenital and acquired colour defects but is seldom used in practice. Despite the name it consists of 85 hue caps contained in four separate racks, in each of which the two end caps are fixed while the others are loose so they can be randomized by the examiner (Fig. 1.31d).
   a. The subject is asked to rearrange the loose randomized caps 'in their natural' order in one box.
   b. The box is then closed, turned upside down and then opened so that the markers on the inside of the caps become visible.
   c. The findings are then recorded in a simple cumulative manner on a circular chart.
   d. Each of the three forms of dichromatism is characterized by failure in a specific meridian of the chart (Fig. 1.32).
5. **Farnsworth D15 hue discrimination** test is similar to the Farnsworth–Munsell 100-hue test but utilizes only 15 caps.

ELECTROPHYSICAL TESTS

Electroretinography

Principles

The electroretinogram (ERG) is the record of an action potential produced by the retina when it is stimulated by light of adequate intensity. The recording may be made between an active electrode either in contact with the cornea or a skin electrode placed just below the lower eyelid margin, and a reference electrode on the forehead. The potential between the two electrodes is then amplified and displayed (Fig. 1.33). The normal ERG is biphasic (Fig. 1.34).

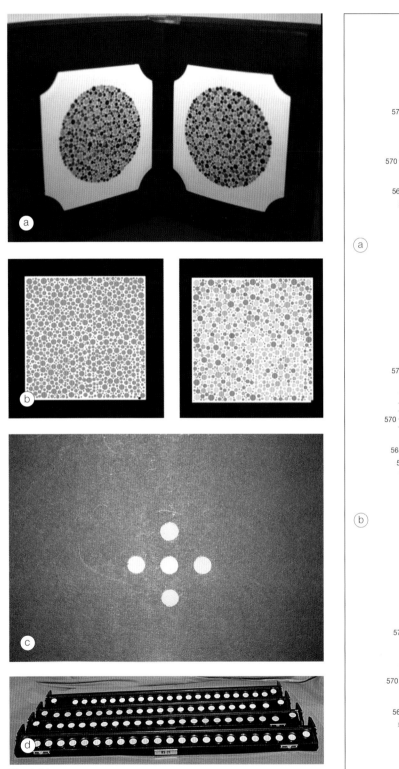

Fig. 1.31
Colour vision tests. **(a)** Ishihara; **(b)** Hardy–Rand–Rittler; **(c)** City University; **(d)** Farnsworth–Munsell 100-hue test (Courtesy of T Waggoner – fig. b)

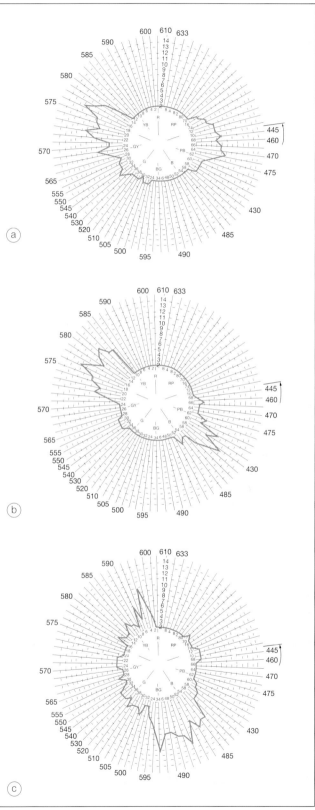

Fig. 1.32
Examples of Farnsworth–Munsell results of colour deficiencies.
(a) Protan; **(b)** deuteran; **(c)** tritan

1. **The a-wave** is the initial fast negative deflection directly generated by photoreceptors.
2. **The b-wave** is the next slower positive deflection with larger amplitude. Although it is generated from fluxes of potassium ions within and surrounding Müller cells, it is directly dependent on functional photoreceptors and its magnitude makes it a convenient measure of photoreceptor integrity. The amplitude of the b-wave is measured from the trough of the a-wave to the peak of the b-wave, and increases with both dark adaptation and increased light stimulus. The b-wave consists of b-1 and b-2 subcomponents. The former probably represents both rod and cone activity and the latter mainly cone activity. It is possible to single out rod and cone responses with special techniques.

Normal ERG

The normal ERG consists of five recordings. The first three are elicited after 30 minutes of dark adaptation (scotopic), and the last two after 10 minutes of adaptation to moderately bright diffuse illumination (photopic) (Fig. 1.35). In children it can be difficult to dark adapt for 30 minutes and therefore dim light (mesopic) conditions can be utilized to evoke predominantly rod mediated responses to low intensity white or blue light stimuli.

1. **Scotopic ERG**
   a. Rod responses are elicited with a very dim flash of white light or a blue light resulting in a large b-wave and a small or non-recordable a-wave.
   b. Combined rod and cone responses are elicited with a very bright white flash resulting in a prominent a-wave and a b-wave.
   c. Oscillatory potentials are elicited by using a bright flash and changing the recording parameters. The oscillatory wavelets occur on the ascending limb of the b-wave and are generated by cells in the inner retina.
2. **Photopic ERG**
   a. Cone responses are elicited with a single bright flash, resulting in an a-wave and a b-wave with small oscillations.
   b. Cone flicker is used to isolate cones by using a flickering light stimulus at a frequency of 30Hz to which rods cannot respond. It provides a measure of the amplitude and implicit time of the cone b-wave. Cone responses can be elicited in normal eyes up to 50Hz, after which point individual responses are no longer recordable (critical flicker fusion).

Multifocal ERG

Multifocal ERG is a method of producing topographical maps of retinal function (Fig. 1.36). The stimulus is scaled for variation in photoreceptor density across the retina; at the

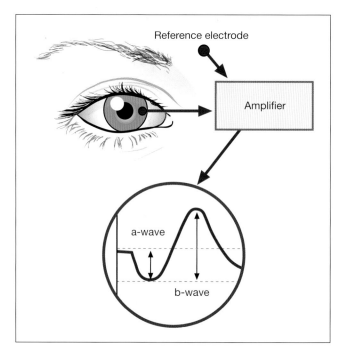

Fig. 1.33
Principles of electroretinography

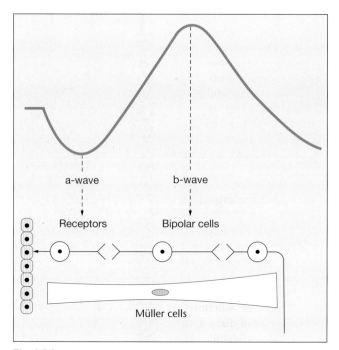

Fig. 1.34
Components and origins of the electroretinogram

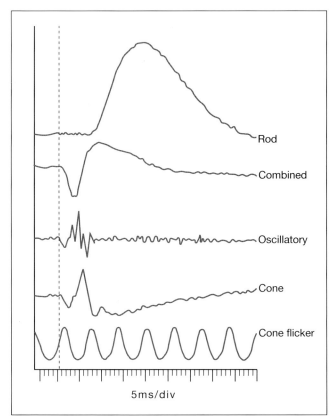

Fig. 1.35
Normal electroretinographic recordings

Rod
Combined
Oscillatory
Cone
Cone flicker

5ms/div

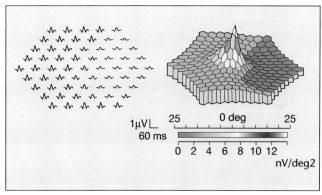

Fig. 1.36
Multifocal electroretinogram

1µVL
60 ms
25   0 deg   25
0 2 4 6 8 10 12
nV/deg2

a. The electrodes are attached to the skin near the medial and lateral canthi.
b. The patient is asked to look rhythmically from side to side, making excursions of constant amplitude. Each time the eye moves the cornea makes the nearest electrode positive with respect to the other.
c. The potential difference between the two electrodes is amplified and recorded.

fovea, where the density of receptors is high, a smaller stimulus element is used than in the periphery where receptor density is lower. As with conventional ERG, many types of measurements can be made at individual locations; both the amplitude and timing of the troughs and peaks can be measured and reported. The information can be summarized in the form of a three-dimensional plot which resembles the hill of vision. The technique can be used for almost any disorder which affects retinal function.

Electro-oculography

1. **Principle.** The electro-oculogram (EOG) measures the standing potential between the electrically positive cornea and the electrically negative back of the eye (Fig. 1.37). It reflects the activity of the RPE and the photoreceptors. This means that an eye blinded by lesions proximal to the photoreceptors will have a normal EOG. In general, diffuse or widespread disease of the RPE is needed to affect the EOG response significantly.
2. **Technique.** The test is performed in both light- and dark-adapted states.

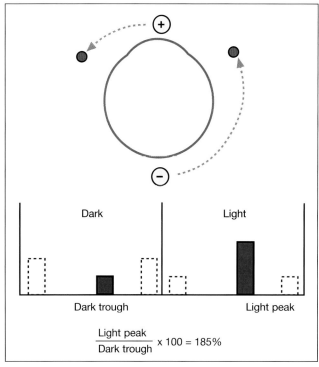

Dark   Light

Dark trough   Light peak

$$\frac{\text{Light peak}}{\text{Dark trough}} \times 100 = 185\%$$

Fig. 1.37
Principles of electro-oculography

3. Interpretation. As there is much variation in EOG amplitude in normal subjects, the result is calculated by dividing the maximal height of the potential in the light (light peak) by the minimal height of the potential in the dark (dark trough). This is expressed as a ratio (Arden ratio) or as a percentage. The normal value is over 1.85 or 185%.

Visual evoked potential

1. Principle. The visual evoked potential (VEP) is a recording of electrical activity of the visual cortex created by stimulation of the retina. The main indications are monitoring of visual function in babies and the investigation of optic neuropathy, particularly when associated with demyelination. It can also be used to monitor macular pathway function.

2. Technique. The stimulus is either a flash of light (flash VEP) or a black-and-white checker-board pattern, which periodically reverses polarity on a screen (pattern VEP) (Fig. 1.38). Several tests are performed and the average potential is calculated by a computer.

3. Interpretation. Both latency (delay) and amplitude of the VEP are assessed. In optic neuropathy both parameters are affected, with prolongation of latency and decrease in amplitude. The use of threshold VEP (by using different sized checks), early or subclinical dysfunction can be detected as the smaller check size responses may become abnormal earlier while larger check-size responses may remain within normal limits.

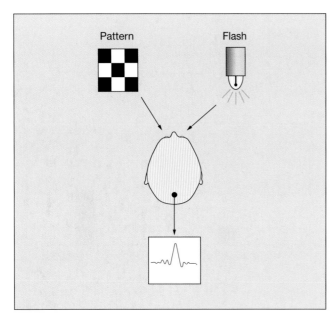

Fig. 1.38
Principles of visually evoked potential

PERIMETRY

Definitions

1. The visual field may be described as an island of vision surrounded by a sea of darkness. It is not a flat plane but a three-dimensional structure akin to a hill of vision (Fig. 1.39). The outer aspect of the visual field extends approximately 60° superiorly, 60° nasally, 80° inferiorly and 90° temporally. Visual acuity is sharpest at the very top of the hill (i.e. the fovea) and then declines progressively towards the periphery, the nasal slope being steeper than the temporal. The blind spot is located temporally between 10° and 20°.

2. An isopter. As the size and luminance of a target is decreased, the area within which it can be perceived becomes smaller, so that a series of ever-diminishing circles called isopters is formed. Isopters therefore resemble the contour lines on a map which enclose an area within which a target of a given size is visible. An erosion of the 'coastline' of the island will therefore cause an indentation of all isopters in the affected area.

3. An absolute scotoma represents an area of total visual loss in which even the largest and brightest target cannot be perceived.

4. A relative scotoma is an area of partial visual loss within which brighter or larger targets can be seen and smaller or dimmer ones cannot. A scotoma may have sloping edges so that an absolute scotoma is surrounded by a relative scotoma.

5. Luminance is the intensity or 'brightness' of a light stimulus, measured in apostilb (asb). A decibel (dB) is a non-specific unit of luminance based on a logarithmic scale (one-tenth of a log unit).

6. Differential light sensitivity represents the degree by which the luminance of a target requires to exceed background luminance in order to be perceived by the eye. The visual field is therefore a three-dimensional representation of differential light sensitivity at different points.

7. Visible threshold is the luminance of a given stimulus (measured in asb or dB) at which it is perceived 50% of the time when presented statically (Fig. 1.40). The threshold is determined by increasing the intensity of the stimulus by 0.1 log unit steps. The human eye needs about a 10% change in brightness to discern a difference between light stimuli. For example, at a background illumination of 0.1asb, the eye can detect a light stimulus that is 0.01asb brighter, while at a background illumination of 1000asb the eye requires a light that is 100asb brighter to detect a difference. The threshold sensitivity (differential light sensitivity) is highest at the fovea and decreases progressively towards the periphery. After the age of 20 years the sensitivity decreases by 1dB per 10 years. For example, at age 20 years the sensitivity at the fovea is

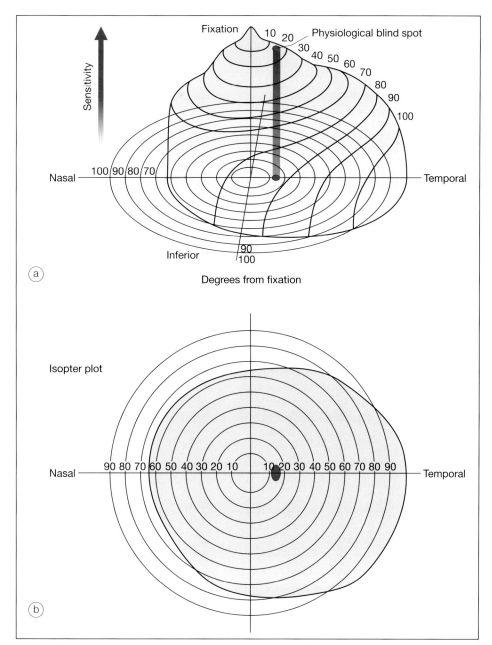

Fig. 1.39
(a) Island of vision; **(b)** island of vision from above

35dB, at age 30 years it will be 34dB, and at age 70 years it will be 30dB.

Types of perimetry

Perimetry involves evaluation of the visual field. Because of the subjective variability of patients' responses, efforts have been made to standardize the many aspects of testing in an endeavour to eliminate as many variables as possible.

Nevertheless, when interpreting a visual field defect, it is important to take into account patient reliability.

Kinetic

Kinetic perimetry is a two-dimensional assessment of the boundary of the hill of vision. It involves the presentation of a moving stimulus of fixed size and intensity from a non-seeing area to a seeing area until it is perceived (Fig. 1.41a). The stimulus is moved at a steady speed along various

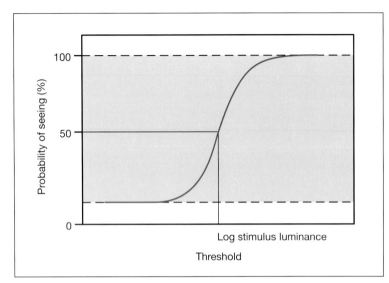

Fig. 1.40
Threshold graph (see text)

meridians (clock hours) and the point of perception is recorded on a chart. By joining these points along different meridians an isopter is plotted for that stimulus intensity. Using stimuli of different intensities a contour map of the visual field with several different isopters can be plotted. Kinetic perimetry can be performed by simple confrontation, the tangent screen, the Lister perimeter and the Goldmann perimeter.

Static

Static perimetry is a more difficult concept to perceive but once grasped forms the basis of modern glaucoma assessment. It is a three-dimensional assessment of the height (differential light sensitivity) of a pre-determined area of the hill of vision. Static perimetry involves the presentation of non-moving stimuli of varying luminance in the same position to obtain a vertical boundary of the visual field (Fig. 1.41b). Static perimetry can be performed using the Henson perimeter, the Octopus perimeter and the Humphrey perimeter.

Suprathreshold

Suprathreshold perimetry is used mainly for screening. It involves the presentation of visual stimuli at luminance levels above expected normal threshold values (suprathreshold) in various locations in the visual field. Detected targets indicate grossly normal visual function, whereas missed targets reflect areas of decreased visual sensitivity. Missed points can later be quantified (i.e. threshold measured). Selecting appropriate suprathreshold intensity is important; if too high, subtle early defects may be missed and if too low, close to threshold, a large number of normal individuals will miss stimuli.

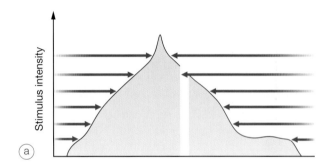

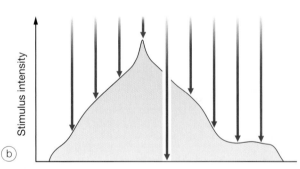

Fig. 1.41
Comparison of static and kinetic perimetry. **(a)** Kinetic perimetry – an object of fixed size and intensity is moved from the non-seeing to a seeing area; **(b)** static perimetry – stimuli of varying intensities are presented in a number of pre-determined locations

Threshold

Threshold perimetry is used for detailed assessment of the hill of vision by plotting the threshold luminance value in various locations in the visual field and comparing the results with age-matched 'normal' values. In Humphrey perimetry,

Fig. 1.42
Determination of threshold (see text)

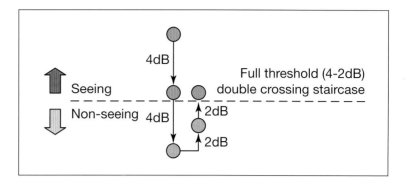

the intensity of a stimulus is increased by 4dB steps until threshold is crossed. Threshold is then re-determined by decreasing the intensity by 2dB steps (Fig. 1.42). Because threshold perimetry represents quantitative assessment it is the most accurate method of monitoring glaucomatous visual field defects. Printouts of a test contain geographic (i.e. grey scale) and numerical results. The latter generally includes the raw data (i.e. sensitivity in dB at each test location), the difference between the patient's results and that expected of a patient of similar age, and summary data (visual field indices). These indices include an assessment of diffuse field loss, localized defects and patient reliability.

Sources of error

The skill of the perimetrist in setting up the test, explaining the procedure to the patient, reassuring the patient and monitoring performance is fundamental to obtaining an accurate field. However, errors may still occur as a result of one or more of the following factors:

1. **Miosis** decreases threshold sensitivity in the peripheral field and increases variability in the central field in both normal and glaucomatous eyes. Pupils less than 3mm in diameter should therefore be dilated prior to perimetry.
2. **Lens opacities** have a profound effect on the visual field, which is exaggerated by miosis.
3. **Uncorrected refractive error** can cause a significant decrease of central sensitivity. If a hypermetropic patient who usually wears contact lenses is tested wearing spectacles, this will have the effect of magnifying and enlarging any scotomas as compared to contact lenses.
4. **Spectacles** can cause rim scotomas if small aperture lenses are used or if incorrectly dispensed.
5. **Ptosis**, even if mild, can result in suppression of the superior visual field.
6. **Inadequate retinal adaptation** may also lead to error if perimetry is performed soon after ophthalmoscopy.

Humphrey perimetry

The Humphrey consists of a hemispherical bowl on to which a target can be projected into any location of the visual field (Fig. 1.43). A monitor, on the side of the instrument, presents a series of menus. Background luminance of 31.5asb, the lower end of photopic illumination, and target luminance can be varied between 0.08asb and 10,000asb brighter than background which equates to a decibel range of 51 to 0. Variation in stimulus intensity is achieved by altering target size or luminance. Stimulus size is set prior to the test; only luminance is altered, while the test is in progress, in order to determine the threshold level for each point tested in the visual field.

Programs

The Humphrey has a range of suprathreshold and full threshold strategies (e.g. 30–1, 24–2). The number before the dash (24– or 30–) indicates the area of the tested field, in degrees from fixation. The 24° strategy tests 54 points and the 30° tests 76 points. The number after the dash (–1 or –2) describes the pattern of the points tested. The –2 strategy involves a grid of test points spaced 6° apart, offset from the vertical and horizontal meridians whereas the –1 includes points along the vertical and horizontal meridians.

1. **Suprathreshold** strategies are rapid (6 minutes per eye) qualitative programs. An 88-point screening test using a three-zone strategy may be used initially as it is fast and less demanding than full threshold formats. An absolute defect is indicated with a black square and a relative defect with a cross.
2. **Full-threshold strategy** is the gold-standard for monitoring glaucoma but has lost appeal for the following reasons:
   • The test time is long (over 13 minutes per eye).
   • Patients find it demanding.
   • There is a significant learning effect and often the

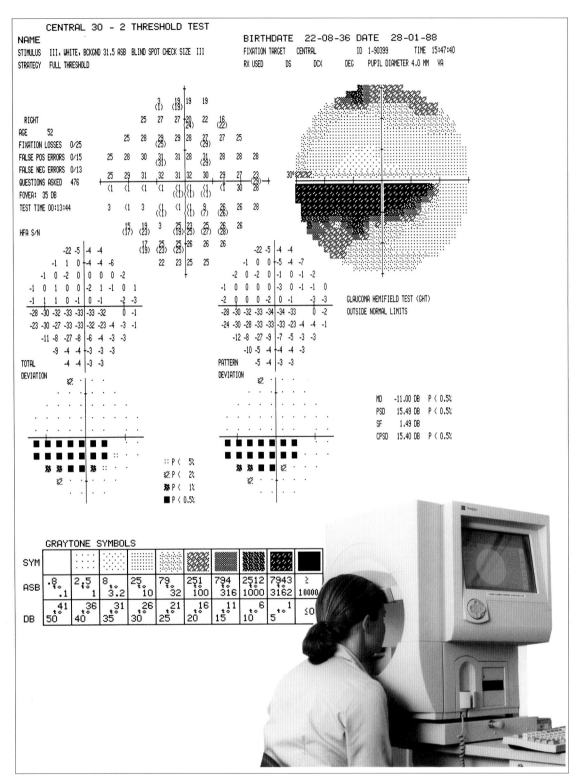

Fig. 1.43
Humphrey perimeter and display

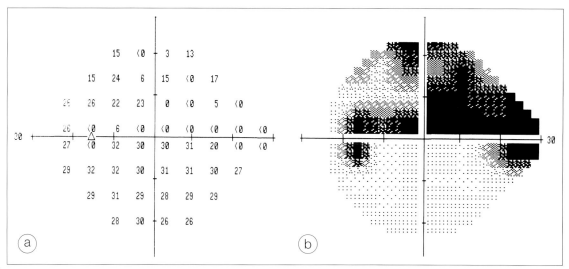

Fig. 1.44
Humphrey display. **(a)** Numerical; **(b)** grey scale

results of the first test may need to be disregarded for the purpose of detecting progression of visual field loss.
- Poor repeatability may occur, particularly in locations where there is some loss of sensitivity.
- The most commonly performed central full threshold strategy is 24–2. Initially four points are tested to determine threshold levels which are then used as a starting level for neighbouring points and so on until the entire field has been tested. Points where the anticipated response is out by 5dB of that expected are re-tested a second time; the second response is indicated in brackets on the final printout.

3. **SITA** (Swedish Interactive Thresholding Algorithm) strategy is one of the latest developments in automated perimetry which is available in both a standard and a faster version. The algorithm is similar to a full-threshold program but does not use a conventional staircase method to establish thresholds, thereby allowing the test to be much faster and more user-friendly. Standard SITA also shows greater sensitivity than full-threshold perimetry in detecting early visual field loss. The fast SITA is quicker but less sensitive than standard SITA.

Displays

1. **Numerical** display gives the threshold (dB) for all points checked (Fig. 1.44a). The figures in brackets indicate threshold at the same point checked a second time, if on initial testing it was at least 5dB less sensitive than expected.
2. **Grey scale** in which decreasing sensitivity is represented by darker tones is the simplest to interpret (Fig. 1.44b). The scale at the bottom of the chart shows corresponding

values of the grey tone symbols in abs and dB. Each change in grey scale tone is equivalent to 5dB change in threshold.
3. **Total deviation** (Fig. 1.45 left) represents the deviation of the patient's result from that of age-matched controls. The upper numerical display illustrates the differences in dB and the lower display exhibits these differences as grey symbols.
4. **Pattern deviation** (Fig. 1.45 right) is similar to total deviation except that it is adjusted for any generalized depression in the overall field which might be caused by other factors such as lens opacities or miosis.
5. **Probability values** (P) indicating the significance of the defects is shown as $< 5\%$, $< 2\%$, $< 1\%$ and $< 0.5\%$ (Fig. 1.45 bottom). The lower the P value the greater its clinical significance and the lesser the likelihood of the defect having occurred 'by chance'.

Reliability indices

Reliability indices reflect the extent to which the patient's results are reliable and should be analysed first. If grossly unreliable, further evaluation of a visual field printout is pointless.

1. **Fixation losses** indicate steadiness of gaze during the test. They are detected by presenting stimuli in the physiological blind spot. If the patient responds, a fixation loss is recorded. The lower the number of losses the more reliable is the test. A high fixation loss score may occur if the instrument has incorrectly plotted the blind spot.
2. **False positives** are detected when a stimulus is accompanied by a sound. If the sound alone is presented

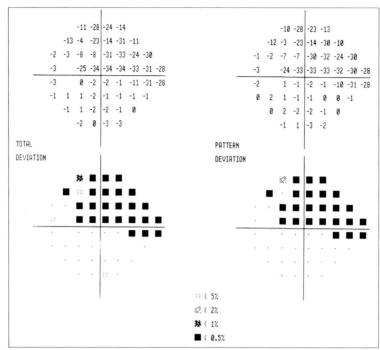

Fig.1.45
Total deviation, pattern deviation and probability indices

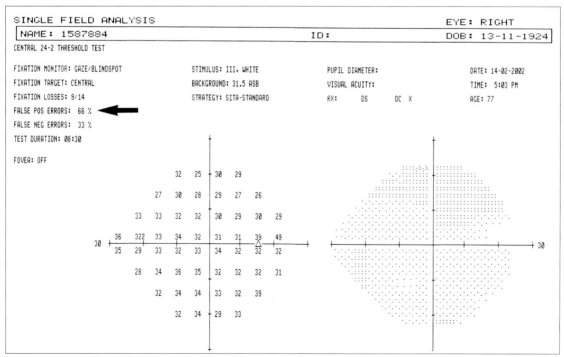

Fig. 1.46
High false-positive score (arrow) with an abnormally pale grey scale display

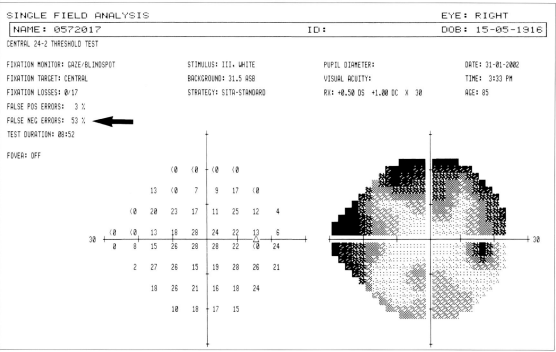

Fig. 1.47
High false-negative score (arrow) with a clover leaf-shaped grey scale display

(without an accompanying light stimulus) and the patient still responds, a false positive is recorded. False positive responses do not increase in damaged visual fields and a visual field with more than one false positive response is usually unreliable. A high false positive score suggests a 'trigger happy' patient. The grey scale printout appears abnormally pale (Fig. 1.46). Fixation losses are also frequently high and the glaucoma hemifield test shows abnormally high sensitivity.

3. **False negatives** are detected by presenting a stimulus much brighter than threshold at a location where sensitivity has already been recorded. If the patient fails to respond a false negative is recorded. A high false negative score indicates inattention or tiredness. It may also be due to short-term fluctuation that is associated with glaucoma, and may be an indicator of disease severity rather than patient unreliability. The greyscale printout in individuals with high false negative responses has a clover leaf shape (Fig. 1.47).

NB In patients who constantly fail to achieve good reliability indices it may be useful to switch to a suprathreshold strategy.

Global indices

Global indices summarize the results in a single number and are principally used to monitor progression of glaucomatous damage rather than for initial diagnosis.

1. **Mean deviation** (MD) (elevation or depression) is a measure of the overall field loss.
2. **Pattern standard deviation** (PSD) is a measure of focal loss or variability within the field taking into account any generalized depression in the hill of vision. An increased PSD is therefore a more specific indicator of glaucomatous damage than MD.
3. **Short-term fluctuation** (SF) is an indication of the consistency of responses. It is assessed by measuring threshold twice at ten pre-selected points and is calculated on the difference between the first and second measurements.
4. **Corrected pattern standard deviation** (CPSD) is a measure of variability within the field after correcting for short-term fluctuation (intra-test variability).

NB The last two indices are not available on SITA.

Frequency-doubling contrast test (FDT)

1. **Physiological principles.** Ganglion (M) cells with relatively large diameter axons comprise 25% of the ganglion cell population. They are particularly susceptible to glaucomatous damage and appear to be preferentially lost in early glaucoma. A loss of a small number of these cells therefore has a considerable effect on visual function. Psychophysiological tests designed to target visual function provided by this magnocellular pathway in the detection of early glaucoma have been devised.

2. **Frequency-doubling illusion** is produced when a low spatial frequency sinusoidal grating (less than one cycle per degree) undergoes high temporal frequency counter phase flicker (> 15Hz). The rapid alternation in which the light bars become dark and vice versa produces the illusion of the grating having doubled its frequency.

3. **The perimeter** is a tabletop instrument which can be used under normal room lighting and requires no patching, since the viewing canopy automatically covers the eye not being tested. The device requires minimal training and is relatively portable.

4. **Stimuli** are presented in 17 or 19 sectors in the central 20° or 30° depending on the program used, screening or full threshold.

5. **Testing time** is short with full threshold programs taking about 5 minutes per eye and screening procedures between 45 and 90 seconds per eye. Because of this most patients prefer the FDT test to conventional perimetry.

6. **Results** are displayed and printed together with reliability indices, probabilities, mean deviation and pattern standard deviation (Fig. 1.48). FDT has high sensitivity both in screening to differentiate healthy individuals from those with glaucoma and for quantifying glaucomatous damage. The results are minimally affected by refractive error of up to 6D and not at all by pupil size. The device has an age-adjusted normative database, as well as a statistical analysis package for immediate evaluation of results.

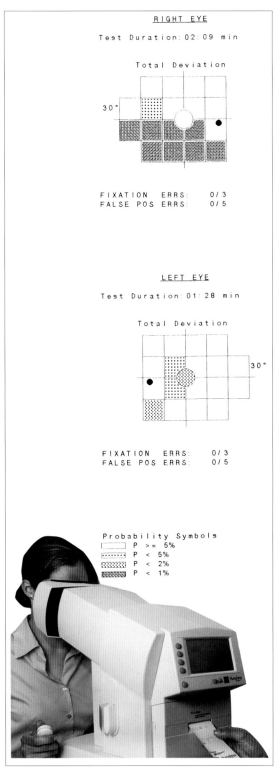

Fig. 1.48
Frequency-doubling perimeter and display

IMAGING TECHNIQUES

CORNEA

Specular microscopy

Specular microscopy is a study of the changes in different layers of the cornea under magnification which is 100 times greater than slit-lamp biomicroscopy. It is principally used to photograph the corneal endothelium. The image can then be analysed with respect to cellular size, shape, density and distribution. The normal endothelial cell is a regular hexagon (Fig. 2.1a). The normal cell density is about 3000 cells/mm^2; counts below 1000 are associated with a significant risk of endothelial decompensation.

I. Physics
- Light striking an optical surface can be reflected, transmitted or absorbed. Usually there is a combination of all three.
- When a light beam of the specular photomicroscope passes through the cornea, it encounters a series of interfaces between optically distinct regions.
- Some light is reflected specularly (i.e. like a mirror) back towards the photomicroscope when the angle of reflection is the same as the angle of incidence.

- This specular light is captured by the photomicroscope and forms an image which can be photographed and analysed.

2. Indications
- Evaluating the functional reserve of the corneal endothelium prior to intraocular surgery is the most important. A clear cornea with normal pachymetry (i.e. thickness) is not necessarily associated with normal endothelial morphology or cell density. Corneal oedema is likely to occur when preoperative cell density is reduced to between 300 and 700 cells/mm^2 and unlikely to occur when cell density is at least 1000 cells/mm^2.
- Evaluation of donor corneas regarding suitability for penetrating keratoplasty.
- To demonstrate various corneal disease states and dystrophies, particularly cornea guttata (Fig. 2.1b), Descemet membrane irregularities and posterior polymorphous dystrophy.

Corneal topography

I. Physics. Topography is the specular reflection of the image of an object by the tear film. Corneal topography

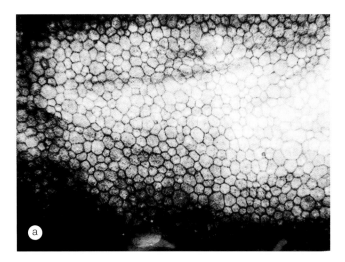

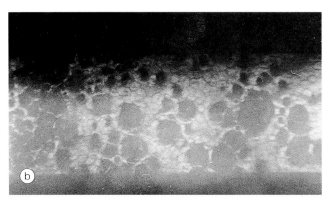

Fig. 2.1
Specular photomicrograph. **(a)** Normal corneal endothelium;
(b) cornea guttata with marked loss of endothelial mosaic
(Courtesy of T A Casey, K W Sharif, from *A Colour Atlas of Corneal Dystrophies and Degenerations*, Wolfe, 1991 – fig. b)

provides a colour-coded map of the corneal surface. The power in dioptres of the steepest and flattest meridians and their axes are calculated and displayed (Figs 2.2 and 2.3).

2. **Indications**
   - To quantify irregular astigmatism and corneal warping associated with contact lens wear.
   - To diagnose early keratoconus.
   - To evaluate changes in corneal shape after refractive surgery, corneal grafting or cataract extraction.

3. **Scales**
   - Steep curvatures (high dioptres) are coloured orange and red.
   - Flat curvatures (low dioptres) are coloured violet and blue.
   - Most normal corneas remain within the yellow-green spectrum of the scale.
   - Absolute scales have fixed end-points and each individual colour represents a specific power interval in dioptres.
   - An absolute scale should always be used to facilitate comparison over time and between patients.
   - Relative (normalized) scales are not fixed and vary according to the range in dioptres of the individual cornea.
   - It is very important to look carefully at the scale before interpreting the map.

4. **Interpretation** can be acquired only with practice; questions to be answered are:
   - What does the scale show?
   - Is the scale appropriate?
   - Is the map reliable?
   - What is the position of the pupil in relation to the curvature pattern display?

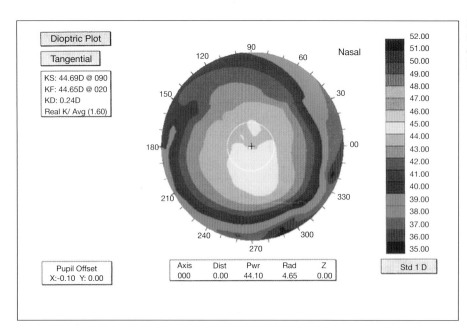

Fig. 2.2
Corneal map of a normal spherical cornea in an absolute scale ranging from 34D to 54D (Courtesy of E Morris)

Fig. 2.3
Normal relative scale map shows 3.5D of with-the-rule astigmatism and a typical bow-tie pattern (Courtesy of E Morris)

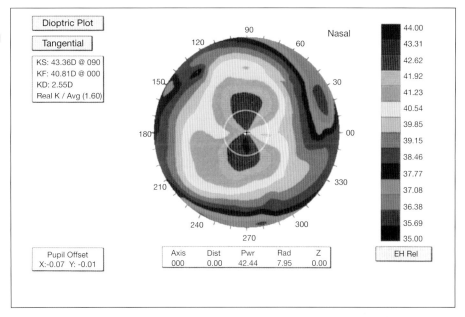

FUNDUS ANGIOGRAPHY

Fluorescein angiography

Principles

1. **Fluorescein** is an orange water-soluble dye that, when injected intravenously, remains largely intravascular and circulates in the blood stream.
2. **Fluorescein angiography** (FA) involves photographic surveillance of the passage of fluorescein through the retinal and choroidal circulations following intravenous injection (Fig. 2.4).
3. **Fluorescein binding.** On intravenous injection, 70–85% of fluorescein molecules bind to serum proteins (bound fluorescein); the remainder remain unbound (free fluorescein) (Fig. 2.5a).
4. **The outer blood–retinal barrier.** The major choroidal vessels are impermeable to both bound and free fluorescein. However, the walls of the choriocapillaris are extremely thin and contain multiple fenestrations through which free fluorescein molecules escape into the extravascular space (Fig 2.5b). They then pass across Bruch membrane but on reaching the retinal pigment epithelium (RPE) encounter tight junctional intercellular complexes termed zonula occludens, which prevent the passage of free fluorescein molecules across the RPE (Fig. 2.6).
5. **The inner blood–retinal barrier** is composed of the tight junctions between retinal capillary endothelial cells across which neither bound nor free fluorescein can pass (Fig. 2.7a); fluorescein is therefore confined within the lumen of the retinal capillaries. The basement membrane and pericytes play only a minor role in this regard. Disrup-

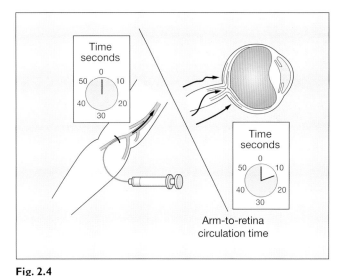

Fig. 2.4
Injection of fluorescein into the antecubital vein and its passage

tion of the inner blood–retinal barrier will permit leakage of both bound and free fluorescein into the extravascular space (Fig. 2.7b).

6. **Fluorescence** is the property of certain molecules to emit light of a longer wavelength when stimulated by light of a shorter wavelength. The excitation peak for fluorescein is about 490nm (blue part of the spectrum) and represents the maximal absorption of light energy by fluorescein. Molecules stimulated by this wavelength will be excited to a higher energy level and will emit light of a longer wavelength at about 530nm (green part of the spectrum) (Fig. 2.8).

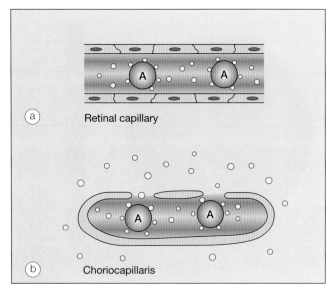

Fig. 2.5
Fluorescein binding and permeability

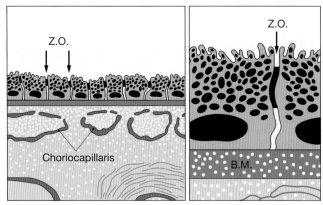

Fig. 2.6
The outer blood–retinal barrier (ZO = zonula occludens; BM = Bruch membrane)

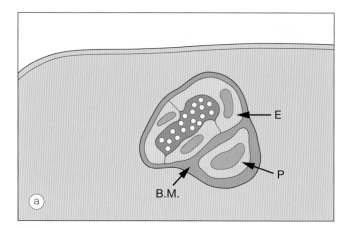

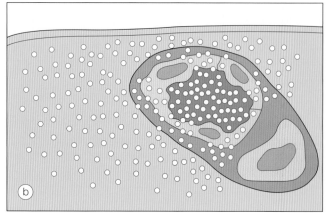

Fig. 2.7
The inner blood–retinal barrier

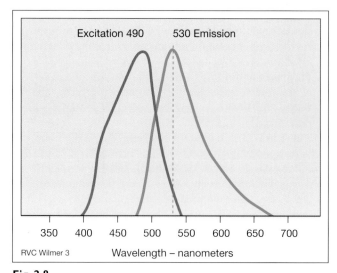

Fig. 2.8
Excitation and emission of fluorescence

7. **Filters** of two types are used to ensure that blue light enters the eye and only yellow-green light enters the camera (Fig. 2.9).
   a. A blue excitation filter through which passes white light from the camera. The emerging blue light enters the eye and excites the fluorescein molecules in the retinal and choroidal circulations, which then emit light of a longer wavelength (yellow-green).
   b. A yellow-green barrier filter then blocks any reflected blue light from the eye, allowing only yellow-green light to pass through unimpaired to be recorded.

Technique

A good quality angiogram requires adequate pupillary dilation and clear media.

a. The patient is seated in front of the fundus camera.
b. Fluorescein, usually 5ml of a 10% solution, is drawn up into a syringe. In eyes with opaque media, 3ml of a 25%

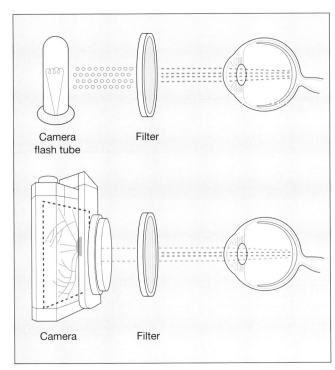

Fig. 2.9
Photographic principles of fluorescein angiography

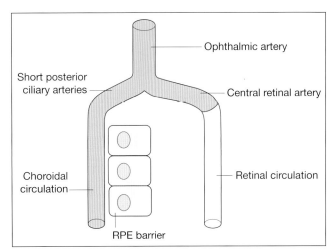

Fig. 2.10
Entry of fluorescein into the choroidal and retinal circulations

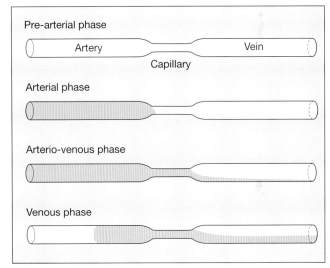

Fig. 2.11
Four phases of the fluorescein angiogram

solution may afford better results.

c. A 'red-free' image is captured.

d. Fluorescein is injected intravenously over a few seconds.

e. Images are taken at approximately 1-second intervals, 5–25 seconds after injection.

f. After the transit phase has been photographed in one eye, control pictures are taken of the opposite eye. If appropriate, late photographs may also be taken after 10 minutes and, occasionally, 20 minutes if leakage is anticipated.

Adverse effects

Discoloration of skin and urine is invariable. Mild side effects include nausea, vomiting, flushing of the skin, itching, hives and excessive sneezing. Serious but rare problems include syncope, laryngeal oedema, bronchospasm and anaphylactic shock.

> **NB** It is very important to have arrangements in place for managing these eventualities.

Phases of the angiogram

Fluorescein enters the eye through the ophthalmic artery, passing into the choroidal circulation through the short posterior ciliary arteries and into the retinal circulation through the central retinal artery. Because the route to the retinal circulation is slightly longer than that to the choroidal, the latter is filled about one second before the former (Fig. 2.10). In the choroidal circulation, precise details are often not discernible, mainly because of rapid leakage of free fluorescein from the choriocapillaris and also because the melanin in the RPE cells blocks choroidal fluorescence. The angiogram consists of the following overlapping phases (Fig. 2.11): (a) *choroidal (pre-arterial)*, (b) *arterial*, (c) *arteriovenous (capillary)*, (d) *venous* and (e) *late (elimination)*.

Normal angiogram

1. The choroidal (pre-arterial) phase occurs 8–12 seconds after dye injection and is characterized by patchy filling of

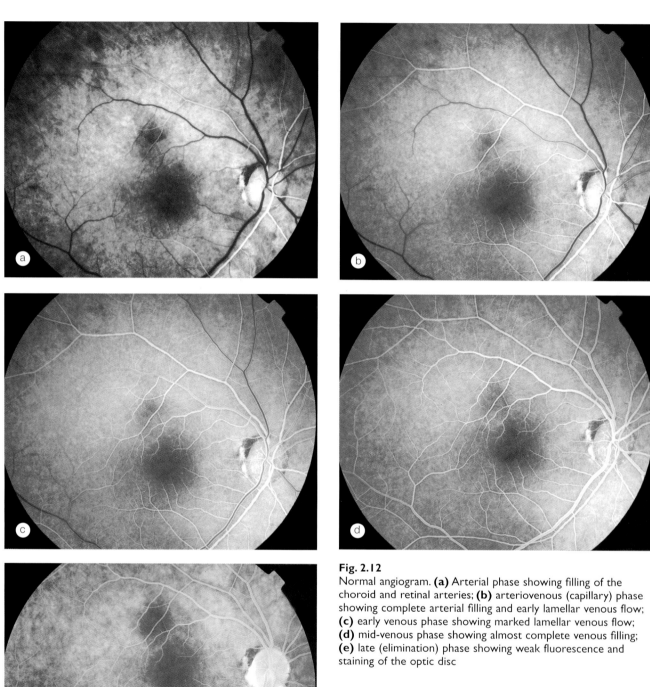

Fig. 2.12
Normal angiogram. **(a)** Arterial phase showing filling of the
choroid and retinal arteries; **(b)** arteriovenous (capillary) phase
showing complete arterial filling and early lamellar venous flow;
(c) early venous phase showing marked lamellar venous flow;
(d) mid-venous phase showing almost complete venous filling;
(e) late (elimination) phase showing weak fluorescence and
staining of the optic disc

the choroid due to leakage of free fluorescein through the fenestrated choriocapillaris. A cilioretinal artery, if present, will fill at this time because it is derived from the posterior ciliary circulation.

2. **The arterial** phase shows arterial filling and the continuation of choroidal filling (Fig. 2.12a).
3. **The arteriovenous** (capillary) phase shows complete filling of the arteries and capillaries with early laminar flow in the veins in which the dye appears to line the venous wall, leaving an axial hypofluorescent strip (Fig. 2.12b). Choroidal filling continues and background choroidal fluorescence increases as free fluorescein continues to leak from the choriocapillaris into the extravascular space. In hypopigmented eyes, this may be so marked that details of the retinal capillaries may obscured. In highly pigmented eyes, background choroidal fluorescence will be less obvious.
4. **The venous** phase
   a. **The early** phase exhibits complete arterial and capillary filling, and more marked laminar venous flow (Fig. 2.12c).
   b. **The mid-** phase displays almost complete venous filling (Fig. 2.12d).
   c. **The late** phase shows complete venous filling with reducing concentration of dye in the arteries.
5. **The late** (elimination) phase demonstrates the effects of continuous recirculation, dilution and elimination of the dye. With each succeeding wave, the intensity of fluorescence becomes weaker. Late staining of the disc is a normal finding (Fig. 2.12e). Fluorescein is absent from the angiogram after 5–10 minutes and is usually totally eliminated from the body within several hours.
6. **The dark appearance of the fovea** (Fig. 2.13a) is caused by three phenomena (Fig. 2.13b):

a. Absence of blood vessels in the foveal avascular zone.
b. Blockage of background choroidal fluorescence due to increased density of xanthophyll at the fovea.
c. Blockage of background choroidal fluorescence by the RPE cells at the fovea, which are larger and contain more melanin than elsewhere.

Hyperfluorescence

Increased fluorescence may be due to enhanced visualization of a normal density of fluorescein in the fundus, or an absolute increase in the fluorescein content of the tissues.

1. **A transmission** (window) defect is caused by atrophy or absence of the RPE (Fig. 2.14a) as in atrophic age-related macular degeneration. This results in unmasking of normal background choroidal fluorescence, characterized by early hyperfluorescence which increases in intensity and then fades without changing size or shape (Fig. 2.14b and c).
2. **Pooling** of dye in an anatomical space occurs due to breakdown of the outer blood–retinal barrier (RPE tight junctions):
   a. In the subretinal space as in central serous retinopathy (Fig. 2.15a). This is characterized by early hyperfluorescence which increases in both size and intensity (Fig. 2.15b and c).
   b. In the sub-RPE space as in a pigment epithelial detachment (PED – Fig. 2.16a). This is characterized by early hyperfluorescence which increases in intensity but not in size (Fig. 2.16b and c).
3. **Leakage** of dye may occur from abnormal choroidal vasculature such as choroidal neovascularization (CNV), breakdown of the inner blood–retinal barrier as in cystoid

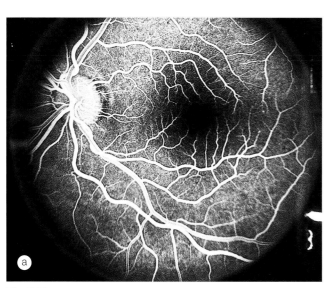
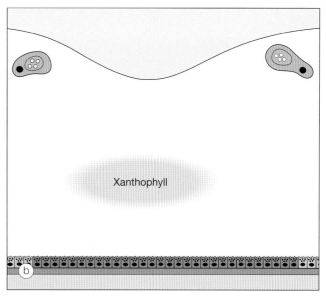

Fig. 2.13
Reasons for the dark appearance of the fovea on fluorescein angiography

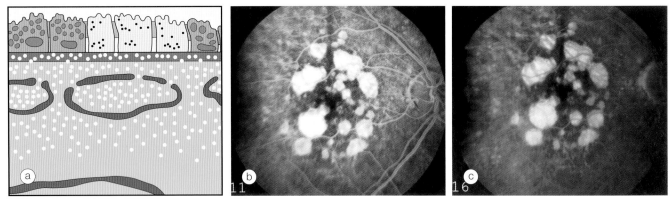

Fig. 2.14
Hyperfluorescence caused by a transmission (window) defect associated with atrophic age-related macular degeneration

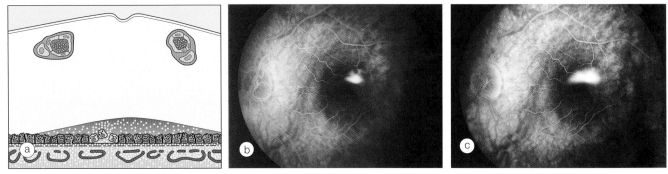

Fig. 2.15
Hyperfluorescence due to pooling of dye in the subretinal space in central serous retinopathy

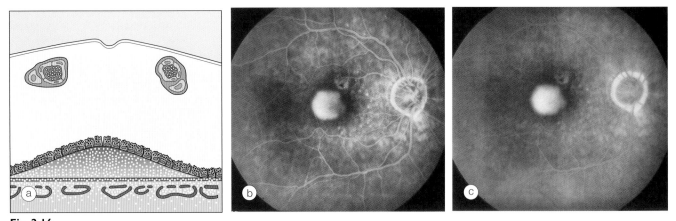

Fig. 2.16
Hyperfluorescence due to pooling of dye in the sub-retinal pigment epithelial space in pigment epithelial detachment

macular oedema, and retinal neovascularization as in proliferative diabetic retinopathy.

4. **Staining** of tissue as a result of prolonged retention of dye (e.g. drusen, fibrous tissue, exposed sclera) may be seen in the late (elimination) phase of the angiogram after the dye has left the choroidal and retinal circulations.

Hypofluorescence

Reduction or absence of fluorescence may be due to: (a) optical obstruction (masking) of normal density of fluorescein in a tissue (Fig. 2.17) or (b) inadequate perfusion of tissue with resultant low fluorescein content.

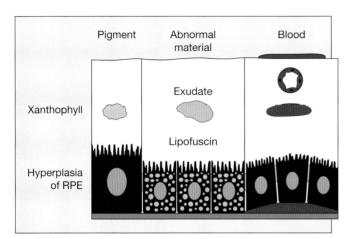

Fig. 2.17
Causes of blocked fluorescence

1. **Blockage of retinal fluorescence** may be caused by lesions anterior to the retina. Preretinal lesions such as blood will block all fluorescence (Fig. 2.18). Deep retinal lesions such as intraretinal haemorrhages and hard exudates will block only capillary fluorescence.
2. **Blockage of background choroidal fluorescence** is caused by all conditions that block retinal fluorescence as well as the following which block only choroidal fluorescence: (a) subretinal or sub-RPE lesions (e.g. blood), (b) increased density of the RPE (e.g. congenital hypertrophy – Fig. 2.19) and (c) choroidal lesions (e.g. naevi).
3. **Filling defects** may result from: (a) vascular occlusion which may involve the choroidal circulation or the retinal arteries, veins or capillaries (capillary drop-out) and (b) loss of the vascular bed (e.g. severe myopic degeneration).

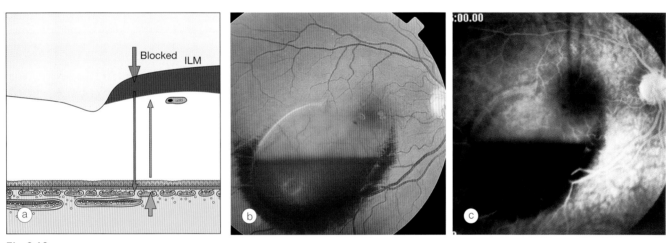

Fig. 2.18
Hypofluorescence due to blockage of all fluorescence by a preretinal haemorrhage

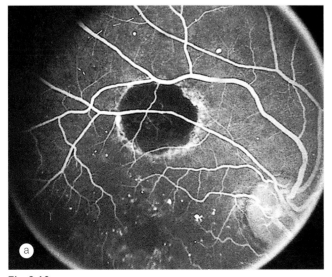
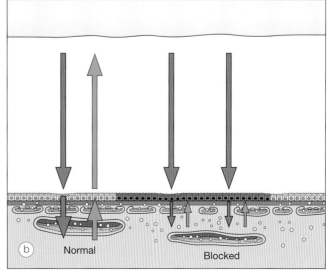

Fig. 2.19
Hypofluorescence due to blockage of background choroidal fluorescence by congenital hypertrophy of the retinal pigment epithelium

Step-wise approach to reporting angiograms

A fluorescein angiogram should be interpreted systematically to optimize diagnostic accuracy, as follows:

a. Indicate whether images of right, left or both eyes have been taken.
b. Comment on the red-free images.
c. Indicate any delay in filling as well as hyper- or hypofluorescence.
d. Indicate any characteristic features such as a smoke-stack or lacy filling pattern (see later).
e. Indicate any evolution through the course of the angiogram in the area or intensity of fluorescence.

NB It is important to take into consideration the patient's history and ophthalmoscopic findings before drawing conclusions from the angiogram.

Indocyanine green angiography

Principles

Whilst FA is an excellent method of demonstrating the retinal circulation against the uniform dark background of the RPE, it is not helpful in delineating the choroidal circulation. In contrast, indocyanine green (ICG) angiography is of particular value in studying the choroidal circulation and can be a useful adjunct to FA in the investigation of macular disease in some circumstances.

1. **ICG binding.** About 98% of ICG molecules bind to serum proteins (mainly albumin) on entering the circulation. This phenomenon reduces the passage of ICG through the fenestrations of the choriocapillaris, which are impermeable to the larger protein molecules.
2. **Fluorescence** of ICG is only 1/25 that of fluorescein. The excitation peak is at 805nm and emission at 835nm, in the near-infrared spectrum. The filters used are infrared barrier and excitation. Infrared light absorbed and emitted by the dye readily penetrates ocular pigments such as melanin and xanthophyll, as well as exudates or thin layers of subretinal blood. Additionally, the near-infrared light is scattered less than visible light, making ICG superior to FA in eyes with media opacities.

Technique

a. ICG powder is mixed with aqueous solvent to provide 40mg in 2ml.
b. The patient is seated in front of the imaging system with one arm outstretched.
c. A 'red-free' image is captured.
d. Between 25–40mg of dye is injected intravenously.
e. Rapid serial photographs are taken initially and then subsequent images are taken at about 3, 10 and 30 minutes.

f. Late phases yield the most useful information in ICG angiography because the dye remains in neovascular tissue after leaving the retinal and choroidal circulations.

If necessary, ICG angiography may be performed at exactly the same time or sequentially to FA. ICG videoangiography (ICG-VA) is commonly used as a supplementary test to FA in the diagnosis and treatment of occult CNV. The two angiographic systems used in performing ICG-VA are the high-resolution digital fundus camera and the scanning laser ophthalmoscope. The scanning laser ophthalmoscope is better at detecting the vascular net in the very early transit phase of the ICG-VA.

Adverse effects

Adverse effects are less common than with FA. Because ICG contains 5% iodine it should not be given to patients allergic to iodine. Its use is also contraindicated in pregnancy. The most common side effects are staining of stools, nausea, vomiting, sneezing and pruritus. Less common manifestations include syncope, skin eruptions, pyrexia, back ache and skin necrosis at the injection site.

Normal angiogram

1. **Early phase** (within 2–60sec of injection – Fig. 2.20a)
   - Hypofluorescence of the optic disc associated with poor perfusion of the watershed zone.
   - Prominent filling of choroidal arteries and early filling of choroidal veins.
   - Retinal arteries are visible but not veins.
2. **Early mid-phase** (1–3min – Fig. 2.20b)
   - Filling of the watershed zone.
   - Fading of choroidal arteries with increased prominence of choroidal veins.
   - Both retinal veins and arteries are visible.
3. **Late mid-phase** (3–15min – Fig. 2.20c)
   - Fading of filling of choroidal vessels.
   - Diffuse hyperfluorescence as the result of diffusion of dye from the choriocapillaris.
   - Retinal vessels are still visible.
4. **Late phase** (15–30min – Fig. 2.20d)
   - Hypofluorescence of choroidal vasculature against a background of hyperfluorescence resulting from staining of extrachoroidal tissue.
   - Decreased visibility of retinal vasculature.
   - The dye may remain in neovascular tissue after it has left the choroidal and retinal circulations.

Abnormal fluorescence

1. **Hyperfluorescence**
   - RPE 'window' defect.
   - Leakage from the retinal or choroidal circulations, or the optic nerve head.
   - Abnormal blood vessels.

Fig. 2.20
Normal indocyanine angiogram.
(a) Early phase; **(b)** early mid-phase;
(c) late mid-phase; **(d)** late phase
(Courtesy of S Milewski)

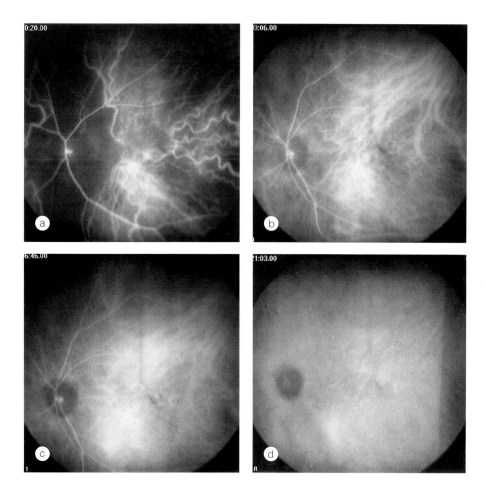

2. Hypofluorescence
- Blockage of fluorescence by pigment, blood or exudate.
- Obstruction of the circulation.
- Loss of vascular tissue.
- PED (hyperfluorescent on FA).

Clinical indications

1. **Exudative age-related macular degeneration.** Whilst FA remains the method of choice for the identification of classic CNV, ICG may be helpful in the following situations:
   - Occult CNV in which FA in the early frames may show a suspicion of CNV and the later frames merely show multiple foci of punctate or diffuse hyperfluorescence. This presumed occult CNV can be identified more clearly with ICG as a focal hyperfluorescent 'hot spot', a plaque or a combination of both. Whilst plaques have a poor visual prognosis, 'hot-spots' are potentially treatable.
   - CNV associated with PED, and subretinal or sub-RPE blood.
   - Recurrent CNV adjacent to laser scars.
   - Identification of feeder vessels.
2. **Other indications** in which ICG may help establish a diagnosis include the following:
   - Polypoidal choroidal vasculopathy in which ICG is superior to FA.
   - Chronic central serous retinopathy in which it is often difficult to interpret the area or areas of leakage on FA. However, ICG shows choroidal leakage and the presence of dilated choroidal vessels. Previously unidentified lesions are also frequently visible using ICG.
   - Breaks in Bruch membrane such as lacquer cracks in myopic eyes are more numerous and longer on ICG than on FA. Angioid streaks are more obvious and appear longer on ICG than on FA.

ULTRASONOGRAPHY

Principles

1. **Definitions.** Ultrasound is defined as sound that is beyond the range of human hearing. Ultrasonography uses high frequency sound waves to produce echoes as they strike interfaces between acoustically distinct structures.
2. **The transducer** consists of a piezoelectric crystal which when stimulated with an electric current vibrates at such a frequency as to emit ultrasonic waves. If the crystal is hit by ultrasonic waves it produces an electric current. Ultrasonic waves reflected by tissues return through the probe and are absorbed by the crystal, which produces a proportional electric current that is sent to the receiver. The signal is then processed and displayed as an echo on the screen. Amplification displays differences in the strengths of reflected echoes. Electric current is passed through the crystal and then switched off repeatedly in order that ultrasound may be emitted and then absorbed.

A-scan

A-scan ultrasonography is performed with a single ultrasound source. It produces a one-dimensional time-amplitude evaluation in the form of vertical spikes along a baseline (Fig. 2.21a). The height of the spikes is proportional to the strength of the echo. The greater the distance to the right, the greater the distance between the source of the sound and the reflecting surface. The distance between individual spikes can be precisely measured. It is used mainly to measure anterior chamber depth, lens thickness and axial length (Fig. 2.22).

B-scan

B-scan ultrasonography may be performed with a vector probe or a linear probe. In a vector probe one main source of ultrasound oscillates back and forth to produce a sweep of ultrasound (see Fig. 2.21b). In a linear probe multiple sources of ultrasound are aligned in a grid to cover a specific area. The amount of reflected sound is portrayed as a dot of light. The more sound reflected, the brighter the dot. B-scan two-dimension ultrasonography provides topographic information concerning the size, shape and quality of a lesion as well as its relationship to other structures. Three-dimensional imaging is also available and can be used to measure tumour volume and enhance localization of a radioactive plaque over a tumour. The addition of a Doppler facility allows the evaluation of blood flow. The frequency of the transducer determines which part of the globe or orbit is examined.

1. **Low frequency** transducers are particularly useful in detecting orbital pathology (Fig. 2.23).

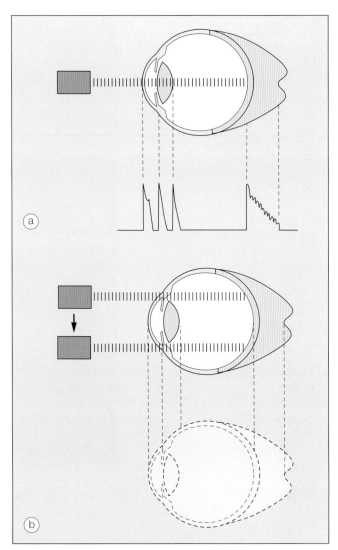

Fig. 2.21
Principles of ultrasonography. **(a)** A-scan; **(b)** B-scan

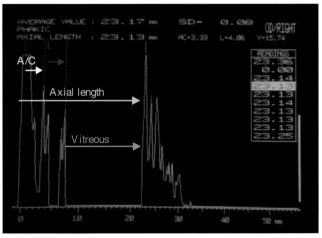

Fig. 2.22
A-scan display (Courtesy of D Michalik and J Bolger)

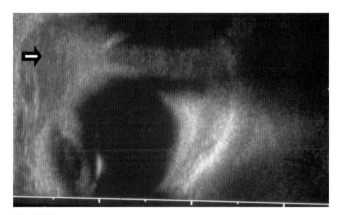

Fig. 2.23
Low frequency ultrasonography shows a capillary haemangioma involving the anterior orbit (arrow) (Courtesy of K Nischal)

2. **Moderate frequency** (7–10MHz) is used to examine the globe. The main indications are: (a) evaluation of eyes with opaque media for retinal detachment (Fig. 2.24a), (b) evaluation of posterior intraocular tumours (Fig. 2.24b) and (c) detection of calcification as in retinoblastoma and optic disc drusen.

3. **High frequency** utilizes 30–50MHz and allows high-definition imaging of the anterior segment but only to a depth of 5mm (Fig. 2.25a and b). It is of particular value in the evaluation of congenital corneal opacification (Fig. 2.25c and d).

Technique of B-scan ultrasonography of the globe

Each probe has a marker for orientation that correlates with a point on the display screen, usually the left.

1. **Technique**
   a. Anaesthetic drops are instilled and the patient placed in the supine position.
   b. The examiner should sit behind the patient's head and hold the probe with the dominant hand.
   c. Methylcellulose or an ophthalmic gel is placed on the tip of the probe to act as a coupling agent.
   d. Vertical scanning is performed with the marker on the probe superiorly orientated (Fig. 2.26a).
   e. Horizontal scanning is performed with the marker pointing towards the nose (Fig. 2.26b).
   f. The eye is then examined with the patient looking straight ahead, up, down, left and right. For each position a vertical and horizontal scan can be performed.
   g. The examiner then moves the probe in the opposite direction to the movement of the eye. For example when examining the right eye the patient looks to the left and the probe is moved to the patient's right, the nasal fundus anterior to the equator is scanned and vice-versa.

2. **Dynamic scanning** is performed by moving the eye but not the probe.

3. **Gain** adjusts the amplification of the echo signal, similar to volume control of a radio. Higher gain increases the sensitivity of the instrument in displaying weak echoes such as vitreous opacities. Lower gain only allows display of strong echoes such as the retina and sclera as well as improving resolution because it narrows the beam.

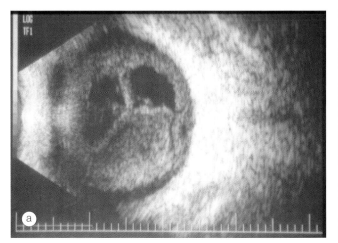
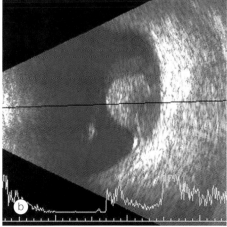

Fig. 2.24
Ultrasonography of the globe. **(a)** Vitreous haemorrhage and flat retina; **(b)** 'collar stud' choroidal melanoma (Courtesy of M Hamza)

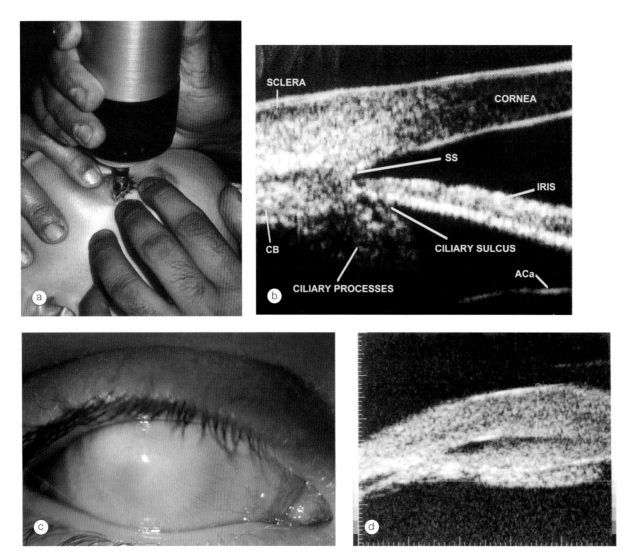

Fig. 2.25
High frequency ultrasonography of the anterior segment. **(a)** Method of scanning; **(b)** normal appearance; **(c)** severe corneal opacification; **(d)** scan shows virtual absence of the anterior chamber (Courtesy of K Nischal)

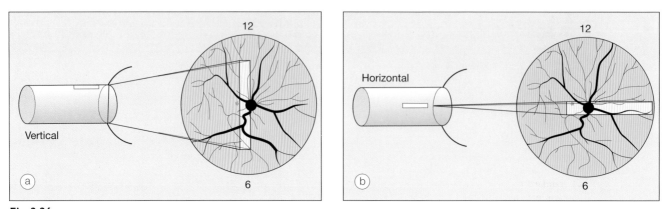

Fig. 2.26
Technique of ultrasound scanning of the globe. **(a)** Vertical with the marker pointing towards the brow; **(b)** horizontal with the marker pointing towards the nose

OPTICAL COHERENCE TOMOGRAPHY

1. **Physics.** Optical coherence tomography (OCT) is a non-invasive, non-contact imaging system which provides high resolution cross-sectional images of the retina, vitreous and optic nerve. Imaging of the anterior segment is also possible. OCT is analogous to B-scan ultrasonography but uses light instead of sound waves. The image is acquired by assessing the intensity of reflected light in conjunction with the intensity of reflectivity of different structures. Cross-sectional images are generated by scanning the optical beam in the transverse direction, thus yielding a two-dimensional data set that can be displayed as a false-colour or grey scale image.

2. **Indications**
   - Diagnosis of macular pathology such as holes, cystoid oedema, epiretinal membranes, vitreomacular traction and central serous retinopathy.
   - To monitor progression of disease processes and response to treatment.
   - Differentiation between long-standing retinal detachment and retinoschisis.
   - Analysis of the optic nerve head and retinal nerve fibre layer thickness.

3. **Normal appearance.** High reflectivity structures are depicted with bright colours (red and white), while those with low reflectivity are represented by darker colours (black and blue). Those with intermediate reflectivity appear green. In general, the nerve fibre layer and plexiform layers are seen as red, yellow or bright green. The inner and outer nuclear layers are seen as blue or black. The inner and outer plexiform layers can be seen as bright green (Fig. 2.27a). Ultrahigh resolution OCT (Fig. 2.27b) has the ability to identify fine retinal structures such as the external limiting membrane and ganglion cell layer which are not visualized as clearly on standard resolution OCT. The junction between the photoreceptor inner and outer segments is a thin red feature in the outer retina, anterior to the RPE and

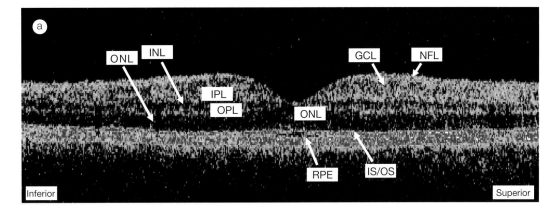

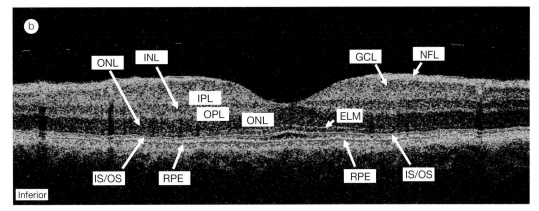

Fig. 2.27
OCT displays. **(a)** Standard resolution of a normal macula in which most of the major intraretinal layers can be visualized and correlated with intraretinal anatomy; **(b)** ultrahigh resolution improves visualization of smaller structures such as the external limiting membrane (ELM) and ganglion cell layer (GCL); (INL = inner nuclear layer; IPL = inner plexiform layer; IS/OS = photoreceptor inner and outer segment junction; NFL = nerve fibre layer; ONL = outer nuclear layer; OPL = outer plexiform layer; RPE = retinal pigment epithelium) (Courtesy of J Fujimoto)

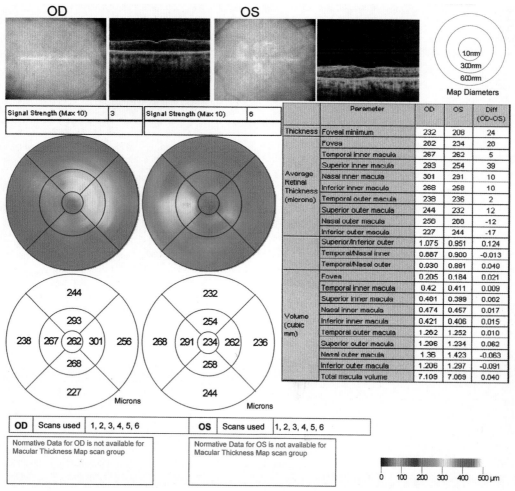

Fig. 2.28
Stratus OCT numerical and false colour display of macular thickness in both eyes (Courtesy of S Milewski)

choriocapillaris. Detailed quantitative information on retinal thickness is displayed numerically and in a false-colour topographical map (Fig. 2.28).

IMAGING IN GLAUCOMA

Confocal scanning laser tomography

1. Physics. The Heidelberg Retinal Tomograph (HRT) is a scanning laser ophthalmoscope that can interpret differences in the profile of the optic nerve head and peripapillary retinal nerve fibre layer (NFL) a to produce a computerized three-dimensional topographical image. This profile is then compared to a regression analysis derived profile.

2. Indications
- To distinguish normal from glaucomatous eyes.
- To monitor disease progress.

3. Display
- Images of the disc and peripapillary retina are shown at the top of the display (Fig. 2.29).
- In the topographic image (top left) the cup is represented in red, the neuroretinal rim in green and the slope in blue.
- The reflectivity image (top right) is divided into six sectors. A green tick within a sector indicates within normal limits, a yellow exclamation mark borderline and a red cross abnormal.
- The two cross-section images (top centre and middle left) show the amount of cupping in the vertical and horizontal planes. Two lines represent the edge of the optic disc and the single red line represents the

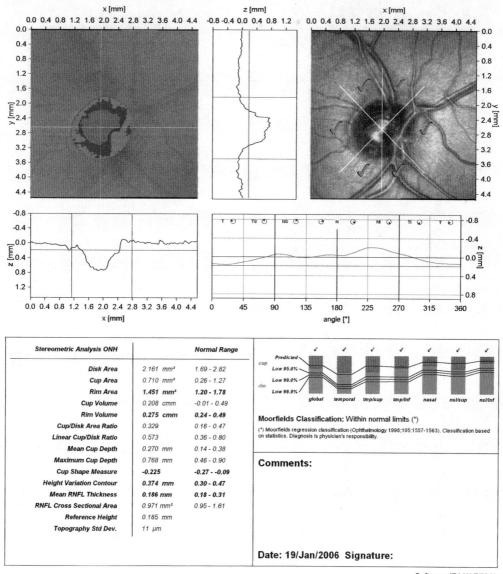

Fig. 2.29
Heidelberg Retinal Tomograph of a normal eye

arbitrary reference plane (which is normally 50μm below the plane of the retina).

- The graph (centre right) displays the height variation of the retinal surface along the contour line (green). The reference line (red) below this shows the position of the separation surface between the cup and the neuroretinal rim. This reference plane is parallel to the peripapillary retinal surface and is located 50μm below the retinal surface at the contour line and on the peripapillary bundle. It is thus approximately located at

the lower extent of the NFL. The display of the retinal surface height variation along the contour line begins temporally at 0 degrees. The height profile is plotted in a clockwise direction for a right eye and a counter-clockwise direction for a left eye. The graph largely corresponds to the course of the NFL thickness along the disc margin.

- The Moorfields regression analysis is depicted as a seven colour bar graph, one bar for each segment and one global bar (bottom right). If the top of the green bar lies

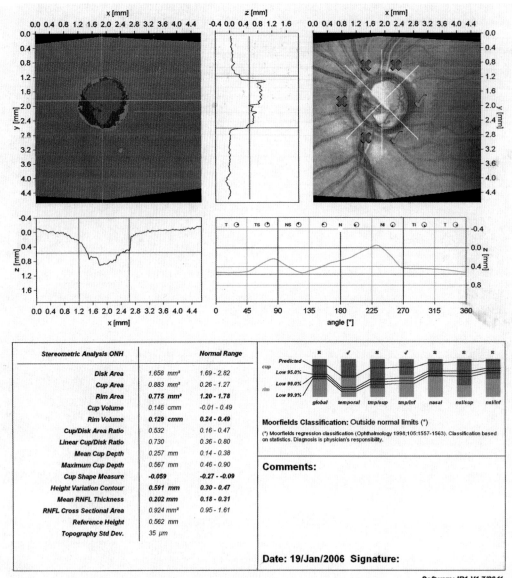

Fig. 2.30
HRT of glaucomatous eye

above the 95.0% prediction interval then the corresponding disc segment is classified as within normal limits, if it lies between the 95.0% and 99.9% it is borderline and if it lies below 99.9% it is outside normal limits.

- Detailed stereometric data are presented in a table (bottom left). Readings outside normal are indicated with an asterisk (Fig. 2.30).

Scanning laser polarimetry

1. **Physics.** The GDxVCC (glaucoma diagnosis variable corneal compensation) retinal nerve fibre layer analyser measures the change in polarization caused by the birefringence of NFL axons. The degree of polarization is assessed over an area of 1.75 disc diameters concentric to the disc and the profile of the density of the NFL established; the thicker the RNFL the greater the polarization.

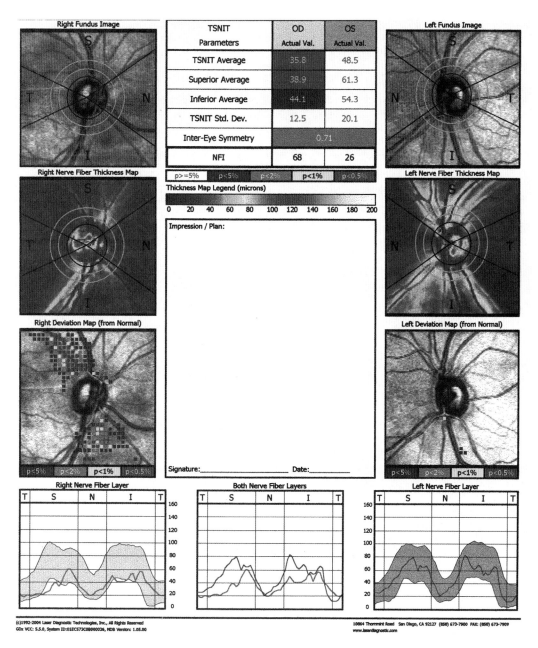

Fig. 2.31
GDxVCC shows reduction retinal nerve fibre density in the right eye and abnormal parameters (Courtesy of J Salmon)

2. **Indications**
   - To distinguish normal from glaucomatous eyes.
   - To monitor disease progress.
3. **Display** provides colour images of the optic nerve head and RNFL maps in the four quadrants (Fig. 2.31):
   - The fundus image of the left and right eyes at the top is useful in identifying image quality.
   - The thickness maps are presented in a colour-coded spectrum from blue to red. Red followed by yellow indicates a thick RNFL whereas blue followed by green shades are consistent with thin RNFL. The map has an hourglass appearance because the RNFL is thickest superiorly and inferiorly.
   - The deviation maps show the location and magnitude of RNFL defects as tiny colour coded squares (pixels).
   - The TSNIT (temporal-superior-inferior-temporal) graph is displayed at the bottom. It shows the actual values for that eye along with a shaded area that represents the 95% normal range for that age. The curve in a healthy eye should fall within the shaded area and has a double hump pattern because the superior and inferior fibres are thickest. The central printout shows the values for both eyes together.
   - Parameters for each eye are displayed in a table (top centre). The nerve fibre indicator (NFI) at the bottom of the table indicates a global value based on the entire thickness map and is the optimal parameter for discriminating normal from glaucoma. Normal is 1–30, borderline is 31–50 and abnormal is 51–100.

NEUROIMAGING

Imaging techniques for visualizing the brain and orbit are evolving and improving and there are now a wide variety of tests available. It is very important to match the appropriate imaging study to the clinical findings so that it is paramount for the ophthalmologist to provide the radiologist with the suspected differential diagnosis and localization of the presumed lesion.

Computed tomography

Physics

Computed tomography (CT) uses X-ray beams to obtain tissue density values from which detailed cross-sectional images are formed by a computer. Tissue density is represented by a grey scale, white being maximum density (e.g. bone) and black being minimum density (e.g. air). It is important to view images of the orbit in at least two planes; usually axial and coronal images are sufficient. Recent technical advance in CT has led to the wider use of multidetector ('multislice')

scanners. These have the ability to acquire thinner slices leading to improved spatial resolution and faster examination times without a proportionate increase in radiation dose. Images are acquired in an axial form and can be viewed in any plane using computer reconstruction. This multiplanar information can be an advantage over magnetic resonance imaging (MR) with regard to anatomical detail.

Contrast

Iodinated contrast material improves sensitivity and specificity but is contraindicated in patients allergic to iodine and those with renal failure. Contrast is not indicated in the assessment of acute haemorrhage, bony injury or localization of foreign bodies because it may mask visualization of these high density structures.

Indications

CT is widely available, easy to perform, relatively inexpensive, takes only a few minutes and is generally well tolerated by claustrophobic patients. However, unlike MR it exposes the patient to ionizing radiation. The main indications for CT are as follows.

1. **Orbital trauma,** for the detection of bony lesions such as fractures (Fig. 2.32a) and erosions, and demonstration of skull anatomy. Foreign bodies as well as blood, herniation of extraocular muscles into the maxillary sinus and surgical emphysema can also be assessed.
2. **Evaluation of the extraocular muscles** in thyroid eye disease (Fig. 2.32b). Although MR may also be of use, CT is usually sufficient.
3. **Bony involvement of orbital tumours** is better assessed using CT rather than MR.
4. **Orbital cellulitis** for assessment of intraorbital extension and subperiosteal abscess formation,
5. **Detection of intraorbital calcification** as in optic disc drusen, meningioma and retinoblastoma.
6. **Detection of acute cerebral or subarachnoid haemorrhage** (Fig. 2.32c and d) because this is harder to visualize on MR in the first few hours.
7. **Visual loss.** As a quick and easily available first-line investigation in the assessment of visual loss in order to exclude a compressive lesion of the optic nerve.
8. **When MR is contraindicated** (e.g. patients with ferrous foreign bodies).

Magnetic resonance imaging

Physics

MRI depends on the rearrangement of hydrogen nuclei (protons – positively charged) when a tissue is exposed to a

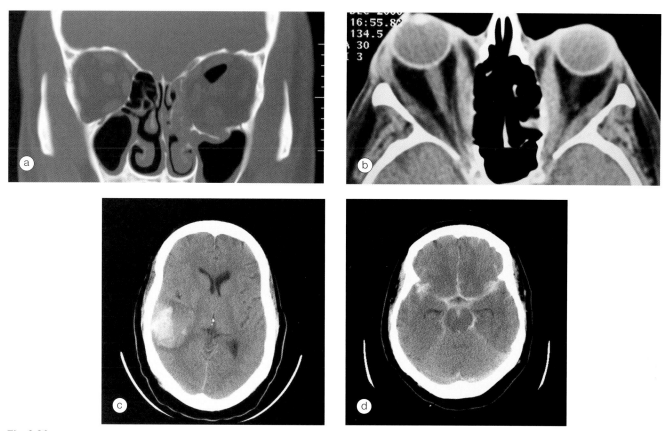

Fig. 2.32
CT scans. **(a)** Coronal image shows a left blowout fracture of the floor and medial wall as well as orbital emphysema; **(b)** axial image shows enlargement of extraocular muscles and right proptosis in thyroid eye disease; **(c)** axial image shows an acute parenchymal haematoma in the right temporal lobe; **(d)** axial image shows extensive subarachnoid blood in the basilar cisterns, and Sylvian and anterior interhemispheric fissures (Courtesy of N Sibtain – figs a, c and d; A Pearson – fig. b)

short electromagnetic pulse. When the pulse subsides, the nuclei return to their normal position, re-radiating some of the energy they have absorbed. Sensitive receivers pick up this electromagnetic echo. Unlike CT, it does not subject the patient to ionizing radiation. Exposed tissues produce radiation with characteristic intensity and time patterns. The signals are analysed, computed and displayed as a cross-sectional image which may be: (a) *axial* (b) *coronal* or (c) *sagittal*.

Imaging sequences

T1- and T2-weighted images are routinely acquired in MR imaging of the brain. Weighting refers to two methods of

measuring the relaxation times of the excited protons after the magnetic field has been switched off. Various body tissues have different relaxation times so that a given tissue may be T1- or T2-weighted (i.e. best visualized on that particular type of image). In practice both types of scans are usually performed.

1. **T1-weighted** images are best for normal anatomy. Hypointense (dark) structures include CSF and vitreous. Hyperintense (bright) structures include fat, blood and contrast agents (Fig. 2.33a, c and e).
2. **T2-weighted** images are useful for viewing pathological changes because water is hyperintense. Therefore oedematous pathological tissue (e.g. inflammation) will be of brighter signal than normal surrounding tissue. CSF and

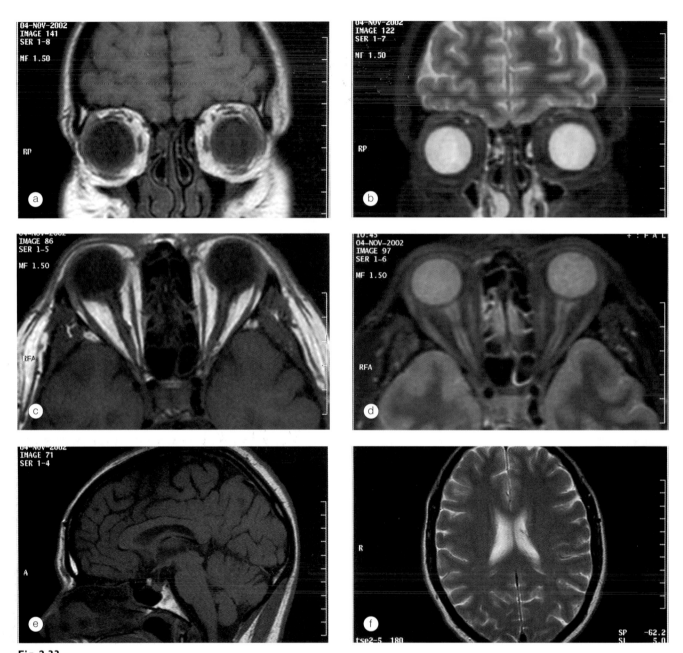

Fig. 2.33
MR scans. **(a)** T1-weighted coronal image through the globes – vitreous is hypointense (dark) and orbital fat is hyperintense (bright); **(b)** T2-weighted image – vitreous is hyperintense; **(c)** T1-weighted axial image through the globes and optic nerves – vitreous and CSF around the optic nerves are hypointense and orbital fat is hyperintense; **(d)** T2-weighted axial image – vitreous and CSF are hyperintense; **(e)** T1-weighted midline sagittal image through the brain – CSF in the third ventricle is hypointense; **(f)** T2-weighted axial image through the brain – CSF in the lateral ventricles is hyperintense

vitreous are hyperintense as they have high water content. Blood vessels appear black on T2 imaging unless they are occluded (Fig. 2.33b, d and f).

NB Bone and calcification are poorly visualized on MR.

Enhancement

1. **Gadolinium** is a substance which acquires magnetic moment when placed in an electromagnetic field. Administered intravenously, it remains intravascular unless there is a breakdown of the blood–brain barrier. It is only visualized on T1-weighted images, and enhancing lesions such as tumours and areas of inflammation will appear bright on these images. Ideally MR is performed both before (Fig. 2.34a) and after (Fig. 2.34b) administration of gadolinium. Special head or surface coils can also be used to improve spatial definition of the image. Gadolinium is safer than iodine; adverse effects are uncommon and usually relatively innocuous (e.g. nausea, hives and headache). Gadolinium does not show up on T2-weighted studies.
2. **Fat-suppression techniques** are applied for imaging the orbit because the bright signal of orbital fat on conventional T1-weighted imaging frequently obscures other orbital contents. Fat-suppression eliminates this bright signal and better delineates normal structures (optic nerve and extraocular muscles) as well as tumours, inflammatory lesions and vascular malformations. The two types of fat suppression sequences used for orbital imaging are:
   a. *T1 fat saturation* which is used with gadolinium. This allows areas of abnormal enhancement (e.g. optic nerve sheath) to be visualized as the T1 high signal of the surrounding orbital fat is suppressed (Fig. 2.34c and d).
   b. *STIR* (Short T1 Inversion Recovery) is considered the optimal sequence for detecting intrinsic lesions of the intraorbital optic nerve (e.g. optic neuritis – Fig. 2.34e). STIR images have very low signal from fat but still have high signal from water. They can therefore be described as a fat suppressed pathology sequence.
3. **FLAIR** (fluid attenuation inversion recovery) sequences suppress the bright cerebrospinal fluid on T2-weighted images to allow better visualization of adjacent pathological tissue such as periventricular plaques of demyelination (Fig. 2.34f).

Limitations

- It does not image bone (which appears black), although this is not necessarily a disadvantage.
- It does not detect recent haemorrhage and is therefore inappropriate in patients with acute intracranial bleeding.
- It cannot be used in patients with magnetic foreign objects (e.g. cardiac pacemakers, intraocular foreign bodies and ferromagnetic aneurysm clips).
- It requires the patient to cooperate and remain motionless.
- It is difficult to perform on claustrophobic patients.

Specific neuro-ophthalmic indications

MR is the technique of choice for lesions of the intracranial pathways. It is important to submit an accurate clinical history to the radiologist and direct attention to specific areas of potential pathology, in order to ensure appropriate imaging.

1. **The optic nerve** is best visualized on coronal STIR images in conjunction with coronal and axial T1 fat saturation post-gadolinium images (Fig. 2.34e). Axial T1 images are useful for displaying normal anatomy. MR can detect lesions of the intraorbital part of the optic nerve (e.g. neuritis, gliomas) as well as intracranial extension of optic nerve tumours.
2. **Optic nerve sheath lesions** (e.g. meningiomas) are of similar signal intensity on T1- and T2-weighted images but enhance avidly with gadolinium (Fig. 2.34a).
3. **Sellar masses** (e.g. pituitary tumours) are best visualized by T1-weighted contrast-enhanced studies (Fig. 2.34b). Coronal images optimally demonstrate the contents of the sella turcica as well as the suprasellar and parasellar regions and are usually supplemented by sagittal images.
4. **Cavernous sinus pathology** is best demonstrated on coronal images and contrast may be required.
5. **Intracranial lesions of the visual pathway** (e.g. inflammatory, demyelinating, neoplastic, vascular). MR allows further characterization of these lesions as well as better anatomical localization, and may be indicated in situations where CT is normal but the clinical picture suggests otherwise.
6. **Intracranial aneurysms** may sometimes be visualized by conventional MR in which case magnetic resonance angiography may also be performed, although this is not the technique of choice in the primary evaluation of suspected aneurysm (see below).

NB It is easy to tell the difference between a CT scan and an MR scan as bone will appear white on a CT scan and will not be clearly demonstrated on MR.

Angiography

Magnetic resonance angiography

Magnetic resonance angiography (MRA) is a non-invasive method of imaging the intra- and extracranial carotids and

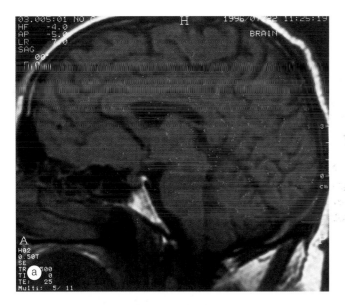
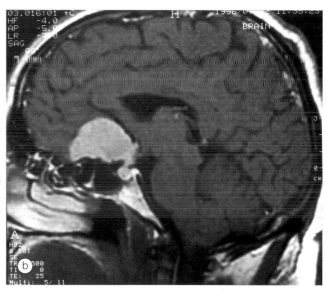
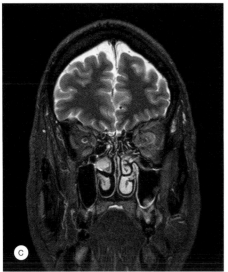
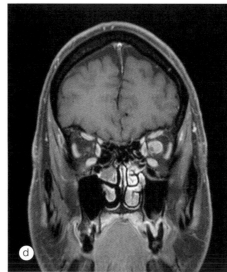
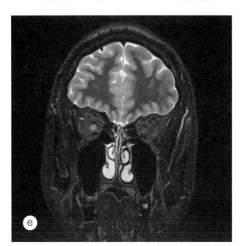
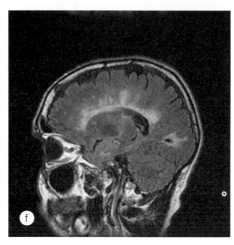

Fig. 2.34
Enhancement techniques. **(a)** Pre-gadolinium coronal T1-weighted sagittal image of a meningioma; **(b)** post-contrast image of the same patient shows enhancement of the tumour; **(c)** coronal STIR image shows an intermediate signal intensity mass surrounding the left optic nerve, consistent with an optic nerve sheath meningioma; **(d)** T1-weighted coronal fat saturation image of the same patient shows avid homogeneous enhancement of a left optic nerve sheath meningioma; **(e)** coronal STIR image of right optic neuritis shows a high signal within the optic nerve with enlargement of the optic nerve-sheath complex; **(f)** sagittal FLAIR image shows multiple periventricular plaques of demyelination (Courtesy of D Thomas – figs a and b; N Sibtain – figs c, d, e and f)

vertebrobasilar circulations (Fig. 2.35a) to demonstrate stenosis, dissection, occlusion, arteriovenous malformations and aneurysms. Typically, this technique uses the motion sensitivity of MR to visualize blood flow within vessels and does not require contrast. However because it relies on flow, thrombosed aneurysms may be missed and turbulent flow may lead to difficulties in interpretation. Furthermore MRA is unreliable at detecting very small aneurysms.

Magnetic resonance venography

Magnetic resonance venography (MRV) is indicated in the diagnosis of venous sinus thrombosis. It may also be of use in benign intracranial hypertension in conjunction with conventional MR, as it may show evidence of chronically thrombosed veins. As with MRA this study does not require contrast and depends on detection of flow within veins, although parameters are adjusted to ensure that the slower blood flow velocities of venous sinuses are detected.

Computed tomography angiography

Computed tomography angiography (CTA) is emerging as the method of choice in the investigation of intracranial aneurysms (Fig. 2.35b). It enables acquisition of extremely thin slice images of the brain following intravenous contrast. Images of the vessels can be reconstructed in three dimensions and viewed in any direction on a workstation. The investigation is safe and quick and without the 1% risk of stroke that is carried with conventional catheter angiography.

Computed tomography venography

Computed tomography venography (CTV) may be useful when MR is contraindicated or there are difficulties in distinguishing slow flow from thrombus on MR. The technique is similar to CTA, only images are acquired in the venous phase of contrast enhancement (Fig. 2.35c). However it is not as sensitive as MR in detecting associated parenchymal changes and this usually limits its use to equivocal cases.

Conventional catheter angiography

Conventional intra-arterial catheter angiography is usually performed under a local anaesthetic. A catheter is passed via the femoral artery into the internal carotid and vertebral arteries in the neck under fluoroscopic guidance. Following contrast injection images are taken in rapid succession. Digital subtraction results in images of the contrast-filled vessels without any background structure such as bone (Fig. 2.35d). Until recently, this technique was the first-line investigation in the diagnosis of intracranial aneurysms. This remains true in some centres where CTA is a relatively new technique and in cases where CTA is equivocal or negative. Other indications include assessment of vascular malformations and tumour vascularity where preoperative embolization is being considered.

Positron emission tomography

Positron emission tomography (PET/CT) is a new diagnostic imaging tool that uses radioactive glucose that accumulates within malignant cells because of their high rate of metabolism. Following injection the patient is imaged on a whole body scanner to reveal tumours that may have been overlooked by conventional CT or MR. It is a sensitive tool for the detection and staging of hepatic and extra-hepatic metastatic choroidal melanoma.

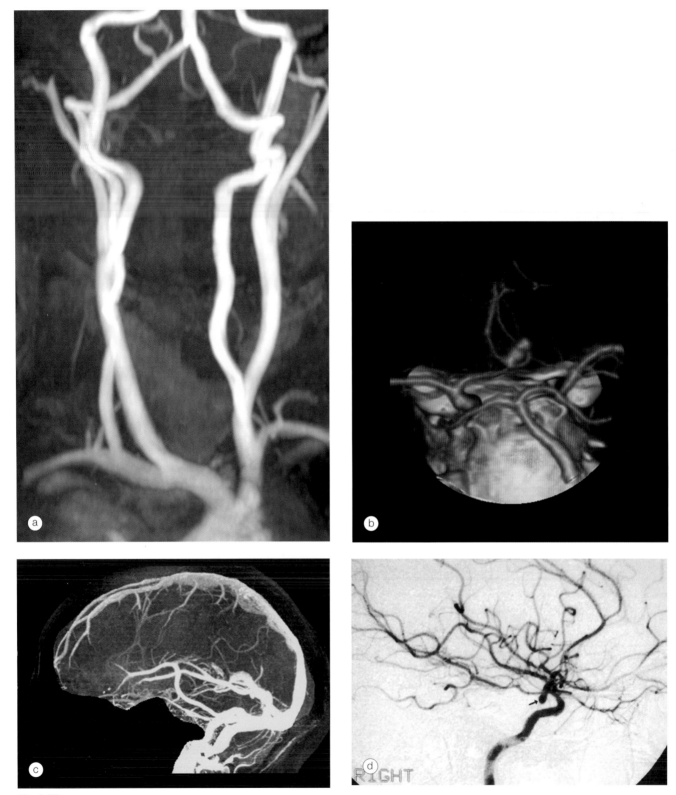

Fig. 2.35
Angiography. **(a)** Normal MRA of the external carotid and vertebral circulation; **(b)** CT angiogram shows an anterior communicating artery complex aneurysm that has a lobulated outline and points superiorly; **(c)** normal CT venogram; **(d)** conventional catheter angiogram with subtraction shows a posterior communicating aneurysm at the junction with the internal carotid artery (Courtesy of N Sibtain – figs a, b and c; S Cudlip – fig. d)

CHAPTER 3

DEVELOPMENTAL MALFORMATIONS AND ANOMALIES

EYELIDS

Epicanthic folds

Epicanthic folds are bilateral vertical folds of skin that extend from the upper or lower lids towards the medial canthi. They may give rise to a pseudo-esotropia.

1. **Signs**
   a. *Palpebralis* The folds are symmetrically distributed between the upper and lower lids (Fig. 3.1a); this is the most common type in Caucasians.
   b. *Tarsalis*. The folds originate in the medial aspects of the upper lids and extend medially before dissipating (Fig. 3.1b); this is the most common type in Orientals.
   c. *Inversus* is associated with the blepharophimosis syndrome. The folds start in the lower lids and extend upwards to the medial canthal areas (Fig. 3.1c).
   d. *Superciliaris*. The folds arise above the brow and extend downwards to the lateral aspect of the nose.
2. **Treatment** of small folds is by Y-V plasty, whilst large folds require a Mustarde Z-plasty.

Telecanthus

Telecanthus is an uncommon condition that may occur in isolation or in association with blepharophimosis syndrome (see Fig. 3.3).

1. **Signs.** Increased distance between the medial canthi as a result of abnormally long medial canthal tendons (Fig. 3.2). It should not be confused with hypertelorism in which there is wide separation of the orbits.
2. **Treatment** involves shortening and refixation of the medial canthal tendons to the anterior lacrimal crest or insertion of a transnasal suture.
3. **Associated systemic syndromes** include Waardenburg, Möbius, Treacher Collins, Rubinstein–Taybi and Turner.

Blepharophimosis syndrome

1. **Inheritance.** The blepharophimosis syndrome (BPS) is a rare, AD disorder. BPS1 (with premature ovarian failure) and BPS2 (without premature ovarian failure) are caused by mutations in FOXL2 gene on chromosome 3.
2. **Signs** (Fig. 3.3)
   • Moderate to severe symmetrical ptosis with poor levator function.
   • Short horizontal palpebral aperture.
   • Telecanthus and epicanthus inversus.
   • Lateral ectropion of lower lids.
   • Poorly developed nasal bridge and hypoplasia of the superior orbital rims.

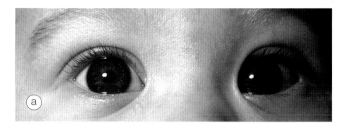
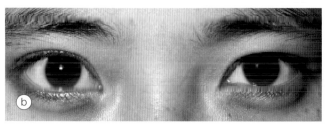
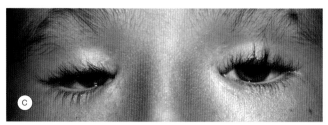

Fig. 3.1
Epicanthic folds. **(a)** Palpebralis; **(b)** tarsalis; **(c)** inversus

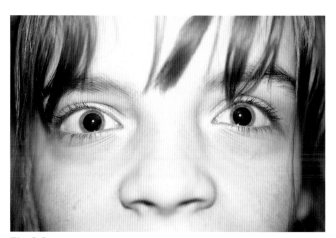

Fig. 3.2
Telecanthus

3. **Treatment** initially involves correction of epicanthus and telecanthus followed a few months later by bilateral frontalis suspension. It is also important to treat amblyopia which is present in about 50% of cases.

Epiblepharon

Epiblepharon is very common in Orientals and should not be confused with the much less common congenital entropion.

I. Signs
- An extra horizontal fold of skin stretches across the anterior lid margin and the lashes are directed vertically, especially in the medial part of the lid (Fig. 3.4a and b).
- When the fold of skin is pulled down the lashes turn out and the normal location of the lid becomes apparent (Fig. 3.4c).
2. **Treatment** is not required in the majority of cases because spontaneous resolution with age is the rule. Persistent cases are treated by excising a strip of skin and muscle, and fixation of the skin crease to the tarsal plate (Hotz procedure – Fig. 3.4d, e and f)

Congenital entropion

Upper lid entropion

Upper lid entropion is usually secondary to mechanical effects of microphthalmos which cause variable degrees of upper lid inversion.

Lower lid entropion

Lower lid entropion is caused by improper development of the inferior retractor aponeurosis.

I. Signs
- In-turning of the entire lower eyelid and lashes with absence of the lower lid crease (Fig. 3.5).
- When downward pressure is applied to the lid, the entire lid becomes pulled away from the globe.
2. **Treatment** involves the Hotz procedure.

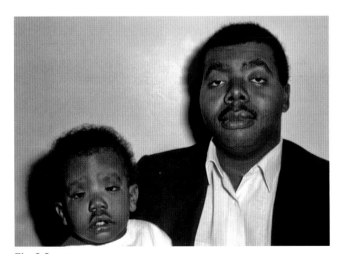

Fig. 3.3
Blepharophimosis syndrome

Coloboma

A coloboma is an uncommon, unilateral or bilateral, partial or full-thickness eyelid defect. It occurs when eyelid development is incomplete, due to either failure of migration of lid ectoderm to fuse the lid folds or to mechanical forces such as amniotic bands.

1. **Upper lid** colobomas occur at the junction of the middle and inner thirds and may occasionally be associated with Goldenhar syndrome (Fig. 3.6a).
2. **Lower lid** colobomas occur at the junction of the middle and outer thirds and are frequently associated with systemic conditions, most notably Treacher Collins syndrome (Fig. 3.6b) and amniotic band syndrome.
3. **Treatment** of small defects involves primary closure, while large defects require skin grafts and rotation flaps.

Euryblepharon

1. **Signs**
- Horizontal enlargement of the palpebral fissure with associated lateral canthal malposition and lateral ectropion (Fig. 3.7).
- In severe cases it may result in lagophthalmos and exposure keratopathy.
2. **Associations** include lateral displacement of the proximal lacrimal drainage system, a double row of meibomian gland orifices, telecanthus and strabismus.
3. **Treatment** involves lateral canthal tightening or tarsorrhaphy.

Microblepharon

Microblepharon is characterized by small eyelids, often associated with anophthalmos (see Fig. 3.30a).

Ablepharon

1. **Signs.** Deficiency of the anterior lamellae of the eyelids.
2. **Treatment** involves reconstructive skin grafting.
3. **Systemic anomalies.** Ablepharon-macrostomia syndrome characterized by an enlarged fish-like mouth due to fusion defects, ear and genital anomalies, and redundant skin (Fig. 3.8).

Cryptophthalmos

1. **Signs.** In complete cryptophthalmos the lids are replaced by a layer of skin which is fused with a microphthalmic eye (Fig. 3.9a). Incomplete cryptophthalmos is characterized

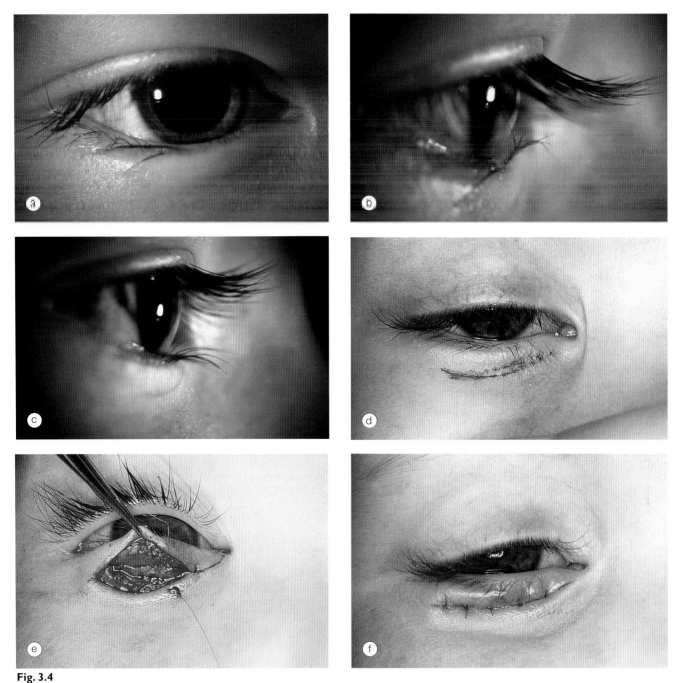

Fig. 3.4
(a) Epiblepharon; **(b)** lashes pointing upwards; **(c)** normal position following manual correction; **(d)** incisions marked on the medial two-thirds of the lid; **(e)** skin sutures passed deeply through the inferior tarsal border; **(f)** skin cease created by skin sutures attached to the tarsal plate (Courtesy of A G Tyers, J R O Collin, from Colour Atlas of Ophthalmic Plastic Surgery, Butterworth-Heinemann, 2001 – figs d, e and f)

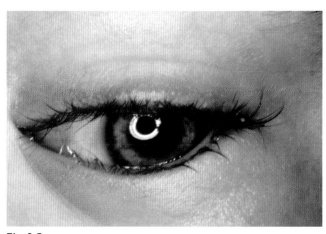

Fig. 3.5
Congenital entropion

by microphthalmos, rudimentary lids and a small conjunctival sac (Fig. 3.9b).

2. **Systemic association.** Fraser syndrome is an AD condition characterized by syndactyly, urogenital anomalies, malformations of the upper airway and craniofacial structures and mental handicap. It is caused by mutations in FRAS-1 gene or the structurally similar FRAS-2 gene on chromosome 13.

Congenital upper lid eversion

Congenital upper lid eversion is a rare condition more frequently seen in black infants, Down syndrome and in collodion skin disease (Fig. 3.10). It is typically bilateral and

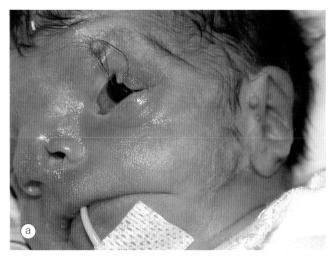

Fig. 3.6
(a) Upper lid coloboma in Goldenhar syndrome – note preauricular tags; **(b)** lower lid coloboma in Treacher Collins syndrome (Courtesy of A Pearson – fig. a)

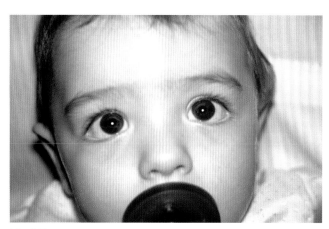

Fig. 3.7
Euryblepharon

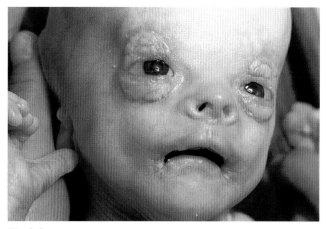

Fig. 3.8
A patient following reconstructive surgery who has the ablepharon-macrostomia syndrome – note the enlarged, fish-like mouth (Courtesy of H Mroczkowska)

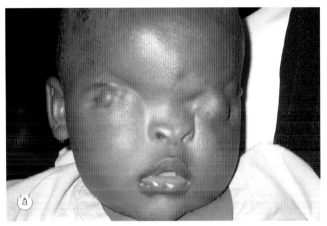 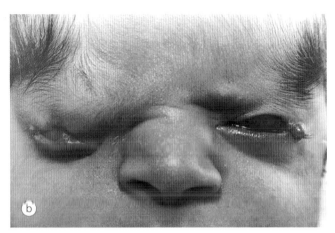

Fig. 3.9
Cryptophthalmos. **(a)** Complete; **(b)** partial in Fraser syndrome (Courtesy of D Meyer – fig. a)

symmetrical and may either resolve spontaneously with conservative treatment or may require surgery.

CRANIOSYNOSTOSES

Crouzon syndrome

Crouzon syndrome is caused primarily by premature fusion of the coronal and sagittal sutures.

1. **Inheritance** is AD, but 25% of cases represent a fresh mutation. The gene (FGFR2) has been isolated to chromosome 10.
2. **Systemic features**
   - Short anteroposterior head distance and wide cranium due to premature fusion.
   - Midfacial hypoplasia and curved 'parrot-beak' nose which gives rise to a 'frog-like' facies and mandibular prognathism
   - Inverted V-shaped palate.
   - Acanthosis nigricans.
3. **Ocular features**
   - Proptosis due to shallow orbits is the most conspicuous feature (Fig. 3.11a).
   - Hypertelorism (wide separation of the orbits).
   - V pattern exotropia (Fig. 3.11b).
   - Ametropia and amblyopia.
   - Vision-threatening complications include exposure keratopathy and optic atrophy, due to compression at the optic foramen.
4. **Ocular associations** include aniridia, blue sclera, cataract, ectopia lentis, glaucoma, coloboma, megalocornea and optic nerve hypoplasia.

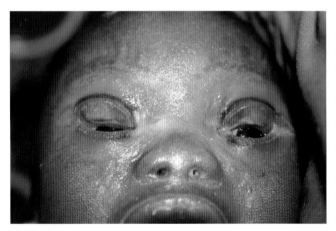

Fig. 3.10
Congenital upper lid eversion in a patient with collodion skin disease (Courtesy of D Meyer)

Apert syndrome

Apert syndrome (acrocephalosyndactyly) is the most severe of the craniosynostoses and may involve all the cranial sutures.

1. **Inheritance** is AD, but the majority of cases are sporadic and are associated with older paternal age.
2. **Systemic features**
   - Oxycephaly with flattened occiput and steep forehead.
   - Horizontal groove above the supraorbital ridge.
   - Midfacial hypoplasia with a 'parrot-beak' nose and low-set ears (Fig. 3.12a).
   - High-arched palate, cleft palate and bifid uvula.
   - Syndactyly of the hands (Fig. 3.12b) and feet.

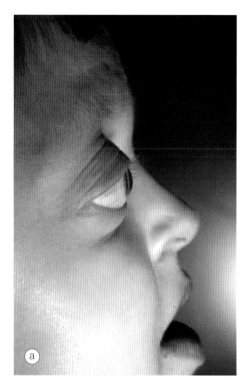

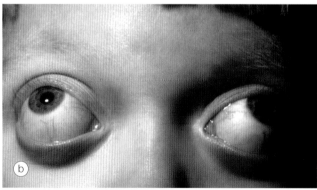

Fig. 3.11
Crouzon syndrome. **(a)** Proptosis, midfacial hypoplasia and mandibular prognathism; **(b)** 'V' exotropia

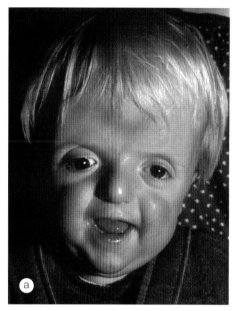

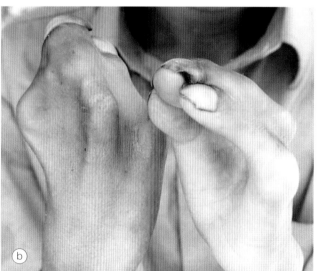

Fig. 3.12
Apert syndrome. **(a)** Mild shallow orbits, midfacial hypoplasia, 'parrot-beak' nose and antimongoloid slant of the palpebral fissures; **(b)** syndactyly of the hands (Courtesy of N Raik – fig. b)

- Anomalies of the heart, lungs and kidneys.
- Acneiform skin eruptions on the trunk and extremities.
- Mental handicap in 30% of cases.

3. Ocular features
- Shallow orbits, proptosis and hypertelorism are generally less pronounced than in Crouzon syndrome.
- Exotropia.
- Antimongoloid slant of the palpebral apertures.
- Vision-threatening complications include corneal exposure and optic atrophy.

4. Ocular associations include keratoconus, ectopia lentis and congenital glaucoma.

Pfeiffer syndrome

1. Inheritance is AD.

2. Systemic features
- Midfacial hypoplasia and down-slanting palpebral fissures (Fig. 3.13a).
- Broad thumbs and great toes (Fig. 3.13b), and soft tissue syndactyly.
- Elbow ankylosis.
- Occasionally clover-leaf skull.
- Mental handicap is uncommon.

3. Ocular features include shallow orbits and hypertelorism similar to Apert syndrome.

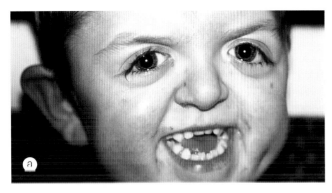

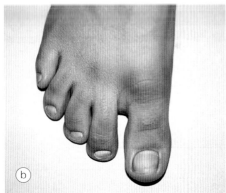

Fig. 3.13
Pfeiffer syndrome. **(a)** Midfacial hypoplasia and down-slanting palpebral fissures; **(b)** broad great toe (Courtesy of K Nischal)

MANDIBULOFACIAL DYSOSTOSES

Treacher Collins syndrome

Treacher Collins syndrome is characterized by malformation of derivatives of the first and second branchial arches.

1. **Inheritance** is AD with high penetrance and variable expressivity, although 60% of cases occur with no family history and are thought to arise by *de novo* mutation.
2. **Systemic features**
   - Bilateral hypoplasia of the mandible and zygoma and beaked nose (Fig. 3.14a).
   - Micrognathia and malformed ears (Fig. 3.14b).
   - Conductive deafness.
3. **Ocular features**
   - Antimongoloid slanting of the palpebral apertures.
   - Colobomas of the lateral lower eyelids (see Fig. 3.6b).
   - Cataract.
   - Microphthalmos.
   - Atresia of the lacrimal passages.

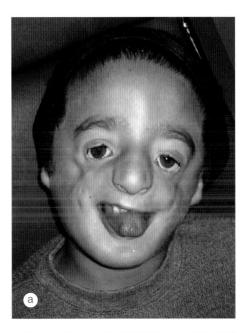

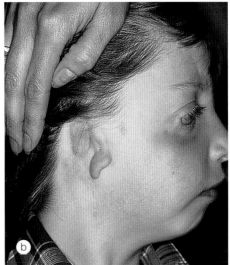

Fig. 3.14
Treacher Collins syndrome. **(a)** Bilateral hypoplasia of the maxilla and zygoma and beaked nose; **(b)** micrognathia and malformed ear

Goldenhar syndrome

Goldenhar syndrome (oculo-auriculo-vertebral spectrum) is usually sporadic. It is thought that hemifacial microsomia and Goldenhar syndrome are part of the same spectrum of anomaly.

1. **Systemic features**
   - Hypoplasia of the malar, maxillary and mandibular regions which may be bilateral (Fig. 3.15a).
   - Macrostomia and microtia (Fig. 3.15b).
   - Preauricular and facial skin tags (Fig. 3.15c).
   - Hemivertebrae, usually cervical.

- Incidence of mental deficiency increases with presence of microphthalmos.

2. Ocular features

- Epibulbar dermoid and upper-lid notch or coloboma (Fig. 3.15d).
- Microphthalmos.
- Disc coloboma.

Hallermann–Streiff–François syndrome

1. Systemic features

- Short stature.
- Beak-shaped nose, micrognathia and hypotrichosis (sparse hair) (Fig. 3.16a and b).
- Dental anomalies (Fig. 3.16c).
- Narrow upper respiratory airway which may necessitate tracheostomy in early infancy.

2. Ocular features

- Bilateral microphthalmos.

- Cataract which may be membranous.
- Nystagmus and strabismus.
- Disc coloboma.
- Blue sclera.

CORNEA

Microcornea

Microcornea is a rare AD, unilateral or bilateral condition.

1. Signs

- The adult horizontal corneal diameter is 10mm or less (Fig. 3.17a).
- Hypermetropia, shallow anterior chamber but other dimensions are normal.

2. Ocular associations include glaucoma (initially closed angle, later open angle), congenital cataract, leukoma

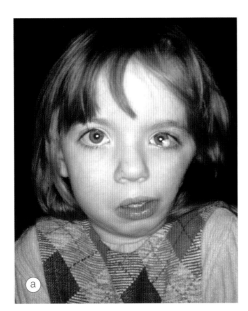
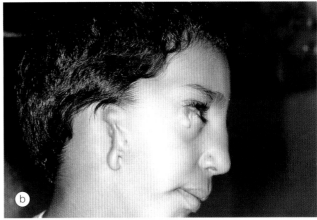
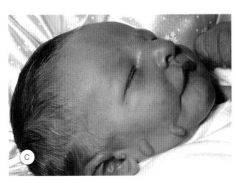
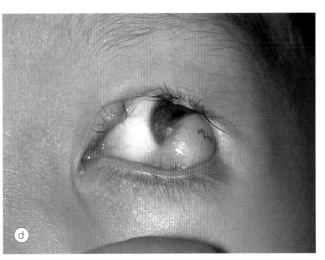

Fig. 3.15
Goldenhar syndrome. **(a)** Malar, maxillary and mandibular hypoplasia, and limbal dermoid; **(b)** microtia; **(c)** skin tags; **(d)** upper lid coloboma and limbal dermoid (Courtesy of U Raina – fig. c; N Rogers – fig. d)

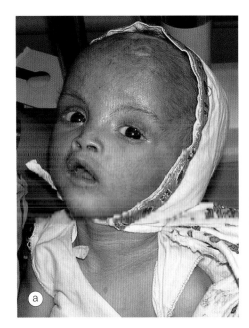
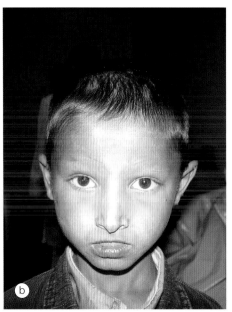
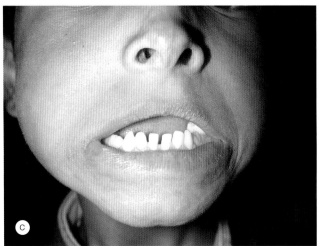

Fig. 3.16
Hallermann–Streiff–François syndrome. **(a)** Beak-shaped nose and severe hypotrichosis; **(b)** beak-shaped nose, micrognathia and mild hypotrichosis; **(c)** dental anomalies (Courtesy of M Parulekar – fig. a; N Rogers – figs b and c)

(Fig. 3.17b), cornea plana, Rieger anomaly, microphakia and optic nerve hypoplasia.

3. **Syndromic systemic associations** include fetal alcohol, Ehlers–Danlos, Weill–Marchesani, Waardenburg, Nance–Horan and Cornelia de Lange.

Megalocornea

Megalocornea is a rare, bilateral, non-progressive condition thought to be due to defective growth of the optic cup.

1. **Inheritance** is usually X-linked recessive so that 90% of affected individuals are males. The condition maps to Xq21.3-q22. The remaining cases are AD and rarely AR.

2. **Signs**
   - Normal intraocular pressure.
   - Large corneal diameter, ≥13mm, and a very deep anterior chamber (Fig. 3.18a).
   - High myopia and astigmatism but normal visual acuity.
   - Pigment dispersion with Krukenberg spindle, trabecular hyperpigmentation (Fig. 3.18b) and iris transillumination.
   - Lens subluxation may occur due to zonular stretching.

3. **Systemic associations** include Alport syndrome, Marfan syndrome, Ehlers–Danlos syndrome, Down syndrome, osteogenesis imperfecta, progressive facial hemiatrophy, renal carcinoma and megalocornea-mental retardation syndrome.

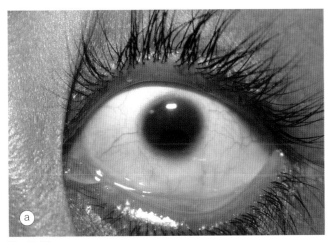
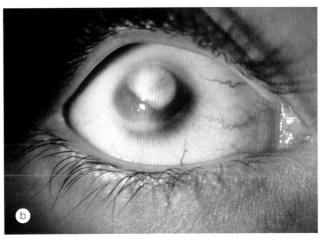

Fig. 3.17
(a) Severe microcornea; **(b)** microcornea and corneal opacity (Courtesy of S Fogla – fig. a)

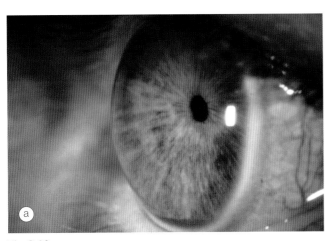
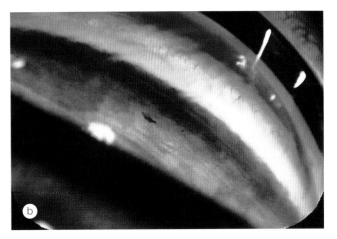

Fig. 3.18
(a) Megalocornea and a very deep anterior chamber; **(b)** gonioscopy shows a very wide angle and trabecular hyperpigmentation due to pigment dispersion

Sclerocornea

Sclerocornea is a rare, usually bilateral condition, characterized by variable opacification and vascularization of the cornea. It may occur in isolation or in association with Peters anomaly and cornea plana.

- If this is restricted to the periphery, the resulting 'scleralization' makes the cornea appear small (Fig. 3.19a).
- In some cases virtually the entire cornea may be affected (Fig. 3.19b).

Cornea plana

Cornea plana is a rare bilateral condition.

1. Inheritance
- The AD form is a relatively mild disorder in which the refractive power of the cornea is reduced to 38–42D.
- The AR form results in significant impairment of visual acuity as corneal refractive power is reduced to 25–35D.

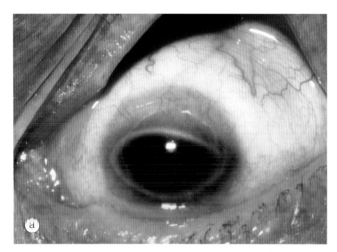

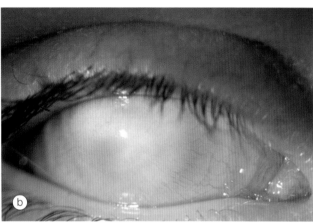

Fig. 3.19
Sclerocornea. **(a)** Mild; **(b)** severe (Courtesy of J Salmon – fig. a; K Nischal – fig. b)

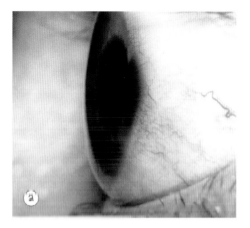

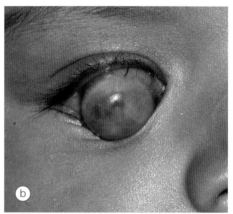

Fig. 3.20
(a) Cornea plana; **(b)** keratectasia (Courtesy of R Visser – fig. a; R Fogla – fig. b)

2. Signs
- Severe decrease in corneal curvature with a K reading of 20–30D (Fig. 3.20a).
- Hypermetropia, shallow anterior chamber and predisposition to angle closure glaucoma.

3. Ocular associations include microcornea, sclerocornea, microphthalmos and Peters anomaly.

Keratectasia

Keratectasia is a very rare usually unilateral condition thought to be the result of intrauterine keratitis and perforation. It is characterized by protuberance between the eyelids or a severely opacified and sometimes vascularized cornea (Fig. 3.20b). It is often associated with raised intraocular pressure.

Posterior keratoconus

Posterior keratoconus is an uncommon, sporadic, unilateral, non-progressive increase in curvature of the posterior corneal surface. The anterior surface is normal and visual acuity unimpaired because of the similar refractive indices of the cornea and aqueous humour. Two types are recognized:

1. **Generalis,** in which there is an increase in curvature of the entire posterior corneal surface.
2. **Conscriptus,** which is characterized by a localized paracentral or central posterior corneal indentation (Fig. 3.21).

LENS

Lenticonus and lentiglobus

Anterior lenticonus

1. **Signs.** Bilateral axial projection of the anterior surface of the lens into the anterior chamber (Fig. 3.22a).

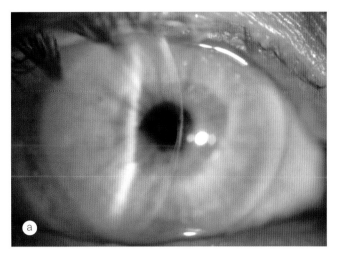

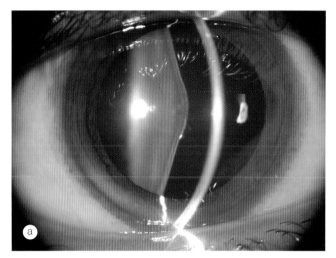

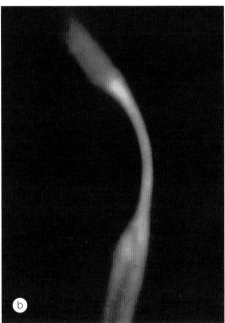

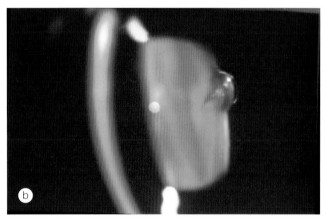

Fig. 3.22
(a) Anterior lenticonus; **(b)** posterior lenticonus (Courtesy of S Fogla – fig. a)

Fig. 3.21
(a) Posterior keratoconus; **(b)** magnified view (Courtesy of S Johns – fig. a; S Boruchoff – fig. b)

- It may be associated with opacification of the posterior capsule and hyaloid remnants.
- With age, the bulge progressively increases in size and the lens cortex may opacify. Progression of cataract is variable, but many cases present with an acutely opacified white lens in infancy or early childhood.

Lentiglobus

Lentiglobus is a very rare, usually unilateral, generalized hemispherical deformity of the lens which may be associated with posterior polar lens opacity.

Microspherophakia and microphakia

Microspherophakia

1. **Signs.** The lens is small and spherical (Fig. 3.23a).
2. **Causes** include AD microspherophakia which is not associated with systemic defects, Marfan syndrome,

2. **Association.** About 90% of patients have Alport syndrome which may also be associated with cataract, retinal flecks and posterior polymorphous corneal dystrophy.

Posterior lenticonus

1. **Inheritance.** Most cases are unilateral, sporadic and not associated with systemic abnormalities. Rarely bilateral cases may be familial.
2. **Signs**
   - A round or conical bulge of the posterior axial zone of the lens into the vitreous associated with local thinning or absence of the capsule (Fig. 3.22b).

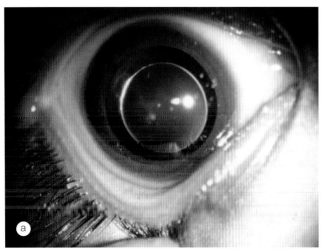 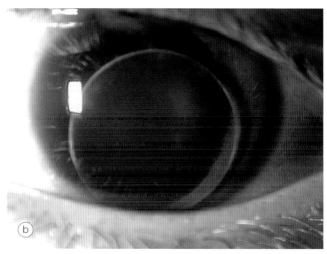

Fig. 3.23
(a) Microspherophakia; **(b)** dislocation into the anterior chamber (Courtesy of U Raina – fig. a)

Weill–Marchesani syndrome, hyperlysinaemia and congenital rubella.
3. **Ocular associations** include Peters anomaly and familial ectopia lentis et pupillae.
4. **Complications** include lenticular myopia, subluxation and total dislocation into the anterior chamber (Fig. 3.23b).

Microphakia

1. **Sign.** A lens with a smaller than normal diameter.
2. **Association.** Lowe syndrome, in which the lens is not only small but also disc-like.

Coloboma

A coloboma is characterized by notching (segmental agenesis) at the inferior equator (Fig. 3.24a) with corresponding absence of zonular fibres. It is not a true coloboma as there is no focal absence of a tissue layer due to failure of closure of the optic fissure. Occasionally a lens coloboma may be associated with a coloboma of the iris (Fig. 3.24b) or fundus.

IRIDOCORNEAL DYSGENESIS

Posterior embryotoxon

Posterior embryotoxon is an isolated innocuous finding in 6% of the general population.

1. **Signs**
   - Thin grey-white, arcuate ridge on the inner surface of the cornea, adjacent to the limbus (Fig. 3.25a and b).

   - It comprises a prominent and anteriorly displaced Schwalbe line, the junction of Descemet membrane and the uveal trabecular meshwork.
2. **Associations**
   a. **Axenfeld–Rieger anomaly** is always associated with posterior embryotoxon.
   b. **Alagille syndrome** is associated with posterior embryotoxon in 95% of cases. It is characterized by paucity of intrahepatic bile ducts, cardiopulmonary malformations, peculiar facies and vertebral defects. Optic disc drusen is also common.

Axenfeld–Rieger syndrome

Pathogenesis and genetics

Axenfeld–Rieger syndrome is a spectrum of disorders designated in current nomenclature by the following eponyms: (a) *Axenfeld anomaly*, (b) *Rieger anomaly* and (c) *Rieger syndrome*. Chromosomal loci have been mapped to 4q25 (PITX2 gene), 6p25 (FKHL7 gene) and 13q14. The two genes regulate the expression of other genes during embryogenesis. This regulatory function explains the ability of mutation in these genes to cause diverse anomalies. All patients with Axenfeld–Rieger syndrome, irrespective of ocular manifestations, share the following features:
- Bilateral developmental ocular anomalies which are not necessarily symmetrical.
- Frequently a family history with AD inheritance.
- No gender predilection.
- Frequent presence of systemic developmental defects.
- Associated glaucoma.

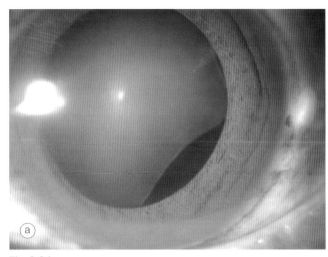 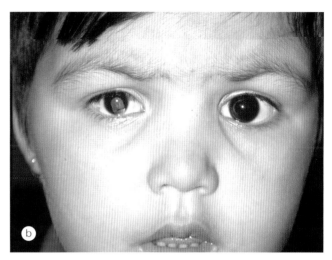

Fig. 3.24
(a) Lens coloboma; **(b)** coloboma of the lens and iris in a microphthalmic eye (Courtesy of R Fogla – fig. a; N Rogers – fig. b)

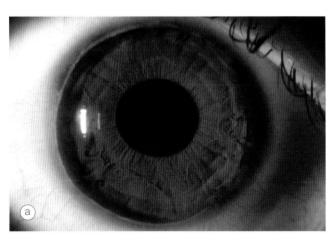 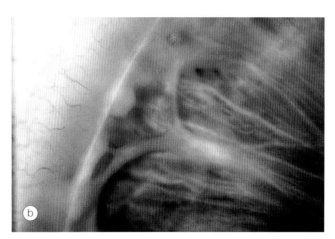

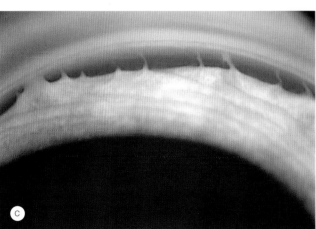

Fig. 3.25
(a) Posterior embryotoxon; **(b)** magnified view; **(c)** Axenfeld anomaly (Courtesy of P Gili – fig. a; L MacKeen – fig. c)

Axenfeld anomaly

Axenfeld anomaly is characterized by posterior embryotoxon with attachment of strands of peripheral iris tissue (Fig. 3.25c).

Rieger anomaly

1. Slit-lamp biomicroscopy
- Posterior embryotoxon; Schwalbe line may become detached into the anterior chamber.

- Iris stromal hypoplasia and ectropion uveae (Fig. 3.26a).
- Corectopia (displacement of the pupil) and full-thickness iris defects (Fig. 3.26b and c).
- Microcornea and corneal opacity are uncommon.

2. **Gonioscopy** in mild cases shows Axenfeld anomaly. In severe cases, broad leaves of the iris stroma adhere to the cornea anterior to Schwalbe line (Fig. 3.26d).

3. **Glaucoma** develops in about 50% of cases, usually during early childhood or early adulthood due to an associated angle anomaly or secondary synechial angle

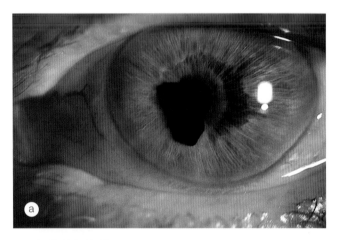

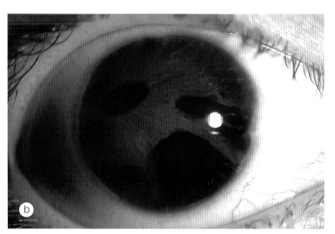

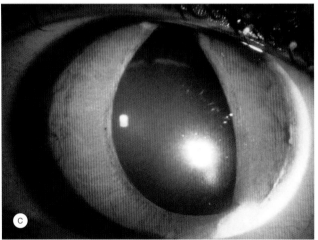

Fig. 3.26
Rieger anomaly and syndrome. **(a)** Iris stromal hypoplasia and ectropion uveae; **(b)** corectopia and full-thickness iris defects; **(c)** severe iris atrophy; **(d)** gonioscopy shows extensive peripheral anterior synechiae; **(e)** facial and dental anomalies in Rieger syndrome (Courtesy of K Nischal – fig. c; P Gili – fig. d; U Raina – fig. e)

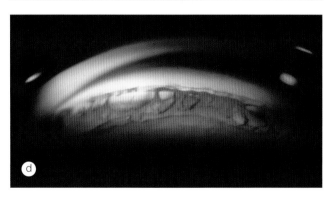

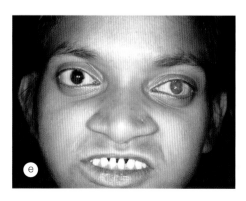

closure. The elevation of IOP should be initially managed medically, although surgery may be required subsequently.

Rieger syndrome

Rieger syndrome is linked to the region of the epidermal growth factor gene on chromosome 4. It is characterized by Rieger anomaly in association with the following extraocular malformations:

1. **Dental** anomalies consisting of hypodontia (few teeth) and microdontia (small teeth – Fig. 3.26e).
2. **Facial** anomalies include maxillary hypoplasia, broad nasal bridge, telecanthus (increased distance between the medial canthi) and hypertelorism (increased interorbital distance) (Fig. 3.26e).
3. **Other** anomalies include redundant paraumbilical skin and hypospadias. Hearing loss, hydrocephalus, cardiac and renal anomalies and congenital hip dislocation are rare.

Peters anomaly

Peters anomaly is an extremely rare but serious condition which is bilateral in 80% of cases. It is the result of defective neural crest cell migration in the sixth to eighth weeks of fetal development, during which time the anterior segment of the eye is formed. It is not a homogeneous condition and may vary from mild to severe.

1. **Inheritance.** Most cases are sporadic, although AR inheritance and chromosomal defects have been described.
2. **Signs**
   - Central corneal opacity of variable density.
   - Underlying defect involving the posterior stroma, Descemet membrane and endothelium with or without iridocorneal (Fig. 3.27a) or kerato-lenticular (Fig. 3.27b) adhesions.
3. **Investigations.** In severe cases (Fig. 3.27c) high-frequency ultrasonography (Fig. 3.27d) is used to determine associated pathology prior to contemplating penetrating keratoplasty.
4. **Ocular associations** occasionally present include Axenfeld–Rieger anomaly, aniridia, microphthalmos, persistent fetal vasculature and retinal dysplasia.
5. **Glaucoma** occurs in about 50% of cases as a result of an associated angle anomaly in which there is incomplete development of the trabecular meshwork and Schlemm canal. Elevation of IOP is usually evident in infancy but may occasionally develop in childhood or even later. Treatment of glaucoma is very difficult and the prognosis is much worse than that of primary congenital glaucoma.
6. **Systemic associations** include craniofacial anomalies, central nervous system anomalies, fetal alcohol syndrome, chromosome abnormalities, and Peters-plus syndrome (short-limbed dwarfism, cleft lip/palate and learning difficulties).

Aniridia

Genetics

Aniridia (AN) is a rare bilateral condition that may have life-threatening associations. It occurs as a result of abnormal neuroectodermal development secondary to a mutation in the PAX6 gene linked to 11p13. This gene controls the development of a number of structures, hence the broad nature of ocular and systemic manifestations.

Classification

1. **AN-1** is AD and accounts for 66% of cases and has no systemic implications. Penetrance is complete but expressivity variable.
2. **AN-2** (Miller syndrome) is sporadic and accounts for 33% of cases. It carries a 30% risk of Wilm tumour developing before the age of 5 years. Some patients may also manifest genitourinary abnormalities and mental handicap.
3. **AN-3** (Gillespie syndrome) is AR and accounts for the remainder. It is associated with mental handicap and cerebellar ataxia.

NB All patients with sporadic aniridia should have abdominal ultrasonography (to detect Wilm tumour) every 3 months until 5 years of age, then every 6 months until 10 years of age and then annually until 16 years of age or until molecular genetic analysis confirms an intragenic mutant without extragenic involvement.

Diagnosis

1. **Presentation** is typically at birth with nystagmus and photophobia. The parents may have noticed absence of irides or 'dilated pupils'.
2. **Aniridia** is variable in severity, ranging from minimal (detectable only by retroillumination) to partial (Fig. 3.28a) and total (Fig. 3.28b).
3. **Gonioscopy** even in eyes with 'total' aniridia usually shows a hypoplastic or rudimentary frill iris tissue (Fig. 3.28c).
4. **Lids** often show meibomian gland dysfunction.
5. **Cornea**
   - Tear film instability, dry eye and epithelial defects are common.
   - Limbal stem cell deficiency may result in 'conjunctivalization' of the peripheral cornea.

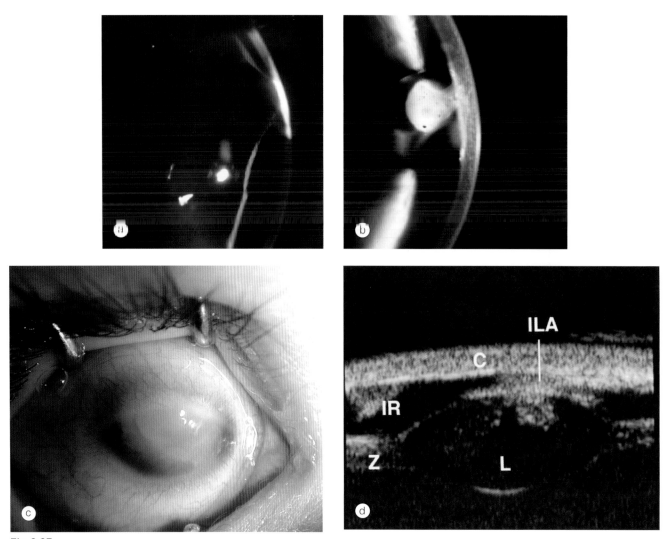

Fig. 3.27
Peters anomaly. **(a)** Corneal opacity with iris adhesions; **(b)** corneal opacity with lenticular adhesions; **(c)** severe corneal opacification; **(d)** high frequency ultrasonography shows keratolenticular apposition (Courtesy of K Nischal – figs c and d)

- Total corneal central stromal scarring and vascularization may occur in end-stage disease.
- Other lesions include opacity, epibulbar dermoids, microcornea, sclerocornea and keratolenticular adhesions.
6. **Lens** changes include cataract, subluxation (usually superiorly – Fig. 3.28d), congenital aphakia and persistent pupillary membranes.
7. **Fundus** may exhibit foveal hypoplasia (Fig. 3.28e), optic nerve hypoplasia and choroidal coloboma.

Glaucoma

Glaucoma occurs in approximately 75% of patients and usually presents in late childhood or adolescence. It is caused by synechial angle closure secondary to the pulling forward of rudimentary iris tissue by contraction of pre-existing fibres that bridge the angle (Fig. 3.28f). Treatment is difficult and the prognosis guarded.

1. **Medical** treatment is usually the initial approach although it is usually eventually inadequate.
2. **Goniotomy** may prevent subsequent rise in IOP if performed before the development of irreversible synechial angle closure.
3. **Combined trabeculectomy-trabeculotomy** may be successful although trabeculectomy alone is seldom beneficial.
4. **Artificial filtering shunts** may be effective in established cases.
5. **Diode laser cycloablation** may be necessary if other modalities fail.

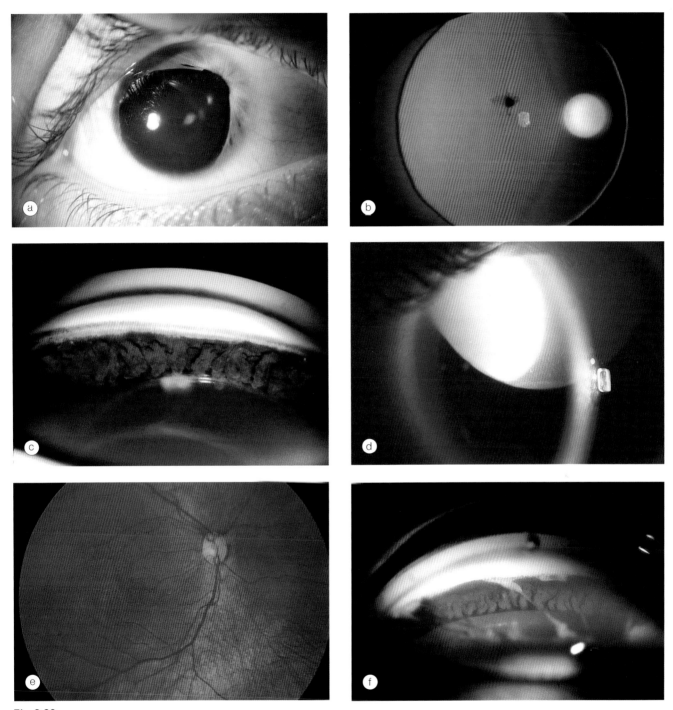

Fig. 3.28
Aniridia. **(a)** Partial; **(b)** total; **(c)** gonioscopy shows an open angle and remnants of the iris root; **(d)** superior subluxation of a cataract; **(e)** foveal hypoplasia; **(f)** gonioscopy shows a closed angle (Courtesy of R Curtis – fig c; L MacKeen – fig. e)

NB Central corneal thickness is increased in eyes with aniridia which may result in incorrect measurement of IOP.

Treatment of aniridia

1. **Opaque contact lenses** may be used to create an artificial pupil and improve vision and cosmesis.
2. **Lubricants** are frequently required for tear film instability.
3. **Cataract surgery** is often required. Care must be taken to minimize trauma to the limbus and preserve stem cell function.
4. **Limbal stem cell transplantation** with or without keratoplasty may be required.

GLOBE

Microphthalmos

Microphthalmos is the result of developmental arrest of ocular growth, defined as total axial length (TAL) at least 2 standard deviations below age-similar controls. The TAL is reduced because of stunted growth of the anterior or posterior segment, or both. Microphthalmos may be unilateral or bilateral.

1. **Simple** microphthalmos is not associated with other major ocular malformations (Fig. 3.29a).
2. **Complex** (colobomatous) microphthalmos is associated with coloboma, usually of the iris (Fig. 3.29b).

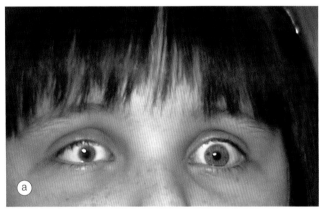
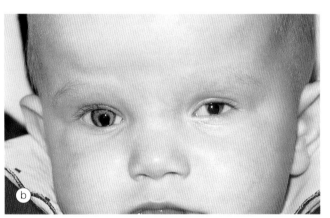

Fig. 3.29
Microphthalmos. **(a)** Simple right microphthalmos; **(b)** left microphthalmos and bilateral iris colobomas

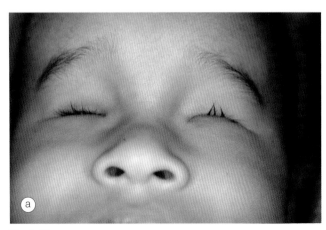
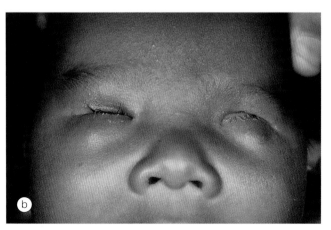

Fig. 3.30
Anophthalmos. **(a)** Bilateral simple anophthalmos; **(b)** bilateral anophthalmos with cyst (Courtesy of U Raina)

3. **Microphthalmos with cyst** is caused by failure of the optic fissure to close leading to the formation of an orbital cyst that communicates with the eye. Although it is usually an isolated sporadic condition it can occur in association with systemic abnormalities notably clefting syndrome, oculo-cerebro-cutaneous syndrome and branchio-oculo-facial syndrome.
4. **Posterior** microphthalmos is a rare subset in which TAL is reduced in the setting of normal corneal diameter, resulting in high hypermetropia and papillomacular retinal folds. This differs from nanophthalmos, which is characterized by microphthalmos, microcornea and a tendency toward uveal effusions.

Anophthalmos

1. **Simple** anophthalmos is caused either by complete failure of budding of the optic vesicle or early arrest in its development. It is associated with other abnormalities such as absence of extraocular muscles, a short conjunctival sac and microblepharon (Fig. 3.30a).
2. **Anophthalmos with cyst** (congenital cystic eyeball) is a condition in which the globe is replaced by a cyst (Fig. 3.30b).

RETINA AND CHOROID

Choroidal coloboma

In the fully developed eye the embryonic fissure is inferior and slightly nasal, and extends from the optic nerve to the margin of the pupil (anterior part of the optic cup). A coloboma is the absence of part of an ocular structure as a result of incomplete closure of the embryonic fissure that may involve the entire length of the fissure (complete coloboma) or only part (i.e. iris, ciliary body, retina and choroid or the optic disc). A chorioretinal coloboma may be unilateral or bilateral and usually occurs sporadically in otherwise normal individuals.

1. **Signs**
   - Sharply circumscribed, white area largely devoid of blood vessels, in the inferior fundus (Fig. 3.31a).
   - A large coloboma may also involve the disc (Fig. 3.31b), and give rise to leukocoria (Fig. 3.31c).
   - Other ocular colobomas may also be present.
2. **Complications.** Retinal detachment may occur due to a break within or outside the coloboma. The former break is difficult to visualize because of lack of contrast between the break and retina due to absence of choroidal background.

Myelinated nerve fibres

In normal eyes, optic nerve myelination stops at the cribriform plate. In eyes with myelinated nerve fibres the ganglion cells retain a myelin sheath.

1. **Signs.** White feathery streaks running within the retinal nerve fibre layer towards the disc (Fig. 3.32a and b). Only one eye is affected in the vast majority of cases.
2. **Ocular associations** of extensive nerve fibre myelination (Fig. 3.32c) include high myopia, anisometropia and amblyopia.
3. **Systemic associations** include neurofibromatosis-1 and Gorlin (multiple basal cell naevus) syndrome.

Aicardi syndrome

1. **Inheritance** is XLD; the condition is lethal *in utero* for males.
2. **Signs.** Bilateral, multiple depigmented 'chorioretinal lacunae' clustered around the disc that may be hypoplastic, colobomatous or pigmented (Fig. 3.33).
3. **Associated features** include microphthalmos, iris colobomas, persistent pupillary membranes and cataract.
4. **Systemic features** include infantile spasms, agenesis of the corpus callosum, skeletal malformations and psychomotor retardation. Other serious CNS malformations may also be present and death usually occurs within the first few years of life.

Retinal macrovessel

1. **Signs.** A unilateral, large, aberrant retinal vessel, usually a vein, is present in the posterior pole and may cross the foveal region and horizontal raphe (Fig. 3.34a). Because arteriovenous anastomoses are often present the condition may be considered to be a variant of racemose angiomatosis. The visual prognosis is excellent.
2. **FA** may show early filling and delayed emptying and a dilated surrounding capillary bed. Areas of capillary non-perfusion and foveal cysts may also be seen.

Arteriovenous communications

Congenital arteriovenous communications usually present on routine examination, with unilateral involvement of single or multiple sites of the same fundus. They have a predilection for the papillomacular bundle and the superotemporal quadrant. Occasionally reported complications include haemorrhage, exudation and vascular occlusion. Some patients may harbour similar systemic lesions. The malformations can be divided into the following three types on the basis of severity.

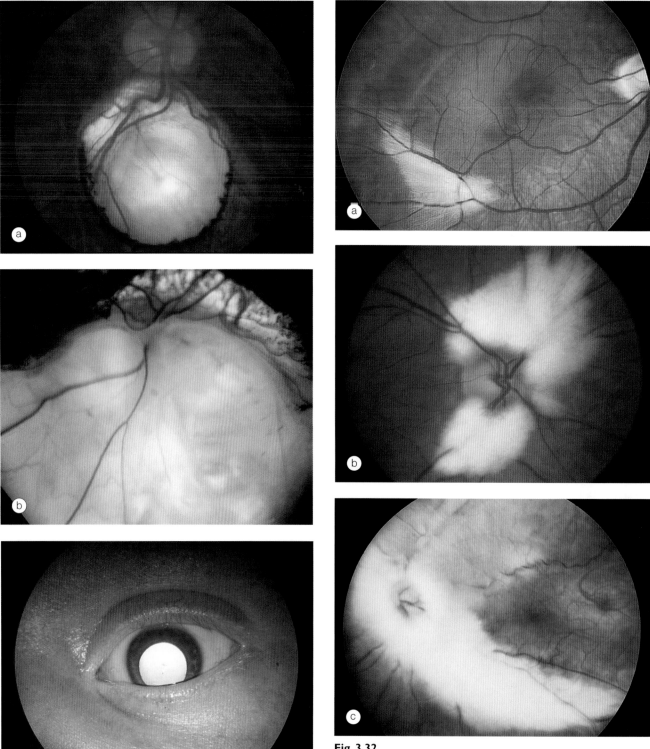

Fig. 3.31
Choroidal coloboma. **(a)** Small coloboma; **(b)** large coloboma
also involving the disc; **(c)** leukocoria

Fig. 3.32
Myelinated nerve fibres. **(a)** Peripheral; **(b)** peripapillary;
(c) extensive

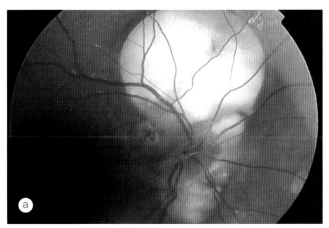

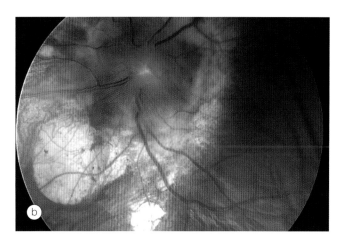

Fig. 3.33
Fundus in Aicardi syndrome. **(a)** Right eye; **(b)** left eye

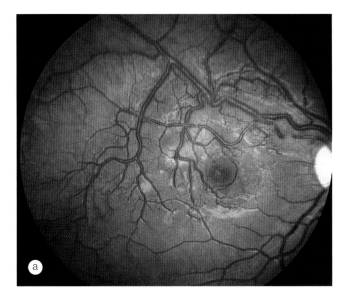

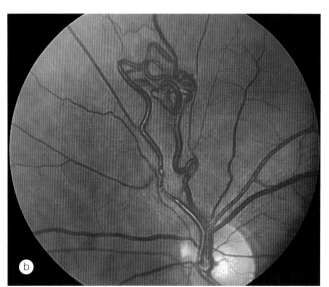

Fig. 3.34
Retinal vascular anomalies. **(a)** Retinal macrovessel;
(b) arteriovenous communication; **(c)** FA shows filling but lack of
leakage (Courtesy of C Barry – figs b and c)

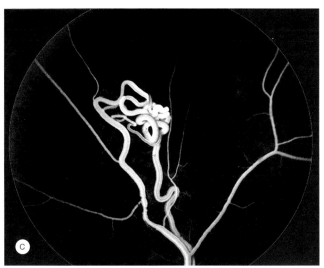

Group 1 consists of an anastomosis between a small arteriole and venule with the interposition of an abnormal capillary or arteriolar plexus. It is non-progressive and associated with good visual acuity.

Group 2 demonstrates direct arteriovenous communications between a branch retinal artery and vein (Fig. 3.34b and c).

Group 3 consists of diffuse marked dilatation of the vascular tree with many large calibre anastomosing channels.

OPTIC NERVE

Prepapillary loop

1. **Signs.** A unilateral vascular loop extending from the disc into the vitreous cavity (Fig. 3.35a).
2. **Complications** Obstruction in the distribution of the retinal artery supplying the loop occurs in 10% of cases. Vitreous haemorrhage is rare.

Bergmeister papilla

Bergmeister papilla is an uncommon unilateral anomaly that is derived from avascular remnants of the hyaloid system and is characterized by raised glial tissue on the disc surface (Fig. 3.35b).

Tilted disc

A tilted optic disc is a common, usually bilateral, anomaly caused by an oblique entry of the optic nerve into the globe. This results in pseudo-rotation of the superior pole of the disc, angulation of the optic cup axis and elevation of the neuroretinal rim.

1. **Signs**
   - Small, oval or D-shaped disc in which the axis is most frequently directed inferonasally but sometimes horizontally or nearly vertically (Fig. 3.36a).
   - The disc margin is indistinct where the retinal nerve fibres are elevated.
   - Situs inversus in which the temporal vessels deviate nasally before turning temporally.
   - Associated findings include inferonasal chorioretinal thinning (Fig. 3.36b) and myopic astigmatic refractive error.
2. **Perimetry** may show superotemporal defects that do not respect the vertical midline.
3. **Complications,** which are uncommon, include CNV and sensory macular detachment.

Optic disc pit

Diagnosis

1. **Signs**
   - VA is normal in the absence of complications.
   - The disc is larger than normal and contains a round or oval pit of variable size that is usually located in the temporal aspect of the disc (Fig. 3.37a) but may occasionally be central.
   - Visual field defects are common and may mimic those due to glaucoma.
2. **Serous macular detachment** develops in about 45% of eyes with non-central disc pits (median age 30 years). The subretinal fluid is thought to be derived from the vitreous; less likely sources are the subarachnoid space and leakage from abnormal vessels within the base of the pit.

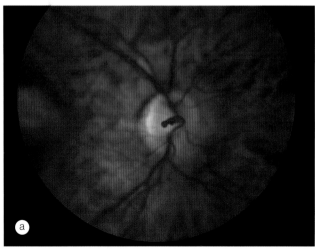
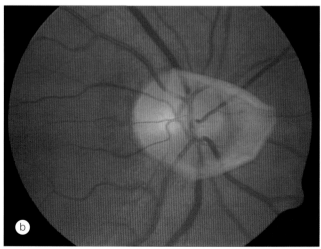

Fig. 3.35
(a) Prepapillary loop; **(b)** Bergmeister papilla (Courtesy of P Gili – fig. b)

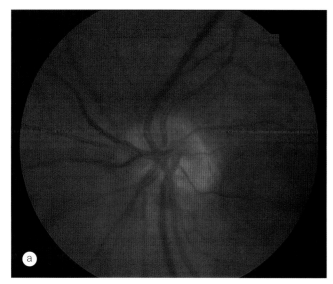

Fig. 3.36
(a) Tilted disc; (b) inferonasal chorioretinal thinning

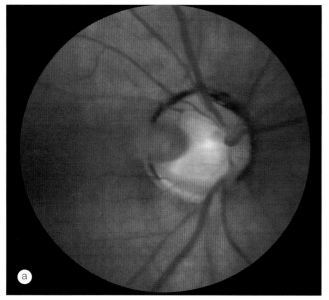

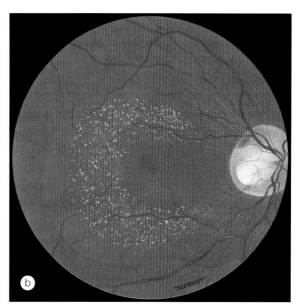

Fig. 3.37
(a) Optic disc pit; (b) serous macular detachment associated with subretinal deposits

- Initially, there is a schisis-like separation of the inner layers of the retina which communicates with the pit.
- This is followed by serous detachment of the outer retinal layers which may be associated with subretinal deposits (Fig. 3.37b). This appearance may be mistaken for central serous retinopathy.

NB It is important to examine the optic disc carefully in all patients with suspected central serous retinopathy.

Treatment

1. **Observation** at 3-monthly intervals for evidence of spontaneous resolution of the detachment which occurs in up to 25% of cases.
2. **Laser photocoagulation** may be considered if visual acuity is deteriorating. The burns are applied along the temporal aspect of the disc. The success rate is 25–35%.
3. **Vitrectomy** with air–fluid exchange and postoperative prone positioning may be considered if laser alone is unsuccessful. The success rate is very good.

Optic disc drusen

Optic disc drusen (hyaline bodies) are composed of hyaline-like calcific material within the substance of the optic nerve head. Clinically, they are present in about 0.3% of the population and are often bilateral. Although only a minority of relatives exhibit disc drusen nearly half exhibit anomalous disc vessels and absence of the optic cup.

Signs

1. **Buried drusen.** In early childhood drusen may be difficult to detect because they lie deep beneath the surface of the disc (Fig. 3.38a). In this setting the appearance may mimic papilloedema. Signs suggestive of disc drusen are:
   * Elevated disc with a scalloped margin without a physiological cup.
   * Hyperaemia is absent and the surface vessels are not obscured, despite the disc elevation.
   * Anomalous vascular patterns such as early branching, increased number of major retinal vessels and tortuosity.
   * Spontaneous venous pulsation is present in 80% of cases.
2. **Exposed drusen.** During the early teenage years drusen usually emerge at the surface of the disc as waxy pearl-like irregularities that transilluminate by oblique ophthalmoscopic illumination or with the slit-lamp beam (Fig. 3.38b).
3. **Associations** include retinitis pigmentosa, angioid streaks and Alagille syndrome.
4. **Complications,** which are rare, include juxtapapillary CNV, disc neovascularization, central retinal arterial and venous occlusion; progressive but limited loss of visual field with a nerve fibre bundle pattern may occur.

Imaging

Imaging may be necessary for the definitive diagnosis of disc drusen, particularly when buried.

1. **FA**
   * Exposed drusen show the phenomenon of auto-fluorescence prior to dye injection (Fig. 3.38c) and then progressive hyperfluorescence due to staining without leakage of dye (Fig. 3.38d).
   * Buried drusen show more subtle findings because of attenuation from the overlying tissue.
2. **US** is the most readily available and reliable method because of its ability to detect calcific deposits that show high acoustic reflectivity (Fig. 3.38e).
3. **CT** shows disc calcification (Fig. 3.38f) but is less sensitive than ultrasonography and may miss small lesions. Drusen may however, be detected incidentally on CT, when performed in the course of investigation of other pathology.

NB FA in papilloedema shows increasing hyperfluorescence and late leakage.

Optic disc coloboma

Disc colobomas are usually sporadic, although AD inheritance has been described. They may be unilateral or bilateral.

Diagnosis

1. **Signs**
   * VA is often decreased.
   * The disc shows a discrete, focal, glistening, white, bowl-shaped excavation, decentred inferiorly so that the inferior neuroretinal rim is thin or absent and normal disc tissue is confined to a small superior wedge (Fig. 3.39a).
   * The optic disc itself may be enlarged but the retinal vasculature is normal.
2. **FA** shows hypofluorescence of the coloboma as compared with the superior disc remnant (Fig. 3.39b).
3. **Perimetry** shows a superior defect which, in conjunction with the disc appearance, may be mistaken for normal-tension glaucoma.
4. **Ocular associations** include microphthalmos and colobomas of iris and fundus.
5. **Complications**
   * Serous retinal detachment at the macula may occur.
   * Progressive enlargement of the excavation and neural rim thinning despite normal intraocular pressure has been described.
   * Peripapillary CNV is rare.

Systemic associations

Systemic associations are numerous; the most notable are:

1. **Chromosomal anomalies** include Patau syndrome (trisomy 13), Edward syndrome (trisomy 18) and Cat-eye syndrome (trisomy 22).
2. **'CHARGE'** association comprises Coloboma, Heart defects, choanal Atresia, Retarded growth and development, Genital and Ear anomalies.
3. **Other syndromes** include Meckel–Gruber, Goltz, Walker–Warburg, Goldenhar, Aicardi, Dandy–Walker cyst and linear sebaceous naevus.
4. **Central nervous system anomalies.**

Morning glory anomaly

Morning glory anomaly is a very rare, usually unilateral sporadic condition that shows a spectrum of severity. Bilateral cases, which are rarer still, may be hereditary.

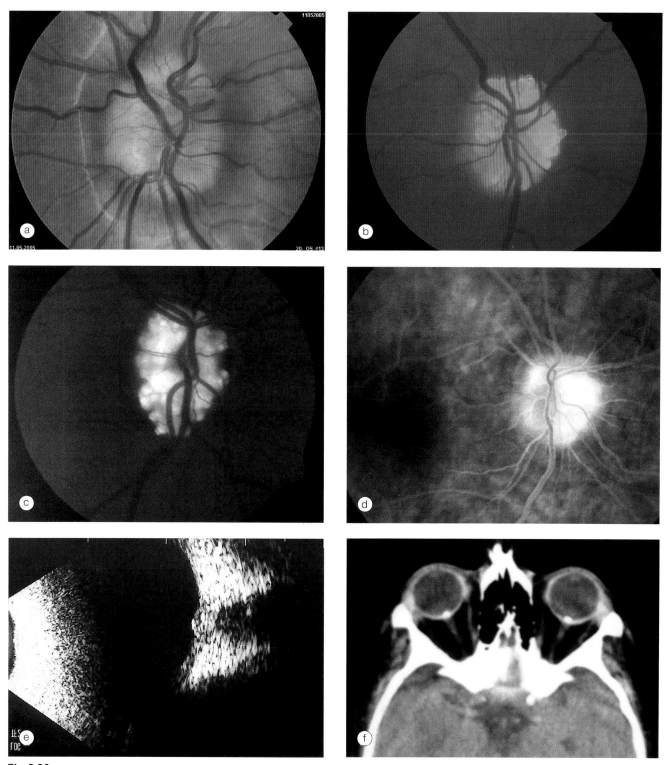

Fig. 3.38
Optic disc drusen. **(a)** Buried; **(b)** exposed; **(c)** autofluorescence; **(d)** FA late phase shows hyperfluorescence but absence of leakage; **(e)** B-scan shows high acoustic reflectivity; **(f)** axial CT shows bilateral drusen (Courtesy of P Gili – fig. c)

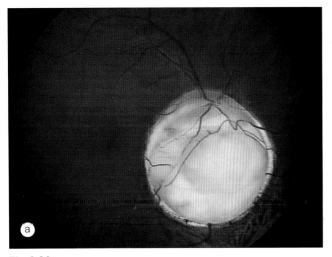
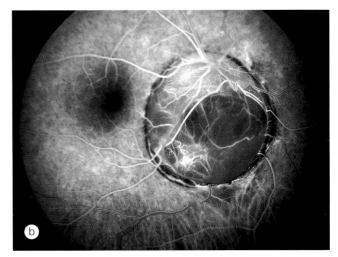

Fig. 3.39
(a) Optic disc coloboma; **(b)** FA shows hypofluorescence of the cavity (Courtesy of P Gili)

Diagnosis

1. Signs
- VA may be normal or impaired to a variable extent.
- A large disc with a funnel-shaped excavation surrounded by an annulus of chorioretinal disturbance (Fig. 3.40a).
- A white tuft of glial tissue overlies the central portion and represents persistent hyaloid remnants.
- The blood vessels emerge from the rim of the excavation in a radial pattern like the spokes of a wheel. They are increased in number and it is difficult to distinguish arteries from veins.

2. Complications
- Serous retinal detachment develops in about 30% of cases (Fig. 3.40b).
- CNV is less common and may develop adjacent to the lesion (Fig. 3.40c).

Systemic associations

Systemic associations, which are uncommon, include the following:

1. **Frontonasal dysplasia,** the most important, is characterized by the following:
   - Mid-facial anomalies consisting of hypertelorism, flat nasal bridge (Fig. 3.40d) a midline notch in the upper lip and occasionally a midline cleft in the soft palate.
   - Basal encephalocele resulting from a defect in the base of the skull (Fig. 3.40e).
   - Absent corpus callosum (Fig. 3.40f) and pituitary deficiency.
2. **Neurofibromatosis type 2** is much less common.
3. **PHACE syndrome,** which is characterized by posterior fossa brain malformations, large facial haemangiomas and cardiovascular anomalies. It almost exclusively affects females.

Optic nerve hypoplasia

The hypoplastic optic nerve, unilateral or bilateral, is characterized by a diminished number of nerve fibres. It may occur as an isolated anomaly in an otherwise normal eye, in a grossly malformed eye or in association with a heterogeneous group of disorders most commonly involving the midline structures of the brain.

Predispositions

Predispositions include specific agents used by the mother during gestation such as excess alcohol, LSD, quinine, protamine zinc insulin, steroids, diuretics, cold remedies and anticonvulsants. Superior segmental hypoplasia may be associated with maternal diabetes.

Diagnosis

1. Presentation
- Blindness in early infancy with roving eye movements and sluggish or absent pupillary light responses is uncommon. Less severe bilateral involvement may cause minor visual defects or squint at any time in childhood.
- Unilateral cases usually present with squint, a relative afferent pupillary conduction defect and unsteady fixation in the affected eye. In mild cases visual acuity may improve with patching of the normal eye.

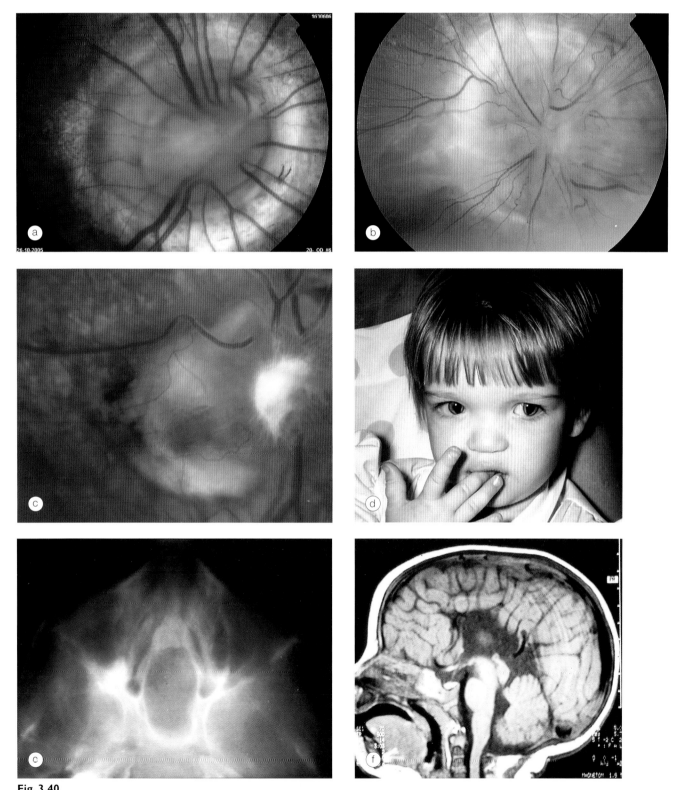

Fig. 3.40
(a) Morning glory anomaly; **(b)** serous retinal detachment over and surrounding the lesion; **(c)** scarring due to CNV; **(d)** hypertelorism and flat nasal bridge – note bilateral iris colobomas; **(e)** defect in the base of the skull; **(f)** sagittal MR shows absence of the corpus callosum (Courtesy of Moorfields Eye Hospital – fig. e; K Nischal – fig. f)

2. **Signs**
   - VA may be normal or impaired to a variable degree, even to no light perception.
   - Small grey disc surrounded by a yellow halo of hypopigmentation caused by concentric chorioretinal atrophy (double-ring sign – Fig. 3.41a); the outer ring represents what would have been the normal disc margin.
   - The distance from the fovea to the temporal border of the optic disc often equals or exceeds three times the disc diameter – this strongly suggests disc hypoplasia.
   - Despite the small size of the disc, the retinal blood vessels are of normal calibre, although they may be tortuous (Fig. 3.41b).
   - Occasionally the disc may show hyperpigmentation.
3. **Other features** vary considerably, depending on severity. They include astigmatism, field defects, dyschromatopsia, afferent pupillary defect, foveal hypoplasia, aniridia, microphthalmos, strabismus and nystagmus. Mild cases can be easily overlooked.

Systemic associations

Optic disc hypoplasia is often associated with a wide variety of midline developmental brain defects. The most common is de Morsier syndrome (septo-optic dysplasia) which is present in about 10% of cases. In addition to bilateral optic nerve hypoplasia, it is characterized by the following:
- Absence of the septum pellucidum and thinning or agenesis of the corpus callosum (see Fig. 3.40f).
- Hypopituitarism with low growth hormone levels is common; if recognized early, the hormone deficiency can be corrected and normal growth resumed. It has been suggested that retinal venous tortuosity in patients with bilateral optic nerve hypoplasia may be a marker for potential endocrine dysfunction.

Miscellaneous anomalies

1. **Megalopapilla,** in which the horizontal and vertical disc diameters are 2.1mm or more (Fig. 3.42a).
2. **Peripapillary staphyloma** is a sporadic, usually unilateral condition in which a relatively normal disc sits at the base of a deep excavation whose walls, as well as the surrounding choroid and retinal pigment epithelium (RPE), show atrophic changes (Fig. 3.42b). Visual acuity is markedly reduced and local retinal detachment may be present. Unlike other excavated optic disc anomalies it is rarely associated with other congenital defects or systemic diseases.
3. **Optic disc dysplasia** is a descriptive term for a markedly deformed disc that does not conform to any recognizable category described above (Fig. 3.42c).
4. **Papillorenal (renal-coloboma) syndrome** is an AD condition characterized by renal abnormalities. The discs are normal in size and may be surrounded by variable pigmentary disturbance. Unlike colobomatous discs the excavation is central, and the disc appears 'vacant', with replacement of the central retinal vasculature by vessels of cilioretinal origin.
5. **Optic nerve aplasia** is an extremely rare condition in which the optic disc is absent or rudimentary and retinal vessels are absent or few in number and abnormal. There may be a retinal pigmentary disturbance, especially at the site where the optic disc might have been. Other ocular and systemic developmental defects may be present.

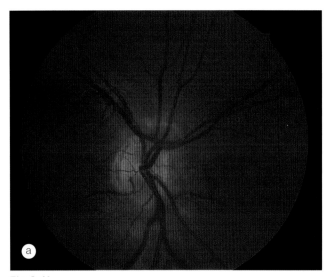 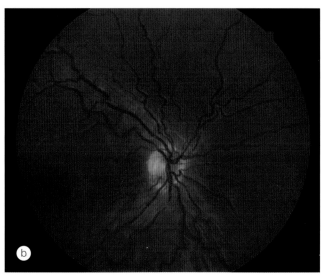

Fig. 3.41
(a) Mild optic disc hypoplasia; **(b)** severe optic disc hypoplasia with vascular tortuosity

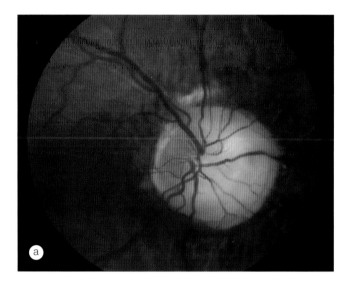

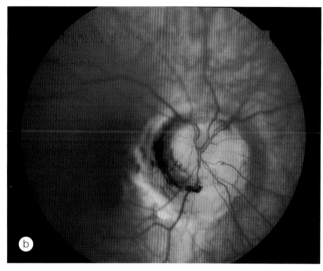

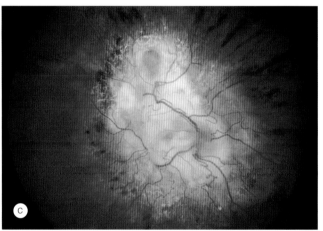

Fig. 3.42
Miscellaneous congenital optic disc anomalies. **(a)** Megalopapilla; **(b)** peripapillary staphyloma; **(c)** dysplastic disc (Courtesy of C Barry – fig. c)

6. **Optic disc pigmentation** may occur in isolation or in association with optic disc hypoplasia.

VITREOUS

Persistent hyaloid artery

Persistent hyaloid artery is a unilateral condition seen in 95% of premature infants but rarely in adults.

1. **Signs**
   * Glial remnants extending from the disc to the lens (Cloquet canal – Fig. 3.43a).
   * The artery may contain blood (Fig. 3.43b) at its point of attachment to the posterior lens capsule forming a white ('Mittendorf') dot.
2. **Complications.** Vitreous haemorrhage is very rare.
3. **Ocular associations** include posterior vitreous cyst, optic disc coloboma and optic nerve hypoplasia.

Persistent fetal vasculature

Persistent fetal vasculature (PFV) is an uncommon, sporadic, unilateral condition, caused by failure of regression of the primary vitreous. It is typically associated with mild microphthalmos. In the past it was referred to as persistent hyperplastic primary vitreous.

Persistent anterior fetal vasculature

The abnormality is confined to the anterior segment and often involves the lens.

1. **Presentation** is typically with unilateral leukocoria (Fig. 3.44a).
2. **Signs**
   * Retrolental mass into which elongated ciliary processes are inserted (Fig. 3.44b and c).
   * With time the mass contracts and pulls the ciliary processes centrally so that they become visible through the pupil.

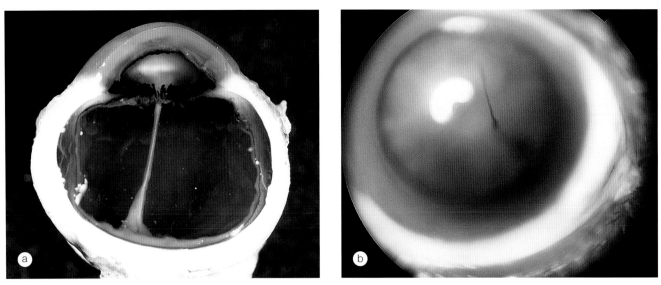

Fig. 3.43
Persistent hyaloid artery; **(a)** Post-mortem specimen; **(b)** artery filled with blood near to its attachment to the lens (Courtesy of J Harry and G Misson, from Clinical Ophthalmic Pathology, Butterworth-Heinemann, 2001 – fig. a)

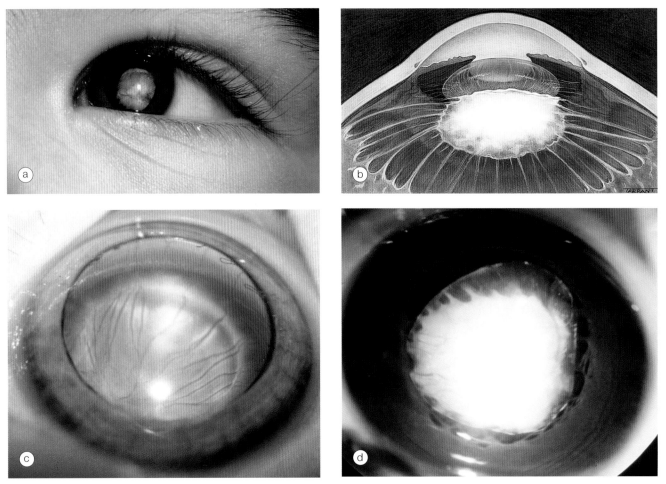

Fig. 3.44
Persistent anterior fetal vasculature. **(a)** Leukocoria; **(b)** retrolental mass with insertion of ciliary processes; **(c)** early involvement; **(d)** advanced case with cataract (Courtesy of K Nischal – figs c and d)

3. **Complications** include cataract (Fig. 3.44d) formation due to a capsular dehiscence.
4. **Treatment** involving vitreoretinal surgery may be successful in selected early cases in salvaging some vision.

Persistent posterior fetal vasculature

The abnormality is confined to the posterior segment and the lens is usually clear.

1. **Presentation** is with leukocoria, strabismus or nystagmus.
2. **Signs.** A dense white membrane or a prominent retinal fold extends from the optic disc to the ora serrata, associated with retinal detachment (Fig. 3.45).
3. **Treatment** is not possible.

Vitreoretinal dysplasia

Vitreoretinal dysplasia is caused by faulty differentiation of the retina and vitreous. It may occur in isolation or in association with systemic abnormalities most notably Norrie disease, incontinentia pigmenti (Bloch–Sulzberger syndrome) and Warburg syndrome.

1. **Signs**
   - Congenital blindness with roving eye movements in bilateral cases.
   - Pink or white retrolental masses (Fig. 3.46a) resulting in leukocoria (Fig. 3.46b).
   - Microphthalmos, shallow anterior chamber and elongated ciliary processes.
2. **Norrie disease** is an XL recessive disorder in which affected males are blind at birth or early infancy. Systemic features include cochlear deafness and mental retardation.
3. **Incontinentia pigmenti** is an XL dominant condition that is lethal in utero for boys. It is characterized by a vesiculobullous rash on the trunk and extremities (Fig. 3.46c) which is later replaced by linear pigmentation (Fig. 3.46d). Other features include malformation of teeth, hair, nails, bones and CNS.

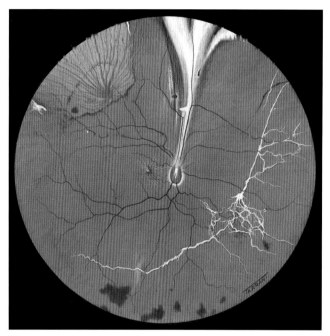

Fig. 3.45
Persistent posterior fetal vasculature with shallow retinal detachment

4. **Warburg syndrome** is an AR condition characterized by congenital muscular dystrophy, absence of cortical gyri and cerebellar malformations that may be associated with hydrocephalus and encephalocele. Neonatal death is common and survivors suffer severe developmental delay.

Vitreous cyst

Vitreous cysts are rare congenital remnants of the primary hyaloidal system or ciliary body pigment epithelium (Fig. 3.47). Most are asymptomatic although some may cause intermittent symptoms. Treatment is seldom required, although laser photocystotomy or vitrectomy have been suggested in patients with annoying symptoms.

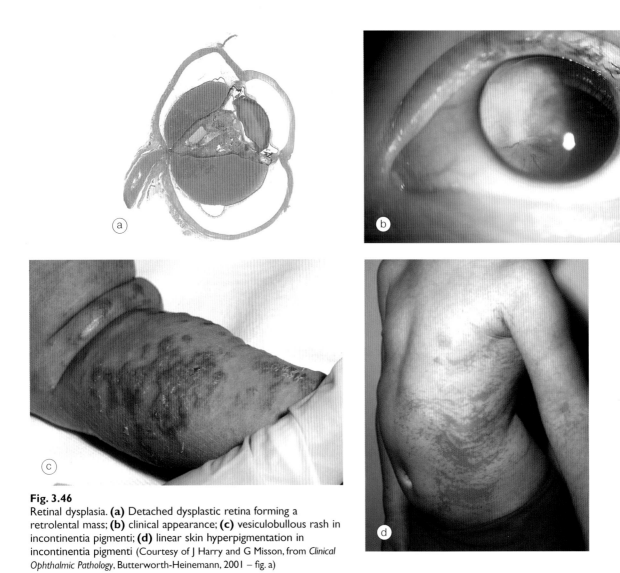

Fig. 3.46
Retinal dysplasia. **(a)** Detached dysplastic retina forming a retrolental mass; **(b)** clinical appearance; **(c)** vesiculobullous rash in incontinentia pigmenti; **(d)** linear skin hyperpigmentation in incontinentia pigmenti (Courtesy of J Harry and G Misson, from *Clinical Ophthalmic Pathology*, Butterworth-Heinemann, 2001 – fig. a)

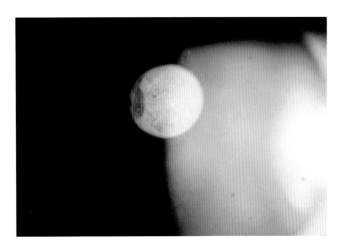

Fig. 3.47
Congenital vitreous cysts (Courtesy of W Lisch)

CHAPTER 4

EYELIDS

INTRODUCTION

Anatomy

The skin consists of the epidermis, dermis and appendages composed of a wide variety of cell types capable of proliferation and neoplastic transformation (Fig. 4.1). The number of cutaneous tumours is thus very extensive ranging from common papillomas and basal cell carcinomas to much rarer skin appendage and soft tissue tumours in the dermis. Both benign and malignant tumours are classified according to their cell of origin as well as their location. This chapter is restricted to those of interest to ophthalmologists.

Epidermis

The epidermis consists of four layers of keratin-producing cells (keratinocytes). It also contains melanocytes, Langerhans cells and Merkel cells. From superficial to deep the four layers of the epidermis are:

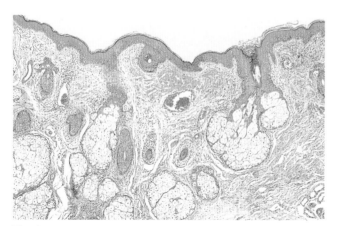

Fig. 4.1
Normal eyelid skin. Keratinized stratified epithelium covers the surface, pilosebaceous elements are conspicuous in the dermis and a few blood vessels and sweat glands are seen (Courtesy of J Harry)

1. **Keratin** (horny) layer is very thin and consists of flat, dead cells devoid of nuclei.
2. **Granular cell** layer consists of one or two layers of diamond-shaped or flattened cells containing keratohyaline granules.
3. **Squamous cell** layer is approximately five cells in thickness. The cells are polygonal and have abundant eosinophilic cytoplasm. Their free borders are united by intercellular bridges (desmosomes); hence the term 'prickle' cell layer.
4. **Basal cell** layer comprises a single row of columnar-shaped cells that give rise to more superficial cells. Basal cells contain melanin derived from adjacent melanocytes.

Dermis

The dermis is much thicker than the epidermis. It is composed of connective tissue and contains blood vessels, lymphatics and nerve fibres in addition to fibroblasts, macrophages and mast cells. Upward dermal projections (papillae) interdigitate with downward epidermal projections (rete ridges). In the eyelid the dermis lies on the orbicularis muscle. Skin appendages (adnexa) lie deep in the dermis or within the tarsal plates. They contain specialized cells that may give rise to solid or cystic proliferations.

1. **Sebaceous (holocrine) glands** are located in the caruncle and within eyebrow hairs. Tiny sebaceous glands are associated with the thin (vellus) hairs covering periocular skin.
2. **Meibomian glands** are modified sebaceous glands located in the tarsal plate. They empty through a single row of about 30 openings on each lid. Each gland consists of a central duct with multiple acini, the cells of which synthesize lipids (meibum) that pass into the duct and form the outer layer of the precorneal tear film.
3. **Glands of Zeis** are modified sebaceous glands associated with lash follicles.
4. **Glands of Moll** are modified apocrine sweat glands which open into a lash follicle. They are more numerous in the lower lid.

5. **Eccrine sweat glands** are distributed throughout the eyelid skin and are not confined to the lid margin, unlike apocrine glands.
6. **Pilosebaceous units** comprise hair follicles together with their sebaceous glands.

Terminology

Clinical

1. **Macule** is a localized area of colour change without infiltration or elevation. It may be pigmented (freckle), hypopigmented (vitiligo) or erythematous (capillary haemangioma).
2. **Papule** is a small solid elevation of skin which may be flat-topped or dome-shaped.
3. **Vesicle** is a circumscribed lesion containing fluid.
4. **Pustule** is a collection of pus.
5. **Crust** is a dried skin exudate.
6. **Nodule** is a solid area of raised skin.
7. **Cyst** is a nodule consisting of an epithelial-lined cavity filled with fluid or semi-solid material.
8. **Plaque** is a palpable flat elevation of the skin, usually more than 2cm in diameter.
9. **Scale** consists of thickening of the horny keratin layer in the form of readily detached fragments.
10. **Papilloma** is a nipple-like projection from the skin surface.
11. **Ulcer** is a circumscribed area of skin loss that extends through the epidermis into the dermis.

Histological

1. **Hyperkeratosis** is an increase in thickness of the keratin layer and appears clinically as white flaky skin. Hyperkeratosis may be a feature of both benign and malignant epithelial tumours.
2. **Acanthosis** is thickening of the squamous cell layer.
3. **Dysplasia** is the alteration of the size, morphology and organization of cellular components of a tissue. It is characterized by increased cell growth and histological features including loss of cell polarity (Fig. 4.2a), cellular atypia with pleomorphism and nuclear hyperchromatism. Dysplastic epidermal and epithelial surfaces may also exhibit dyskeratosis and parakeratosis.
4. **Dyskeratosis** is keratinization other than on the surface (Fig. 4.2b).
5. **Parakeratosis** is the retention of nuclei into the keratin layer (Fig. 4.2c).
6. **Carcinoma *in situ*** (intraepidermal carcinoma, Bowen disease) exhibits dysplastic changes throughout the thickness of the epidermis and marked hyperkeratosis – Fig. 4.2d).

General considerations

Benign skin lesions are much more varied and common than malignancies

1. **Classification** is based on the structure of origin: epidermal, adnexal or dermal.
2. **Diagnosis.** The clinical characteristics of benign lesions are lack of induration and ulceration, uniform colour, lack of or very slow growth, regular outline and preservation of normal lid margin structures. In the vast majority of cases diagnosis is straightforward although occasionally biopsy may be required if the appearance is unusual.
   - An incisional (shave) biopsy using a knife removes a portion of the lesion for histology and is usually employed for large superficial lesions such as seborrhoeic keratosis. In some cases the bulk of the lesion is also removed and no further treatment is required, provided histology confirms a benign lesion.
   - An excision biopsy is performed on small tumours and fulfils both diagnostic and treatment objectives.
3. **Treatment** options include:
   - Excision of the entire lesion and a small surrounding portion of normal tissue.
   - Marsupialization involves the removal of the top of a cyst allowing drainage of its contents and subsequent epithelialization.
   - Other options include ablation with laser or cryotherapy.

BENIGN NODULES AND CYSTS

Chalazion

Pathogenesis

A chalazion (meibomian cyst) is a chronic, sterile, granulomatous inflammatory lesion caused by retained sebaceous secretion leaking from the meibomian glands or other sebaceous glands into adjacent stroma. A chalazion secondarily infected with *S. aureus* is referred to as an internal hordeolum. Patients with meibomian gland disease or rosacea are at increased risk of chalazion formation which may be multiple or recurrent.

Histology

Histology shows a lipogranulomatous inflammatory reaction containing epithelioid cells and multinucleated giant cells intermixed with lymphocytes and plasma cells, and on occasion neutrophils and eosinophils (Fig. 4.3a).

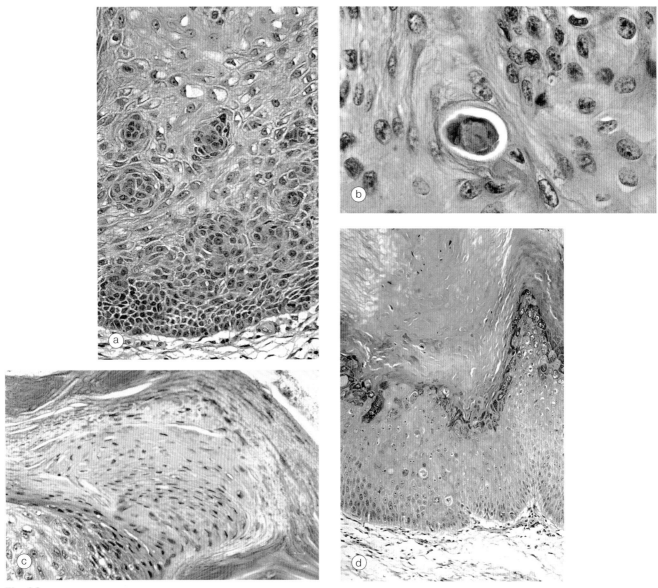

Fig. 4.2
Histology of dysplasia **(a)** Loss of cell polarity; **(b)** dyskeratosis – an epithelial cell not on the surface producing keratin; **(c)** parakeratosis – retention of cell nuclei into the surface keratin layer; **(d)** carcinoma *in-situ* – dysplastic changes throughout the thickness of the epidermis and marked hyperkeratosis (Courtesy of J Harry and G Misson, from *Clinical Ophthalmic Pathology*, Butterworth-Heinemann, 2001)

Diagnosis

1. **Presentation** is at any age with a gradually enlarging painless nodule. Very occasionally a large upper lid chalazion may press on the cornea, induce astigmatism and cause blurred vision.
2. **Signs**
   - A non-tender, roundish, nodule within the tarsal plate (Fig. 4.3b).
   - Eversion of the lid may show an associated polypoidal granuloma if the lesion has ruptured through the tarsal conjunctiva.

- A 'marginal' chalazion is similar except that it involves a gland of Zeis and is therefore located not in the tarsal plate but on the anterior lid margin.

Treatment

Treatment may not be required because about a third of chalazia resolve spontaneously and an internal hordeolum may discharge and disappear. Persistent lesions may be treated as follows:

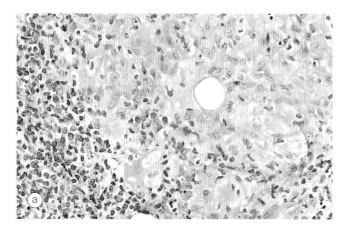

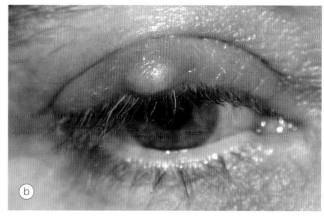

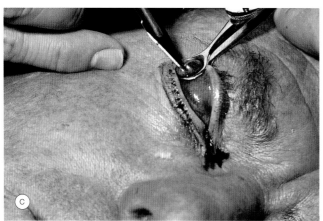

Fig. 4.3
Chalazion. **(a)** Histology shows a lipogranuloma; the large pale cells are epithelioid cells and the well-demarcated empty space is from where fat was dissolved out during processing; **(b)** chalazion involving the upper lid; **(c)** incision of chalazion (Courtesy of J Harry and G Misson, from *Clinical Ophthalmic Pathology*, Butterworth-Heinemann, 2001 – fig. a)

1. **Surgery.** The eyelid is everted with a special clamp, the cyst is incised vertically and its contents curetted through the tarsal plate (Fig. 4.3c).
2. **Steroid injection** into the lesion is preferable for lesions close to the lacrimal punctum because of the risk of damage.
   - Between 0.1–0.2ml triamcinolone diacetate aqueous suspension diluted with lignocaine (or equivalent) to a concentration of 5mg/ml is injected through the conjunctiva into the tissue around the lesion with a 30-gauge needle.
   - The success rate following one injection is about 80%. In unresponsive cases a second injection can be given 2 weeks later. Local skin depigmentation has been reported.
   - There is little to distinguish between surgical drainage and steroid injection in terms of effect.
3. **Systemic tetracycline** may be required as prophylaxis in patients with recurrent chalazia, particularly if associated with acne rosacea.

NB It is very important not to mistake a sebaceous gland carcinoma for 'recurrent chalazion'. In doubtful cases, the lesion should be biopsied and examined histologically.

Epidermoid cyst

Epidermoid (keratinous) cysts are uncommon. The term 'sebaceous' cyst is often used to describe these lesions but is incorrect because the cysts are lined by keratinized stratified squamous epithelium and contain keratin, as well as retained sebaceous secretion. Epidermoid cysts are the result of implantation of surface epidermis during trauma or surgery; a minority of similar cysts are developmental and occur along embryonic lines of closure.

1. **Histology** shows a keratin-filled cavity within the dermis lined by stratified squamous epithelium (Fig. 4.4a).

2. Signs
- Firm, round, mobile lesion which is superficial or subcutaneous (Fig. 4.4b).
- Rupture of the cyst may result in a foreign body reaction and secondary infection.

3. Treatment involves marsupialization or excision.

Miscellaneous cysts and nodules

1. **Cyst of Zeis** is a small, non-translucent cyst on the anterior lid margin (Fig. 4.5a).
2. **Cyst of Moll** (apocrine hidrocystoma) is a small retention cyst that appears as a round, non-tender, translucent fluid-filled lesion on the anterior lid margin that may have a bluish tinge (Fig. 4.5b).
3. **Eccrine hidrocystoma** is less common but similar in appearance to a cyst of Moll except that it is usually located along the medial or lateral aspects of the lid and is close to but does not involve the lid margin itself (Fig. 4.5c).
4. **Syringoma** is a cellular proliferation of intraepidermal duct eccrine sweat gland epithelium. It is characterized by multiple, small papules (Fig. 4.5d).
5. **Milia** are caused by occlusion of pilosebaceous units resulting in retention of keratin and represent tiny epidermoid cysts. They are characterized by tiny, white, round, superficial papules which tend to occur in crops (Fig. 4.5e).
6. **Comedones** occur in patients with acne vulgaris and consist of a plug of keratin and sebum within the dilated orifice of a hair follicle. They may be either open (blackheads) containing a plug of melanin-containing keratin (Fig. 4.5f), or closed (white heads) which are cream coloured papules.

BENIGN TUMOURS

Squamous cell papilloma

A squamous cell papilloma (fibroepithelial polyp) is a very common condition that has a variable clinical appearance but common histological features.

1. **Histology** shows finger-like projections of fibrovascular connective tissue covered by irregular acanthotic and hyperkeratotic, stratified squamous epithelium (Fig. 4.6a).
2. **Signs**
- A flesh-coloured, narrow-based, pedunculated lesion (skin tag – Fig. 4.6b).
- A broad-based (sessile) lesion which may exhibit a raspberry-like surface (Fig. 4.6c).
- A hyperkeratotic filiform lesion similar to a cutaneous horn (Fig. 4.6d).
3. **Treatment** involves simple excision.
4. **Differential diagnosis** includes viral wart, seborrhoeic keratosis and intradermal naevus.

Basal cell papilloma

Basal cell papilloma (seborrhoeic keratosis, seborrhoeic wart, senile verruca) is a common, slow-growing condition found on the face, trunk and extremities of elderly individuals.

1. **Histology** shows expansion of the squamous epithelium of the epidermis by a proliferation of basal cells. The acanthotic epidermis may show keratin-filled cystic inclusions which may be either horn cysts within the mass or

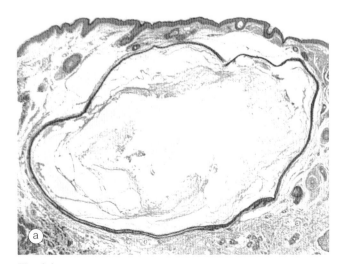

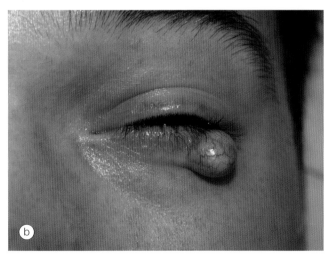

Fig. 4.4
Epidermoid cyst. **(a)** Histology shows a cavity containing keratin lined by keratinized stratified squamous epithelium; **(b)** clinical appearance (Courtesy of J Harry – fig. a; A Pearson – fig. b)

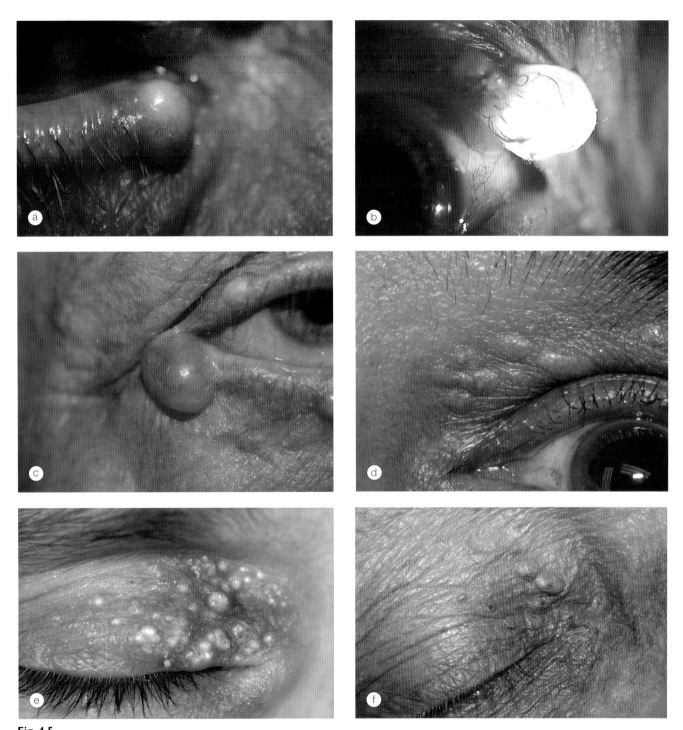

Fig. 4.5
Miscellaneous cysts. **(a)** Cyst of Zeis; **(b)** cyst of Moll; **(c)** eccrine hidrocystoma; **(d)** syringomas; **(e)** milia; **(f)** comedones (Courtesy of A Pearson – figs a, d and f)

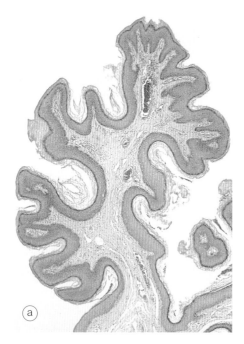

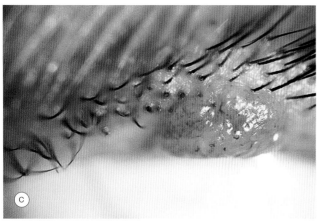

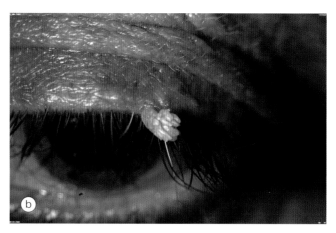

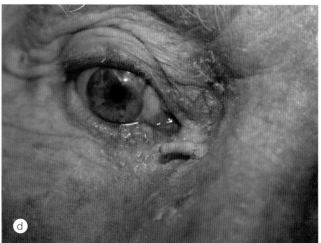

Fig. 4.6
Squamous cell papilloma. **(a)** Histology shows finger-like projections of fibrovascular connective tissue covered by irregular acanthotic and hyperkeratotic squamous epithelium; **(b)** skin tag; **(c)** sessile lesion with a raspberry-like surface; **(d)** hyperkeratotic filiform lesion (Courtesy of J Harry – fig. a; A Pearson – fig. d)

invaginations of surface keratin forming pseudohorn cysts (Fig. 4.7a).
2. **Signs.** A discrete, greasy, brown plaque with a friable verrucous surface and a 'stuck-on' appearance (Fig. 4.7b).
3. **Treatment** involves shave excision from the skin surface of flat lesions and excision of pedunculated lesions.
4. **Differential diagnosis** includes pigmented basal cell carcinoma, naevus and melanoma.

Inverted follicular keratosis

Inverted follicular keratosis (irritated seborrhoeic keratosis, irritated basal cell papilloma) is an uncommon condition usually found on the face.

1. **Histology** resembles seborrhoeic keratosis but also shows zones of squamous cells arranged in whorls (squamous eddies) and extension into the dermis (Fig. 4.8a).
2. **Signs.** A non-pigmented papillomatous lesion on the lid margin that may grow rapidly (Fig. 4.8b).
3. **Treatment** involves complete excision because recurrence is common if incomplete.

Actinic keratosis

Actinic (solar, senile) keratosis is a common, slow-growing, lesion that rarely develops on the eyelids. It typically affects elderly, fair-skinned individuals who have been exposed to excessive sunlight and most frequently occurs on the

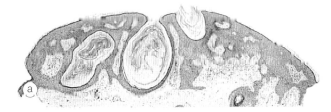

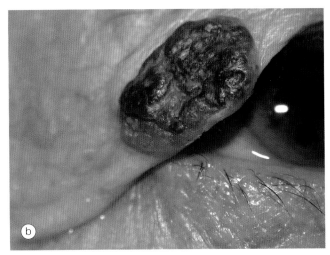

Fig. 4.7
Basal cell papilloma. **(a)** Histology shows an elevated expansion of the epidermis by a proliferation from basal cells; horn cysts and pseudohorn cysts are evident; **(b)** typical 'stuck-on' appearance (Courtesy of J Harry – fig. a; A Pearson – fig. b)

forehead and backs of the hands. It has a potential for transformation into squamous cell carcinoma.

1. **Histology** shows irregular dysplastic epidermis with hyperkeratosis, parakeratosis and a developing cutaneous horn (Fig. 4.9a).
2. **Signs**
   - Hyperkeratotic plaque with distinct borders with a scaly surface that may become fissured (Fig. 4.9b).
   - Occasionally the lesion is nodular or wart-like and may be give rise to a cutaneous horn.
3. **Treatment** involves biopsy followed by either excision or cryotherapy, especially for multiple lesions.

Keratoacanthoma

Keratoacanthoma (molluscum sebaceum) is a rare, rapidly growing tumour which usually occurs in fair-skinned individuals with a history of chronic sun exposure. It is found more frequently than would be expected by chance in patients on immunosuppressive therapy following renal transplants. Keratoacanthoma may have a similar appear-

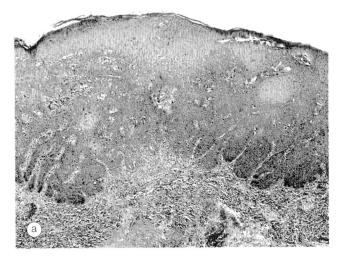

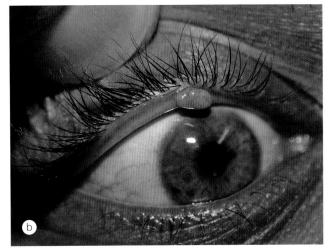

Fig. 4.8
Inverted follicular keratosis. **(a)** Histology shows irregular expansion of the epidermis with rounded extensions into the underlying inflamed dermis; **(b)** clinical appearance (Courtesy of L Horton – fig. a)

ance to squamous cell carcinoma, particularly in immunosuppressed individuals. Histologically keratoacanthoma is regarded as part of the spectrum of squamous cell carcinoma.

1. **Histology** shows irregular thickened epidermis surrounded by acanthotic squamous epithelium. The sharp transition from the thickened to normal adjacent epidermis is referred to as shoulder formation. A keratin-filled crater may be seen (Fig. 4.10a and b).
2. **Signs** in chronological order:
   - A pink, rapidly growing lesion, often on the lower lid (Fig. 4.10c), which may double or treble in size (Fig. 4.10d).

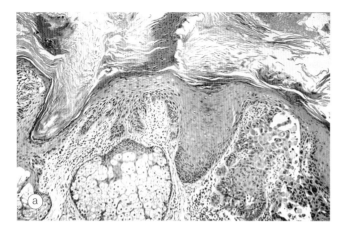

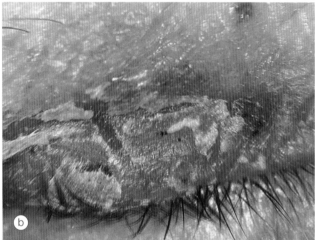

Fig. 4.9
Actinic keratosis. **(a)** Histology shows irregular dysplastic epidermis with hyperkeratosis, parakeratosis and a developing cutaneous horn; **(b)** clinical appearance (Courtesy of J Harry – fig. a)

- The lesion stops growing and remains static for 2–3 months, after which time it starts to involute spontaneously but the diagnosis cannot always be made with confidence until this phenomenon has been observed.
- During the period of regression the central part of the lesion becomes hyperkeratotic and a keratin-filled crater may develop (Fig. 4.10e).
- Complete involution may take up to a year and usually leaves a residual ugly scar.

3. **Treatment** involves complete excision. Other options include radiotherapy, cryotherapy and topical or intralesional 5-fluorouracil.

4. **Differential diagnosis** includes squamous cell carcinoma and basal cell carcinoma.

Acquired melanocytic naevus

A naevus is composed of naevus cells (naevocytes) which are derived either from epidermal melanocytes (junctional, compound and intradermal naevi) or from dermal melanocytes (blue naevi).

1. **Classification,** clinical appearance and potential for malignant transformation of naevi are determined by their histological location within the skin as follows:
   a. *Junctional* naevus occurs in young individuals as a uniformly brown macule or plaque (Fig. 4.11a). The naevus cells are located at the junction of the epidermis and dermis and have low potential for malignant transformation (Fig. 4.11b).
   b. *Compound* naevus occurs in middle-age as a raised papular lesion. The shade of pigment varies from light tan to dark brown but tends to be relatively uniform throughout (Fig. 4.11c). The naevus cells extend from the epidermis into the dermis (Fig. 4.11d) and have low malignant potential which is related to the junctional component.
   c. *Intradermal* naevus, the most common, typically occurs in old age. It is a papillomatous lesion with little, if any, pigmentation, that may show dilated vessels and protruding lashes (Fig. 4.11e). Histologically the naevus cells are confined to the dermis and have no malignant potential (Fig. 4.11f).
   d. *Histological variants* of naevi include balloon cell naevi, halo naevi, Spitz naevi (juvenile melanomas) and dysplastic naevi (atypical moles). Multiple dysplastic naevi constitute the dysplastic naevus syndrome (atypical mole syndrome – AMS) which carries an increased risk of conjunctival and uveal naevi as well as cutaneous, conjunctival and uveal melanomas.

2. **Treatment** is indicated for cosmetic reasons or concern about malignancy. Excision must be complete because it may be difficult to differentiate recurrence following incomplete removal, from melanoma both clinically and histologically.

Congenital melanocytic naevus

Congenital naevi are uncommon and may range in size from a few millimetres to covering a large area of the body. Histologically they resemble their conventional acquired counterparts.

1. **Signs**
   - The colour is generally uniform and numerous hairs may be present.
   - A kissing or split naevus is a rare type that equally involves the upper and lower eyelid (Fig. 4.12).

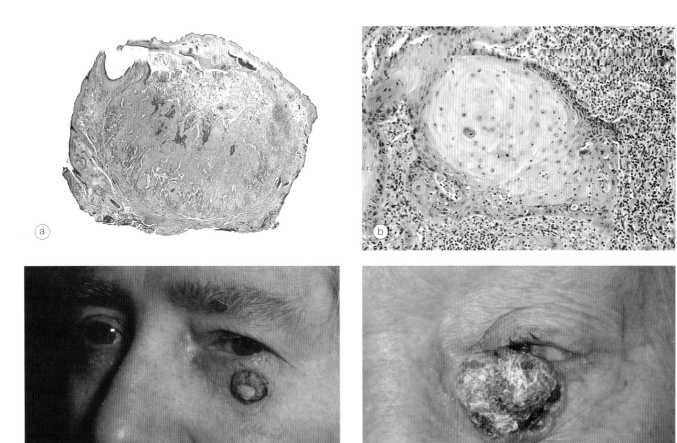

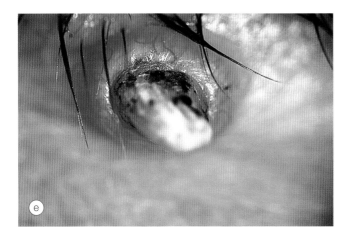

Fig. 4.10
Keratoacanthoma. **(a)** Histology shows irregularly thickened epidermis with a keratin-containing cup and well-marked shoulder formation; **(b)** the dermis shows irregular islands of dysplastic squamous epithelium associated with a heavy inflammatory cellular infiltrate; **(c)** hyperkeratotic lesion; **(d)** fast-growing tumour; **(e)** keratin-filled crater during involution (Courtesy of J Harry – fig. a; L Horton – fig. b; A Pearson – fig. e)

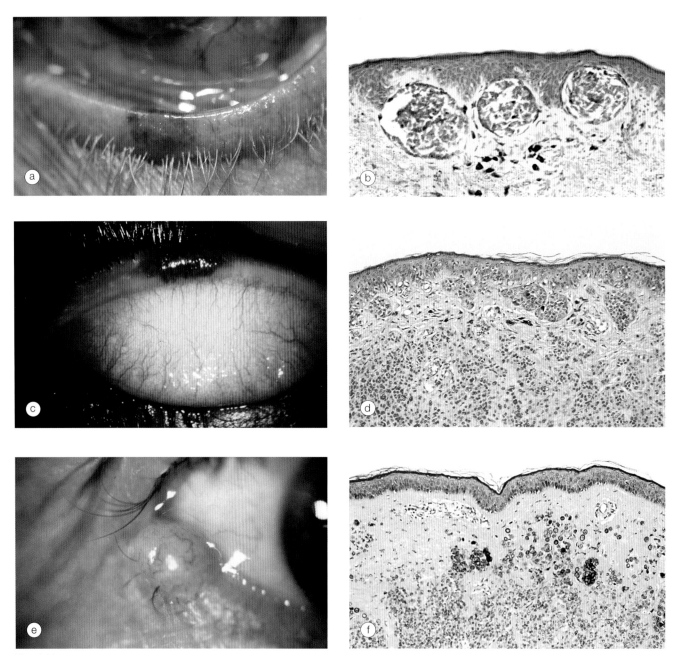

Fig. 4.11
Acquired melanocytic naevus. (a) Junctional naevus; (b) histology shows heavily pigmented naevus cells at the epidermal/dermal junction. (c) Compound naevus; (d) histology shows naevus cell at the epidermal/dermal junction and within the dermis. (e) Intradermal naevus; (f) histology shows naevus cells within the dermis separated by a clear zone from the epidermis (Courtesy of J Harry – figs b, d and f)

- The lesion is frequently cosmetically objectionable and may cause ptosis
2. **Treatment** involves excision and reconstruction with split or full thickness skin grafts.

Capillary haemangioma

Capillary haemangioma (strawberry naevus), although rare is one of the most common tumours of infancy and presents shortly after birth. The female to male ratio is 3:1. Eyelid haemangiomas have a predilection for the upper lid and may have orbital extensions. Occasionally the lesion may also involve the skin of the face and some patients have strawberry naevi on other parts of the body. It is important to be aware of the association between multiple cutaneous lesions and visceral haemangiomas.

1. **Histology** shows proliferation of varying-sized vascular channels in the dermis and subcutaneous tissue (Fig. 4.13a).
2. **Signs.** Unilateral, raised bright red lesion (Fig. 4.13b) which blanches on pressure and may swell on crying. A large lesion on the upper lid may cause mechanical ptosis (Fig. 4.13c).
3. **Treatment** of periocular and orbital haemangiomas is described in Chapter 6.

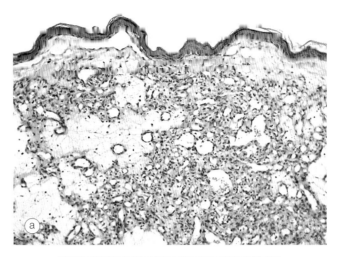
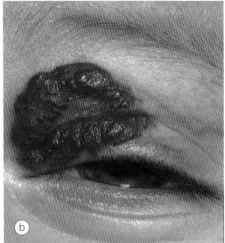
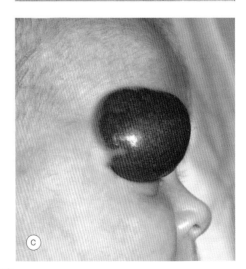

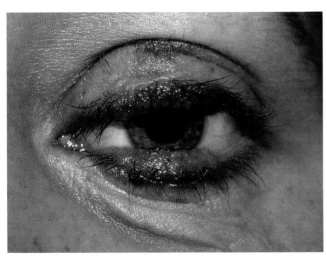

Fig. 4.12
'Kissing' congenital melanocytic naevus (Courtesy of A Pearson)

Fig. 4.13
Capillary haemangioma. **(a)** Histology shows varying-sized small vascular channels within the dermis and subcutaneous tissue; **(b)** small haemangioma; **(c)** mechanical ptosis due to a large lesion (Courtesy of J Harry – fig. a; K Nischal – figs b and c)

Port-wine stain

A port-wine stain (naevus flammeus) is a rare congenital, subcutaneous lesion consisting of large ectatic vessels of varying calibre. It most frequently occurs on the face and is usually unilateral and segmental but may be bilateral.

1. **Histology** shows dilated blood-filled spaces separated by thin fibrous septae (Fig. 4.14a).
2. **Signs**
   • A sharply demarcated, soft, pink patch which does not blanch with pressure (Fig. 4.14b).

   • With age, the lesion does not grow but darkens to red or purple (Fig. 4.14c).
   • The overlying skin may become hypertrophied, coarse, nodular and friable and may bleed or become infected (Fig. 4.14d).
3. **Associations** in patients with extensive lesions involving the first and second divisions of the trigeminal nerve are ipsilateral glaucoma (in about 30%), diffuse ipsilateral choroidal haemangioma and Sturge–Weber syndrome in 5% of cases (see Chapter 24).
4. **Treatment** with an erbium laser, if undertaken during early life, is effective in decreasing the amount of skin

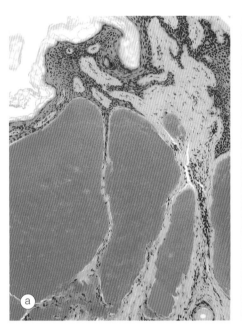
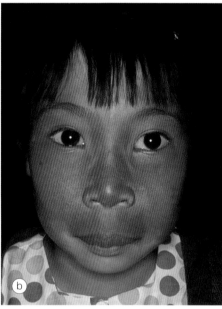
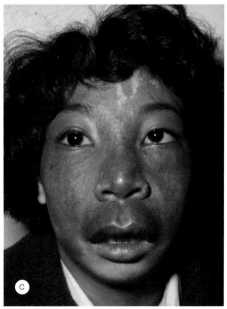
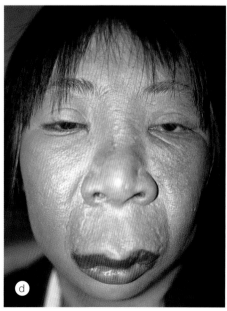

Fig. 4.14
Port-wine stain. **(a)** Histology shows widely dilated blood-filled spaces separated by fibrous septae; **(b–d)** progression (Courtesy of L Horton – fig. a)

discoloration in relatively flat or mildly hypertrophic lesions.

Pyogenic granuloma

A pyogenic granuloma is a fast-growing proliferation of granulation tissue which is usually antedated by surgery, trauma or infection, although some cases are idiopathic.

1. **Histology** shows granulation tissue composed of wide, thin-walled vascular channels and inflammatory cells infiltrating a loose stroma (Fig. 4.15a).
2. **Signs.** A painful, rapidly growing, vascular polypoidal lesion which may bleed following relatively trivial trauma (Fig. 4.15b).
3. **Treatment** involves excision.

Xanthelasma

Xanthelasma is a common, frequently bilateral condition which is usually found in middle-aged and elderly individuals. Xanthelasma and corneal arcus may be associated with increased levels of serum cholesterol and low density lipoprotein cholesterol, especially in younger males.

1. **Histology** shows lipid-laden histiocytes in the dermis (Fig. 4.16a).
2. **Signs.** Multiple, yellowish, subcutaneous plaques usually located at the medial aspects of the eyelids (Fig. 4.16b).
3. **Treatment** for cosmetic reasons is either by excision or preferably destruction with a carbon dioxide or argon laser. Patients with the highest recurrence rate are those with persistent elevated cholesterol levels. A case has been reported in which oral cholesterol lowering agents resulted in regression.

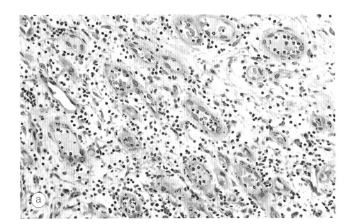
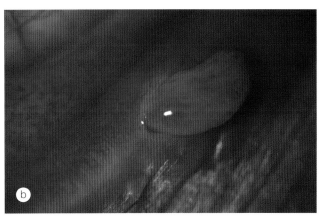

Fig. 4.15
Pyogenic granuloma. **(a)** Histology shows inflamed vascularized connective tissue; **(b)** clinical appearance (Courtesy of J Harry and G Misson, from *Clinical Ophthalmic Pathology*, Butterworth-Heinemann, 2001 – fig. a)

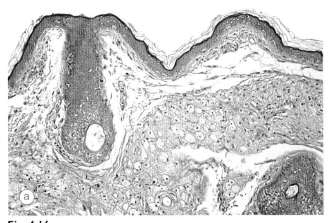
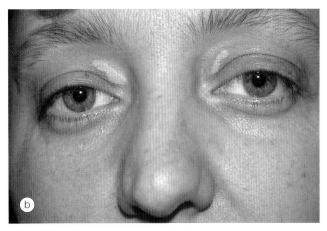

Fig. 4.16
Xanthelasma. **(a)** Histology shows foamy histiocytes within the dermis; **(b)** clinical appearance (Courtesy of J Harry – fig. a; A Pearson – fig. b)

Pilomatricoma

Pilomatricoma (pilomatrixoma, calcifying epithelioma of Malherbe) is derived from the germinal matrix cells of the hair bulb. It typically affects young females and is the commonest hair follicle proliferation seen by ophthalmologists.

1. **Histology** shows irregular epithelial islands exhibiting viable basophilic cells at the periphery and degenerate shadow cells more centrally. Calcification is frequently present and there is often a foreign body giant cell reaction (Fig. 4.17a).
2. **Signs.** A deep, dermal nodule that may be hard due to calcification (Fig. 4.17b).
3. **Treatment** involves excision.

Other less common hair follicle proliferations include trichofolliculoma, trichoepithelioma and trichilemmoma.

Neurofibroma

Plexiform neurofibromas typically affect children with neurofibromatosis-1. Solitary neurofibromas tend to occur in adults, 25% of whom have associated neurofibromatosis-1.

1. **Histology** shows proliferation of Schwann cells, fibroblasts and nerve axons (Fig. 4.18a).
2. **Signs.** Neurofibromas typically affect the upper lid and give rise to a characteristic S-shaped deformity (Fig. 4.18b).
3. **Treatment** of solitary lesions involves simple excision but removal of plexiform lesions may be difficult, especially if they are diffuse.

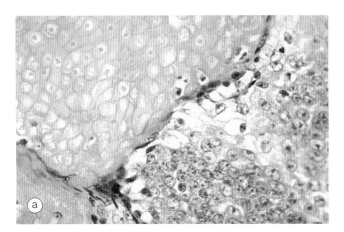

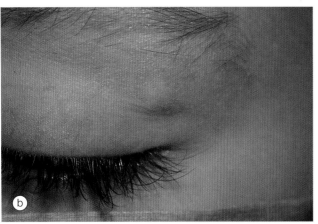

Fig. 4.17
Pilomatricoma **(a)** Histology shows viable basophilic cells to the right and degenerate shadow cells to the left; **(b)** clinical appearance (Courtesy of J Harry and G Misson, from *Clinical Ophthalmic Pathology*, Butterworth-Heinemann, 2001 – fig. a; A Pearson – fig. b)

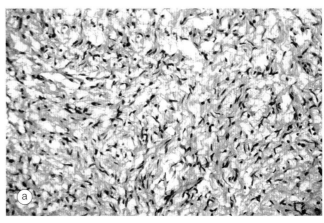

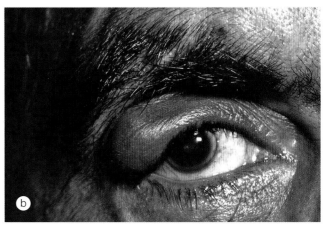

Fig. 4.18
Neurofibroma. **(a)** Histology shows proliferation of Schwann cells, fibroblasts and nerve axons, and wavy collagen fibres; **(b)** characteristic S-shaped deformity (Courtesy of J Harry – fig. a)

MALIGNANT TUMOURS

Rare predisposing conditions

Young patients who suffer from one of these conditions may develop eyelid malignancies.

1. **Xeroderma pigmentosum** is an AR disease characterized by skin damage on exposure to natural sunlight which gives rise to progressive cutaneous pigmentation abnormalities (Fig. 4.19a). Affected patients have a bird-like facies and a great propensity to the development of skin basal cell carcinoma (BCC), squamous cell carcinoma (SCC) and melanoma, which may be multiple (Fig. 4.19b). Conjunctival malignancies have also been reported.
2. **Gorlin–Goltz syndrome** (naevoid basal cell carcinoma syndrome) is a rare AD disorder characterized by extensive congenital deformities of the eye, face, bone and CNS. Many patients develop multiple, small BCC during the second decade of life (Fig. 4.19c). They are also predisposed to other malignancies including medulloblastoma, breast carcinoma and Hodgkin lymphoma.
3. **Muir–Torre syndrome** is a rare AD condition that predisposes to cutaneous and systemic malignancies. Cutaneous tumours include BCC, sebaceous gland carcinoma (SGC) and keratoacanthoma. Colorectal and genitourinary carcinoma is the most common systemic tumour.
4. **Other** predispositions include immunosuppression, retinoblastoma survival and albinism.

Basal cell carcinoma

General features

BCC is the commonest human malignancy and typically affects elderly patients. Important risk factors are fair skin, inability to tan and chronic exposure to sunlight. Ninety per cent of cases occur in the head and neck and about 10% of these involve the eyelid. BCC is by far the most prevalent malignant eyelid tumour, accounting for 90% of all cases. The majority arise from the lower eyelid, followed in relative frequency by the medial canthus, upper eyelid and lateral canthus. The tumour is slow growing and locally

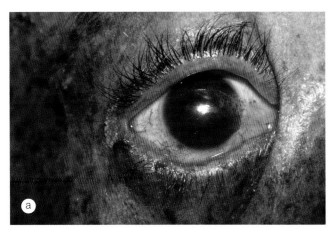

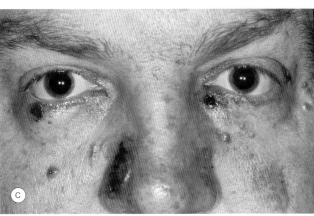

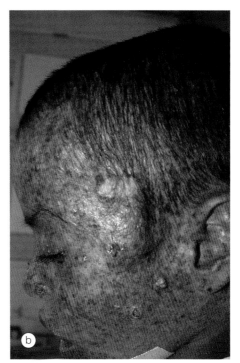

Fig. 4.19
Xeroderma pigmentosum. **(a)** Pigmentary skin changes; **(b)** multiple malignancies on the face; **(c)** Gorlin–Goltz syndrome shows hypertelorism, broad nasal bridge and multiple basal cell carcinomas (Courtesy of K Nischal – figs a and b; Krachmer, Mannis and Holland, from *Cornea*, Mosby, 2005 – fig. c)

invasive but non-metastasizing. Tumours located near the medial canthus are more prone to invade the orbit and sinuses, and are more difficult to manage than those arising elsewhere and carry the greatest risk of recurrence. Tumours that recur following incomplete treatment tend to be more aggressive and difficult to treat.

Histology

The tumour arises from pluripotent basal cells of the epidermis. The cells proliferate downwards (Fig. 4.20a) and exhibit palisading at the periphery (Fig. 4.20b). Squamous differentiation with the production of keratin results in a

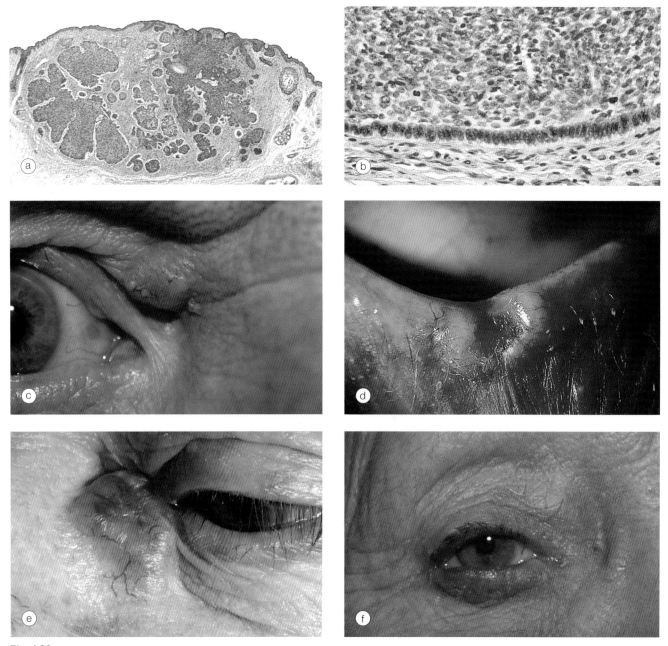

Fig. 4.20
Basal cell carcinoma. **(a)** Histology shows downward proliferation of basal cells; **(b)** histology shows palisading of cells at the periphery of a tumour lobule; **(c)** nodular tumour; **(d)** rodent ulcer; **(e)** large rodent ulcer; **(f)** sclerosing tumour (Courtesy of J Harry – figs a and b)

keratotic type of BCC. There can also be sebaceous and adenoid differentiation with the development of cystic and adenoid cystic types, while the growth of elongated strands and islands of cells embedded in a dense fibrous stroma results in a sclerosing (morphoeic) tumour.

Clinical types

> **NB** The main clinical features of epidermal malignancy are ulceration, lack of tenderness, induration, irregular borders and destruction of lid margin architecture.

1. **Nodular** BCC is a shiny, firm, pearly nodule with small dilated blood vessels on its surface. Initially, growth is slow and it may take the tumour 1–2 years to reach a diameter of 0.5cm (Fig. 4.20c).
2. **Noduloulcerative** (rodent ulcer) has central ulceration, pearly raised rolled edges (Fig. 4.20d) and dilated and irregular blood vessels (telangiectasis) over its lateral margins (Fig. 4.20e); with time it may erode a large portion of the eyelid.
3. **Sclerosing** BCC (morphoeic) is less common and may be difficult to diagnose because it infiltrates laterally beneath the epidermis as an indurated plaque (Fig. 4.20f). The margins of the tumour may be impossible to delineate clinically and the lesion tends to be much more extensive on palpation than inspection. On cursory examination a sclerosing BCC may simulate a localized area of unilateral 'chronic blepharitis'.
4. **Other types** of BCC not usually found on the lid are cystic, adenoid, pigmented and multiple superficial.

> **NB** Patients with BCC frequently show signs of actinic damage of facial skin.

Squamous cell carcinoma

General features

SCC is a much less common, but potentially more aggressive tumour than BCC with metastasis to regional lymph nodes in about 20% of cases. Careful surveillance of regional lymph nodes is therefore an important aspect of initial assessment. The tumour may also exhibit perineural spread to the intracranial cavity via the orbit. SCC accounts for 5–10% of eyelid malignancies and may arise *de novo* or from pre-existing actinic keratosis or carcinoma *in situ* (Bowen disease - Fig. 4.2d). Immunocompromised patients with AIDS and those with renal transplants are at increased risk. The tumour has a predilection for the lower eyelid and the lid margin. It occurs most commonly in elderly individuals with

a fair complexion and a history of chronic sun exposure and skin damage. The diagnosis of SCC may be difficult because keratoacanthoma and cutaneous horn may reveal histological evidence of invasive SCC at deeper levels of sectioning.

Histology

The tumour arises from the squamous cell layer of the epidermis. It is composed of variable sized groups of atypical epithelial cells with prominent nuclei and abundant eosinophilic cytoplasm within the dermis (Fig. 4.21a). Well differentiated tumours may show characteristic keratin 'pearls' and intercellular bridges (desmosomes – Fig. 4.21b).

Clinical types

The clinical types are variable and there are no pathognomonic characteristics. Clinically, SCC may be indistinguishable from BCC but surface vascularization is usually absent, growth is more rapid and hyperkeratosis is often present.

1. **Nodular** SCC is characterized by a hyperkeratotic nodule which may develop crusting erosions and fissures (Fig. 4.21c).
2. **Ulcerating** SCC has a red base and sharply defined, indurated and everted borders but pearly margins and telangiectasia are not usually present (Fig. 4.21d and e).
3. **Cutaneous horn** with underlying invasive SCC (Fig. 4.21f).

Sebaceous gland carcinoma

General features

Sebaceous glands are located in the periocular skin, the caruncle and eyebrow skin follicles. SGC is a very rare slow-growing tumour which most frequently affects the elderly, with a predisposition for females. It usually arises from the meibomian glands, although on occasion it may arise from the glands of Zeis or sebaceous glands in the caruncle. In contrast to BCC and SCC, the tumour occurs more commonly on the upper eyelid where meibomian glands are more numerous. In about 5% of cases there is simultaneous involvement of both lids probably due to intraepithelial spread or spontaneous development of multiple primaries.

The clinical diagnosis of SGC is frequently difficult because, in its early stages, external signs of malignancy may be subtle so that the tumour may resemble a less aggressive lesion such as a chalazion or chronic blepharitis. However, the presence of yellowish material within the tumour is highly suggestive of SGC. Because of frequent difficulties in diagnosis and delay in

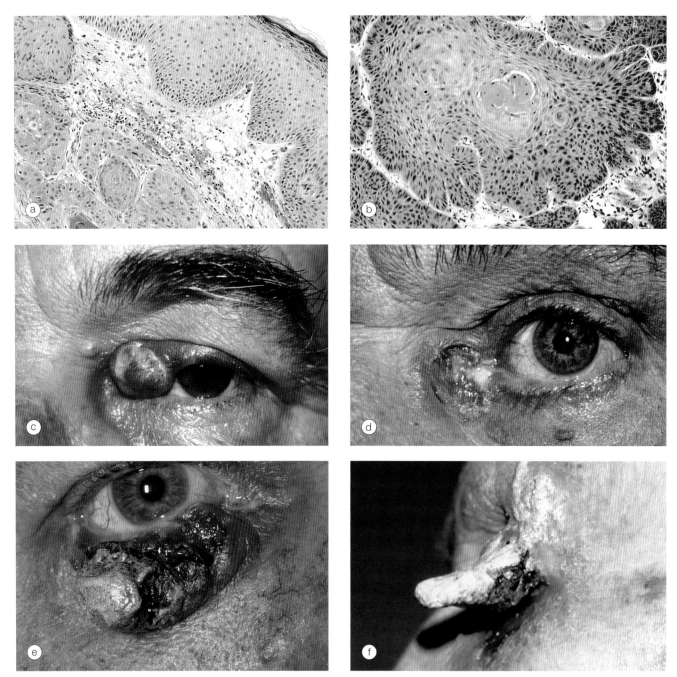

Fig. 4.21
Squamous cell carcinoma. **(a)** Histology shows acanthotic squamous epithelium (top right); islands of dysplastic squamous epithelium are seen within the dermis; **(b)** histology shows pleomorphic squamous cells with a central keratin 'pearl'; **(c)** nodular tumour with surface keratosis; **(d)** ulcerating tumour; **(e)** large ulcerating tumour with surface hyperkeratosis; **(f)** cutaneous horn with underlying carcinoma (Courtesy of L Horton – figs a and b; H Frank – figs c and d; L Merin – fig. e)

treatment, the overall mortality rate is about 5–10%. Adverse prognostic features are upper lid involvement, tumour size of 10mm or more and duration of symptoms of over 6 months. SGC that arises from the glands of Zeis is thought to have a more favourable prognosis.

Histology

The tumour consists of lobules of cells with pale foamy vacuolated cytoplasm and large hyperchromatic nuclei (Fig. 4.22a). They cells stain positive for lipid (Fig. 4.22b).

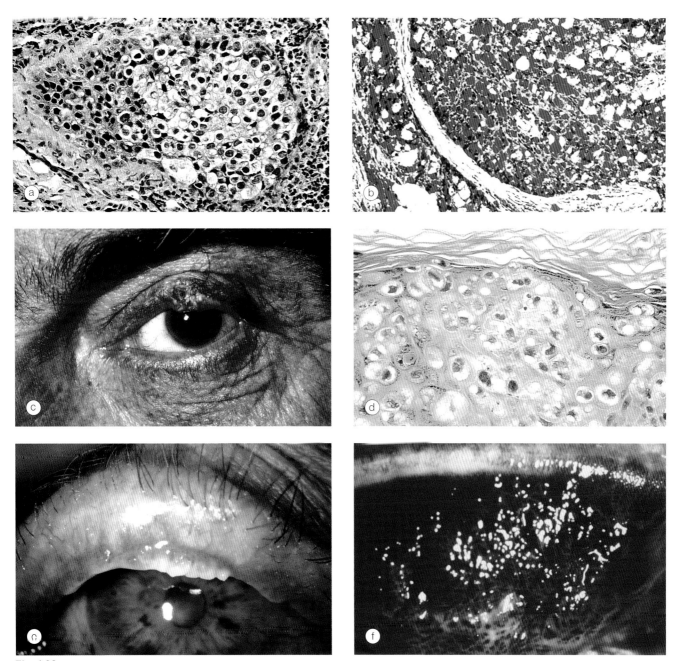

Fig. 4.22
Sebaceous gland carcinoma. **(a)** Histology shows cells with large hyperchromatic nuclei and vacuolated cytoplasm; **(b)** histology shows lipid globules (red); oil red O stain; **(c)** nodular tumour; **(d)** histology of a spreading tumour shows malignant sebaceous cells infiltrating the epidermis (pagetoid spread); **(e)** spreading tumour; **(f)** conjunctival intraepithelial involvement (Courtesy of A Garner – figs a and b; A Frank – fig. c; J Harry and G Misson, from *Clinical Ophthalmic Pathology*, Butterworth-Heinemann, 2001 – fig. d; S Tuft – fig. e)

Clinical types

Although SGC does not have a characteristic clinical appearance it may present with the following:

1. **Nodular** SGC is a discrete, hard, immobile nodule most commonly within the upper tarsal plate that may exhibit yellow discoloration because of the presence of lipid (Fig. 4.22c). Because the lesion may masquerade as a 'chalazion' it is recommended that any chalazion of an unusual consistency should undergo full-thickness resection and histological examination.
2. **Spreading** SGC is characterized by diffuse infiltration of the epidermis (pagetoid spread – Fig. 4.22d) that causes a diffuse thickening of the lid margin (Fig. 4.22e) and may result in loss of lashes and be mistaken for 'chronic blepharitis'. Occasionally the tumour may diffusely infiltrate the conjunctival epithelium in a similar way (Fig. 4.22f) and may be mistaken for an inflammatory condition such as unilateral chronic blepharoconjunctivitis, superior limbic keratoconjunctivitis or cicatricial pemphigoid (masquerade syndrome).

Lentigo maligna and melanoma

Melanoma rarely develops on the eyelids but is potentially lethal. Although pigmentation is a hallmark of skin melanomas, half of lid melanomas are non-pigmented and this may give rise to diagnostic difficulties. Features suggestive of melanoma include irregular margins, asymmetrical shape, colour change or presence of multiple colours and size greater than 6mm in diameter.

Lentigo maligna

Lentigo maligna (melanoma *in-situ*, intraepidermal melanoma and Hutchinson freckle) is a relatively uncommon condition that develops in sun-damaged skin in elderly individuals that may subsequently infiltrate the dermis and become malignant.

1. **Histology** shows intraepidermal proliferation of usually spindle-shaped atypical melanocytes that replace the basal layer of the epidermis (Fig. 4.23a).
2. **Signs.** A very slowly expanding pigmented macule with an irregular border (Fig. 4.23b). Nodular thickening and areas of irregular pigmentation are highly suggestive of malignant transformation (4.23c).

Melanoma

1. **Histology** shows melanoma cells within the epidermis and dermis (Fig. 4.24a).

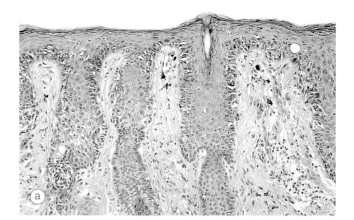
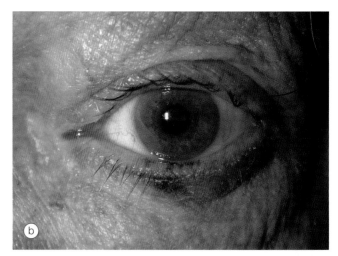
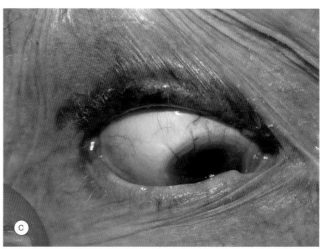

Fig. 4.23
Melanoma *in situ*. **(a)** Histology shows melanoma cells proliferating within the basal layers of the epidermis; **(b)** lentigo maligna; **(c)** melanoma arising from lentigo maligna (Courtesy of L Horton – fig. a; S Delva – figs b and c)

2. Signs

  a. **Superficial spreading** melanoma is characterized by a plaque with an irregular outline and variable pigmentation (Fig. 4.24b).

  b. **Nodular** melanoma is characterized by a blue-black nodule surrounded by normal skin (Fig. 4.24c).

NB Any skin lesion may be pigmented and most pigmented lesions are not melanomas.

Merkel cell carcinoma

Merkel cell (cutaneous neuroendocrine) carcinoma is a fast-growing tumour which typically affects the elderly. Although Merkel cells lie within the epidermis the tumour appears to arise from the dermis. Its rarity may lead to difficulty in diagnosis and delay in treatment. The tumour is highly malignant and potentially lethal and many patients have metastatic spread at presentation.

1. **Histology** shows sheets of cells with scanty cytoplasm, round or oval nuclei and numerous mitotic figures (Fig. 4.25a).

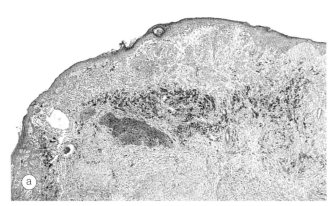
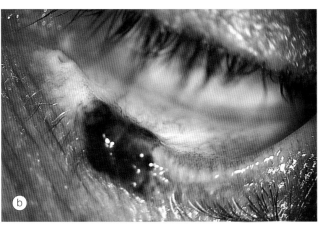
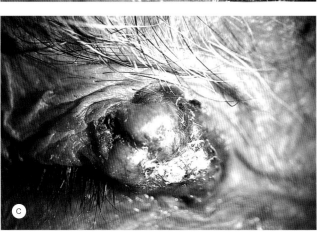
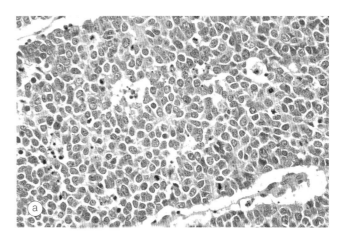
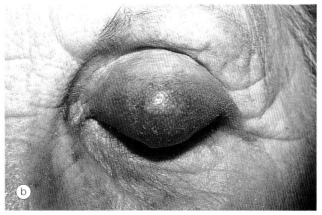

Fig. 4.24
Melanoma. **(a)** Histology shows melanoma cells within the epidermis and dermis; **(b)** superficial spreading melanoma; **(c)** nodular melanoma (Courtesy of J Harry – fig. a)

Fig. 4.25
Merkel cell carcinoma. **(a)** Histology shows a sheet of Merkel cells; **(b)** clinical appearance (Courtesy of J Harry and G Misson, from *Ocular Ophthalmic Pathology*, Butterworth-Heinemann, 2001 – fig. a)

2. **Signs.** A violaceous, well demarcated nodule with intact overlying skin, most frequently involving the upper eyelid (Fig. 4.25b).
3. **Treatment** is by excision which is frequently combined with chemotherapy.

Kaposi sarcoma

Kaposi sarcoma is a vascular tumour which typically affects patients with AIDS in whom the vascular endothelium becomes infected by Kaposi sarcoma virus (KSV) which is the same as human herpesvirus 8 *(HHV-8)*. Many patients have advanced systemic disease although in some instances the tumour may be the sole manifestation.

1. **Histology** shows proliferating spindle cells, vascular channels, mitotic figures and inflammatory cells within the dermis (Fig. 4.26a).

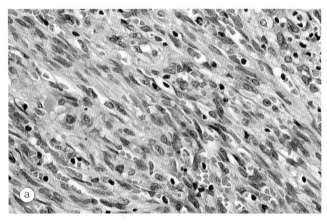

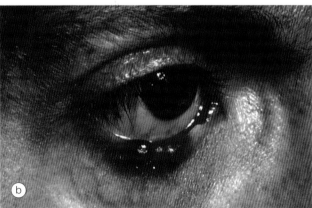

Fig. 4.26
Kaposi sarcoma. **(a)** Histology shows a proliferation of predominantly spindle-shaped cells; vascular channels and a few mitotic figures are evident; **(b)** clinical appearance (Courtesy of J Harry – fig. a)

2. **Signs.** The tumour is a pink, red-violet to brown lesion which may be mistaken for a haematoma or a naevus (Fig. 4.26b).
3. **Treatment** is by radiotherapy or excision.

Treatment of malignant tumours

Biopsy

The two types of biopsy are incisional, in which only part of the lesion is removed, and excisional, in which the entire lesion is removed. The two types of incisional biopsy are:

1. **Shave** biopsy is performed with a knife and involves removal of the superficial part of the lesion. It may be used in the diagnosis of benign lesions but is not appropriate if malignancy is suspected.
2. **Punch** biopsy is performed using a skin dermatome similar to a corneal trephine. Histological examination of the deep part of the lesion is possible.

Surgical excision

The entire tumour should be removed with preservation of as much of normal tissue as possible. Most small BCC can be cured by excision of the tumour together with a 4mm margin of tissue which looks clinically normal. More radical surgical excision is required for large BCC and aggressive tumours such as SCC and SGC. Frozen section control by either a standard method or micrographic surgery can further improve the success rate.

1. **Standard frozen section** involves histological examination of the margins of the excised specimen at the time of surgery to ensure that they are tumour-free. If no tumour cells are detected, the eyelid is reconstructed; if some are present in a particular area, further excision is performed until the specimen is tumour-free.
2. **Mohs' micrographic surgery** involves excision with operative analysis of serial horizontal frozen sections from the under-surface of the tumour. The sections are then colour coded or mapped to identify any remaining areas of tumour. Although time-consuming, this maximizes the chances of total tumour excision with minimal sacrifice of normal tissue. This is a particularly useful technique for tumours that grow diffusely and have indefinite margins with finger-like extensions, such as sclerosing BCC, SCC, recurrent tumours and those involving the medial or lateral canthi.

Reconstruction

The technique of eyelid reconstruction depends on the extent of tissue removed and whether it is full-thickness. It is important to reconstruct both anterior and posterior lamellae. If one of the lamellae has been sacrificed during excision of the tumour, it must be reconstructed with similar tissue. Anterior lamellar defects may be closed directly or with a local flap or skin graft. Full thickness defects may be repaired as follows.

1. **Small** defects involving less than one-third of the eyelid can usually be closed directly, provided the surrounding tissue is sufficiently elastic to allow approximation of the cut edges (Fig. 4.27). If necessary, a lateral cantholysis can be fashioned to mobilize additional tissue if the defect cannot be reapproximated
2. **Moderate** size defects involving up to half of the eyelid may require a Tenzel semicircular flap for closure (Fig. 4.28).
3. **Large** defects involving over half of the eyelid may be closed by one of the following techniques:
   a. ***Posterior lamellar reconstruction*** may involve an upper lid free tarsal graft, buccal mucous membrane or hard palate graft, or a Hughes flap from the upper lid (Fig. 4.29).
   b. ***Anterior lamellar reconstruction*** may involve skin advancement, a local skin flap or a free skin graft (Fig. 4.30).

Radiotherapy

1. **Indications**
   a. Small BCC which does not involve the medial canthal area in patients who are either unsuitable for or refuse surgery.
   b. Kaposi sarcoma because it is radiosensitive.
2. **Contraindications**
   a. Medial canthal BCC because radiotherapy would damage the canaliculi and result in epiphora.
   b. Upper eyelid tumours because subsequent keratinization results in a chronically uncomfortable eye.
   c. Aggressive tumours such as sclerosing BCC, SCC and SGC.
3. **Complications**
   a. Skin damage and madarosis.
   b. Nasolacrimal duct stenosis following irradiation to the medial canthal area.
   c. Conjunctival keratinization, dry eye, keratopathy and cataract
   d. Retinopathy and optic neuropathy.

NB Many of these complications can be avoided if the globe is protected by a special eye shield during irradiation. However, the recurrence rate is higher than after surgery, and radiotherapy does not allow histological confirmation of tumour eradication. Recurrences following radiotherapy are difficult to treat surgically because of the poor healing properties of irradiated tissue.

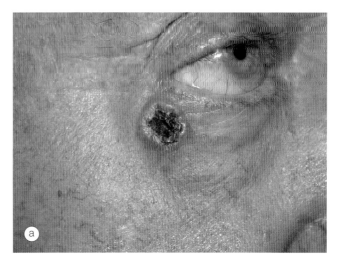
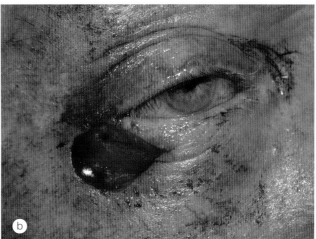
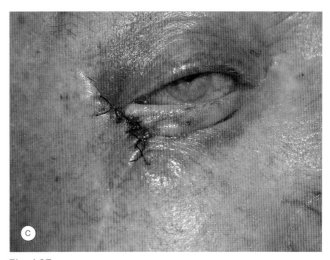

Fig. 4.27
Direct closure. **(a)** Preoperative appearance of a basal cell carcinoma; **(b)** appearance following excision; **(c)** direct closure of defect (Courtesy of A Pearson)

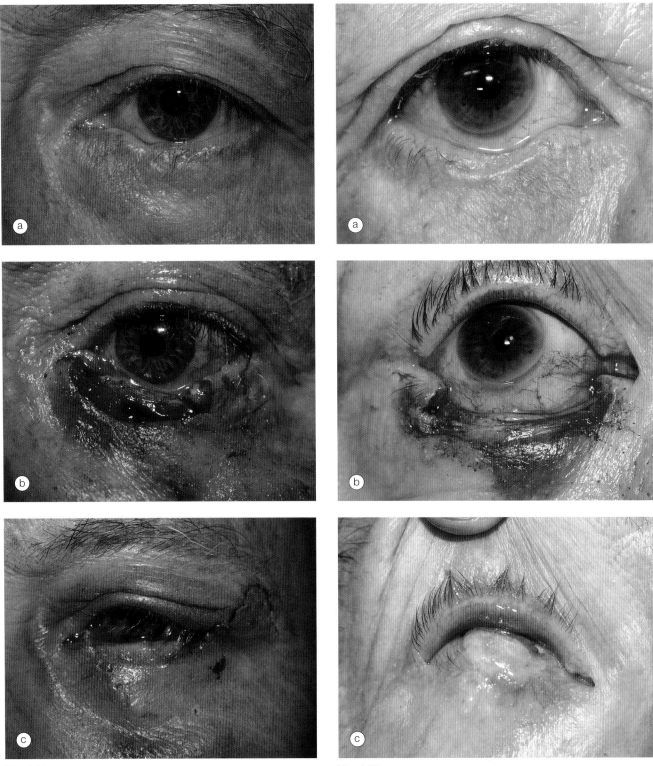

Fig. 4.28
Tenzel flap. **(a)** Preoperative appearance; **(b)** appearance
following excision; **(c)** appearance following closure of the flap
(Courtesy of A Pearson)

Fig. 4.29
Posterior lamellar reconstruction with a Hughes upper lid flap.
(a) Preoperative appearance; **(b)** appearance following excision;
(c) postoperative appearance with the flap yet to be divided
(Courtesy of A Pearson)

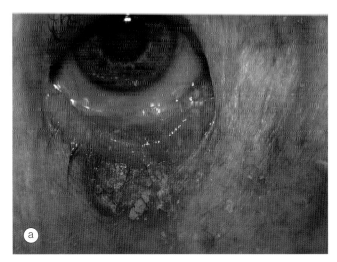

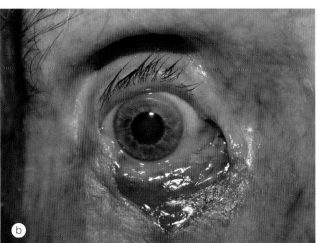

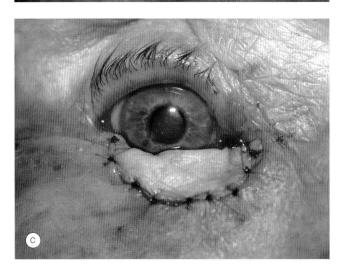

Fig. 4.30
Anterior lamellar reconstruction with a free skin graft.
(a) Preoperative appearance; **(b)** appearance following excision;
(c) skin graft in place (Courtesy of A Pearson)

Cryotherapy

1. **Indications** Small superficial BCC
2. **Contraindications** are similar to those of radiotherapy, although cryotherapy may be a useful adjunct to surgery in patients with epibulbar pagetoid extensions of SGC, thus sparing the patient an exenteration.
3. **Complications** are skin depigmentation, madarosis and conjunctival overgrowth.

Laissez-faire

The wound edges are approximated as far as possible and the defect is allowed to granulate and heal by secondary intention. Even large defects with time can achieve a satisfactory outcome.

DISORDERS OF LASHES

Anatomy

The lashes are slightly more numerous in the upper (approximately 100) than in the lower lid. The lash roots lie against the anterior surface of the tarsus between the pretarsal orbicularis oculi muscle and the muscle of Riolan. The cilia pass between the orbicularis oculi and the muscle of Riolan and exit the skin at the anterior lid margin and curve away from the globe. Scarring of the tarsal plate and conjunctiva can alter their position and direction. Following intense inflammation abnormal lashes can grow from meibomian gland openings (distichiasis).

Trichiasis

Trichiasis is a very common acquired condition which may occur in isolation or as a result of scarring of the lid margin secondary to conditions such as chronic blepharitis and herpes zoster ophthalmicus. Trichiasis should not be mistaken for pseudo-trichiasis secondary to entropion because in some cases the in-turning of the eyelid may be intermittent and the condition may be mistaken for true trichiasis and inappropriately treated.

Signs

Trichiasis is characterized by posterior misdirection of lashes arising from normal sites of origin (Fig. 4.31a and b). Trauma to the corneal epithelium may cause punctate epithelial erosions and ocular irritation made worse on blinking. Corneal ulceration and pannus formation may occur in severe long-standing cases.

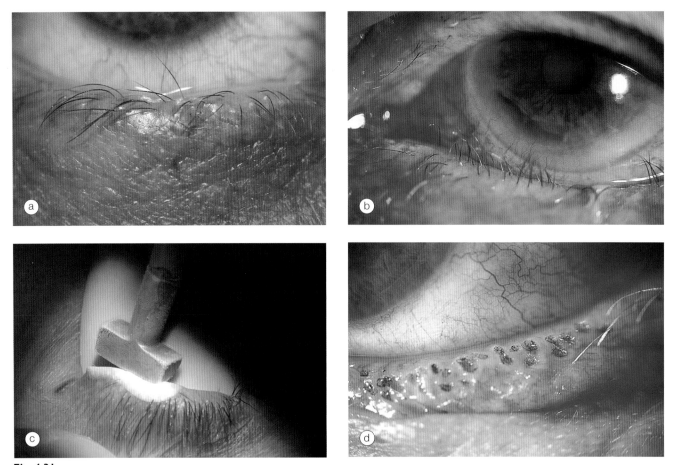

Fig. 4.31
Trichiasis. **(a)** Mild; **(b)** very severe; **(c)** cryotherapy; **(d)** appearance following laser ablation (Courtesy of A Pearson – fig a)

Treatment

1. **Epilation** with forceps is simple and effective but recurrences within 4–6 weeks are inevitable.
2. **Electrolysis** is useful for a few isolated lashes but is tedious and frequently multiple treatments are required to obtain a satisfactory result. An electrocautery needle is inserted down the shaft of the lash root and current applied until coagulated tissue bubbles to the surface. The lash is then removed. Retreatment for recurrences is required in about 40% of cases and can cause scarring.
3. **Cryotherapy** is very effective in eliminating many lashes (Fig. 4.31c). With a special cryoprobe a double freeze-thaw cycle at −20°C is applied. Potential complications include skin necrosis, depigmentation in dark-skinned individuals, damage to meibomian glands, which may adversely affect the precorneal tear film, and shallow notching of the lid margin.
4. **Argon laser ablation** is useful for a few scattered lashes and is performed as follows:

a. The initial settings are 50μm, 0.2 seconds and 1000mW.
b. The laser is fired at the root of the lash and a small crater formed.
c. The spot size is increased to 200μm and the crater deepened to reach the follicle (Fig. 4.31d).
d. About a dozen applications are required and most patients are cured by one or two sessions.
5. **Surgery** involving full-thickness wedge resection or anterior lamellar excision may be useful for a localized crop of lashes resistant to other methods of treatment.

Congenital distichiasis

Congenital distichiasis is a rare condition that occurs when a primary epithelial germ cell destined to differentiate into a specialized sebaceous gland (meibomian gland) of the tarsus develops into a complete pilosebaceous unit. The condition is frequently inherited in an AD manner with high penetrance but variable expressivity. The majority of patients also manifest primary lymphoedema of the legs (lymphoedema distichiasis syndrome Fig. 4.32a).

1. **Signs.** A partial or complete second row of lashes emerging at or slightly behind the meibomian gland orifices. The aberrant lashes tend to be thinner and shorter and than normal cilia and are often directed posteriorly (Fig. 4.32b). They are usually well tolerated during infancy and may not become symptomatic until the age of 5 years

2. **Treatment** of the lower lid is with cryotherapy. Distichiasis of the upper lid involves lamellar eyelid division and cryotherapy, which is performed as follows:
    a. An incision is made along the grey line dividing the lid into anterior and posterior lamellae (Fig. 4.32c).
    b. The posterior lamella and lash follicles are frozen with a double freeze-thaw cycle to −20°C (Fig. 4.32d).
    c. The lamellae are surgically re-apposed.

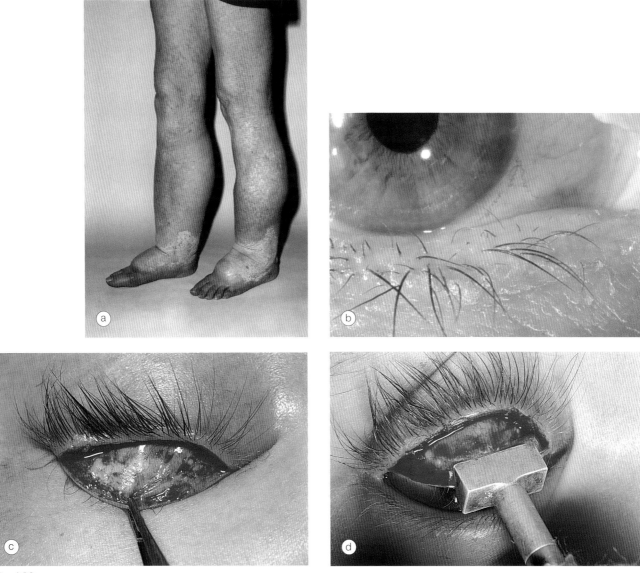

Fig. 4.32
Congenital distichiasis. **(a)** Lymphoedema; **(b)** severe distichiasis; **(c)** lamellar eyelid division; **(d)** cryotherapy to the posterior lamella
(Courtesy of A Pearson – fig. b; A G Tyers and J R O Collin, from *Colour Atlas of Ophthalmic Plastic Surgery*, Butterworth-Heinemann, 2001 – figs c and d)

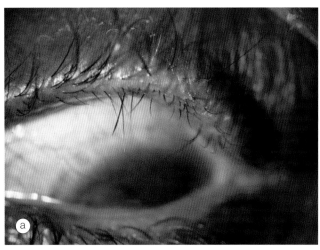
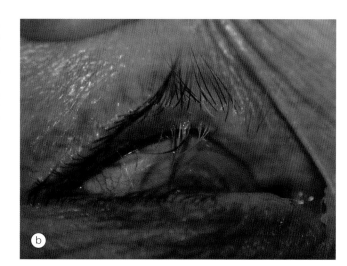

Fig. 4.33
Acquired distichiasis **(a)** Mild; **(b)** severe

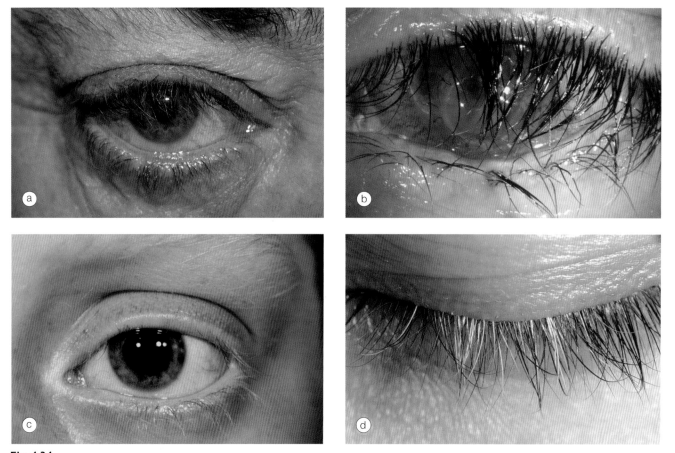

Fig. 4.34
Miscellaneous eyelash disorders. **(a)** Eyelash ptosis; **(b)** trichomegaly; **(c)** madarosis; **(d)** poliosis (Courtesy of A Pearson – fig. a; L Merin – fig. b)

Acquired distichiasis

Acquired distichiasis (metaplastic lashes) is caused by metaplasia and dedifferentiation of the meibomian glands to become hair follicles. The most important cause is late stage cicatrizing conjunctivitis associated with chemical injury, Stevens–Johnson syndrome and ocular cicatricial pemphigoid.

1. **Signs.** Variable number of lashes which originate from meibomian gland orifices (Fig. 4.33). Unlike congenital distichiasis, the cilia tend to be non-pigmented and stunted, and are usually symptomatic.
2. **Treatment** of mild cases is as for trichiasis. Severe cases require lamellar eyelid division and cryotherapy to the posterior lamella.

Eyelash ptosis

Eyelash ptosis is a downward sagging of upper eyelid lashes (Fig. 4.34a). The condition may be idiopathic or associated with the floppy eyelid syndrome, dermatochalasis with anterior lamellar slip or long-standing facial palsy.

Trichomegaly

Trichomegaly is excessive eyelash growth (Fig. 4.34b). The main causes are listed in Table 4.1.

Madarosis

Madarosis is a decrease in the number of lashes (Fig. 4.34c). The main causes are shown in Table 4.2.

Table 4.1 Causes of trichomegaly

1. *Acquired*
   - Drug-induced – phenytoin, ciclosporin and topical prostaglandin analogues
   - Malnutrition
   - AIDS
   - Porphyria
   - Hypothyroidism
   - Familial
2. *Congenital*
   - Oliver–McFarlane syndrome – pigmentary retinopathy, dwarfism and mental handicap
   - Cornelia de Lange syndrome – synophrys, low hairline and developmental and musculoskeletal abnormalities
   - Goldstein–Hutt syndromes – cataract and hereditary spherocytosis
   - Hermansky–Pudlak syndrome – albinism and bleeding diathesis
   - Oculocutaneous albinism type I

Table 4.2 Causes of madarosis

1. *Local*
   - Chronic anterior lid margin disease
   - Infiltrating lid tumours
   - Burns
   - Radiotherapy or cryotherapy of lid tumours
2. *Skin disorders*
   - Generalized alopecia
   - Psoriasis
3. *Systemic diseases*
   - Myxoedema
   - Systemic lupus erythematosus
   - Acquired syphilis
   - Lepromatous leprosy
4. *Following removal*
   - Iatrogenic for trichiasis
   - Trichotillomania – psychiatric disorder of hair removal

Table 4.3 Causes of poliosis

1. *Ocular*
   - Chronic anterior blepharitis
   - Sympathetic ophthalmitis
2. *Systemic*
   - Vogt–Koyanagi–Harada syndrome
   - Waardenburg syndrome
   - Vitiligo
   - Marfan syndrome
   - Tuberous sclerosis

Poliosis

Poliosis is a premature localized whitening of hair, which may involve the lashes and eyebrows (Fig. 4.34d). The main causes are shown in Table 4.3.

ALLERGIC DISORDERS

Acute allergic oedema

Acute allergic oedema is usually caused by insect bites, angioedema and urticaria, and occasionally drugs.

1. **Signs.** Sudden onset of bilateral pitting periorbital oedema (Fig. 4.35a).
2. **Treatment** with systemic antihistamines may be helpful.

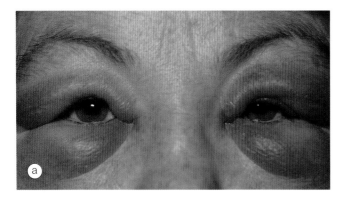

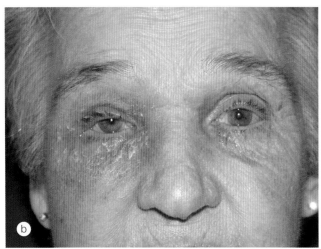

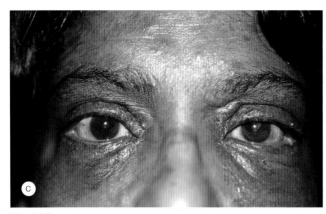

Fig. 4.35
Allergic disorders. **(a)** Acute allergic oedema; **(b)** contact dermatitis; **(c)** atopic dermatitis (Courtesy of A Pearson – fig. b)

Contact dermatitis

Contact dermatitis is an inflammatory response that usually follows exposure to a medication or preservative, cosmetics or metals. The individual is sensitized on first exposure and develops an immune reaction on further exposure. Reaction is mediated by a delayed type IV hypersensitivity response.

1. **History** of exposure and re-exposure to a potential allergen.
2. **Symptoms** include itching and tearing following exposure.
3. **Signs**
   - Lid oedema, scaling, angular fissuring and tightness (Fig. 4.35b).
   - Chemosis, redness and papillary conjunctivitis.
   - Punctate corneal epithelial erosions.
4. **Treatment**
   - Stopping exposure to the allergen, if it can be identified.
   - Use of non-preserved drops, if sensitivity to preservatives is suspected.
   - Cold compress for symptomatic relief.
   - Topical steroids may be helpful but are rarely required.
   - Oral antihistamine for severe cases.
   - Care to avoid re-exposure (record in notes).

Atopic dermatitis

Atopic dermatitis (eczema) is a very common, idiopathic condition frequently associated with asthma and hay fever. Eyelid involvement is relatively infrequent but when present is invariably associated with generalized dermatitis.

1. **Signs.** Thickening, crusting and vertical fissuring of the lids associated with staphylococcal blepharitis and madarosis (Fig. 4.35c).
2. **Treatment** is with emollients to hydrate the skin and the judicious use of mild topical steroids such as hydrocortisone 1%. It is also important to treat associated infection.
3. **Ocular associations**
   a. *Common.* Vernal disease in children and chronic keratoconjunctivitis in adults.
   b. *Uncommon.* Keratoconus, presenile cataract and retinal detachment.

BACTERIAL INFECTIONS

External hordeolum

An external hordeolum (stye) is an acute staphylococcal abscess of a lash follicle and its associated gland of Zeis. It is more common in children and young adults.

1. **Signs**
   - A tender swelling in the lid margin pointing anteriorly through the skin with usually a lash at the apex (Fig. 4.36a).
   - Multiple lesions may be present and occasionally minute abscesses may involve the entire lid margin.
2. **Treatment** involves topical antibiotics, hot compresses and epilation of the associated lash to hasten resolution.

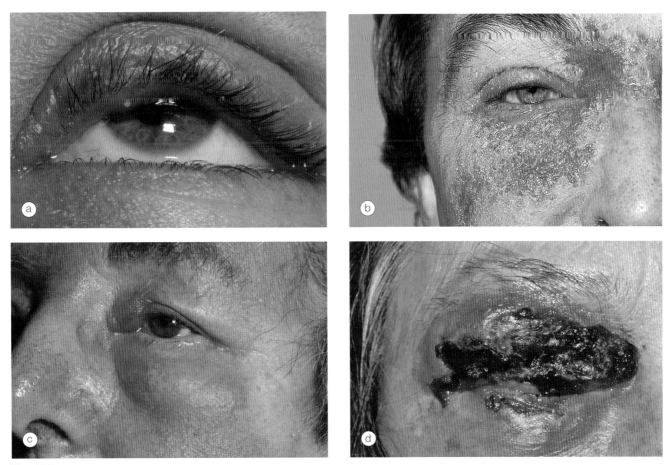

Fig. 4.36
Bacterial infections. **(a)** External hordeolum; **(b)** impetigo; **(c)** erysipelas; **(d)** necrotizing fasciitis (Courtesy of S Tuft – fig. a)

Impetigo

Impetigo is an uncommon, superficial skin infection caused by *S. aureus* or *S. pyogenes* which most frequently affects children. Involvement of the eyelids is usually associated with painful infection of the face.

1. **Signs.** Erythematous macules which rapidly develop into thin-walled blisters which produce golden-yellow crusts on rupturing (Fig. 4.36b).
2. **Treatment** is with topical antibiotics and oral flucloxacillin or erythromycin.

Erysipelas

Erysipelas (St. Anthony fire) is an uncommon, acute subcutaneous spreading cellulitis usually caused by *S. pyogenes* through a site of minor skin trauma.

1. **Signs**
   - An expanding, well-defined, indurated, erythematous, subcutaneous plaque (Fig. 4.36c).
   - Primary lid involvement, when it occurs, is usually severe and may result in secondary contracture.
2. **Treatment** is with oral phenoxymethylpenicillin.

Necrotizing fasciitis

Necrotizing fasciitis is an extremely rare rapidly progressive necrosis initially involving subcutaneous soft tissues and later the skin. It is usually caused by *S. pyogenes* and occasionally *S. aureus*. The most frequent sites of involvement are the extremities, trunk and perineum, as well as postoperative wound sites. Unless treatment is early and appropriate, death may result. Periocular infection is rare and may be secondary to trauma or surgery.

1. **Signs.** Periorbital redness and oedema leading to formation of large bullae and black discoloration of skin due to gangrene secondary to underlying thrombosis (Fig. 4.36d).
2. **Complications** include ophthalmic artery occlusion, lagophthalmos and disfigurement.
3. **Treatment** involves intravenous benzylpenicillin, debridement of necrotic tissue and reconstructive surgery.

VIRAL INFECTIONS

Molluscum contagiosum

Molluscum contagiosum is a skin infection caused by a human-specific double-stranded DNA poxvirus which typically affects otherwise healthy children, with a peak incidence between 2 and 4 years. Transmission is by contact with infected people and then by autoinoculation. Multiple, and occasionally confluent, lesions may develop in immunocompromised patients. A distribution in the chin-strap region is common in HIV positive patients.

1. **Histology** shows a central pit on the skin surface and lobules of hyperplastic epidermis proliferating downwards (Fig. 4.37a). The epidermal cells are enlarged and contain eccentrically placed intracytoplasmic inclusions (molluscum bodies).
2. **Signs**
   - Single or multiple, pale, waxy, umbilicated nodule (Fig. 4.37b).
   - Lesions on the lid margin may shed virus into the tear film and give rise to secondary, ipsilateral, chronic, follicular conjunctivitis. Unless the lid margin is examined

carefully the causative molluscum lesion may be overlooked.
   - White cheesy material consisting of infected degenerate cells can be expressed from the lesion.
3. **Treatment** may not be necessary unless the lesion is very close to the lid margin. Options include shave excision or destruction of the lesion by cauterization, cryotherapy or laser.

Herpes zoster ophthalmicus

Herpes zoster ophthalmicus (HZO) is a common, unilateral infection caused by varicella-zoster virus. It typically affects the elderly but may occur at an earlier age and be more severe in immunocompromised individuals.

Diagnosis

1. **Presentation** is with pain in the distribution of the first division of the trigeminal nerve.
2. **Signs**
   - A maculopapular rash on the forehead (Fig. 4.38a).
   - Progression through vesicles, pustules to crusting (Fig. 4.38b).
   - Periorbital oedema may spread to the other side, giving the erroneous impression that the condition is bilateral.
3. **Ocular complications** (see Chapter 9).

Treatment

1. **Systemic** valaciclovir 1g t.i.d. or famciclovir 250mg t.i.d. or 750mg once daily, for 7 days,
2. **Topical** aciclovir or penciclovir cream, and a steroid-antibiotic combination such as Fucidin-H (hydrocortisone 1%, fusidic acid 2%) or Terra-Cortil (hydrocortisone 1%, oxytetracycline 3%) t.i.d. until the crusts have separated.

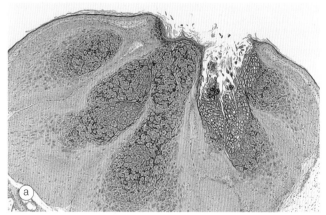 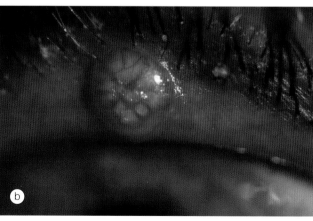

Fig. 4.37
Molluscum contagiosum. **(a)** Histology shows a surface pit, hyperplastic epidermis and molluscum bodies which are small and eosinophilic near the surface and larger and basophilic deeper; **(b)** molluscum nodule (Courtesy of J Harry – fig. a)

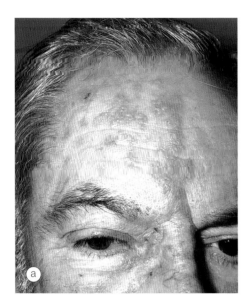

- Associated papillary conjunctivitis, discharge and lid swelling.
- Dendritic corneal ulcers can develop, especially in atopic patients.
- Gradual resolution over 6 to 8 days.
- Involvement can be very severe in atopic patients (eczema herpeticum – Fig. 4.39b).

3 Treatment
- Topical antiviral (aciclovir) 5 times daily for 3 days. This tends to be messy when rubbed on the skin.
- Oral aciclovir 400mg 5 times daily for 3 days is usually better tolerated than topical treatment.

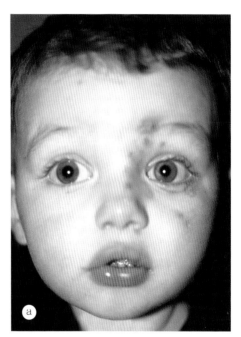

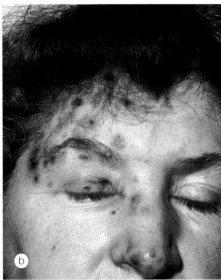

Fig. 4.38
Herpes zoster ophthalmicus **(a)** Maculopapular rash; **(b)** vesicles and crusts

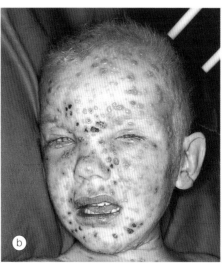

Fig. 4.39
Herpes simplex. **(a)** Blepharitis; **(b)** eczema herpeticum

NB Talc and calamine lotion should be avoided.

Herpes simplex

1. **Pathogenesis.** Reactivation of herpes simplex virus previously dormant in the trigeminal ganglion.
2. **Diagnosis**
   - Prodromal facial and lid tingling lasting about 24 hours.
   - Eyelid and periorbital vesicles on the lid margin that break down over 48 hours (Fig. 4.39a).

- Add flucloxacillin (500mg q.i.d) or erythromycin (250mg q.i.d) if there is eczema herpeticum (to treat secondary staphylococcal infection).

BLEPHARITIS

Chronic anterior blepharitis

Chronic blepharitis is a very common cause of ocular discomfort and irritation. Involvement is usually bilateral and symmetrical. Blepharitis may be subdivided into anterior and posterior although there is often considerable overlap in symptoms; features of both are often present. The poor correlation between symptoms and signs, the uncertain aetiology and mechanisms of the disease process, conspire to make management difficult.

> **NB** Some signs of blepharitis (e.g. lid margin telangiectasis, pouting of meibomian gland orifices) may occur as a part of the normal ageing process in asymptomatic individuals.

Pathogenesis

Anterior blepharitis affects the area surrounding the bases of the eyelashes and may be staphylococcal or seborrhoeic. The former is thought to be the result of an abnormal cell mediated response to components of the cell wall of *S. aureus* which may also be responsible for the red eye reaction and the peripheral corneal infiltrates seen in some patients. Seborrhoeic blepharitis is often associated with generalized seborrhoea that may involve the scalp, nasolabial folds, behind the ears, and the sternum.

> **NB** Because of the intimate relationship between the lids and ocular surface, chronic blepharitis may cause secondary inflammatory and mechanical changes in the conjunctiva and cornea.

Diagnosis

1. **Symptoms** do not provide a reliable clue to the type of blepharitis and are caused by disruption of normal ocular surface function and reduction in tear stability.
   - Burning, grittiness and mild photophobia with remissions and exacerbations are characteristic.
   - Symptoms are usually worse in the mornings although in patients with associated dry eye they may increase during the day.

> **NB** Because of poor correlation between the severity of symptoms and clinical signs it can be difficult to objectively assess the benefit of treatment.

2. **Signs**
   a. Staphylococcal blepharitis
   - Hard scales and crusting mainly located around the bases of the lashes (collarettes – Fig. 4.40a).
   - Mild papillary conjunctivitis (Fig. 4.40b) and chronic conjunctival hyperaemia are common.
   - Scarring and notching (tylosis) of the lid margin (Fig. 4.40c), madarosis, trichiasis (Fig. 4.40d) and poliosis in severe long-standing cases.
   - Secondary changes include stye formation, marginal keratitis and occasionally phlyctenulosis.
   - Associated tear film instability and dry eye are common.
   b. Seborrhoeic blepharitis
   - Hyperaemic and greasy anterior lid margins with sticking together of lashes (Fig. 4.41a).
   - The scales are soft and located anywhere on the lid margin and lashes (Fig. 4.41b)

Treatment

There is little evidence to support any particular treatment protocol for anterior blepharitis. Patients should be advised that lifelong treatment may be necessary and that a permanent cure is unlikely, but control of symptoms is usually possible.

1. **Lid hygiene**
   - A warm compress applied for several minutes to soften crusts at the bases of the lashes.
   - Lid cleaning to mechanically remove crusts involves scrubbing the lid margins once or twice daily with a cotton bud dipped in a dilute solution of baby shampoo or sodium bicarbonate.
   - Commercially produced soap/alcohol impregnated pads for lid scrubs are available but care should be taken not to induce mechanical irritation.
   - The eyelids can also be cleaned with diluted shampoo when washing the hair.
   - Gradually, lid hygiene can be performed less frequently as the condition is brought under control but blepharitis often recurs if it is stopped completely.

2. **Antibiotics**
   a. Topical sodium fusidic acid, bacitracin or chloramphenicol is used to treat acute folliculitis but is of limited value in long-standing cases. Following lid hygiene the ointment should be rubbed onto the anterior lid margin with a cotton bud or clean finger.

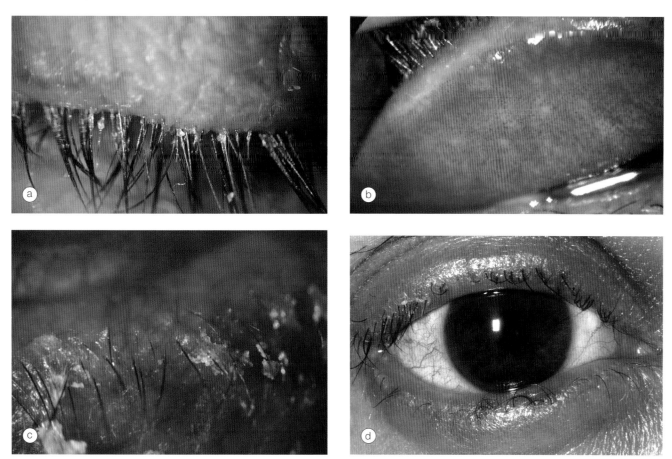

Fig. 4.40
Chronic staphylococcal blepharitis. **(a)** Collarettes; **(b)** papillary conjunctivitis; **(c)** scarring of the lid margin; **(d)** madarosis and trichiasis (Courtesy of S Tuft – figs b and d)

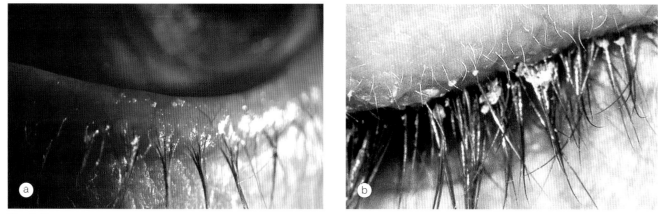

Fig. 4.41
Chronic seborrhoeic blepharitis. **(a)** Greasy lid margin with sticky lashes; **(b)** soft scales (Courtesy of J Silbert, from *Anterior Segment Complications of Contact Lens Wear*, Butterworth-Heinemann, 1999 – fig. b)

*b. **Oral*** azithromycin (500mg daily for 3 days) may be helpful to control ulcerative lid margin disease.

3. **Weak topical steroid** such as fluorometholone 0.1% q.i.d. for one week is useful in patients with severe papillary conjunctivitis, marginal keratitis and phlyctenulosis, although repeated courses may be required.

4. **Tear substitutes** are required for associated tear film instability and dry eye.

> **NB** In long-standing cases several weeks of intensive treatment may be needed to achieve improvement.

Chronic posterior blepharitis

Pathogenesis

Posterior blepharitis is caused by meibomian gland dysfunction and alterations in meibomian gland secretions. Bacterial lipases may result in the formation of free fatty acids. This increases the melting point of the meibum preventing its expression from the glands, contributing to ocular surface irritation and possibly enabling growth of *S. aureus*. Loss of the tear film phospholipids that act as surfactants results in increased tear evaporation and osmolarity, and an unstable tear film.

Diagnosis

There is a poor correlation between the severity of symptoms and the clinical signs.

1. **Symptoms** are similar to anterior blepharitis.
2. **Signs** of meibomian gland dysfunction:
   - Excessive and abnormal meibomian gland secretion which may manifest as capping of meibomian gland orifices with oil globules (Fig. 4.42a).
   - Pouting, recession, or plugging of the meibomian gland orifices with hyperaemia and telangiectasis of the posterior lid margin (Fig. 4.42b).
   - Pressure on the lid margin results in expression of meibomian fluid that may be turbid or appear like toothpaste (Fig. 4.42c); in severe cases the secretions become so inspissated that expression is impossible.
   - Lid transillumination may show gland loss and cystic dilatation of meibomian ducts.
   - The tear film is oily and foamy and froth may accumulate on the lid margins or inner canthi (Fig. 4.42d).
   - Secondary changes include papillary conjunctivitis and inferior corneal punctate epithelial erosions.

Treatment

It is very important to inform the patient that cure is unlikely.

Although remission may be achieved recurrence is common, particularly if treatment is stopped.

1. **Lid hygiene**
   - Warm compresses and hygiene performed as for anterior blepharitis except the emphasis is on massaging the lid to express accumulated meibum.
   - Massaging toward the lid margin edge to 'milk' meibum and physical expression of the glands by the physician is of uncertain benefit.
2. **Systemic tetracyclines** are the mainstay of treatment.
   - The rationale for the use of tetracyclines is their ability to block staphylococcal lipase production at concentrations well below the minimum inhibitory concentration.
   - Tetracyclines are particularly indicated in patients with recurrent phlyctenulosis and marginal keratitis although repeated courses of treatment may be needed.

> **NB** Tetracyclines should not be used in children under the age of 12 years (erythromycin is an alternative) or in pregnant or breast-feeding women because they are deposited in growing bone and teeth, and may cause staining of teeth and dental hypoplasia.

   *a. **Oxytetracycline*** 250mg b.d. for 6–12 weeks.
   *b. **Doxycycline*** 100mg b.d. for one week and then daily for 6–12 weeks.
   *c. **Minocycline*** 100mg daily for 6–12 weeks; skin pigmentation may develop after prolonged use.
   *d. **Erythromycin*** 250mg daily or b.d. may be used in children.
3. **Topical therapy** involves antibiotics, steroids and tear substitutes for evaporative dry eye.

Conditions associated with chronic blepharitis

1. **Tear film instability and dry eye** is found in 30–50% of patients, probably as a result of imbalance between the aqueous and lipid components of the tear film allowing increased evaporation. Tear film break up time is typically reduced.
2. **Chalazion formation,** which may be multiple and recurrent, is common, particularly in patients with posterior blepharitis.
3. **Epithelial basement membrane disease** and recurrent epithelial erosion may be exacerbated by posterior blepharitis.
4. **Cutaneous**
   *a. **Acne rosacea*** is often associated with meibomian gland dysfunction.

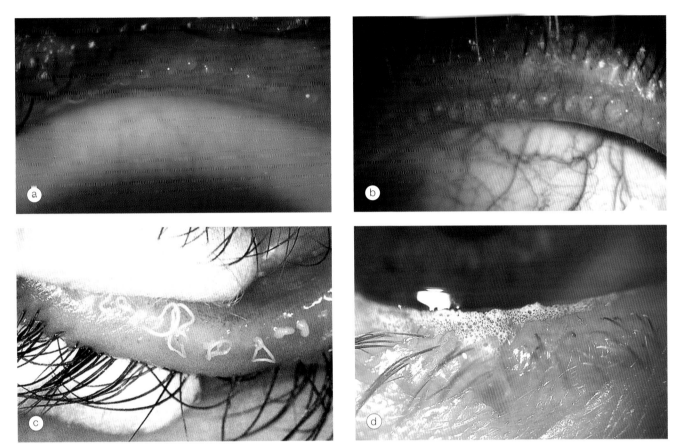

Fig. 4.42
Posterior blepharitis. **(a)** Capping of meibomian gland orifices by oil globules; **(b)** plugging of meibomian gland orifices and telangiectasis; **(c)** expressed toothpaste-like plaques; **(d)** froth on the lid margin (Courtesy of J Silbert, from *Anterior Segment Complications of Contact Lens Wear*, Butterworth-Heinemann, 1999 – fig. c)

    *b. **Seborrhoeic dermatitis*** is present in > 90% of patients with seborrhoeic blepharitis.

    *c. **Acne vulgaris*** treatment with isotretinoin is associated with the development of blepharitis in about 25% of patients; it subsides when the treatment is stopped.

5. **Bacterial keratitis** is associated with ocular surface disease secondary to chronic blepharitis.

6. **Atopic keratoconjunctivitis** is often associated with staphylococcal blepharitis. Treatment of the blepharitis often helps the symptoms of allergic conjunctivitis and vice versa.

7. **Contact lens intolerance.** Long-term contact lens wear is associated with posterior lid margin disease. Inhibition of lid movement and the normal expression of meibomian oil may be the cause. There may also be associated giant papillary conjunctivitis making comfortable lens wear difficult. Blepharitis is also a risk factor for contact lens associated bacterial keratitis.

The characteristics of chronic blepharitis are summarized in Table 4.4.

Phthiriasis palpebrarum

Pathogenesis

The crab louse *Phthirus pubis* is adapted to living in pubic hair (Fig. 4.43a). An infested person may transfer the lice to another hairy area such as the chest, axillae or eyelids. Phthiriasis palpebrarum is an infestation of lashes which typically affects children living in poor hygienic conditions.

Diagnosis

1. **Symptoms** consist of chronic irritation and itching of the lids.

2. **Signs**
   - The lice are anchored to the lashes by their claws (Fig. 4.43b).
   - The ova and their empty shells appear as oval, brownish, opalescent pearls adherent to the base of the cilia (Fig. 4.43c).
   - Conjunctivitis is uncommon.

Table 4.4 Summary of characteristics of chronic blepharitis

	Feature	Anterior blepharitis		Posterior blepharitis
		Staphylococcal	*Seborrhoeic*	
Lashes	Deposit	Hard	Soft	
	Loss	++	+	
	Distorted or trichiasis	++	+	
Lid margin	Ulceration	+		
	Notching	+		++
Cyst	Hordeolum	++		
	Meibomian			++
Conjunctiva	Phlyctenule	+		
Tear film	Foaming			++
	Dry eye	+	+	++
Cornea	Punctate erosions	+	+	++
	Vascularization	+	+	++
	Infiltrates	+	+	++
Associated disease		Atopic dermatitis	Seborrhoeic dermatitis	Acne rosacea

Treatment

1. **Mechanical removal** of the lice and associated lashes with fine forceps.
2. **Topical** yellow mercuric oxide 1% or petroleum jelly applied to the lashes and lids twice a day for 10 days.
3. **Delousing** of the patient, family members, clothing and bedding is important to prevent recurrences.

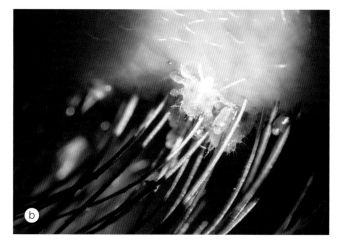

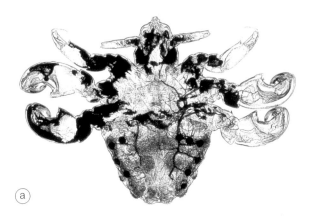

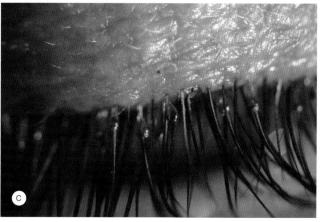

Fig. 4.43
Phthiriasis palpebrarum. **(a)** *Phthirus pubis*; **(b)** lice anchored to lashes; **(c)** ova and shells (Courtesy of J Harry and G Misson, *Ophthalmic Pathology*, Butterworth-Heinemann, 2001 – fig. a)

NB One third of patients with pubic lice have a sexually transmitted disease.

Angular blepharitis

Angular blepharitis involves the lateral parts of the lids and is associated with fissuring of the skin at the lateral and median canthus. Similar changes may be seen in patients with severe allergic conjunctivitis.

1. **Pathogenesis.** The infection is usually caused by *Moraxella lacunata* or *S. aureus* although other bacteria, and rarely herpes simplex, have also been implicated.
2. **Signs**
   • Often unilateral red, scaly, macerated skin at the canthus (Fig. 4.44).
   • Associated papillary and follicular conjunctivitis may occur.
3. **Treatment** involves topical chloramphenicol, bacitracin or erythromycin cream.

Childhood blepharokeratoconjunctivitis

Childhood blepharokeratoconjunctivitis is a poorly defined condition which tends to be more severe in Asian and Middle Eastern populations.

1. **Presentation** is usually at about 6 years of age with recurrent episodes of redness (Fig. 4.45a) and irritation that results in constant eye rubbing and photophobia which may be misdiagnosed as allergic eye disease.
2. **Signs**
   • Chronic anterior or posterior blepharitis which may be associated with recurrent styes or meibomian cysts.
   • Conjunctival changes include diffuse hyperaemia, bulbar phlyctens and follicular or papillary hypertrophy.
   • Corneal changes include superficial punctate keratopathy, marginal keratitis, peripheral vascularization (Fig. 4.45b) and axial subepithelial haze.
3. **Treatment**
   • Lid hygiene and topical antibiotic ointment at bedtime.
   • Topical low dose steroids (prednisolone 0.1% or fluorometholone 0.1%).
   • Oral erythromycin syrup 125mg daily for 4–6 weeks.

PTOSIS

Classification

Ptosis is an abnormally low position of the upper lid which may be congenital or acquired. An anatomical classification is shown in Table 4.5.

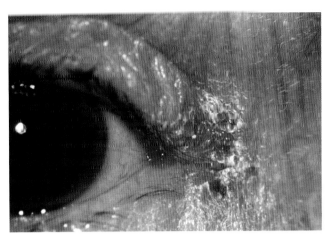

Fig. 4.44
Angular blepharitis

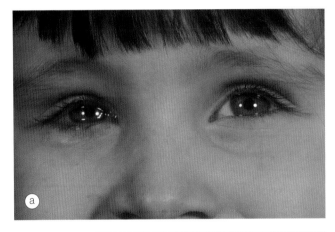

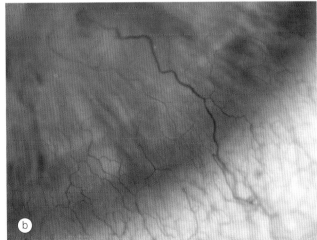

Fig. 4.45
Childhood blepharokeratoconjunctivitis. **(a)** Right blepharoconjunctivitis; **(b)** peripheral vascularization
(Courtesy of S Tuft)

1. **Neurogenic** ptosis is caused by innervational defect such as third nerve and oculosympathetic palsy (Horner syndrome) (see Chapter 21).
2. **Myogenic** ptosis is caused by a myopathy of the levator muscle itself, or by impairment of transmission of impulses at the neuromuscular junction (neuromyopathic). Acquired myogenic ptosis occurs in myasthenia gravis, myotonic dystrophy (see Chapter 24) and progressive external ophthalmoplegia (see Chapter 21).
3. **Aponeurotic** ptosis is caused by a defect in the levator aponeurosis.
4. **Mechanical** ptosis is caused by gravitational effect of a mass or scarring.

Clinical evaluation

History

The age at onset of ptosis and its duration will usually distinguish congenital from acquired cases. If the history is ambiguous, old photographs may be helpful. It is also important to enquire about symptoms of possible underlying systemic disease, such as associated diplopia, variability of ptosis during the day and excessive fatigue.

Pseudoptosis

A false impression of ptosis may be caused by the following:

1. **Lack of support** of the lids by the globe may be due to an orbital volume deficit associated with an artificial

Table 4.5 Classification of ptosis

1. Neurogenic
- Third nerve palsy
- Horner syndrome
- Marcus Gunn jaw-winking syndrome
- Third nerve misdirection

2. Myogenic
- Myasthenia gravis
- Myotonic dystrophy
- Ocular myopathy
- Simple congenital
- Blepharophimosis syndrome

3. Aponeurotic
- Involutional
- Postoperative

4. Mechanical
- Dermatochalasis
- Tumours
- Oedema
- Anterior orbital lesions
- Scarring

eye (Fig. 4.46a), microphthalmos, phthisis bulbi or enophthalmos.
2. **Contralateral lid retraction,** which is detected by comparing the levels of the upper lids remembering that the margin of the upper lid normally covers the superior 2mm of the cornea (Fig. 4.46b).
3. **Ipsilateral hypotropia,** because the upper lid follows the globe downwards (Fig. 4.46c). The pseudoptosis will disappear when the hypotropic eye assumes fixation on covering the normal eye.
4. **Brow ptosis** due to excessive skin on the brow or seventh nerve palsy which is diagnosed by manually elevating the eyebrow (Fig. 4.46d).
5. **Dermatochalasis** in which there is excessive skin on the upper lids (see Fig. 4.68).

Measurements

1. **Margin–reflex distance** is the distance between the upper lid margin and the corneal reflection of a pen torch held by the examiner, at which the patient is directly looking (Fig. 4. 47); normal is 4–4.5mm.
2. **Palpebral fissure height** is the distance between the upper and lower lid margins, measured in the pupillary plane (Fig. 4.48). The upper lid margin normally rests about 2mm below the upper limbus and the lower 1mm above the lower limbus. This measurement is less in males (7–10mm) than in females (8–12 mm). Unilateral ptosis can be quantified by comparison with the contralateral side. Ptosis is may be graded as mild (up to 2mm), moderate (3mm) and severe (4mm or more).
3. **Levator function** (upper lid excursion) is measured by placing a thumb firmly against the patient's brow to negate the action of the frontalis muscle, with the eyes in down-gaze (Fig. 4.49a). The patient then looks up as far as possible and the amount of excursion is measured with a rule (Fig. 4.49b). Levator function is graded as normal (15mm or more), good (12–14mm), fair (5–11mm) and poor (4mm or less).
4. **Upper lid crease** is the vertical distance between the lid margin and the lid crease in down-gaze. In females it measures about 10mm and in males 8mm. Absence of the crease in a patient with congenital ptosis is indirect evidence of poor levator function, whereas a high crease suggests an aponeurotic defect. The skin crease is also used as a guide to the initial incision.
5. **Pretarsal show** is the distance between the lid margin and the skin fold with the eyes in the primary position.

Associated signs

1. **Increased innervation** may flow to the levator muscle of a unilateral ptosis, particularly in up-gaze. Associated increased innervation to the contralateral normal levator will result in lid retraction. The examiner should therefore manually elevate the ptotic lid and look for a droop

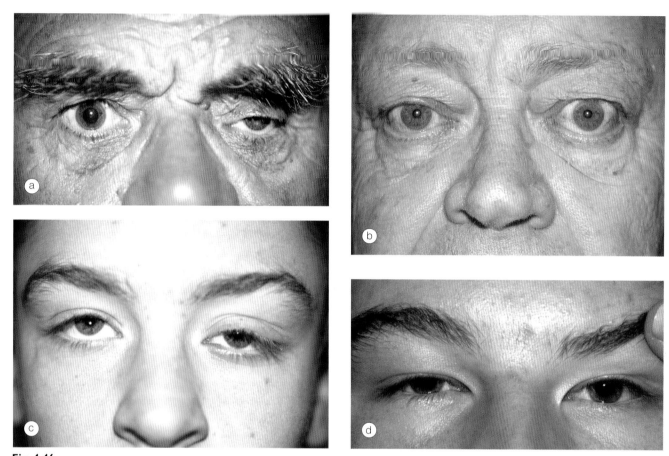

Fig. 4.46
Causes of pseudoptosis. **(a)** Lack of lid support by a prosthesis; **(b)** contralateral lid retraction; **(c)** ipsilateral hypotropia; **(d)** bilateral brow ptosis (Courtesy of S Webber – figs c and d)

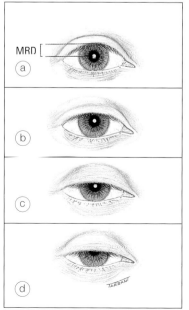

Fig. 4.47
Margin–reflex distance. **(a)** Normal; **(b)** mild ptosis; **(c)** moderate ptosis; **(d)** severe ptosis

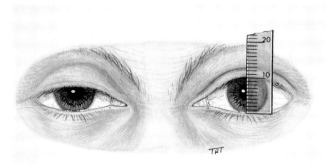

Fig. 4.48
Measurement of vertical fissure height

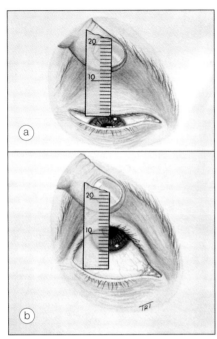

Fig. 4.49
Measurement of levator function

of the opposite lid. If this occurs, the patient should be warned that surgical correction may induce ptosis in the opposite lid.

2. **Fatigability** is tested by asking the patient to look up without blinking for 30 seconds. Progressive drooping of one or both lids, or inability to maintain up-gaze, is suggestive of myasthenia. Myasthenic ptosis may show an overshoot of the upper lid on saccade from down-gaze to the primary position (Cogan twitch sign) and also a 'hop' on side-gaze.

3. **Ocular motility defects,** particularly of the superior rectus, must be evaluated in patients with congenital ptosis. Correction of an ipsilateral hypotropia may improve the degree of ptosis.

4. **Jaw-winking phenomenon** can be detected by asking the patient to chew and move the jaws from side to side (see below).

5. **Bell phenomenon** is tested by manually holding the lids open, asking the patient to try to shut the eyes and observing upward rotation of the globe. A weak Bell phenomenon carries a risk of postoperative exposure keratopathy, particularly following large levator resections or suspension procedures.

Simple congenital ptosis

Simple congenital ptosis is probably caused by failure of neuronal migration or development with muscular sequelae. A minority of cases are hereditary.

Signs

- Unilateral or bilateral ptosis of variable severity (Fig. 4.50).
- Absent upper lid crease and poor levator function.
- In down-gaze the ptotic lid is higher than the normal because of poor relaxation of the levator muscle. This is in contrast with acquired ptosis in which the affected lid is either level with or lower than the normal lid on down-gaze.

NB Following surgical correction the lid lag in down-gaze may worsen.

Associations

- Superior rectus weakness may be present because of its close embryological association with the levator.
- Compensatory chin elevation in severe bilateral cases.
- Refractive errors are common and more frequently responsible for amblyopia than the ptosis itself.

Treatment

Treatment should be carried out during the preschool years when accurate measurements can be obtained, although it may be considered earlier in severe cases to prevent amblyopia. Most cases require levator resection.

Marcus Gunn jaw-winking syndrome

About 5% of all cases of congenital ptosis manifest the Marcus Gunn jaw-winking phenomenon. The vast majority of cases are unilateral. Although the exact aetiology is unclear, it has been postulated that a branch of the mandibular division of the fifth cranial nerve is misdirected to the levator muscle.

Signs

- Retraction of the ptotic lid in conjunction with stimulation of the ipsilateral pterygoid muscles by chewing, sucking, opening the mouth (Fig. 4.51) or contralateral jaw movement.
- Less common stimuli to winking include jaw protrusion, smiling, swallowing and clenching of teeth.
- Jaw-winking does not improve with age, although patients may learn to mask it.

Treatment

Surgery should be considered if jaw-winking or ptosis represents a significant functional or cosmetic problem. Although no surgical treatment is entirely satisfactory possible approaches include:

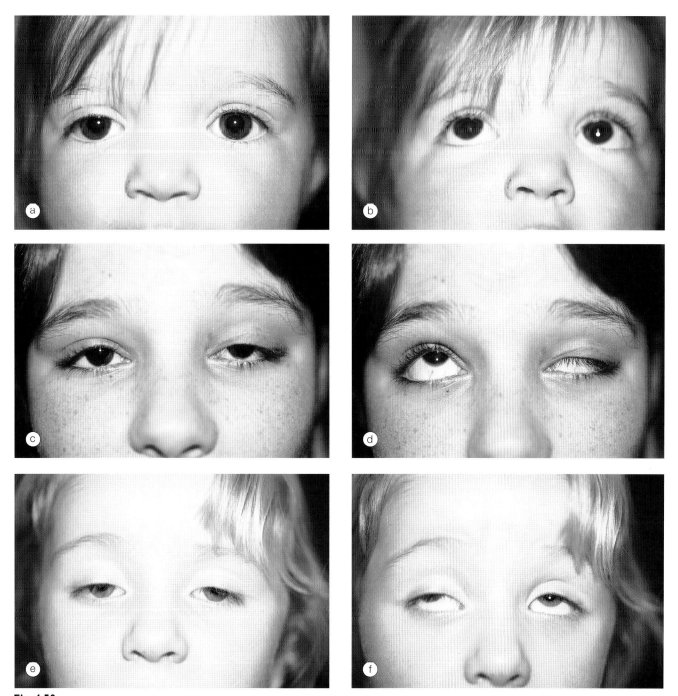

Fig. 4.50
Congenital ptosis. **(a)** Mild right ptosis; **(b)** good levator function; **(c)** severe left ptosis with absent lid crease; **(d)** very poor levator function; **(e)** severe bilateral ptosis; **(f)** very poor levator function

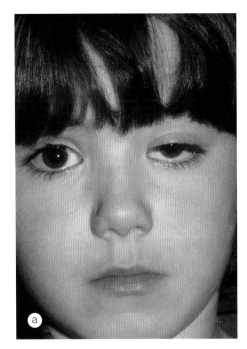
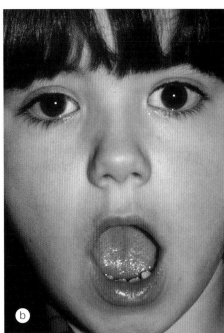

Fig. 4.51
Marcus Gunn jaw-winking syndrome.
(a) Moderate left ptosis;
(b) retraction of the lid on opening the mouth

1. **Unilateral levator resection** for mild cases with levator function 5mm or better.
2. **Unilateral levator disinsertion** and part resection with ipsilateral brow (frontalis) suspension for more severe cases.
3. **Bilateral levator disinsertion** and part resection with bilateral brow suspension to produce a symmetrical result.

Third nerve misdirection syndromes

Third nerve misdirection syndromes may be congenital, or more frequently, follow acquired third nerve palsies.

1. **Signs.** Bizarre movements of the upper lid which accompany various eye movements (Fig. 4.52).
2. **Treatment** is by levator disinsertion and brow suspension.

> **NB** Ptosis may also occur following aberrant facial nerve regeneration.

Involutional ptosis

Involutional ptosis is an age-related condition caused by dehiscence, disinsertion or stretching of the levator aponeu-

rosis which restricts transmission of force from a normal levator muscle to the upper lid.

1. **Signs**
   - Variable, usually bilateral ptosis with a high upper lid crease.
   - In severe cases the upper lid crease may be absent, the eyelid above the tarsal plate very thin and the upper sulcus deep (Fig. 4.53a).
   - Levator function is usually reasonably good (Fig. 4.53b).

> **NB** Involutional ptosis should not be confused with myasthenic ptosis because it frequently worsens towards the end of the day. This is because of fatigue of Müller muscle, which has to work harder to keep the lid elevated.

2. **Treatment** options include levator resection, reinsertion or anterior levator repair.

Mechanical ptosis

Mechanical ptosis is the result of impaired mobility of the upper lid. It may be caused by dermatochalasis, large tumours such as neurofibromas, scarring, severe oedema and anterior orbital lesions.

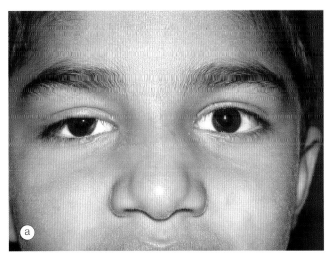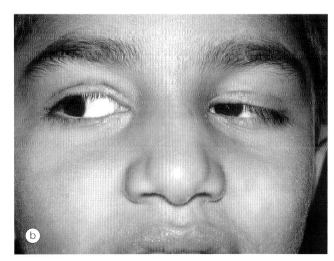

Fig. 4.52
Third nerve misdirection. **(a)** Moderate right ptosis; **(b)** retraction of the lid on right gaze (Courtesy of A Pearson)

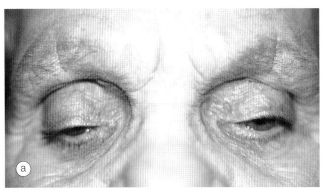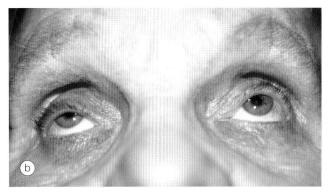

Fig. 4.53
(a) Severe bilateral involutional ptosis with absent upper lid creases and deep sulci; **(b)** reasonable levator function particularly on the left

Surgery

Anatomy

1. **The levator aponeurosis** fuses with the orbital septum about 4mm above the superior border of the tarsus (Fig. 4.54). Its posterior fibres insert into the lower third of the anterior surface of the tarsus. The medial and lateral horns are expansions that act as check ligaments. Surgically, the aponeurosis can be approached through the skin or conjunctiva.
2. **Müller muscle** is inserted into the upper border of the tarsus and can be approached transconjunctivally.
3. **The inferior tarsal aponeurosis** consists of the capsulopalpebral expansion of the inferior rectus muscle and is analogous to the levator aponeurosis.
4. **The inferior tarsal muscle** is analogous to Müller muscle.

Conjunctival Müller resection

1. **Indications** are cases of mild ptosis with levator function of at least 10mm such as most cases of Horner syndrome and very mild congenital ptosis.
2. **Technique.** Müller muscle and overlying conjunctiva are excised and the resected edges re-attached (Fig. 4.55). The maximal lift is 2–3mm.

Levator resection

1. **Indications** are ptosis of any cause provided levator function is at least 5mm. The amount of resection is determined by the amount of levator function and the severity of ptosis.
2. **Technique** involves shortening of the levator complex through either an anterior (skin – Fig. 4.56) or posterior (conjunctival) approach.

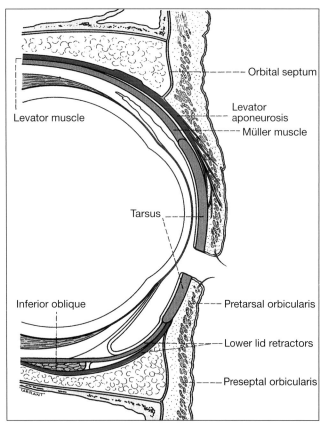

Fig. 4.54
Anatomy

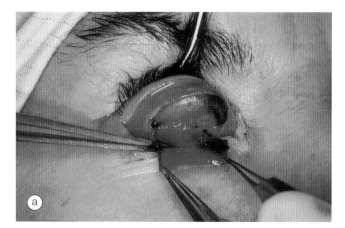

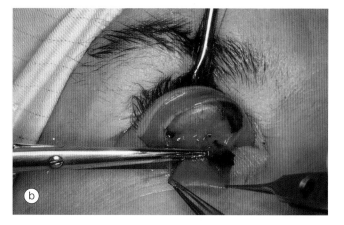

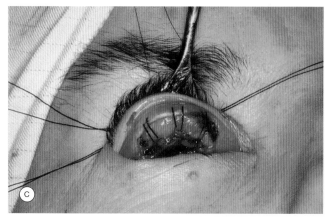

Fig. 4.55
Conjunctival-Müller resection. **(a)** Dissection of conjunctiva and Müller muscle; **(b)** excision; **(c)** attachment of resected edge
(Courtesy of R Khooshebah)

Brow suspension

1. **Indications**
   - Severe ptosis (> 4mm) with very poor levator function (< 4mm).
   - Marcus Gunn jaw-winking syndrome.
   - Ptosis associated with aberrant regeneration of the third nerve.
   - Blepharophimosis syndrome.
   - Ptosis associated with third nerve palsy.
   - Unsatisfactory result from previous levator resection.
2. **Technique** involves suspension of the tarsus from the frontalis muscle with a sling consisting of autologous fascia lata (Fig. 4.57) or non-absorbable material such as prolene or silicone.

ECTROPION

Involutional ectropion

Involutional (age-related) ectropion affects the lower lid of elderly patients. It results in epiphora and in long-standing cases the tarsal conjunctiva may become chronically inflamed, thickened and keratinized (Fig. 4.58).

Pathogenesis

The following age-related changes are contributory:

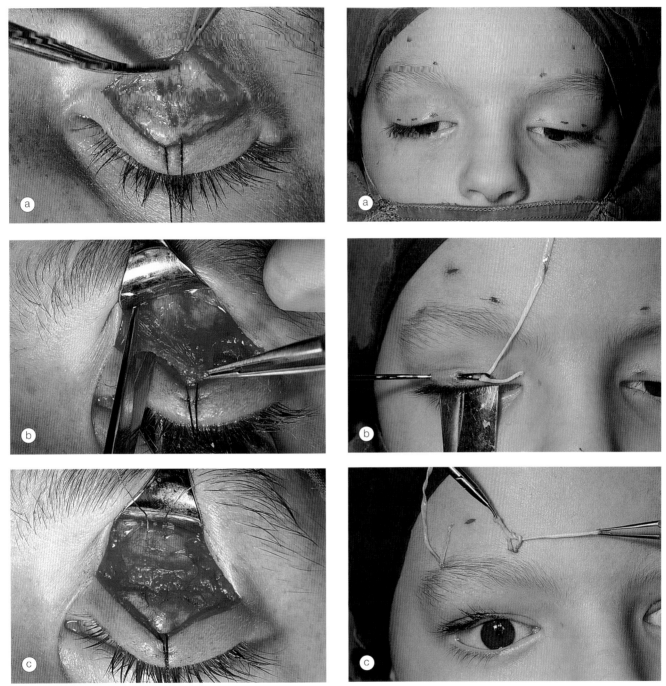

Fig. 4.56
Anterior levator resection. **(a)** Skin incision; **(b)** dissection and resection of levator aponeurosis; **(c)** levator reattachment to the tarsal plate (Courtesy of A G Tyers and J R O Collin, from *Colour Atlas of Ophthalmic Plastic Surgery*, Butterworth-Heinemann, 2001)

Fig. 4.57
Brow suspension. **(a)** Site of incisions marked; **(b)** threading of fascia lata strips; **(c)** tightening and tying of strips (Courtesy of A G Tyers and J R O Collin, from *Colour Atlas of Ophthalmic Plastic Surgery*, Butterworth-Heinemann, 2001)

1. **Horizontal lid laxity,** which is demonstrated by pulling the central part of the lid 8mm or more from the globe and its failure to snap back to its normal position on release without the patient first blinking (Fig. 4.59a).
2. **Medial canthal tendon laxity,** which is demonstrated by pulling the lower lid laterally and observing the position of the inferior punctum. If the lid is normal the punctum should not be displaced more than 1–2mm. If laxity is mild the punctum reaches the limbus, and if severe it reaches the pupil (Fig. 4.59b).
3. **Lateral canthal tendon laxity,** which is characterized by a rounded appearance of the lateral canthus and the ability to pull the lower lid medially more than 2mm (Fig. 4.59c).
4. **Disinsertion of lower lid retractors** is occasionally relevant.

Treatment

The methods of repair depend on the underlying aetiology and the predominant location of the ectropion as follows:

1. **Generalized** ectropion is treated with horizontal lid shortening where the ectropion is most marked (Fig. 4.60). This is usually combined with a lateral canthal sling procedure (see Fig. 4.63b).
2. **Medial** ectropion may be treated with a medial tarso-conjunctival diamond excision, usually combined with lateral canthal sling as horizontal laxity often coexists.
3. **Medial canthal tendon laxity,** if marked, requires stabilization prior to horizontal shortening to avoid excessive dragging of the punctum laterally.

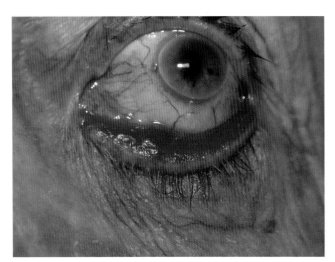

Fig. 4.58
Severe longstanding ectropion with keratinization of the tarsal conjunctiva (Courtesy of A Pearson)

Cicatricial ectropion

Cicatricial ectropion is caused by scarring or contracture of the skin and underlying tissues which pulls the eyelid away from the globe (Fig. 4.61a). If the skin is pushed over the orbital margin with a finger the ectropion will be relieved and the lids will close. Opening the mouth tends to accentuate the ectropion. Depending on the cause, both lids may be involved

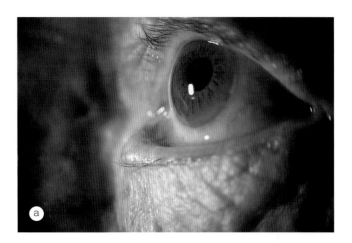

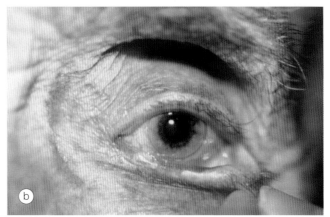

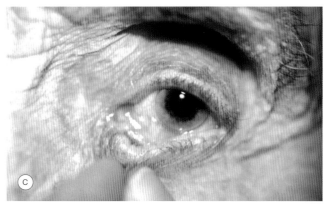

Fig. 4.59
Pathogenesis of involutional ectropion. **(a)** Horizontal lid laxity; **(b)** medial canthal tendon laxity; **(c)** lateral canthal tendon laxity

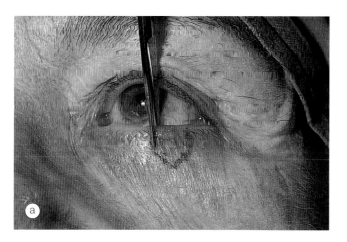

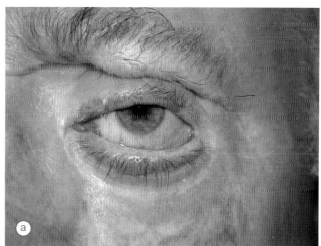

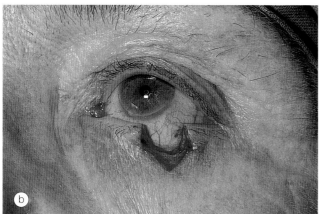

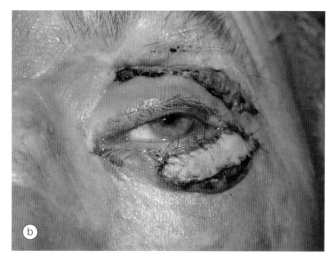

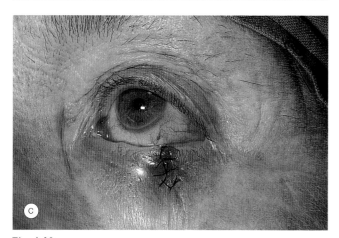

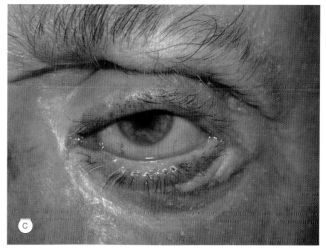

Fig. 4.60
Horizontal lid shortening to correct ectropion. **(a)** Vertical cut; **(b)** excision of a pentagon; **(c)** closure (Courtesy of A G Tyers and J R O Collin, from *Colour Atlas of Ophthalmic Plastic Surgery*, Butterworth Heinemann 2001)

Fig. 4.61
Correction of cicatricial ectropion. **(a)** Preoperative appearance; **(b)** free-skin graft in place; **(c)** postoperative appearance (Courtesy of A Pearson)

and the defect may be local (e.g. trauma) or general (e.g. burns, dermatitis and ichthyosis).

1. **Mild localized** cases are treated by excision of the offending scar tissue combined with a procedure that lengthens vertical skin deficiency such as Z-plasty.
2. **Severe generalized** cases require transposition flaps or free skin grafts (Fig. 4.61b and c). Sources of skin include upper lids, as well as posterior auricular, preauricular and supraclavicular areas.

Paralytic ectropion

Paralytic ectropion is caused by ipsilateral facial nerve palsy (Fig. 4.62a) and is associated with retraction of the upper and lower lids and brow ptosis; the latter may cause narrowing of the palpebral aperture.

Complications

1. **Exposure keratopathy** is caused by a combination of lagophthalmos (Fig. 4.62b) and inadequate resurfacing of the tear film over the cornea by the lids.
2. **Epiphora** is caused by malposition of the inferior lacrimal punctum, failure of the lacrimal pump mechanism and an increase in tear production resulting from corneal exposure.

Temporary treatment

Temporary treatment is aimed at protecting the cornea in anticipation of spontaneous recovery of facial nerve function.

1. **Lubrication** with tear substitutes during the day and instillation of ointment and taping shut of the lids during sleep are usually adequate in mild cases.
2. **Botulinum toxin injection** into the levator to induce temporary ptosis.
3. **Temporary tarsorrhaphy,** a procedure in which the lateral aspect of the upper and lower lids are sutured together, may be necessary in patients with a poor Bell phenomenon in which the cornea remains exposed when the patient attempts to blink.

Permanent treatment

Permanent treatment should be considered when there is permanent damage to the facial nerve as may occur following removal of an acoustic neuroma, or when no further improvement is likely after Bell's palsy. Treatment is aimed at reducing horizontal and vertical dimensions of the palpebral aperture by one of the following procedures:

1. **Medial canthoplasty** may be performed if the medial canthal tendon is intact. The eyelids are sutured together medial to the lacrimal puncta (Fig. 4.63a) so that the puncta become inverted and the fissure at the inner canthus is shortened.
2. **Lateral canthal sling** may be used to correct residual ectropion and raise the lateral canthus (Fig. 4.63b).
3. **Gold weights** implanted to the upper lid.

Mechanical ectropion

Mechanical ectropion is caused by tumours on or near the lid margin which mechanically evert the lid. Treatment involves

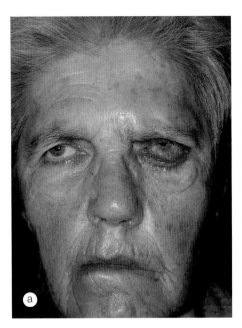
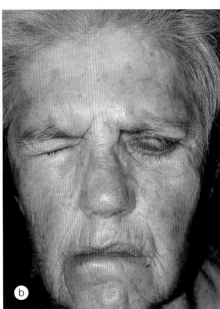

Fig. 4.62
Paralytic ectropion. **(a)** Left facial palsy and severe ectropion; **(b)** lagophthalmos (Courtesy of A Pearson)

removal of the cause, if possible, and correction of significant horizontal lid laxity.

ENTROPION

Involutional entropion

Involutional (age-related) entropion affects mainly the lower lid because the upper has a broader tarsus and is more stable. The constant rubbing of the lashes on the cornea in long-standing entropion (pseudotrichiasis – Fig.4.64a) may cause irritation, corneal punctate epithelial erosions and, in severe cases, ulceration and pannus formation.

Pathogenesis

The pathogenesis involves age-related degeneration of elastic and fibrous tissues within the eyelid resulting in the following:

1. **Horizontal lid laxity** caused by stretching of the canthal tendons and tarsal plate.
2. **Vertical lid instability** caused by attenuation, dehiscence or disinsertion of the lower lid retractors. Weakness of the latter is recognized by decreased excursion of the lower lid in down-gaze.

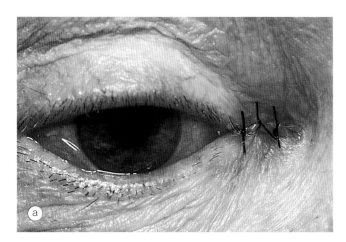

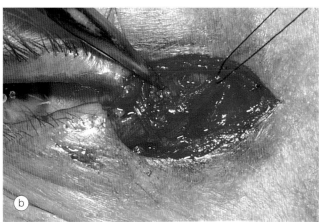

Fig. 4.63
Permanent treatment of paralytic ectropion. **(a)** Medial canthoplasty; **(b)** lateral canthal sling – refashioned canthal tendon from the lower lid is passed through a button hole in the tendon from the upper lid (Courtesy of A G Tyers and J R O Collin, from *Colour Atlas of Ophthalmic Plastic Surgery*, Butterworth-Heinemann, 2001)

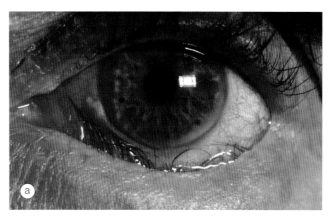

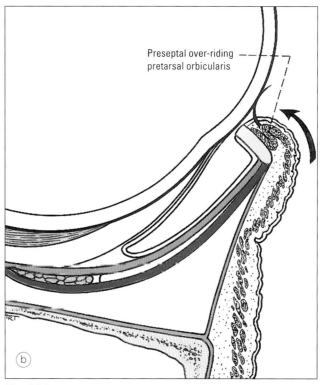

Preseptal over-riding pretarsal orbicularis

Fig. 4.64
(a) Involutional entropion; **(b)** pathogenesis

3. **Over-riding** of the pretarsal by the preseptal orbicularis during lid closure tends to move the lower border of the tarsus anteriorly, away from the globe, and the upper border towards the globe, thus tipping the lid inwards (Fig. 4.64b).

Treatment

Temporary treatment is with lubricants, taping, soft bandage contact lenses or orbicularis chemodenervation with botulinum toxin injection. Surgical treatment aims to correct the underlying problems as follows:

1. **Horizontal lid laxity** is usually present and is corrected with a lateral canthal sling or a full-thickness wedge excision.
2. **Over-riding and disinsertion**
   a. *Transverse everting sutures* prevent over-riding and provide temporary correction lasting several months (Fig. 4.65).
   b. *Wies procedure* gives a more lasting correction. It consists of full-thickness horizontal lid-splitting and insertion of everting sutures (Fig. 4.66). The scar creates a barrier between the preseptal and pretarsal orbicularis, and the everting suture transfers the pull of the lower lid retractors from the tarsus to the skin and orbicularis.
   c. *Jones procedure* tightens the lower lid retractors, thus increasing their pull and creating a barrier between the preseptal and pretarsal orbicularis (Fig. 4.67). It can be performed as primary treatment but is frequently reserved for recurrences.

NB Surgery may involve a combination of more than one procedure.

Cicatricial entropion

Pathogenesis

Cicatricial entropion is caused by severe scarring of the palpebral conjunctiva, which pulls the upper or lower lid margin towards the globe. Causes include cicatrizing conjunctivitis, trachoma, trauma and chemical injuries.

Treatment

1. **Medical** treatment is aimed at keeping the lashes away from the cornea by bandage contact lenses.
2. **Surgical** treatment of mild cases is by transverse tarsotomy (tarsal fracture) with anterior rotation of the lid margin. Treatment of severe cases is difficult and is directed at replacing deficient or keratinized conjunctiva and replacing the scarred and contracted tarsus with composite grafts.

MISCELLANEOUS ACQUIRED DISORDERS

Dermatochalasis

Dermatochalasis is a very common, usually bilateral condition which typically affects elderly patients.

1. **Signs**
   - Baggy lids with indistinct creases and pseudoptosis (Fig. 4.68a).
   - Redundant upper lid skin (Fig. 4.68b) which may be associated with herniation of orbital fat through a weak orbital septum.

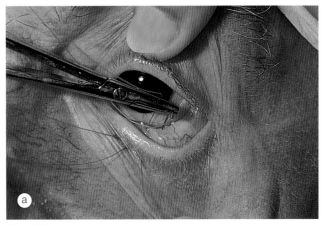
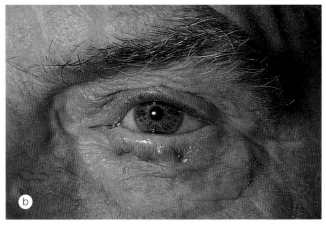

Fig. 4.65
Lid everting suture for entropion. **(a)** Three double-armed sutures are passed below the tarsal plate; **(b)** sutures are tied (Courtesy of A G Tyers and J R O Collin, from *Colour Atlas of Ophthalmic Plastic Surgery*, Butterworth-Heinemann, 2001)

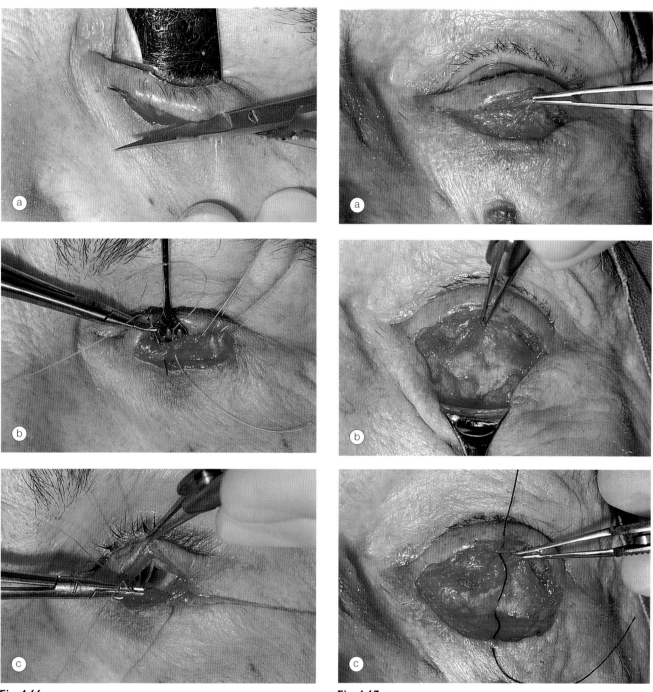

Fig. 4.66
Wies procedure for entropion. **(a)** Full-thickness incision;
(b) sutures are passed through the conjunctiva and lower lid
retractors; **(c)** sutures are passed anterior to the tarsal plate to
exit inferior to the lashes (Courtesy of A G Tyers and J R O Collin,
from *Colour Atlas of Ophthalmic Plastic Surgery*, Butterworth-Heinemann,
2001)

Fig. 4.67
Jones procedure for entropion. **(a)** Incision exposes the lower
border of the tarsal plate; **(b)** reflection of the orbital septum
and fat pad to expose the lower lid retractors; **(c)** tightening of
retractors by plication (Courtesy of A G Tyers and J R O Collin, from
Colour Atlas of Ophthalmic Plastic Surgery, Butterworth-Heinemann, 2001)

2. **Treatment** of severe cases involves excision of redundant skin (blepharoplasty).

Blepharochalasis

Blepharochalasis is an uncommon condition characterized by recurrent episodes of painless, non-pitting oedema of both upper lids which usually resolves spontaneously after a few days.

1. **Presentation** is usually around puberty; with time the episodes become less frequent.
2. **Signs**
   - A hypertrophic form with orbital fat herniation and an atrophic form with absorption of orbital fat have been described.

- Redundant, wrinkled and atrophic lid skin resembling wrinkled cigarette paper.
- Severe cases may also give rise to stretching of the canthal tendons and levator aponeurosis resulting in ptosis (Fig. 4.69).
- Lacrimal gland prolapse may occur.

3. **Differential diagnosis** includes drug-induced urticaria and angioedema.
4. **Treatment** involves blepharoplasty for redundant upper lid skin and correction of ptosis.

Floppy eyelid syndrome

Floppy eyelid syndrome is an uncommon, unilateral or bilateral condition, which is often misdiagnosed. It typically affects middle-aged, obese men who sleep face down with their lids everted by the pillow. Nocturnal exposure and poor contact of the lax lid with the globe in combination with tear film abnormalities result in keratoconjunctivitis. Keratoconus and sleep apnoea are reported associations.

1. **Signs**
   - Redundant upper lid skin (Fig. 4.70a), and loose and rubbery tarsal plates that readily evert with gentle pressure on the skin below the brow (Fig. 4.70b).
   - Chronic, intense micropapillary conjunctivitis of the superior tarsal conjunctiva.
   - Punctate keratopathy, filamentary keratitis and superior superficial vascularization may be present.
   - Other findings include eyelash ptosis, lacrimal gland prolapse, ectropion and aponeurotic ptosis.
2. **Associations** include eyelid imbrication syndrome (see below), keratoconus, skin hyperelasticity and joint hypermobility, obstructive sleep apnoea, diabetes and mental retardation.

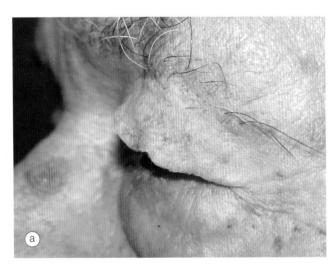

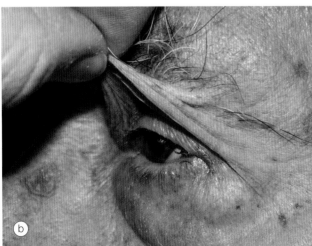

Fig. 4.68
Dermatochalasis. **(a)** Baggy upper lid skin with indistinct crease and pseudoptosis; **(b)** redundant skin (Courtesy of A Pearson)

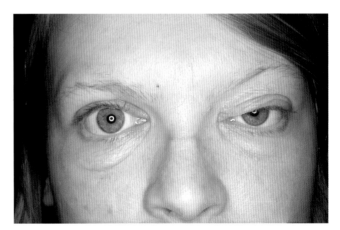

Fig. 4.69
Left aponeurotic ptosis and very thin upper lid skin resulting from blepharochalasis

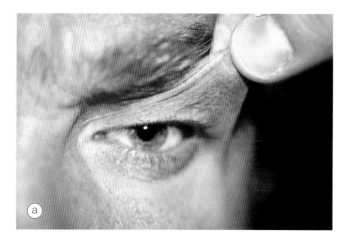

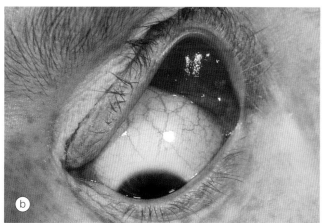

Fig. 4.70
Floppy eyelid syndrome. **(a)** Redundant upper lid skin; **(b)** easily eversible lid with papillary conjunctivitis of the upper tarsal conjunctiva (Courtesy of S Tuft – fig. b)

3. **Treatment** of mild cases involves lubrication and nocturnal eye shields or taping of the lids. Severe cases require horizontal lid shortening to stabilize both eyelid and ocular surface to prevent nocturnal lagophthalmos.

Eyelid imbrication syndrome

1. **Signs**
   - Eyelid imbrication syndrome is an uncommon disorder in which the upper lid overlaps the lower.
   - It may be unilateral or bilateral, affects both genders equally and causes ocular irritation.
   - Associated signs include chronic papillary conjunctivitis of the upper tarsal conjunctiva and staining with rose bengal of the upper lid margins.
2. **Associations** include floppy eyelid syndrome, eyelid tumours, mucous membrane disease, surgical trauma and self-inflicted behaviour.

3. **Treatment** may involve full-thickness upper lid wedge resection, lateral canthal tendon plication, and lower lid horizontal shortening using a tarsal strip procedure.

Eyelid retraction

Lid retraction is suspected when the upper lid margin is either level with or above the superior limbus (Fig. 4.71); the causes are listed in Table 4.6.

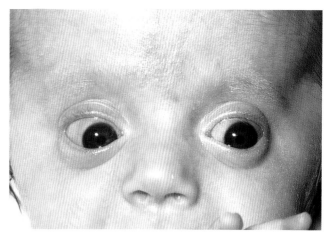

Fig. 4.71
Bilateral lid retraction and 'sunset' eye position in infantile hydrocephalus

Table 4.6

Causes of lid retraction

1. *Thyroid eye disease*

2. *Neurogenic*
   - Contralateral unilateral ptosis
   - Unopposed levator action due to facial palsy
   - Third nerve misdirection
   - Marcus Gunn jaw-winking syndrome
   - Collier sign of the midbrain (Parinaud syndrome)
   - Infantile hydrocephalus (setting sun sign)
   - Parkinsonism
   - Sympathomimetic drops

3. *Mechanical*
   - Surgical over-correction of ptosis
   - Scarring of upper lid skin

4. *Congenital*
   - Isolated
   - Duane retraction syndrome
   - Down syndrome
   - Transient 'eye popping' reflex in normal infants

5. *Miscellaneous*
   - Prominent globe (pseudo-lid retraction)
   - Uraemia (Summerskill sign)

CHAPTER 5

LACRIMAL DRAINAGE SYSTEM

Anatomy

The lacrimal drainage system consists of the following structures (Fig. 5.1).

1. **The puncta** are located at the posterior edge of the lid margin, at the junction of the lash-bearing lateral five-sixths (pars ciliaris) and the medial non-ciliated one-sixth (pars lacrimalis). Normally they face slightly posteriorly and can be inspected by everting the medial aspect of the lids. Treatment of watering caused by punctal stenosis or malposition is relatively straightforward.
2. **The canaliculi** pass vertically from the lid margin (the ampullae) for about 2mm. They then turn medially and run horizontally for about 8mm to reach the lacrimal sac. The superior and inferior canaliculi most often unite to form the common canaliculus which opens into the lateral wall of the lacrimal sac. In some individuals, each canaliculus opens separately. A small flap of mucosa (valve of Rosenmüller) overhangs the junction of the common canaliculus and the lacrimal sac, and prevents reflux of tears into the canaliculi. Treatment of canalicular obstruction is frequently complicated.
3. **The lacrimal sac** is about 10mm long and lies in the lacrimal fossa between the anterior and posterior lacrimal crests. The lacrimal bone and the frontal process of the maxilla separate the lacrimal sac from the middle meatus of the nasal cavity. In a dacryocystorhinostomy (DCR) an anastomosis is created between the sac and the nasal mucosa to bypass an obstruction in the nasolacrimal duct.
4. **The nasolacrimal duct** is about 12mm long and is the continuation of the lacrimal sac. It descends and angles slightly laterally and posteriorly to open into the inferior nasal meatus, lateral to and below the inferior turbinate. The opening of the duct is partially covered by a mucosal

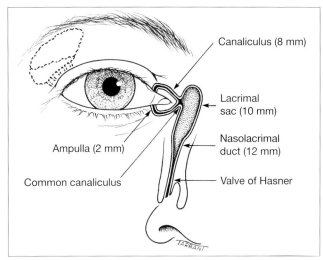

Fig. 5.1
Anatomy of the lacrimal drainage system

fold (valve of Hasner). Obstruction of the duct may cause secondary distension of the sac.

Physiology

Tears secreted by the main and accessory lacrimal glands pass laterally across the ocular surface. A variable amount of the aqueous component of the tear film is lost by evaporation. This is related to the size of the palpebral aperture, the blink rate, ambient temperature and humidity. The remainder of the tears drain as follows (Fig. 5.2):

a. Tears flow along the upper and lower marginal strips and enter the upper and lower canaliculi by capillarity and also

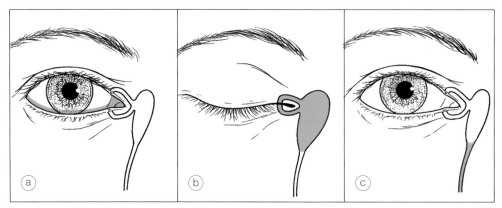

Fig. 5.2
Physiology of the lacrimal drainage system

possibly by suction (Fig. 5.2a). About 70% of tears drain through the lower canaliculus and the remainder through the upper.

b. With each blink, the pretarsal orbicularis oculi compresses the ampullae, shortens the horizontal canaliculi and moves the puncta medially (Fig. 5.2b). Simultaneously, the lacrimal part of the orbicularis oculi, which is attached to the fascia of the lacrimal sac, contracts and expands the sac, thereby creating a negative pressure which sucks the tears from the canaliculi into the sac.

c. When the eyes open the muscles relax, the sac collapses and a positive pressure is created which forces the tears down the nasolacrimal duct into the nose (Fig. 5.2c). Gravity also plays a role. The puncta move laterally, and the canaliculi lengthen and fill with tears.

Causes of a watering eye

Overflow of tears (epiphora) may be caused by the following.

1. **Hypersecretion** (lacrimation) secondary to ocular inflammation or surface disease. In these cases watering is associated with symptoms of the underlying cause and treatment is usually medical.
2. **Defective drainage** due to compromise of the lacrimal drainage system. It is exacerbated by a cold and windy atmosphere, and is least in a warm, dry room. It may be caused by:
   a. Malposition of the lacrimal puncta (e.g. secondary to ectropion).
   b. Obstruction anywhere along the lacrimal drainage system, from the puncta to the nasolacrimal duct.
3. **Lacrimal pump failure,** which may occur secondarily to lower lid laxity or weakness of the orbicularis muscle (e.g. facial nerve palsy).

Evaluation

External examination

1. **The puncta and eyelids** are best examined on the slit-lamp for evidence of the following conditions:
   • Ectropion causing malposition of the punctum, often associated with secondary stenosis (Fig. 5.3a).
   • Punctal obstruction by an eyelash (Fig. 5.3b) or a fold of redundant conjunctiva (conjunctivochalasis – Fig. 5.3c).
   • A large caruncle displacing the punctum away from the globe (Fig. 5.3d).
   • A pouting punctum is typical of canaliculitis (Fig. 5.3e).
   • Centurion syndrome is characterized by anterior malposition of the medial part of the lid with displacement of puncta out of the lacus lacrimalis due to a prominent nasal bridge (Fig. 5.3f).
2. **The lacrimal sac** should then be palpated. Punctal reflux of mucopurulent material on compression is indicative of a mucocele with a patent canalicular system, but with an obstruction either at, or distal to, the lower end of the lacrimal sac. In acute dacryocystitis palpation and compression are painful and should be avoided. Rarely, palpation will reveal a stone or a tumour.

Fluorescein disappearance test

The marginal tear strip of both eyes should be examined on the slit-lamp prior to any manipulation of the eyelids or instillation of topical medication, which may prejudice the clinical picture. Many patients do not have obvious overflow of tears onto the face but merely show a high marginal tear strip on the affected side. The fluorescein disappearance test is performed by instilling fluorescein 2% drops into both conjunctival fornices. Normally, little or no dye remains after

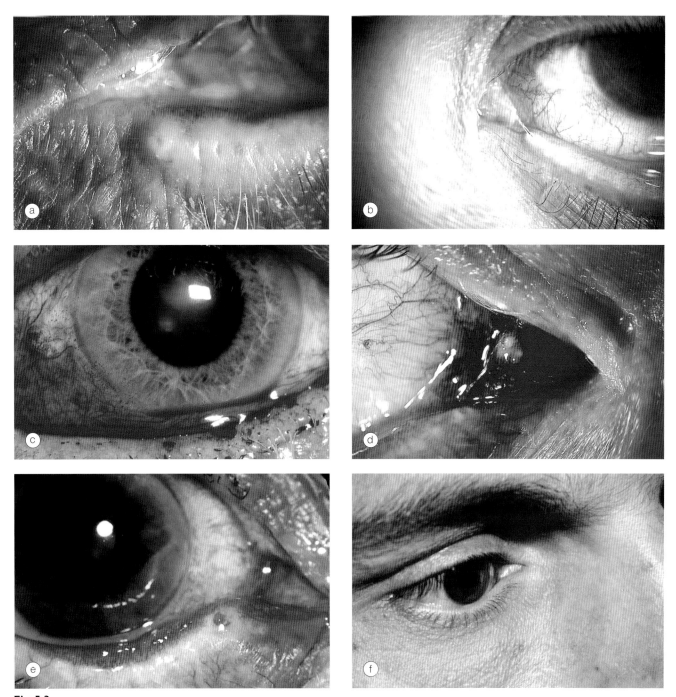

Fig. 5.3
(a) Punctal ectropion; (b) punctal obstruction by an eyelash; (c) conjunctivochalasis; (d) large caruncle; (e) pouting punctum; (f) centurion syndrome

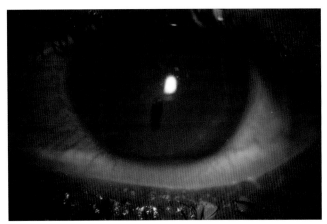

Fig. 5.4
High marginal tear strip stained with fluorescein

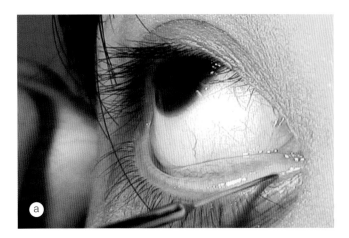

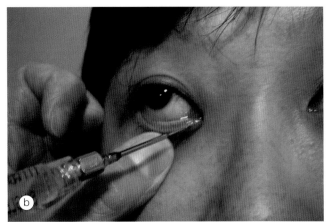

Fig. 5.5
(a) Dilatation of the inferior punctum; **(b)** irrigation (Courtesy of K Nischal)

3 minutes. Prolonged retention is indicative of inadequate lacrimal drainage and can be graded 1–4 (Fig. 5.4).

Probing and irrigation

Probing and irrigation are performed only after ascertaining punctal patency:
a. Local anaesthetic is instilled into the conjunctival sac.
b. The punctum is dilated (Fig. 5.5a).
c. A gently curved, blunt tipped lacrimal cannula on a 2ml saline-filled syringe is inserted into the lower punctum and advanced a few mm following the contour of the canaliculus prior to irrigation (Fig. 5.5b).
d. If obstruction is encountered, an attempt can be made to enter the lacrimal sac, the medial wall of which lies against the bone of the lacrimal fossa.
e. The cannula can come either to a hard stop or to a soft stop.
1. **A hard stop** occurs if the cannula enters the lacrimal sac but comes to a stop at the medial wall of the sac, through which can be felt the rigid lacrimal bone (Fig. 5.6a). This excludes complete obstruction of the canalicular system. The examiner places a finger over the lacrimal fossa and irrigates. If the saline passes into the nose the patient has a patent lacrimal drainage system, which may, however, be stenosed; alternatively there may be subtle lacrimal pump failure. Failure of saline to reach the nose is indicative of total obstruction of the nasolacrimal duct. In this situation, the lacrimal sac will become distended during irrigation and there will also be reflux through the upper punctum. The regurgitated material may be clear, mucoid, muco-purulent or frankly purulent, depending on the contents of the lacrimal sac.
2. **A soft stop** is experienced if the cannula stops at or proximal to the junction of the common canaliculus and the lacrimal sac, i.e. at the lateral wall of the sac. The sac

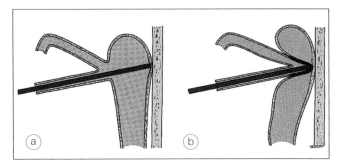

Fig. 5.6
Probing. **(a)** Hard stop; **(b)** soft stop

is thus not entered – a spongy feeling is experienced as the cannula presses the soft tissue of the common canaliculus and the lateral wall against the medial wall of the sac and the lacrimal bone behind it (Fig. 5.6b). Irrigation will therefore not cause the sac to distend. In the case of lower canalicular obstruction, there will be reflux of saline through the lower punctum. Reflux through the upper punctum indicates patency of both upper and lower canaliculi, but obstruction of the common canaliculus.

Jones dye testing

Dye testing is rarely needed and is only indicated in patients with suspected partial obstruction of the drainage system. These patients manifest epiphora, but the lacrimal system can be successfully syringe irrigated. Dye testing is of no value in the context of total obstruction.

1. **The primary test** (Fig. 5.7a) differentiates partial obstruction of the lacrimal passages from primary hypersecretion of tears. First, a drop of 2% fluorescein is instilled into the conjunctival sac. After about 5 minutes, a cotton-tipped bud moistened in a local anaesthetic is inserted under the inferior turbinate at the nasolacrimal duct opening. The results are interpreted as follows:
   a. *Positive*: fluorescein recovered from the nose indicates patency of the drainage system. Watering is due to primary hypersecretion and no further tests are necessary.

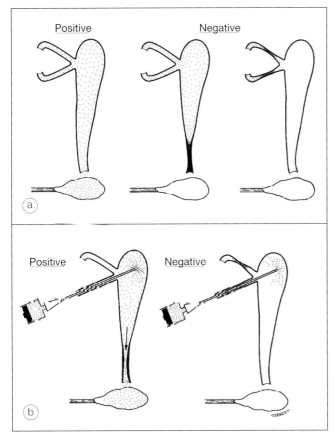

(a)
(b)

Fig. 5.7
Jones dye testing. **(a)** Primary; **(b)** secondary

   b. *Negative*: no dye recovered from the nose indicates a partial obstruction (site unknown) or failure of the lacrimal pump mechanism. In this situation the secondary dye test is performed immediately.
2. **The secondary** (irrigation) test (Fig. 5.7b) identifies the probable site of partial obstruction, on the basis of whether the topical fluorescein instilled for the primary test entered the lacrimal sac. Topical anaesthetic is instilled and any residual fluorescein washed out. The drainage system is then irrigated with saline with a cotton bud under the inferior turbinate.
   a. *Positive*: fluorescein-stained saline recovered from the nose indicates that fluorescein entered the lacrimal sac, thus confirming functional patency of the upper lacrimal passages. Partial obstruction of the nasolacrimal duct is inferred.
   b. *Negative*: unstained saline recovered from the nose indicates that fluorescein did not enter the lacrimal sac. This implies partial obstruction of the puncta, canaliculi or common canaliculus, or a defective lacrimal pump mechanism.

Contrast dacryocystography

Dacryocystography (DCG) involves injection of radio-opaque dye into the canaliculi and taking magnified images. The test is usually performed on both sides simultaneously.

1. **Indications**
   • To confirm the site of obstruction, especially prior to lacrimal surgery.
   • To aid diagnosis of diverticula, fistulae and filling defects caused by stones or tumours.

   NB A DCG is not necessary if the site of obstruction is obvious such as in the case of a regurgitating mucocele. It should also not be performed in a patient with acute dacryocystitis.

2. **Technique**
   a. The inferior puncta are dilated with a Nettleship punctum dilator.
   b. Plastic catheters are inserted into the inferior canaliculi on both sides (alternatively the upper puncta may be used).
   c. Contrast medium, usually 1–2ml of Liptodol, is simultaneously injected on both sides and posteroanterior radiographs are taken.
   d. Ten minutes later an erect oblique film is taken to assess the effect of gravity on tear drainage. Digital subtraction DCG provides a higher quality image.
3. **Interpretation**
   • Failure of dye to reach the nose indicates an anatomical obstruction, the site of which is usually evident (Fig. 5.8a, b and c).

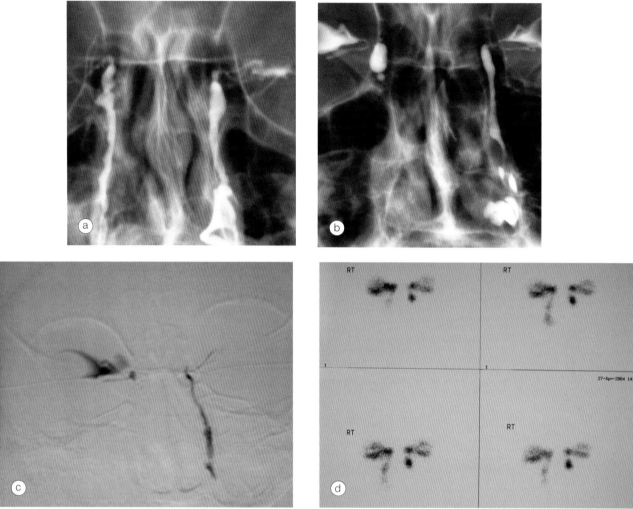

Fig. 5.8
Dacryocystography (DCG). **(a)** Conventional DCG without subtraction shows normal filling on both sides; **(b)** normal left filling and obstruction at the junction of the right sac and nasolacrimal duct; **(c)** digital subtraction DCG shows similar findings: **(d)** nuclear lacrimal scintigraphy shows passage of tracer in the right lacrimal system but hold-up in the left nasolacrimal duct (Courtesy of A Pearson)

- A normal dacryocystogram in the presence of epiphora indicates either functional obstruction or lacrimal pump failure, especially if contrast is retained on the late film.

Nuclear lacrimal scintigraphy

Scintigraphy is a sophisticated test which assesses tear drainage under more physiological conditions than a DCG. Although it does not provide the same detailed anatomical visualization as DCG, it is more sensitive in assessing incomplete blocks, especially in the upper part of the lacrimal system. The test is performed as follows:

a. Radionuclide technetium-99 is delivered by a micropipette to the lateral conjunctival sac as a 10μl drop. The tears are thus labelled with this gamma-emitting radioactive substance.

b. The tracer is imaged by a gamma camera focused on the inner canthus and a sequence of images is recorded over 20 minutes (Fig. 5.8d).

Acquired obstruction

Primary punctal stenosis

Primary stenosis occurs in the absence of punctal eversion.

1. Causes in order of frequency are:
- Chronic blepharitis.

- Idiopathic primary stenosis.
- Herpes simplex and herpes zoster lid infection.
- Following irradiation of malignant lid tumours.
- Cicatrizing conjunctivitis and trachoma.
- Systemic cytotoxic drugs such as 5 fluorouracil and docetaxel.
- Rare systemic conditions such as porphyria cutanea tarda and acrodermatitis enteropathica.

2. Treatment
- Dilatation of the punctum with a Nettleship dilator can be tried but rarely gives long-term benefit (Fig. 5.9).
- Punctoplasty is usually required. It involves removal of the posterior wall of the ampulla by a two- or three-snip technique (Fig. 5.10a and b).

Secondary punctal stenosis

1. Cause. Secondary stenosis is caused by punctal eversion (see Fig. 5.3a).

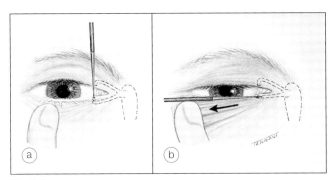

Fig. 5.9
Technique of dilating the inferior punctum

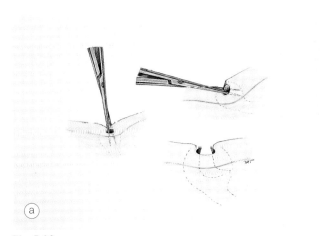

Fig. 5.10
Punctoplasty. **(a)** Technique; **(b)** postoperative appearance

2. Treatment
- ***a. Ziegler cautery*** can be used for pure punctal eversion. Burns are applied to the palpebral conjunctiva, 5mm below the punctum. Subsequent shrinkage of the cauterized tissue should invert the punctum.
- ***b. Medial conjunctivoplasty*** can be used in medial ectropion not associated with lid laxity. A diamond shaped piece of tarsoconjunctiva is excised, about 4mm high and 8mm wide, parallel with and inferolateral to the canaliculus and punctum, followed by approximation of the superior and inferior wound margins with sutures (Fig. 5.11). Incorporation of the lower lid retractors in the sutures further aids punctal inversion. Once the punctum is restored to its normal position, it is dilated so that it will remain open when normal tear flow is established. If stenosis recurs, treatment is the same as for primary stenosis.
- ***c. Lower lid tightening***, usually with a lateral canthal sling, is used to correct lower lid laxity and may be combined with medial conjunctivoplasty where there is significant medial ectropion.

Canalicular obstruction

1. Causes include congenital, trauma, herpes simplex infection, drugs and irradiation. Chronic dacryocystitis can cause a thin membrane to form at the common canalicular opening.

2. Treatment depends on the site and degree of obstruction.
- ***a. Partial*** obstruction of the common or individual canaliculi, or indeed anywhere in the nasolacrimal drainage system, may be treated by intubation. Two ends of a length of silicone tubing are threaded via the superior and inferior puncta, through the lacrimal sac down to the nose, where they are tied (or secured with a Watzke sleeve) and left in situ for 3–6 months (Fig. 5.12).

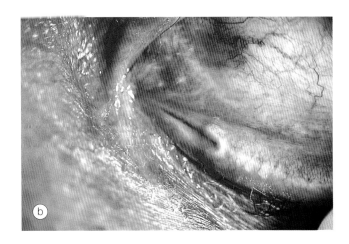

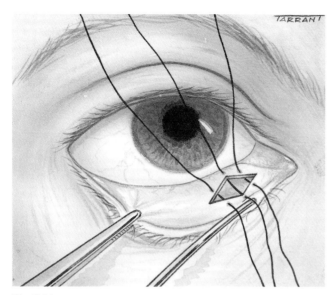

Fig. 5.11
Medial conjunctivoplasty

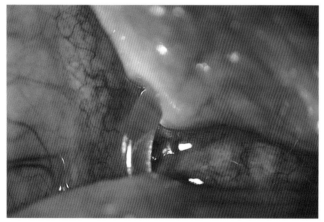

Fig. 5.12
Silicone tube *in situ*

b. ***Total individual canalicular obstruction***, with
6–8mm of patent normal canaliculus between the
punctum and obstruction, is treated by anastomosis
of the patent part of the canaliculus into the lacrimal
sac (canaliculodacryocystorhinostomy – CDCR) and
intubation. When it is not possible to anastomose the
remaining canaliculi to the sac treatment involves
conjunctivodacryocystorhinostomy and the insertion
of a special (Lester Jones) tube (see below).

Nasolacrimal duct obstruction

1. Causes
- Idiopathic stenosis is by far the most common.

- Naso-orbital trauma and previous nasal and sinus
  surgery.
- Granulomatous disease such as Wegener granulomatosis and sarcoidosis.
- Infiltration by nasopharyngeal tumours.

2. Treatment is with DCR. Other techniques include
intubation, stents and balloon dilatation.

Dacryolithiasis

Dacryoliths (lacrimal stones) may occur in any part of the
lacrimal system. Although the pathogenesis is unclear, it has
been proposed that tear stagnation secondary to
inflammatory obstruction and squamous metaplasia of the
lacrimal sac epithelium may be responsible.

1. Presentation is often in late adulthood in a variety of
ways including intermittent epiphora, recurrent attacks of
acute dacryocystitis and lacrimal sac distension.

2. Signs
- The lacrimal sac is distended and relatively firm, but is
  not inflamed and tender as in acute dacryocystitis.
- Mucus reflux on pressure may be present.

3. Treatment involves DCR.

Congenital obstruction

Nasolacrimal duct obstruction

Duct obstruction is perhaps better termed delayed canalization since it often resolves spontaneously. The lower end of
the nasolacrimal duct (at the valve of Hasner) is the last
portion of the lacrimal drainage system to canalize, complete
canalization usually occurring soon after birth. Epiphora
affects approximately 20% of neonates, but spontaneous
resolution occurs in 96% of cases within the first 12 months.

1. Signs
- Epiphora and matting of lashes (Fig. 5.13) may be
  constant or intermittent when the child has a cold or
  upper respiratory tract infection.
- Gentle pressure over the lacrimal sac causes reflux of
  purulent material from the puncta.
- Acute dacryocystitis is uncommon (Fig 5.14).

2. Differential diagnosis includes other congenital causes
of a watering eye such as punctal atresia and fistulae
between the sac and skin (Fig. 5.15).

NB It is important to exclude congenital glaucoma in an
infant with a watering eye.

3. Treatment
a. ***Massage*** of the lacrimal sac increases the hydrostatic

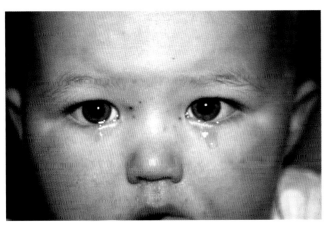

Fig. 5.13
Severe bilateral epiphora (Courtesy of K Nischal)

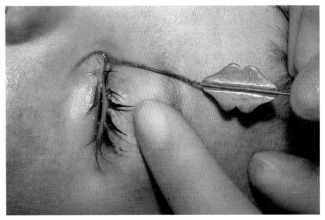

Fig. 5.16
Probing of the nasolacrimal duct (Courtesy of K Nischal)

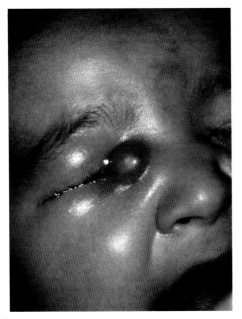

Fig. 5.14
Acute dacryocystitis

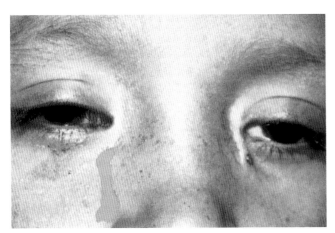

Fig. 5.15
Fluorescein-stained tears in a congenital fistula between the skin and lacrimal sac

pressure and may rupture the membranous obstruction. In performing this manoeuvre, the index finger is placed over the common canaliculus to block reflux through the puncta and then massaged firmly downwards. Ten strokes should be applied four times a day. Massage should be accompanied by lid hygiene but topical antibiotics should be reserved for superadded bacterial conjunctivitis, which is surprisingly uncommon.

b. Probing of the lacrimal system (Fig. 5.16) should be delayed until the age of 12–18 months because spontaneous canalization occurs in 96% of cases. Probing performed within the first 1–2 years of life has a very high success rate, but thereafter the efficacy decreases. It should be carried out under a general anaesthetic. The rationale is to manually overcome the obstructive membrane at the Hasner valve. After probing, the lacrimal system is irrigated with saline labelled with fluorescein. If fluorescein can be recovered by aspiration from the pharynx, successful probing is confirmed. Postoperative steroid-antibiotic drops are used q.i.d. for up to 3 weeks. If, after 6 weeks, there is no improvement, repeat probing can be arranged. Nasal endoscopic monitoring of probing is recommended, especially for repeated probing, to detect anatomical abnormalities and ensure correct probe position.

4. **Results** are usually excellent and 90% of children are cured by the first probing and a further 6% by the second. Failure is usually the result of abnormal anatomy, which can usually be recognized by difficulty in passing the probe and subsequent non-patency of the lacrimal drainage system on irrigation. If symptoms persist despite one to two technically satisfactory probings temporary intubation with fine Silastic tubes with or without balloon dilatation of the nasolacrimal duct may effect a cure.

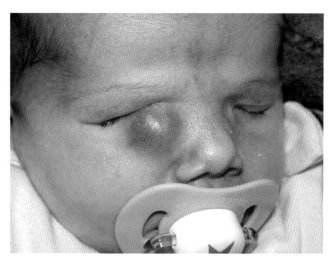

Fig. 5.17
Congenital dacryocele (Courtesy of A Pearson)

Patients who fail to respond to such measures can be treated with DCR performed between the ages of 3 and 4 years, provided the obstruction is distal to the lacrimal sac.

Congenital dacryocele

A congenital dacryocele (amniontocele) is a collection of amniotic fluid or mucus in the lacrimal sac caused by an imperforate Hasner valve.

1. **Presentation** is perinatal with a bluish cystic swelling at or below the medial canthal area, accompanied by epiphora (Fig. 5.17).

2. **Signs.** A tense lacrimal sac which is initially filled with mucus but may become secondarily infected.

> **NB** It should not be mistaken for an encephalocele which is characterized by a pulsatile swelling above the medial canthal tendon.

3. **Treatment** is initially conservative but if this fails probing should not be delayed.

Lacrimal surgery

Conventional dacryocystorhinostomy

Dacryocystorhinostomy (DCR) is indicated for obstruction beyond the medial opening of the common canaliculus (i.e. the canalicular system is patent). In principle this operation involves anastomosing the lacrimal sac to the nasal mucosa of the middle nasal meatus. The procedure is performed under general hypotensive anaesthesia.

1. **Technique**
   a. The blood vessels in middle nasal mucosa are constricted with ribbon gauze or cotton-buds lightly wetted with 1:1000 adrenaline or cocaine 4–10% solution.
   b. A straight vertical incision is made 10mm medial to the inner canthus, avoiding the angular vein (Fig. 5.18a).
   c. The anterior lacrimal crest is exposed by blunt dissection and the superficial portion of the medial palpebral ligament divided.

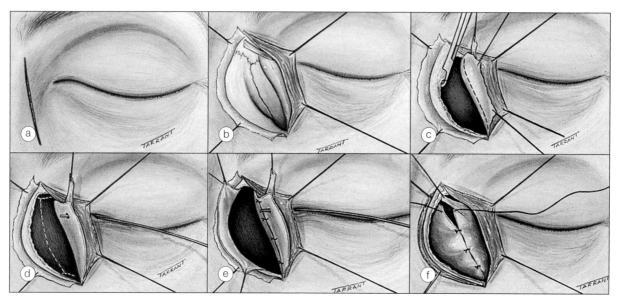

Fig. 5.18
Dacryocystorhinostomy (see text)

d. The periosteum is divided from the spine on the anterior lacrimal crest to the fundus of the sac and reflected forwards. The sac is reflected laterally from the lacrimal fossa (Fig. 5.18b).

e. The anterior lacrimal crest and the bone from the lacrimal fossa are removed (Fig. 5.18c).

f. A probe is introduced into the lacrimal sac through the lower canaliculus and the sac is incised in an 'H-shaped' manner to create two flaps.

g. A vertical incision is made in the nasal mucosa to create anterior and posterior flaps (Fig. 5.18d).

h. The posterior flaps are sutured (Fig. 5.18e).

i. Silicone intubation tubes may be inserted.

j. The anterior flaps are sutured (Fig. 5.18f).

k. The medial canthal tendon is re-sutured to the periosteum and the skin incision closed with interrupted sutures.

2. **Results** are excellent with a success rate of over 90%.

3. **Causes of failure** include inadequate size and position of the ostium, unrecognized common canalicular obstruction, scarring and the 'sump syndrome', in which the surgical opening in the lacrimal bone is too small and too high. There is thus a dilated lacrimal sac lateral to and below the level of the inferior margin of the ostium, in which secretions collect, unable to gain access to the ostium and thence the nasal cavity.

4. **Complications** include cutaneous scarring, injury to medial canthal structures, haemorrhage, cellulitis and cerebrospinal fluid rhinorrhoea, if the subarachnoid space is inadvertently entered.

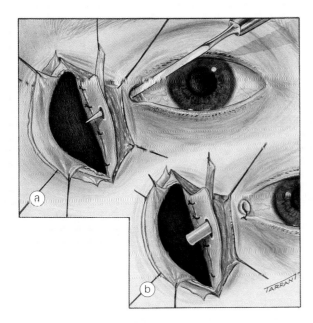

Fig. 5.19
Insertion of Lester Jones tube (see text)

Lester Jones tube

Primary Lester Jones tube insertion is indicated when there is either canalicular obstruction less than 8mm from the puncta, or lacrimal pump failure. Secondary placement may be undertaken for failed DCR. For primary placement the technique is as follows:

a. A DCR is performed as far as suturing the posterior flaps.

b. The caruncle is partially excised.

c. A stab incision is made with a Graefe knife from a point about 2mm behind the inner canthus (under the former caruncle) in a medial direction, so that the tip of the knife emerges just behind the anterior flap of the lacrimal sac (Fig. 5.19a).

d. The tract is enlarged sufficiently with dilators to allow the introduction of a Lester Jones tube (Fig. 5.19b).

e. The incision is sutured as for a DCR.

NB If the tube falls out it should be replaced as soon as possible to prevent stenosis.

Endoscopic surgery

Endoscopic DCR may be considered for obstruction beyond the medial opening of the common canaliculus, particularly following failed conventional DCR. The procedure can be performed either under general anaesthesia (without hypotension) or local anaesthesia. Advantages over conventional DCR include the lack of skin incision, shorter operating time, minimal blood loss and less risk of cerebrospinal fluid rhinorrhoea. Disadvantages include lower success rates, difficulty in examining the lacrimal sac mucosa and common canalicular opening, and possible need for additional procedures to allow adequate visualization such as correction of deviated nasal septum.

1. **Technique.** A slender light pipe is passed through the lacrimal puncta and canaliculi into the lacrimal sac and viewed from within the nasal cavity with an endoscope. The remainder of the procedure is performed from within the nasal cavity.

a. The mucosa over the frontal process of the maxilla is stripped.

b. A part of the nasal process of the maxilla is removed.

c. The lacrimal bone is broken off piecemeal.

d. The lacrimal sac is opened.

e. Silicone tubes are passed through the upper and lower puncta, pulled out through the ostium and tied within the nose.

2. **Results.** The success rate is about 80–85%.

Endolaser DCR

Performed with a Holmium:YAG or KTP laser, this is a quick

procedure which can be carried out under local anaesthesia. It is therefore particularly suitable for elderly patients. The success rate is only about 70% but because normal anatomy is not disrupted it does not prejudice subsequent surgical intervention in the cases that fail.

Balloon dacryocystoplasty

Dacryocystoplasty has been used in children with congenital nasolacrimal duct obstruction and in adults with partial nasolacrimal duct obstruction. The success rate in adults is approximately 50%.

Chronic canaliculitis

Chronic canaliculitis is an uncommon condition, frequently caused by *Actinomyces israelii* which is an anaerobic Gram-positive bacterium (Fig. 5.20a). While a diverticulum or obstruction of the canaliculus can promote anaerobic bacterial growth secondary to stasis, in most cases there is no identifiable predisposition.

Diagnosis

1. **Presentation** is with unilateral epiphora associated with chronic mucopurulent conjunctivitis (Fig. 5.20b), refractory to conventional treatment.

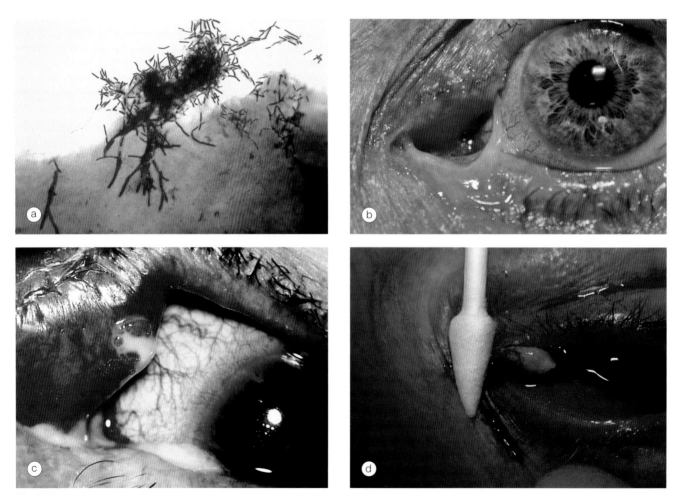

Fig. 5.20
Canaliculitis. **(a)** Gram stain of *Actinomyces israelii;* **(b)** oedema of the upper canaliculus and mucopurulent discharge; **(c)** mucopurulent discharge from the upper canaliculus on pressure; **(d)** expressed sulphur concretions (Courtesy of J Harry – fig. a; A Pearson – figs b and d)

2. Signs

- A 'pouting' punctum is a diagnostic clue in mild cases (see Fig. 5.3e).
- Pericanalicular inflammation is characterized by oedema of the canaliculus and mucopurulent discharge on pressure over the canaliculus (Fig. 5.20c).
- Concretions consisting of sulphur granules can be expressed on canalicular compression with a glass rod (Fig. 5.20d) or become evident following canaliculotomy.

NB In contrast to dacryocystitis, there is no nasolacrimal duct obstruction or lacrimal sac distension.

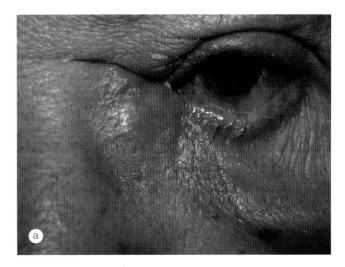

Treatment

1. **Topical antibiotics** such as ciprofloxacin q.i.d for 10 days may be tried initially but are rarely curative.
2. **Canaliculotomy** involving a linear incision into the conjunctival side of the canaliculus is the most effective treatment, although occasionally it may result in scarring and interference with canalicular function.

Differential diagnosis

1. **The 'giant fornix syndrome'** may also cause chronic relapsing purulent conjunctivitis. This is due to retained debris in the upper fornix that is colonized by *S. aureus*, usually in elderly patients with levator disinsertion. Secondary corneal vascularization is common. Treatment involves thorough cleaning of the fornix and topical and systemic antibiotics.
2. **Other conditions** that may cause similar symptoms are a lacrimal diverticulum and a dacryolith.

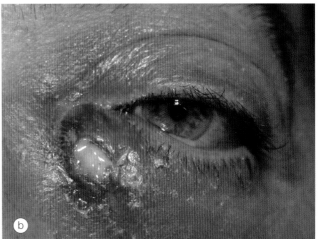

Dacryocystitis

Infection of the lacrimal sac is usually secondary to obstruction of the nasolacrimal duct. It may be acute or chronic and is most commonly staphylococcal or streptococcal.

Acute dacryocystitis

1. **Presentation** is with subacute onset of pain, redness and swelling at the medial canthus, and epiphora.
2. **Signs**
   - Very tender, red, tense swelling at the medial canthus that may be associated with mild preseptal cellulitis (Fig. 5.21a).
   - Abscess formation may occur in severe cases.

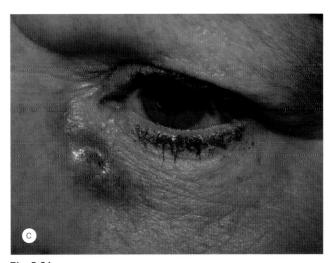

Fig. 5.21
(a) Acute dacryocystitis; **(b)** discharging lacrimal abscess; **(c)** lacrimal fistula (Courtesy of A Pearson)

3. Treatment
a. Initial treatment involves the application of local warmth and oral antibiotics such as flucloxacillin or augmentin.

> **NB** Irrigation and probing should not be performed.

b. Incision and drainage may be considered if pus points and the abscess is about to drain spontaneously (Fig. 5.21b). This however, carries a risk of the development of a lacrimal fistula, which may serve as a conduit for tears from the lumen of the lacrimal sac to the skin surface (Fig. 5.21c).

c. DCR is usually necessary after the acute infection has been controlled and should not be delayed because of the risk of recurrent infection.

Chronic dacryocystitis

1. Presentation is with epiphora which may be associated with a chronic or recurrent unilateral conjunctivitis.

2. Signs
- A painless swelling at the inner canthus caused by a mucocele (Fig. 5.22a).
- Obvious swelling may be absent, although pressure over the sac commonly still results in reflux of mucopurulent material through the canaliculi (Fig. 5.22b).

> **NB** It is often wise to postpone intraocular surgery till lacrimal infection has been treated, owing to the grave risk of endophthalmitis.

3. Treatment is with DCR.

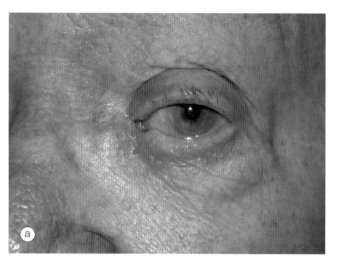
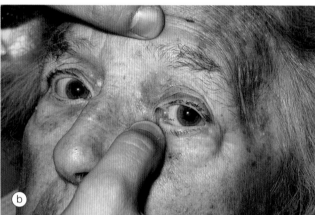

Fig. 5.22
(a) Mucocele; **(b)** expression of mucopurulent material

CHAPTER 6

ORBIT

INTRODUCTION

Anatomy

The orbit is a pear-shaped cavity, the stalk of which is the optic canal (Fig. 6.1). The intraorbital portion of the optic nerve is longer (25mm) than the distance between the back of the globe and the optic canal (18mm). This allows for significant forward displacement of the globe (proptosis) without excessive stretching of the optic nerve.

1. **The roof** consists of two bones: the lesser wing of the sphenoid and the orbital plate of the frontal. It is located subjacent to the anterior cranial fossa and frontal sinus. A defect in the orbital roof may cause pulsatile proptosis as a result of transmission of cerebrospinal fluid pulsation to the orbit.
2. **The lateral wall** also consists of two bones: greater wing of the sphenoid and zygomatic. The anterior half of the globe is vulnerable to lateral trauma since it protrudes beyond the lateral orbital margin.

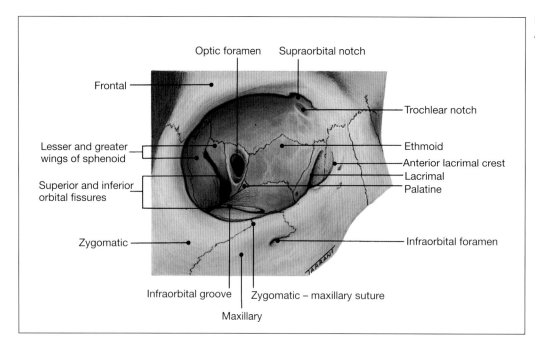

Fig. 6.1
Anatomy of the orbit

Optic foramen   Supraorbital notch

Frontal

Trochlear notch

Lesser and greater
wings of sphenoid

Ethmoid
Anterior lacrimal crest
Lacrimal
Palatine

Superior and inferior
orbital fissures

Zygomatic

Infraorbital foramen

Infraorbital groove | Zygomatic – maxillary suture

Maxillary

3. **The floor** consists of three bones: zygomatic, maxillary and palatine. The posteromedial portion of the maxillary bone is relatively weak and may be involved in a 'blowout' fracture. The orbital floor also forms the roof of the maxillary sinus so that maxillary carcinoma invading the orbit may displace the globe upwards.

4. **The medial wall** consists of four bones: maxillary, lacrimal, ethmoid and sphenoid. The lamina papyracea, which forms part of the medial wall, is paper-thin and perforated by numerous foramina for nerves and blood vessels. Orbital cellulitis is therefore frequently secondary to ethmoidal sinusitis.

5. **The superior orbital fissure** is a slit between the greater and lesser wings of the sphenoid bone through which pass the following important structures from the cranium to the orbit:
   - The superior portion contains the lacrimal, frontal and trochlear nerves, and the superior ophthalmic vein.
   - The inferior portion contains the superior and inferior divisions of the oculomotor nerve, the abducens, the nasociliary and sympathetic fibres.

NB Inflammation of the superior orbital fissure and apex (Tolosa–Hunt syndrome) may therefore result in a multitude of signs including ophthalmoplegia and venous outflow obstruction.

Clinical signs

Soft tissue involvement

1. **Signs** include lid and periorbital oedema, ptosis, chemosis (oedema of the conjunctiva and caruncle) and epibulbar injection (Fig. 6.2a).

2. **Causes** include thyroid eye disease, orbital inflammatory diseases and obstruction to venous drainage.

Proptosis

Proptosis describes an abnormal protrusion of the globe which may be caused by retrobulbar lesions or, less frequently, a shallow orbit. Asymmetrical proptosis is best detected by looking down at the patient from above and behind (Fig. 6.2b). The following characteristics are relevant.

1. **Direction** of proptosis may indicate the possible pathology. For example, space-occupying lesions within the muscle cone, such as cavernous haemangiomas and optic nerve tumours, cause axial proptosis, whereas extraconal lesions usually give rise to eccentric proptosis, the direction of which is governed by the site of the mass.

2. **Severity** of proptosis can be measured with a plastic rule resting on the lateral orbital margin (Fig. 6.3a) or an exophthalmometer, by means of which the corneal apices

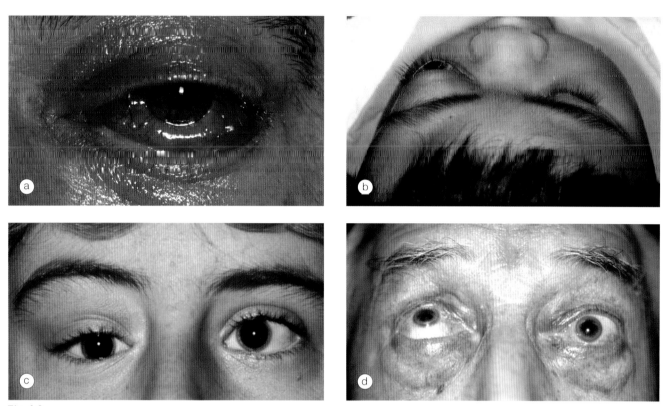

Fig. 6.2
General signs of orbital disease. **(a)** Soft tissue involvement; **(b)** proptosis; **(c)** dystopia; **(d)** ophthalmoplegia

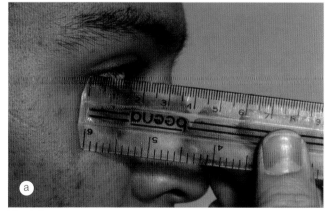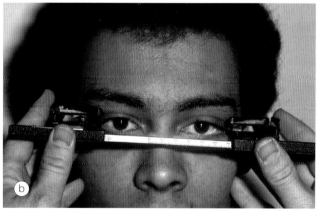

Fig. 6.3
Measurement of proptosis. **(a)** With a plastic rule; **(b)** with a Hertel exophthalmometer

are visualized in the mirrors and the degree of ocular protrusion is read from a scale (Fig. 6.3b). Ideally, measurements should be taken in both erect and supine positions. Readings greater than 20mm are indicative of proptosis and a difference of 2mm between the two eyes is

suspicious regardless of the absolute value. Proptosis is graded as mild (21–23mm), moderate (24–27mm) and severe (28mm or more). The dimensions of the palpebral apertures and any lagophthalmos should also be noted.

3. Pseudo-proptosis (false impression of proptosis) may be due to facial asymmetry, severe ipsilateral enlargement of the globe (e.g. high myopia or buphthalmos), ipsilateral lid retraction or contralateral enophthalmos.

Enophthalmos

Enophthalmos implies recession of the globe within the orbit. Often subtle, it may be caused by the following mechanisms:
- Structural abnormalities of the orbital walls may be post-traumatic, such as blowout fractures of the orbital floor, or congenital.
- Atrophy of orbital contents that may be due to radio-therapy, scleroderma or eye poking (oculodigital sign) in blind infants.
- Sclerosing orbital lesions such as metastatic schirrous car-cinoma and chronic inflammatory orbital disease.

NB Pseudo-enophthalmos may be caused by micro-phthalmos or phthisis bulbi.

Dystopia

Dystopia implies displacement of the globe in the coronal plane, usually due to an extraconal orbital mass such as a lacrimal gland tumour (see Fig. 6.2c). It may coexist with proptosis or enophthalmos. Horizontal displacement is measured from the midline (nose) to the nasal limbus while vertical dystopia is read from a vertical scale perpendicular to a horizontal rule placed over the bridge of the nose. In the context of coexistent strabismus, it is essential to establish that the eye is fixating, if necessary by occluding the fellow eye, while measuring dystopia.

Ophthalmoplegia

Defective ocular motility may be caused by one or more of the following:

1. **An orbital mass.**
2. **Restrictive myopathy** in thyroid eye disease or orbital myositis (see Fig. 6.2d).
3. **Ocular motor nerve** involvement associated with lesions in the cavernous sinus, orbital fissures or posterior orbit (e.g. carotid-cavernous fistula, Tolosa–Hunt syndrome and malignant lacrimal gland tumours).
4. **Tethering** of extraocular muscles or fascia in a blowout fracture.
5. **Splinting** of the optic nerve by an optic nerve sheath meningioma.

Restrictive versus neurological

The following tests may be used to differentiate a restrictive from a neurological motility defect.

1. **The forced duction test.**
   a. Topical anaesthetic drops are instilled.
   b. A cotton pledget soaked in anaesthetic solution is inserted into both eyes over the muscles to be tested and left for about 5 minutes.
   c. The insertion of the muscle in the involved eye is grasped with forceps and the globe is rotated in the direction of limited mobility.
   d. The test is repeated in the unaffected eye.
      - Positive result: difficulty or inability to move the globe indicates a restrictive problem such as thyroid myopathy or muscle entrapment in an orbital floor fracture. In the opposite eye, no such resistance will be encountered unless pathology is bilateral.
      - Negative result: no resistance will be encountered in either eye if the muscle is paretic as a result of a neurological lesion.
2. **The differential intraocular pressure test.** The intra-ocular pressure is measured in the primary position of gaze and then with the patient attempting to look into the direction of limited mobility.
      - Positive result: an increase of $\geq 6\,mmHg$ denotes resistance transmitted to the globe by muscle restriction.
      - Negative result: an increase of $< 6\,mmHg$ suggests a neurological lesion.

NB The advantage of this test over the forced duction is less discomfort and an end-point that is objective rather than subjective.

3. **Saccadic eye movements** in neurological lesions are reduced in velocity, while restrictive defects manifest normal saccadic velocity with 'sudden halting' of ocular movement.

Dynamic properties

The following dynamic features may give clues as to the probable pathology.

1. **Increasing venous pressure** by dependent head position, Valsalva manoeuvre or jugular compression may induce or exacerbate proptosis in patients with orbital venous anomalies or infants with capillary orbital haemangiomas.
2. **Pulsation** is caused either by an arteriovenous com-munication or a defect in the orbital roof:
   - In the latter the pulsation is transmitted from the brain by the cerebrospinal fluid and there is no associated bruit.
   - In the former pulsation may be associated with a bruit depending on the size of the communication.

NB Mild pulsation is best detected on the slit-lamp, particularly when performing applanation tonometry.

5. A bruit is a sign of carotid-cavernous fistula. It is best heard with the bell of the stethoscope and is lessened or abolished by gently compressing the ipsilateral carotid artery in the neck.

Fundus changes

1. **Optic disc swelling** may be the initial feature of compressive optic neuropathy (Fig. 6.1a).
2. **Optic atrophy** (Fig. 6.4b), which may be preceded by swelling, is a feature of severe compressive optic neuropathy. Important causes include thyroid eye disease and optic nerve tumours.

3. **Opticociliary collaterals** consist of enlarged pre-existing peripapillary capillaries which divert blood from the central retinal venous circulation to the peripapillary choroidal circulation when there is obstruction of the normal drainage channels. On ophthalmoscopy the vessels appear as large tortuous channels most frequently on the temporal side which disappear at the disc margin (Fig. 6.4c). Although rare, they may be associated with orbital or optic nerve tumours which compress the intraorbital optic nerve and impair blood flow through the central retinal vein. The most common tumour associated with shunts is the optic nerve sheath meningioma but they may also occur with optic nerve glioma, cavernous haemangioma, central retinal vein occlusion, idiopathic intracranial hypertension, and glaucoma.
4. **Choroidal folds** are a series of roughly parallel alternating light and dark delicate lines or striae which

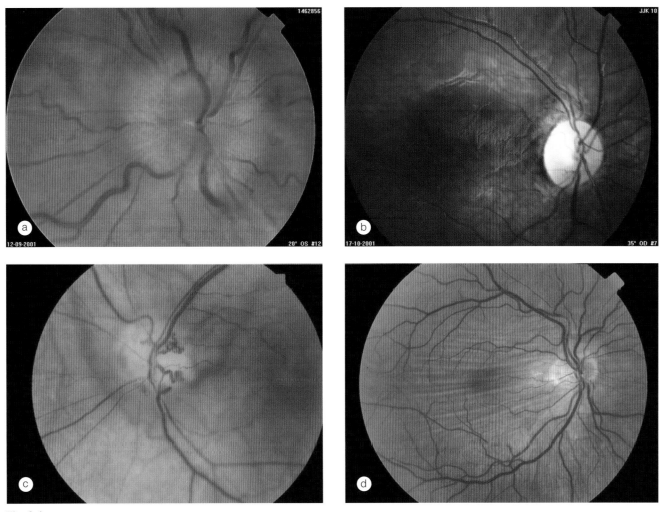

Fig. 6.4
Fundus changes in orbital disease. **(a)** Disc swelling; **(b)** optic atrophy; **(c)** opticociliary vessels; **(d)** choroidal folds

most frequently involve the posterior pole (Fig. 6.4d). Choroidal folds may occur in a wide variety of orbital lesions including tumours, dysthyroid ophthalmopathy, inflammatory conditions and mucoceles. The folds are usually asymptomatic and do not cause visual loss although some patients develop an increase in hypermetropia. Although choroidal folds tend to be more common with greater amounts of proptosis and anteriorly located tumours, in some cases, their presence can precede the onset of proptosis.

Special investigations

1. **CT** is useful for depicting bony structures and the location and size of space-occupying lesions. It is of particular value in patients with orbital trauma because it can detect small fractures, foreign bodies, blood, herniation of extraocular muscle and emphysema. It is, however, unable to distinguish different pathological soft tissue masses which are radiologically isodense.
2. **MR** can image orbital apex lesions and intracranial extension of orbital tumours. Serial short tau inversion recovery (STIR) scans are valuable in assessing inflammatory activity in thyroid eye disease.
3. **Fine needle biopsy,** performed under CT guidance using a 23-gauge needle, is valuable in patients with suspected orbital metastases and in those with orbital invasion by neoplasms from contiguous structures. Potential problems are haemorrhage and ocular penetration.

THYROID EYE DISEASE

Introduction

Thyrotoxicosis

Thyrotoxicosis (Graves disease) is an autoimmune disorder which usually presents in the third to fourth decades of life and affects women more commonly than men (see Chapter 24). Thyroid eye disease (TED) affects 25–50% of patients with Graves disease, of which 5% have severe involvement. TED may precede, coincide with or follow hyperthyroidism and bears no relationship to the severity of thyroid dysfunction. It may vary from being merely a nuisance, to blindness secondary to exposure keratopathy or optic neuropathy.

Risk factors

Once a patient has Graves disease, the major clinical risk factor for developing TED is smoking. The greater the number of cigarettes smoked per day, the greater the risk, and giving up smoking seems to reduce the risk. Women are five times more

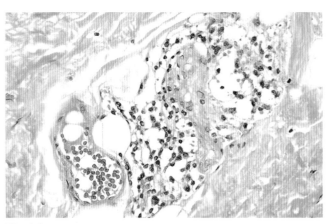

Fig. 6.5
Inflammatory cells in vascularized fibro-fatty orbital tissue in thyroid eye disease (Courtesy of J Harry and G Misson, from *Clinical Ophthalmic Pathology*, Butterworth-Heinemann, 2001)

likely to be affected by TED than men, but this largely reflects the increased incidence of Graves disease in women. Radioactive iodine used to treat hyperthyroidism can worsen TED.

Pathogenesis

Thyroid ophthalmopathy involves an organ-specific autoimmune reaction in which a humoral agent (IgG antibody) produces the following changes:

1. **Inflammation of extraocular muscles** which is characterized by pleomorphic cellular infiltration, associated with increased secretion of glycosaminoglycans and osmotic imbibition of water. The muscles become enlarged, sometimes up to eight times their normal size, and may compress the optic nerve. Subsequent degeneration of muscle fibres eventually leads to fibrosis, which exerts a tethering effect on the involved muscle, resulting in restrictive myopathy and diplopia.
2. **Inflammatory cellular infiltration** with lymphocytes, plasma cells, macrophages and mast cells of interstitial tissues, orbital fat (Fig. 6.5) and lacrimal glands associated with accumulation of glycosaminoglycans and retention of fluid. This causes increase in the volume of orbital contents and secondary elevation of intraorbital pressure, which may itself cause further fluid retention within the orbit.

Clinical manifestations

The five main clinical manifestations of TED are: (a) *soft tissue involvement*, (b) *lid retraction*, (c) *proptosis*, (d) *optic neuropathy* and (e) *restrictive myopathy*. There are two stages in the development of the disease.

1. **Congestive** (inflammatory) stage, in which the eyes are red and painful, tends to remit within 3 years and only 10% of patients develop serious long-term ocular problems.
2. **Fibrotic** (quiescent) stage in which the eyes are white, although a painless motility defect may be present.

Soft tissue Involvement

Diagnosis

1. **Symptoms** include grittiness, photophobia, lacrimation and retrobulbar discomfort.
2. **Signs**
   • Epibulbar hyperaemia is a sensitive sign of inflammatory activity. Intense focal hyperaemia may outline the insertions of the horizontal recti (Fig. 6.6a).
   • Periorbital swelling is caused by oedema and infiltration behind the orbital septum which may be associated with chemosis and prolapse of retro-septal fat into the eyelids (Fig. 6.6b).
   • Superior limbic keratoconjunctivitis (Fig. 6.6c).
   • Keratoconjunctivitis sicca secondary to infiltration of the lacrimal glands.

Treatment

1. **Lubricants** for superior limbic keratoconjunctivitis, corneal exposure and dryness.
2. **Head elevation** with three pillows during sleep to reduce periorbital oedema.
3. **Eyelid taping** during sleep may alleviate mild exposure keratopathy.

Lid retraction

Pathogenesis

Retraction of upper and lower lids occurs in about 50% of patients with Graves disease as a result of the following postulated mechanisms:

1. **Fibrotic contracture** of the levator associated with adhesions with the overlying orbital tissues causes lid retraction to be worse on down-gaze. Fibrosis of the inferior rectus muscle may similarly induce retraction of the lower eyelid via its capsulo-palpebral head.
2. **Secondary overaction of the levator-superior rectus complex** in response to hypotropia produced by fibrosis and tethering of the inferior rectus muscle, evidenced by increased lid retraction from down-gaze to up-gaze. Retraction of the lower eyelid resulting from overaction of the inferior rectus may also occur secondary to fibrosis of the superior rectus muscle.

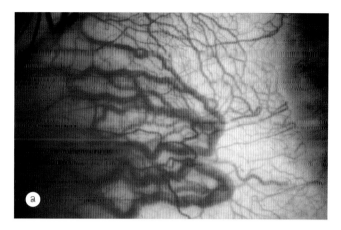
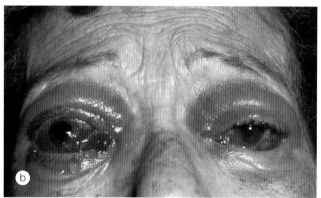
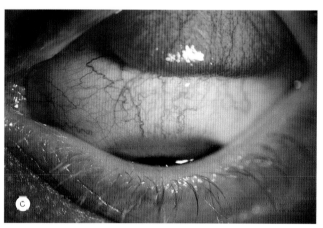

Fig. 6.6
Soft tissue involvement in thyroid eye disease. **(a)** Epibulbar hyperaemia overlying a horizontal rectus muscle; **(b)** periorbital oedema, chemosis and prolapse of fat into the eyelids; **(c)** superior limbic keratoconjunctivitis

3. **Humorally-induced overaction of Müller muscle** as a result of sympathetic overstimulation secondary to high levels of thyroid hormones. Supporting this hypothesis is the observation that lid retraction may sometimes be lessened by a topical sympatholytic drug such as guanethidine; against it is the absence of associated

pupillary dilatation and the fact that lid retraction may occur without hyperthyroidism.

Signs

The upper lid margin normally rests 2mm below the limbus (Fig. 6.7a, right eye). Lid retraction is suspected when the margin is either level with or above the superior limbus, allowing sclera to be visible ('scleral show') (Fig. 6.7a, left eye). Likewise, the lower eyelid normally rests at the inferior limbus; retraction is suspected when sclera shows below the limbus. Lid retraction may occur in isolation (Fig. 6.7b) or in association with proptosis, which exaggerates its severity.

1. **Dalrymple sign** is lid retraction in primary gaze.
2. **Kocher sign** describes a staring and frightened appearance of the eyes which is particularly marked on attentive fixation (Fig. 6.7c).
3. **von Graefe sign** signifies retarded descent of the upper lid on down-gaze (lid lag) (Fig. 6.7d).

Management

Mild lid retraction does not require treatment because it frequently improves spontaneously. Surgery to decrease the vertical dimensions of the palpebral fissures may be considered in patients with significant but stable lid retrac-

tion, but only after addressing proptosis and strabismus. In general therefore, the sequence of surgical procedures in TED is: (a) *orbital*, (b) *strabismus* and (c) *eyelid*. The rationale for this sequence is that orbital decompression may affect both ocular motility and eyelid position, and extraocular muscle surgery may also influence eyelid position. The main surgical procedures for lid retraction are:

1. **Müllerotomy** (disinsertion of Müller muscle) for mild lid retraction. More severe cases may also require recession/disinsertion of the levator aponeurosis and the suspensory ligament of the superior conjunctival fornix.
2. **Recession of lower lid retractors,** with or without a hard palate graft, when retraction of the lower lid is 2mm or more.
3. **Botulinum toxin injection** aimed at the levator aponeurosis and Müller muscle may be used as a temporary measure in patients awaiting definitive correction.

Proptosis

Signs

Proptosis is axial, unilateral or bilateral, symmetrical or asymmetrical (Fig. 6.8), and frequently permanent. Severe proptosis may compromise lid closure with resultant

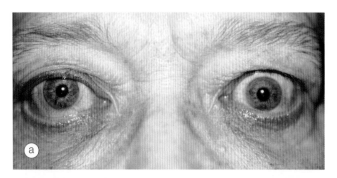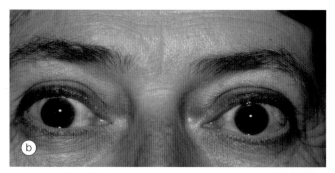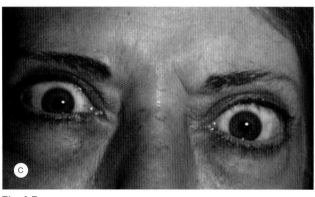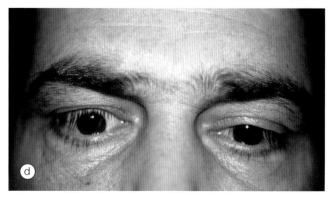

Fig. 6.7
Lid signs in thyroid eye disease. **(a)** Mild left lid retraction; **(b)** mild bilateral symmetrical lid retraction without proptosis; **(c)** severe bilateral lid retraction; **(d)** right lid lag on down-gaze (Courtesy of G Rose – fig. b)

exposure keratopathy, corneal ulceration and infection (Fig. 6.9).

Management

Management is controversial. Some favour early surgical decompression whereas others consider surgery only when non-invasive methods have failed or are inappropriate.

1. **Systemic steroids** may be used in rapidly progressive and painful proptosis during the congestive phase, unless contraindicated (e.g. tuberculosis or peptic ulceration).

   a. Oral prednisolone 60–80mg/day is given initially. Reduction in discomfort, chemosis and periorbital oedema usually occurs within 48 hours, at which point the dose should be tapered. Maximal response is usually achieved within 2–8 weeks. Ideally steroid therapy

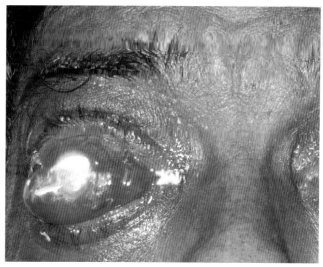

Fig. 6.9
Bacterial keratitis due to exposure in severe thyroid eye disease
(Courtesy of S Kumar Puri)

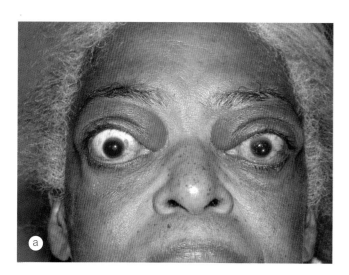

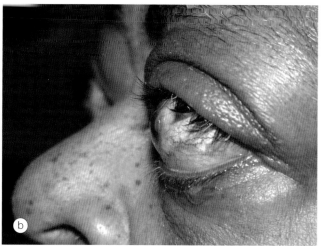

Fig. 6.8
Severe asymmetrical proptosis in thyroid eye disease. **(a)** Frontal view; **(b)** side view (Courtesy of A Pearson)

should be discontinued after about 3 months, although long-term low-dose maintenance may be necessary.

   b. Intravenous methylprednisolone 0.5g in 200ml isotonic saline given over 30 minutes, which may be repeated after 48 hours, may also be effective but is usually reserved for compressive optic neuropathy. This is because of potential cardiovascular risks which mandate careful supervision by a physician.

2. **Radiotherapy** may be used in addition to steroids or when steroids are contraindicated or ineffective. A positive response is usually evident within 6 weeks, with maximal improvement by 4 months.

3. **Combined therapy** with irradiation, azathioprine and low-dose prednisolone may be more effective than steroids or radiotherapy alone.

4. **Surgical decompression** may be considered either as primary treatment or when non-invasive methods are ineffective, such as for cosmetically unacceptable proptosis in the quiescent phase. Decompression, which may be performed via an external or endoscopic approach, may involve:

   a. Two-wall (antral-ethmoidal), involves removal of a part of the floor and the posterior portion of the medial wall. This affords 3–6mm of retroplacement of the globe.

   b. Three-wall, involves an antral-ethmoidal decompression and removal of the lateral wall. The amount of retroplacement achieved is 6–10 mm.

   c. Four-wall, involves a three-wall decompression, removal of the lateral half of the orbital roof and a large portion of the sphenoid at the apex of the orbit. This affords 10–16mm of retroplacement and is reserved for very severe proptosis.

Restrictive myopathy

Diagnosis

Some 30–50% of patients with TED develop ophthalmoplegia which may be permanent. Ocular motility is restricted initially by inflammatory oedema and later by fibrosis. Intraocular pressure may increase in up-gaze due to ocular compression by a fibrotic inferior rectus. Occasionally there may be a sustained increase in the intraocular pressure through compression of the globe by a combination of fibrotic extraocular muscles and increased intraorbital pressure. In order of frequency the four ocular motility defects are:

1. **Elevation** defect caused by fibrotic contracture of the inferior rectus (Fig. 6.10), which may mimic superior rectus palsy.
2. **Abduction** defect due to fibrosis of the medial rectus, which may simulate sixth nerve palsy.
3. **Depression** defect secondary to fibrosis of the superior rectus.
4. **Adduction** defect caused by fibrosis of the lateral rectus.

Treatment

1. **Surgery**
   a. **The indication** is diplopia in the primary or reading positions of gaze, provided the disease is quiescent and the angle of deviation has been stable for at least 6 months. Until these criteria are met, diplopia may be alleviated, if possible, with prisms.
   b. **The goal** is to achieve binocular single vision in the primary and reading positions. Restrictive myopathy, which causes incomitant strabismus, often precludes binocularity in all positions of gaze. However, with time the field of binocular single vision may enlarge as a result of increasing vergences.
   c. **The technique** most commonly involves recession of the inferior and/or medial recti, for best results on adjustable sutures. The suture is adjusted on the first postoperative day to obtain optimal alignment, and the patient is encouraged to practise achieving single vision with a distant target such as a television.
2. **Botulinum toxin injection** into the involved muscle may be useful in selected cases.

NB A rectus muscle should never be resected but only recessed.

Optic neuropathy

Optic neuropathy is an uncommon but serious complication caused by compression of the optic nerve or its blood supply at the orbital apex by the congested and enlarged recti (Fig. 6.11). Such compression, which may occur in the absence of significant proptosis, may lead to severe, permanent, but preventable visual impairment.

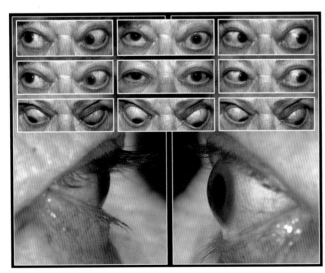

Fig. 6.10
Restrictive thyroid myopathy resulting in mainly defective elevation of both eyes; also note left superior limbic keratoconjunctivitis (Courtesy of C Barry)

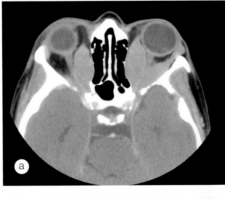
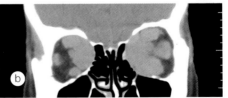

Fig. 6.11
CT shows muscle enlargement in thyroid eye disease. **(a)** Axial view; **(b)** coronal view – note sparing of the right lateral rectus muscle (Courtesy of N Sibtain)

Diagnosis

1. **Presentation** is with impairment of central vision. In order to detect early involvement, patients should be advised to monitor their own visual function by alternatively occluding each eye and reading small print and assessing the intensity of colours (e.g., on a television screen).
2. **Signs**
   - Visual acuity is usually reduced, but not invariably, and is associated with a relative afferent pupillary defect, colour desaturation and diminished light brightness appreciation.
   - Visual field defects may be central or paracentral, and may be combined with nerve fibre bundle defects. These findings, associated with elevated intraocular pressure, may be confused with primary open-angle glaucoma.
   - The optic disc is usually normal, occasionally swollen and rarely atrophic.

NB It is important not to attribute disproportionate visual loss to minor corneal complications and miss optic neuropathy.

Treatment

Initial treatment is usually with intravenous methylprednisolone. Orbital decompression may be considered if this is ineffective or inappropriate.

INFECTIONS

Preseptal cellulitis

Preseptal cellulitis is an infection of the subcutaneous tissues anterior to the orbital septum. Although not strictly an orbital disease, it is included here because it must be differentiated from the much less common but more serious orbital cellulitis. Occasionally rapid progression to orbital cellulitis may occur.

1. **Causes**
   a. **Skin trauma** such as laceration or insect bites. The offending organism is usually *S. aureus* or *S. pyogenes*.
   b. **Spread of local infection,** such as from an acute hordeolum or dacryocystitis.
   c. **From remote infection** of the upper respiratory tract or middle ear by haematogenous spread.
2. **Signs.** Unilateral, tender and red periorbital oedema (Fig. 6.12a).
3. **CT** shows opacification anterior to the orbital septum (Fig. 6.12b).

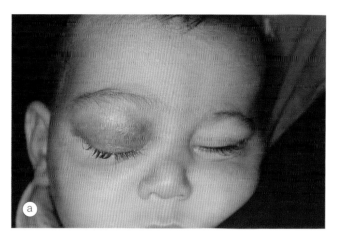

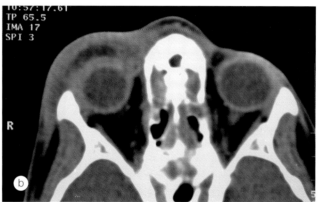

Fig. 6.12
(a) Right preseptal cellulitis; **(b)** axial CT shows opacification anterior to the orbital septum (Courtesy of K Nischal)

NB Unlike orbital cellulitis proptosis and chemosis are absent; visual acuity, pupillary reactions and ocular motility are unimpaired.

3. **Treatment** is with oral co-amoxiclav 250mg every 6 hours. Very severe infection may require intramuscular benzylpenicillin 2.4–4.8mg in four divided doses and oral flucloxacillin 250–500mg every 6 hours.

Bacterial orbital cellulitis

Bacterial orbital cellulitis is a life-threatening infection of the soft tissues behind the orbital septum. It can occur at any age but is more common in children. The most prevalent causative organisms are *S. pneumoniae, S. aureus, S. pyogenes* and *H. influenzae.*

Pathogenesis

1. **Sinus-related,** most commonly ethmoidal, typically affects children and young adults.

2. **Extension of preseptal cellulitis** through the orbital septum.
3. **Local spread** from adjacent dacryocystitis, and mid-facial or dental infection. The last condition may cause orbital cellulitis via an intermediary maxillary sinusitis.
4. **Haematogenous spread.**
5. **Post-traumatic** develops within 72 hours of an injury that penetrates the orbital septum. The typical clinical features may be masked by associated laceration or haematoma.
6. **Post-surgical** may complicate retinal, lacrimal or orbital surgery.

Diagnosis

1. **Presentation** is with a rapid onset of severe malaise, fever, pain and visual impairment.
2. **Signs**
   - Unilateral, tender, warm and red periorbital oedema.
   - Proptosis, which is often obscured by lid swelling, is most frequently lateral and downwards.
   - Painful ophthalmoplegia (Fig. 6.13a).
   - Optic nerve dysfunction.
3. **CT** shows preseptal and orbital opacification (Fig. 6.13b).

Complications

1. **Ocular** complications include exposure keratopathy, raised intraocular pressure, occlusion of the central retinal artery or vein, endophthalmitis and optic neuropathy.
2. **Intracranial** complications, which are rare, include meningitis, brain abscess and cavernous sinus thrombosis. The last is a rare but extremely serious complication which should be suspected when there is evidence of bilateral involvement, rapidly progressive proptosis and congestion of the facial, conjunctival and retinal veins. Additional features include abrupt progression of clinical signs associated with prostration, severe headache, nausea and vomiting.
3. **Subperiosteal abscess** is most frequently located along the medial orbital wall. It is a serious problem because of the potential for rapid progression and intracranial extension.
4. **Orbital abscess** is relatively rare in sinus-related orbital cellulitis but may occur in post-traumatic or postoperative cases.

Treatment

1. **Hospital admission** with frequent ophthalmic and otolaryngological assessment is mandatory. Intracranial abscess formation may necessitate drainage.
2. **Antimicrobial therapy** involves intramuscular cef-tazidime 1g every 8 hours and oral metronidazole 500mg every 8 hours to cover anaerobes. Intravenous van-comycin is a useful alternative in the context of penicillin

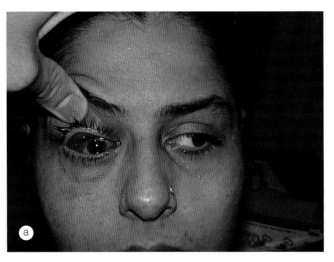

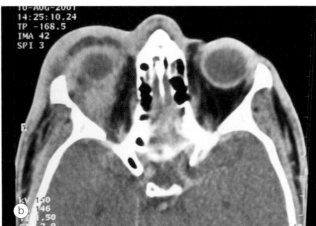

Fig. 6.13
Right orbital cellulitis. **(a)** Ophthalmoplegia; **(b)** axial CT shows preseptal and orbital opacification

allergy. Therapy should be continued until the patient is apyrexial for 4 days.
3. **Monitoring of optic nerve function** every 4 hours by testing pupillary reactions, visual acuity, colour vision and light brightness appreciation.
4. **Investigations,** where appropriate, include the following:
   - White cell count.
   - Blood culture.
   - CT of the orbit, sinuses and brain. Orbital CT is useful in the differentiation between severe preseptal cellulitis and orbital cellulitis (see above).
   - Lumbar puncture if meningeal or cerebral signs develop.
5. **Surgical intervention** should be considered in the following circumstances:
   - Unresponsiveness to antibiotics.
   - Decreasing vision.
   - Orbital or subperiosteal abscess.
   - Atypical picture, which may merit a biopsy.

NB It is usually necessary to drain the infected sinuses as well as the orbit.

Rhino-orbital mucormycosis

Mucormycosis is a very rare opportunistic infection caused by fungi of the family Mucoraceae, which typically affects patients with diabetic ketoacidosis or immunosuppression. This aggressive and potentially fatal infection is acquired by the inhalation of spores, which give rise to an upper respiratory infection. The infection then spreads to the contiguous sinuses and subsequently to the orbit and brain. Invasion of blood vessels by the hyphae results in occlusive vasculitis with ischaemic infarction of orbital tissues.

1. **Presentation** is with gradual onset facial and periorbital swelling, diplopia and visual loss.
2. **Signs**
   • Ischaemic infarction superimposed on septic necrosis is responsible for the black eschar which may develop on the palate, turbinates, nasal septum, skin and eyelids (Fig. 6.14).
   • Ophthalmoplegia.
   • Progression is slower than in bacterial orbital cellulitis.
3. **Complications** include retinal vascular occlusion, multiple cranial nerve palsies and cerebrovascular occlusion.
4. **Treatment**
   • Intravenous amphotericin.
   • Daily packing and irrigation of the involved areas with amphotericin.
   • Wide excision of devitalized and necrotic tissues.
   • Adjunctive hyperbaric oxygen may be helpful.
   • Correction of the underlying metabolic defect, if possible.
   • Exenteration may be required in severe unresponsive cases.

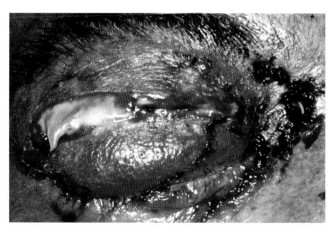

Fig. 6.14
Necrosis of the eyelid in rhino-orbital mucormycosis

INFLAMMATORY DISEASE

Idiopathic orbital inflammatory disease

Idiopathic orbital inflammatory disease (IOID), previously referred to as orbital pseudotumour, is an uncommon disorder characterized by non-neoplastic, non-infectious, space-occupying, orbital lesions. The inflammatory process may involve any or all of the orbital soft tissues, resulting in, for example, myositis, dacryoadenitis, optic perineuritis or scleritis. Histopathological analysis reveals pleomorphic cellular inflammatory infiltration followed by reactive fibrosis, but has thus far shown no correlation between clinicopathological features and the subsequent course of the disease. Unilateral disease is the rule in adults, although in children bilateral involvement may occur. Simultaneous orbital and sinus involvement is a rare but distinct entity.

Diagnosis

1. **Presentation** is in the third to sixth decades with acute periorbital redness, swelling and pain (Fig. 6.15a).
2. **Signs**
   • Congestive proptosis and ophthalmoplegia may occur in severe cases.
   • Optic nerve dysfunction if the inflammation involves the posterior orbit.
3. **CT** shows ill-defined orbital opacification and loss of definition of contents (Fig. 6.15b and c).
4. **Course.** This follows one of the following patterns:
   • Spontaneous remission after a few weeks without sequelae.
   • Prolonged intermittent episodes of activity with eventual remission.
   • Severe prolonged inflammation eventually leading to progressive fibrosis of orbital tissues, resulting in a 'frozen orbit' characterized by ophthalmoplegia, which may be associated with ptosis and visual impairment caused by optic nerve involvement (Fig. 6.16).

Treatment

1. **Observation,** for relatively mild disease, in anticipation of spontaneous remission.
2. **Biopsy** may be required in persistent cases to confirm the diagnosis and to rule out neoplasia.
3. **Oral non-steroidal anti-inflammatory agents** are often effective and should precede steroid therapy.
4. **Systemic steroids** should be administered only after the diagnosis has been confirmed as they may mask other pathology such as infection and Wegener granulomatosis. Oral prednisolone, initially 60–80mg/day, is later tapered and discontinued, depending on clinical response, although it may need to be reintroduced in the event of recurrence.

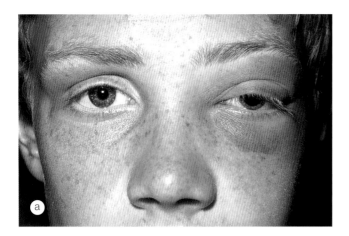

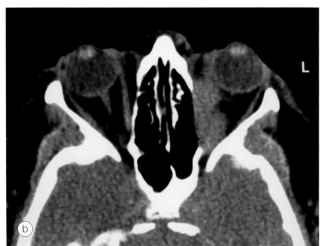

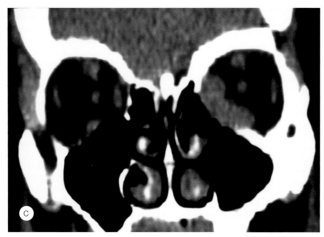

Fig. 6.15
(a) Idiopathic orbital inflammatory disease. **(b)** CT axial view shows ill-defined orbital opacification; **(c)** CT coronal view (Courtesy of A Pearson)

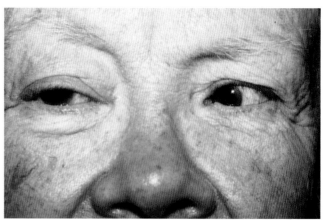

Fig. 6.16
Right ophthalmoplegia and ptosis due to a 'frozen orbit' (Courtesy of G Rose)

5. **Radiotherapy** may be considered if there has been no improvement after 2 weeks of adequate steroid therapy. Even a low dose treatment (i.e. 10Gy) may produce long-term, and sometimes permanent, remission.
6. **Antimetabolites** such as methotrexate or mycophenolate mofetil may be necessary in the context of resistance to both steroids and radiotherapy.
7. **Systemic infliximab,** a tumour necrosis factor inhibitor, may be effective in recurrent or recalcitrant cases that have failed to respond to conventional therapy.

Differential diagnosis

1. **Bacterial orbital cellulitis** should be considered when the anterior orbital tissues are markedly inflamed. A trial of systemic antibiotics may be necessary before the correct diagnosis becomes apparent.
2. **Severe acute TED** shares many features with IOID, but is commonly bilateral while IOID is usually unilateral.
3. **Systemic disorders** such as Wegener granulomatosis, polyarteritis nodosa and Waldenström macroglobulinaemia may manifest orbital involvement similar to IOID.
4. **Malignant orbital tumours,** particularly metastatic.
5. **Ruptured dermoid cyst** may evoke a secondary painful granulomatous inflammatory reaction.

Acute dacryoadenitis

Lacrimal gland involvement occurs in about 25% of patients with IOID. More commonly however, dacryoadenitis occurs in isolation, resolves spontaneously and does not require treatment.

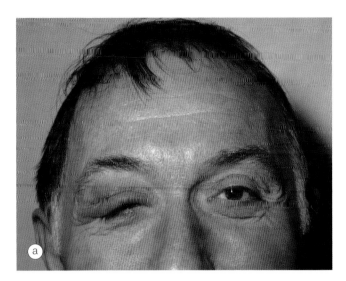

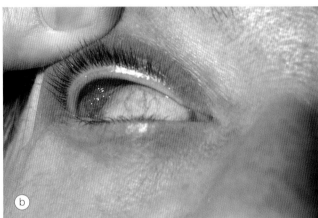

Fig. 6.17
Acute dacryoadenitis. **(a)** Swelling on the lateral aspect of the eyelid and an S-shaped ptosis; **(b)** injection of the palpebral portion of the lacrimal gland and adjacent conjunctiva

Diagnosis

1. **Presentation** is with acute discomfort in the region of the lacrimal gland.
2. **Signs**
   - Swelling of the lateral aspect of the eyelid giving rise to a characteristic S-shaped ptosis and mild downward and inward dystopia (Fig. 6.17a).
   - Tenderness over the lacrimal gland fossa.
   - Injection of the palpebral portion of the lacrimal gland and adjacent conjunctiva (Fig. 6.17b).
   - Lacrimal secretion may be reduced.

Differential diagnosis

1. **Lacrimal gland infection** caused by mumps, infectious mononucleosis and, less commonly, bacteria.

2. **Ruptured dermoid cyst** may cause localized inflammation in the region of the lacrimal gland.
3. **Malignant lacrimal gland tumours** may cause pain but the onset is not usually acute.

Orbital myositis

Orbital myositis is an idiopathic, non-specific inflammation of one or more extraocular muscles and is considered a subtype of IOID.

Histology

Histology shows a chronic inflammatory cellular infiltrate in relation to muscle fibres (Fig. 6.18a).

Diagnosis

1. **Presentation** is usually in early adult life with acute pain, exacerbated by eye movement, and diplopia.
2. **Signs**
   - Lid oedema, ptosis and chemosis.
   - Worsening of pain on attempted gaze into the field of action of the involved muscle(s) usually associated with diplopia due to under-action.
   - Vascular injection over the involved muscle.
   - Mild proptosis may be present.
   - In chronic cases the affected muscle may become fibrosed and cause permanent restrictive myopathy (Fig. 6.18b).
3. **CT** shows fusiform enlargement of the affected muscles, with or without involvement of tendons (Fig. 6.18c).
4. **Differential diagnosis** includes orbital cellulitis, dysthyroid myopathy and Tolosa–Hunt syndrome.
5. **Course**
   - Acute non-recurrent involvement which resolves spontaneously within 6 weeks.
   - Chronic disease characterized by either a single episode persisting for longer than 2 months (often for years) or recurrent attacks.

Treatment

Treatment is aimed at relieving discomfort and dysfunction, shortening the course and preventing recurrences.

1. **NSAIDs** may be adequate in mild disease.
2. **Systemic steroids** are generally required and usually produce dramatic improvement, although recurrences affect 50% of cases.
3. **Radiotherapy** is also effective, particularly in limiting recurrence.

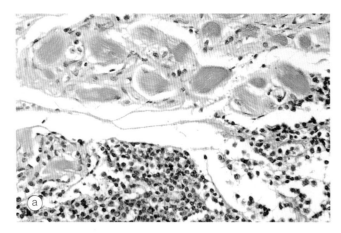

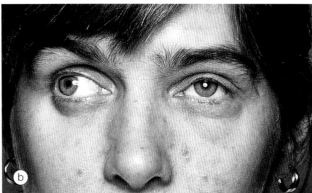

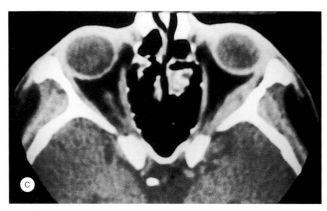

Fig. 6.18
Orbital myositis. **(a)** Histology shows a chronic inflammatory cellular infiltrate in relation to muscle fibres; **(b)** restriction of left adduction and narrowing of the palpebral fissure; **(c)** axial CT shows fusiform enlargement of the left lateral rectus (Courtesy of J Harry and G Misson, from *Clinical Ophthalmic Pathology*, Butterworth-Heinemann, 2001 – fig. a)

Tolosa–Hunt syndrome

Tolosa–Hunt syndrome is a diagnosis of exclusion. It is a rare condition caused by non-specific granulomatous inflam-mation of the cavernous sinus, superior orbital fissure and/or orbital apex. The clinical course is characterized by remissions and recurrences.

1. **Presentation** is with diplopia associated with ipsilateral periorbital or hemicranial pain.
2. **Signs**
   • Proptosis, if present, is usually mild.
   • Ocular motor nerve palsies, often with involvement of the pupil.
   • Sensory loss along the distribution of the first and second divisions of the trigeminal nerve.
3. **Treatment** is with systemic steroids.

Wegener granulomatosis

Wegener granulomatosis (see Chapter 24) involves the orbit, often bilaterally, usually by contiguous spread from the paranasal sinuses or nasopharynx. Primary orbital involvement is less common. The possibility of Wegener granulomatosis should be considered in any patient with bilateral orbital inflammation, particularly if associated with sinus pathology. The antineutrophilic cytoplasmic antibody (cANCA) is a very useful serological test.

1. **Signs**
   • Proptosis, orbital congestion and ophthalmoplegia.
   • Dacryoadenitis and nasolacrimal duct obstruction.
   • Coexistent manifestations include scleritis and peripheral ulcerative keratitis.
2. **Treatment**
   a. **Systemic** cyclophosphamide and steroids are highly effective. In resistant cases ciclosporin, azathioprine, antithymocyte globulin or plasmapheresis may be useful.
   b. **Surgical** orbital decompression may be required for severe orbital involvement.

VASCULAR MALFORMATIONS

Varices

Varices consist of weakened segments of the orbital venous system, of variable length and complexity. Intrinsic to the circulation, they enlarge with increased venous pressure, their distensibility varying with the residual thickness and strength of their walls. Most cases are unilateral and involve the upper nasal quadrant. CT and plain radiographs show phleboliths in about 20% of cases.

Diagnosis

1. **Presentation** ranges from early childhood to late middle age
2. **Signs**
   - Intermittent proptosis without external signs. The proptosis is non-pulsatile and is not associated with a bruit. As the orbital veins are devoid of valves, rapidly reversible proptosis may be precipitated or accentuated by increasing venous pressure through coughing, straining, Valsalva manoeuvre (Fig. 6.19), assuming the dependent position or external compression of the jugular veins.
   - Visible lesions in the eyelid which may also be accentuated by performing the Valsalva procedure (Figs 6.20 and 6.21a).
   - Conjunctival varices (Fig. 6.21b).
   - A combination of visible lesions and proptosis (the most common).

3. **CT** and plain radiographs may show phleboliths (Fig. 6.22a).
4. **Angiography** may be useful in identifying the vascular pattern (Fig. 6.22b).

Complications

Complications include acute haemorrhage and thrombosis. Patients with long-standing lesions may develop atrophy of surrounding fat and enophthalmos associated with a deepened superior sulcus in the resting position (Fig. 6.23), reversible with increase in venous pressure.

Treatment

Treatment by surgical excision is technically difficult and often incomplete because the lesions are friable and bleed easily. Indications include recurrent thrombosis, pain, severe proptosis and optic nerve compression.

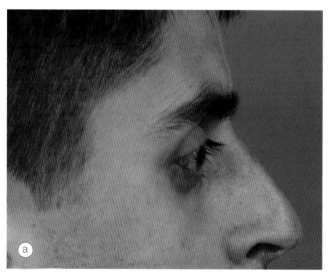
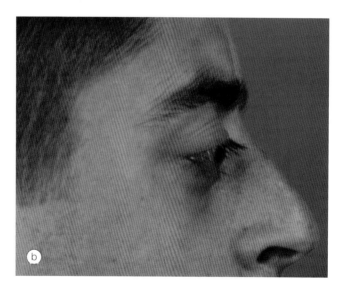

Fig. 6.19
Orbital varices. **(a)** Before Valsalva; **(b)** with Valsalva

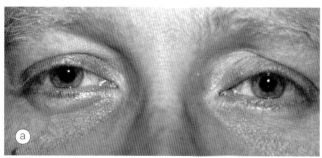
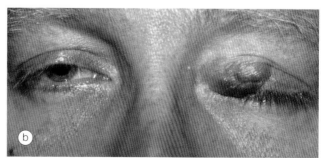

Fig. 6.20
Eyelid varices. **(a)** Before Valsalva; **(b)** with Valsalva (Courtesy of G Rose)

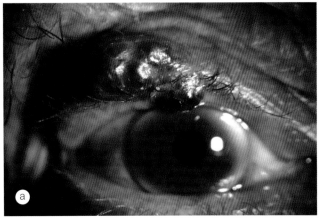

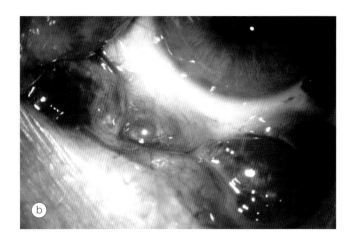

Fig. 6.21
(a) Severe eyelid varices; (b) conjunctival varices

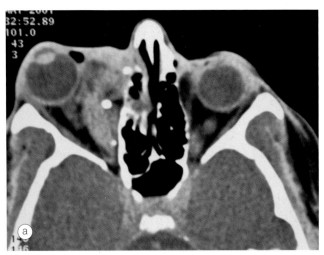

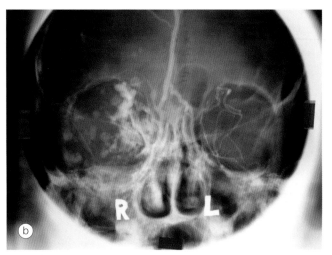

Fig. 6.22
Orbital varices. (a) Axial CT shows medical opacification and phleboliths; (b) angiogram showing severe involvement and phleboliths
(Courtesy of A Pearson)

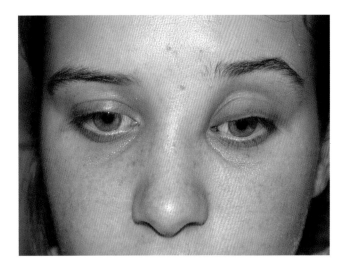

Fig. 6.23
Left orbital fat atrophy and a deep superior sulcus associated with long-standing orbital varices (Courtesy of A Pearson)

Lymphangioma

Lymphangiomas are not neoplasms but abortive, non functional, benign, vascular malformations. Although haemodynamically isolated from the circulation, bleeding into the lumen may occur with resultant blood-filled 'chocolate' cysts. Lymphangiomas may be confused with orbital venous anomalies and haemangiomas.

Diagnosis

1. **Presentation** is usually in early childhood
2. **Signs**
   - Anterior lesions typically manifest several soft bluish masses in the upper nasal quadrant with an associated cystic conjunctival component (Fig. 6.24).
   - Posterior lesions may cause slowly progressive proptosis, or initially may lie dormant and later present with sudden onset of painful proptosis secondary to spontaneous haemorrhage which may be associated with optic nerve compression (Fig. 6.25).
   - The blood subsequently becomes encysted with the formation of 'chocolate cysts' which may regress spontaneously with time.
   - Involvement of the oropharynx may be present.

Treatment

Surgical excision is difficult because the lesions are friable, not encapsulated, bleed easily and may infiltrate normal orbital tissues. Persistent sight-threatening 'chocolate cysts'

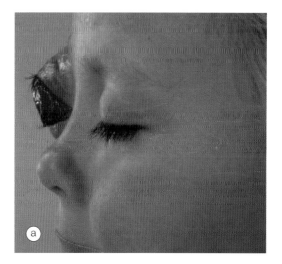

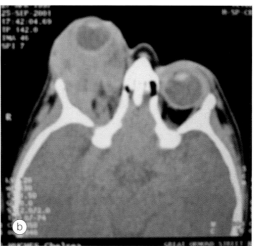

Fig. 6.25
(a) Severe proptosis due to bleeding from a posterior lymphangioma; **(b)** axial CT shows proptosis and orbital opacification (Courtesy of A Pearson)

should be drained or removed sub-totally by controlled vaporization using a carbon dioxide laser.

Direct carotid-cavernous fistula

Introduction

An arteriovenous fistula is an abnormal communication between an artery and a vein. The blood within the affected vein becomes 'arterialized', the venous pressure rises, and venous drainage may be altered in both rate and direction. The arterial pressure and perfusion are also reduced. A carotid-cavernous fistula is one such communication between the carotid artery and the cavernous sinus. When arterial blood flows anteriorly into the ophthalmic veins, ocular manifestations occur because of venous and arterial

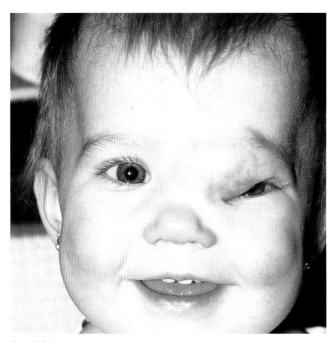

Fig. 6.24
Anterior orbital lymphangioma with typical bluish discoloration

stasis around the eye and orbit, increased episcleral venous pressure and decrease in arterial blood flow to the cranial nerves within the cavernous sinus. Carotid-cavernous fistulae can be classified on the basis of: (a) *aetiology* (spontaneous and traumatic), (b) *haemodynamics* (high and low flow) and (c) *anatomy* (direct and indirect).

Causes

Direct carotid-cavernous fistulae account for 50% of all cases. They are high-flow shunts in which carotid artery blood passes directly into the cavernous sinus through a defect in the wall of the intracavernous portion of the internal carotid artery as a result of the following:

1. **Trauma** is responsible for 75% of cases. A basal skull fracture may cause a tear in the intracavernous internal carotid artery with sudden and dramatic onset of symptoms and signs.
2. **Spontaneous** rupture of an intracavernous carotid aneurysm or an atherosclerotic artery accounts for the remainder. Post-menopausal hypertensive women are at particular risk. Spontaneous fistulae usually have lower flow rates and less severe symptoms than traumatic cases.

Diagnosis

1. **Presentation** may be days or weeks after head injury with the classic triad of pulsatile proptosis, chemosis and a whooshing noise in the head.
2. **Signs** are usually ipsilateral to the fistula but may be bilateral or even contralateral because of the vascular connections across the midline between the two cavernous sinuses.
   - Severe epibulbar injection (Fig. 6.26a).
   - Ptosis and haemorrhagic chemosis (Fig. 6.26b). The presence of ptosis may be helpful in differentiation from acute thyroid eye disease.
   - Pulsatile proptosis associated with a bruit and a thrill, both of which can be abolished by ipsilateral carotid compression in the neck. A cephalic bruit may also be present.
   - Increased intraocular pressure from elevated episcleral venous pressure and orbital congestion.
   - Anterior segment ischaemia characterized by corneal epithelial oedema, aqueous cells and flare, iris atrophy, cataract and rubeosis iridis.
   - Ophthalmoplegia occurs in 60–70% of cases due to ocular motor nerve damage caused by the initial trauma, the intracavernous aneurysm or the fistula itself. The sixth nerve is most frequently affected because of its free-floating location within the cavernous sinus. The third and fourth nerves, situated in the lateral wall of the sinus, are less commonly involved. Engorgement and swelling of extraocular muscles may also contribute to defective ocular motility.

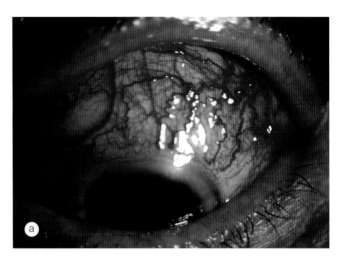

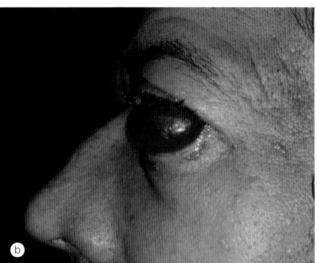

Fig. 6.26
Direct carotid-cavernous fistula. **(a)** Severe epibulbar injection; **(b)** haemorrhagic chemosis

   - Fundus examination shows optic disc swelling, venous dilatation and intraretinal haemorrhages from venous stasis and impaired retinal blood flow. Preretinal or vitreous haemorrhages are rare.
3. **Vision.** Immediate visual loss may be due to coincidental ocular or optic nerve damage at the time of head trauma. Delayed visual loss may occur as a result of exposure keratopathy, secondary glaucoma, central retinal vein occlusion, anterior segment ischaemia or ischaemic optic neuropathy.
4. **Special investigations.** CT and MR will show prominence of the superior ophthalmic vein and diffuse enlargement of extraocular muscles. Definitive diagnosis involves arterial angiography with selective injection of both internal and external carotid arteries, and the vertebral circulation.

Treatment

Most carotid-cavernous fistulae are not life-threatening; the major organ at risk is the eye. Surgery is indicated if spontaneous closure secondary to thrombosis of the cavernous sinus does not occur. A post-traumatic fistula is much less likely to close on its own than a spontaneous one because of higher blood flow.

1. **Indications** for treatment are secondary glaucoma, diplopia, intolerable bruit or headache, severe proptosis causing exposure keratopathy and anterior segment ischaemia.
2. **Interventional radiology** involves detachable balloon occlusion of the fistula. The balloon is introduced into the cavernous sinus either by an arterial route, through the tear in the internal carotid artery, or by a venous route, through the inferior petrosal sinus or the superior ophthalmic vein.

Indirect carotid-cavernous fistula

In an indirect carotid-cavernous fistula (dural shunt) the intracavernous portion of the internal carotid artery remains intact. Arterial blood flows through the meningeal branches of the external or internal carotid arteries indirectly into the cavernous sinus. Due to slow blood flow, the clinical features are more subtle than in a direct fistula. The condition may therefore be misdiagnosed or missed altogether.

1. **Types**
   - Between meningeal branches of the internal carotid artery and the cavernous sinus.
   - Between meningeal branches of the external carotid artery and the cavernous sinus.
   - Between meningeal branches of both the external and internal carotid arteries and the cavernous sinus.
2. **Causes**
   a. **Congenital malformations,** in which the onset of symptoms is precipitated by intracranial vascular thrombosis.
   b. **Spontaneous rupture,** which may be precipitated by minor trauma or straining, especially in hypertensive patients.
3. **Presentation** is with gradual onset of redness of one or both eyes caused by vascular engorgement.
4. **Signs** are variable:
   - Mild epibulbar injection (Fig. 6.27a).
   - Exaggerated ocular pulsation best detected on applanation tonometry.
   - Raised intraocular pressure.
   - Mild proptosis occasionally associated with a soft bruit.
   - Ophthalmoplegia caused by sixth nerve palsy (Fig. 6.27b) or swelling of extraocular muscles.

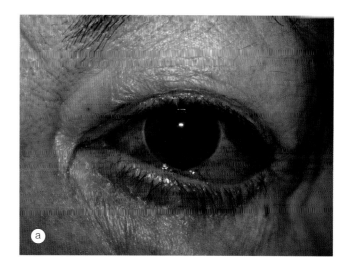

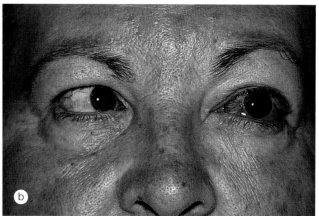

Fig. 6.27
Indirect carotid-cavernous fistula. **(a)** Mild epibulbar injection and chemosis; **(b)** sixth nerve palsy (Courtesy of J Yanguela)

   - Fundus may be normal or manifest moderate venous dilatation.
5. **Differential diagnosis** includes chronic conjunctivitis, thyroid eye disease, glaucoma and orbital arteriovenous malformations which may mimic dural shunts.
6. **Treatment** involves 'interventional radiology' to occlude the feeding arteries, although some patients recover spontaneously.

CYSTIC LESIONS

Dacryops

A dacryops is a ductal cyst of the lacrimal gland. It is the most common orbital cystic lesion and is frequently bilateral.

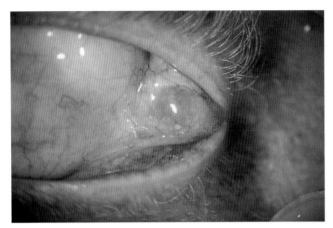

Fig. 6.28
Dacryops

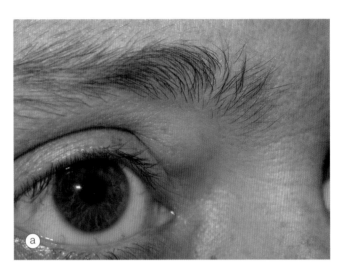

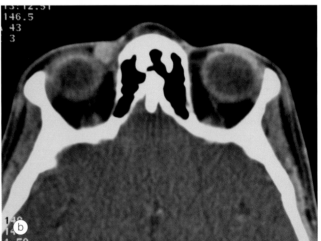

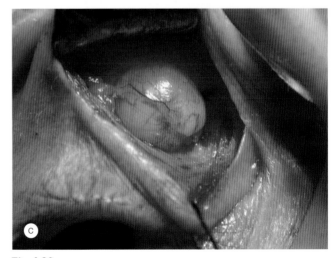

Fig. 6.29
(a) Superficial dermoid cyst; **(b)** axial CT shows a well-circumscribed heterogeneous lesion; **(c)** appearance at surgery (Courtesy of A Pearson)

1. **Signs.** A round, cystic lesion originating from the palpebral portion of the lacrimal gland which protrudes into the superior fornix (Fig. 6.28).
2. **Treatment** involves simple aspiration.

Dermoid cyst

A dermoid cyst is a choristoma derived from displacement of ectoderm to a subcutaneous location along embryonic lines of closure. Dermoids are lined by keratinized stratified squamous epithelium (like skin), have a fibrous wall and contain dermal appendages such as sweat glands, sebaceous glands and hair follicles. Epidermoid cysts do not contain such adnexal structures. Dermoids may be (a) *superficial* or (b) *deep*, located anterior or posterior to the orbital septum respectively.

Superficial dermoid cyst

1. **Presentation** is in infancy with a painless nodule most commonly located in the supero-temporal and occasionally the supero-nasal part of the orbit.
2. **Signs**
   • A firm, round, smooth, non-tender, subcutaneous mass 1–2cm in diameter which is freely mobile (Fig. 6.29a).
   • The posterior margins are easily palpable denoting lack of deeper origin or extension.
3. **CT** shows a heterogeneous well-circumscribed lesion (Fig. 6.29b).
4. **Treatment** is by excision *in toto* (Fig. 6.29c), taking care not to rupture the lesion, since leaking of keratin into the surrounding tissue results in a severe foreign body reaction.

Deep dermoid cyst

1. **Presentation** is in adolescence or adult life.
2. **Signs**
   - Proptosis, dystopia or a mass lesion with indistinct posterior margins (Fig. 6.30a).
   - Some deep dermoids, associated with bony defects, may extend into the inferotemporal fossa or intracranially.
3. **CT** shows a well-circumscribed cystic lesion (Fig. 6.30b)
4. **Treatment** by excision *in toto* is advisable because deep dermoids enlarge and may leak their contents into adjacent tissues. This induces a painful foreign body reaction, often followed by fibrosis. If incompletely excised, they may recur and cause persistent low-grade inflammation.

Sinus mucocele

A mucocele develops when the drainage of normal paranasal sinus secretions is obstructed due to infection, allergy, trauma, tumour or congenital narrowing. A slowly expanding cystic accumulation of mucoid secretions and epithelial debris develops and gradually erodes the bony walls of the sinuses, causing symptoms by encroaching upon surrounding tissues. Orbital invasion occurs usually from frontal or ethmoidal mucoceles; and rarely from those arising in the maxillary sinus.

1. **Presentation** is in adult life with proptosis or dystopia (Fig. 6.31a), diplopia or epiphora. Pain is uncommon unless secondary infection develops (mucopyocele).
2. **CT** shows a soft tissue mass with thinning of the bony walls of the sinus (Fig. 6.31b).
3. **Treatment** involves complete removal of the mucocele, with re-establishment of normal sinus drainage or obliteration of the sinus cavity.

Encephalocele

An encephalocele is formed by herniation of intracranial contents through a congenital defect of the base of the skull. A meningocele contains only dura whilst a meningoencephalocele also contains brain tissue. Orbital encephalocele

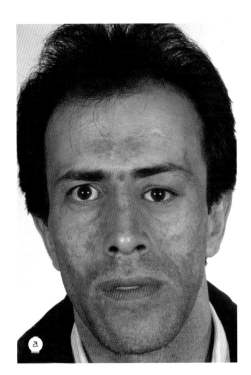
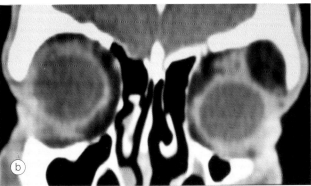

Fig. 6.30
(a) Left deep orbital dermoid cyst causing dystopia; (b) coronal CT shows a well-circumscribed cystic lesion and bone re-modelling (Courtesy of A Pearson)

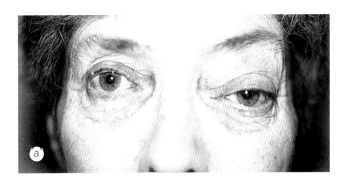
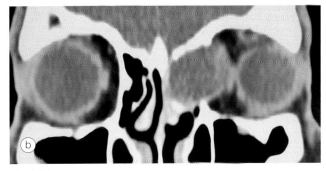

Fig. 6.31
(a) Left ethmoidal sinus mucocele causing dystopia; (b) coronal CT shows orbital involvement and indentation of the medial rectus

may be (a) *anterior* (fronto-ethmoidal) or (b) *posterior* which is associated with dysplasia of the sphenoid bone.

Diagnosis

1. **Presentation** is usually during infancy.
2. **Signs**
   - Anterior encephaloceles involve the superomedial part of the orbit and displace the globe forwards and laterally (Fig. 6.32a).
   - Posterior encephaloceles displace the globe forwards and downwards (Fig. 6.32b).
   - The cyst increases in size on straining or crying and may be reduced by manual pressure.
   - Pulsating proptosis may occur due to communication with the subarachnoid space but, because the communication is not vascular, there is neither a thrill nor a bruit.

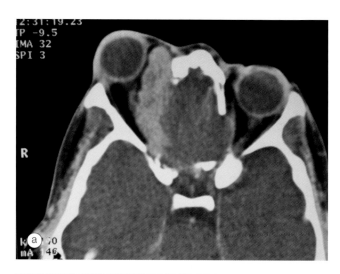

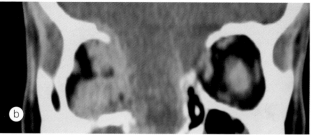

Fig. 6.33
CT of posterior encephalocele showing a large bony defect.
(a) Axial view; **(b)** coronal view (Courtesy of A Pearson)

3. **CT** shows the bony defect responsible for the herniation (Fig. 6.33).

Differential diagnosis

1. **Of anterior encephalocele** includes other causes of medial canthal swellings such as dermoid cysts and amniontoceles of the lacrimal sac.
2. **Of posterior encephalocele** includes other orbital lesions that present during early life such as capillary haemangioma, juvenile xanthogranuloma, teratoma and microphthalmos with cyst.

Associations

1. **Other bony abnormalities** such as hypertelorism, broad nasal bridge and cleft palate (Fig. 6.34a and b).
2. **Ocular** associations include microphthalmos, orbital varices, colobomas and the morning glory syndrome (Fig. 6.34c).
3. **Neurofibromatosis-1** is frequently associated with posterior encephalocele.

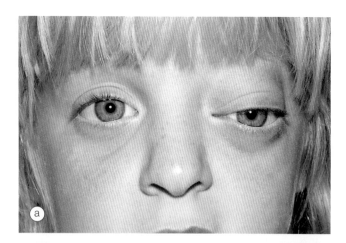

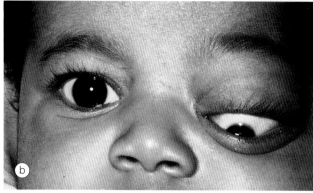

Fig. 6.32
(a) Anterior superomedial encephalocele causing proptosis and down and out dystopia; **(b)** posterior encephalocele causing proptosis and inferior dystopia

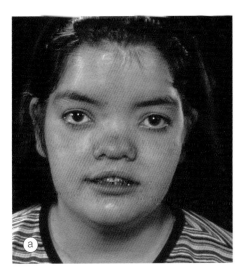

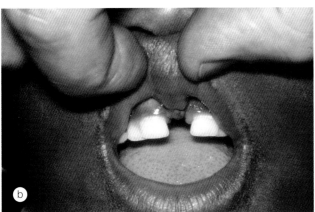

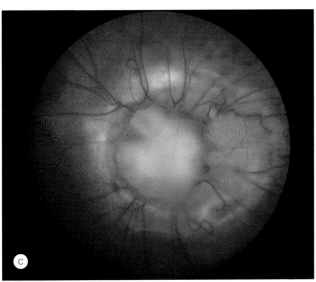

Fig. 6.34
Associations of encephalocele **(a)** Hypertelorism; **(b)** cleft palate; **(c)** morning glory anomaly (Courtesy of K Nischal – fig. a; Moorfields Eye Hospital – figs b and c)

TUMOURS

Capillary haemangioma

Capillary haemangioma, a hamartoma, is the most common tumour of the orbit and periorbital areas in childhood. Girls are affected more commonly than boys. The tumour may present as a small isolated lesion of minimal clinical significance or as a large disfiguring mass that can cause visual impairment and systemic complications.

Histology

The tumour is composed of varying-sized small vascular channels without true encapsulation (Fig. 6.35a).

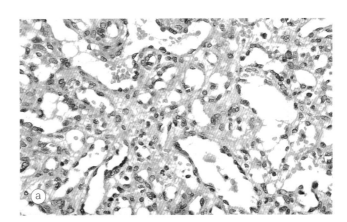

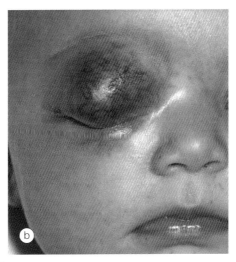

Fig. 6.35
Capillary haemangioma. **(a)** Histology shows irregular capillary channels of varying size; **(b)** large preseptal tumour causing ptosis and purple cutaneous discoloration (Courtesy of J Harry – fig. a; K Nischal – fig. b)

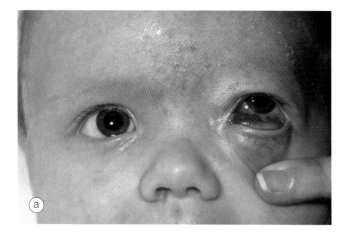

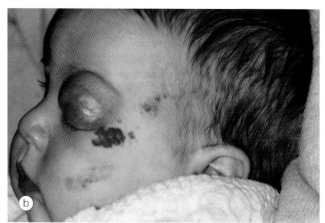

Fig. 6.36
Capillary haemangioma. **(a)** Involvement of the forniceal conjunctiva; **(b)** preseptal and cutaneous involvement; **(c)** very severe involvement

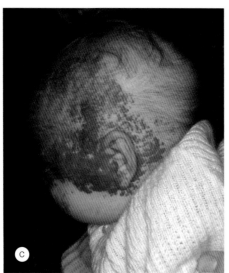

Diagnosis

The tumour is classified according to its location with respect to the skin and orbital septum as follows: (a) *cutaneous*; (b) *purely preseptal*, (c) *preseptal with an extraconal element* and (d) *combination* of preseptal, extraconal and intraconal.

1. **Presentation** is usually in the first few weeks of life (approximately 30% are present at birth).
2. **Signs**
   - Superficial cutaneous lesions are bright red.
   - Preseptal tumours appear dark blue or purple through the overlying skin and most frequently located superiorly (Fig. 6.35b).
   - A large tumour may enlarge and change in colour to a deep blue during crying or straining, but both pulsation and a bruit are absent.
   - Deep orbital tumours give rise to unilateral proptosis without skin discoloration.
   - Haemangiomatous involvement of the palpebral or forniceal conjunctiva is common and may be an important diagnostic clue (Fig. 6.36a).
   - Coexisting haemangiomas on the eyelids (Fig. 6.36b) or elsewhere are common (Fig. 6.36c).
3. **CT or MR** may be required for deep lesions when the diagnosis is not apparent on inspection. The lesion appears as a homogeneous enhancing soft tissue mass in the anterior orbit or as an extraconal mass with 'finger-like' posterior expansions (Fig. 6.37a). The orbital cavity may show enlargement but there is no bony erosion.
4. **US and Doppler** is essential in determining the anatomical relations and extent of the tumour, guiding treatment choice (Fig. 6.37b).
5. **Course** is characterized by rapid growth 3–6 months after diagnosis (Fig. 6.38), followed by a slower phase of natural resolution in which 30% of lesions resolve by the age of 3 years and 70% by the age of 7 years.

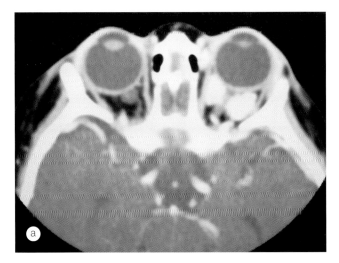

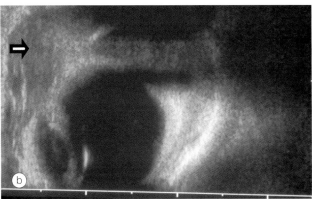

Fig. 6.37
Imaging of capillary haemangioma. **(a)** Axial enhanced CT shows a homogeneous intraconal orbital soft tissue mass; **(b)** US of a preseptal lesion with an intraorbital component (Courtesy of A Pearson – fig. a; K Nischal – fig. b)

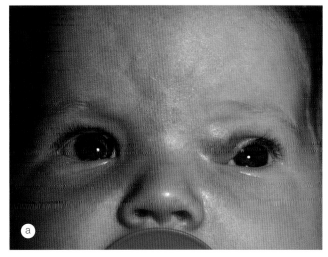

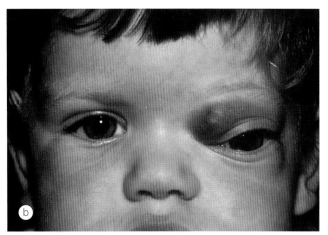

Fig. 6.38
Growth of capillary haemangioma. **(a)** At presentation; **(b)** several months later

Treatment

1. **Indications**
   - Amblyopia, most commonly secondary to induced astigmatism and anisometropia.
   - Optic nerve compression.
   - Exposure keratopathy.
   - A severe cosmetic blemish, necrosis or infection.
2. **Laser** treatment may be used to close blood vessels in superficial skin lesions less than 2mm in thickness.
3. **Steroid injection** of triamcinolone acetonide 40mg/ml and betamethasone 4mg/ml into the lesion, if cutaneous or preseptal, is very effective during the early active stage (Fig. 6.39a and b). A maximum of 1–2ml should be injected using multiple entry sites. The tumour usually begins to regress within 2 weeks but, if necessary, a second and third injection can be given after about 2 months. It is advisable not to inject deep into the orbit for fear of causing occlusion of the central retinal artery due to raised intraorbital pressure. Other complications of steroid injection include retrograde forcing of the solution into the central retinal artery, skin depigmentation and necrosis, bleeding and fat atrophy. Adrenal suppression and failure to thrive have also been reported.
4. **Systemic steroids** administered daily over several weeks may be used, particularly if there is a large orbital component.
5. **Subcutaneous injection of interferon alpha-2b** is a good option for treatment of steroid-resistant, organ interfering and/or life-threatening giant haemangiomas.
6. **Local resection** with cutting cautery (Fig. 6.39c) may reduce the bulk of an anterior circumscribed tumour, but is usually reserved for the late inactive stage.

Systemic associations

Children with large capillary haemangiomas may have the following conditions:

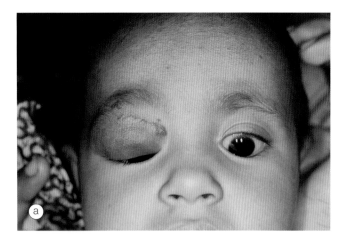

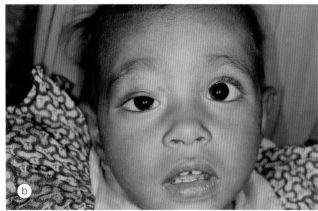

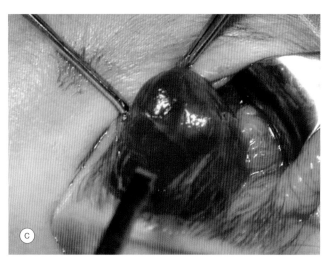

Fig. 6.39
Treatment of capillary haemangioma. Steroid injection **(a)** before and **(b)** after; **(c)** local resection – note the tumour is not encapsulated (Courtesy of U Raina – figs a and b; K Nischal – fig. c)

1. **High-output heart failure** may occur in a small minority of patients with very large fast-growing visceral haemangiomas.
2. **Kasabach–Merritt syndrome** which is characterized by thrombocytopenia, anaemia and low levels of coagulant factors may also occur in children with large visceral tumours.
3. **Maffuci syndrome** which is characterized by skin haemangiomas, enchondromata of hands, feet and long bones, as well as bowing of long bones.

Cavernous haemangioma

Cavernous haemangioma is the most common benign orbital tumour in adults, with a female preponderance of 70%. Although it may develop anywhere in the orbit, it most frequently occurs within the lateral part of the muscle cone just behind the globe.

1. **Histology** shows endothelial-lined vascular channels of varying size separated by fibrous septae (Fig. 6.40a).
2. **Presentation** is in the fourth to fifth decades with slowly progressive unilateral proptosis. Growth may be accelerated by pregnancy.
3. **Signs**
   - Axial proptosis (Fig. 6.40b) which may be associated with optic disc oedema and choroidal folds.
   - A lesion at the orbital apex may compress the optic nerve without causing significant proptosis.
   - Gaze-evoked transient blurring of vision may occur.
4. **CT** shows a well-circumscribed oval lesion with slow contrast enhancement (Fig. 6.40c).
5. **Treatment.** Surgical excision is required in most cases because the lesion gradually enlarges. The cavernous haemangioma, unlike its capillary counterpart, is usually well encapsulated and relatively easy to remove (Fig. 6.40d).

Pleomorphic lacrimal gland adenoma

Pleomorphic adenoma (benign mixed-cell tumour) is the most common epithelial tumour of the lacrimal gland and is derived from the ducts and secretory elements including myoepithelial cells.

1. **Histology.** The inner layer of cells forms glandular tissue that may be associated with squamous differentiation and keratin production (Fig. 6.41a); the outer cells undergo metaplastic change leading to the formation of myxoid tissue (Fig. 6.41b).
2. **Presentation** is in the second to fifth decades with a painless, slowly progressive proptosis or swelling in the supero-lateral part of the orbit, usually of more than a year's duration. Old photographs may reveal their presence for many years prior to presentation.
3. **Signs of an orbital lobe tumour**
   - Smooth, firm, non-tender mass in the lacrimal gland fossa with inferonasal dystopia (Fig. 6.41c).
   - Posterior extension may cause proptosis, ophthalmoplegia and choroidal folds.

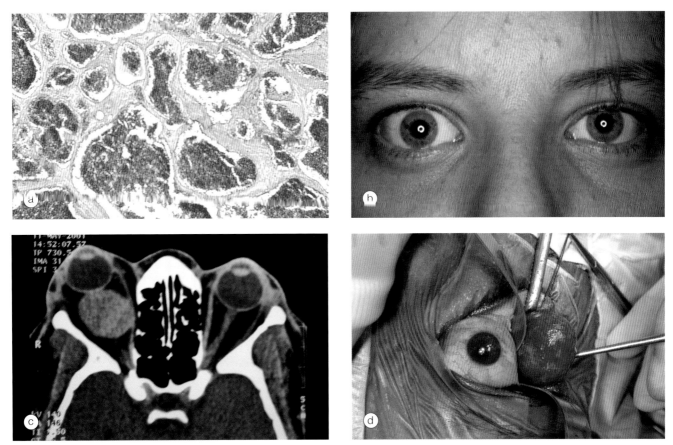

Fig.6.40
Cavernous haemangioma. **(a)** Histology shows congested varying-sized endothelial-lined vascular channels separated by fibrous septae; **(b)** right axial proptosis; **(c)** axial CT shows a well-circumscribed retrobulbar oval lesion and proptosis; **(d)** the tumour is encapsulated and easy to remove (Courtesy of J Harry and G Misson, from *Clinical Ophthalmic Pathology*, Butterworth-Heinemann, 2001 – fig. a; A Pearson – figs b, c and d)

- CT shows a round or oval mass, with a smooth outline with indentation but not destruction of the lacrimal gland fossa (Fig. 6.41d). The lesion may also indent the globe and show calcification.
4. **Signs of a palpebral lobe tumour**
   - This is less common and tends to grow anteriorly, causing upper lid swelling without dystopia (Fig. 6.42a).
   - The lesion may be visible to inspection (Fig. 6.42b).
5. **Treatment** involves surgical excision. If the diagnosis is strongly suspected, it is wise to avoid prior biopsy, to avoid tumour seeding into adjacent orbital tissue – although this may not always be possible in the context of diagnostic uncertainty. Tumours of the palpebral lobe are usually resected, along with a margin of normal tissue, through an anterior (trans-septal) orbitotomy. Those of the

orbital portion are excised through a lateral orbitotomy (Fig. 6.43).
6. **Prognosis** is excellent provided excision is complete and without disruption of the capsule. Incomplete excision or preliminary incisional biopsy may result in seeding of the tumour into adjacent tissues, with recurrences which may later turn malignant.

Lacrimal gland carcinoma

Lacrimal gland carcinomas are rare tumours which carry a high morbidity and mortality. In order of frequency the main histological types are: (a) *adenoid cystic*, (b) *pleomorphic adenocarcinoma*, (c) *mucoepidermoid* and (d) *squamous cell*.

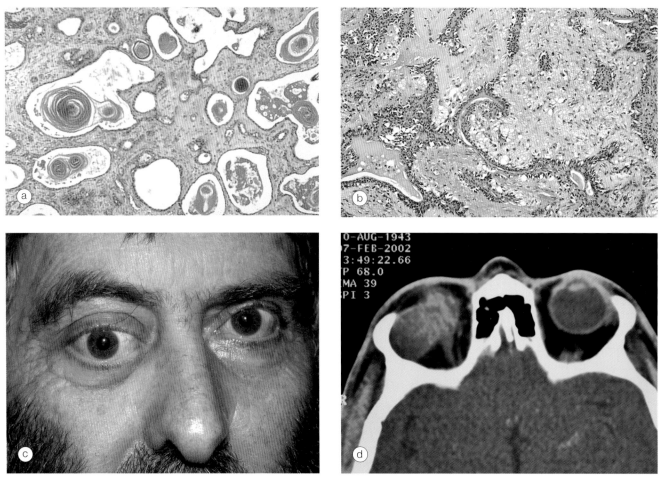

Fig. 6.41
Pleomorphic lacrimal gland adenoma. **(a)** Histology shows glandular tissue and squamous differentiation with keratin formation; **(b)** histology shows epithelial and myoepithelial proliferation with the formation of myxoid tissue; **(c)** inferonasal dystopia due to a tumour arising from the orbital lobe; **(d)** axial CT shows an oval mass that indents the lacrimal gland fossa (Courtesy of J Harry and G Misson, from *Clinical Ophthalmic Pathology*, Butterworth-Heinemann, 2001 – figs a and b; A Pearson – figs c and d)

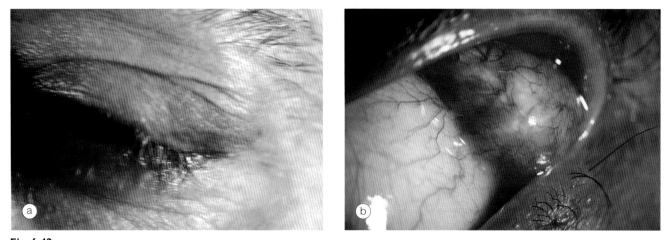

Fig. 6.42
Pleomorphic lacrimal gland adenoma arising from the palpebral lobe. **(a)** Eyelid swelling without dystopia; **(b)** eversion of the upper eyelid reveals the tumour

Fig. 6.43
Lateral orbitotomy. **(a)** Incision of temporalis muscle; **(b)** drilling of underlying bone for subsequent wiring; **(c)** removal of the lateral orbital wall and the tumour; **(d)** repair of the lateral orbital wall and temporalis muscle

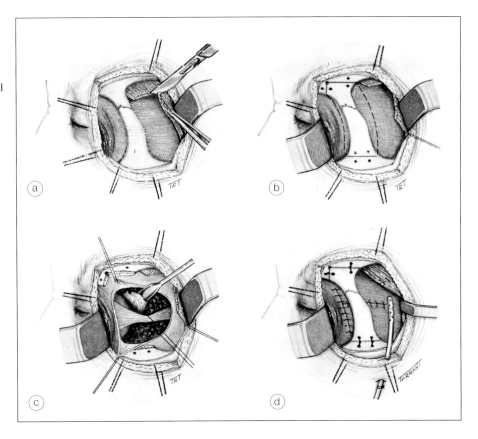

1. **Histology** of adenoid cystic carcinoma is characterized by nests of basaloid cells with numerous mitoses (Fig. 6.44a).
2. **Presentation** is in the fourth to fifth decades with a history shorter than that of a benign tumour. Pain is a frequent feature of malignancy but may also occur with inflammatory lesions. An adenoid cystic carcinoma may present in three main clinical settings:
   - After incomplete or piecemeal excision of a benign pleomorphic adenoma, followed by one or more recurrences over a period of several years with eventual malignant transformation.
   - As a long-standing proptosis (and/or a swollen upper lid) which suddenly starts to increase.
   - Without a previous history of a pleomorphic adenoma as a rapidly growing lacrimal gland mass (usually of several months' duration).
3. **Signs**
   - A mass in the lacrimal area causing infero-nasal dystopia.
   - Posterior extension with involvement of the superior orbital fissure may give rise to epibulbar congestion, proptosis, periorbital oedema and ophthalmoplegia (Fig. 6.44b).
   - Hypoaesthesia in the region supplied by the lacrimal nerve.
   - Optic disc swelling and choroidal folds.
4. **CT** shows a globular lesion with irregular serrated edges, often with contiguous erosion or invasion of bone (Fig. 6.44c). Calcification in the tumour is commonly seen.
5. **Biopsy** is necessary to establish the histological diagnosis. Subsequent management depends on the extent of tumour invasion of adjacent structures as seen on imaging studies.
6. **Neurological assessment** is mandatory because adenoid-cystic carcinoma exhibits perineural spread and may extend into the cavernous sinus.
7. **Treatment** involves excision of the tumour and adjacent tissues. Extensive tumours may require orbital exenteration (Fig. 6.44d) or mid-facial resection but the prognosis for life is frequently poor. Radiotherapy combined with local resection may prolong life and reduce pain.

Optic nerve glioma

Optic nerve glioma is a slow-growing, pilocytic astrocytoma which typically affects children, girls more often than boys. Approximately 30% of patients have associated neurofibromatosis-1 and in these patients the prognosis is better (see Chapter 24).

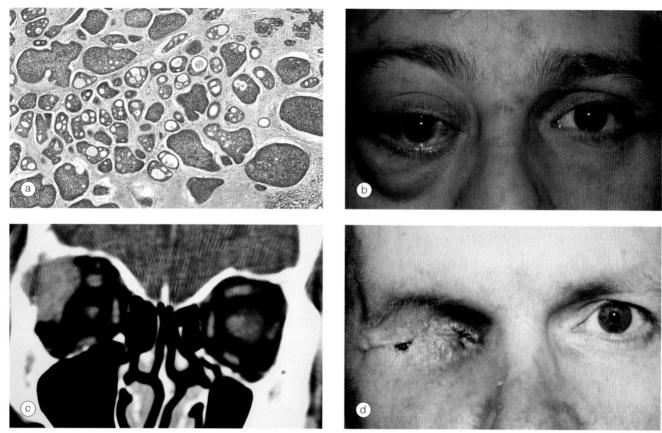

Fig. 6.44
Lacrimal gland carcinoma. **(a)** Histology of adenoid cystic carcinoma shows nests of basaloid cells with solid and cribriform areas;
(b) dystopia, proptosis, periorbital oedema and epibulbar congestion due to extension to involve the superior orbital fissure;
(c) coronal CT shows contiguous erosion of bone and spotty calcification in the tumour; **(d)** appearance following lid-sparing
exenteration (Courtesy of J Harry and G Misson, from *Clinical Ophthalmic Pathology*, Butterworth-Heinemann, 2001 – fig. a; G Rose – fig. b; A Pearson –
figs c and d)

1. **Histology** shows spindle-shaped pilocytic astrocytes and glial filaments (Fig. 6.45a).
2. **Presentation** is most frequently in the first decade of life (median age 6.5 years) with slowly-progressive visual loss, followed later by proptosis, although this sequence may occasionally be reversed. Acute loss of vision as a result of haemorrhage into the tumour is uncommon.
3. **Signs**
   - Proptosis often with inferior dystopia (Fig. 6.45b).
   - The optic nerve head is initially swollen and subsequently becomes atrophic.
   - Opticociliary collaterals and central retinal vein occlusion are occasionally seen.
   - Intracranial spread to the chiasm and hypothalamus may develop.
4. **CT** in patients with associated NF-1 shows a fusiform enlargement of the optic nerve with a clear cut margin produced by the intact dural sheath (Fig. 6.45c). In patients without NF-1 the nerve is more irregular and shows low-density areas. In some cases the optic canal is enlarged but this does not necessarily indicate intracranial extension.
5. **MR** shows gliomas to be hypointense to isointense on T1-weighted images and hyperintense on T2-weighted scans (Fig. 6.45d). MR may also show intracranial extension (Fig. 6.45e).
6. **Treatment** may not be required in patients with no evidence of growth, good vision and no cosmetic deformity. Surgical excision (Fig. 6.45f) with preservation of the globe is required for large or growing tumours that are confined to the orbit, particularly if vision is poor and proptosis significant. Radiotherapy may be combined with chemotherapy for tumours with intracranial extension.
7. **Prognosis** for life is variable. Some tumours have an indolent course with little growth, while others may extend intracranially and threaten life.

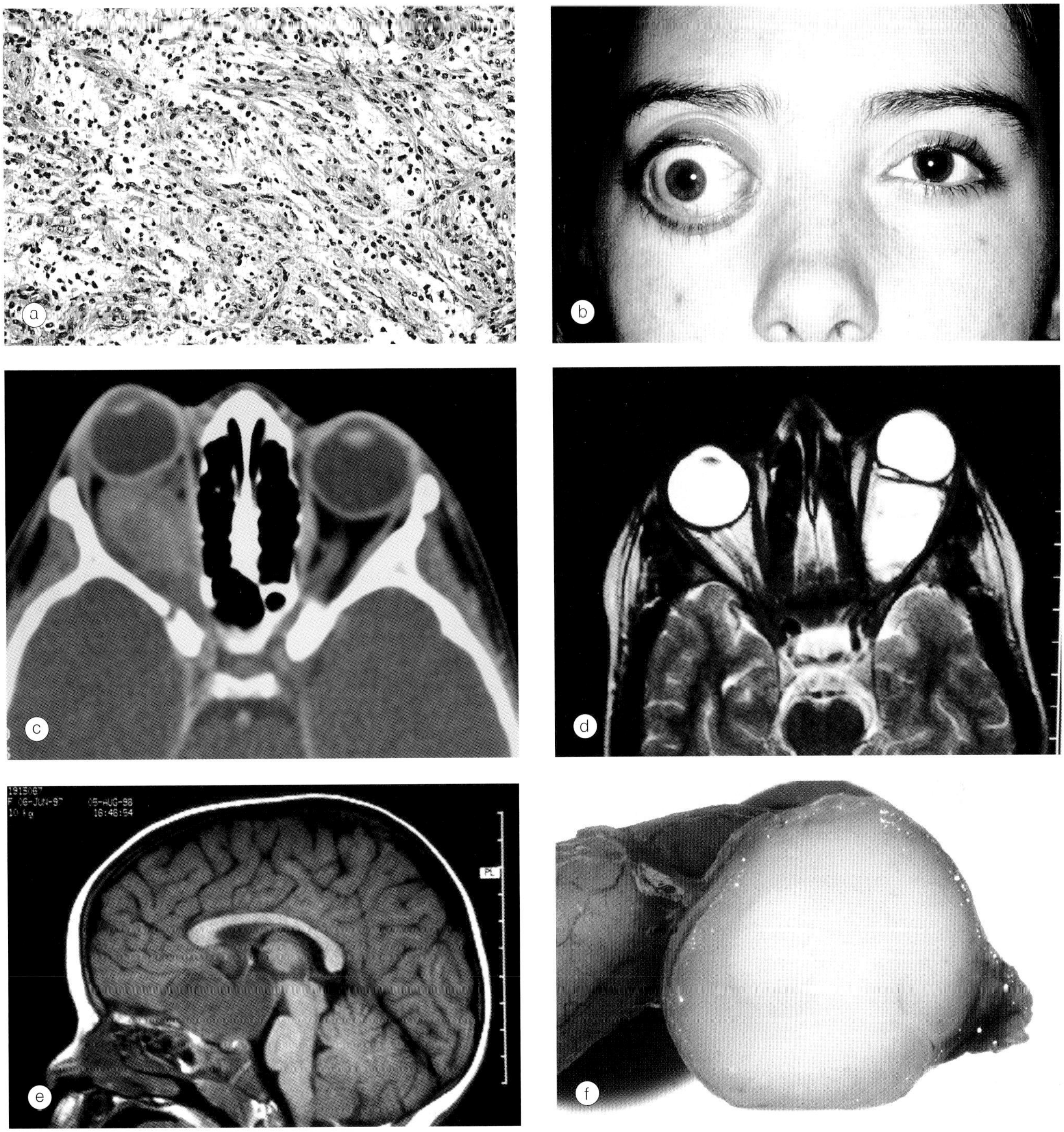

Fig. 6.45
Optic nerve glioma. **(a)** Histology shows spindle-shaped pilocytic astrocytes and glial filaments; **(b)** proptosis with inferior dystopia; **(c)** axial CT shows fusiform optic nerve enlargement; **(d)** axial T2-weighted MR in a different case shows a hyperintense mass; **(e)** sagittal T1-weighted MR shows invasion of the hypothalamus by an optic nerve glioma; **(f)** the cut surface of a surgical specimen is homogeneous (Courtesy of J Harry – figs a and f; A Pearson – figs c and d; D Armstrong – fig. e)

NB Malignant gliomas are rare and almost always occur in adults. The prognosis is very poor with almost certain death within one year of diagnosis.

Optic nerve sheath meningioma

Optic nerve sheath meningiomas arise from meningothelial cells of the arachnoid villi surrounding the intraorbital or, less commonly, the intracanalicular portion of the optic nerve. In some cases the tumour merely encircles the optic nerve whilst in others it invades the nerve by growing along the fibrovascular pial septae. Primary optic nerve sheath meningiomas are less common than optic nerve gliomas and, as with other meningiomas, typically affect middle-aged women.

1. **Histology** shows two main types – the meningothelial is characterized by varying-sized irregular lobules of meningothelial cells separated by fibrovascular strands; (Fig. 6.46a); the psammomatous shows psammoma bodies among proliferating meningothelial cells (Fig. 6.46b).
2. **Presentation** is with gradual unilateral visual impairment. Transient obscurations of vision may be the presenting symptom.
3. **Signs.** The classical triad is (a) visual loss; (b) optic atrophy; (c) opticociliary shunt vessels. However, the simultaneous occurrence of all three signs in one individual is uncommon. The sequence of involvement is as follows:
   - Optic nerve dysfunction and chronic disc swelling followed by atrophy.
   - Opticociliary collaterals (see Fig. 6.4c), found in about 30% of cases, regress as optic atrophy supervenes.
   - Restrictive motility defects, particularly in up-gaze, because the tumour may 'splint' the optic nerve.
   - Proptosis caused by intraconal spread – usually develops after the onset of visual loss.

NB This sequence is the opposite of that seen with tumours outside the dural sheath, in which proptosis develops long before optic nerve compression.

4. **CT** shows thickening and calcification of the optic nerve (Fig. 6.46c).
5. **MR** more clearly detects smaller tumours and those around the optic canal (Fig. 6.46d).
6. **Treatment** may not be required in middle-aged patients with slow-growing tumours because the prognosis is good. Surgical excision is required in young patients with aggressive tumours, particularly if the eye is also blind.

Fractionated stereotactic radiotherapy may be appropriate in selected cases or as adjunctive treatment following surgery.
7. **Prognosis** for life is good in adults, although the tumour may be more aggressive and sometimes fatal in children.

Secondary meningioma

Secondary meningiomas arise intracranially, usually from the sphenoidal ridge, tuberculum sellae or olfactory groove and subsequently invade the optic canal and orbit (see Chapter 21).

Plexiform neurofibroma

Plexiform neurofibroma is the most common peripheral neural tumour of the orbit and occurs almost exclusively in association with neurofibromatosis-1 (see Chapter 24).

1. **Presentation** is in early childhood with periorbital swelling.
2. **Signs**
   - Diffuse involvement of the orbit with disfiguring hypertrophy of periocular tissues (Fig. 6.47).
   - Involvement of the eyelids causes mechanical ptosis with a characteristic S-shaped deformity.
   - On palpation the involved tissues feel like a bag of worms.
3. **Treatment** is often unsatisfactory and complete surgical removal is extremely difficult. Orbital surgery should be avoided if at all possible because of the intricate relationship between the tumour and important orbital structures.

Isolated neurofibroma

Isolated (localized) neurofibroma is less common and is associated with neurofibromatosis-1 in about 10% of cases.

1. **Presentation** is in the third to fourth decades with insidious mildly painful proptosis unassociated with visual impairment or ocular motility dysfunction.
2. **Treatment** by excision is usually straightforward because the tumour is well-circumscribed and relatively avascular.

Lymphoma

Lymphomas of the ocular adnexae constitute approximately 8% of all extranodal lymphomas. They represent one end of the spectrum of lymphoproliferative lesions, at the other end of which lies benign reactive lymphoid hyperplasia. Accurate diagnosis of the type of lymphoma has improved

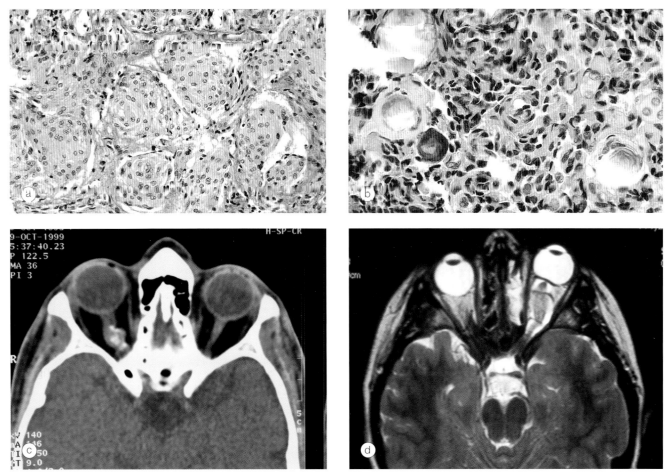

Fig. 6.46
Optic nerve meningioma. **(a)** Histology of meningothelial type; **(b)** histology of psammomatous type; **(c)** axial CT of a small tumour shows slight thickening and calcification; **(d)** axial T2-weighted MR in a more advanced case shows fusiform enlargement of the optic nerve and proptosis (Courtesy of J Harry and G Misson, from *Clinical Ophthalmic Pathology*, Butterworth-Heinemann, 2001 – figs a and b; A Pearson – figs c and d)

considerably with the introduction of immunological staining methods.

1. **Classification** is complex and is based on the overall histological appearance (diffuse or nodular) and the cell type (B, T and NK cells). The currently used classification is the WHO-REAL (World Health Organization – Revised European/American Lymphoma) classification. Most orbital lesions are extranodal marginal B cell lymphomas and many are derived from lacrimal gland-associated MALT (Mucosa-Associated Lymphoid Tissue) (Fig. 6.48a).
2. **Presentation** is insidious and usually in old age.
3. **Signs**
   • Any part of the orbit may be affected and occasionally involvement is bilateral (Fig. 6.48b and c).
   • Anterior lesions may be palpated and have a rubbery consistency (Fig. 6.48d).

   • Occasionally the lymphoma may be confined to the conjunctiva or lacrimal glands, sparing the orbit.
4. **Systemic investigations** in patients with lymphoid lesions of the orbit include chest radiographs, serum immunoprotein electrophoresis, thoraco-abdominal CT to detect possible retroperitoneal involvement and, if necessary, bone marrow aspiration.
5. **Course** is variable and may be unpredictable. In some patients histological features raise suspicion of malignancy and yet the lesion resolves spontaneously or with the help of steroids. Conversely, what appears to be a benign reactive lymphoid hyperplasia may be followed several years later by the development of lymphoma. Small lymphoproliferations and those involving the conjunctiva have the best prognosis.
6. **Treatment** involves radiotherapy for localized lesions and chemotherapy for disseminated disease.

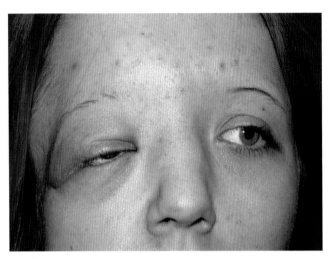

Fig. 6.47
Plexiform neurofibroma causing periorbital involvement and facial disfigurement (Courtesy of A Pearson)

Embryonal sarcoma

Embryonal sarcoma (traditionally designated 'rhabdomyosarcoma') is the most common primary orbital malignancy of childhood. The tumour is derived from undifferentiated mesenchymal cell rests, which have the potential to differentiate into striated muscle. They do not arise from striated muscle, and the term rhabdomyosarcoma is appropriate only if there is evidence of differentiation into muscle. The main role of the ophthalmologist is confined to diagnosis by incisional biopsy followed by prompt referral to a paediatric oncologist.

1. **Histology.** Undifferentiated tumours show a mass of loosely arranged mesenchymal cells (Fig. 6.49a). Differentiated tumours contain elongated and strap-like cells with a 'tadpole' or 'tennis-racket' configuration (rhabdomyoblasts – Fig. 6.49b) with or without cross-striations (Fig. 6.49c).

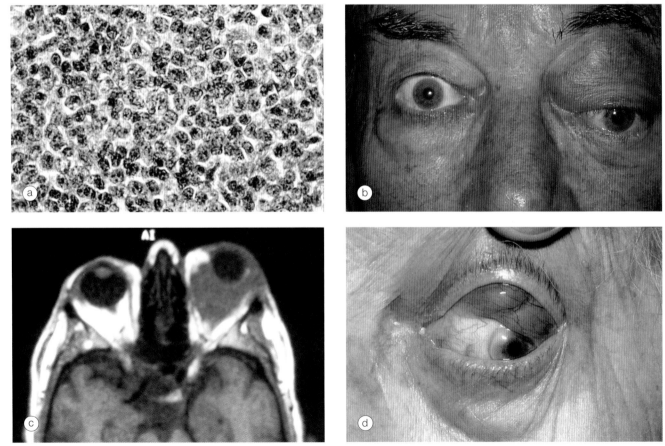

Fig. 6.48
Orbital lymphoma. **(a)** Histology shows neoplastic lymphoid cells; **(b)** involvement of the superior orbit causing proptosis and inferior dystopia; **(c)** axial T1-weighted MR of the same patient shows a large orbital soft tissue mass and proptosis; **(d)** anterior lesion
(Courtesy of J Harry – fig. a; A Pearson – figs b and c)

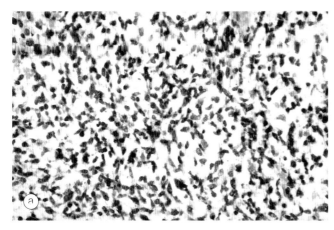

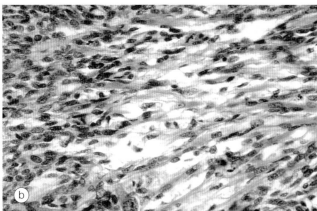

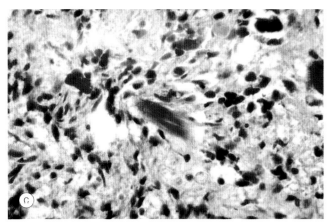

Fig. 6.49
Histology of embryonal sarcoma. **(a)** Undifferentiated tumour with loosely-arranged proliferation of mesenchymal cells; **(b)** differentiated tumour shows many elongated strap-like cells with eosinophilic cytoplasm (rhabdomyoblasts); **(c)** differentiated tumour in which the rhabdomyoblast in the centre of the field has cross-striations; Masson trichrome stain (Courtesy of J Harry and G Misson, from *Clinical Ophthalmic Pathology*, Butterworth-Heinemann, 2001)

2. **Presentation** is in the first decade (average 7 years) with rapidly progressive unilateral proptosis which may initially mimic an inflammatory process.
3. **Signs**
   - The tumour is most frequently superonasal or retrobulbar followed by superior and inferior (Fig. 6.50a).
   - A palpable mass and ptosis are present in about one-third of cases.
   - Swelling and injection of overlying skin develop later but the skin is not warm (Fig. 6.50b).
   - In advanced cases tumour spread to the sinuses may be seen (Fig. 6.50c).
4. **MR** shows a poorly defined mass of homogeneous density, often with adjacent bony destruction (Fig. 6.50d).
5. **Systemic investigations** for evidence of metastatic spread include chest x-ray, liver function tests, bone marrow biopsy, lumbar puncture and skeletal survey. The most common sites for metastases are lung and bone.
6. **Treatment** involves radiotherapy and chemotherapy with vincristine, actinomycin and cyclophosphamide. Surgical excision is reserved for the rare recurrent or radio-resistant tumour.
7. **Prognosis** is dependent on the stage and location of disease at the time of diagnosis. Patients with tumours localized to the orbit have a 95% cure rate.
8. **Differential diagnosis** includes orbital cellulitis which typically presents in children with similar acute signs although in embryonal sarcoma the skin is not warm. Other tumours such as metastatic neuroblastoma and myeloid sarcoma may also present similarly with a rapidly growing orbital mass (see below).

Adult metastatic tumours

Orbital metastases are an infrequent cause of proptosis and are much less common than metastases to the choroid. If the orbit is the initial manifestation of the tumour, the ophthalmologist may be the first person to see the patient. In order of frequency the most common primary sites are breast, bronchus, prostate, skin melanoma, gastrointestinal tract and kidney.

1. **Presentation**
   - A mass causing dystopia and proptosis is the most common (Fig. 6.51a).
   - Infiltration of orbital tissues characterized by ptosis, diplopia, brawny indurated periorbital skin and a firm orbit, characterized by resistance to manual retropulsion of the globe.
   - Enophthalmos with scirrhous tumours.
   - Chronic orbital inflammation.
   - Primarily with involvement of the cranial nerves (II, III, IV, V, VI) at the orbital apex and only mild proptosis.

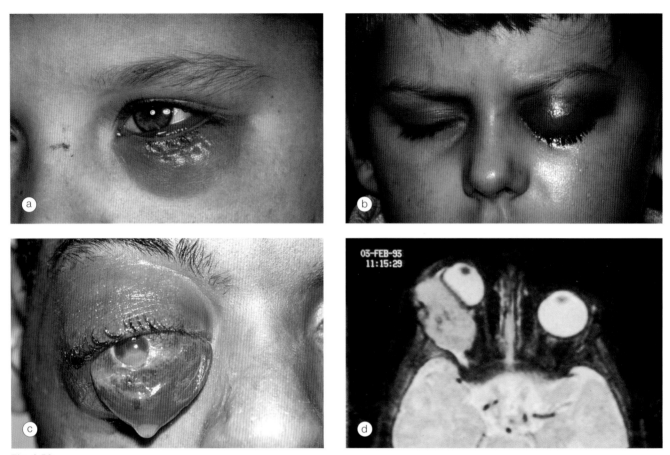

Fig. 6.50
Embryonal sarcoma. **(a)** Early anterior involvement; **(b)** more advanced involvement with redness of overlying eyelid skin; **(c)** very advanced tumour; **(d)** axial T2-weighted MR shows a poorly defined mass which indents the globe and causes proptosis (Courtesy of M Szreter – fig. b; A Pearson – fig. d)

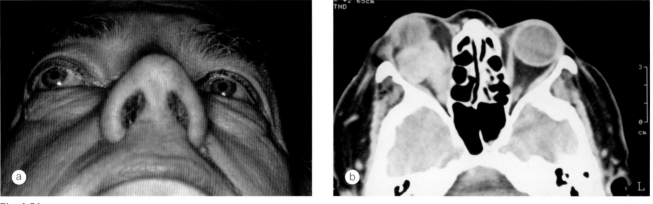

Fig. 6.51
Metastatic carcinoma. **(a)** Proptosis and dystopia; **(b)** axial CT shows a non-encapsulated retrobulbar mass (Courtesy of A Pearson – fig. b)

2. **Fine needle biopsy** under CT control (Fig. 6.51b) is useful for histological confirmation. If this fails, open biopsy may be required.

3. **Treatment** is aimed at preserving vision and relieving pain because most patients die within a year. Radiotherapy is the mainstay of treatment. Orbital exenteration rarely may be required if other modalities fail to control intolerable symptoms.

Childhood metastatic tumours

Neuroblastoma

Neuroblastoma is one of the most common childhood malignancies. It arises from primitive neuroblasts of the sympathetic chain, most commonly in the abdomen, followed by the thorax and pelvis. Presentation is usually in early childhood; in almost half the cases the tumour is disseminated at diagnosis with an appalling prognosis. Orbital metastases may be bilateral and typically present with an abrupt onset of proptosis accompanied by a superior orbital mass and lid ecchymosis (Fig. 6.52a).

Myeloid sarcoma

Myeloid sarcoma, previously referred to as granulocytic sarcoma and chloroma, is a localized tumour composed of malignant cells of myeloid origin. Because the tumour may exhibit a characteristic green colour it was formerly referred to as chloroma. Granulocytic sarcoma may occur as a manifestation of established myeloid leukaemia or it may precede the disease. Presentation is most frequently at about age 7 years with rapid onset of proptosis, sometimes bilateral, which may be associated with ecchymosis and lid oedema (Fig. 6.52b). When orbital involvement precedes systemic leukaemia the diagnosis may be difficult.

Langerhans cell granulomatosis

Langerhans cell granulomatosis is a rare, poorly understood, multisystem disease characterized by destructive inflammatory lesions that primarily involve bone. Soft tissues are less commonly involved, but cutaneous and visceral involvement may occur. Patients with solitary lesions (usually eosinophilic granuloma) have a benign course and respond well to treatment. Orbital involvement consists of unilateral or bilateral osteolytic lesions and soft-tissue

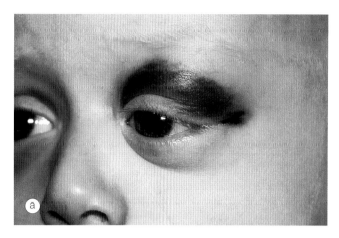
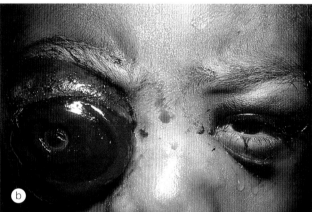
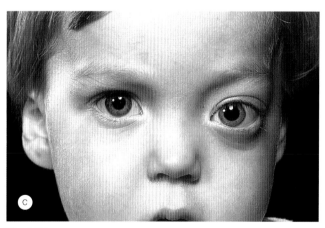

Fig. 6.52
Childhood orbital metastatic tumours. **(a)** Neuroblastoma; **(b)** advanced myeloid sarcoma; **(c)** Langerhans-cell histiocytosis (Courtesy of D Taylor – fig. c)

involvement, typically in the supero-temporal quadrant (Fig. 6.52c).

Orbital invasion by sinus tumours

Malignant tumours of the paranasal sinuses, although rare, may invade the orbit and carry a poor prognosis unless diagnosed early. It is therefore important to be aware of both their otolaryngological and ophthalmic features.

1. **Maxillary carcinoma** is by far the most common sinus tumour to invade the orbit (Fig. 6.53).
   - Otolaryngological manifestations include facial pain and swelling, epistaxis and nasal discharge.
   - Ophthalmic features include upward dystopia, diplopia and epiphora.
2. **Ethmoidal carcinoma** may cause lateral dystopia.
3. **Nasopharyngeal carcinoma** may spread to the orbit through the inferior orbital fissure; proptosis is a late finding.

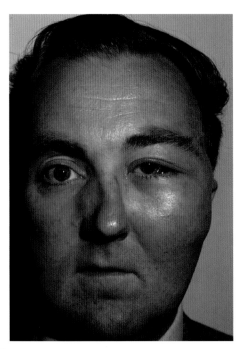

Fig. 6.53
Advanced maxillary carcinoma showing facial swelling and upward dystopia

DRY EYE DISORDERS

Definitions

Dry eye occurs when there is inadequate tear volume or function resulting in an unstable tear film and ocular surface disease.

1. **Keratoconjunctivitis sicca** (KCS) refers to any eye with some degree of dryness.
2. **Xerophthalmia** describes a dry eye associated with vitamin A deficiency.
3. **Xerosis** refers to extreme ocular dryness and keratinization that occurs in eyes with severe conjunctival cicatrization.
4. **Sjögren syndrome** is an autoimmune inflammatory disease which is usually associated with dry eyes.

Physiology

Tear film constituents

The tear film has three layers (Fig. 7.1):

1. **Lipid** layer secreted by the meibomian glands.
2. **Aqueous** layer secreted by the lacrimal glands.
3. **Mucin** layer secreted principally by conjunctival goblet cells.

Spread of the tear film

The tear film is mechanically spread over the ocular surface through a neuronally controlled blinking mechanism. Three factors are required for effective resurfacing of the tear film:
• Normal blink reflex.
• Contact between the external ocular surface and eyelids.
• Normal corneal epithelium.

Outer lipid layer

1. **Composition**
   • The outer lipid layer is composed of a polar phase containing phospholipids adjacent to the aqueous-mucin phase, and a non-polar phase containing waxes, cholesterol esters and triglycerides.
   • The polar lipids are bound to lipocalins within the aqueous layer which are small secreted proteins that have the ability to bind hydrophobic molecules and may also contribute to tear viscosity.
   • Lid movement during blinking is important in releasing lipids from the glands. The thickness of the layer can be increased by forced blinking and conversely reduced by infrequent blinking.
2. **Functions**
   • To prevent evaporation of the aqueous layer and maintain tear film thickness.
   • To act as a surfactant allowing spread of the tear film.
   • Deficiency results in evaporative dry eye.

Middle aqueous layer

1. **Secretion**
   • The main lacrimal glands produce about 95% of the aqueous component of tears; the accessory lacrimal glands of Krause and Wolfring produce the remainder.
   • Secretion of tears has basic (resting) and much greater reflex components. The latter occurs in response to corneal and conjunctival sensory stimulation, tear break-up and ocular inflammation mediated via the fifth cranial nerve. It is reduced by topical anaesthesia and during sleep. Secretion can increase 500% in response to injury.
2. **Composition**
   • Water, electrolytes, dissolved mucins and proteins.

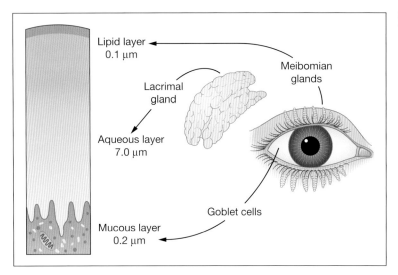

Fig. 7.1
The three layers of the tear film

- Growth factors derived from the lacrimal gland, production of which increases in response to injury.
- Pro-inflammatory interleukin cytokines which accumulate during sleep when tear production is reduced.

3. **Functions**
- To provide atmospheric oxygen to the corneal epithelium.
- Antibacterial function due to the presence of proteins such as IgA, lysozyme and lactoferrin.
- To wash away debris and noxious stimuli and allow the passage of leucocytes after injury.
- To provide a smooth optical surface to the cornea by abolishing minute irregularities of the anterior corneal surface.

Inner mucin layer

1. **Composition**
- Mucins are high molecular weight glycoproteins that may be transmembrane or secretory.
- Secretory mucins are further classified as gel-forming or soluble. They are principally produced by the conjunctival goblet cells and also by the lacrimal glands.
- The superficial epithelial cells of the cornea and conjunctiva produce transmembrane mucins that form the glycocalyx.
- Epithelial staining with rose bengal indicates that the transmembrane and gel mucin layer is absent and the cell surface exposed. Damage to the epithelial cells will prevent normal tear film adherence.

2. **Functions**
- To permit wetting by converting the corneal epithelium from a hydrophobic to a hydrophilic surface.
- Lubrication.

NB Deficiency of the mucin layer may be a feature of both aqueous deficiency and evaporative states. Goblet cell loss is associated with cicatrizing conjunctivitis, vitamin A deficiency, chemical burns and toxicity to medications.

Regulation of tear film components

1. **Hormonal**
- Androgens are the prime hormones that regulate lipid production.
- Oestrogen and progesterone receptors in conjunctiva and lacrimal gland are essential for normal function of these tissues.
2. **Neural** fibres adjacent to the lacrimal gland and goblet cells result in aqueous and mucus secretion.

Mechanism of disease

Inflammation in the conjunctiva and accessory glands is present in 80% of patients with KCS and may be the cause and consequence of dry eye, amplifying and perpetuating disease. The presence of inflammation is the rationale for steroid therapy. Hyperosmolarity of tears is also a key mechanism of disease and may be the major pathway for epithelial cell damage.

Classification

The following classification is usually applied although most individuals have considerable overlap between mechanisms (Table 7.1). Table 7.2 shows the causes of non-Sjögren KCS and Table 7.3 the causes of evaporative KCS.

Table 7.1   Classification of KCS

Aqueous layer deficiency
- Sjögren syndrome
- Non-Sjögren

Evaporative
- Meibomian gland disease
- Exposure
- Defective blinking
- Contact lens associated
- Environmental factors

Sjögren syndrome

Sjögren syndrome is a systemic autoimmune condition characterized by lymphocytic infiltration of the exocrine glands and mucous membranes resulting in a secondary reduction in secretion, leading to abnormalities in the tear film and ocular surfaces disease. The primary features are KCS and dry eye with dry mouth (xerostomia).

NB Detection of associated disease is important because patients are also at risk of developing keratitis and scleritis or a life threatening systemic vasculitis.

1. **Diagnostic criteria**
   a. *Symptomatic*
      - Ocular symptoms or the use of artificial tear substitutes.
      - Oral symptoms of xerostomia, swollen salivary glands or frequent need to drink.
   b. *Objective*
      - Objective evidence of KCS (see below).
      - Positive involvement of minor salivary gland on labial biopsy.
      - Salivary involvement demonstrated by sialography or scintigraphy.
      - Laboratory evaluation for extractable nuclear antigens, anti-nuclear antibody (ANA) or rheumatoid factor (RF).
2. **Primary** Sjögren syndrome may have systemic manifestations (arthralgia, myalgia and fatigue) that do not constitute a readily classifiable disease (see Chapter 24). Diagnostic criteria require histology or serology to be positive with a total of four criteria fulfilled, or three of the four objective criteria.
3. **Secondary** Sjögren syndrome is associated with an underlying distinct autoimmune disease. Examples include rheumatoid arthritis, systemic lupus erythematosus, scleroderma, dermatomyositis and polymyositis, mixed connective disease, relapsing polychondritis and primary biliary cirrhosis. Diagnostic criteria require confirmation of disease and two other objective criteria.

Table 7.2   Causes of non-Sjögren KCS

1. **Primary age-related hyposecretion**
2. **Lacrimal tissue destruction**
   - Tumour
   - Inflammation (e.g. pseudotumour or sarcoidosis)
3. **Absence or reduction of lacrimal gland tissue**
   - Surgical removal
   - Rarely congenital
4. **Conjunctival scarring with obstruction of lacrimal gland ductules**
   - Chemical burns
   - Cicatricial pemphigoid
   - Stevens–Johnson syndrome
   - Old trachoma
5. **Neurological lesions with sensory or motor reflex loss**
   - Familial dysautonomia (Riley–Day syndrome)
   - Parkinson's disease
   - Reduced sensation may also contribute to dry eye after refractive surgery and contact lens wear
6. **Vitamin A deficiency**

Table 7.3   Causes of evaporative KCS

1. **Meibomian gland dysfunction**
   - Posterior blepharitis
   - Rosacea
   - Atopic keratoconjunctivitis
   - Congenital meibomian gland absence
2. **Lagophthalmos**
   - Severe proptosis
   - Facial nerve palsy
   - Eyelid scarring
   - Following blepharoplasty
3. **Miscellaneous**
   - Contact lens wear
   - Environmental factors such as air conditioning

NB Exclusion criteria for Sjögren syndrome include head or neck irradiation, hepatitis C infection, AIDS, lymphoma, sarcoidosis, graft versus host disease and the use of anticholinergic drugs.

Clinical features

Symptoms

The most common symptoms are feelings of dryness, grittiness and burning that characteristically worsen during the day. Stringy discharge, transient blurring of vision, redness and crusting of the lids are also common. Lack of emotional or reflex tearing is, however, uncommon.

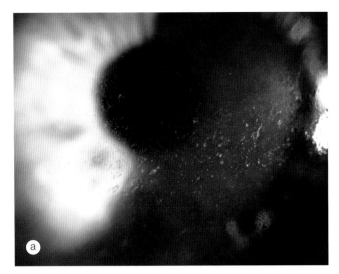

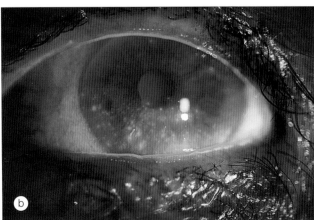

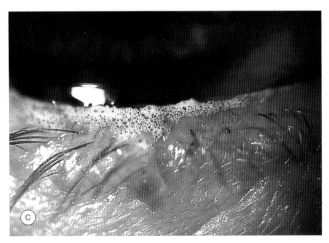

Fig. 7.2
Tear film abnormalities in dry eye. **(a)** Mucous debris; **(b)** thin marginal tear meniscus and inferior punctate erosions stained with fluorescein; **(c)** foam on the lid margin

NB The symptoms of KCS are frequently exacerbated on exposure to conditions associated with increased tear evaporation (e.g. air-conditioning, wind and central heating) or prolonged reading, when blink frequency is reduced.

Signs

1. **Posterior blepharitis** and meibomian gland dysfunction may be present.
2. **Conjunctiva** may show mild keratinization and redness.
3. **Tear film**
   - In the normal eye, as the tear film breaks down, the mucin layer becomes contaminated with lipid but is washed away. In the dry eye, the lipid-contaminated mucin accumulates in the tear film as particles and debris that move with each blink (Fig. 7.2a).
   - The marginal tear meniscus is a crude measure of the volume of aqueous in the tear film. In the normal eye the meniscus is about 1mm in height, while in dry eye the tear meniscus becomes thin (Fig. 7.2b) or absent.
   - Froth in the tear film or along the eyelid margin occurs in meibomian gland dysfunction (Fig. 7.2c).
4. **Cornea**
   - Punctate epithelial erosions that stain with fluorescein involving the interpalpebral and inferior cornea (see Fig. 7.2b).
   - Filaments consist of mucus strands lined with epithelium attached at one end to the corneal surface (Fig. 7.3a) that stain well with rose bengal (Fig. 7.3b).
   - Mucus plaques consist of semi-transparent, white-to-grey, slightly elevated lesions of various sizes. They are composed of mucus, epithelial cells and proteinaceous and lipoidal material and are usually seen in association with corneal filaments (Fig. 7.3c).
5. **Complications** in very severe cases include peripheral superficial corneal neovascularization, epithelial breakdown, melting (Fig. 7.4a) and perforation, and bacterial keratitis (Fig. 7.4b).

Special investigations

The aim of investigation is to confirm and quantify the diagnosis of dry eye. Unfortunately, although the repeatability of symptoms is good that of clinical tests is poor, as is the correlation between symptoms and tests. The reliability of tests improves as the severity of dry eye increases. The tests measure the following parameters:
- Stability of the tear film (break-up time).
- Tear production (Schirmer, fluorescein clearance and tear osmolarity).
- Ocular surface disease (corneal stains and impression cytology).

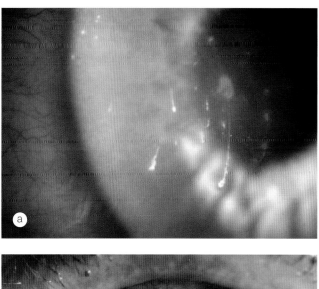

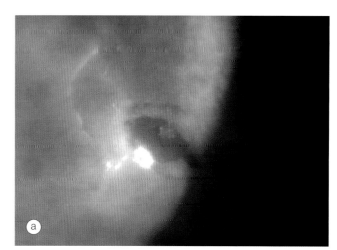

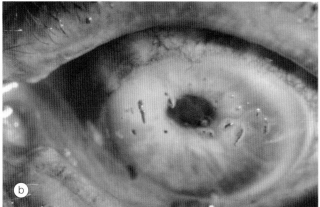

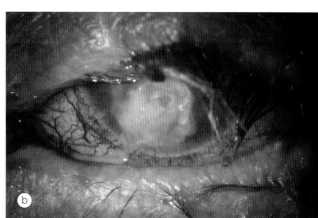

Fig. 7.4
Severe corneal complications of dry eye. **(a)** Melting;
(b) bacterial infection (Courtesy of S Tuft)

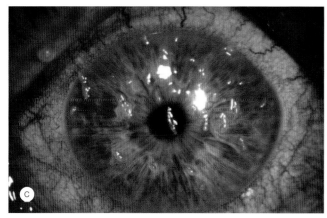

Fig. 7.3
Filamentary keratitis. **(a)** Several fine filaments; **(b)** filaments
stained with rose bengal; **(c)** filaments and mucus plaques
(Courtesy of S. Tuft – figs a and c; W Wykes – fig. b)

NB There is no clinical test to confirm the diagnosis of
evaporative dry eye. It is therefore a presumptive diagnosis
based on the presence of meibomian gland disease. Tarsal
transillumination to visualize the meibomian glands can
give an indication of gland drop-out

It is suggested the tests are performed in the following order
because the Schirmer strip paper can damage the ocular
surface and cause staining.

Tear film break-up time

The tear film break-up time (BUT) is abnormal in aqueous tear
deficiency and meibomian gland disorders. It is measured as
follows:

a. Fluorescein 2% or an impregnated fluorescein strip
   moistened with non-preserved saline is instilled into the
   lower fornix.
b. The patient is asked to blink several times.
c. The tear film is examined with a broad beam and a cobalt
   blue filter. After an interval of time, black spots or lines
   appear in the fluorescein stained film, indicating the
   formation of dry areas (Fig. 7.5a).

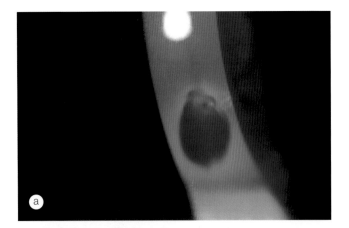

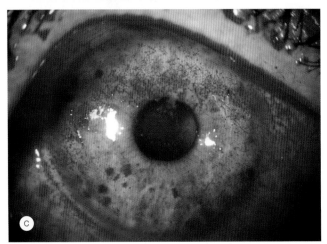

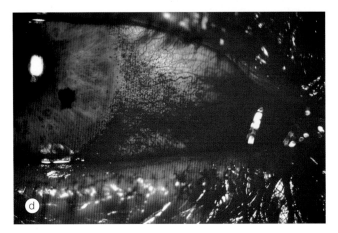

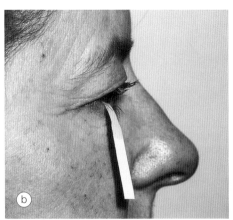

Fig. 7.5
Diagnostic tests in dry eye. **(a)** Tear film break-up time; a dry spot is shown in a fluorescein-stained tear film; **(b)** Schirmer test; **(c)** corneal staining with rose bengal; **(d)** conjunctival staining with rose bengal (Courtesy of S Tuft – fig. c)

Schirmer test

Schirmer test is a useful assessment of aqueous tear production. The test involves measuring the amount of wetting of a special (no. 41 Whatman) filter paper, 5mm wide and 35mm long. The test can be performed with or without topical anaesthesia. In theory, when performed with an anaesthetic (Schirmer 1) it measures basic secretion whereas without anaesthetic and with nasal stimulation (Schirmer 2) it measures maximum basic and reflex secretion. In practice, however, topical anaesthesia cannot abolish all sensory and psychological stimuli for reflex secretion. The test is performed as follows:

a. The eye is gently dried of excess tears. If topical anaesthesia is applied the excess should be removed from the inferior fornix with filter paper.
b. The filter paper is folded 5mm from one end and inserted at the junction of the middle and outer third of the lower lid, taking care not to touch the cornea or lashes (Fig. 7.5b).
c. The patient is asked to keep the eyes gently closed.
d. After 5 minutes the filter paper is removed and the amount of wetting from the fold measured.
e. Less than 10mm of wetting after 5 minutes without anaesthesia and less than 6mm with anaesthesia is considered abnormal.

d. The BUT is the interval between the last blink and the appearance of the first randomly distributed dry spot. A BUT of less than 10 seconds is abnormal.

NB The development of dry spots always in the same location may indicate a local corneal surface abnormality (e.g. epithelial basement membrane disease) rather than an intrinsic instability of the tear film.

NB Results can be variable and a single Schirmer test should not be used as the sole criterion for diagnosing dry eye but repeatedly abnormal tests are highly supportive.

Ocular surface staining

1. **Fluorescein** stains corneal and conjunctival epithelium where there is sufficient damage to allow the dye to enter the tissues. In intensely dry eyes there may be no apparent staining due to dye quenching; staining can then be demonstrated by adding a drop of saline to the inferior fornix.
2. **Rose bengal** is a dye that has an affinity for dead or devitalized epithelial cells that have a lost or altered mucous layer. Corneal filaments and plaques are also shown up more clearly by the dye and the use of a red free filter may help visualization. A 1% solution of rose bengal or a moistened impregnated strip can be used.

NB Rose bengal may cause intense stinging that can last for up to a day, particularly in patients with severe KCS. To minimize irritation a very small drop should be used, immediately preceded by a drop of topical anaesthetic, and the excess washed out with saline.

3. **The pattern** of staining may aid diagnosis as follows:
   - Interpalpebral staining of the cornea and conjunctiva is common in aqueous tear deficiency (Fig. 7.5c and d).
   - Superior conjunctival stain may indicate superior limbic keratoconjunctivitis.
   - Inferior corneal and conjunctival stain is often seen in patients with blepharitis or exposure.

Other tests

The following tests are rarely performed in clinical practice.

1. **Fluorescein clearance test** and the tear function index may be assessed by placing 5µl of fluorescein on the ocular surface and measuring the residual dye in a Schirmer strip placed on the lower lateral lid margin at intervals of 1, 10, 20 and 30 minutes. The presence of fluorescein on each strip is examined under blue light and compared to a standard scale or measured using fluorophotometry. In normal eyes the value will have fallen to zero after 20 minutes. Delayed clearance is observed in all dry eye states.
2. **Lactoferrin** is the major protein secreted by the lacrimal gland. Tear lactoferrin is decreased in Sjögren syndrome and other lacrimal gland diseases. Commercially available immunoassay kits are available to measure lactoferrin in body fluids.
3. **Phenol red thread test** uses a thread impregnated with a pH sensitive dye. The end of the thread is placed over the lower lid and the length that is wet (dye changes yellow to red in tears) is measured after 15 seconds. A value of 6mm

is abnormal. It is comparable with the Schirmer test but takes less time.
4. **Tear meniscometry** is a technique to quantify the height and thus the volume of the lower lid meniscus.
5. **Tear film osmolarity** measurement techniques are available as research tools.
6. **Impression cytology** to determine goblet cell numbers.

Treatment

Dry eye is generally not curable and management is therefore structured around the control of symptoms and prevention of surface damage. The choice of treatment depends on the severity of the disease and involves one or more of the following measures alone or in combination.

Patient education

- Establishment of a realistic expectation of outcome and emphasis on the importance of compliance.
- Avoidance of toxic drugs or environmental factors and discontinuation of toxic topical medication if possible.
- Review of work environment.
- Emphasis on the importance of blinking whist reading or using VDU.
- Aids should be provided for patients with a loss of dexterity (e.g. rheumatoid arthritis). Plastic dropper bottles can be held in a nut-cracker as small unit dispensers may not be appropriate.
- Caution against laser refractive surgery.
- Discussion of management of contact lens intolerance.

Tear substitutes

Tear substitutes have a relatively simple formulation that cannot approximate the complex number of components and structure of the normal tear film (Table 7.4). Their delivery is also periodic rather than continuous. Almost all are based on replacement of the aqueous phase of the tear film. There are no mucus substitutes, and paraffin is only an approximation to the action of tear lipids.

1. **Drops and gels**
   - Cellulose derivatives are appropriate for mild cases.
   - Carbomers cling to the eyelids and are longer lasting.
   - Polyvinyl alcohol increases the persistence of the tear film and is useful in mucin deficiency.
   - Sodium hyaluronate may be useful in promoting conjunctival and corneal epithelial healing.
   - Autologous serum may be used in very severe cases.
   - Povidone and sodium chloride.
2. **Ointments** containing petrolatum mineral oil can be used at bedtime.

Table 7.4 Tear substitutes

Formulation	Name	Product and manufacturer	Disadvantage
Cellulose derivatives	Carboxymethylcellulose sodium 1% drops	Celluvisc (Allergan)	Deposits on lashes
	Hydroxypropylmethylcellulose drops	Hypromellose 0.3% (Generic) Hypromellose 0.5% (Isopto Plain – Alcon) Hypromellose 1% (Isopto Alkaline)	Poor contact time
	Hydroxyethylcellulose 0.44% and sodium chloride 0.35% drops	Minims Artificial Tears (Chauvin)	Short duration of action
	Dextran 70 0.1% and hypromellose 0.3% drops	Tears Naturale (Alcon)	Preservative limits frequency, lash deposits
Carbomers (polyacrylic acid)	Carbomer 980 0.2% gel	GelTears (Chauvin) Liposic (B & L) Viscotears (Novartis)	Preservative limits frequency
	Carbomer 974 0.25% gel	Liquivisc (Allergan)	
Polyvinyl alcohol	Polyvinyl alcohol (PVA) 1% drops Polyvinyl alcohol (PVA) 1.4% drops	Hypotears (Novartis) Liquifilm Tears (Allergan) Sno Tears (Chauvin)	
Povidone	Polyvinylpyrrolidone 5% drops	Oculotect (Novartis)	
Sodium chloride	Sodium chloride 0.9% drops	Minims Sodium Chloride (Chauvin)	
Sodium hyaluronate	Sodium hyaluronate 0.1% or 0.15%	Vismed Vislube	
Lipids and oils	Soft paraffin, liquid paraffin and wool fat	Simple (Generic) Lacri-Lube (Allergan) Lubri-Tears (Alcon)	
Acetylcysteine (mucolytic)	Acetylcysteine 5% and hypromellose 0.35%	Ilube (Alcon)	Stinging

NB The preservatives are a potential source of toxicity, especially after punctal occlusion. Non-preserved drops should therefore be used whenever possible.

Mucolytic agents

Acetylcysteine 5% drops (Ilube) q.i.d. may be useful in patients with corneal filaments and mucous plaques but may cause irritation following instillation. Acetylcysteine is also malodorous and has a limited bottle life so that it can only be used for up to 2 weeks. Debridement of filaments may also be useful.

Punctal occlusion

Punctal occlusion reduces drainage and thereby preserves natural tears and prolongs the effect of artificial tears. It is of greatest value in patients with moderate to severe KCS who have not responded to frequent use of topical treatment.

1. **Temporary** occlusion can be achieved by inserting collagen plugs into the canaliculi that dissolve in 1–2 weeks (Fig. 7.6a). The main aim is to ensure that epiphora

does not occur following permanent occlusion.
- Initially the inferior puncta are occluded and the patient is reviewed after one or two weeks.
- If the patient is now asymptomatic and without epiphora the plugs are removed and the inferior canaliculi are permanently occluded (see below).
- In severe KCS the inferior and superior canaliculi are plugged.

2. **Reversible** prolonged occlusion can be achieved with silicone or long-acting collagen plugs that dissolve in 2–6 months.
- Problems include extrusion, granuloma formation and distal migration.
- Plugs that pass into the horizontal portion of the canaliculus cannot be visualized and although they can usually be flushed out with saline, if they cause epiphora, this is not always possible.

3. **Permanent** occlusion should be undertaken only in patients with severe dry eye with repeated Schirmer test values of 5mm or less, and who have had a positive response to temporary plugs without epiphora. It should not be performed, if possible, in young patients who may have reversible pathology.

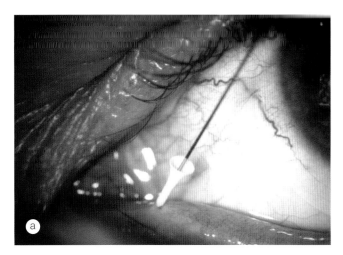

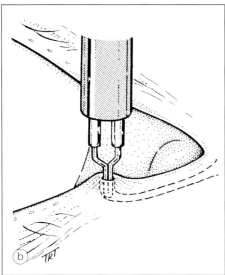

Fig. 7.6
Punctal occlusion. **(a)** Insertion of a silicone plug;
(b) cauterization (Courtesy of S Tuft – fig. a)

- Permanent occlusion is performed following punctal dilatation by coagulating the proximal canaliculus with cautery (Fig. 7.6b); following successful occlusion, it is important to watch for signs of recanalization.
- Diode laser cautery is less effective than thermal coagulation with higher rates of recanalization.

NB All four puncta should not be occluded at the same session.

Anti-inflammatory agents

1. **Low dose topical steroids** are effective supplementary treatment for acute exacerbations. The risks of long-term treatment must be balanced against the potential benefits of increased comfort.
2. **Topical ciclosporin** (0.05%, 0.1%) reduces T-cell mediated inflammation of lacrimal tissue, resulting in increase in the number of goblet cells and reversal of squamous metaplasia of the conjunctiva.
3. **Systemic tetracyclines** may control associated blepharitis and reduce inflammatory mediators in the tears.

Contact lenses

Although long-term contact lens wear may increase tear film evaporation, reduce tear flow and increase the risk of infection, these effects can be outweighed by the reservoir effect of fluid trapped behind the lens.

1. **Low water** content HEMA lenses may be successfully fitted to moderately dry eyes.
2. **Silicone** rubber lenses that contain no water and readily transmit oxygen are effective in protecting the cornea in extreme tear film deficiency. Deposition of debris on the surface of the lens can blur vision and be problematic. The continued availability of these lenses is in doubt.
3. **Occlusive** gas permeable scleral contact lenses provide a reservoir of saline over the cornea. They can be worn on an extremely dry eye with exposure.

Conservation of existing tears

1. **Reduction of room temperature,** by avoiding central heating, to minimize evaporation of tears.
2. **Room humidifiers** may be tried but are frequently disappointing because the apparatus is incapable of significantly increasing the relative humidity of an average-sized room. A temporary local increase in humidity can be achieved with moist chamber goggles or side shields to glasses but they may be cosmetically unacceptable.

Other options

1. **Tarsorrhaphy** diminishes surface evaporation by reducing the palpebral aperture.
2. **Botulinum toxin injection** to the orbicularis muscle may help control the blepharospasm in severe dry eye. Injected at the median canthus it reduces tear drainage, presumably by blocking lid movement.
3. **Oral cholinergic agonists** such as pilocarpine (5mg q.i.d) may reduce the symptoms of dry eye and dry mouth in patients with Sjögren syndrome. They may also cause blurred vision and intolerable sweating.
4. **Zidovudine,** an anti-retroviral agent, may be beneficial in primary Sjögren syndrome.
5. **Submandibular gland transplantation** for extreme dry eye requires extensive surgery and tends to produce unacceptable levels of mucus in the tear film.

CONJUNCTIVA

INTRODUCTION

Anatomy

The conjunctiva is a transparent mucous membrane lining the inner surface of the eyelids and surface of the globe as far as the limbus. It has a dense lymphatic supply and an abundance of immunocompetent cells. Mucus from the goblet cells and secretions from the accessory lacrimal glands are essential components of the tear film. The conjunctiva is part of the defensive barrier against infection. The lymphatic drainage is to the preauricular and submandibular nodes, which corresponds to the drainage of the eyelids. The conjunctiva may be subdivided into the following:

1. **The palpebral** conjunctiva starts at the mucocutaneous junction of the lid margins and is firmly attached to the posterior tarsal plates. The underlying tarsal blood vessels can be seen passing vertically from the lid margin and fornix.
2. **The forniceal** conjunctiva is loose and redundant and may be thrown into folds.
3. **The bulbar** conjunctiva covers the anterior sclera and is continuous with the corneal epithelium at the limbus. Radial ridges at the limbus form the palisades of Vogt. The stroma is loosely attached to the underlying Tenon capsule except at the limbus where the two layers fuse. A plica semilunaris (semilunar fold) is present nasally.

Histology

1. **The epithelium** is non-keratinizing and about five cell layers thick (Fig. 8.1). Basal cuboidal cells evolve into flattened polyhedral cells before they are shed from the

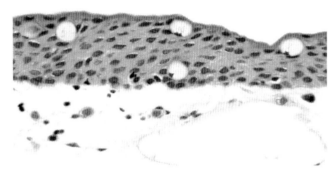

Fig. 8.1
Histology of the conjunctiva (Courtesy of J Harry)

surface. Goblet cells are located within the epithelium. They are most dense inferonasally and in the fornices, where they may account for 5–10% of the basal cells.
2. **The stroma** (substantia propria) consists of richly vascularized loose connective tissue. The adenoid superficial layer does not develop until about 3 months after birth, hence the inability of the newborn to produce a follicular conjunctival reaction. The deep fibrous layer merges with the tarsal plates. The accessory lacrimal glands of Krause and Wolfring are located deep within the stroma.

Features of conjunctival inflammation

Clinical features of particular relevance to the differential diagnosis of conjunctival inflammation are: symptoms, discharge, conjunctival reaction, membranes, associated keratopathy and lymphadenopathy.

Symptoms

Non-specific symptoms include lacrimation, gritty irritation, stinging and burning. Itching is the hallmark of allergic conjunctivitis, although it may also occur to a lesser extent in blepharitis and dry eye. Pain, photophobia and foreign body sensation suggest associated corneal involvement.

Discharge

1. **Watery** discharge is composed of a serous exudate and tears and occurs in acute viral or acute allergic conjunctivitis.
2. **Mucoid** discharge is typical of chronic allergic conjunctivitis and dry eye.
3. **Mucopurulent** discharge occurs in acute bacterial or chlamydial infections.
4. **Purulent** discharge is typical of gonococcal infection.

NB Patients often remove excessive discharge prior to examination.

Conjunctival reaction

1. **Conjunctival injection** that is diffuse, beefy-red and more intense away from the limbus is typical of bacterial infection (Fig. 8.2a).
2. **Haemorrhagic conjunctivitis** often occurs with viral infections and occasionally bacterial infections caused by *S. pneumoniae*, *H. influenzae* and *N. meningitidis* (Fig. 8.2b).
3. **Chemosis** may occur when the conjunctiva is severely inflamed producing a translucent swelling which may protrude through the closed lids (Fig. 8.2c). Acute chemosis usually indicates a hypersensitivity response whereas chronic oedema suggests orbital outflow constriction.
4. **Membranes**
   a. **Pseudomembranes** consist of coagulated exudate adherent to the inflamed conjunctival epithelium; they can be easily peeled leaving the epithelium intact (Fig. 8.2d).
   b. **True membranes** infiltrate the superficial layers of the conjunctival epithelium; attempted removal may be accompanied by tearing of the epithelium and bleeding.
   c. **Causes**
      – Severe adenoviral conjunctivitis.
      – Gonococcal conjunctivitis.
      – Ligneous conjunctivitis.
      – Acute Stevens–Johnson syndrome.
      – Bacterial infection (*Streptococcus* spp., *Corynebacterium diphtheriae*).

NB The distinction between a true membrane and a pseudomembrane is rarely clinically helpful; both can leave scarring following resolution.

5. **Infiltration** represents cellular recruitment to the site of chronic inflammation and typically accompanies a papillary response. It is recognized by loss of detail of the normal tarsal vessels, especially on the upper lid (Fig. 8.2e).
6. **Subconjunctival scarring** may occur in trachoma and cicatrizing disease (Fig. 8.2f). Severe scarring may cause loss of goblet cells and cicatricial entropion.
7. **Follicular reaction**
   a. **Signs.** Multiple, discrete, yellowish, slightly elevated lesions, most prominent in the fornices (Fig. 8.3a). The size of the lesions is related to severity and duration of disease. Vessels normally pass over the surface of the follicle and as it increases in size, they are displaced peripherally.

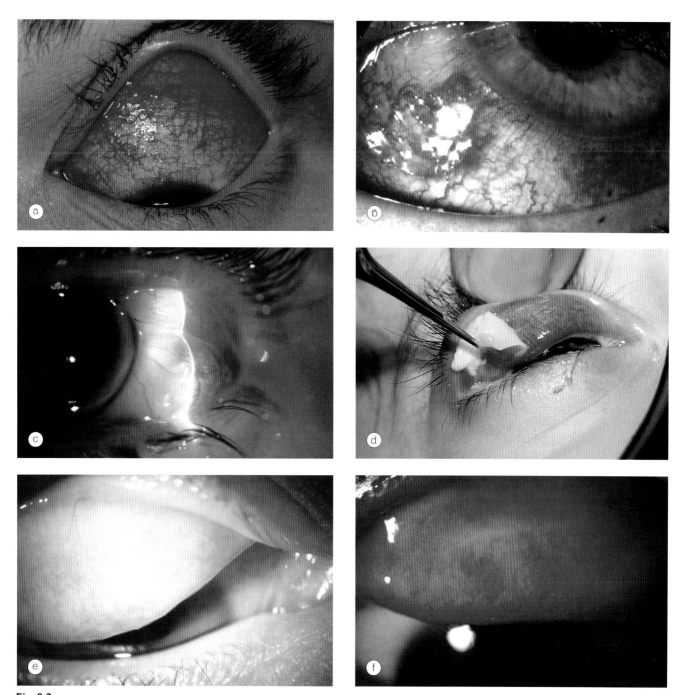

Fig. 8.2
Signs of conjunctival inflammation. **(a)** Injection; **(b)** haemorrhages; **(c)** chemosis; **(d)** pseudomembrane; **(e)** infiltration; **(f)** subconjunctival scarring (Courtesy of P Saine – fig. a; S Tuft – fig. b; J Dart – fig. d)

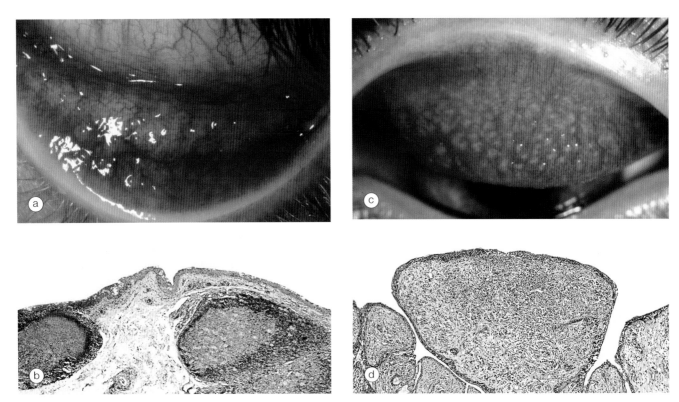

Fig. 8.3
(a) Conjunctival follicles; **(b)** histology shows two subepithelial germinal centres with immature lymphocytes centrally and mature cells peripherally; **(c)** conjunctival macropapillae; **(d)** histology shows folds of hyperplastic conjunctival epithelium with a fibrovascular core and subepithelial stromal infiltration with inflammatory cells (Courtesy of S Tuft – figs a and c; J Harry – figs b and d)

b. Histology shows a subepithelial germinal centre with immature lymphocytes centrally and mature cells peripherally (Fig. 8.3b).

c. Causes
  – Viral conjunctivitis.
  – Chlamydial conjunctivitis.
  – Parinaud oculoglandular syndrome.
  – Hypersensitivity to topical medications.

NB Small follicles are a normal finding in childhood (folliculosis), as are those in the fornices and at the margin of the upper tarsal plate in adults.

8. Papillary reaction
  a. Signs. Papillae can only develop in the palpebral conjunctiva and the limbal bulbar conjunctiva where it is attached to the deeper fibrous layer.
  – Micropapillae form a mosaic-like pattern of elevated red dots as a result of the central vascular channel.
  – Macropapillae (< 1mm) (Fig. 8.3c) and giant papillae (> 1mm) develop with prolonged inflammation.
  – Apical staining with fluorescein or the presence of mucus between giant papillae indicates active disease.

  – Limbal papillae have a more gelatinous appearance; Trantas dots may develop at the apex in chronic allergic conjunctivitis.
  b. Histology shows folds of hyperplastic conjunctival epithelium with a fibrovascular core and subepithelial stromal infiltration with inflammatory cells (Fig. 8.3d). Late changes include superficial stromal hyalinization, scarring and the formation of crypts containing goblet cells.
  c. Causes
  – Chronic blepharitis.
  – Allergic conjunctivitis.
  – Bacterial conjunctivitis.
  – Contact lens wear.
  – Superior limbic keratoconjunctivitis.
  – Floppy eyelid syndrome.

NB Keratinization of the caruncle is a common early sign of mucous membrane pemphigoid.

Lymphadenopathy

Causes of lymphadenopathy are viral, chlamydial and gonococcal infection, and Parinaud oculoglandular syndrome.

BACTERIAL CONJUNCTIVITIS

Acute bacterial conjunctivitis

Acute bacterial conjunctivitis is a common and usually self-limiting condition caused by direct eye contact with infected secretions. The most common isolates are *H. influenzae, S. pneumoniae, S. aureus,* and *Moraxella catarrhalis.*

Diagnosis

1. Symptoms
- Acute onset of redness, grittiness, burning and discharge.
- Involvement is usually bilateral although one eye may become affected 1–2 days before the other.
- On waking, the eyelids are frequently stuck together and difficult to open.

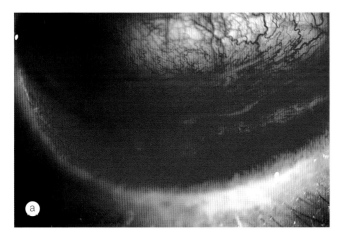

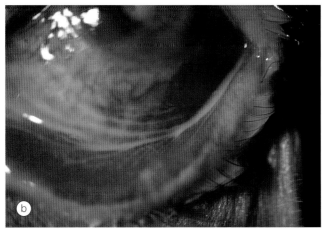

Fig. 8.4
Bacterial conjunctivitis. **(a)** Injection, mild papillary changes and mucus strands in the inferior fornix; **(b)** mucopurulent exudate

2. Signs
- Diffuse conjunctival injection and an intense papillary reaction over the tarsal plates (Fig. 8.4a).
- The discharge is initially watery, mimicking viral conjunctivitis, but later it becomes mucopurulent (Fig. 8.4b).
- Superficial corneal punctate epithelial erosions are common.

3. Investigations are not routinely performed.

Treatment

About 60% of cases resolve within 5 days without treatment. Antibiotics are frequently administered to speed recovery and prevent re-infection. In adults broad-spectrum antibiotic drops should be administered every 2 hours during waking hours for 5–7 days. Compliance in children is often better when using a gel or ointment. There is no evidence that any topical antibiotic is best at achieving clinical or microbiological cure.

> **NB** Before using topical antibiotics it is important to clean the eyelids of discharge.

1. **Fusidic acid** is a viscous gel which is useful for staphylococcal infections but not for most Gram-negative bacteria.
2. **Drops** include chloramphenicol, ciprofloxacin, ofloxacin, lomefloxacin, gatifloxacin, moxifloxacin, gentamicin, neomycin, framycetin and polymyxin B (in combination with bacitracin or trimethoprim).
3. **Ointments** provide higher concentrations for longer periods than drops but daytime use is limited because of blurred vision. Antibiotics available in ointment form include chloramphenicol, gentamicin, tetracycline, framycetin and polymyxin B (in combination with bacitracin or trimethoprim).

> **NB** Although the majority of cases of acute bacterial conjunctivitis are benign, children with *H. influenzae* conjunctivitis have a 25% risk of developing otitis.

Gonococcal keratoconjunctivitis

Gonorrhoea is a venereal genitourinary tract infection caused by *N. gonorrhoeae* which is capable of invading the intact corneal epithelium.

Diagnosis

1. Presentation is with acute, profuse, conjunctival discharge.
2. Signs
- Severe eyelid oedema and tenderness (Fig. 8.5a).

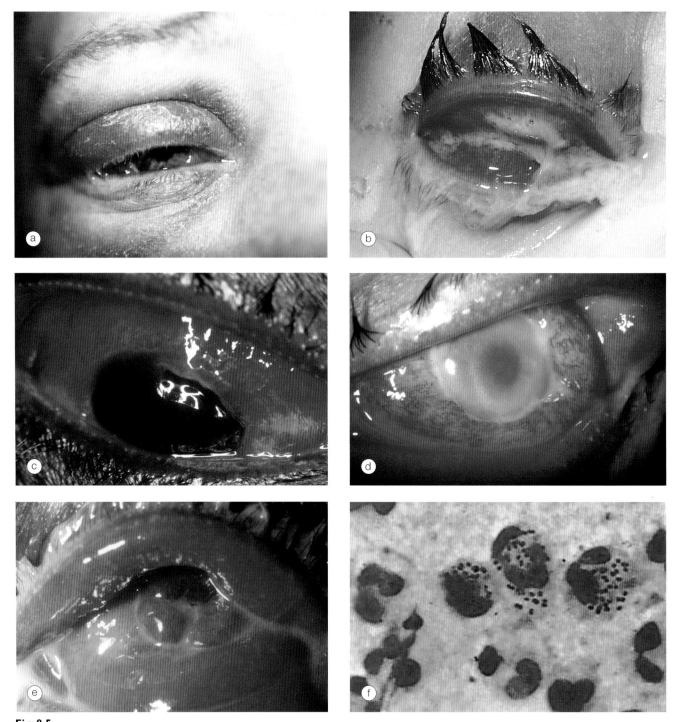

Fig. 8.5
Gonococcal keratoconjunctivitis. **(a)** Severe lid oedema and erythema; **(b)** profuse purulent discharge; **(c)** peripheral corneal ulceration; **(d)** central spread of keratitis; **(e)** perforation; **(f)** Gram stain shows kidney-shaped diplococci (Courtesy of S Tuft – fig. c; S Lewallen – fig. e)

- Intense conjunctival hyperaemia, chemosis, profuse purulent discharge (Fig. 8.5b).
- Pseudomembrane formation.
- Lymphadenopathy is prominent and, in severe cases, suppuration may occur.
- Peripheral corneal ulceration ensues if conjunctivitis is not treated appropriately (Fig. 8.5c).
- Central extension of ulceration (Fig. 8.5d).
- Perforation and endophthalmitis (Fig. 8.5e).
3. **Laboratory investigations**
   - Gram stain shows Gram-negative kidney-shaped diplococci (Fig. 8.5f).
   - Culture on enriched media such as chocolate agar or Thayer–Martin medium

Treatment

The patient must be hospitalized if there is corneal ulceration.

1. **Topical** gentamicin or bacitracin is initially administered every hour.
2. **Systemic**
   - Intramuscular ceftriaxone 250mg daily for 3 days or 1g stat. Patients with keratitis require more aggressive treatment (up to 2g intravenously for 3 days) than those with only conjunctival involvement.
   - Intramuscular spectinomycin 1g stat is an alternative on a named patient basis.
   - Because of problems with multi-drug resistance it is important to determine local guidelines regarding antibiotic susceptibility and recommended treatment.

NB Patients must be referred to a genitourinary department to be screened for associated chlamydial infection and contact tracing. Chlamydial co-infection is treated with doxycycline 200mg daily for 1 week or azithromycin 1g stat.

Meningococcal conjunctivitis

Pathogenesis

About 35% of the population are asymptomatic carriers of *N. meningitidis*. Meningococcal conjunctivitis is usually seen in children and is very rare in adults. It may be primary or secondary.

1. **Primary** conjunctivitis may appear as:
   - Non-invasive disease.
   - Invasive disease characterized by systemic symptoms of fever, septicemia and meningitis, which is fatal in 10–15% of cases. The risk of developing invasive disease increases 10–20 times if prophylactic systemic antibiotics are not given acutely.

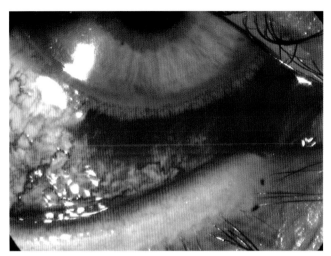

Fig. 8.6
Haemorrhagic meningococcal conjunctivitis (Courtesy of S Tuft)

2. **Secondary** conjunctivitis can be spread to the eye during end-stage septicaemia but is extremely rare.

Diagnosis

- Acute conjunctivitis which may be associated with subconjunctival haemorrhages (Fig. 8.6) and preauricular lymphadenopathy.
- Keratitis develops in 30% of cases and may lead to ulceration and perforation.

Treatment

1. **Topical** penicillin or cefotaxime drops.
2. **Systemic prophylaxis** should be given to reduce the risk of meningitis.
   - Patients with conjunctivitis should receive oral ciprofloxacin 750mg stat; alternatives include intramuscular ceftriaxone 250mg or cefotaxime 500mg.
   - Close contacts of patients with invasive disease should receive oral ciprofloxacin 500mg stat but prophylactic treatment of contacts of patients with primary conjunctivitis is not required.

Adult chlamydial conjunctivitis

Pathogenesis

Chlamydia spp. are small, obligate intracellular bacteria but they cannot replicate extracellularly and hence depend on host cells. They exist in two forms: a robust infective extracellular elementary body and a fragile intracellular replicating reticular body. Adult chlamydial (inclusion) conjunctivitis is an oculogenital infection caused by serotypes D–K of *C. trachomatis*. Transmission is by autoinoculation from genital secretions although eye-to-eye spread may account for about 10% of cases. The incubation period is about 1 week.

Urogenital infection

1. **In males** chlamydial infection is the most common cause of non-specific urethritis (NSU) and 'non-gonococcal urethritis' (NGU). It may also cause epididymitis and act as a trigger for Reiter disease.
2. **In females** chlamydial infection may cause dysuria, pelvic inflammatory disease and perihepatitis (Fitz-Hugh-Curtis syndrome). Chronic salpingitis may result in infertility.

Diagnosis

1. **Presentation** is with a subacute onset of unilateral or bilateral redness, watering, and discharge. Untreated, the conjunctivitis becomes chronic and may persist for several months.
2. **Signs**
   - Watering or mucopurulent discharge.
   - Large follicles are often most prominent in the inferior fornix (Fig. 8.7a) and may also involve the upper tarsal conjunctiva.
   - Peripheral corneal infiltrates may appear 2–3 weeks after the onset of conjunctivitis (Fig. 8.7b).
   - Tender preauricular lymphadenopathy.
   - Neglected cases have less prominent follicles and develop mild conjunctival scarring and a superior pannus.
3. **Special investigations**
   - PCR to detect chlamydial DNA is the investigation of choice.
   - Direct monoclonal fluorescent antibody microscopy of conjunctival smears is rapid and inexpensive (Fig. 8.7c).
   - Standard single-passage McCoy cell culture shows glycogen-positive inclusion bodies but requires at least 3 days (Fig. 8.7d).

NB In view of the venereal nature of the disease, referral to a genitourinary clinic is mandatory for investigation and treatment of other possible sexually transmitted diseases.

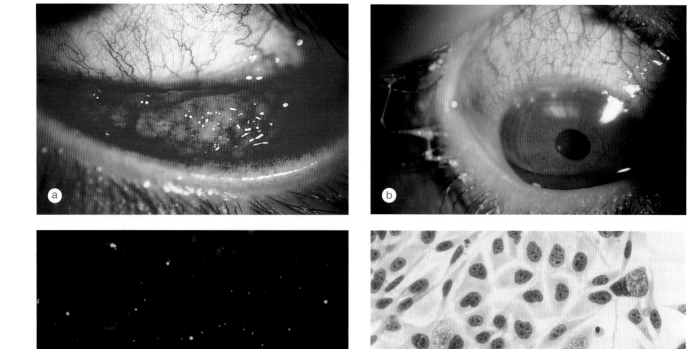

Fig. 8.7
Adult chlamydial conjunctivitis. **(a)** Large forniceal follicles; **(b)** peripheral corneal infiltrates; **(c)** elementary bodies seen on direct immunofluorescence; **(d)** McCoy cell culture shows glycogen-positive inclusion bodies (Courtesy of J Harry and G Misson, from *Clinical Ophthalmic Pathology*, Butterworth-Heinemann, 2001 – fig. c)

Treatment

1. **Topical** erythromycin or tetracycline ointment can be used initially for symptomatic relief.
2. **Systemic** therapy is with one of the following:
   - Doxycycline 100mg b.d. for 10 days.
   - Azithromycin 1g as a single dose is particularly effective because it acts intracellularly.

NB Systemic therapy should not be started prior to GU investigations.

Trachoma

Pathogenesis

Trachoma is chronic conjunctival inflammation caused by infection with serotypes A, B, Ba, and C of *C. trachomatis*. Initial infection is self-limiting and resolves without scarring but repeated infection, particularly if associated with bacterial conjunctivitis, can lead to blindness (Table 8.1). Trachoma is associated with poverty, overcrowding, and poor hygiene. Sharing living space is also a risk factor, and there may be direct transmission from eye or nasal discharge. The fly is an important vector. Currently trachoma is the leading cause of preventable blindness in the world.

Diagnosis

1. **Active disease**
   - Mixed follicular/papillary conjunctivitis associated with a mucopurulent discharge (Fig. 8.8a); in children under the age of 2 years the papillary component may predominate.
   - Superior conjunctival follicles at the upper limbus may resolve to leave a row of shallow depressions (Herbert pits Fig. 8.8b).
   - Superior epithelial keratitis and pannus formation (Fig. 8.8c).

Table 8.1   Modified WHO grading of trachoma

TF	=	trachoma follicles with five or more (> 0.5mm) on the superior tarsus
TI	=	trachomatous inflammation diffusely involving the tarsal conjunctiva, which obscures 50% or more of the normal deep tarsal vessels
TS	=	trachomatous conjunctival scarring
TT	=	trachomatous trichiasis (at least one lash) touching the globe
CO	=	corneal opacity over the pupil sufficient to blur iris details

2. **Chronic disease**
   - Linear or stellate conjunctival scars in mild cases (Fig. 8.8d), or broad confluent scars (Arlt lines) (Fig. 8.8e) in severe disease.
   - The entire conjunctiva is involved but the effects are most prominent on the upper tarsus.
3. **Complications**
   - Trichiasis, distichiasis, corneal vascularization and cicatricial entropion (Fig. 8.8f).
   - Severe corneal opacification.
   - Dry eye caused by destruction of goblet cells and the ductules of the lacrimal gland.

Management

1. **Prevention** involves regular face washing and control of flies by spraying.
2. **Antibiotics**
   - A single dose of azithromycin 20mg/kg up to 1g reduces rates of active trachoma, but may need to be repeated after one year.
   - Erythromycin 500mg b.d. for 14 days is an alternative for women of childbearing age.
   - Topical 1% tetracycline is less effective than oral treatment.
3. **Surgery** is aimed at relieving trichiasis and maintaining complete lid closure.

NB The acronym **SAFE** is based on four major aspects of trachoma control: **S**urgery for trachoma trichiasis, **A**ntibiotics for active disease, **F**ace washing, and **E**nvironmental improvements.

Ophthalmia neonatorum

Pathogenesis

Ophthalmia neonatorum (neonatal conjunctivitis) develops within 2 weeks of birth as the result of infection transmitted from mother to infant during delivery. It is serious because of the lack of immunity in the infant and immaturity of the ocular surface (no lymphoid tissue and relatively poor tear film).

1. ***N. gonorrhoeae*** is now an uncommon although serious cause in developed countries.
2. ***C. trachomatis*** accounts for the majority of cases in developed countries and may also cause pneumonitis, otitis and rhinitis.
3. **Other pathogens** include *S. aureus, S. pneumoniae, H. influenzae* and *Enterobacteriaceae (Bacillus* spp., *E. coli, and Klebsiella* spp.). Herpes simplex virus (typically HSV-2) is a rare cause and usually associated with generalized virus infection including encephalitis.

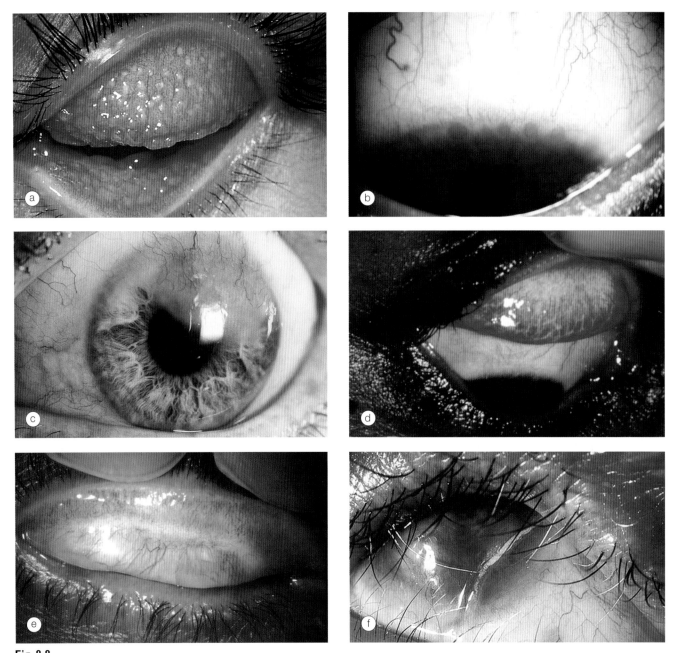

Fig. 8.8
Trachoma. **(a)** Mixed follicular-papillary conjunctivitis; **(b)** Herbert pits; **(c)** pannus; **(d)** linear scars; **(e)** Arlt line; **(f)** trichiasis and cicatricial entropion

Prophylaxis

Povidone-iodine 2.5% is a cheap and effective agent against all of the common pathogens that cause ophthalmia neonatorum. It appears that a single application at birth is sufficient. Erythromycin 0.5% ointment or tetracycline 1% ointment is used by some.

Diagnosis

1. **Presentation** is usually between 3 and 19 days after birth.
2. **Signs**
   - Usually bilateral eyelid oedema which may be severe in gonococcal infection (Fig. 8.9a).
   - Discharge which is initially sero-sanguineous and later mucopurulent.
   - A papillary conjunctival reaction which may occasionally be associated with pseudomembranes (Fig. 8.9b).
   - Corneal complications are more severe with *N. gonorrhea* infection and include corneal ulcer and perforation. *C. trachomatis*, if untreated, can cause conjunctival scarring and peripheral corneal pannus.
3. **Investigation**
   - Gram stain of exudate for diplococci (gonorrhoea) and Giemsa stain for inclusion bodies (chlamydia – Fig. 8.9c).
   - Cultures on chocolate agar or Thayer–Martin plates for *N. gonorrhoeae*.
   - Immunofluorescence tests for chlamydia.
   - PCR for chlamydia and neisserial DNA.

Treatment

Urgent treatment is indicated in association with paediatric infectious diseases specialist.

1. **Chlamydial** infection is treated with oral erythromycin ethyl succinate for 2 weeks. If pneumonitis is suspected treatment should be for 3 weeks. Erythromycin or tetracycline ointment is used in addition but not as sole therapy.
2. **Gonococcal** infection requires ceftriaxone intravenously or intramuscularly, or cefotaxime.
3. **Other bacterial** infections are treated with chloramphenicol or neomycin ointment q.i.d. Systemic antibiotics may be considered in severe cases.
4. **Herpes simplex** infection requires systemic aciclovir for 14 days and topical aciclovir 5 times daily.

NB If chlamydia or gonorrhoea is confirmed the parents and their partners must be investigated and treated by a genitourinary physician.

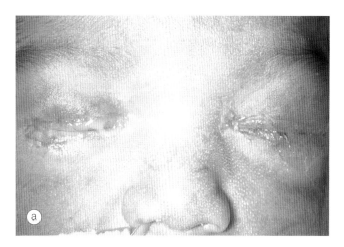
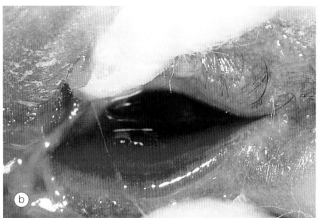
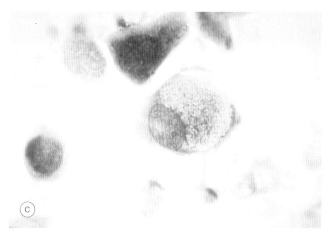

Fig. 8.9
Ophthalmia neonatorum. **(a)** Lid oedema and discharge; **(b)** papillary conjunctivitis; **(c)** Giemsa stain shows an oval structure adjacent to the nucleus of an epithelial cell which is an intracytoplasmic inclusion body (Courtesy of J Harry and G Misson, from *Clinical Ophthalmic Pathology*, Butterworth-Heinemann, 2001 – fig. c)

VIRAL CONJUNCTIVITIS

Adenoviral keratoconjunctivitis

Pathogenesis

Adenoviruses are icosahedral-shaped, unenveloped viruses with a linear, double-stranded DNA genome. There are 51 subtypes that affect humans and many cause clinical infection. Viral subtyping permits epidemiological tracing of outbreaks.

1. **Adenoviral keratoconjunctivitis** is the most common external ocular viral infection that may be sporadic or occur in epidemics in hospitals, schools and factories. The spread of infection is facilitated by the ability of the virus to survive on dry surfaces and the fact that viral shedding may occur for 4–10 days before clinical disease is apparent.
2. **Transmission** of this highly contagious virus is by respiratory or ocular secretions, and dissemination is by contaminated towels or equipment such as tonometer heads. Following the onset of conjunctivitis the virus is shed for about 12 days.
3. **Precautions** must be taken to avoid transmission following examination of patients with suspected adenovirus infection. Thorough washing of hands is important, as is meticulous disinfection of ophthalmic instruments. In addition, infected hospital personnel should not come in contact with patients and busy eye departments should have a separate 'red eye room' for management of patients with conjunctivitis.

   NB It is an occupational hazard for ophthalmologists.

Spectrum of infection

The spectrum of adenoviral eye infection varies from mild and almost subclinical disease to full-blown infection with significant morbidity.

1. **Pharyngoconjunctival fever (PCF)** is caused mainly by serotypes 3, 7 and 11. It is spread by droplets within families with upper respiratory tract infection. Keratitis develops in about 30% of cases but is seldom severe.
2. **Epidemic keratoconjunctivitis (EKC)** is caused mainly but not exclusively by serotypes 8, 19 and 37. The virus is usually transmitted by hand to eye contact, instruments and solutions. Keratitis, which may be severe, develops in about 80% of cases.

Conjunctivitis

1. **Presentation** is usually with unilateral watering, redness, discomfort and photophobia; the contralateral eye is typically affected 1–2 days later, but less severely.
2. **Signs**
   - Eyelid oedema and tender pre-auricular lymphadenopathy.
   - Follicular conjunctivitis (Fig. 8.10a).
   - Severe infection may result in conjunctival haemorrhages, chemosis and pseudomembranes (Fig. 8.10b).
   - Tender pre-auricular lymphadenopathy.
   - The pseudomembranes resolve but may result in mild conjunctival scarring (Fig. 8.10c).

Keratitis

1. **Stage 1** occurs within 7–10 days of the onset of symptoms and is characterized by a punctate epithelial keratitis that resolves within 2 weeks (Fig. 8.10d).
2. **Stage 2** is characterized by focal, white, subepithelial opacities that develop beneath the fading epithelial lesions that are thought to represent immune response to the virus (Fig. 8.10e).
3. **Stage 3** is characterized by anterior stromal infiltrates that gradually fade over months or years (Fig. 8.10f).

Treatment

1. **Conjunctivitis** is treated symptomatically with artificial tears and cold compresses until spontaneous resolution occurs within 3 weeks. Topical steroids may be required for severe membranous conjunctivitis.
2. **Keratitis** responds well to topical steroids. Unfortunately, they do not shorten the natural course of the disease but merely suppress the corneal inflammation so that the lesions tend to recur if steroid therapy is discontinued prematurely.

Molluscum contagiosum conjunctivitis

Pathogenesis

Molluscum contagiosum is a skin infection caused by a human specific double stranded DNA poxvirus which typically affects otherwise healthy children with a peak incidence between 2 and 4 years (Fig. 8.11a). Transmission is by contact with infected people and then by autoinoculation. Multiple, and occasionally confluent, lesions may develop in immunocompromised patients. A distribution in the chin-strap region is common in HIV positive patients.

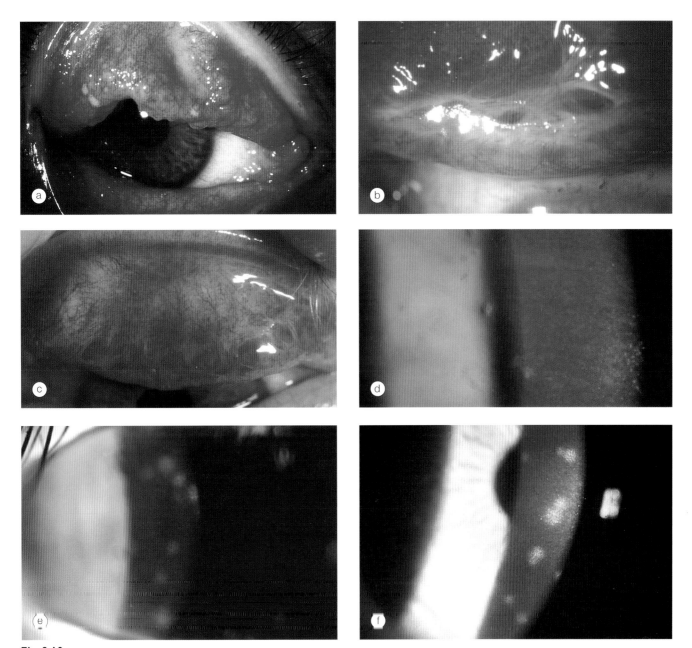

Fig. 8.10
Adenoviral keratoconjunctivitis. **(a)** Follicular conjunctivitis; **(b)** pseudomembrane; **(c)** mild residual scarring; **(d)** stage 1 keratitis;
(e) stage 2 keratitis; **(f)** stage 3 keratitis (Courtesy of S Tuft – figs b, c and d)

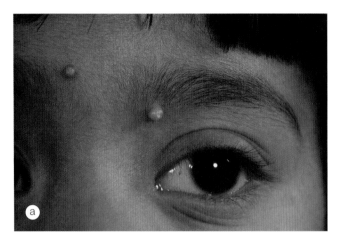

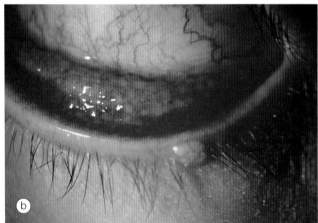

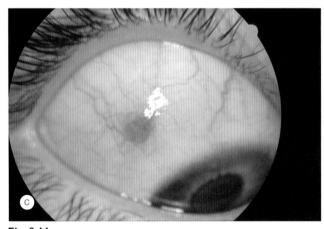

Fig. 8.11
(a) Molluscum lesions; **(b)** follicular conjunctivitis associated with a molluscum lesion; **(c)** molluscum lesion on the bulbar conjunctiva (Courtesy of R Murray – fig. c)

Diagnosis

1. **Presentation** is with chronic, unilateral, ocular irritation and a mild discharge.
2. **Signs**
   - A pale, waxy, umbilicated nodule on the lid margin associated with follicular conjunctivitis and mild mucoid discharge (Fig. 8.11b).
   - Bulbar nodules may rarely occur in immunocompromised patients (Fig. 8.11c).
   - Untreated long-standing cases may develop a fine epithelial keratitis or pannus.

NB The lash line should be examined carefully in patients with chronic conjunctivitis so as not to overlook a molluscum lesion.

Treatment

The lesions are self-limiting and removal may only be necessary for cosmetic reasons or secondary conjunctivitis.

1. **Preferred** treatment is by physical expression, which may be facilitated by making a small nick in the skin at the margin of the lesion with the tip of a needle.
2. **Other options** such as phenol ablation, cauterization, cryotherapy or laser are more hazardous and liable to cause scarring, depigmentation, or loss of lashes

Acute haemorrhagic conjunctivitis

Acute haemorrhagic conjunctivitis is caused by enterovirus 70 or coxsackievirus A24. It has a rapid onset and resolution. The infection is spread by direct inoculation and the use of traditional eye medicines rather than the usual faecal–oral route.

1. **Presentation** is with acute onset of usually bilateral burning, watering, discharge and lid swelling. Some patients have a sore throat and malaise.
2. **Signs**
   - Subconjunctival haemorrhages and follicular conjunctivitis.
   - Pre-auricular lymphadenopathy.

NB *N. meningitidis* or herpes simplex infection may also cause sporadic haemorrhagic conjunctivitis.

3. **Treatment.** As there is no antiviral therapy for either agent management involves limitation of infection by education and infection control.

ALLERGIC CONJUNCTIVITIS

Acute allergic rhinoconjunctivitis

Pathogenesis

Atopy is a genetically determined predisposition to mount an allergic response to environmental allergens. Acute rhinoconjunctivitis is the most common form of ocular and nasal allergy affecting about 20% of the population. The following two clinical syndromes have been described, based on the pattern of exacerbations and the likely allergen.

1. **Seasonal allergic conjunctivitis** (hay fever), with onset during the spring and summer, is the commonest form. The most frequent allergens are tree and grass pollens, although the specific allergen varies with geographic location.
2. **Perennial allergic conjunctivitis** causes symptoms throughout the year with exacerbation in the autumn when exposure to house dust mites (*Dermatophagoides pteronyssinus*), animal dander and fungal allergens is greatest. It is less common and milder than seasonal allergic conjunctivitis.

Diagnosis

1. **Presentation** is with transient, acute attacks of redness, watering and itching, associated with sneezing and nasal discharge.
2. **Signs** which resolve completely between attacks are:
   • Lid oedema.
   • Chemosis and a mild papillary reaction (Fig. 8.12).

Treatment

1. **Mast cell stabilizers** (sodium cromoglycate q.i.d., nedocromil sodium b.d. and lodoxamide b.d.) are effective for long-term use. There is no difference in benefit of a particular preparation except frequency of instillation.
2. **Antihistamines** (levocabastine, epinastine, emedastine b.d or q.i.d) when the patient is symptomatic. They are as effective as mast cell stabilizers and there is no difference in benefit between different preparations.
3. **Combined antihistamines and mast cell stabilizers** (olopatadine, ketotifen, azelastine b.d.).
4. **Steroids** are effective but rarely indicated.

Vernal keratoconjunctivitis

Pathogenesis

Vernal keratoconjunctivitis (VKC) is a bilateral, recurrent, disorder in which IgE and cell mediated immune mechanisms

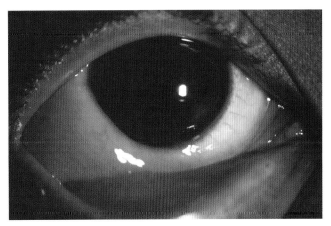

Fig. 8.12
Conjunctival injection and chemosis in acute allergic conjunctivitis

play important roles. It primarily affects boys and usually presents in the first decade of life (mean age 7 years); 95% of cases remit by the late teens and the remainder develops atopic keratoconjunctivitis. VKC is rare in temperate regions but in sub-Saharan regions of Africa it is a significant public health problem. In temperate regions about three-quarters of patients have associated atopy and two-thirds have a family history of atopy. Such patients often develop asthma and eczema in infancy. VKC may occur on a seasonal basis, with a peak incidence over late spring and summer although there may be mild perennial symptoms.

Classification

1. **Palpebral** disease primarily involves the upper tarsal conjunctiva and may be associated with significant corneal disease as a result of the close apposition between the inflamed upper tarsal plates and corneal epithelium.
2. **Limbal** disease typically affects black and Asian patients.
3. **Mixed** has features of both palpebral and limbal disease.

Diagnosis

1. **Symptoms** consist of intense itching, which may be associated with lacrimation, photophobia, a foreign body sensation, burning and thick mucoid discharge. Constant blinking is also common and may be misdiagnosed as neurotic.
2. **Palpebral disease**
   • Diffuse papillary hypertrophy on the superior tarsus (Fig. 8.13a).
   • Macropapillae (> 1mm) have a flat-topped polygonal appearance reminiscent of cobblestones (Fig. 8.13b).
   • Mucus deposition between giant papillae (Fig. 8.13c).
   • Decreased disease activity is characterized by less conjunctival injection and mucus production (Fig. 8.13d).

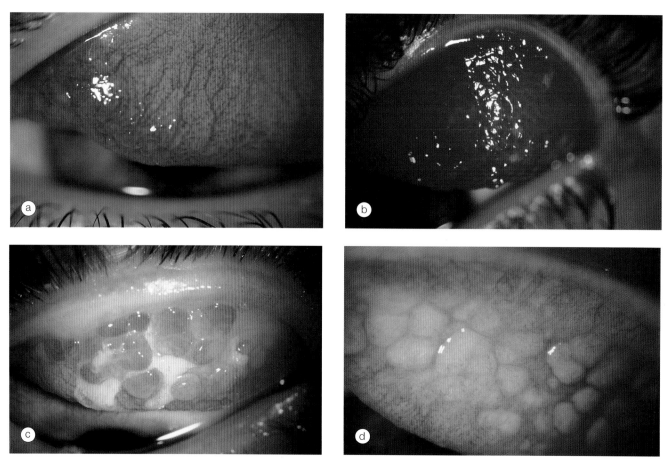

Fig. 8.13
Palpebral vernal disease. **(a)** Diffuse papillary hypertrophy; **(b)** macropapillae; **(c)** giant papillae and mucus; **(d)** relatively inactive disease
(Courtesy of S Tuft – figs b and d)

3. Limbal disease
- Gelatinous papillae on the limbal conjunctiva that may be associated with discrete white spots at their apices (Trantas dots) (Fig. 8.14a–c).
- In tropical regions limbal disease may be very severe (Fig. 8.14d).

4. Keratopathy is more frequent in palpebral disease and may take the following forms:
- Punctate epithelial erosions involving the superior cornea are the earliest findings.
- Epithelial macroerosions resulting from necrosis caused by toxins released from the inflamed conjunctiva (Fig. 8.15a).
- Shield ulcers and plaques (Fig. 8.15b) may develop in palpebral or mixed disease when exposed Bowman layer becomes coated with mucus and calcium phosphate. This may result in poor wetting and delayed re-epithelialization.
- Pseudogerontoxon can develop in recurrent limbal disease. It resembles a local area of arcus senilis

adjacent to a previously inflamed segment of the limbus (Fig. 8.15c).
- Peripheral superficial vascularization, especially superior, may develop following chronic inflammation and mucus deposition in the absence of ulceration (Fig. 8.15d).
- Herpes simplex keratitis can be aggressive and occasionally bilateral.

NB Patients with VKC have an increased incidence of keratoconus which is frequently complicated by hydrops and a strong tendency for vascularization.

Treatment

1. Topical

a. Mast cell stabilizers are rarely effective as sole treatment, but they reduce the need for steroids.

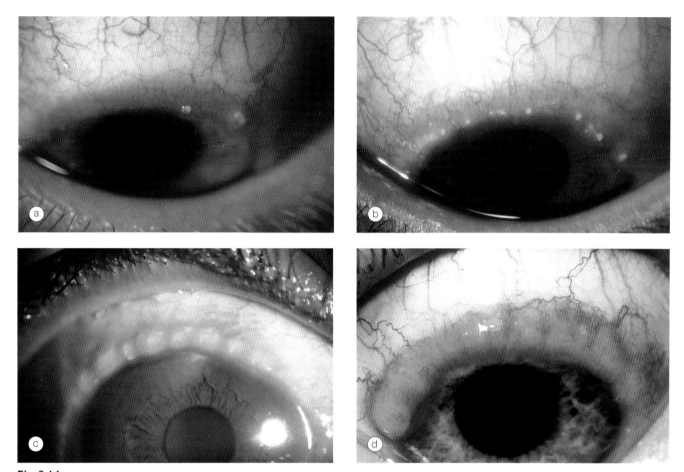

Fig. 8.14
Limbal vernal disease. **(a)** Sparse limbal papillae; **(b)** papillae with Trantas dots; **(c)** extensive papillae; **(d)** extremely severe involvement (Courtesy of S Tuft – fig. b)

Lodoxamide and nedocromil sodium are more effective than sodium cromoglycate.

*b. **Antihistamines*** when used in isolation are as effective as mast cell stabilizers.

*c. **Steroids*** are indicated mainly for keratopathy although they may be required short-term for severe discomfort. Fluorometholone 0.1% is preferred as it has a low risk of causing ocular hypertension. Exacerbations should be treated intensively with prompt tapering. It is often possible to discontinue steroids between attacks.

*d. **Acetylcysteine*** is useful for mucous deposition and early plaque formation.

*e. **Ciclosporin*** q.i.d. may be considered in steroid-resistant cases. Improvement occurs after about 2 weeks of therapy but relapses occur if the drug is stopped suddenly.

2. Supratarsal steroid injection for non-compliant patients and those resistant to conventional therapy. The injection consists of 0.1ml of either dexamethasone 4mg/ml or triamcinolone 40mg/ml after upper lid eversion. There is no clear benefit between the two steroids.

3. Systemic

*a. **Immunosuppressive agents*** (steroids, ciclosporin and azathioprine) may be used in severe unremitting disease unresponsive to maximum tolerated topical therapy.

*b. **Oral antihistamines*** help sleep and reduce nocturnal eye rubbing.

4. Surgery

*a. **Superficial keratectomy*** may be required to remove plaques. The epithelium is removed to the edge of the calcified region and a very superficial dissection performed. Medical treatment must be maintained until the cornea has re-epithelialized to prevent recurrences. Excimer laser phototherapeutic keratectomy is an alternative.

*b. **Amniotic membrane overlay graft*** with tarsorrhaphy or lamellar keratoplasty may be required for severe persistent epithelial defects with ulceration.

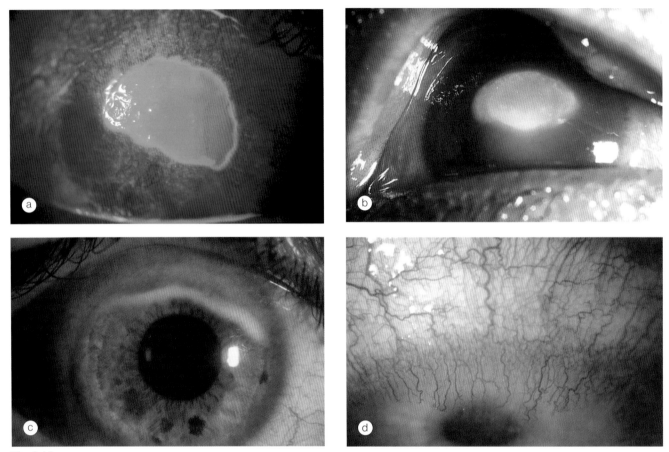

Fig. 8.15
Keratopathy in vernal disease. (a) Macroerosion; (b) shield ulcer and plaque; (c) pseudogerontoxon; (d) superficial vascularization
(Courtesy of S Tuft – figs c and d)

Atopic keratoconjunctivitis

Pathogenesis

Atopic keratoconjunctivitis (AKC) is a rare bilateral and symmetrical disease that typically develops in young men following a long history of severe atopic dermatitis. About 5% of patients have childhood vernal disease. AKC tends to be chronic and unremitting with a low expectation of eventual resolution and is therefore associated with significant visual morbidity. Patients are sensitive to a wide range of environmental airborne allergens.

Diagnosis

The diagnosis is clinical and there is no single laboratory test to distinguish AKC from VKC.

1. Symptoms are similar to VKC but often more severe and unremitting.

2. Eyelids
- Red, thickened, macerated and fissured lids with chronic staphylococcal blepharitis and madarosis (Fig. 8.16a).
- Tightening of the facial skin may cause lower lid ectropion and epiphora.

3. Conjunctiva
- Micropapillary conjunctivitis over the upper and lower tarsal plates and inferior fornix.
- Giant papillae may develop with time.
- Scarring and infiltration of the tarsal conjunctiva results in flattening of giant papillae and featureless appearance (Fig. 8.16b).
- Cicatricial conjunctivitis may develop with inferior forniceal shortening (Fig. 8.16c).
- Symblepharon formation and keratinization of the caruncle (Fig. 8.16d).

4. Keratopathy
- Punctate epithelial erosions over the inferior third of the cornea are common (Fig. 8.16e).

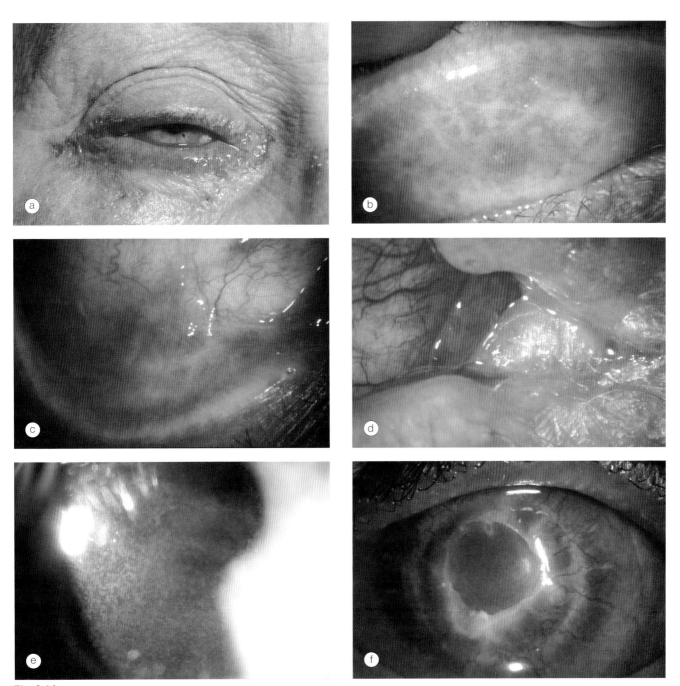

Fig. 8.16
Atopic disease. **(a)** Severe eyelid involvement; **(b)** infiltration and scarring of the tarsal conjunctiva; **(c)** forniceal shortening; **(d)** keratinization of the caruncle; **(e)** punctate epithelial erosions; **(f)** persistent epithelial defect and peripheral corneal vascularization (Courtesy of S Tuft)

- Persistent epithelial defects, plaque formation and peripheral superficial vascularization in response to chronic surface inflammation (Fig. 8.16f).
- Predisposition to keratoconus, secondary bacterial and fungal infection, and aggressive herpes simplex infection.

NB Patients with atopic disease may also develop shield-like presenile cataracts.

Treatment

Guidelines are similar to those of vernal disease although AKC is less responsive and requires prolonged treatment.

1. **Topical**
   a. *Mast cell stabilizers* are effective and should be used throughout the year as prophylaxis against exacerbation and as steroid-sparing agents.
   b. *Ketolorac* combined with a mast cell stabilizer.
   c. *Antihistamines* are less effective than in VKC.
   d. *Steroids* are effective short-term for severe exacerbations and keratopathy. A small number of patients require long-term low dose therapy for reasonable control.
   e. *Acetylcysteine* for corneal mucus deposits.
   f. *Ciclosporin* is an effective steroid-sparing agent in patients with severe disease. However, its efficacy as a first-line agent for long-term therapy warrants further studies.
   g. *Antibiotics* and lid hygiene should be used for associated staphylococcal blepharitis.
2. **Supratarsal steroid injections** should be considered when topical treatment is ineffective.
3. **Systemic**
   a. *Antihistamines* for severe itching.
   b. *Antibiotics* (doxycycline 50–100mg daily for 6 weeks or azithromycin 500mg once daily for 3 days) to reduce inflammation aggravated by blepharitis.
   c. *Ciclosporin* in severe cases.

NB Because of the high carriage of *S. aureus* on the lid margins, cataract surgery carries an increased risk of endophthalmitis.

Giant papillary conjunctivitis

Pathogenesis

Giant papillary conjunctivitis (GPC) was originally described in association with soft contact lens wear, but has subsequently been recognized in association with a variety of mechanical stimuli of the tarsal conjunctiva including ocular prosthesis, exposed sutures and filtering blebs. The risk of developing GPC is increased by deposition of mucous and cellular debris on the contact lens surface (lens spoliation – Fig. 8.17). GPC may develop in patients with mild allergic eye disease that is exacerbated by contact lens wear.

Diagnosis

1. **Symptoms** consist of a foreign body sensation, redness, itching and loss of contact lens tolerance, often worse when the contact lens has been removed.
2. **Signs**
   - Excessive mobility of the contact lens with upper lid lens capture.
   - Increased mucus production and coating of the contact lens.
   - Micropapillae on the superior tarsal conjunctiva.
   - Macropapillae with focal scarring on the apices may develop in advanced cases.

NB In contrast to VKC, keratopathy is rare due to less secretion of toxic cytokines.

Treatment

1. **Removal of the stimulus**
   - Stopping contact lens wear.
   - Removal of exposed sutures, ocular prosthesis etc.
2. **Cleaning contact lens or prosthesis**
   - Use of daily disposable lens.
   - Rigid contact lens may be easier to clean effectively.
   - Protein removing tablets.
   - Polishing of prosthesis and cleaning with a detergent.

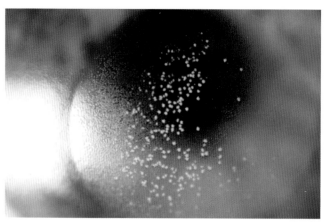

Fig. 8.17
Contact lens deposits

3. Mast cell stabilizers, which should be non-preserved in patients wearing soft contact lenses.

4. Topical steroids are rarely indicated but are safe to treat GPC associated with an ocular prosthesis.

CICATRIZING CONJUNCTIVITIS

Mucous membrane pemphigoid

Mucous membrane pemphigoid is an autoimmune muco-cutaneous blistering disease with a peak age of onset after 70 years of age (see Chapter 24). Conjunctival disease (ocular cicatricial pemphigoid – OCP) is seen in 75% of cases with oral involvement but only 25% of those with skin lesions; occasionally it occurs in isolation. OCP is always bilateral, but frequently asymmetrical with regard to time of onset, severity and rate of progression.

Diagnosis

1. Presentation is with an insidious onset of non-specific conjunctivitis with redness, irritation, burning and tearing.

NB Because of the rarity of the condition the diagnosis is often overlooked and treatment delayed.

2. Conjunctiva
- Papillary conjunctivitis, diffuse hyperaemia and oedema, which in severe cases may be associated with necrosis (Fig. 8.18a).
- Chronic conjunctivitis with fine lines of subconjunctival fibrosis and shortening of the inferior fornices (Fig. 8.18b).
- Flattening of the plica and keratinization of the caruncle (Fig. 8.18c).
- Symblepharon – adhesion between the bulbar and palpebral conjunctiva (Fig. 8.18d).
- The chronically progressive course of the disease may be interrupted by exacerbations.

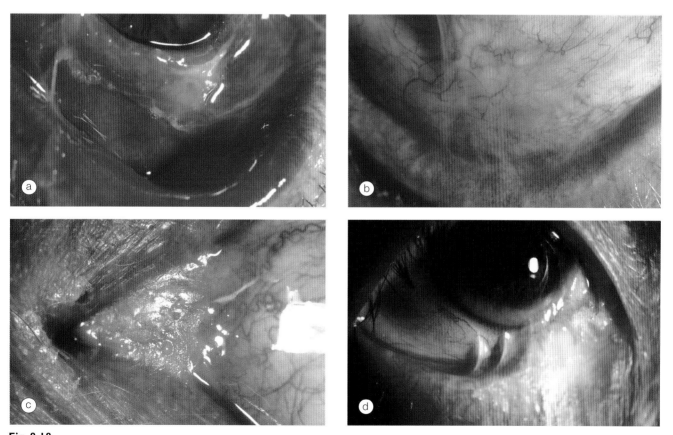

Fig. 8.18
Conjunctivitis in ocular cicatricial pemphigoid. **(a)** Hyperaemia, chemosis and necrosis; **(b)** subretinal fibrosis and forniceal shortening; **(c)** flat plica and keratinized caruncle; **(d)** symblepharon (Courtesy of S Tuft – figs a, b and c)

3. Lids
- Aberrant lashes.
- Blepharitis and keratinization of the lid margin.
- Ankyloblepharon – adhesions at the outer canthus between the upper and lower lids (see Fig. 8.19c).

4. Cornea
- Epithelial defects associated with drying and exposure (Fig. 8.19a).
- Infiltration and peripheral vascularization (Fig. 8.19b).
- Keratinization and 'conjunctivalization' of the cornea surface following damage to the limbus with epithelial stem cell failure (Fig. 8.19c).
- End-stage disease is characterized by total symblepharon and corneal opacification (Fig. 8.19d).

Monitoring disease progress

The depth of the fornices should be measured regularly and the position of adhesions noted. The sum of the three readings for the distance from the inferior limbus to the centre of the lower posterior lid margin in three positions of gaze (up, right, and left) is simple and reliable.

Systemic treatment

Systemic treatment should be introduced incrementally until all signs of active disease have resolved. Initial treatment depends on activity at presentation. Unfortunately, although some patients are cured, about 30% progress inexorably to blindness despite maximum tolerated treatment.

1. Acute disease
- Systemic steroids (prednisolone 1–1.5mg/kg) are essential to control limbitis and conjunctival necrosis but must not be used as sole long-term therapy.
- Cyclophosphamide (1–2mg/kg) should be added to allow the steroid dose to be reduced.

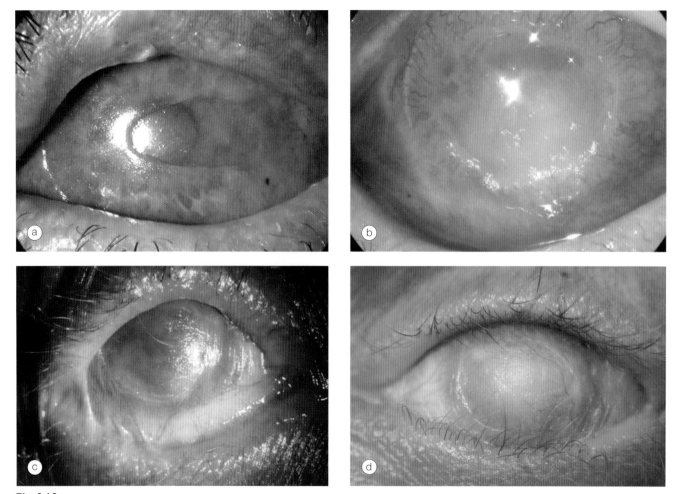

Fig. 8.19
Keratitis in ocular cicatricial pemphigoid. **(a)** Epithelial defect; **(b)** peripheral vascularization and infiltration; **(c)** keratinization and ankyloblepharon; **(d)** end-stage disease (Courtesy of S Tuft)

2. Mild to moderate disease
- Dapsone 50mg daily increasing to 100mg, if tolerated. It is important to check glucose-6-phosphate dehydrogenase and haemoglobin levels before starting therapy.
- Azathioprine or methotrexate if dapsone is contraindicated, although the onset of action is 2–3 weeks.
- Ciclosporin has been used although data to support its effect is lacking.

3. Severe disease
- Cyclophosphamide should not be used for more than 12 months because of the risk of bladder carcinoma.
- Azathioprine or mycophenolate mofetil (CellCept) are suitable for long-term therapy.
- Monoclonal antibodies against Il-2 receptor and intravenous immunoglobulin therapy have shown promising results in some patients.

Local treatment

1. Topical
- Steroids are used as adjunctive treatment.
- Artificial tears for surface drying.
- Retinoic acid to reduce keratinization.

2. Subconjunctival mitomycin C injection if systemic immunosuppression is not possible, but the results in advanced disease are disappointing.

3. Contact lenses
- Silicone rubber contact lenses may be used with caution to protect the cornea from aberrant lashes and drying.
- Rigid scleral contact lenses may be effective in holding a tear film in front of the cornea and protecting it from lid friction and exposure, but do not prevent forniceal scarring and symblepharon formation.

4. Reconstructive surgery should be performed *only* after inflammation is controlled.
- Aberrant lashes can be treated by cryotherapy which may be combined with lid splitting to expose the lash follicles.
- Severe dry eyes may require punctal occlusion if the puncta are not already scarred.
- Large, recurrent, corneal defects may require tarsorrhaphy or botulinum toxin injection into the levator to induce ptosis.
- Entropion is best managed by a technique that does not incise conjunctiva such as retractor plication or Jones procedure.
- Keratinization may be controlled by mucous membrane transplantation. Alternatively amniotic membranes may be used although the long-term success is worse.
- Keratoplasty is a high risk procedure in a dry eye with corneal epithelial failure because of frequent problems with re-epithelialization. Lamellar grafts are preferred for perforations.
- Limbal stem cell transfer may be attempted for conjunctivalization and keratinization.
- Keratoprostheses may be beneficial in end-stage disease.

NB The following cutaneous conditions may occasionally be associated with cicatrizing conjunctivitis: epidermolysis bullosa, pemphigus vulgaris, bullous pemphigoid, dermatitis herpetiformis, lichen planus, porphyria cutanea tarda, xeroderma pigmentosum and Wegener granulomatosis.

Stevens–Johnson syndrome and toxic epidermal necrolysis

Stevens–Johnson syndrome and toxic epidermal necrolysis (Lyell disease) reflect different severities of the same mucocutaneous blistering disease process (see Chapter 24). Both are uncommon but potentially lethal conditions that may be associated with severe ocular complications. They have similar clinical signs, treatment and prognosis, although ocular involvement is much less common in toxic epidermal necrolysis. Males are affected more often than females with a mean age of onset of 25 years.

Diagnosis

1. Acute disease
- Crusty eyelids associated with a transient, self-limiting papillary conjunctivitis (Fig. 8.20a).
- Severe membranous or pseudomembranous conjunctivitis with patchy conjunctival infarction is less common (Fig. 8.20b).

2. Late disease
- Reticular scarring of the upper tarsal plate (Fig. 8.20c).
- Conjunctival keratinization and forniceal shortening (Fig. 8.20d).
- Posterior lid margin disease with opening of the meibomian orifices onto the ocular surface (Fig. 8.20e).
- Conjunctival scarring and symblepharon formation.
- Dry eye resulting from loss of goblet cells and destruction of lacrimal gland ductules.
- Corneal keratinization (Fig. 8.20f).
- Keratopathy secondary to cicatricial entropion, aberrant lashes and infection.

Systemic treatment

Systemic disease is treated by maintaining hydration and debridement, and replacement of sloughing skin, if necessary. Systemic steroids are occasionally prescribed to moderate acute manifestations although their efficacy is debatable. Ciclosporin, thalidomide and immunoglobulins have been advocated but without controls trials to demonstrate a consistent effect.

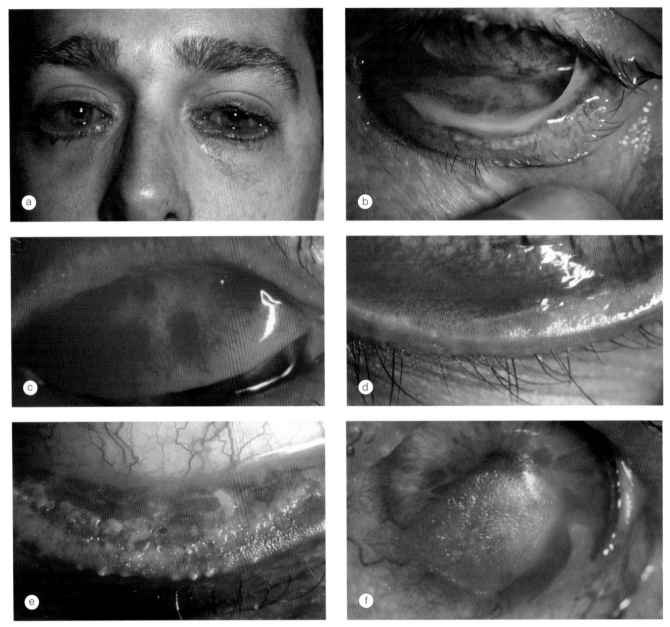

Fig. 8.20
Stevens–Johnson syndrome. **(a)** Acute conjunctivitis; **(b)** pseudomembrane; **(c)** reticular scarring; **(d)** conjunctival keratinization and early forniceal shortening; **(e)** severe posterior lid margin disease and keratinization; **(f)** corneal keratinization (Courtesy of S Tuft figs c–f)

Local treatment

1. Acute disease
- Lubrication and prevention of exposure.
- Topical steroid and antibiotics.
- Lysis of conjunctival adhesions.
- A scleral ring, consisting of a large haptic lens with the central zone removed, may prevent symblepharon formation.

2. Chronic disease
- Lubrication and punctal occlusion for mild disease.
- Topical retinoic acid for keratinization.
- Bandage contact lenses to maintain surface moisture and overcome irregular astigmatism. Gas permeable scleral contact lens for trichiasis and visual rehabilitation.
- Mucous membrane grafting and limbal cell transplantation.
- Lamellar corneal grafting is preferred to penetrating keratoplasty
- Keratoprosthesis in end-stage disease.

NB In contrast to ocular pemphigoid, immunosuppression is not required prior to conjunctival or lid surgery.

MISCELLANEOUS CONJUNCTIVITIS

Superior limbic keratoconjunctivitis

Superior limbic keratoconjunctivitis (SLK) is an uncommon, usually bilateral, chronic disease of the superior limbus and bulbar conjunctiva, with papillary hypertrophy of the superior tarsal conjunctiva. It typically affects middle-aged women who may have abnormal thyroid function, usually hyperthyroidism. SLK is probably under-diagnosed because symptoms are more severe than signs. The course can be prolonged although remission eventually occurs without sequelae.

Pathogenesis

SLK appears to be the result of blink-related mechanical trauma from abnormal forces between the upper lid and superior bulbar conjunctiva, probably precipitated by tear film insufficiency. This results in loss of the ability of the lid to move freely over the conjunctiva and excess of conjunctival tissue. With increased movement of the conjunctiva there is mechanical damage to both the tarsal and conjunctival surfaces.

Diagnosis

1. **Presentation** is with non-specific symptoms such as foreign body sensation, burning, photophobia and mucoid discharge.
2. **Conjunctiva**
   - Papillary hypertrophy of the superior tarsus that may give rise to a diffuse velvety appearance (Fig. 8.21a).
   - Hyperaemia of the superior bulbar conjunctiva and limbal papillary hypertrophy which stains readily with rose bengal (Fig. 8.21b).
   - Light downward pressure on the upper lid results in a fold of redundant conjunctiva crossing the upper limbus (Fig. 8.21c).
   - Limbal palisades may be lost superiorly and petechial haemorrhages may be present.
   - Keratinization can be demonstrated on biopsy or impression cytology.
3. **Cornea**
   - Superior punctate corneal epithelial erosions are common, often separated from the limbus by a zone of normal epithelium.
   - Superior filamentary keratitis develops in about one-third of cases (Fig. 8.21d).
   - A superior arcus may develop in long-standing disease.
4. **Keratoconjunctivitis sicca** is present in only about 50% of cases.

Treatment

The aim is to alter the abnormal mechanical interaction between the upper lid and the superior limbus. Conservative treatment should be tried initially as the condition is usually self-limiting.

1. **Topical**
   - a. *Lubricants* to reduce friction between the lid and bulbar conjunctiva.
   - b. *Mast cell stabilizers* and steroids to reduce any inflammatory component.
   - c. *Ciclosporin* may be effective as primary or adjunctive therapy, particularly in the presence of coexisting keratoconjunctivitis sicca.
   - d. *Acetylcysteine* for filamentary keratitis.
   - e. *Retinoic acid* to prevent keratinization.
2. **Temporary superior punctal occlusion** is simple and usually effective.
3. **Soft contact lenses,** which intervene between the lid and the superior conjunctiva, may be useful. Interestingly, a unilateral lens may provide bilateral relief.
4. **Resection** of the superior limbal conjunctiva and Tenon capsule, either in a zone 2mm from the superior limbus or at the upper margin of rose bengal staining, is usually effective in resistant disease. The mechanism is to remove

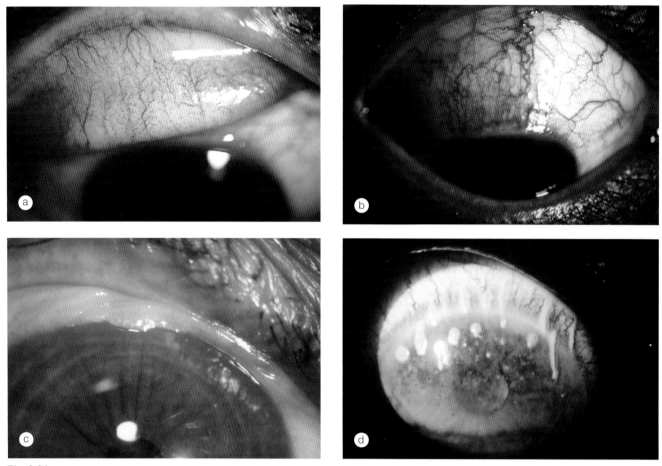

Fig. 8.21
Superior limbic keratoconjunctivitis. **(a)** Papillary hypertrophy; **(b)** bulbar conjunctival injection and limbal papillae; **(c)** redundant conjunctiva; **(d)** superior corneal filaments (Courtesy of S Tuft – fig. c; C Barry – fig. d)

excess conjunctiva and enable the remaining conjunctiva to grow on the sclera and not be mobile.

5. **Other modalities** include transconjunctival thermo-cautery or application of topical silver nitrate to the affected area.

Ligneous conjunctivitis

Ligneous conjunctivitis is a very rare disorder characterized by recurrent, often bilateral, firm, fibrin rich, woody-like pseudomebranous lesions that develop mainly on the tarsal conjunctiva. Lesions may also develop in the periodontal tissue in the mouth, upper and lower respiratory tract, middle ear, and cervix. The disease may be triggered by relatively minor trauma or fever. Histology shows an eosinophilic fibrous coagulum (Fig. 8.22a).

Diagnosis

1. **Presentation** is usually in childhood but may be at any age.
2. **Signs**
   - Gradual onset of conjunctival lesions (Fig. 8.22b).
   - The lesions may be covered by a yellow-white thick mucoid discharge (Fig. 8.22c).
   - Subepithelial deposits of hyaline-like material consisting predominantly of fibrin and granulation tissue.
   - Corneal scarring, vascularization, infection or melting may occur.

Treatment

Treatment is very unsatisfactory although the following measures may be beneficial.

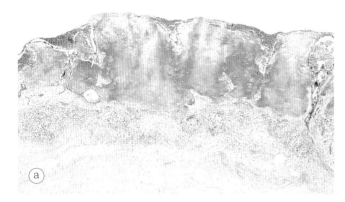

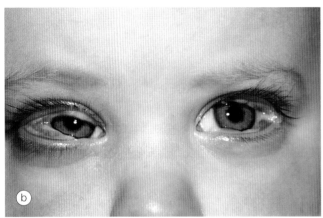

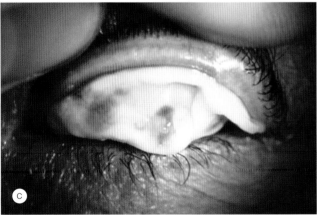

Fig. 8.22
Ligneous conjunctivitis. **(a)** Histology shows eosinophilic
fibrinous coagulum on the conjunctival surface; **(b)** bilateral
involvement in a child; **(c)** thick mucus overlying a ligneous lesion
(Courtesy of J Harry and G Misson, from *Clinical Ophthalmic Pathology*,
Butterworth-Heinemann, 2001 – fig. a; C Barry – fig. b; S Barabino – fig. c)

1. **Surgical** removal with meticulous diathermy of the base
   of the lesion. Simple surgical removal without supplementary therapy results in rapid recurrences in the
   majority of cases.

2. **Topical**
   * Following removal immediate hourly heparin and
     steroids until the wound has re-epithelialized.
   * Subsequently heparin, which is tapered until all signs of
     inflammation have resolved.
   * Re-growth requires long-term ciclosporin and steroids.
3. **Other** modalities include:
   * Intravenous or topical plasminogen prepared from fresh
     frozen plasma.
   * Amniotic membrane transplantation to the conjunc-
     tiva after removal of the lesion.
   * Prophylactic heparin should be used prior to any
     subsequent ocular surgery.

Differential diagnosis

Other causes of conjunctival granulomas include foreign
bodies, amyloid deposits, cat scratch disease, ophthalmia
nodosum, tuberculosis and Kimura disease.

Parinaud oculoglandular syndrome

Parinaud oculoglandular syndrome is a rare condition
characterized by chronic fever, unilateral granulomatous
conjunctivitis with surrounding follicles (Fig. 8.23) and
ipsilateral regional lymphadenopathy. It is virtually
synonymous with cat-scratch disease (see Chapter 24)
although several other agents have been implicated,
including tularaemia, sporotrichosis, tuberculosis, and acute
Chlamydia trachomatis infection.

Factitious conjunctivitis

Self injury (factitious keratitis) is most often intentional.
Corneal injury can also occur inadvertently as in mucous
fishing syndrome and removal of contact lenses. Self injury
may be the result of either mechanical abrasion or
perforation, or self instillation of potentially toxic drops such
as topical anaesthetics and antivirals.

Diagnosis

* Inferior conjunctival injection and staining with rose bengal
  (Fig. 8.24) with a normal superior bulbar conjunctiva.
* Linear corneal abrasions, focal perforations and persistent
  epithelial defect.
* Secondary infection with *Candida*.
* Sterile ring infiltrate and hypopyon.
* Corneal scarring.
* Seeking multiple medical opinions.

Management

* Exclude all other diagnoses.

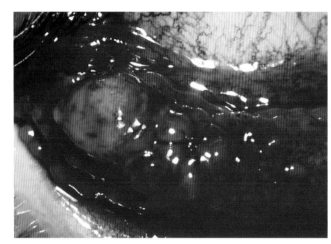

Fig. 8.23
Granulomatous conjunctivitis in Parinaud syndrome

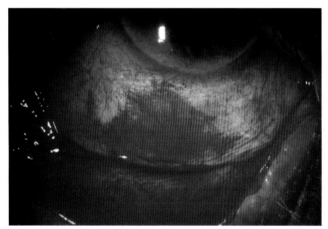

Fig. 8.24
Inferior conjunctival injection and staining with rose bengal in factitious conjunctivitis (Courtesy of S Tuft)

- Close observation may be required.
- Remove supply of medication.
- Immediate confrontation often leads to failure to return for review.

DEGENERATIONS

Pinguecula

A pinguecula is an extremely common, innocuous, usually bilateral and asymptomatic condition.

1. **Signs.** Yellow-white deposits on the bulbar conjunctiva adjacent to the nasal or temporal limbus (Fig. 8.25a).
2. **Treatment** is usually unnecessary because growth is very slow or absent. Occasionally, however, a pinguecula may become acutely inflamed (pingueculitis – Fig. 8.25b) and require a short course of a weak steroid such as fluorometholone.

Pterygium

A pterygium is a triangular fibrovascular subepithelial ingrowth of degenerative bulbar conjunctival tissue over the limbus onto the cornea. Pterygia typically develop in patients who have been living in hot climates and may represent a response to chronic dryness and ultraviolet exposure.

Histology

A pterygium consists of collagenous degenerative changes in vascularized subepithelial stroma (Fig. 8.26a).

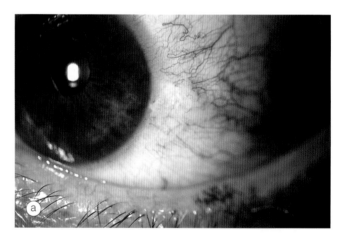

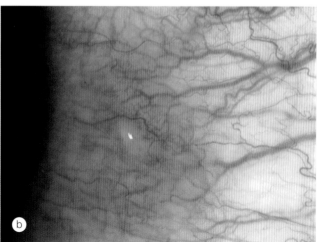

Fig. 8.25
(a) Pinguecula; **(b)** pingueculitis

Clinical features

1. **Type 1** extends less than 2mm onto the cornea (Fig. 8.26b). A deposit of iron (Stocker line) may be seen in the corneal epithelium anterior to the advancing head of the pterygium. The lesion is often asymptomatic, although it may become intermittently inflamed. Patients who wear soft contact lenses may have symptoms earlier because large-diameter lenses rest on the elevated head of the pterygium and cause irritation.
2. **Type 2** involve up to 4mm of the cornea and may be primary or recurrent following surgery (Fig. 8.26c). They may interfere with the precorneal tear film, and induce astigmatism.
3. **Type 3** invade more than 4mm of the cornea and involve the visual axis (Fig. 8.26d). Extensive lesions, particularly if recurrent, may be associated with subconjunctival fibrosis extending to the fornices that may occasionally cause mild restriction in ocular motility.

Treatment

1. **Medical** treatment of symptomatic patients involves tear substitutes, and topical steroids for inflammation. The patient should also be advised to wear sunglasses to reduce ultraviolet exposure and decrease the growth stimulus.
2. **Surgery** is indicated for type 2 and 3 lesions. Simple excision is associated with a high rate of recurrence that may be more aggressive than the initial lesion. Numerous techniques aimed at preventing recurrence have been described. Currently the most widely used technique involves excision of the pterygium and covering of the defect with either a conjunctival autograft or amniotic membrane. Adjunctive treatment with mitomycin C and beta-irradiation may be used to minimize recurrence but may rarely be complicated by late scleral necrosis. Occasionally peripheral lamellar keratoplasty is required for deep extensive lesions.

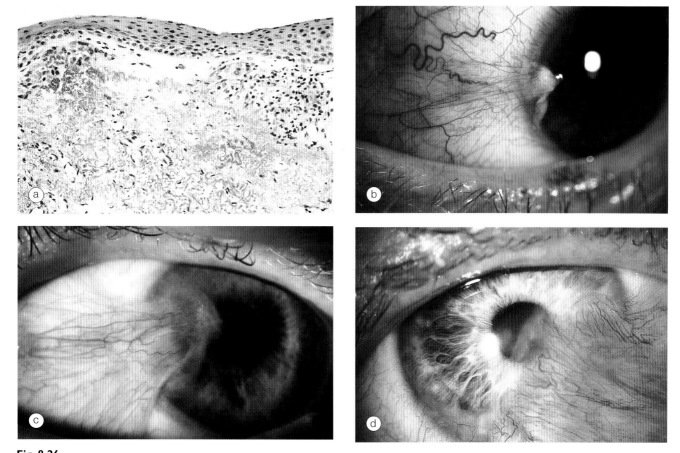

Fig. 8.26
Pterygium. **(a)** Histology shows collagenous degenerative changes in vascularized subepithelial stroma; **(b)** type 1; **(c)** type 2; **(d)** type 3
(Courtesy of J Harry – fig. a)

Differential diagnosis

1. **Pseudopterygium** is caused by the adhesion of a fold of conjunctiva to a peripheral corneal ulcer or area of peripheral thinning, and is fixed only at its apex to the cornea. A true pterygium is adherent to underlying structures throughout.
2. **Conjunctival intraepithelial neoplasia** (see below).

Concretions

Concretions are extremely common lesions which most frequently affect elderly patients and may also occur in chronic meibomian gland disease.

1. **Signs.** Small, often multiple, chalky, yellow-white deposits most commonly seen in the inferior tarsal and forniceal conjunctiva (Fig. 8.27a).
2. **Treatment** is usually unnecessary because concretions are subepithelial and asymptomatic. If a large concretion erodes through the epithelium and causes irritation it can be removed with a needle (Fig. 8.27b).

Conjunctivochalasis

Conjunctivochalasis is probably a normal ageing change that may be exacerbated by posterior lid margin disease. Mechanical stress on the conjunctiva precipitated by dry eye is a potential mechanism.

1. **Symptoms**
   - Watering of the eye by mechanical obstruction of the inferior punctum, interference with the marginal tear meniscus.
   - Foreign body sensation on down-gaze.
2. **Signs**
   - Fold of redundant conjunctiva interposed between the globe and lower eyelid protrudes over the lid margin.
   - Inferior corneal stain with rose bengal (Fig. 8.28).
3. **Treatment**
   - Topical lubricants and treatment of blepharitis (oral doxycycline).
   - Conjunctival resection in severe cases.

Retention cyst

A retention cyst is a very common, usually asymptomatic, thin-walled lesion containing clear fluid (Fig. 8.29a). Small cyst may be arranged in clusters (Fig. 8.29b). Treatment, if appropriate, is by simple puncture with a needle.

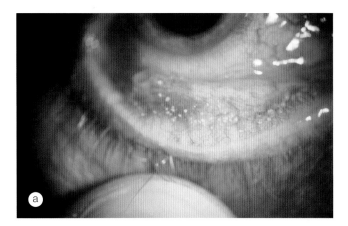

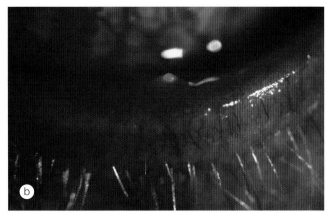

Fig. 8.27
(a) Multiple small concretions; **(b)** large concretion eroding the conjunctival surface

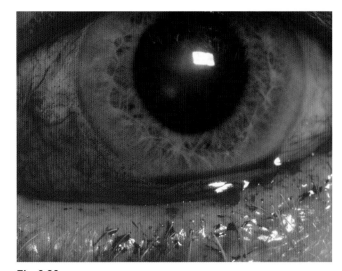

Fig. 8.28
Conjunctivochalasis stained with rose bengal (Courtesy of S Tuft)

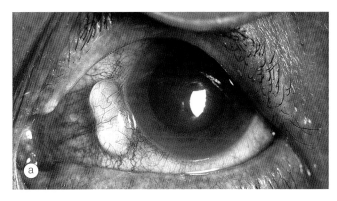

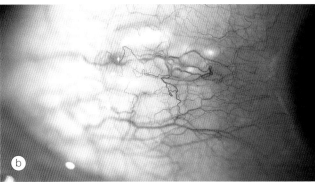

Fig. 8.29
(a) Large solitary conjunctival retention cyst; **(b)** cluster of small cysts

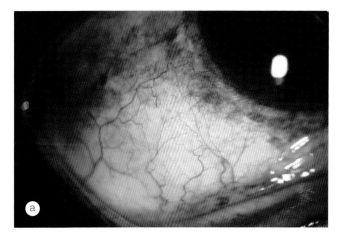

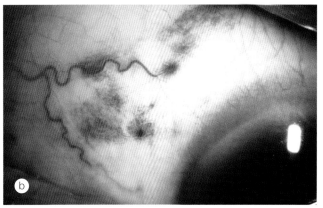

Fig. 8.30
(a) Primary epithelial melanosis; **(b)** associated with an Axenfeld loop

BENIGN PIGMENTED LESIONS

Epithelial melanosis

Primary

Conjunctival (racial) epithelial melanosis is a benign condition due to increased melanin production that is often seen in dark-skinned individuals. Both eyes are affected but the intensity may be asymmetrical.

1. **Presentation** is during the first few years of life. The melanosis becomes static by early adulthood.
2. **Signs**
   - Areas of flat, patchy, brownish pigmentation scattered throughout the conjunctiva but more intense at the limbus (Fig. 8.30a).
   - The lesions may be more intense around the perforating branches of the anterior ciliary vessels or around an intrascleral nerve as they enter the sclera (Axenfeld loop) (Fig. 8.30b).

- Juxtalimbal pigmentation may extend onto the peripheral cornea.
- With the slit-lamp the pigmentation is seen to be within the epithelium and therefore moves freely over the surface of the globe.

Secondary

1. **Mascara deposits** usually accumulate in the inferior fornix (Fig. 8.31a).
2. **Adrenochrome deposits** are tiny clumps of pigment on the tarsal or forniceal conjunctiva associated with the long-term use of adrenaline drops for glaucoma (Fig. 8.31b).

Congenital ocular melanocytosis

Classification

Congenital ocular melanocytosis is an uncommon condition characterized by an increase in number, size and pigmen-

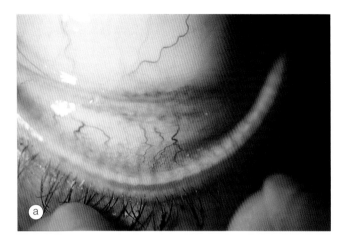

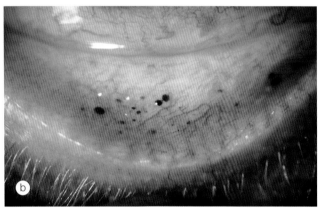

Fig. 8.31
Secondary epithelial melanosis. **(a)** Mascara; **(b)** adrenochrome

tation of melanocytes (Fig. 8.32a). It occurs in the following three clinical settings.

1. **Ocular** melanocytosis, the least common, involves only the eye.
2. **Dermal** melanocytosis involves only the skin and accounts for about one-third of cases.
3. **Oculodermal** melanocytosis (naevus of Ota) which involves both skin and eye is the most frequent type.

Diagnosis

1. **Signs**
   - Multifocal, slate-grey pigmentation in the episclera that cannot be moved over the globe (Fig. 8.32b).
   - Occasionally the peripheral cornea may be involved.
2. **Naevus of Ota** is bilateral in 5% of patients, occurring frequently in Orientals and darker races but rarely in white people.
   - Deep bluish hyperpigmentation of facial skin, most frequently oph the distribution of the first and second divisions of the trigeminal nerve (Fig. 8.32c).

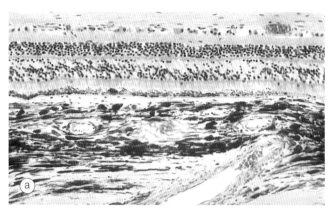

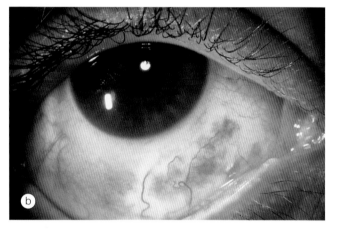

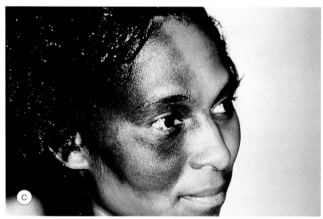

Fig. 8.32
Naevus of Ota. **(a)** Histology shows an increase in the number, size and pigmentation of melanocytes in the inner sclera and choroid; **(b)** ocular melanocytosis; **(c)** dermal melanocytosis.
(Courtesy of J Harry and G Misson, from *Clinical Ophthalmic Pathology*, Butterworth-Heinemann, 2001 – fig. a; P G Watson, B Hazelman, C Pavesio, W R Green, from *The Sclera and Systemic Disorders*, Butterworth-Heinemann, 2004 – fig. c)

- It may be subtle in fair-skinned individuals and is best detected by observation in good lighting.
- Involvement of the third division of the trigeminal nerve and of the nasal and buccal mucosa is uncommon.

Ipsilateral associations

1. **Iris hyperchromia** is common (Fig. 8.33a).
2. **Iris mammillations** which are tiny, regularly spaced, villiform lesions are uncommon (Fig. 8.33b). They may also be found in patients with neurofibromatosis-1, Axenfeld–Rieger anomaly and Peters anomaly.

3. **Fundus hyperpigmentation** can occur (Fig. 8.33c).
4. **Trabecular hyperpigmentation** (Fig. 8.33d), which is associated with glaucoma in about 10% of cases.
5. **Uveal melanoma** may develop in a small minority of white people.

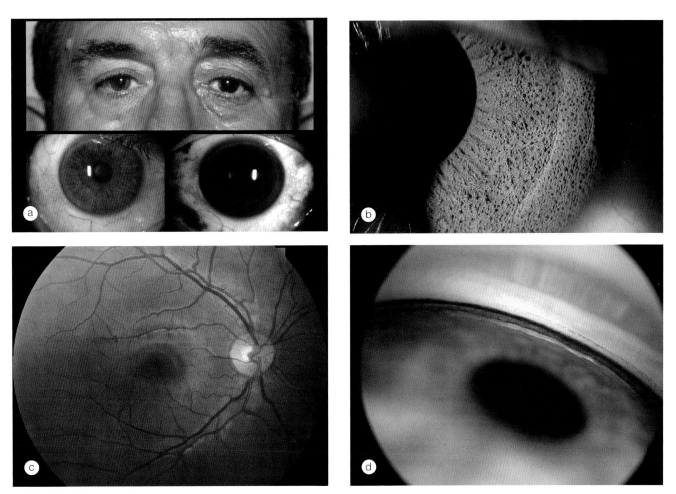

Fig. 8.33
Associations of Naevus of Ota. **(a)** Heterochromia iridis; **(b)** iris mammillations; **(c)** fundus hyperpigmentation; **(d)** trabecular hyperpigmentation (Courtesy of P Gili – fig. a; L MacKeen – fig. d)

CHAPTER 9

CORNEA

INTRODUCTION

Anatomy

The average corneal diameter is 11.5mm (vertical) and 12mm (horizontal). The cornea consists of the following layers (Fig. 9.1):

1. **The epithelium** is stratified, squamous and non-keratinized, and comprises:
   - A single layer of basal columnar cells attached by hemidesmosomes to the underlying basement membrane.
   - Two to three rows of wing cells.
   - Two layers of squamous surface cells.
   - The surface area of the outermost cells is increased by microplicae and microvilli that facilitate the attachment of mucin and the tear film. After a lifespan of a few days the superficial cells are shed into the tear film.

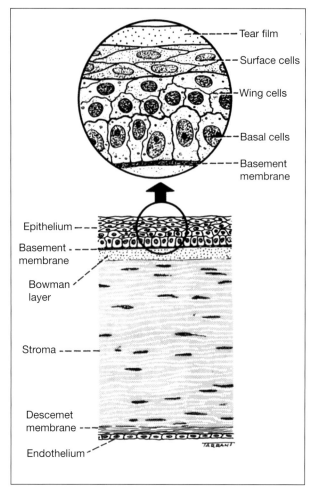

Fig. 9.1
Anatomy of the cornea

- The epithelial stem cells are principally located at the superior and inferior limbus, possibly in the palisades of Vogt, and are indispensable for the maintenance of healthy corneal epithelium. They also act as a junctional barrier, preventing conjunctival tissue from growing onto the cornea.

NB Dysfunction or deficiency of limbal stem cells may result in chronic epithelial defects, overgrowth of conjunctival epithelium onto the corneal surface and vascularization. Some of these problems may be treated by limbal cell transplantation.

2. **Bowman layer** is the acellular superficial layer of the stroma.
3. **The stroma** makes up 90% of corneal thickness. It is principally composed of regularly orientated layers of collagen fibrils whose spacing is maintained by proteoglycan ground substance (chondroitin sulphate and keratan sulphate) with interspersed modified fibroblasts (keratocytes).
4. **Descemet membrane** is composed of a fine latticework of collagen fibrils. It consists of an anterior banded zone that is deposited *in utero* and a posterior non-banded zone laid down throughout life by the endothelium.
5. **The endothelium** consists of a single layer of hexagonal cells that cannot regenerate. It plays a vital role in maintaining corneal deturgescence. The adult cell density is about 2500 cells/mm^2. The number of cells decreases at about 0.6% per year and neighbouring cells enlarge to fill the space as cells die. At a cell density of about 500 cells/mm^2 corneal oedema develops and corneal transparency is reduced.

NB The cornea is the most densely innervated tissue in the body. The sensory supply is via the first division of the trigeminal nerve. There is a subepithelial and a stromal plexus of nerves. In eyes with corneal abrasions or bullous keratopathy, the direct stimulation of these nerve endings causes pain, reflex lacrimation and photophobia.

Signs of corneal inflammation

NB Because definitions vary between clinicians it is recommended that signs are described or drawn wherever possible.

Superficial lesions

1. **Punctate epithelial erosions (PEE).**
   a. **Signs.** Tiny, epithelial defects that stain with fluorescein (Fig. 9.2a) and with rose bengal.

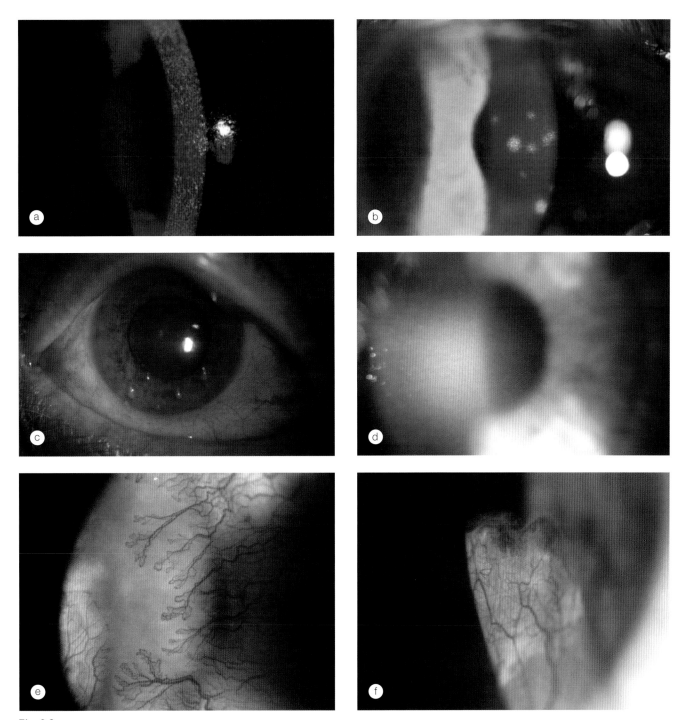

Fig. 9.2
Superficial corneal lesions. **(a)** Punctate epithelial erosions stained with fluorescein; **(b)** punctate epithelial keratitis; **(c)** unstained filaments; **(d)** epithelial oedema; **(e)** superficial neovascularization; **(f)** pannus (Courtesy of A Bacon – fig. a; S Tuft – figs b and c)

b. Causes are non-specific and PEE may develop in response to a wide variety of stimuli. Location may frequently indicate aetiology; for example:
- Superior in vernal disease, superior limbic kerato-conjunctivitis, floppy eyelids and poorly fitting contact lenses.
- Interpalpebral in dry eyes, reduced corneal sensation and exposure to ultraviolet light.
- Inferior in blepharitis, lagophthalmos, toxicity from drops and self-induced.

2. Punctate epithelial keratitis (PEK)

a. Signs. Granular, opalescent, swollen epithelial cells, visible unstained (Fig. 9.2b), which stain well with rose bengal but poorly with fluorescein.

b. Causes
- Adenoviral infection is the most common.
- Chlamydial infections.
- Thygeson superficial punctate keratitis.
- Staphylococcal hypersensitivity.

3. Mucus filaments

a. Signs. Mucus strands lined with epithelium, attached at one end to the corneal surface; the unattached end moves with each blink (Fig. 9.2c). Grey subepithelial opacities may be seen at the site of attachments. They stain well with rose bengal.

b. Causes
- Dry eye is by far the most common.
- Superior limbic keratoconjunctivitis.
- Corneal epithelial instability.
- Neurotrophic keratitis.
- Eye patching.
- Essential blepharospasm.

4. Epithelial oedema is characterized by loss of normal corneal lustre (Fig. 9.2d) and if severe may be associated with vesicles and bullae. It is a sign of endothelial decompensation or severe, acute elevation of intraocular pressure and may be associated with stromal oedema.

5. Superficial neovascularization is a feature of chronic ocular surface irritation or hypoxia as in contact lens wear (Fig. 9.2e).

6. Pannus is a non-specific term that is usually applied to superficial neovascularization accompanied by degenerative subepithelial change extending centrally from the limbus (Fig. 9.2f); it follows chronic surface inflammation.

Deep lesions

1. Infiltrates are focal areas of active stromal inflammation composed of accumulations of leucocytes and cellular debris.

a. Signs. Focal, granular, grey-white opacities usually within the anterior stroma and associated with limbal or conjunctival hyperaemia (Fig. 9.3a). A surrounding halo of less dense infiltration such that individual inflammatory cells may be discernible.

b. Causes
- Non-infectious 'sterile keratitis' is the result of a hypersensitivity response to antigen.
- Suppurative keratitis caused by bacteria, viruses, fungi and protozoa.

NB The **'PEDAL'** mnemonic is useful in distinguishing non-infectious from suppurative infiltrates. The latter are typically associated with more **P**ain, have larger **E**pithelial defects (> 1mm), have purulent **D**ischarge, are associated with **A**nterior chamber reaction (uveitis, hypopyon) and usually have a more central **L**ocation.

2. Ulceration (Fig. 9.3b) is due to melting of the connective tissue in response to the release of enzymes from endogenous sources in response to inflammation or from exogenous organisms (bacteria, amoebae and fungi).

NB Classification of melting disorders into *central* or *peripheral ulcerative keratitis* can be a helpful aid in determining aetiology. In rheumatoid arthritis a central melt is often the result of dry eye, whereas a peripheral melt is often immune mediated.

3. Vascularization (Fig. 9.3c) occurs in response to a wide variety of stimuli. The venous blood vessels are easily seen, whereas the arterial feeding vessels are smaller and require high magnification. Non-perfused, deep vessels appear as 'ghost vessels', best detected by retroillumination (see Fig. 9.18b).

4. Lipid deposition follows chronic inflammation with leakage from corneal new vessels (Fig. 9.3d).

5. Folds in Descemet membrane (striate keratopathy – Fig. 9.3e) may be caused by surgical trauma, ocular hypotony and stromal inflammation.

6. Breaks in Descemet membrane (Fig. 9.3f) may be due to corneal enlargement, birth trauma and keratoconus. They may result in acute influx of aqueous into the corneal stroma.

Documentation of clinical signs

A clinical diagram is useful to document the type and position of each change. The dimensions of epithelial opacities and stromal ulceration, and depth of new vessels and opacities should be recorded. Colour coding can be helpful (Fig. 9.4).

1. Opacities such as scars and degenerations are drawn in black.

2. Epithelial oedema is represented by fine blue circles, stromal oedema as blue shading and folds in Descemet membrane as wavy blue lines.

3. Hypopyon is shown in yellow.

4. Blood vessels are then added in red. Superficial vessels are wavy lines that begin outside the limbus and deep vessels are straight lines that begin at the limbus.

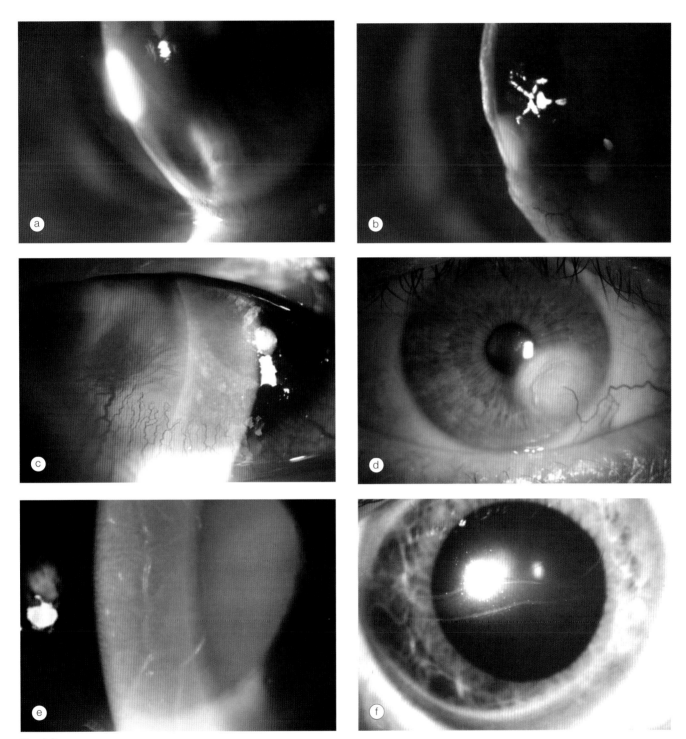

Fig. 9.3
Deep corneal lesions. **(a)** Infiltration; **(b)** ulceration; **(c)** vascularization; **(d)** lipid deposition; **(e)** folds in Descemet membrane; **(f)** breaks in Descemet membrane (Courtesy of S Tuft – fig. d)

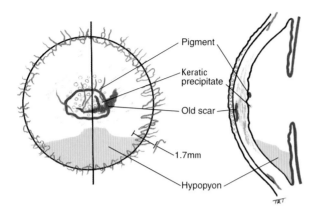

Fig. 9.4
Documentation of corneal lesions

5. **Pigment** such as iron rings and Krukenberg spindle are shown in brown.

Principles of treatment

The aim is to stop the disease process, eliminate any infectious agent, and limit associated corneal damage.

> **NB** Have a working diagnosis on which to base treatment. Try to avoid unguided intervention and be prepared to modify the diagnosis.

Control of infection and inflammation

1. **Antimicrobial agents** should be started as soon as preliminary investigations have been completed. The initial choice of agent is determined by the likely aetiology, which is determined by the clinical examination. Broad spectrum treatment is used initially, with more selective agents introduced if necessary when the results of investigation are available.
2. **Topical steroids** should be used with caution because they may promote microbial growth and suppress corneal repair. They are contraindicated in active herpes simplex epithelial disease without effective antiviral cover.
3. **Systemic immunosuppressive agents** may be useful in certain forms of severe corneal ulceration and melting associated with systemic connective tissue disorders.

Promotion of healing

In eyes with a thin stroma it is important to promote re-epithelialization because thinning seldom progresses if the epithelium is intact. The following are the main methods of promoting re-epithelialization:

1. **Reduction of exposure** to toxic medications and preservatives wherever possible.
2. **Lubrication** with unpreserved artificial tears and ointments.
3. **Eyelid closure** is particularly useful in exposure and neurotrophic keratopathies as well as in eyes with persistent epithelial defects. It can be achieved by one of the following methods:
   - Taping the lids closed temporarily (Fig. 9.5a).
   - Botulinum toxin injection into the levator muscle to induce a temporary ptosis.
   - Lateral tarsorrhaphy (Fig. 9.5b) or medial canthoplasty.
4. **Conjunctival (Gundersen) flap** will cover the corneal ulceration if it is progressive and unresponsive (Fig. 9.5c). This procedure is particularly suitable for chronic unilateral disease in which the prognosis for restoration of useful vision is poor.
5. **Bandage soft contact lenses** (Fig. 9.5d) promote healing by mechanically protecting regenerating corneal epithelium from the constant rubbing of the eyelids.
6. **Amniotic membrane grafting** (Fig. 9.5e) may be necessary for persistent unresponsive epithelial defects.
7. **Tissue adhesive** (cyanoacrylate) glue may be used to limit stromal ulceration and to seal small perforations. It is first applied onto a plastic patch, which is then applied to the area of thinning or perforation and a bandage contact lens inserted (Fig. 9.5f).
8. **Limbal stem cell transplantation** may be required if there is stem cell deficiency following a variety of injuries such as chemical burns or cicatrizing conjunctivitis. The source of the donor tissue may be the fellow eye (autograft) in unilateral disease or from a living or cadaver donor (allograft) when both eyes are affected.

BACTERIAL KERATITIS

Introduction

Pathogens

Bacterial keratitis is very uncommon in a normal eye and usually only develops when the ocular defences have been compromised. Bacteria that can penetrate an apparently normal corneal epithelium are *N. gonorrhoeae, N. meningitidis, C. diphtheriae* and *H. influenzae*. The virulence of the organism and the anatomic site of the infection determine the pattern of disease. The most common pathogens are:

1. *P. aeruginosa* which is a ubiquitous Gram-negative bacillus (rod) that flourishes in soil, vegetation and moist situations in the hospital environment. It is also a commensal of the gastrointestinal tract.
2. *S. aureus* which is a common Gram-positive and coagulase-positive commensal of the nares, skin and conjunctiva.

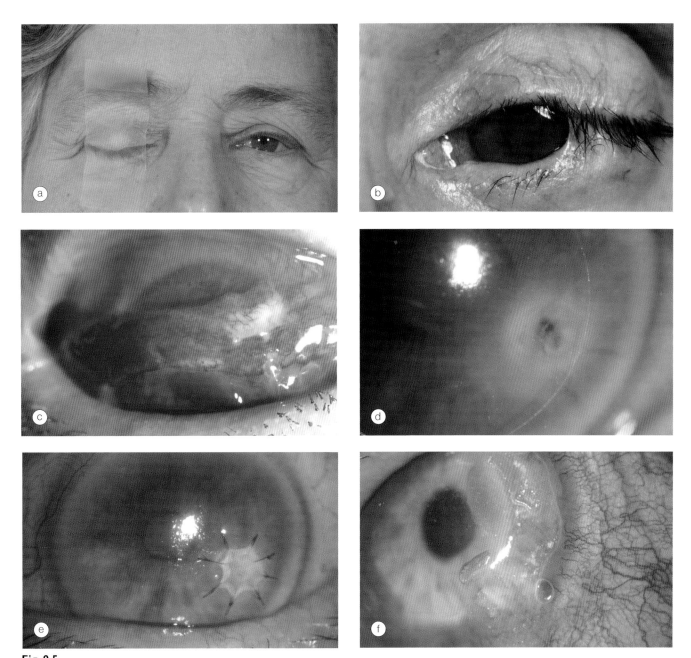

Fig. 9.5
Methods of promoting healing. **(a)** Taping the lids temporarily; **(b)** lateral tarsorrhaphy; **(c)** conjunctival (Gundersen) flap; **(d)** bandage contact lens in an eye with a small perforation; **(e)** amniotic membrane graft over a persistent epithelial defect; **(f)** tissue glue under a bandage contact lens in an eye with severe peripheral thinning (Courtesy of S Tuft – figs a, d, e and f)

3. *S. pyogenes* is a common Gram-positive commensal of the throat and vagina.
4. *S. pneumoniae* (pneumococcus) is a Gram-positive commensal of the upper respiratory tract.

NB Infections with *Pseudomonas* and streptococci are often very aggressive.

Risk factors

1. **Contact lens wear,** particularly of soft lenses worn overnight, is the most important risk factor for bacterial keratitis. *Pseudomonas* spp. account for over 60% of cases. Infection is more likely if there is poor lens hygiene but it can also occur even with apparently meticulous lens care and with daily disposable lenses. Bacteria may multiply in the contact lens case where they are protected from disinfection by bacterial biofilm. A corneal epithelium compromised by hypoxia and trauma is also susceptible to infection. A diagnosis of bacterial keratitis must be considered in any contact lens user with an acutely painful red eye.
2. **Trauma** such as accidental injury, surgical (refractive surgery) and loose sutures. In developing countries agricultural injury is the major risk factor for developing corneal infection.
3. **Ocular surface disease** such as herpetic keratitis, bullous keratopathy, dry eye, chronic blepharitis, trichiasis, exposure, severe allergic eye disease and corneal anaesthesia.
4. **Other factors** include topical or systemic immuno-suppression, diabetes, vitamin A deficiency and measles.

Diagnosis

Clinical features

1. **History** with particular attention paid to risk factors mentioned above.
2. **Presenting symptoms** include pain, photophobia, blurred vision and discharge.
3. **Signs** in chronological order:
   - An epithelial defect associated with an infiltrate around the margin and base associated with circumcorneal injection (Fig. 9.6a).
   - Enlargement of the infiltrate associated with stromal oedema and small hypopyon (Fig. 9.6b).
   - Severe infiltration with enlarging hypopyon (Fig. 9.6d).
   - Progressive ulceration may lead to corneal perforation and endophthalmitis.
   - Scleritis may develop with infections at the limbus.

NB If the cornea is opaque an ultrasound scan should be performed to exclude endophthalmitis.

4. **Differential diagnosis** includes fungal keratitis, acanthamoeba keratitis, necrotic stromal herpes simplex keratitis, marginal keratitis and sterile inflammatory corneal infiltrates associated with contact lens wear. Table 9.1 shows the comparison between marginal and bacterial keratitis.

Microbiology

NB Techniques and preferred culture media vary according to centres; liaison with the microbiologist is essential.

1. **Taking samples**
   - A non-preserved topical anaesthetic is instilled.
   - At the slit-lamp any loose mucus is wiped away from the surface of the ulcer.
   - The margins and base of the lesion are scraped either with a heat sterilized (Kimura) spatula, a blade, or the bent tip of a 21-gauge hypodermic needle.
   - A thin smear is placed on a glass slide for Gram stain and microscopy.

NB Do not use transport media because the sample volume is tiny and isolation is unlikely.

2. **Gram staining**
   - Differentiates bacterial species into Gram-positive and Gram-negative based on the ability of the dye (crystal violet) to penetrate the cell wall.
   - Bacteria that take up crystal violet are Gram-positive (Fig. 9.7a and b) and those that allow the dye to wash off are Gram-negative (Fig. 9.7c).
3. **Culture media.** The samples are plated onto selected media (Fig. 9.7d), taking care not to break the surface of the agar, and placed into an incubator until they are transported to the laboratory.
   - Blood agar (Fig. 9.7e) is suitable for most bacteria and fungi except *Neisseria*, *Haemophilus* and *Moraxella* spp.
   - Chocolate agar (Fig. 9.7f) is used to isolate *Neisseria*, *Haemophilus* and *Moraxella* spp.
   - Cooked meat broth for anaerobic and fastidious organisms.
   - Brain-heart infusion for most aerobic bacteria and fungi.
   - For unresponsive ulcers consider stopping treatment for 24 hours before re-scraping the ulcer. Additional examinations should then include Ziehl–Neelsen stain and Lowenstein–Jensen media.
4. **Sensitivity report.** The plates should be transported to the laboratory as soon as possible to increase the chances of isolating the offending organism. Generally, reports are sent out at 1 or 2 days, 7 days and 2 weeks. When determining drug sensitivity for an isolated organism the results are reported as:

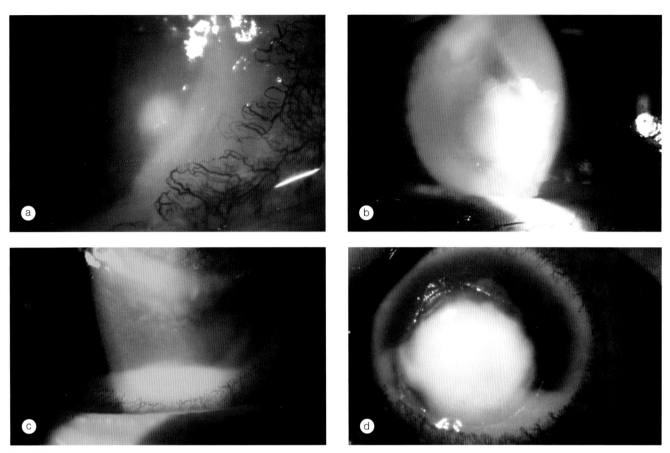

Fig. 9.6
Bacterial keratitis. **(a)** Peripheral infiltration; **(b)** enlargement of infiltrate; **(c)** hypopyon; **(d)** advanced keratitis (Courtesy of S Tuft – fig a)

Table 9.1   Comparison between marginal and bacterial keratitis

	Marginal keratitis	*Bacterial keratitis*
Location	Peripheral	Central
Size	< 1mm	> 1mm
Epithelial defect	Small or absent	Present
Uveitis	Absent	Present

a. Susceptible: the organism is sensitive to the normal dose of the antimicrobial agent.

b. Intermediate: the organism is likely to be sensitive to a high dose of the antimicrobial agent.

c. Resistant: the organism is not sensitive to the antimicrobial agent at the tested dose.

NB Most laboratories report sensitivity using a disc diffusion (Kirby–Bauer) method. The relevance of these results to topical antibiotics that can achieve very high tissue levels is uncertain.

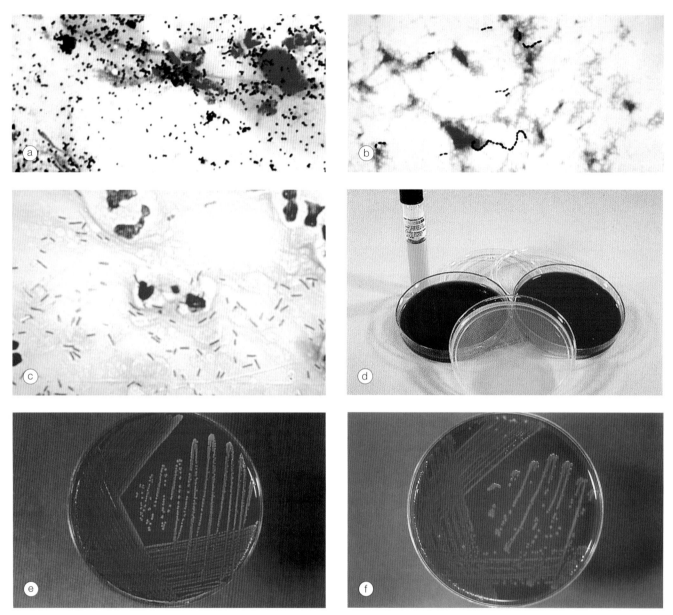

Fig. 9.7
Bacteriology. **(a)** Smear of pus shows Gram-positive spherical cocci mostly arranged in clusters (*S. aureus*); **(b)** smear shows Gram-positive cocci arranged in pairs or chains (*S. pyogenes*); **(c)** smear shows Gram-negative bacilli (*P. aeruginosa*); **(d)** culture media; **(e)** *S. aureus* grown on blood agar forming golden colonies with a shiny surface; **(f)** *N. gonorrhoeae* grown on chocolate agar (Courtesy of J Harry – fig a; J Harry and G Misson from *Clinical Ophthalmic Pathology,* Butterworth-Heinemann, 2001 – figs b–c; Emond, Welsby and Rowland, from *Colour Atlas of Infectious Diseases,* Mosby, 2003 – figs d–f)

Treatment

Bacterial keratitis has the potential to progress rapidly to corneal perforation. Even small axial lesions can cause surface irregularity and scar that can lead to significant loss of vision.

General principles

1. **Decision** to treat is based on clinical grounds but the causative organism cannot be guessed reliably from the appearance of the ulcer. Treatment should be initiated even if Gram stain is negative and before the results of culture are available.

Table 9.2   Antibiotics for treatment of keratitis

Isolate	Antibiotic	Concentration
Empiric treatment	Cefuroxime +	5%
	Gentamicin or	1.4%
	Fluoroquinolone	0.3%
Gram-positive cocci	Cefuroxime	0.3%
	Vancomycin	5%
Gram-negative rods	Gentamicin or	1.4%
	Fluoroquinolone or	0.3%
	Ceftazidime	5%
Gram-negative cocci	Fluoroquinolone	0.3%
	Ceftriaxone	5%
Mycobacteria	Amikacin or	2%
	Clarithromycin	
Nocardia	Amikacin or	2%
	Trimethoprim +	1.6%
	sulphamethoxazole	8%

2. **Topical** therapy can achieve high tissue concentration and initially should involve broad spectrum antibiotics to cover the most common pathogens.
3. **Dual therapy** involves a combination of two fortified antibiotics (an aminoglycoside and a cephalosporin) to cover common Gram-positive and Gram-negative pathogens. It is not commercially available and the antibiotics have to be specially prepared (see below).
4. **Monotherapy** with a fluoroquinolone (e.g ciprofloxacin 0.3% or ofloxacin 0.3%) is commercially available. Although they contain preservatives, toxicity is uncommon, although ciprofloxacin may be associated with white corneal precipitates which may also delay epithelial healing. Table 9.2 lists the antibiotics used in the treatment of keratitis.

NB Increasing resistance to fluoroquinolones has been reported (*Staphylococcus* spp. in the USA, and *Pseudomonas* spp. in India). New generations of fluoroquinolones (e.g. moxifloxacin) have been introduced to address this. MRSA is an uncommon cause of bacterial keratitis and can usually be treated with vancomycin.

Preparation of fortified antibiotics

A standard parenteral or lyophilized antibiotic preparation is combined with a compatible vehicle such that the antibiotic does not precipitate.

1. **Gentamicin** 15mg/ml (1.5%): 2ml of parenteral antibiotic (40mg/ml) is added to 4ml commercially available antibiotic ophthalmic solution (0.3%).

2. **Cefazolin, cefuroxime, or ceftazidime** 50mg/ml (5%): 500mg parenteral antibiotic is diluted with 2.5ml sterile water and added to 7.5ml of preservative-free artificial tears. This is stable for 24 hours at room temperature or 96 hours if kept in a refrigerator.

NB Potential problems with fortified antibiotics include cost, limited availability, possibly decreased sterility, short shelf-life and need for refrigeration.

Treatment regimen

1. **Topical antibiotics** are initially instilled at hourly intervals day and night for 24–48 hours. The frequency can be reduced to 2-hourly during waking hours for a further 48 hours, and then q.i.d. for 1 week. Treatment is continued until the epithelium has healed.

NB It is important not to confuse failure of re-epithelialization (persistent epithelial defect), resulting from toxicity, with continued infection.

2. **Oral antibiotics** (ciprofloxacin 750mg twice daily for 7–10 days) is not usually necessary. Exceptions are threatened or actual corneal perforation, or a peripheral ulcer in which there is scleral extension. Oral therapy is also indicated for isolates for which there are potential systemic complications (e.g. *N. meningitidis*).
3. **Subconjunctival** antibiotics are only indicated if there is poor compliance with topical treatment. Intensive topical treatment and subconjunctival injection achieve similar corneal levels.
4. **When to change antibiotics?** Only if a resistant pathogen is isolated and ulceration is progressing. There is no need to change initial therapy if this has induced a favourable response, *even if cultures show a resistant organism.*
5. **Mydriatics** (atropine 1% or cyclopentolate 1%) are used to prevent the formation of posterior synechiae and to reduce pain from ciliary spasm.
6. **Topical steroids** therapy in established bacterial infection is unproven and the following guidelines apply:
   - They should not be introduced until the sensitivity of the isolate to antibiotics has been demonstrated and fungal infection excluded.
   - They can potentiate coexisting fungal or herpes infection, and may make elimination of acanthamoeba infection more difficult.
   - They reduce inflammation and can rapidly make the eye more comfortable. However, their use probably does not affect the amount of scar formation or the final visual outcome.
   - They may help to prevent rejection following infection of a corneal graft.

Causes of failure

1. **Incorrect diagnosis** caused by inappropriate cultures.
   - The most common causes are unrecognized infection with herpes simplex virus, fungi, acanthamoeba and atypical mycobacteria.
   - The cultures should be repeated using special media such as Lowenstein–Jensen (mycobacteria) and non-nutrient agar seeded with *E. coli* (acanthamoeba).
   - If cultures are still negative, it may be necessary to perform corneal biopsy for histology and culture, or excisional keratoplasty.
2. **Inappropriate choice of antibiotics.**
3. **Drug toxicity,** particularly following frequent instillation of fortified aminoglycosides, may cause conjunctival necrosis and white corneal precipitates (Fig. 9.8) which delay corneal epithelial healing. There may be increasing discomfort, redness and discharge despite eradication of infection.
4. **Gram-negative ulcers** may show increased inflammation during the first 48 hours despite appropriate treatment.

Visual rehabilitation

1. **Lamellar keratoplasty** may be required for residual dense corneal scarring.
2. **Rigid contact lenses** may be required for irregular astigmatism but only 3 months after re-epithelialization of the ulcer.
3. **Cataract surgery** may be required because secondary lens opacities are common following severe inflammation.

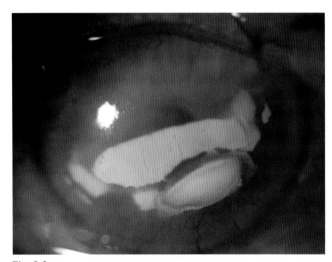

Fig. 9.8
Ciprofloxacin corneal precipitates

FUNGAL KERATITIS

Fungi are micro-organisms that have rigid walls and multiple chromosomes containing both DNA and RNA. The main types are:

1. **Filamentous** fungi (*Aspergillus* spp., *Fusarium solani*, and *Scedosporium* spp.) are multicellular organisms that produce tubular projections known as hyphae. They are the most common pathogens in tropical climates.
2. **Yeasts** (*Candida* spp.) are ovoid unicellular organisms that reproduce by budding and may occasionally form hyphae or pseudo-hyphae. They are responsible for most cases in temperate climates.

Pathogenesis

Fungal keratitis is rare in temperate countries but is a major cause of visual loss in tropical and developing countries. In some hot and humid regions it accounts for 50% of cases. The primary risk factors for infection are trauma (65% of cases in tropical areas) particularly with vegetable matter, chronic ocular surface disease and epithelial defects, diabetes, systemic immunosuppression and hydrophilic contact lenses. Fungal infection can elicit a severe inflammatory response that can cause stromal necrosis and melting. Filamentous fungi can penetrate the intact Descemet membrane and corneal perforation is common. Once in the anterior chamber the infection is very difficult to eradicate and aggressive surgery is usually required.

Clinical features

The diagnosis is often delayed unless there is a high index of suspicion.

1. **Presenting symptoms** are a gradual onset of foreign body sensation, photophobia, blurred vision and discharge. Patients often have a history of trauma or chronic ocular surface disease.
2. **Signs** vary with the infectious agent. In early disease there tends to be less redness and lid swelling than with bacterial infection.
   - *a. Filamentous keratitis*
     - A grey-yellow stromal infiltrate with indistinct margins.
     - Progressive infiltration, often surrounded by satellite lesions, and hypopyon (Fig. 9.9a).
   - *b. Candida keratitis* is characterized by a yellow-white infiltrate associated with dense suppuration (Fig. 9.9b).

Investigations

Laboratory examination should be performed before starting antifungal therapy as it is slowly progressive. Filamentous fungi tend to proliferate anterior to Descemet membrane and

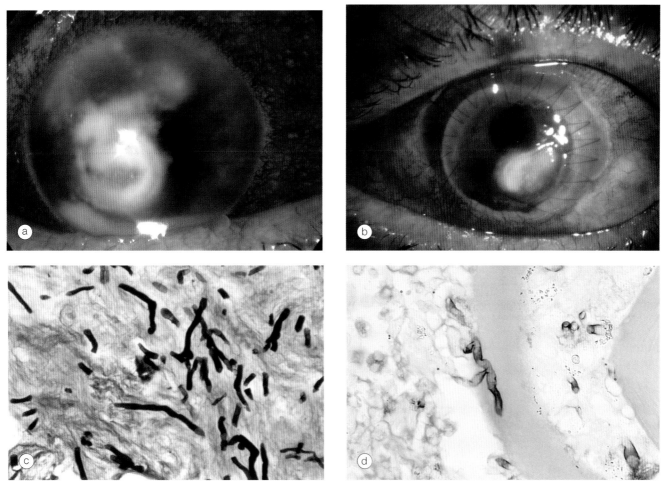

Fig. 9.9
Fungal keratitis. **(a)** Filamentous keratitis with satellite lesions and a small hypopyon; **(b)** *Candida* keratitis following penetrating keratoplasty; **(c)** Gram-stained *Candida* spp. shows pseudohyphae; **(d)** corneal smear stained with Grocott hexamine silver shows *Aspergillus* spp. (Courtesy of S Tuft – fig. a; Hart and Shears – fig. c; J Harry and G Misson, from *Clinical Ophthalmic Pathology*, Butterworth-Heinemann, 2001 – fig. d)

a deep stromal biopsy may be required (similar in technique to performing a trabeculectomy – the excised deep tissue is sent for culture). Sometimes the diagnosis can only be confirmed following anterior chamber tap or excisional keratoplasty.

1. **Gram and Giemsa** staining are equally sensitive (Fig. 9.9c).
2. **Cultures** should be taken and plated on Sabouraud dextrose agar, although most fungi will also grow on blood agar or in enrichment media at 27°C. Sensitivity testing can be performed in reference laboratories but the relevance of these results to clinical effectiveness is uncertain.
3. **Histology** involving periodic acid–Schiff (PAS) stain and Grocott silver stain of corneal tissue are the most sensitive (Fig. 9.9d).

Treatment

1. **Removal of the epithelium** over the lesion enhances penetration of antifungal agents. Similarly, a superficial keratectomy may help de-bulk the lesion.
2. **Topical treatment** should be given intensively: initially hourly for 48 hours and then reducing as signs permit. As most antifungals are only fungistatic topical treatment should be continued for several weeks.
   a. Filamentous infection is treated with natamycin 5% or econazole 1%. Amphotericin B 0.15% and miconazole 1% are alternatives.
   b. Candida infection is usually treated with econazole 1%. Alternatives include natamycin 5%, fluconazole 2%, amphotericin B 0.15% and clotrimazole 1%.

NB A broad spectrum antibiotic should also be used as bacterial co-infection is common.

3. **Subconjunctival** fluconazole may be used in severe cases with hypopyon.
4. **Systemic** anti-fungals may be required for severe keratitis or endophthalmitis. Preferred treatment options are itraconazole 100mg daily or voriconazole 100mg with a loading dose of 200mg.
5. **Excisional penetrating keratoplasty** may be required in unresponsive cases.

VIRAL KERATITIS

Herpes simplex keratitis

Herpetic eye disease is the major cause of unilateral corneal scarring worldwide, and is the most common infectious cause of corneal blindness in developed countries. As many as 60% of corneal ulcers in developing countries may be the result of herpes simplex virus (HSV) and 10 million people worldwide may have herpetic eye disease.

Herpes simplex virus

HSV is enveloped with a cuboidal capsule and a linear double-stranded DNA genome. The two subtypes are *HSV-1* and *HSV-2* which reside in almost all ganglia. *HSV-1* primarily causes infection above the waist that may affect the face, lips and eyes, whereas *HSV-2* causes venereally acquired infection (genital herpes). Rarely *HSV-2* may be transmitted to the eye through infected secretions, either venereally or at birth (ophthalmia neonatorum). HSV transmission is facilitated in conditions of crowding and poor hygiene.

Primary infection

Primary infection (no previous viral exposure) usually occurs by droplet transmission, or less frequently by direct inoculation. Due to protection bestowed by maternal antibodies, it is uncommon during the first 6 months of life. Most cases are probably subclinical or only cause mild fever, malaise and upper respiratory tract symptoms. Children may develop blepharoconjunctivitis (Fig. 9.10) which is usually benign and self-limited although corneal microdendrites develop in a minority of cases.

Recurrent infection

Recurrent disease (reactivation in presence of cellular and humoral immunity) occurs as follows:

1. **After primary infection** the virus is carried to the sensory ganglion for that dermatome (e.g. trigeminal ganglion) where a latent infection is established.
2. **Subclinical reactivation** can periodically occur when HSV is shed and patients are contagious. Stimuli such as

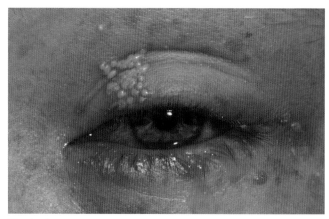

Fig. 9.10
Blepharoconjunctivitis in primary herpes simplex infection

fever, hormonal change, ultraviolet radiation, trauma, and trigeminal injury may cause a clinical reactivation, when the virus replicates and is transported in the sensory axons to the periphery where there is recurrent disease.
3. **The pattern of disease** depends on the site of reactivation, which may be remote from the site of primary disease. Hundreds of reactivations can occur during lifetime.
4. **The rate for ocular recurrence** after one episode is estimated to increase from 10% at 1 year, 23% at 2 years, to about 50% at 10 years. The more the number of previous attacks the greater the risk of recurrence.

   NB Risk factors for severe disease, which may be bilateral and frequently recurrent, include atopic eye disease, children, AIDS, malnutrition, measles, and malaria. Inappropriate use of topical steroids may enhance the development of geographic ulceration (see below).

Clinical features of epithelial keratitis

Epithelial (dendritic, geographic) keratitis is the result of virus replication and is the most common presentation.

1. **Presentation** may be at any age with mild discomfort, watering and blurred vision.
2. **Signs** in chronological order:
   - Opaque epithelial cells arranged in a coarse punctate or stellate pattern.
   - Central desquamation results in a linear-branching (dendritic) ulcer, most frequently located centrally (Fig. 9.11a).
   - The ends of the ulcer have characteristic terminal buds and the bed of the ulcer stains well with fluorescein (Fig. 9.11b).

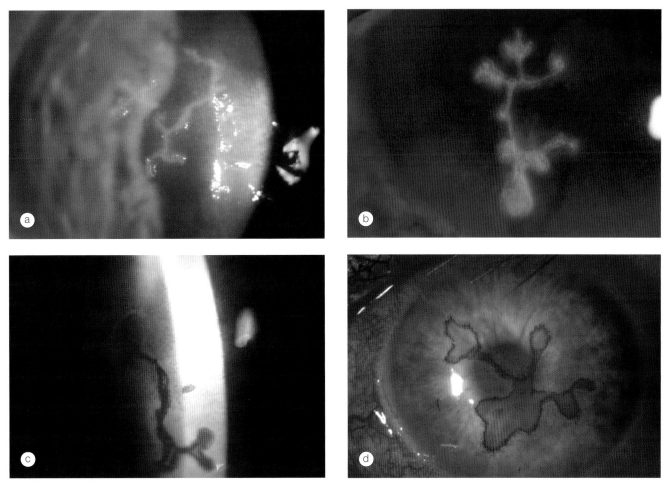

Fig. 9.11
Epithelial herpes simplex keratitis. **(a)** Unstained dendritic ulcer; **(b)** bed of a dendritic ulcer stained with fluorescein; **(c)** margins of a dendritic ulcer stained with rose bengal; **(d)** geographic ulcer (Courtesy of S Tuft – figs a and d)

- The virus-laden cells at the margin of the ulcer stain with rose bengal (Fig. 9.11c).
- Corneal sensation is reduced.
- Inadvertent topical steroid treatment may allow progressive enlargement of the ulcer to a geographical or 'amoeboid' configuration (Fig. 9.11d).
- Following healing, there may be persistent punctate epithelial erosions which resolve spontaneously and should not be mistaken for persistent active infection.
- Mild subepithelial scarring may develop after healing.

3. **Culture** can be taken by debridement of the ulcer. This relies on a characteristic cytopathic effect in tissue culture which can be used to distinguish HSV-1 from HSV-2; PCR is also available.
4. **Differential diagnosis** of dendritic ulceration includes herpes zoster keratitis, healing corneal abrasion (pseudo-dendrite), acanthamoeba keratitis and toxic keratopathies secondary to topical medication.

Treatment of epithelial keratitis

Treatment of HSV disease is with purine or pyrimidine analogues that are incorporated to form abnormal viral DNA. Idoxuridine and vidarabine (Ara-A) are poorly soluble and relatively toxic, but are still used in regions where low cost is essential. Trifluridine (TFT) and aciclovir (Zovirax) have low toxicity and the latter can be used systemically. Both are active against *HSV1* and *HSV2*.

1. **Topical** antiviral agents (trifluorothymidine, aciclovir, vidarabine and ganciclovir) are equally effective. The most frequently used drug in Europe is aciclovir 3% ointment administered five times daily. It is relatively non-toxic, even when given for up to 60 days, because it acts preferentially on virus-laden epithelial cells. Aciclovir penetrates intact corneal epithelium and stroma, achieving therapeutic levels in the aqueous humour, and can therefore be used to

treat stromal herpetic keratitis. On this treatment 99% will be resolved by 2 weeks.

2. **Debridement** may be used for dendritic but not geographic ulcers. The corneal surface is wiped with a sterile cellulose sponge 2mm beyond the edge of the ulcer since pathology extends well beyond the visible dendrite. The removal of the virus-containing cells protects adjacent healthy epithelium from infection and also eliminates the antigenic stimulus to stromal inflammation. An antiviral agent must be used in conjunction to prevent recurrence.

3. **Signs of treatment toxicity** include superficial punctate erosions, follicular conjunctivitis and punctal occlusion.

> **NB** The majority of dendritic ulcers will eventually heal spontaneously without treatment.

Disciform keratitis

The exact aetiology of disciform keratitis (endotheliitis) is controversial. It may be an HSV infection of keratocytes or endothelium, or hypersensitivity reaction to viral antigen in the cornea. A past history of dendritic ulceration is not always present.

1. **Presenting symptoms** are a gradual onset of blurred vision which may be associated by haloes around lights.

2. **Signs**
   - A central zone of stromal oedema often with overlying epithelial oedema (Fig. 9.12a); occasionally the lesion is eccentric.
   - Keratic precipitates underlying the oedema (Fig. 9.12b).
   - Folds in Descemet membrane in severe cases (Fig. 9.12c).
   - A surrounding (Wessely) immune ring of stromal haze signifies deposition of viral antigen and host antibody complexes (Fig. 9.12d).
   - The intraocular pressure may be elevated despite only mild anterior uveitis.
   - Healed lesions often have a faint ring of stromal opacification and thinning.
   - Corneal sensation is reduced.

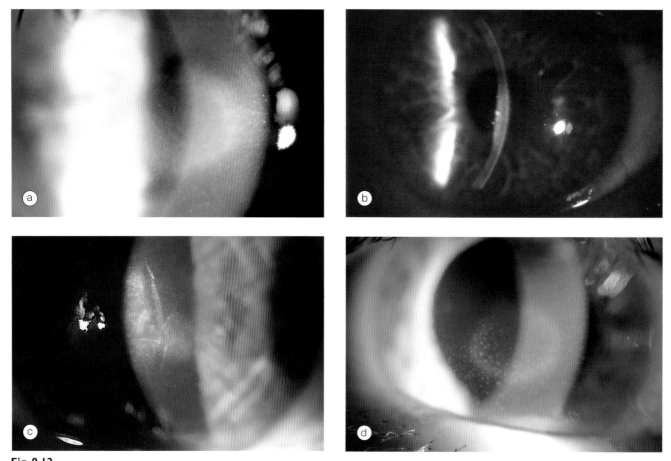

Fig. 9.12
Disciform herpes simplex keratitis. **(a)** Central epithelial and stromal oedema; **(b)** underlying keratic precipitates; **(c)** folds in Descemet membrane; **(d)** Wessely ring and keratic precipitates

3. Treatment

    a. Initial treatment of lesions involving the visual axis is with topical steroids with antiviral cover, both q.i.d. As improvement occurs, the frequency of administration of both is reduced in parallel over not less than 4 weeks.

    b. Subsequently prednisolone 0.5% once daily is generally considered a safe dose at which to stop topical antiviral cover. A small number of patients require a weak steroid such fluorometholone 0.1% on alternate days for several months. Periodic attempts should be made to stop medication altogether.

Stromal necrotic keratitis

Viral antigen is detectable in stromal disease but viral replication is not thought to be an important component. Lymphocytes (Th1), antigen presenting cells and polymorphonuclear neutrophils are critical for viral clearance but they also mediate tissue destruction.

1. Signs

- Stromal necrosis and melting often with profound interstitial opacification (Fig. 9.13a).
- Associated anterior uveitis with keratic precipitates underlying the area of active stromal infiltration.
- If inappropriately treated, scarring, vascularization and lipid deposition may result (Fig. 9.13b).

NB Acute deterioration and melting might indicate secondary microbial infection.

2. Treatment is primarily aimed at achieving epithelial recovery with frequent use of non-preserved tear substitutes. Inflammation should be reduced with topical steroids. Although this may make the eye comfortable more quickly there is no evidence that the final visual outcome is improved. Further strategies to control corneal melting are described below.

Metaherpetic ulceration

Metaherpetic ulceration is caused by failure of re-epithelialization resulting from devitalization of the stroma and epithelial toxicity rather than viral replication.

1. Signs

- A non-healing epithelial defect after prolonged topical treatment (Fig. 9.14).
- There may be stromal ulceration although necrosis is not a major feature.
- The stroma beneath the defect is grey and opaque.

2. Treatment is that of persistent epithelial defects as follows:

- Reduction of exposure to toxic drops and preservatives.
- Frequent topical lubrication with non-preserved drops.
- Minimal use of topical steroid to control an inflammatory component.

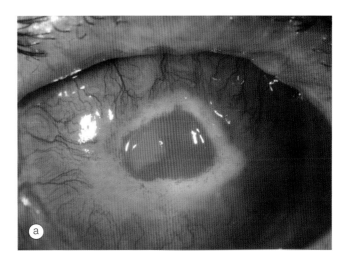
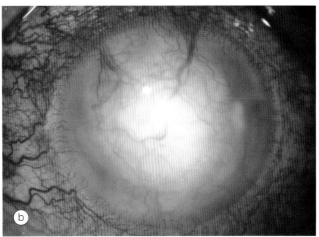

Fig. 9.13
Stromal necrotic herpes simplex keratitis. **(a)** Melting, opacification and peripheral vascularization; **(b)** severe vascularization and lipid deposition in advanced disease (Courtesy of S Tuft)

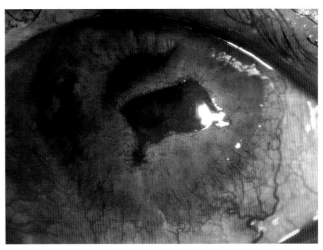

Fig. 9.14
Metaherpetic ulceration stained with rose bengal (Courtesy of S Tuft)

- Bandage contact lens or temporary tarsorrhaphy as necessary.

Prophylaxis

Oral aciclovir (400mg b.d.) reduces the rate of recurrent epithelial and stromal keratitis by about 45% but this effect reduces or even disappears when the drug is stopped. The benefit of prophylaxis is greatest in patients with frequent debilitating recurrences, particularly if bilateral or involving an only eye.

Complications

1. **Secondary infection.** Herpetic eye disease is a major predisposing factor for microbial keratitis.
2. **Secondary glaucoma** which may progress undetected if there is a poor view of the optic disc. Corneal thinning may give rise to a falsely low reading on applanation.
3. **Cataract** secondary to inflammation or prolonged steroid use.
4. **Iris atrophy** secondary to keratouveitis.

Keratoplasty

Recurrence of herpetic eye disease on the graft and rejection threaten the survival of corneal grafts. Survival can be improved by preventing reactivation by prophylactic treatment after surgery.

1. **Topical** antivirals given during a rejection episode may reduce epithelial viral reactivation but may be toxic and delay re-epithelialization.
2. **Oral** aciclovir (400mg b.d.) should be given to patients undergoing penetrating keratoplasty for herpetic eye disease and those with associated severe atopic eye disease. The duration of treatment and the optimum dose is not known. Immunohistochemistry should be performed on the excised tissue to confirm the presence of herpes antigen.

Herpes zoster ophthalmicus

Pathogenesis

The varicella-zoster virus (VZV) causes chickenpox (varicella) and shingles (herpes zoster). VZV and HSV belong to the same subfamily of the herpes virus group and are morphologically identical but antigenically different. After the initial attack of chickenpox the virus travels in a retrograde manner to the dorsal root and cranial nerve sensory ganglia where it may remain dormant for decades. From there it can reactivate to cause shingles after VZV-specific cellular immunity has faded.

Mechanisms of ocular involvement

Ocular damage may be caused by the following mechanisms.

1. **Direct viral invasion** may result in epithelial keratitis and conjunctivitis.
2. **Secondary inflammation** and occlusive vasculitis may cause episcleritis, scleritis, keratitis and uveitis. Inflammation and destruction of the peripheral nerves or central ganglia, or altered signal processing in the CNS, may be responsible for post-herpetic neuralgia.
3. **Reactivation** causes necrosis and inflammation in the affected sensory ganglia causing corneal anaesthesia that may result in neurotrophic keratitis.

Risk of ocular involvement

1. **Hutchinson sign** describes involvement of the external nasal nerve, which supplies the side of the tip, and the side and root of the nose. It correlates significantly with subsequent development of ocular inflammation and corneal denervation because it is the terminal branch of the nasociliary nerve. Eye involvement may rarely occur when the disease affects the maxillary nerve.
2. **Age.** HZO occurs most frequently in the sixth and seventh decades. In the elderly, the signs and symptoms are more severe and last longer.
3. **AIDS** patients tend to have more severe disease. The development of shingles in children or young adults (< 50 years) should prompt a search for immunodeficiency or malignancy.

NB There is no correlation between severity of ocular complications and age and severity of the skin rash.

Clinical features of acute systemic disease

1. **A prodromal phase** precedes the appearance of the rash. It lasts 3–5 days and is characterized by tiredness, fever, malaise and headache. Symptoms involving the dermatome of the ophthalmic nerve vary from a superficial itching, tingling or burning sensation to a severe deep, boring or lancing pain that is either constant or intermittent. Older patients with severe pain and larger area of involvement are at particular risk of post-herpetic neuralgia.
2. **Skin lesions**
   - A painful erythema with a maculopapular rash that may initially be confused with cellulitis or contact dermatitis.
   - Within 24 hours groups of vesicles appear and these become confluent over 2–4 days.
   - The vesicles often pass through a pustular phase before they crust and dry after 2–3 weeks (9.15a).

- Large, deep haemorrhagic lesions are more common in immunodeficiency (Fig. 9.15b).
- The lesions may involve one or more of the cutaneous branches of the trigeminal nerve.
- Residual skin destruction and depigmented scars (Fig. 9.15c).
- Occasionally the rash may become generalized and the patient becomes severely ill within 1–2 weeks. Such patients often have lymphoma or other malignancies, or are immunosuppressed.

NB People with shingles can transmit chickenpox to non-immune individuals. Contact with non-immune or immunosuppressed individuals should be avoided until crusting is complete.

Treatment of acute systemic disease

1. **Oral aciclovir** 800mg five times daily for 3–7 days given within 72 hours of onset is the treatment of choice. Patients presenting with new vesicles after 72 hours should also be treated to reduce the severity of acute HZO and the risk of post-herpetic neuralgia at 6 months. The incidence of late ophthalmic complications is also reduced by about 50%.
2. **Intravenous aciclovir** 5–10mg/kg t.i.d. is only indicated for encephalitis. The duration of treatment should be extended for the elderly or immunosuppressed. Aciclovir resistance has been reported in immunosuppressed patients receiving low-dose therapy to prevent recurrences; foscarnet is then the treatment of choice.
3. **Other oral antiviral agents** such as valaciclovir 1g t.i.d, famciclovir 750mg daily and brivudine 125mg daily are more expensive but have a more convenient dosing and are as effective as aciclovir 800mg five times daily.
4. **Systemic steroids** (prednisolone 40–60mg daily) should be used only in conjunction with systemic antivirals. They have a moderate effect at reducing acute pain and accelerating skin healing but have no effect on the incidence or severity of post-herpetic neuralgia.
5. **Symptomatic** treatment of skin lesions involves drying, antisepsis and cold compresses. The benefit of topical antibiotic/steroid combinations is uncertain.

Acute eye disease

1. **Acute epithelial keratitis** develops in about 50% of patients within 2 days of the onset of the rash and resolves spontaneously within a few days.
   - It is characterized by small, fine, dendritic lesions which, in contrast to herpes simplex dendrites, have tapered ends without terminal bulbs (Fig. 9.16a).
   - The lesions stain with fluorescein and rose bengal.
   - Treatment is with a topical antiviral, if appropriate.

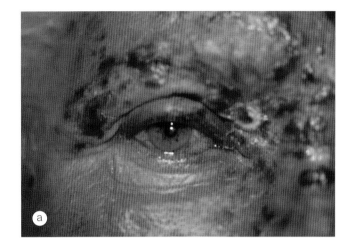
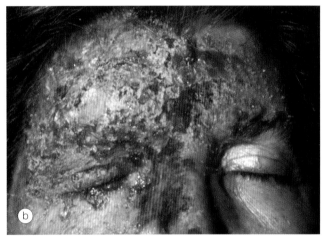
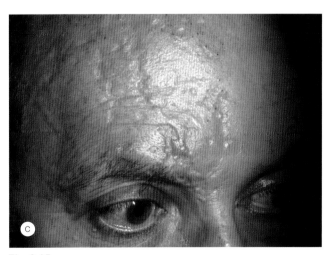

Fig. 9.15
Herpes zoster ophthalmicus. **(a)** Confluent crusting; **(b)** haemorrhagic involvement; **(c)** residual scarring

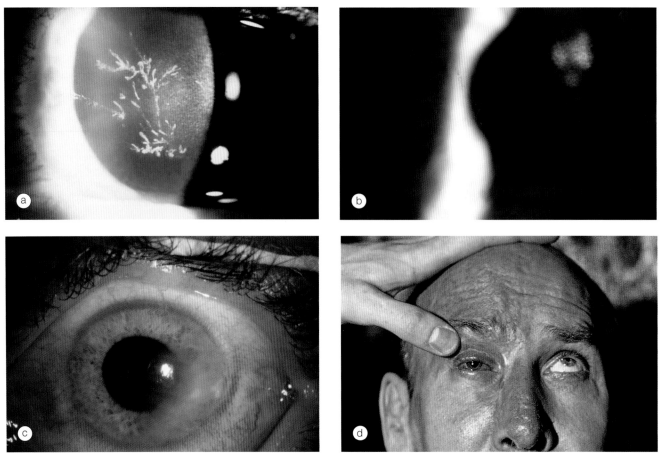

Fig. 9.16
Acute lesions in herpes zoster ophthalmicus. **(a)** Dendritic epithelial lesions with tapered ends; **(b)** nummular keratitis; **(c)** stromal keratitis; **(d)** third nerve palsy (Courtesy of N Rogers – fig. a; S Tuft – fig. b)

2. **Conjunctivitis** is common and always associated with lid margin vesicles. Treatment is not required in the absence of corneal disease.

3. **Episcleritis** occurs at the onset of the rash and usually resolves spontaneously.

4. **Scleritis** and sclerokeratitis are uncommon and may develop at the end of the first week. If indolent, oral flurbiprofen (Froben) 100mg t.i.d. may be required.

5. **Nummular keratitis** usually develops about 10 days after the onset of the rash. It is characterized by fine granular subepithelial deposits surrounded by a halo of stromal haze (Fig. 9.16b). The lesions fade in response to topical steroids but recur if treatment is discontinued prematurely.

6. **Stromal keratitis** develops 3 weeks after the onset of the rash in about 5% of cases (Fig. 9.16c). It responds to topical steroids but often becomes chronic.

7. **Disciform keratitis** is less common than with herpes simplex infection but may lead to corneal decompensation. Treatment is with topical steroids.

8. **Anterior uveitis** is frequently associated with sectoral iris ischaemia and atrophy.

9. **Neurological complications**
   - Cranial nerve palsies affecting the third (most common – Fig. 9.16d), fourth and sixth nerves usually recover within 6 months.
   - Optic neuritis is very rare.
   - Guillain–Barré syndrome and encephalitis are rare and only occur with severe infection.
   - Contralateral hemiplegia is also rare, usually mild and typically develops 2 months after the rash.

Chronic eye disease

1. **Lid scarring** may result in ptosis, cicatricial entropion, trichiasis, madarosis and notching of the lid margin (Fig. 9.17a).

2. **Lipid-filled granulomata** under the tarsal conjunctiva and subconjunctival scarring (Fig. 9.17b).

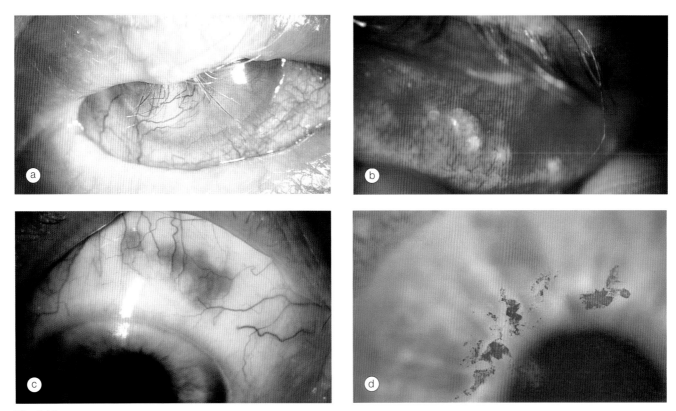

Fig. 9.17
Chronic lesions in herpes zoster ophthalmicus. **(a)** Lid scarring; **(b)** lipid-filled granulomas; **(c)** scleral atrophy; **(d)** mucous plaque keratitis (Courtesy of R Marsh – fig. d)

3. **Scleritis** may become chronic and lead to patchy scleral atrophy (Fig. 9.17c)
4. **Mucous plaque keratitis** develops in about 5% of cases, most commonly between the third and sixth months. It is characterized by the sudden appearance of elevated mucous plaques that stain with rose bengal (Fig. 9.17d). Treatment involves a combination of topical steroids and acetylcysteine. Untreated, plaques resolve after a few months, leaving a faint diffuse corneal haze.
5. **Neurotrophic keratitis** with reduced sensation develops in about 50% of cases. It may rarely lead to severe ulceration, secondary bacterial infection and even perforation.
6. **Lipid degeneration** (see Fig. 9.3d) may develop in eyes with persistent severe nummular or disciform keratitis.

Postherpetic neuralgia

Postherpetic neuralgia is pain that persists after the rash has healed. It develops in up to 75% of patients over 70 years of age. Pain may be constant or intermittent, worse at night and aggravated by minor stimuli (allodynia), touch and heat. It generally improves slowly with time, with only 2% of patients affected after 5 years. Neuralgia may lead to depression, sometimes of sufficient severity to present the danger of suicide, and can significantly impair the quality of life. Patients severely affected should be referred to a special pain clinic. Treatment involves the following:

1. **Topical** treatment with cold compress, topical capsaicin (depletes substance P) or local anaesthetic (lidocaine 5%) creams may be effective.
2. **Systemic** treatment should be increased in steps as follows:
   - Simple analgesics such as paracetamol up to 4g daily.
   - Stronger analgesics such as codeine up to 240mg daily.
   - Amitriptyline 10–25mg at night increasing gradually to 75mg daily if appropriate.
   - Carbamazepine 400mg daily for lancinating pain.

NB NSAIDs are ineffective.

Relapsing eye disease

In the relapsing phase lesions may reappear years after acute disease. On occasions the acute episode may have been forgotten and lid scarring may be the only diagnostic clue. Reactivation of keratitis, episcleritis, scleritis or iritis can occur.

INTERSTITIAL KERATITIS

Interstitial keratitis (IK) is an inflammation of the corneal stroma without primary involvement of the epithelium or endothelium. In developed countries it is most often associated with congenital syphilis but may occur with a wide variety of infective causes such as tuberculosis, Lyme disease, leprosy and viral infection. All patients with IK should have treponemal serology to determine if the patient has congenital syphilis, irrespective of the absence or presence of other clinical features.

Syphilitic IK

Syphilitic IK is due to the spread of infection from the mother to child during primary, secondary, or early latent phases (i.e. within 2 years of maternal primary infection).

Diagnosis

1. **Presentation** is between 5–25 years with acute bilateral pain and severe blurring of vision.
2. **Signs** in chronological order
   - Limbitis associated with deep vascularization of the stroma associated with cellular infiltration and clouding that may obscure the vessels resulting in the characteristic 'salmon-patch' (Fig. 9.18a).
   - Anterior uveitis may be obscured by corneal clouding.
   - After several months the cornea begins to clear and the vessels become non-perfused (ghost vessels – Fig. 9.18b).
   - If the cornea later becomes inflamed, the vessels may re-fill with blood and, rarely, bleed into the stroma (Fig. 9.18c).
   - The healed stage is characterized by 'ghost vessels' and deep stromal scarring and thinning (Fig. 9.18d).

Treatment

Active IK is treated with systemic penicillin, and topical steroids and cycloplegics. All patients with positive treponemal serology should be referred to a genitourinary clinic for evaluation, treatment and screening of siblings, parents and partners.

Cogan syndrome

Cogan syndrome is a rare systemic, autoimmune vasculitis characterized by the combination of intraocular inflammation and vestibulo-auditory dysfunction, particularly neurosensory deafness, which develop within months of each other. The disease primarily occurs in young adults with sexes affected equally. Systemic associations include polyarteritis nodosa and necrotizing vasculitis of the renal, gastrointestinal and cardiovascular systems.

1. **Signs**
   - Redness, pain, photophobia and blurred vision.
   - Early signs are faint bilateral peripheral anterior stromal opacities.
   - Deeper opacities and neovascularization may ensue.
   - Uveitis, scleritis and retinal vasculitis may occasionally develop.
2. **Treatment** is with topical steroids for keratitis. Systemic steroids are usually required for scleritis or retinal vasculitis.

   NB Vestibulo-auditory symptoms require immediate treatment with systemic steroids (1–2g/kg) to prevent hearing loss. Management in conjunction with an otolaryngologist is essential; immunosuppression may also be required.

PROTOZOAN KERATITIS

Acanthamoeba keratitis

Pathogenesis

Acanthamoeba spp. are ubiquitous free-living protozoa commonly found in soil, fresh or brackish water, and the upper respiratory tract. The cystic form (Fig. 9.19) is highly resilient although under appropriate environmental conditions the cysts may turn into trophozoites, which produce a variety of enzymes that aid tissue penetration and destruction. In developed countries keratitis is most frequently associated with contact lens wear, especially if tap water is used for cleaning.

Diagnosis

1. **Presenting symptoms** are blurred vision and pain, which may be severe and disproportionate to the clinical signs.
2. **Signs**
   - In early disease the epithelial surface is irregular and greyish.

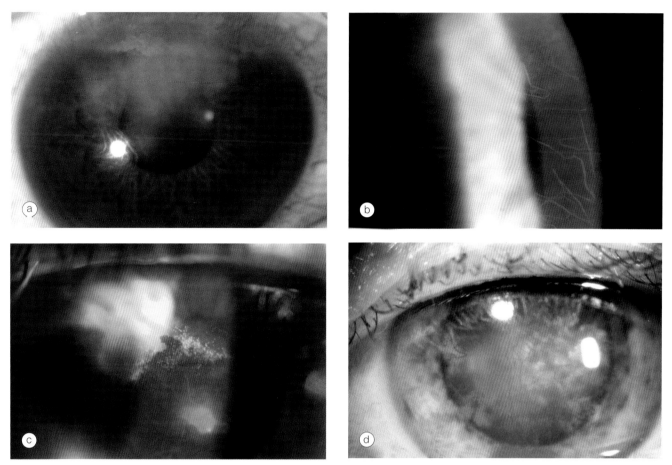

Fig. 9.18
Syphilitic interstitial keratitis. **(a)** 'Salmon patch'; **(b)** 'ghost vessels' in inactive disease; **(c)** intrastromal corneal haemorrhage from re-perfused new vessels; **(d)** patchy residual scarring (Courtesy of Krachmer, Mannis and Holland, from *Cornea*, Mosby, 2005 – fig. a)

- Epithelial pseudodendrites (Fig. 9.20a) that may be mistaken for herpes simplex keratitis.
- Limbitis with diffuse or focal anterior stromal infiltrates (Fig. 9.20b).
- Perineural infiltrates (radial keratoneuritis – Fig. 9.20c) are seen during the first 1–4 weeks and are pathognomonic.
- Gradual enlargement and coalescence of the infiltrates to form a ring abscess (Fig. 9.20d).
- Scleritis may develop without obvious extension of the infection.
- Slowly progressive stromal opacification and vascularization (Fig. 9.20e).
- Corneal melting (Fig. 9.20f) may occur at any stage when there is stromal disease. The melt often develops at the periphery of the area of infiltrate.

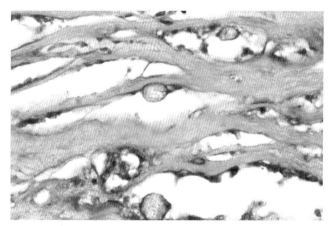

Fig. 9.19
Acanthamoeba cysts in a corneal biopsy (Courtesy of J Harry)

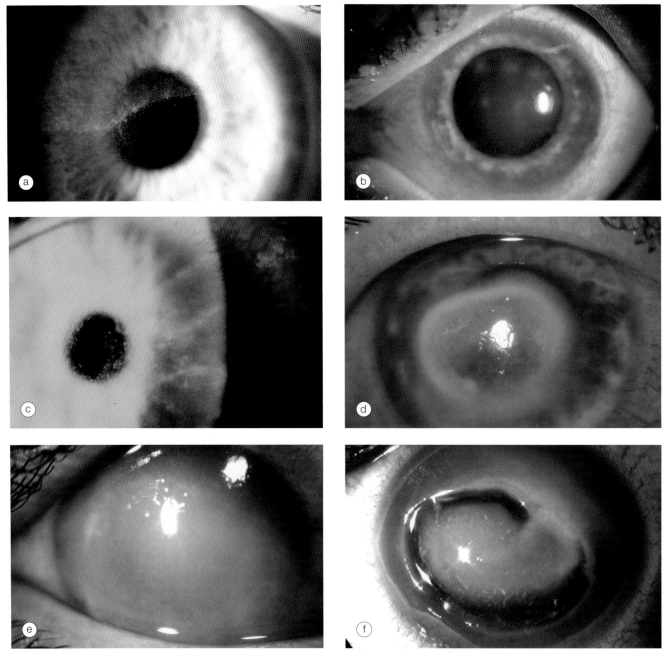

Fig. 9.20
Acanthamoeba keratitis. **(a)** Epithelial pseudodendrites; **(b)** focal anterior stromal infiltrates; **(c)** radial perineuritis; **(d)** ring abscess; **(e)** stromal opacification; **(f)** melting (Courtesy of R Curtis – fig. a; S Tuft – figs d, e and f)

3. Investigations

a. Cultures are performed by scraping the lesion and placing the sample onto non-nutrient agar which is later seeded with dead *E. coli*. Culture of the contact lens case will often yield acanthamoeba and Gram-negative organisms.

b. Staining using periodic acid–Schiff or calcofluor white (a fluorescent dye with an affinity for amoebic cysts and fungi) may also be used.

c. Other investigations include immunohistochemistry and PCR.

NB About 30% of patients are culture negative. If there is a high index of suspicion (non-suppurative keratitis in a contact lens wearer) treatment should be as for acanthamoeba infection.

Treatment

It is important to have a high index of suspicion because the outcome is very much better if treatment is started within 4 weeks of onset of symptoms.

1. **Debridement** to remove infected epithelium for early disease.
2. **Topical amoebicides** given as dual therapy with propamidine isethionate 0.1% (Brolene) and polyhexamethylene biguanide 0.02% drops or hexamidine and chlorhexidine 0.02%. An antibiotic such as ciprofloxacin should be added if there is ulceration to cover potential Gram negative co-infection. Because cysts are difficult to eradicate stromal relapses are common as treatment is tapered. In these cases therapy should be increased and the tapering process re-started.
3. **Topical steroids** should be avoided if possible although low-dose therapy may be useful for persistent inflammation which may be due to acanthamoeba antigen rather than viable organisms. The frequency of steroid administration should be tapered in parallel with anti-amoebic therapy.
4. **Pain control** from corneal disease or scleritis is with an oral non-steroidal anti-inflammatory agent such as flurbiprofen 100mg t.i.d.
5. **Keratoplasty** is occasionally necessary for residual scarring.

Differential diagnosis

In early disease this includes herpetic keratitis and adenovirus keratoconjunctivitis. In advanced disease fungal keratitis should be considered.

Microsporidial keratitis

Pathogenesis

Microsporidia are obligate intracellular, spore-forming protozoa that are opportunistic pathogens of the phylum *Microspora*. Infection occurs when the spores are injected into the host cell by the characteristic polar tube of the spore. Until the advent of AIDS microsporidia were rare human pathogens. The most common general infection is enteritis and the most common ocular manifestation is keratoconjunctivitis.

Diagnosis

1. **Signs**
   - Bilateral chronic diffuse punctate epithelial keratitis (Fig. 9.21a).
   - Slowly progressive deep stromal keratitis may rarely affect immunocompetent patients (Fig. 9.21b).
   - Sclerokeratitis and endophthalmitis are rare.

2. **Biopsy** and histology shows characteristic spores and intracellular parasites.

Treatment

1. **Medical** therapy of epithelial disease is with topical fumagillin. Highly active antiretroviral therapy (HAART) for AIDS may also help resolution. Stromal disease is treated with a combination of topical fumagillin and oral albendazole 400 mg daily for 2 weeks, repeated 2 weeks later with a second course. Patients should be closely monitored for hepatic toxicity.
2. **Keratoplasty** may be indicated although recurrence of disease can occur in the graft periphery; cryotherapy to the residual tissue may reduce this risk.

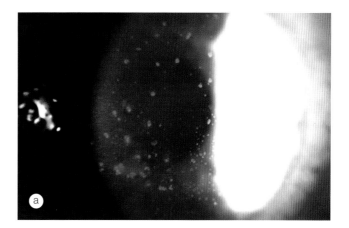

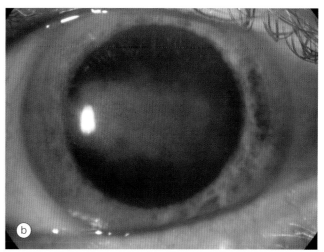

Fig. 9.21
Microsporidia keratitis; **(a)** Diffuse punctate epithelial keratitis; **(b)** deep stromal keratitis (Courtesy of S Tuft)

Onchocercal keratitis

Onchocerciasis or river blindness is caused by infestation with the parasitic helminth *Onchocerca volvulus* (see Chapter 24).

1. **Punctate keratitis** represents white cell infiltrate surrounding dead microfilariae in the cornea. The lesions are most commonly at the 3 and 9 o'clock positions in the anterior third of the stroma.
2. **Sclerosing keratitis** starts at the 3 and 9 o'clock positions (Fig. 9.22a) and progresses slowly to involve the entire cornea. Full thickness scarring has superficial and deep vessels with pigment migration over the surface (Fig. 9.22b).
3. **Treatment** of acute disease is with topical steroids.

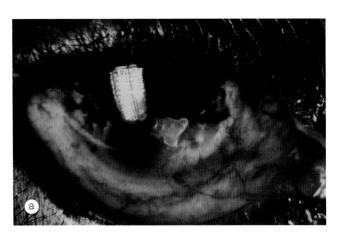

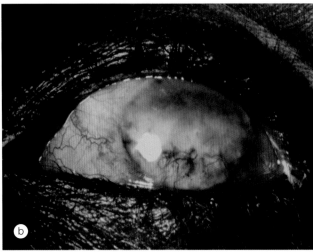

Fig. 9.22
Sclerosing onchocercal keratitis. **(a)** Peripheral involvement;
(b) advanced disease (Courtesy of S Tuft)

BACTERIAL HYPERSENSITIVITY-MEDIATED CORNEAL DISEASE

Marginal keratitis

Pathogenesis

Marginal keratitis is thought to be the result of a reaction against staphylococcal exotoxins and cell wall proteins with deposition of antigen–antibody complexes in the peripheral cornea (antigen diffusing from the tear film, antibody from the blood vessels) with a secondary lymphocytic infiltration. The lesions are culture negative but *S. aureus* can frequently be isolated from the lid margins.

Diagnosis

1. **Symptoms** are mild irritation, lacrimation and discomfort.
2. **Signs**
   - Subepithelial marginal infiltrates separated from the limbus by a clear zone often associated with a focal adjacent area of conjunctivitis and episcleritis (Fig. 9.23a).
   - Coalescence and circumferential spread (Fig. 9.23b).
   - Without treatment resolution occurs in 3–4 weeks leaving slight thinning and a superficial scar, usually without vascularization.
   - Gross corneal infiltration can occur in the presence of modifying factors such as recurrent epithelial erosion or recent LASIK surgery.

Treatment

Coexisting lid margin disease should be treated with hygiene and topical antibiotics. Symptomatic treatment is with topical fluorometholone 0.1% q.i.d for one week. Oral tetracycline may rarely be required for troublesome recurrent disease.

NB If there is a significant epithelial defect (> 1mm) treatment is that of suspected bacterial keratitis.

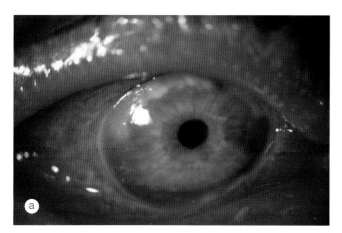

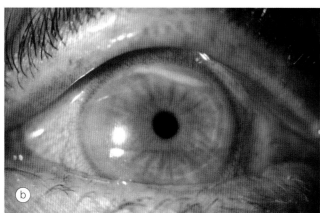

Fig. 9.23
Marginal keratitis. **(a)** Marginal infiltrates; **(b)** coalescence and circumferential spread

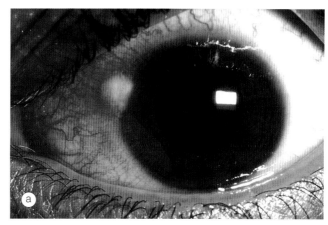

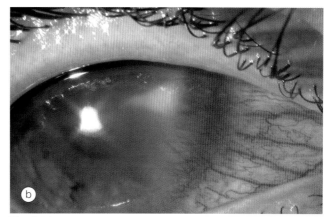

Fig. 9.24
Phlyctenulosis. **(a)** Limbal phlycten; **(b)** corneal phlycten
(Courtesy of J Harry and G Misson, from *Clinical Ophthalmic Pathology*, Butterworth-Heinemann, 2001 – fig. a; S Tuft – fig. b)

Phlyctenulosis

Pathogenesis

Phlyctenulosis is usually a self-limiting disease although rarely it may be severe and even blinding. Most cases seen in developed countries are the result of a presumed delayed hypersensitivity reaction to staphylococcal cell wall antigen. However, in developing countries the majority are associated with tuberculosis or helminth infestation. The most common systemic association is rosacea.

Diagnosis

1. **Presentation** is usually in children or young adults with photophobia, lacrimation and blepharospasm.
2. **Signs**
   • A small white nodule associated with intense local hyperaemia on the conjunctiva or limbus (Fig. 9.24a).

• A limbal phlycten may then extend progressively onto the cornea (Fig. 9.24b).
• A healed corneal phlycten usually leaves a triangular limbal-based scar associated with superficial vascularization and thinning.
• Spontaneous resolution usually occurs in 2–3 weeks, but severe thinning and even perforation can occur.

Treatment

A short course of topical steroids accelerates healing. Recurrent troublesome disease may require oral tetracycline. It is also important to treat associated staphylococcal blepharitis.

NB Mantoux test and chest x-ray is only indicated in tuberculosis endemic areas.

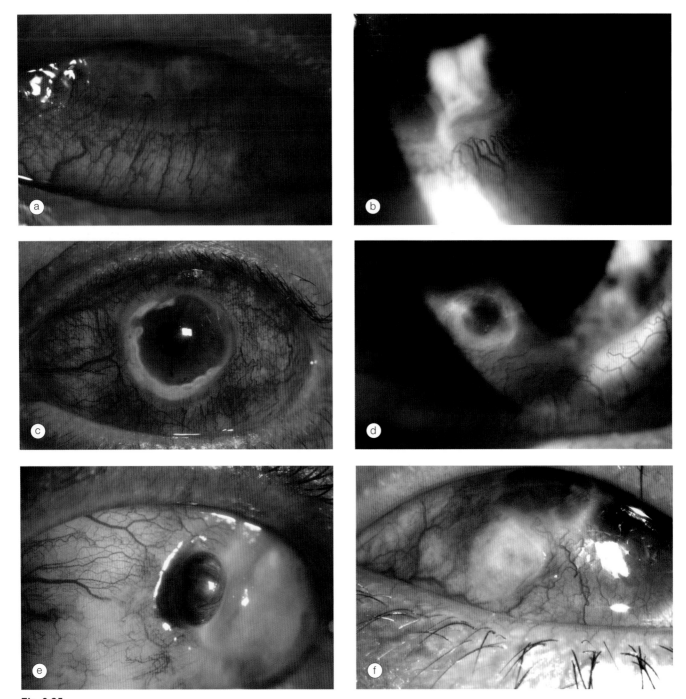

Fig. 9.25
Rosacea keratitis. **(a)** Peripheral vascularization; **(b)** marginal keratitis; **(c)** circumferential peripheral infiltration; **(d)** thinning; **(e)** perforation; **(f)** scarring and vascularization (Courtesy of S Tuft – figs c, e and f)

ROSACEA KERATITIS

Acne rosacea is a common, idiopathic, chronic dermatosis involving the sun-exposed skin of the face and upper neck (see Chapter 24). Between 6–18% of patients with acne rosacea develop ocular complications. Ocular rosacea is a term used to define a spectrum of eye findings in the presence of lid margin telangiectasia, often without significant involvement of the rest of the face.

Diagnosis

1. **Symptoms** are non-specific irritation, burning and lacrimation.
2. **Lid** signs include margin telangiectasia and intractable posterior blepharitis, often associated with recurrent meibomian cyst formation.
3. **Conjunctiva**
   - Conjunctival hyperaemia, especially bulbar.
   - Rarely, cicatricial conjunctivitis, conjunctival granulomas and phlyctenulosis may occur.
4. **Cornea**
   - Inferior punctate erosions.
   - Peripheral vascularization (Fig. 9.25a)
   - Marginal keratitis especially involving the inferonasal and inferotemporal cornea (Fig. 9.25b).
   - Circumferential spread (Fig. 9.25c).
   - Corneal thinning in severe cases (Fig. 9.25d).
   - Perforation may occur as a result of severe peripheral (Fig. 9.25e) or central melting, which may be precipitated by secondary bacterial infection.
   - Corneal scarring and vascularization (Fig. 9.25f).

Treatment

1. **Topical**
   - Hot compresses and lid hygiene for posterior blepharitis.
   - Fusidic acid ointment at bedtime for 4 weeks.
   - Fluorometholone 0.1% as a short-term measure.
2. **Systemic**
   - Oxytetracycline 500mg b.d. suppresses but does not cure the disease; improvement usually lasts for 6 months after cessation of therapy. The therapeutic effect of tetracycline is not related to its antibacterial action.
   - Doxycycline 100mg once daily is an alternative.
   - Severe disease with corneal melt may require immunosuppression (azathioprine).

NB Systemic tetracyclines should not be used in children under the age of 12 years or in pregnant or breast-feeding women because the antibiotic is deposited in teeth (being bound to calcium), and may cause dental hypoplasia and discoloration. Erythromycin can be used in children.

SEVERE PERIPHERAL CORNEAL ULCERATION

Mooren ulcer

Mooren ulcer is a rare, idiopathic disease characterized by progressive, circumferential, peripheral, stromal ulceration with later central spread. The diagnosis depends upon identification of the clinical features and exclusion of other causes of peripheral ulcerative keratitis. Mooren ulcer affects males more commonly than females and is very rare in children. Bilateral disease is present in 30% of cases and is more aggressive than unilateral involvement, which tends to be more slowly progressive and responds better to treatment. The exact aetiology is uncertain. An autoimmune process may be present that is directed against a specific target antigen in the corneal stroma, possibly triggered in genetically susceptible individuals by trauma.

Diagnosis

1. **Symptoms** include severe pain, photophobia and blurred vision due to astigmatism.
2. **Signs** in chronological order:
   - Peripheral ulceration affecting the superficial one-third of clear cornea (Fig. 9.26a).
   - Progressive circumferential and central stromal thinning with an undermined and infiltrated leading edge (Fig. 9.26b).
   - Vascularization involving the bed of the ulcer up to its leading edge but not beyond (Fig. 9.26c).
   - The healing stage is characterized by thinning, vascularization and scarring (Fig. 9.26d).
3. **FA** initially shows capillary closure at the limbus and then leakage from vascularization extending into the base of the ulcer.
4. **Complications** include severe astigmatism, perforation following minor trauma (spontaneous perforation is rare), secondary bacterial infection, cataract and glaucoma.

Treatment

There is no single effective treatment for Mooren ulcer. Untreated, the disease eventually burns itself out over 6–18 months with blindness from thinning and vascularization. Even with treatment vision is reduced to light perception in about 18% of eyes. The response to both topical and systemic immunotherapy is poor. The results of corneal grafting are also unsatisfactory with recurrence of ulceration in the graft. A wide range of therapies has been reported. The following graded therapeutic strategy, governed by the severity of the disease and the response to initial treatment, is recommended.

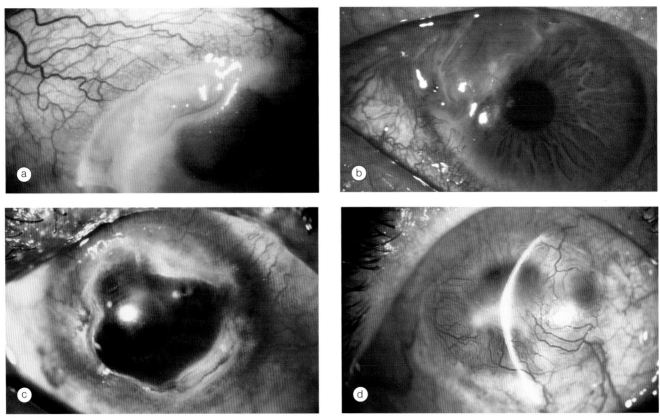

Fig. 9.26
Mooren ulcer. **(a)** Local peripheral ulceration; **(b)** circumferential and central spread; **(c)** advanced disease; **(d)** healed stage (Courtesy of P G Watson, B L Hazelman, C E Pavesio, W R Green, from *The Sclera and Systemic Disorders*, Butterworth-Heinemann, 2004 – fig. a)

1. **Topical** treatment initially involves steroids or ciclosporin 1.0%. Other topical medication includes artificial tears and collagenase inhibitors (acetylcysteine 10%, L-cysteine 0.2 molar).
2. **Conjunctival resection or cryotherapy,** which may be combined with excision of necrotic tissue, may be effective for unilateral but not bilateral disease. Treatment should extend 4mm back from the limbus and 2mm beyond the margins of the lesion.
3. **Systemic** immunosuppression should be instituted earlier for bilateral disease, or if involvement is advanced at first examination. Traditionally treatment has been with cyclophosphamide, but more recently ciclosporin (5mg/kg) has also been shown to be effective.
4. **Surgery**
   - Primary lamellar keratoplasty is generally contra-indicated although there have been some good reports when it is combined with topical ciclosporin.
   - Lamellar dissection of the residual central island in advanced disease may remove the stimulus for further inflammation.
   - Cyanoacrylate glue may be used to treat perforation.
   - Reconstruction should ideally involve lamellar surgery

with systemic immunosuppression cover to reduce the risk of recurrence; without systemic cover recurrence rate is about 25%.

Peripheral ulcerative keratitis

Peripheral ulcerative keratitis (PUK) is a severe condition that may precede or follow the onset of systemic disease. Severe, persistent, peripheral corneal infiltration, ulceration or thinning unexplained by coexistent ocular disease should therefore prompt a search for an associated systemic collagen vascular disorder which may be life-threatening (see below).

Pathogenesis

In patients with an underlying autoimmune disease there is immune complex deposition in peripheral cornea. Diseased epithelium, keratocytes and recruited inflammatory cells may result in release of matrix metalloproteinases that degrade collagen and the extracellular matrix. Auto-antibodies may target sites in the corneal epithelium.

Diagnosis

- Crescent-shaped ulceration and stromal infiltration at the limbus (Fig. 9.27a).
- Limbitis, episcleritis or scleritis are usually present.
- Circumferential and occasionally central spread.

- End stage disease may result in a 'contact lens' cornea (Fig. 9.27b).

NB Unlike Mooren ulcer the process may also extend to involve the sclera.

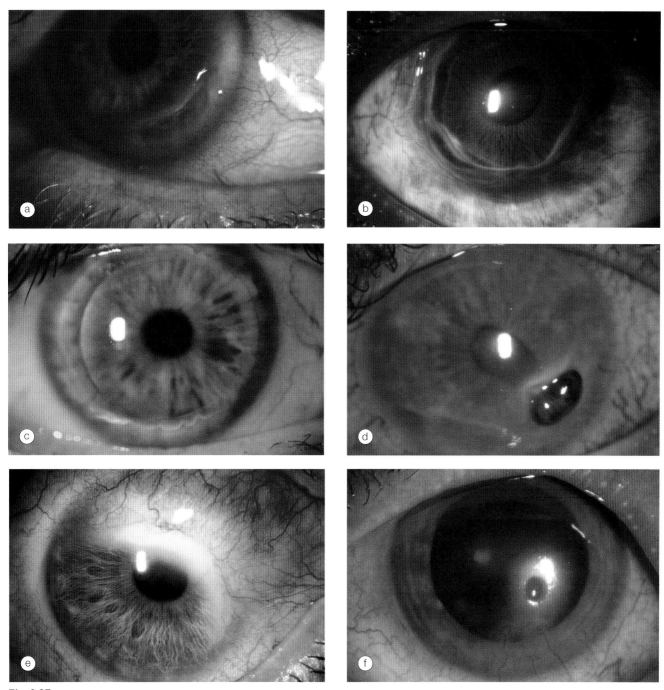

Fig. 9.27
Keratitis in systemic collagen vascular disease. **(a)** Early peripheral ulcerative keratitis; **(b)** 'contact-lens' cornea; **(c)** peripheral stromal thinning; **(d)** peripheral melting; **(e)** sclerosing keratitis; **(f)** acute central melting (Courtesy of S Tuft – fig. d; P G Watson, B L Hazelman, C E Pavesio, W R Green, from *The Sclera and Systemic Disorders*, Butterworth-Heinemann, 2004 – fig. e)

Associated systemic diseases

Rheumatoid arthritis and Wegener granulomatosis account for about 95% of associated disease.

1. **Rheumatoid arthritis** (see Chapter 24) is the commonest systemic association. PUK involves both eyes in 30% of cases and tends to affect patients during the late and advanced vasculitic phase of the disease. Patients with rheumatoid arthritis may also develop the following non-ulcerative types of keratitis:
   a. *Peripheral stromal thinning* characterized by gradual resorption of peripheral stroma leaving the epithelium intact (Fig. 9.27c). Perforation may occur in advanced cases (Fig. 9.27d).
   b. *Sclerosing keratitis* characterized by gradual thickening and opacification of the corneal stroma adjacent to a site of scleritis (Fig. 9.27e).
   c. *Acute central corneal melting* may occur in association with inflammation or severe dry eye (Fig. 9.27f).
2. **Wegener granulomatosis** (see Chapter 24) is the second most common systemic association of PUK. In contrast with rheumatoid arthritis ocular complications are the initial presentation in 50% of cases.
3. **Relapsing polychondritis** (see Chapter 24) is more commonly associated with episcleritis or scleritis than with PUK.
4. **Systemic lupus erythematosus** is a rare association; keratitis is more commonly the result of severe keratoconjunctivitis sicca.

Treatment

PUK associated with a potentially life-threatening systemic vasculitis must be treated with systemic immunosuppressive agents in collaboration with a rheumatologist.

1. **Systemic** high-dose steroids are used to control acute disease. Cytotoxic therapy is required for longer term management to prevent the unacceptable side effects of steroids. Cyclophosphamide is especially useful for Wegener granulomatosis; other options include azathioprine, mycophenolate mofetil and methotrexate.
2. **Keratoplasty.** Emergency keratoplasty (preferably lamellar) may be required for peripheral corneal perforation. Elective keratoplasty (lamellar or penetrating) may be performed subsequently to restore vision.

NEUROTROPHIC KERATITIS

Pathogenesis

Neurotrophic keratopathy occurs when there is loss of the trigeminal innervation to the cornea resulting in partial or complete anaesthesia. Sensory innervation is vital to the health of the corneal epithelium and stroma. The loss of neural influences results in intracellular oedema, exfoliation of the epithelial cells, impairment of epithelial healing and loss of goblet cells, culminating in epithelial breakdown and persistent ulceration. Loss of acetylcholine, substance P, and growth factors from the epithelium appears to be important.

Causes

1. **Acquired.** Damage to the fifth cranial nerve or trigeminal ganglion following surgical ablation for trigeminal neuralgia (tic douloureux), stroke, aneurysm, multiple sclerosis or tumour (acoustic neuroma or neurofibroma).
2. **Systemic diseases** such as diabetes and leprosy.
3. **Ocular disease** such as herpes simplex and herpes zoster keratitis, abuse of topical anaesthetic, chemical burn and refractive corneal surgery.
4. **Congenital** causes include familial dysautonomia (Riley–Day syndrome), Möbius syndrome, Goldenhar syndrome, anhidrotic ectodermal dysplasia and hereditary sensory neuropathy.

Diagnosis

The severity of signs can vary during the course of disease. Some patients develop serious lesions early while others only develop problems after many years.

1. **Corneal sensation** is tested with a wisp of cotton or an anaethesiometer (< 5mm is clinically significant).
2. **Signs**
   • Punctate keratopathy in the interpalpebral zone in which the epithelium appears irregular, slightly opaque and oedematous (Fig. 9.28a).
   • Persistent epithelial defect in which the epithelium at the edge of the lesion appears rolled and thickened, and is poorly attached (Fig. 9.28b).
   • Enlargement of epithelial defect with stromal oedema and infiltration (Fig. 9.28c).
   • Stromal corneal melting (Fig. 9.28d). Perforation is uncommon but can occur rapidly if there is secondary infection.

NB Progression to ulceration may be virtually asymptomatic.

Treatment

1. **Topical** lubricants (non-preserved) for associated dry eye or corneal exposure. Topical insulin-like growth factor-1, substance P, and neurogenic growth factor have been evaluated but are not commercially available.

NB It is also important to eliminate potentially toxic medications already in use.

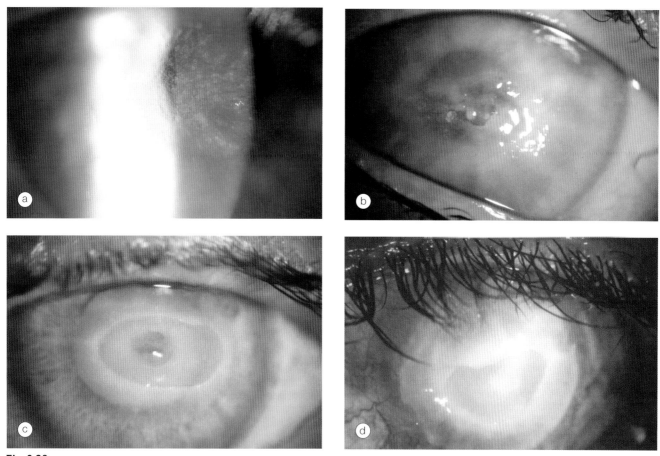

Fig. 9.28
Neurotrophic keratitis. **(a)** Early central epithelial changes; **(b)** small epithelial defect and stromal oedema; **(c)** large epithelial defect and stromal infiltration; **(d)** stromal melting (Courtesy of S Bonini – fig. d)

2. Protection of the ocular surface
 a. ***Simple taping*** of the lids to provide temporary protection.
 b. ***Botulinum toxin injection*** to induce protective ptosis.
 c. ***Tarsorrhaphy*** to prevent drying and reduce exposure, may be temporary or permanent, according to the underlying pathology.
 d. ***Therapeutic silicone contact lenses*** may be fitted provided the eye is carefully monitored for infection.
 e. ***Amniotic membrane*** onlay with temporary central tarsorrhaphy.

EXPOSURE KERATITIS

Pathogenesis

Exposure keratopathy is the result of incomplete lid closure (lagophthalmos) during blinking. Mild exposure during sleep is normal in some individuals but may become symptomatic if there is a poor Bell phenomenon. Lagophthalmos may only be present with blinking or gentle lid closure, but absent on forced lid closure. The result is drying of the cornea despite normal tear production.

Causes

1. Neuroparalytic, especially facial nerve palsy (Fig. 9.29a) which may be idiopathic or the result of surgery for acoustic neuroma or parotid tumour.
2. Reduced muscle tone as in coma or parkinsonism.
3. Mechanical
 • Eyelid scarring associated with cicatricial pemphigoid, burns (Fig. 9.29b) and trauma.
 • Tight facial skin due to eczema, solar keratosis, xeroderma pigmentosum and following blepharoplasty.
4. Abnormality of globe position
 • Severe proptosis resulting in lagophthalmos due to thyroid ophthalmopathy (Fig. 9.29c) or orbital tumour.
 • Severe enophthalmos.

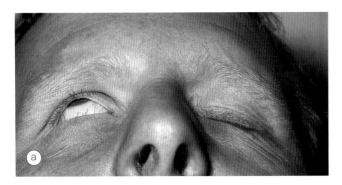

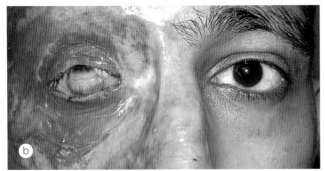

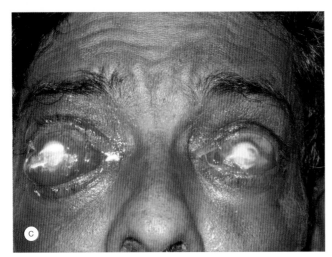

Fig. 9.29
Causes of lagophthalmos. **(a)** Facial nerve palsy; **(b)** eyelid scarring; **(c)** severe proptosis – note bilateral endophthalmitis (Courtesy of S Kumar Puri – fig. c)

Diagnosis

1. **Symptoms** are those of a dry eye.
2. **Signs**
   - Mild punctate epithelial changes involving the inferior third of the cornea (Fig. 9.30a), particularly with nocturnal lagophthalmos.
   - Epithelial breakdown (Fig. 9.30b).
   - Stromal melting (Fig. 9.30c) which may result in perforation.

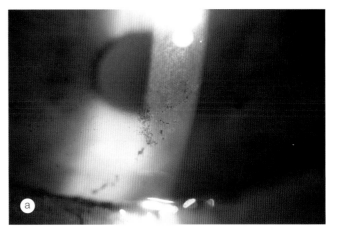

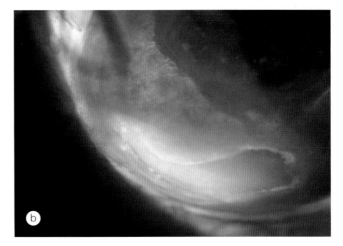

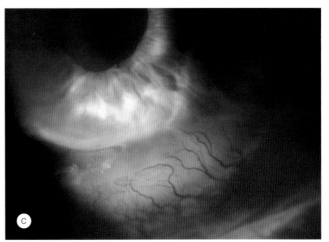

Fig. 9.30
Exposure keratitis. **(a)** Inferior epithelial changes; **(b)** inferior epithelial defect; **(c)** stromal melting

- Secondary infection may supervene at any stage.
- Inferior fibrovascular change with Salzmann degeneration may develop over time.

Treatment

Treatment depends on the severity of exposure and whether recovery is anticipated.

1. Reversible exposure
- Artificial tears (non-preserved) during the day and ointment at night.
- Taping the lid closed at night.
- Bandage silicone rubber or scleral contact lenses.
- Temporary tarsorrhaphy or Frost suture.

2. Permanent exposure
- Permanent lateral or median tarsorrhaphy.
- Gold weights inserted in the upper lid for VII nerve palsy.
- Permanent central tarsorrhaphy and conjunctival flap may be required for severe cases.
- Management of proptosis by orbital decompression if necessary.

NB Combined neuroparalytic and neurotrophic keratopathy is particularly difficult to manage.

MISCELLANEOUS KERATITIS

Infectious crystalline keratitis

Pathogenesis

Infectious crystalline keratitis is a rare, indolent infection usually associated with long-term topical steroid therapy following penetrating keratoplasty. *S. viridans* is most commonly isolated although numerous other bacteria and fungi have been implicated. The mechanism appears to be slow proliferation of low virulence organisms along the plane of stromal lamellae when the inflammatory response has been suppressed. Bacteria may also grow within a protective biofilm (bacterial extracellular matrix), which could explain the lack of inflammation and the relative resistance to therapy.

Diagnosis

1. Signs
- Slowly progressive, grey-white, branching opacities in the anterior or mid stroma (Fig. 9.31a and b).
- Minimal inflammation and usually intact overlying epithelium.

2. Culture or biopsy to determine the organism.

Treatment

Treatment is with topical antibiotics for several weeks. Stopping topical steroid without adequate antibiotic cover can precipitate a rapid increase in inflammation and even suppuration.

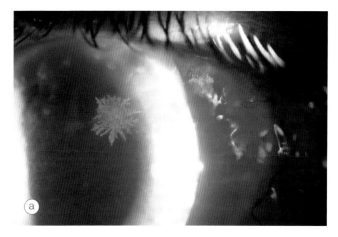

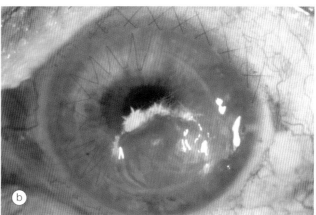

Fig. 9.31
(a) Infectious crystalline keratitis; **(b)** crystalline keratitis on a graft (Courtesy of M Kerr-Muir – fig. a)

Thygeson superficial punctate keratitis

Thygeson superficial punctate keratitis is an uncommon, usually bilateral, idiopathic, condition characterized by exacerbations and remissions. It most commonly affects young adults but may occur at any age and recurrences can continue for decades. Although reports of virus isolation exist these have not been repeatable.

Diagnosis

1. Symptoms are recurrent attacks of irritation, photophobia and tearing.

2. Signs
- Coarse, distinct, granular, greyish, elevated epithelial lesions (Fig. 9.32a).
- A mild subepithelial haze may be present (Fig. 9.32b), especially if topical antivirals have been used.

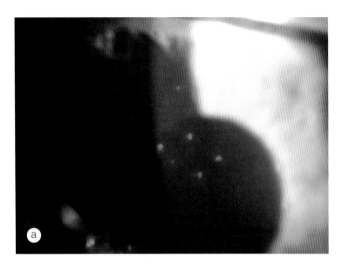

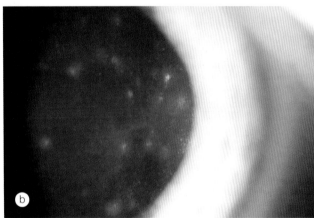

Fig. 9.32
(a) Thygeson superficial punctate keratitis; **(b)** associated subepithelial haze (Courtesy of R Curtis – fig. b)

NB The conjunctiva is uninvolved and vascularization is not a feature. The most common differential diagnosis is staphylococcal hypersensitivity, punctate epitheliopathy or adenoviral keratitis.

Treatment

1. Topical
- Lubricants may suffice in mild cases.
- Steroids (fluorometholone 0.1% b.d.) with gradual tapering. In some cases long-term low-dose therapy (one drop weekly) may be required.
- Ciclosporin is a good alternative to steroids, particularly in patients requiring long-term steroid therapy.

2. Contact lenses (extended wear or daily disposable soft) may be considered if steroids are contraindicated. Most patients can be instructed to manage these themselves.
3. Phototherapeutic keratectomy brings short term relief but eventual recurrence is likely.

Filamentary keratitis

Pathogenesis

Filamentary keratitis is a common condition that can cause considerable discomfort. It is thought that a loose area of epithelium acts as a focus for deposition of mucus and cellular debris. Causes include the following:
- Aqueous deficiency dry eye (KCS) is the most common.
- Corneal epithelial instability (recurrent erosion syndrome, corneal graft, cataract surgery, refractive surgery and drug toxicity).
- Superior limbic keratoconjunctivitis.
- Neurotrophic keratitis.
- Prolonged occlusion as from patching or associated with essential blepharospasm.

Diagnosis

1. **Symptoms** are discomfort and foreign body sensation
2. **Signs**
   - Strands of degenerating epithelial cells and mucus attached at one end to the cornea that moves with blinking (Fig. 9.33a and b). They stain well with rose bengal.
   - A small epithelial defect may be present at the base of a filament.

Management

1. **General**
   - Underlying cause such as dry eye should be treated (see Chapter 7).
   - All unnecessary medications should be stopped.
   - Short-term topical steroids.
   - Non-steroidal anti-inflammatory drops such as diclofenac 0.1% may also be used and they seem to have an anaesthetic effect.
2. **Specific treatment for filaments**
   - Mechanical removal of filaments for short term symptomatic relief.
   - Hypertonic 5% saline to encourage adhesion of loose epithelium.
   - Mucolytic agents such as 5% or 10% acetylcysteine.
   - Bandage contact lenses, to protect the surface of the eye from the shearing action of the lids, are only justified for short term use because of the risk of infection.

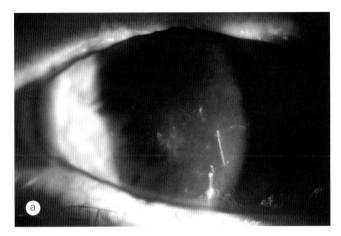

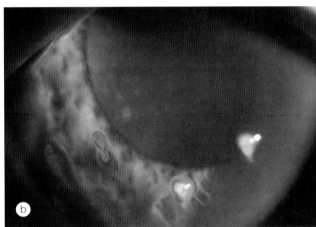

Fig. 9.33
Filamentary keratitis. **(a)** Fine filaments; **(b)** coarse filaments
(Courtesy of S Tuft)

Recurrent corneal epithelial erosions

Pathogenesis

There is an abnormally weak attachment between the basal cells of the corneal epithelium and the basement membrane. Minor injury, such as opening the eye after sleep, can cause shearing forces sufficient to cause movement of the epithelial sheet or tearing of the epithelium. Erosions may be associated with previous trauma, epithelial membrane dystrophy or anterior stromal dystrophy.

Diagnosis

1. **Presentation** is with severe pain, spasm, and watering occurring during the night or on wakening. There may be a prior history of trauma, sometimes years previously.
2. **Signs**
   - Epithelial microcysts or a frank epithelial defect may be present, particularly in the interpalpebral zone and lower half of the cornea (Fig. 9.34).

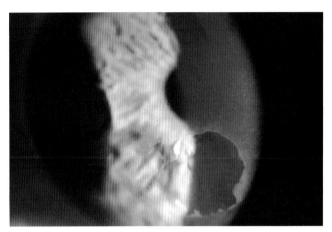

Fig. 9.34
Corneal erosion

- The extent of loose epithelium may be highlighted by pooling with fluorescein.
- Signs of epithelial basement membrane disease, especially fingerprint lines, or stromal dystrophy may be detected in both eyes.

Treatment

1. **Acute symptoms**
   - Simple abrasions heal faster without patching.
   - Pressure patching does not help discomfort.
   - A bandage contact lens may help pain but does not enhance healing.
   - Topical antibiotic and cycloplegia.
   - Topical diclofenac 0.1% to reduce discomfort.
2. **Recurrent symptoms**
   - Topical lubricant gel or ointment at night.
   - Bandage contact lens.
   - Excimer laser ablation after epithelial debridement is probably more effective at reducing recurrences than epithelial debridement alone.
   - Anterior stromal puncture for localized areas not involving the visual axis.

Xerophthalmia

Pathogenesis

Ascorbic acid (vitamin C) is essential for the synthesis of retinal photopigments and conjunctival glycoproteins. It is also required for normal immunity so that deficiency leads to susceptibility to respiratory, intestinal and genitourinary infection. Lack of vitamin A in the diet may be caused by malnutrition, malabsorption, chronic alcoholism or highly selective dieting. Xerophthalmia is a spectrum of ocular disease caused by vitamin A deficiency. It is responsible for up to 100,000 new cases of blindness worldwide each year and is the leading cause of childhood blindness. The risk in infants is increased if their mothers are malnourished and by coexisting diarrhoea or measles (see below).

Diagnosis

1. **Symptoms** are night blindness (nyctalopia) and ocular irritation due to dryness.
2. **Conjunctiva**
   - Xerosis is characterized by dryness of the conjunctiva in the interpalpebral zone with loss of goblet cells, squamous metaplasia and keratinization.
   - Bitot spots are triangular patches of foamy keratinized epithelium in the interpalpebral zone (Fig. 9.35a) thought to be caused by infection with *Corynebacterium xerosis*.

3. **Cornea**
   - Lustreless appearance due to xerosis.
   - Bilateral punctate corneal epithelial erosions in the interpalpebral zone which can progress to epithelial defect but are reversible with treatment.
   - Sterile corneal melting by liquefactive necrosis (keratomalacia) which may result in perforation (Fig. 9.35b).
4. **Retinopathy** characterized by yellowish peripheral dots may occur in advanced cases and is associated with decreased electroretinogram amplitude.
5. **Investigations** are not usually required and the diagnosis is confirmed by response to treatment. Impression cytology shows loss of goblet cells and squamous metaplasia which may detect preclinical xerosis. Serum shows reduced vitamin A and retinol binding proteins.

Table 9.3 shows the World Health Organization grading of xerophthalmia.

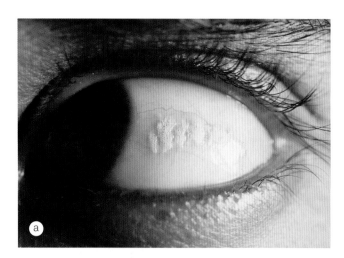

Table 9.3   WHO grading of xerophthalmia

XN	= night blindness
X1	= conjunctival xerosis (X1A) with Bitot spot (X1B)
X2	= corneal xerosis
X3	= corneal ulceration, less than one third (X3A); more than one third (X3B)
XS	= corneal scar
XF	= xerophthalmic fundus

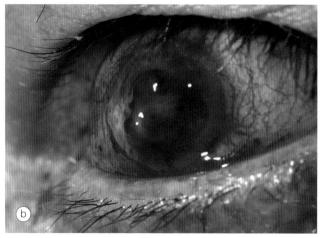

Treatment

Keratomalacia reflects very severe vitamin A deficiency and should be treated as a medical emergency to reduce child mortality.

1. **Systemic** treatment of keratomalacia involves oral or intramuscular vitamin A. Multivitamin supplements and dietary sources of vitamin A are also administered.
2. **Local**
   - Intense lubrication.
   - Topical retinoic acid may promote healing but is not sufficient without systemic supplements.
   - Emergency surgery for corneal perforation may be necessary.

NB Children with keratomalacia and perforation usually cannot tolerate general anaesthesia due to general debility, and are thus untreatable.

Fig. 9.35
Xerophthalmia. **(a)** Bitot spot; **(b)** keratomalacia and perforation
(Courtesy of U Raina – fig. a)

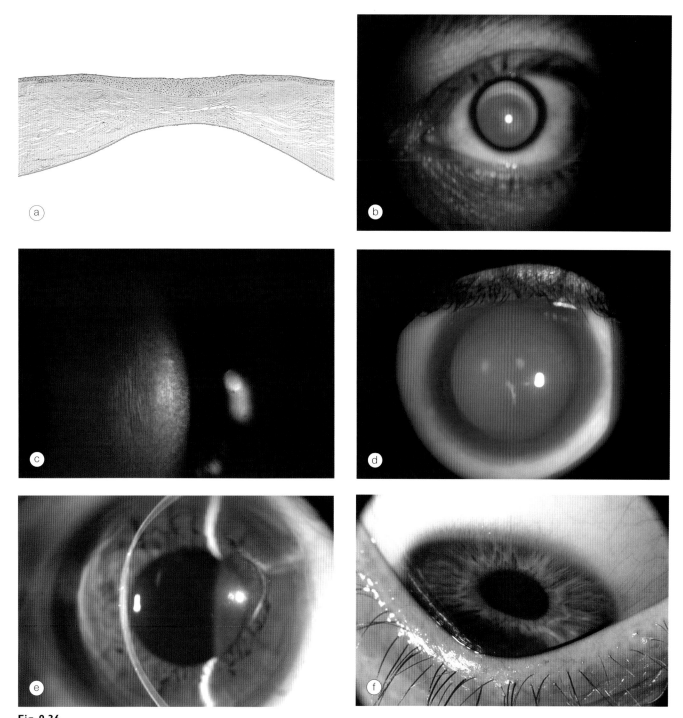

Fig. 9.36
Keratoconus. **(a)** Histology shows central stromal thinning; **(b)** 'oil-droplet' red reflex; **(c)** Vogt striae; **(d)** Fleischer ring; **(e)** advanced thinning; **(f)** Munson sign (Courtesy of J Harry and G Misson, from *Clinical Ophthalmic Pathology*, Butterworth-Heinemann, 2001 – fig. a; S Fogla – figs d and e)

Measles keratitis

Measles (rubeola) is a highly infectious acute exanthematous disease of childhood transmitted by droplets. Although it has been largely eradicated in developed countries, as a result of mass vaccination and good diet, it still remains a major cause of preventable blindness in developing countries. There is a close association between visual loss from measles and vitamin A deficiency (see above). An attack of measles may also precipitate keratomalacia in borderline cases of vitamin A deficiency. Innocuous ocular manifestations of measles include conjunctivitis, subconjunctival haemorrhage and punctate epithelial keratitis.

CORNEAL ECTASIAS

Keratoconus

Keratoconus is a progressive disorder in which the cornea assumes a conical shape secondary to stromal thinning and protrusion (Fig. 9.36a). The onset is around puberty with slow progression thereafter until the third or fourth decades of life, when it usually arrests, although the ectasia can become stationary at any time. Both eyes are affected, if only topographically, in almost all cases. It appears that patients with severe disease also tend to have more asymmetrical involvement. The role of heredity has not been clearly defined and most patients do not have a positive family history. Offspring appear to be affected in only about 10% of cases and an AD transmission with incomplete penetrance has been proposed.

Presentation

Presentation is typically during puberty with unilateral impairment of vision due to progressive myopia and astigmatism, which subsequently becomes irregular. The patient may report frequent changes in spectacle prescription or decreased tolerance to contact lens wear. As a result of the asymmetrical nature of the condition, the fellow eye usually has normal vision with negligible astigmatism at presentation. Approximately 50% of normal fellow eyes will progress to keratoconus within 16 years; the greatest risk is within the first six years of onset.

Diagnosis

The hallmark of keratoconus is central or paracentral stromal thinning, apical protrusion and irregular astigmatism. It can be graded by keratometry according to severity as mild (< 48D), moderate (48–54D) and severe (> 54D).

1. **Signs**
   - Direct ophthalmoscopy from a distance of one foot shows an 'oil droplet' reflex (Fig. 9.36b).
   - Retinoscopy shows an irregular 'scissor' reflex.
   - Slit-lamp biomicroscopy shows fine, vertical, deep stromal striae (Vogt lines – Fig. 9.36c) which disappear with external pressure on the globe.
   - Epithelial iron deposits may surround the base of the cone (Fleischer ring) – best seen with a cobalt blue filter (Fig. 9.36d).
   - Progressive corneal thinning, to as little as one-third of normal thickness (Fig. 9.36e) associated with poor visual acuity resulting from marked irregular myopic astigmatism with steep keratometry (K) readings.
   - Bulging of the lower lid in down-gaze (Munson sign – Fig. 9.36f).
2. **Corneal topography** shows irregular astigmatism and is the most sensitive method of detecting early keratoconus and in monitoring progression (Fig. 9.37).

Acute hydrops

Acute hydrops is caused by a rupture in Descemet membrane (Fig. 9.38a) that allows an influx of aqueous into the cornea (Fig. 9.38b and c). This causes a sudden drop in visual acuity associated with discomfort and watering. Although the break usually heals within 6–10 weeks and the corneal oedema clears, a variable amount of stromal scarring may develop (Fig. 9.38d). Acute episodes are initially treated with hypertonic saline and patching or a soft bandage contact lens. Healing may result in improved visual acuity as a result of scarring and flattening of the cornea. Keratoplasty should be deferred till the oedema has resolved.

Associations

1. **Systemic** disorders include Down, Turner, Ehlers–Danlos and Marfan syndromes, atopy, osteogenesis imperfecta, mitral valve prolapse and mental retardation.
2. **Ocular** associations include vernal keratoconjunctivitis, blue sclera, aniridia, ectopia lentis, Leber congenital amaurosis, retinitis pigmentosa and persistent eye rubbing.

Treatment

1. **Spectacles** in early cases to correct regular and mild irregular astigmatism.
2. **Rigid contact lenses** are required for higher degrees of astigmatism to provide a regular refracting surface. Advances in both lens design and material have increased the proportion of keratoconus patients who can use contact lenses.
3. **Keratoplasty,** penetrating or deep lamellar, is indicated in patients with advanced progressive disease, especially with significant corneal scarring. Although clear grafts are obtained in over 85% of cases, optical outcomes may be compromised by residual astigmatism and anisometropia, necessitating contact lens correction for best acuity.

Fig. 9.37
Relative scale corneal maps showing advanced keratoconus in the right eye and an early paracentral cone in the left (Courtesy of E Morris)

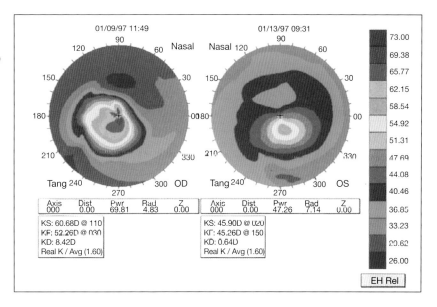

Fig. 9.38
Advanced keratoconus. **(a)** Histology shows a defect in Descemet membrane; **(b)** acute hydrops; **(c)** histology shows oedema of basal epithelial cells and partial loss of Bowman layer; **(d)** apical scarring (Courtesy of J Harry and G Misson, from *Clinical Ophthalmic Pathology*, Butterworth-Heinemann, 2001 – figs a and c)

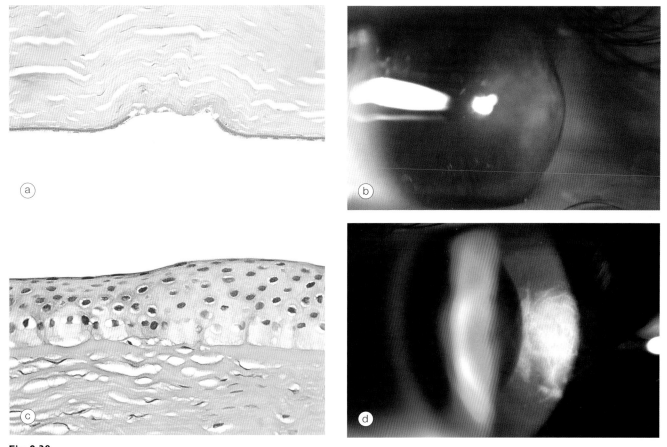

Pellucid marginal degeneration

Pellucid marginal degeneration is a rare, progressive, peripheral corneal thinning disorder typically involving the inferior portion although rarely the superior cornea may be involved. Occasionally it may coexist with keratoconus and keratoglobus. Like keratoconus, pellucid marginal degeneration is bilateral, although eyes may be asymmetrically affected.

Diagnosis

1. **Presentation** is in the fourth to fifth decades with reduced visual acuity due to high increasing astigmatism.
2. **Signs**
   - Bilateral, slowly progressive, crescent-shaped band of inferior corneal thinning extending from 4 to 8 o'clock, 1mm from the limbus (Fig. 9.39a).
   - The area of thinning usually measures 1–2mm in width and is separated from the limbus by normal cornea.
   - The epithelium is intact, and the cornea above the thinned out area is ectatic. Flattening in the vertical meridian results in severe irregular against-the-rule astigmatism.
   - Unlike keratoconus Fleischer rings and Vogt striae do not occur.
   - Acute hydrops and spontaneous perforation are rare complications.
3. **Corneal topography** map shows a classical 'butterfly' pattern associated with severe astigmatism and diffuse steepening of the inferior cornea (Fig. 9.39b).

Treatment

1. **Spectacles** usually fail very early as irregular astigmatism increases.
2. **Contact lenses.** In early disease soft toric lenses are adequate but in more advanced cases rigid gas permeable contact lenses are often the best option.
3. **Surgical options,** none of which are ideal, in patients intolerant to contact lenses include large eccentric penetrating keratoplasty, thermocauterization, crescentic lamellar keratoplasty, wedge resection of diseased tissue, epikeratoplasty and intracorneal ring implantation.

Keratoglobus

Keratoglobus is an extremely rare condition in which the entire cornea is abnormally thin. Possibly related to keratoconus, it may be associated with Leber congenital amaurosis and blue sclera.

1. **Onset** is at birth.
2. **Signs**
   - In contrast with keratoconus ectasia is generalized (Fig. 9.40a).

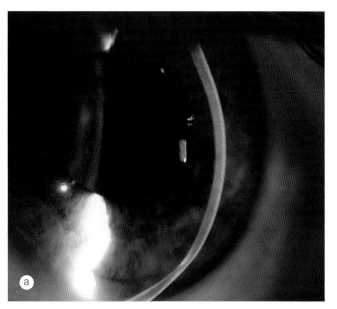

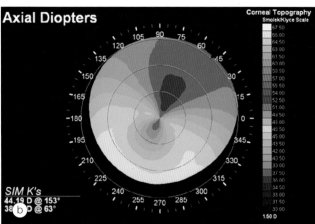

Fig. 9.39
(a) Pellucid marginal degeneration; **(b)** topography shows severe astigmatism and diffuse steepening of the inferior cornea
(Courtesy of R Visser – fig. a; S Fogla – fig. b)

- Acute hydrops (Fig. 9.40b) occurs less commonly than in either keratoconus or pellucid marginal degeneration but the cornea is more prone to rupture on relatively mild trauma.
3. **Corneal topography** shows generalized steepening (Fig. 9.40c).
4. **Management** is with scleral contact lenses because the results of surgery are very poor.

CORNEAL DYSTROPHIES

The corneal dystrophies are a group of progressive, usually bilateral, mostly genetically determined, non-inflammatory, opacifying disorders. The age at presentation varies between

Recent advances in molecular genetics have identified the responsible gene defects for most of the dystrophies.

Epithelial dystrophies

Epithelial basement membrane dystrophy

Epithelial basement membrane dystrophy, also known as Cogan microscystic or map-dot-fingerprint, is the most common dystrophy seen in clinical practice. Despite this it is frequently misdiagnosed due to its variable appearance.

1. **Inheritance.** The condition is usually sporadic and rarely AD with incomplete penetrance.
2. **Onset** is in the second decade. About 10% of patients develop recurrent corneal erosions in the third decade. The remainder are asymptomatic throughout life. Simultaneous bilateral recurrent erosions suggest epithelial basement membrane dystrophy.
3. **Signs.** The following lesions may be seen in isolation or combination and are best visualized by retroillumination or scleral scatter.
   - Dot-like opacities (Fig. 9.41a).
   - Epithelial microcysts (Fig. 9.41b).
   - Subepithelial map-like patterns surrounded by a faint haze (Fig. 9.41c).
   - Whorled fingerprint-like lines (Fig. 9.41d).

   NB Over time one pattern frequently changes to another and the distribution of the lesions may also vary.

4. **Histology** shows thickening of the basement membrane with deposition of fibrillary protein between it and Bowman layer (Fig. 9.41e). There is also absence of hemidesmosomes of the basal epithelial cells which is responsible for recurrent corneal erosions.
5. **Treatment** is that of recurrent corneal erosions.

Meesmann dystrophy

Meesmann dystrophy is a very rare innocuous condition.

1. **Inheritance** is AD with the gene locus on 12q13 or 17q12.
2. **Onset** is in the first two years of life with ocular irritation.
3. **Signs**
   - Myriads of tiny intraepithelial cysts of uniform size but variable density are maximal centrally and extend towards but do not reach the limbus (Fig. 9.42a).
   - The cornea may be slightly thinned and sensation reduced.
4. **Histology** shows irregular thickening of the epithelial basement membrane and intraepithelial cysts (Fig. 9.42b).
5. **Treatment** other than lubrication is not normally required.

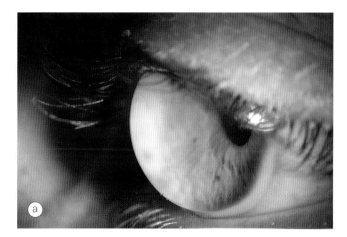
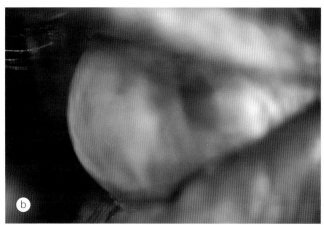
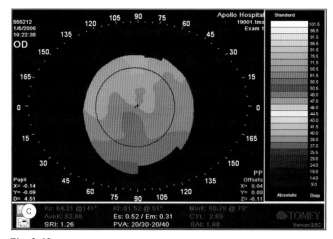

Fig. 9.40
(a) Keratoglobus; **(b)** acute hydrops; **(c)** topography shows generalized steepening (Courtesy of S Fogla – fig. c)

the first and fourth decades depending on the relative frequency of secondary recurrent epithelial erosions and visual impairment. Based on biomicroscopic and histopathological features, corneal dystrophies are classified into: (a) *epithelial*, (b) *Bowman layer*, (c) *stromal* and (d) *endothelial*.

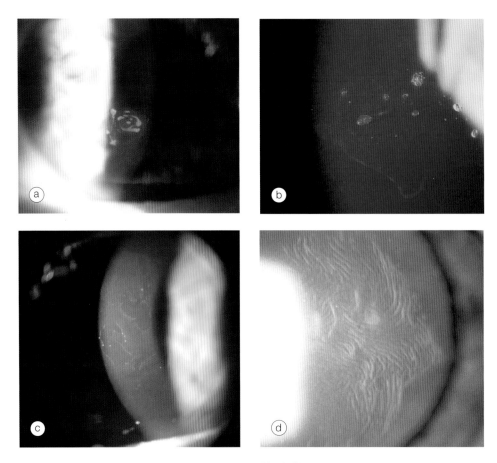

Fig. 9.41
Epithelial basement membrane dystrophy of Cogan. **(a)** Dots; **(b)** multiple microcysts; **(c)** map-like patterns; **(d)** fingerprint lines seen on retroillumination; **(e)** histology shows intraepithelial extension of the basement membrane above the intraepithelial cyst – toluidine blue stain (Courtesy of S Fogla – fig. c; Krachmer, Mannis and Holland, from *Cornea*, Mosby, 2005 – fig. d; J Harry and G Misson, from *Clinical Ophthalmic Pathology*, Butterworth-Heinemann, 2001 – fig. e)

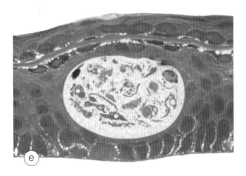

Lisch dystrophy

1. **Inheritance** is AD or XLD with the gene locus on Xp22.3.
2. **Signs**
   - Grey bands with a whorled configuration (Fig. 9.43a).
   - Retroillumination shows densely packed microcysts (Fig. 9.43b).

Bowman layer dystrophies

Reis–Bückler dystrophy (Bowman layer 1 or corneal dystrophy of Bowman – CDB1)

1. **Inheritance** is AD with the gene locus on 5q31.
2. **Onset** is in first to second decades with painful recurrent corneal erosions.

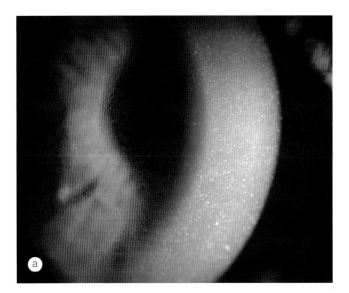

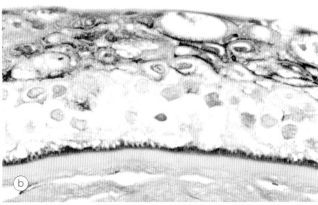

Fig. 9.42
Meesmann dystrophy. **(a)** Myriads of intraepithelial cysts;
(b) histology shows thickening of the epithelial basement
membrane and intraepithelial cysts – PAS stain (Courtesy of S Fogla
– fig. a; J Harry and G Misson, from *Clinical Ophthalmic Pathology*,
Butterworth-Heinemann, 2001 – fig. b)

3. Signs

- Grey-white, fine, round and polygonal opacities in Bowman layer, most dense centrally (Fig. 9.44a and b).
- The changes increase in density with age resulting in a reticular pattern due to the laying down of irregular bands of collagen replacing Bowman layer.
- Corneal sensation is reduced and visual impairment may occur due to scarring at Bowman layer.

4. Histology
shows replacement of Bowman layer and the epithelial basement membrane with fibrous tissue (Fig. 9.44c).

5. Treatment
is mainly by excimer laser keratectomy. Lamellar keratoplasty may be required in some cases but is associated with a high incidence of recurrence of the dystrophy on the graft, which may develop rapidly.

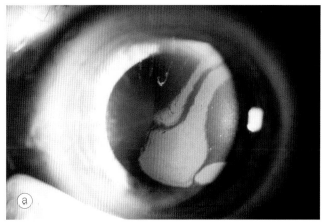

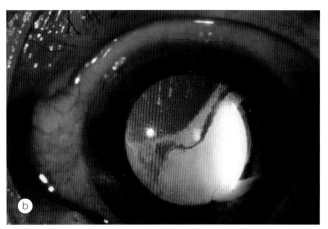

Fig. 9.43
Lisch dystrophy. **(a)** Grey bands with a whorled configuration;
(b) retroillumination shows clear, densely crowded microcysts
(Courtesy of W Lisch)

Thiel–Behnke dystrophy (Bowman layer 2 or corneal dystrophy of Bowman – CDB2)

1. **Inheritance** is AD with the gene locus on 10q24.
2. **Onset** is at the end of the first decade with recurrent erosions.
3. **Signs** are similar to Reis–Bückler dystrophy except that the opacities assume more of a honeycomb pattern (Fig. 9.45).
4. **Histology** shows 'curly fibres' in Bowman layer.
5. **Treatment** may not be necessary because visual impairment is less than in Reis–Bückler dystrophy.

Central Schnyder (crystalline) dystrophy

Crystalline dystrophy is a disorder of corneal lipid metabolism which is associated with raised serum cholesterol in approximately 50% of patients.

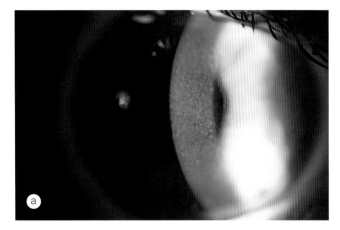

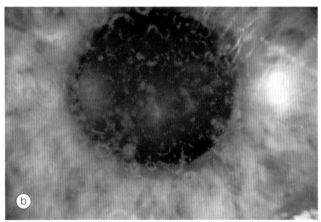

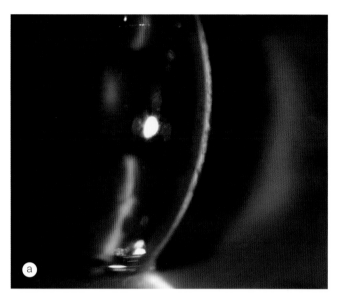

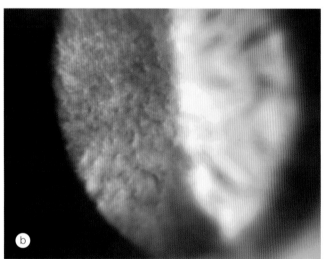

Fig. 9.45
(a) Thiel–Behnke dystrophy; slit view showing location of lesions; **(b)** magnified view

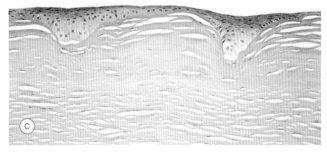

Fig. 9.44
(a) Reis–Bückler dystrophy; **(b)** magnified view; **(c)** histology shows replacement of Bowman layer and epithelial basement membrane by fibrous tissue (Courtesy of W Lisch – fig. b; J Harry and G Misson, from *Clinical Ophthalmic Pathology*, Butterworth-Heinemann, 2001 – fig. c)

1. **Inheritance** is AD with the gene locus on 1p36.
2. **Onset** is in the second decade with visual impairment and glare.
3. **Signs**
   - Central, oval, subepithelial 'crystalline' opacity (Fig. 9.46a).

- Diffuse corneal haze and prominent corneal arcus by the third decade (Fig. 9.46b).
4. **Histology** shows deposits of phospholipids and cholesterol.
5. **Treatment** involves excimer laser keratectomy.

Stromal dystrophies

Lattice dystrophy type 1 (Biber–Haab–Dimmer)

1. **Inheritance** is AD with the gene locus on 5q31.
2. **Onset** is at the end of the first decade with recurrent

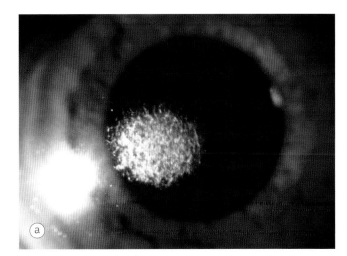

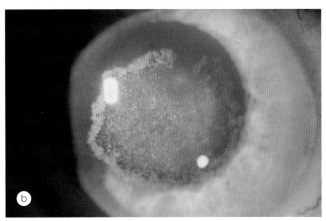

Fig. 9.46
Schnyder dystrophy. **(a)** Central crystalline opacity; **(b)** diffuse corneal haze (Courtesy of K Nischal – fig. a; W Lisch – fig. b)

erosions which precede typical stromal changes. It may therefore be initially missed.

3. **Signs** in chronological order:
- Anterior stromal, glassy, refractile dots (Fig. 9.47a).
- Coalescence into fine lattice lines best seen on retroillumination (Fig. 9.47b).
- Deep and outward spread sparing the periphery (Fig. 9.47b).
- Generalized stromal haze that progressively impairs vision and may obscure the lattice lines (Fig. 9.47c).

4. **Histology** shows amyloid that stains with Congo red (Fig. 9.47d). When viewed with a polarized filter amyloid deposits show characteristic green birefringence (Fig. 9.47e).

5. **Treatment** by penetrating or deep lamellar keratoplasty is frequently required before the sixth decade.

Lattice dystrophy type 2 (Meretoja syndrome)

Lattice type 2 is associated with systemic amyloidosis.

1. **Inheritance** is AD with the gene locus on 9q34.
2. **Onset** is in the third decade with recurrent erosions, but less frequently than in type 1 lattice.
3. **Signs.** Randomly scattered, short, fine lattice lines which are sparse, more delicate and more radially orientated (Fig. 9.48) than in type 1 lattice dystrophy.
4. **Histology** shows amyloid deposits in the corneal stroma and other involved sites.
5. **Treatment** by penetrating or deep lamellar keratoplasty may be required in the seventh decade but may be complicated by recurrent infection consequent to exposure keratopathy.
6. **Systemic features** include progressive bilateral cranial and peripheral neuropathy, dysarthria, dry and extremely lax itchy skin, a characteristic 'mask-like' facial expression due to bilateral facial palsy, protruding lips and pendulous ears. Amyloidosis may also involve the kidneys and heart.

Lattice dystrophy type 3 and 3A

1. **Inheritance** of type 3 is presumed to be AR; type 3A is AD with the gene locus on 5q31 in both.
2. **Onset** of type 3 is between the fourth and sixth decades with visual impairment but recurrent erosions are uncommon; type 3A presents later.
3. **Signs**
- Thick, ropy lines extending from limbus to limbus with minimal intervening haze (Fig. 9.49).
- There may be gross asymmetry or the lesions may be unilateral for a time.
- Progression is rapid if the cornea is subjected to trauma, however minor.
4. **Treatment** by penetrating or deep lamellar keratoplasty is invariably required.

Granular dystrophy type 1

1. **Inheritance** is AD with the gene locus on 5q31.
2. **Onset** is in the first decade but vision is usually not affected in the early stage of the disease although some patients may have mild photophobia from light scattering. Recurrent erosions are uncommon.
3. **Signs** in chronological order:
- Small, white, sharply demarcated deposits resembling crumbs, rings or snowflakes in the central anterior stroma (Fig. 9.50a).
- The overall pattern of deposition is radial or disc shaped, or it may be in the form of a Christmas tree.
- Initially the corneal stroma between the opacities is clear.
- Gradual increase in number and size of the deposits with deeper and outward spread but not reaching the limbus (Fig. 9.50b).
- Gradual confluence and diffuse haze of intervening stroma causes visual impairment (Fig. 9.50c).
- Corneal sensation is impaired.

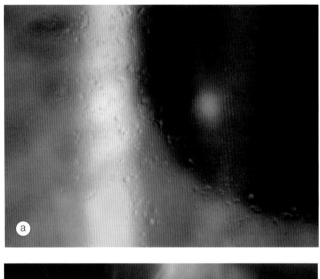

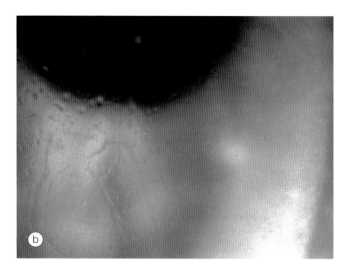

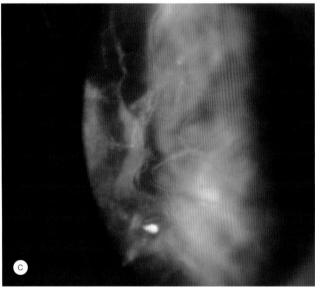

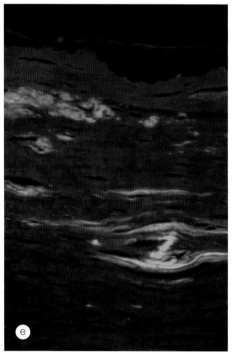

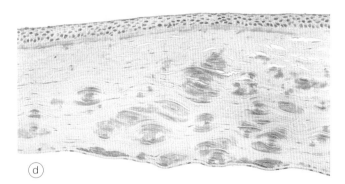

Fig. 9.47
Lattice dystrophy type 1. **(a)** Glassy dots in the anterior stroma;
(b) fine lattice lines seen on retroillumination; **(c)** prominent
lattice lines and stromal haze; **(d)** histology shows amyloid that
stains with Congo red; **(e)** characteristic green birefringence of
amyloid viewed with polarized light – thioflavine T (Courtesy of
J Harry – fig. d; J Harry and G Misson, from *Clinical Ophthalmic Pathology*,
Butterworth-Heinemann, 2001 – fig. e)

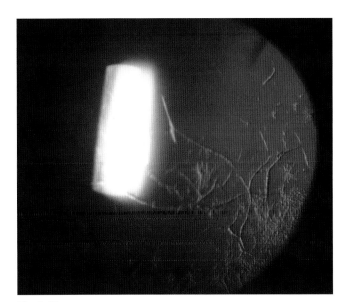

Fig. 9.48
Lattice dystrophy type 2 – fine sparse lines

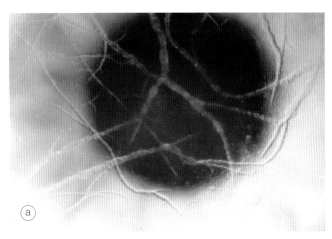

(a)

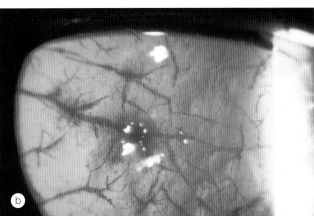

(b)

Fig. 9.49
Lattice dystrophy type 3 and 3a. **(a)** Thick, ropy lines; **(b)** view on retroillumination

4. **Histology** shows amorphous hyaline deposits which stain bright red with Masson trichrome (Fig. 9.50d).
5. **Treatment** by penetrating or deep lamellar keratoplasty is usually required by the fifth decade. Superficial recurrences may require repeated excimer laser keratectomy.

Granular dystrophy type 2 (Avellino)

1. **Inheritance** is AD with the gene locus on 5q31.
2. **Onset** is in the second decade. Recurrent erosions are rare, and if present, mild so that some patients may be unaware of their disease.
3. **Signs.** Superficial, fine, opacities that resemble rings, discs stars or snowflakes, most dense centrally (resembling those seen in granular dystrophy type 1) associated with deeper linear opacities reminiscent of lattice dystrophy (Fig. 9.51).
4. **Histology** shows both hyaline and amyloid in the stroma that stains with Masson trichrome and Congo red.
5. **Treatment** is usually not required.

NB Mutations in TGFBI on chromosome 5 cause CDB1, CDB2, lattice type 1, lattice type 3A, Avellino, and granular dystrophy. These are therefore allelic variants.

Macular dystrophy

Macular dystrophy is the least common stromal dystrophy in which a systemic inborn error of keratan sulphate metabolism has only corneal manifestations. It has been divided into clinically indistinguishable types I, IA and II depending on the presence or absence of antigenic keratan sulphate in the serum and cornea.

1. **Inheritance** is AR with the gene locus on 16q22.
2. **Onset** is towards the end of the first decade with gradual visual deterioration.
3. **Signs** in chronological order:
   - Anterior stromal haze, initially involves the central cornea.
   - Greyish-white, dense, focal, poorly delineated spots in the anterior stroma centrally and posterior stroma in the periphery (Fig. 9.52a).
   - Superficial deposits may produce an irregularity of the corneal surface, although recurrent erosions are unusual.
   - Increasing opacification (Fig. 9.52b).
   - Eventual involvement of full-thickness stroma up to the limbus associated with corneal thinning (Fig. 9.52c).
4. **Histology** shows abnormally close packing of collagen in the corneal lamellae and abnormal aggregations of glycosaminoglycans which stain with Prussian blue and colloidal iron (Fig. 9.52d).
5. **Treatment** by penetrating keratoplasty is generally successful but late recurrence on the graft may occur.

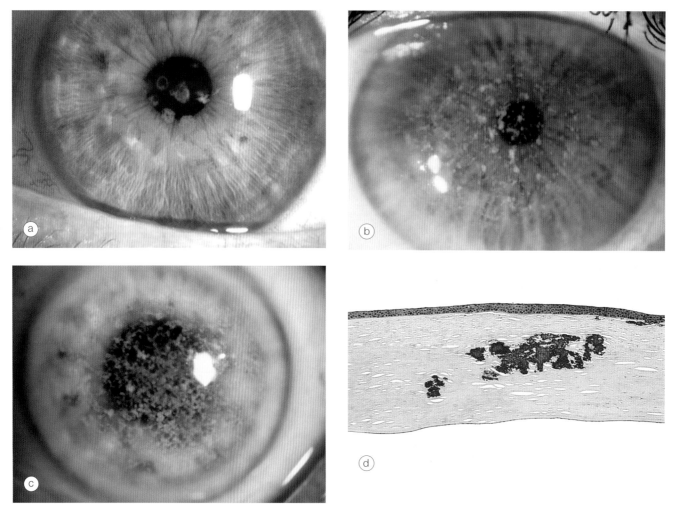

Fig. 9.50
Granular dystrophy type 1. **(a)** Sharply demarcated crumbs; **(b)** increase in number and outward spread; **(c)** confluence; **(d)** histology shows red-staining material with Masson trichrome (Courtesy of B Tompkins – fig. a; A Ridgway – fig. c; J Harry – fig. d)

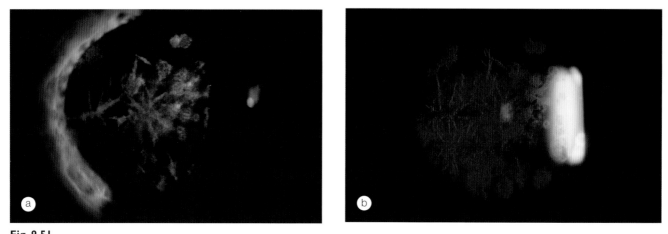

Fig. 9.51
Granular dystrophy type 2 (Avellino). **(a)** Superficial stromal rings, stars or snowflakes associated with deeper linear opacities; **(b)** view on retroillumination (Courtesy of W Lisch)

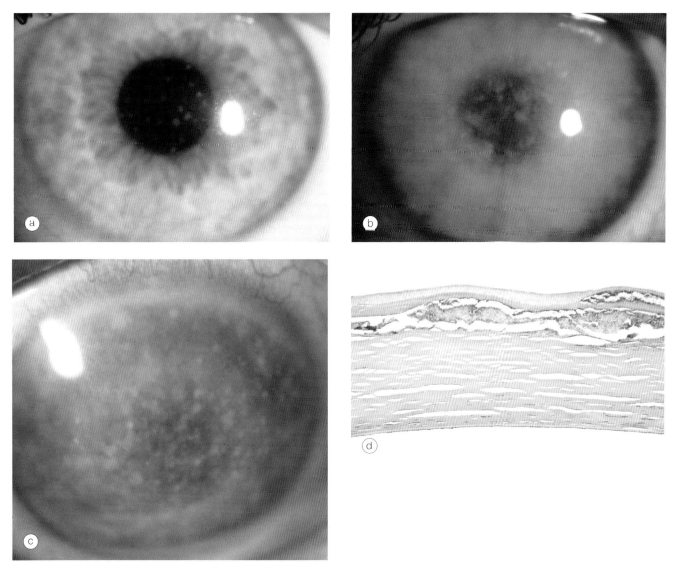

Fig. 9.52
Macular dystrophy (a) Poorly delineated spots; (b) increase in size and stromal haze; (c) extensive involvement; (d) histology shows deposits of abnormal glycosaminoglycans that stain a Prussian blue colour with colloidal iron stain (Courtesy of A. Ridgway – figs a, b and c; J Harry – fig. d)

Gelatinous drop-like dystrophy

Gelatinous dystrophy is a rare disorder which is also known as familial subepithelial amyloidosis of the cornea. Most reported cases have been from Japan.

1. **Inheritance** is AR.
2. **Onset** is in the first to second decades with severe photophobia, watering and visual impairment.
3. **Signs** in chronological order:
   - Grey subepithelial nodules.
   - Gradual confluence, stromal involvement and increase in size giving rise to a mulberry-like appearance (Fig. 9.53a).
3. **Histology** shows subepithelial and anterior stromal accumulation of amyloid (Fig. 9.53b).
4. **Treatment** is with repeated superficial keratectomy because of early recurrences on corneal grafts.

Central cloudy dystrophy of François

1. **Inheritance** is AD.
2. **Signs.** Polygonal, cloudy grey opacities separated by relatively clear spaces, in the posterior stroma most

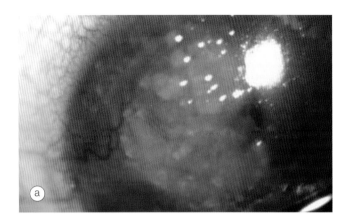

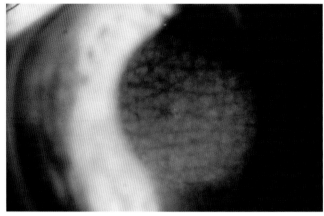

Fig. 9.54
Central cloudy dystrophy of François (Courtesy of W Lisch)

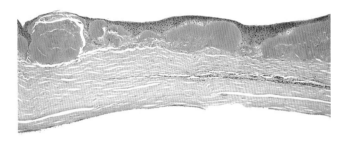

Fig. 9.53
(a) Gelatinous drop-like dystrophy; **(b)** histology shows irregular anterior stromal amyloid deposits (Courtesy of Xin Tian – fig. a; J Harry and G Misson, from *Clinical Ophthalmic Pathology*, Butterworth-Heinemann, 2001 – fig. b)

prominent centrally, creating a leather-like appearance (Fig. 9.54).
3. Treatment is not required.

NB Cloudy dystrophy is similar to crocodile shagreen but is differentiated by its posterior location and AD inheritance.

Endothelial dystrophies

Fuchs endothelial dystrophy

Fuchs endothelial dystrophy is a bilateral disease characterized by accelerated corneal endothelial cell loss. It is more common in women and is associated with a slightly increased prevalence of primary open-angle glaucoma.

1. Inheritance may occasionally be AD although the majority are sporadic.
2. Onset of this slowly progressive disease is in old age.

3. Staging
   a. Stage 1 (cornea guttata).
      – Irregular warts or excrescences of Descemet membrane secreted by abnormal endothelial cells (Fig. 9.55a).
      – Specular reflection shows tiny dark spots caused by disruption of the regular endothelial mosaic (Fig. 9.55b).
      – In more advanced cases, there is a 'beaten metal' appearance which may be associated with melanin deposition (Fig. 9.55c).
   b. Stage 2
      – Endothelial decompensation resulting in central stromal oedema and blurred vision, initially worse in the morning, which clears later in the day.
      – Epithelial oedema develops when stromal thickness has increased by about 30%.
   c. Stage 3 is characterized by persistent epithelial oedema resulting in the formation of microcysts and bullae (bullous keratopathy – Figs 9.55d and e), which causes pain and discomfort on rupture due to exposure of naked nerve endings.
4. Treatment
   a. Topical sodium chloride 5% drops or ointment.
   b. Bandage contact lenses provide comfort by protecting exposed nerve endings and flattening the bullae.
   c. Penetrating keratoplasty has a high success rate and should not be delayed.
   d. Other options in eyes with poor visual potential include conjunctival flaps and amniotic membrane transplants.
5. Cataract surgery may accelerate endothelial cell loss and result in decompensation. Intraoperative soft-shell viscoelastic technique to protect the endothelium should be used in eyes with hard nuclei. A triple procedure (cataract surgery, lens implantation and keratoplasty) should be considered in eyes with corneal epithelial

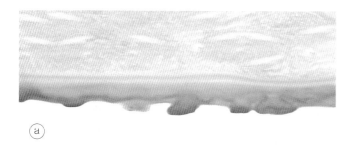

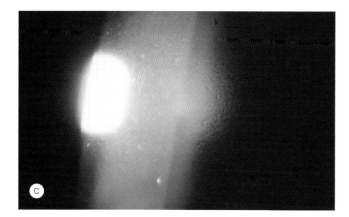

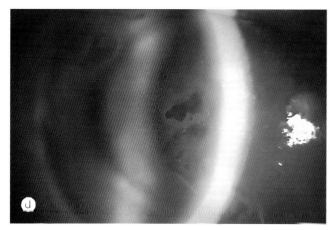

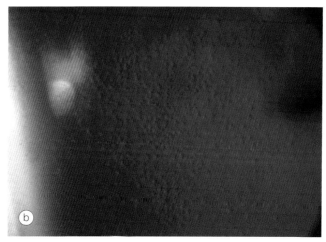

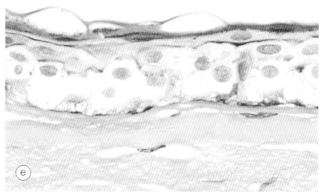

Fig. 9.55
Fuchs endothelial dystrophy. **(a)** Histology of cornea guttata shows irregular excrescences of Descemet membrane – PAS stain; **(b)** cornea guttata seen on specular reflection; **(c)** 'beaten-bronze' endothelium; **(d)** bullous keratopathy; **(e)** histology of bullous keratopathy shows severe epithelial oedema with surface bullae – PAS stain (Courtesy of J Harry – figs a and e)

oedema or when preoperative pachymetry measurement is more than 640μm. If corneal thickness is less than 640μm, a good visual outcome is to be expected.

Posterior polymorphous dystrophy

Posterior polymorphous dystrophy is a rare, innocuous and asymptomatic condition in which corneal endothelial cells display characteristics similar to epithelium.

1. **Inheritance** is usually AD with the gene locus on chromosome 20.
2. **Onset** is at birth or soon thereafter, although it is most frequently identified by chance in later life.
3. **Signs** consist of subtle vesicular endothelial patterns (Fig. 9.56a) that may become confluent (Fig. 9.56b), band-like lesions (Fig. 9.56c) or diffuse opacities (Fig. 9.56d) which may be asymmetrical.
4. **Associations** include iris membranes, peripheral anterior synechiae, ectropion uveae, corectopia, polycoria and glaucoma, reminiscent of iridocorneal endothelial syndrome. It has therefore been speculated that the two clinical pictures may represent points on a spectrum of one disease. There is also an association with Alport syndrome.
5. **Treatment** is not required.

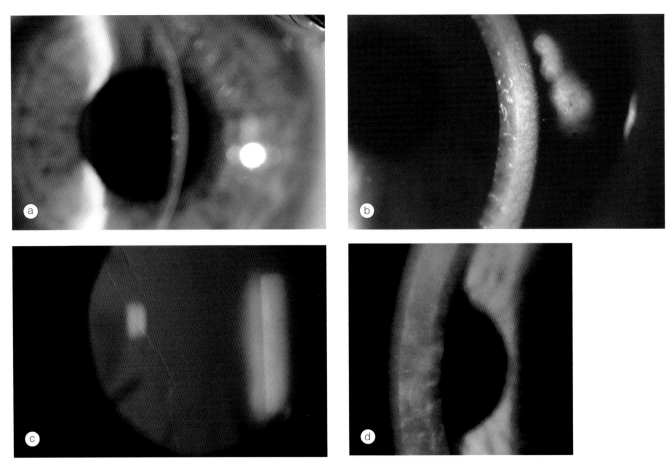

Fig. 9.56
Posterior polymorphous dystrophy. **(a)** Vesicles; **(b)** confluent vesicles; **(c)** band-like lesions; **(d)** diffuse opacities (Courtesy of W Lisch – figs b and c; T Casey and K Sharif, from *Corneal Dystrophies and Degenerations*, Wolfe, 1991 – fig. d)

Congenital hereditary endothelial dystrophy

Congenital hereditary endothelial dystrophy (CHED) is a rare dystrophy in which there is focal or generalized absence of corneal endothelium. There are two main forms CHED1 and CHED2, the latter being more severe.

1. **Inheritance** of CHED1 is AD with the gene locus on 20p11.2-q11.2. CHED2 is AR with the gene locus on 20p13.
2. **Onset** is perinatal.
3. **Signs**
   - Bilateral, symmetrical, diffuse corneal oedema.
   - Corneal appearance varies from a blue-grey, ground-glass appearance (Fig. 9.57a) to total opacification (Fig. 9.57b).

   - Visual impairment is variable; acuity may surpass that expected from corneal appearance.
4. **Treatment** by penetrating keratoplasty has a reasonable chance of success when performed early but is risky and technically more difficult than in adults. Undue delay in surgical intervention carries the risk of dense amblyopia.
5. **Differential diagnosis** includes other causes of neonatal corneal opacification such as congenital glaucoma, mucopolysaccharidoses, birth trauma, rubella keratitis and sclerocornea.

   NB Pedigrees of families with CHED may have individuals who also manifest posterior polymorphous dystrophy, suggesting that the two conditions may be part of the same spectrum.

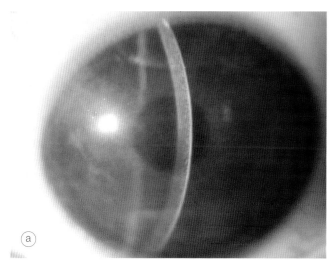

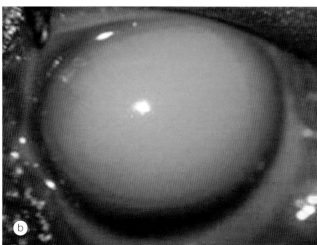

Fig. 9.57
Congenital hereditary endothelial dystrophy. **(a)** Mild; **(b)** very severe (Courtesy of Krachmer, Mannis and Holland, from *Cornea*, Mosby, 2005 – fig. a; K Nischal – fig. b)

CORNEAL DEGENERATIONS

Age-related degenerations

Arcus senilis

1. **Systemic implications.** Arcus senilis is the most common peripheral corneal opacity, which frequently occurs without predisposing systemic conditions in elderly individuals. Occasionally arcus may be associated with familial and non-familial dyslipoproteinaemias. Hyperlipoproteinaemia, most notably type II, is frequently associated with bilateral arcus, with less common association in types III, IV and V. Unilateral arcus is a rare

entity that may be associated with carotid disease or ocular hypotony. Arcus has also been noted in patients with Schnyder crystalline corneal dystrophy.

2. **Signs**
   * Lipid stromal deposition which starts in the superior and inferior perilimbal cornea and then progresses circumferentially to form a band about 1mm wide (Fig. 9.58a).
   * The band is usually wider in the vertical than horizontal meridian.
   * The central border of the band is diffuse; the peripheral edge is sharp and separated from the limbus by a clear zone.
   * This lucid interval may occasionally undergo mild thinning (senile furrow).

Vogt limbal girdle

Vogt limbal girdle is a common, innocuous, age-related finding characterized by bilateral, narrow, crescentic lines composed of chalk-like flecks running in the interpalpebral fissure along the nasal and temporal limbus (Fig. 9.58b). Type 1 is separated from the limbus by a clear interval but type 2 is not.

Cornea farinata

Corneal farinata is an innocuous condition characterized by minute, usually bilateral, flour-like deposits in the deep corneal stroma, most prominent centrally (Fig. 9.58c).

Crocodile shagreen

Crocodile shagreen is characterized by usually asymptomatic, greyish-white, polygonal stromal opacities separated by relatively clear spaces (Fig. 9.58d). The opacities most frequently involve the anterior two-thirds of the stroma.

Lipid keratopathy

1. **Primary** lipid keratopathy is rare and occurs spontaneously. It is characterized by white or yellowish stromal deposits consisting of cholesterol, fats and phospholipids and is not associated with vascularization (Fig. 9.59a).
2. **Secondary** lipid keratopathy is much more common and is associated with previous ocular injury or disease which has resulted in corneal vascularization (Fig. 9.59b). The most common causes are herpes simplex and herpes zoster disciform keratitis.
3. **Treatment** is primarily aimed at medical control of the underlying inflammatory disease. Other treatment options include:
   a. Argon laser photocoagulation to the arterial 'feeder'

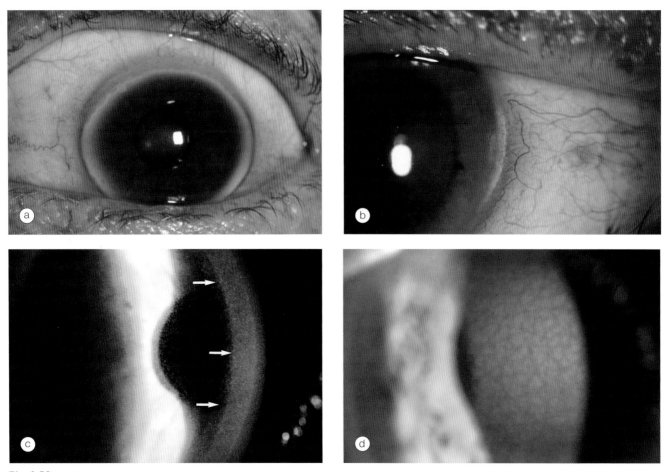

Fig. 9.58
Age-related degenerations. **(a)** Arcus senilis; **(b)** Vogt limbal girdle; **(c)** cornea farinata; **(d)** crocodile shagreen

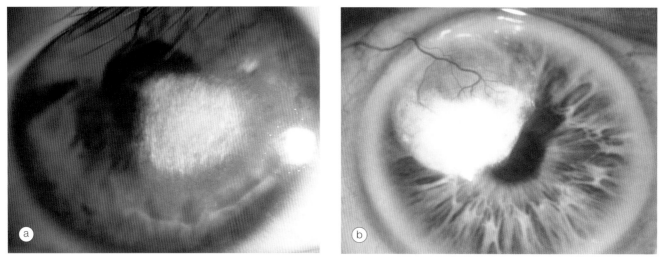

Fig. 9.59
Lipid keratopathy. **(a)** Primary; **(b)** secondary to vascularization (Courtesy of S Tuft – fig. b)

vessels may induce resorption of the lipid infiltrate provided they can be identified by fluorescein angiography.

b. *Needle point cautery* may also be successful. It is performed by grasping a suture needle in thermal cautery forceps and applying the hot tip to the feeder vessels at the limbus under microscopic control.

c. *Penetrating keratoplasty* may be required in advanced but quiescent disease, although vascularization, thinning and hypoaesthesia may prejudice the outcome.

Band keratopathy

Band keratopathy is a common condition characterized by the deposition of calcium salts in Bowman layer, epithelial basement membrane and anterior stroma (Fig. 9.60a).

Causes

1. **Ocular** causes, the most common, include chronic anterior uveitis (particularly in children), phthisis bulbi, silicone oil in the anterior chamber, chronic corneal oedema and severe chronic keratitis.
2. **Age-related** band keratopathy affects otherwise healthy individuals.
3. **Metabolic** causes (metastatic calcification), which are rare, include increased serum calcium and phosphorus, hyperuricaemia and chronic renal failure.
4. **Hereditary** causes include familial cases and ichthyosis.

Signs

- Peripheral interpalpebral calcification with clear cornea separating the sharp peripheral margins of the band from the limbus (Fig. 9.60b).
- Gradual central spread to form a band-like chalky plaque

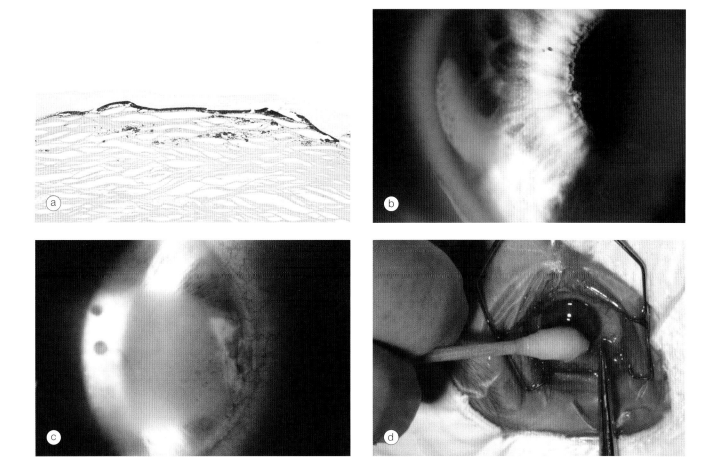

Fig. 9.60
Band keratopathy. **(a)** Histology shows black calcium deposits – von Kossa stain; **(b)** early involvement; **(c)** advanced; **(d)** chelation
(Courtesy of J Harry and G Misson, from *Clinical Ophthalmic Pathology*, Butterworth-Heinemann, 2001 – fig. a)

containing transparent small holes and occasionally clefts (Fig. 9.60c).
- Advanced lesions may become nodular and elevated with considerable discomfort due to epithelial breakdown.

Treatment

Treatment is indicated if vision is threatened or if the eye is uncomfortable.

1. **Chelation** is simple and effective for relatively mild cases and is performed under the operating microscope.
   a. Large chips of calcium can be scraped off the cornea with forceps.
   b. The corneal epithelium overlying the opacity and any solid layer of calcification is scraped off with a No. 15 blade.
   c. The cornea is rubbed with a cotton-tipped bud dipped in a solution of ethylenediaminetetraacetic acid (EDTA) until all calcium has been removed (Fig. 9.60d).
   d. Re-epithelialization takes about 7 days, much longer than the 2–3 days of a similar-sized corneal abrasion in a normal eye.
   e. Recurrence is possible, particularly in patients with an underlying systemic condition or persistent uveitis.
2. **Other modalities** include the use of a diamond burr, Nd:YAG laser, lamellar keratoplasty and phototherapeutic keratectomy.

   NB It important to recognize and treat any underlying conditions to prevent recurrences.

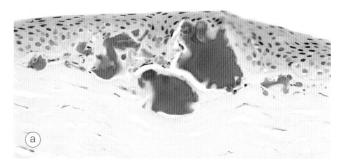

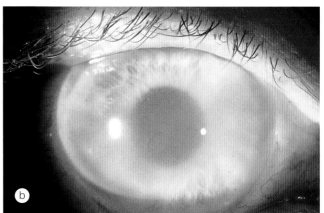

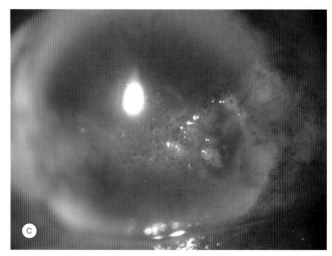

Fig. 9.61
Spheroidal degeneration. **(a)** Histology shows dark red proteinaceous deposits in the anterior stroma that replace Bowman layer; **(b)** early involvement; **(c)** advanced involvement (Courtesy of J Harry and G Misson, from *Clinical Ophthalmic Pathology*, Butterworth-Heinemann, 2001 – fig. a; R Fogla – fig. c)

Spheroidal degeneration

Spheroidal degeneration has many eponyms including corneal elastosis, Labrador keratopathy, climatic droplet keratopathy and Bietti nodular dystrophy. It is a bilateral, degenerative condition of unknown cause which typically occurs in men whose working lives are spent outdoors. The main postulated predisposing factor is ultraviolet exposure, since severity correlates closely with the length of time spent outdoors. The condition is relatively innocuous although visual impairment may occur rarely.

1. **Histology** shows irregular proteinaceous deposits in the anterior stroma that replace Bowman layer (Fig. 9.61a).
2. **Signs**
   - Amber-coloured granules in the superficial stroma of the peripheral interpalpebral cornea.
   - Increasing opacification, coalescence and central spread (Fig. 9.61b).
   - Advanced lesions are nodular and the surrounding stroma often hazy (Fig. 9.61c).
3. **Treatment** options include protection against ultraviolet damage with sunglasses, superficial keratectomy to improve vision and lamellar keratoplasty for visually incapacitating cases.

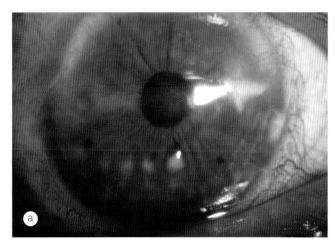

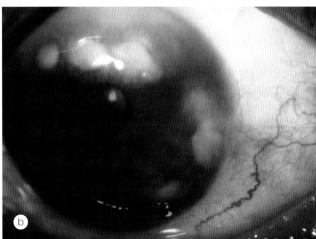

Fig. 9.62
Salzmann nodular degeneration. **(a)** Early; **(b)** advanced

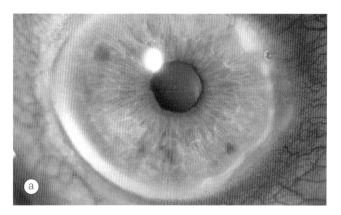

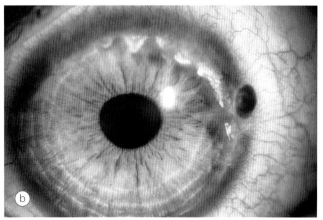

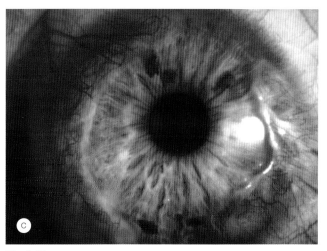

Fig. 9.63
Terrien marginal degeneration. **(a)** Peripheral stromal opacification; **(b)** small corneal perforation at 3 o'clock; **(c)** pseudopterygia (Courtesy of P G Watson, B L Hazelman, C E Pavesio and W R Green, from *The Sclera and Systemic Disorders*, Butterworth-Heinemann, 2004 – fig. b)

Salzmann nodular degeneration

Salzmann nodular degeneration is secondary to chronic keratitis, especially trachoma.

1. Signs
- Discrete, elevated grey or blue-grey, nodular, superficial stromal opacities (Fig. 9.62).
- The lesions are located in scarred cornea or at the edges of transparent cornea.
- The base of a nodule may be surrounded by epithelial iron deposits.
- Recurrent epithelial erosions may occur.
2. Treatment is similar to that of spheroidal degeneration.

Terrien marginal degeneration

Terrien disease is an uncommon, idiopathic, non-inflammatory thinning of the peripheral cornea. About 75%

of affected patients are males and the condition is usually bilateral although involvement may be asymmetrical.

Diagnosis

1. **Presentation** is usually after the fourth decade with initially asymptomatic peripheral corneal lesions.
2. **Signs**
   - Fine, yellow-white, punctate stromal opacities frequently associated with mild superficial vascularization, usually start superiorly, spread circumferentially and are separated from the limbus by a clear zone (Fig. 9.63a).
   - On cursory examination they may resemble arcus senilis. This stage is usually asymptomatic and progression is extremely slow.
   - Progressive circumferential thinning results in a peripheral gutter, the outer slope of which shelves gradually, while the central part rises sharply.
   - Perforation may rarely occur either spontaneously or following blunt trauma (Fig. 9.63b).
   - Gradual visual deterioration occurs as a result of increasing corneal astigmatism.
   - A few patients develop recurrent episodes of disabling pain and inflammation.
   - Pseudopterygia may develop in long-standing cases at positions other than the 9 o'clock and 3 o'clock meridians (Fig. 9.63c).

Treatment

Treatment of significant astigmatism is primarily with gas permeable scleral contact lenses. While surgery involving crescent-shaped excision of the gutter with suturing of the 'healthier' margins is possible, the results are not ideal and contact lenses are usually necessary to achieve best acuity.

METABOLIC KERATOPATHIES

Cystinosis

Cystinosis is a rare AR disorder characterized by widespread tissue deposition of non-protein cystine crystals as a result of a defect in lysosomal transport.

1. **Systemic features** include severe growth retardation, early-onset renal failure, hepatosplenomegaly and hypothyroidism. Patients with the most severe nephropathic form usually succumb before the second decade. Treatment with systemic cysteamine may forestall renal disease.
2. **Keratopathy** is present by 1 year of age and is characterized by progressive deposition of cystine crystals in the conjunctiva and cornea which cause epithelial erosions, intense photophobia, blepharospasm and visual disability by the end of the first decade of life. Peripherally, crystals involve the entire stromal thickness, whereas centrally only the anterior two-thirds are affected (Fig. 9.64a). Later, involvement of the iris, lens capsule and retina may further affect vision.
3. **Treatment** with topical cysteamine 0.2% for several weeks can reverse corneal crystal deposition.

Mucopolysaccharidoses

The mucopolysaccharidoses (MPS) comprise a group of inherited deficiencies of catabolic glycosidase necessary for hydrolysis of mucopolysaccharides. The altered metabolite accumulates in intracellular vacuoles in various tissues and organs, and may also be detected in the urine.

1. **Inheritance** is AR except for the two subtypes of Hunter syndrome which are X-linked recessive.
2. **Systemic features,** which vary with the type of MPS, include facial coarseness, skeletal anomalies, mental retardation and heart disease.
3. **Keratopathy** is characterized by punctate corneal opacification and diffuse stromal haze (Fig. 9.64b). It occurs in all MPS except Hunter and Sanfilippo. In Hurler and Scheie syndromes corneal deposits are most severe and present at birth. Corneal clouding in this setting should be differentiated from that secondary to congenital glaucoma, rubella keratopathy, congenital hereditary endothelial dystrophy and birth trauma.
4. **Other ocular features**
   a. **Pigmentary retinopathy** occurs in all except Morquio and Maroteaux–Lamy.
   b. **Optic atrophy** occurs in all six MPS and is most severe in Hurler.
   c. **Glaucoma** is uncommon.

Wilson disease

Wilson disease (hepatolenticular degeneration) is a rare condition caused by deficiency of caeruloplasmin resulting in widespread deposition of copper in the tissues.

1. **Presentation** is with liver disease, basal ganglia dysfunction or psychiatric disturbances.
2. **Keratopathy** is present in nearly all patients and is very useful in diagnosis. It is characterized by a zone of copper granules in the peripheral part of Descemet membrane (Kayser–Fleischer ring) which change colour under different types of illumination (Fig. 9.64c). The deposits are preferentially distributed in the vertical meridian and may disappear with penicillamine therapy.

NB An early Keiser–Fleischer ring is best detected on gonioscopy.

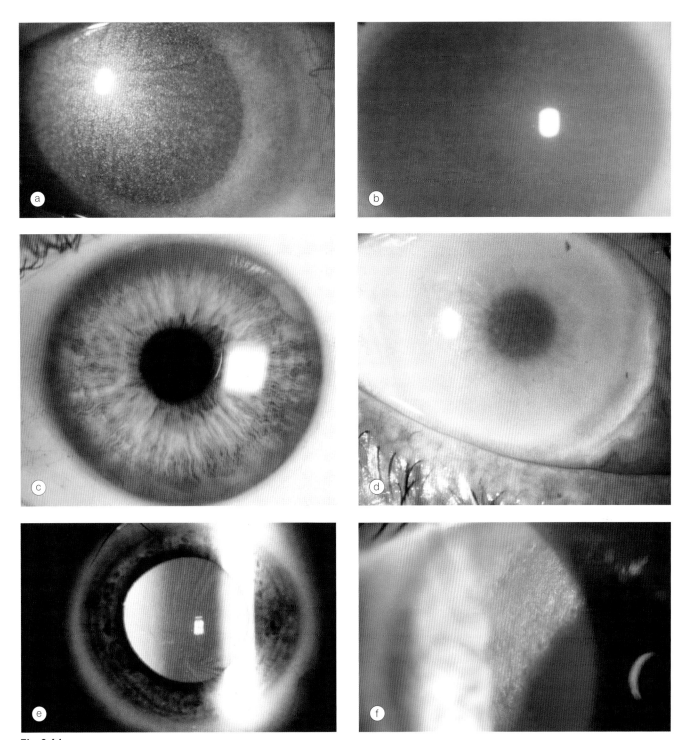

Fig. 9.64
Metabolic keratopathies. **(a)** Cystinosis; **(b)** mucopolysaccharidoses; **(c)** Wilson disease; **(d)** Norum disease; **(e)** Fabry disease; **(f)** immunoprotein deposits (Courtesy of K Nischal – figs a and b; W Lisch – fig. e)

3. Anterior capsular 'sunflower' cataract is seen in some patients.

Lecithin-cholesterol-acyltransferase deficiency (Norum disease)

This is an AR disease characterized by hyperlipidaemia, early atheroma, anaemia and renal disease. Keratopathy is characterized by numerous, minute, greyish dots throughout the stroma, often concentrated in the periphery in an arcus-like configuration (Fig. 9.64d).

Fabry disease (angiokeratoma corporis diffusum)

This is an X-linked lysosomal storage disorder caused by deficiency of alpha-galactosidase A. Systemic features include periodic burning pain in the extremities, purple cutaneous telangiectasis (angiokeratoma corporis diffusum), hypertrophic cardiomyopathy and renal disease. Keratopathy is characterized by faint but extensive vortex changes similar to those induced by chloroquine (Fig. 9.64e). Other ocular manifestations include wedge-shaped cataract, conjunctival vascular tortuosity, retinal vascular tortuosity (especially venous), third nerve palsy and nystagmus.

Tyrosinaemia type 2 (Richner–Hanhart syndrome)

This is a rare AR disease in which there is deficiency of hepatic cytosolic tyrosine aminotransferase with resultant increase in plasma tyrosine levels. Ocular involvement may occasionally be the presenting feature.

1. **Systemic features** include painful, palmar and plantar hyperkeratotic lesions, and variable central nervous system involvement which may cause mental retardation, nystagmus, tremor, ataxia and convulsion.
2. **Ocular signs.** Recalcitrant pseudodendritic keratitis with crystalline edges. In contrast with true herpetic ulcers the lesions are usually bilateral and inferotemporal, corneal sensation is normal, there is a lack of response to antiviral therapy, typical terminal bulbs are absent and staining with fluorescein is poor.

Immunoprotein deposits

Diffuse or focal immunoprotein deposition is a relatively uncommon manifestation of several systemic diseases, including multiple myeloma, Waldenström macroglobulinaemia, monoclonal gammopathy of unknown cause, certain lymphoproliferative disorders and leukaemia. Corneal involvement may be the earliest manifestation of the disease.

1. **Signs.** Gradual bilateral development of a band of multiple, punctate, flake-like opacities mostly at the level of the posterior stroma (Fig. 9.64f).
2. **Treatment** should address the underlying systemic disease with cytotoxic chemotherapy or steroids. Severe corneal involvement may require penetrating keratoplasty.

CONTACT LENSES

Therapeutic uses

The risks of fitting a contact lens to an already compromised eye are greater than with lens wear for cosmetic reasons. The balance between benefit and risk should therefore be carefully considered. Close monitoring is vital to ensure early diagnosis and treatment of complications. The choice of lens type is dictated by the nature of ocular pathology.

Optical

Optical indications are aimed at improving visual acuity when this cannot be achieved by spectacles in the following conditions:

1. **Irregular astigmatism** associated with keratoconus can be corrected with rigid contact lenses long after spectacles have failed and long before corneal grafting becomes necessary. Patients with astigmatism following corneal grafting may also benefit.
2. **Superficial corneal irregularities** can be neutralized by rigid contact lenses by providing a smoother and optically more regular surface. Visual acuity can thus be improved, provided the irregularities are not too severe.
3. **Anisometropia** in which binocular vision cannot be achieved by spectacles, due to aniseikonia and prismatic effects, as may occur following cataract surgery.

Promotion of epithelial healing

1. **Persistent epithelial defects** often heal if the regenerating corneal epithelium is protected from constant rubbing action of the lids. This allows the development of attachments of hemidesmosomes to the basement membrane.
2. **Recurrent corneal erosions,** if associated with basement membrane dystrophy, may require long-term contact lens wear. In post-traumatic cases, lens wear can usually be discontinued after a few weeks.

Pain relief

1. **Bullous keratopathy** can be managed with soft bandage lenses which relieve pain by protecting the exposed corneal nerve endings from the shearing forces of the

lids during blinking. The lens may also flatten bullae into diffuse fine epithelial oedema. Installation of hypertonic 5% saline may further osmotically reduce oedema and improve vision. As the bullae gradually subside and scarring supervenes the patient can be weaned off lens wear.

2. **Wet filamentary keratitis** associated with profuse lacrimation, as seen in patients with brain stem strokes and essential blepharospasm, can be treated with soft contact lenses and preservative-free acetylcysteine.
3. **Other indications** include Thygeson superficial punctate keratitis and protection of the corneal epithelium from aberrant lashes.

Preservation of corneal integrity

1. **A descemetocele** can be temporarily capped with a tight-fitting, large-diameter soft or scleral lens to prevent perforation and allow natural healing to occur.
2. **Splinting** and apposition of the edges of a small corneal wound can be achieved by a contact lens which supports the cornea during healing. Examples include trauma, graft dehiscence and leaking trabeculectomy. Slightly larger perforations may be sealed with glue followed by insertion of a bandage contact lens to protect the glue and prevent irritation of the lids from the glue's rough surface.

Miscellaneous indications

1. **Ptosis props** to support the upper lids in patients with ocular myopathies.
2. **Maintenance of the fornices** to prevent symblepharon formation in eyes with cicatrizing conjunctivitis.
3. **Drug delivery** can be enhanced by a hydrogel lens impregnated with topical medication which increases exposure to the drug.

Complications

Most of the oxygen for corneal metabolism is supplied from the atmosphere and diffuses from the tear film. The endothelium is supplied from the aqueous. A contact lens lies within the tear film and is a barrier to the diffusion of oxygen to the cornea. Lens movement and circulation of oxygenated tears behind the lens is an important mechanism of providing oxygen to the cornea. The presence of a contact lens may modify the normal circulation of tears, cause mechanical and hypoxic damage to the tissues, and bind proteins and debris that are then kept in contact with the ocular surface. Contact lens care products can be associated with both acute and chronic keratopathy. Extended wear contact lenses, poor lens hygiene and inappropriate lens fit are particular risk factors for complications. After long-term contact lens wear the epithelium becomes thinner and less sensitive to touch. The wearing of contact lenses may also exacerbate pre-existing disease. Contact lens associated giant papillary conjunctivitis is described in Chapter 8.

Mechanical and hypoxic keratitis

The oxygen transmission through the lens (Dk/t value) may be insufficient. A tightly fitting contact lens, which does not move with blinking, will impair tear circulation under the lens. This is exacerbated by lid closure if the lens is worn during sleep. Hypoxia leads to anaerobic metabolism and lactic acidosis that inhibits the normal barrier and pump mechanisms of the cornea. The cornea may be abraded by the contact lens or by a foreign body trapped by the lens.

1. **Superficial punctate keratitis** is the most common complication. The pattern may give a clue as to the aetiology. For example, staining at 3 and 9 o'clock is associated with incomplete blinking and drying in rigid lens wearers.
2. **The tight lens syndrome** is characterized by indentation and staining of the conjunctival epithelium in a ring around the cornea.
3. **Acute hypoxia** is characterized by epithelial microcysts (Fig. 9.65a), necrosis and endothelial blebs. Very painful macroerosions may develop only several hours after lenses are removed following a period of overwear.
4. **Chronic hypoxia** may result in vascularization and lipid deposition (Fig. 9.65b).
5. **Treatment** depends on the cause and may involve the following:
   - Increasing oxygen permeability by refitting with a thinner lens or one with a higher DK/t value such as a gas permeable rigid lens or silicone hydrogel soft lens.
   - Modifying lens fit to increase movement
   - Reducing lens wearing time.

NB Superficial peripheral neovascularization of < 1.5mm is common in myopic contact lens wearers and can be monitored.

Immune response keratitis

Contact lens-related acute red eye (CLARE) may be associated with marginal corneal infiltrates which are thought to be the result of sensitization to bacterial toxins. The mechanism is similar to the development of marginal infiltrates associated with blepharitis.

1. **Signs.** Red eye associated with marginal infiltrates with no or minimal epithelial defects (Fig. 9.65c).
2. **Management.** Contact lens wear should be stopped until resolution occurs. Topical antibiotics and steroids may be used in severe cases but if the diagnosis is uncertain treatment should be that of bacterial keratitis. It is also important to review lens fit and hygiene.

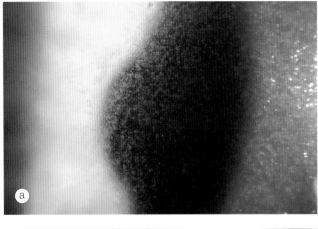

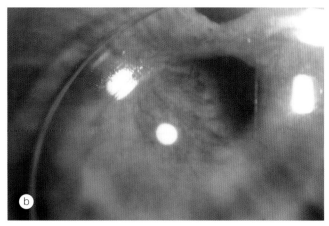

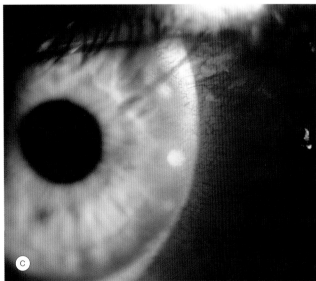

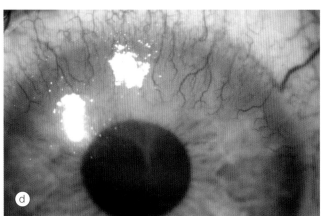

Fig. 9.65
Complications of contact lens wear. **(a)** Epithelial microcysts from acute hypoxia; **(b)** lipid deposition from chronic hypoxia; **(c)** marginal infiltrates in immune response keratitis; **(d)** vascularization and scarring in chronic toxic keratitis
(Courtesy of S Tuft – figs a and b; J Dart – fig. d)

Toxic keratitis

Acute chemical injury may be caused by placing a contact lens on the eye without neutralizing hydrogen peroxide or surfactant cleaners. Chronic toxicity can result from long-term exposure to disinfecting agents such as thiomersal or benzalkonium chloride. The mechanism of thiomersal keratopathy may have been partly an induced hyper-sensitivity response resulting in apparent corneal epithelial stem cell failure.

1. **Signs**
   • Acute pain, redness, and chemosis on lens insertion which may take 48 hours to resolve completely.
   • Vascularization and scarring of the cornea and limbal conjunctiva in chronic cases (Fig. 9.65d).
2. **Management.** Daily disposable contact lenses should be fitted and a non-preserved disinfectant used such as hydrogen peroxide or heat.

NB In some patients with persistent problems associated with contact lens wear refractive corneal surgery is an alternative for visual correction.

Suppurative keratitis

Contact lens wear is the greatest risk factor for the development of bacterial keratitis. The risk is least for rigid contact lenses. Bacteria in the tear film are normally unable to bind to the corneal epithelium. Following an abrasion and hypoxia bacteria can attach and penetrate the epithelium with the potential to cause infection. Bacteria and amoebae may also be introduced onto the corneal surface by poor lens hygiene or the use of tap water. *P. aeruginosa* and *Acanthamoeba* spp. are significantly more associated with soft contact lens wear.

CORNEAL AND REFRACTIVE SURGERY

KERATOPLASTY

Keratoplasty (corneal transplantation, grafting) is an operation in which abnormal corneal host tissue is replaced by healthy donor cornea. A corneal graft may be (a) *full-thickness* (penetrating) or (b) *partial-thickness* (lamellar or deep lamellar).

Penetrating keratoplasty

Indications

1. **Optical** keratoplasty is performed to improve vision. Important indications include bullous keratopathy, keratoconus, dystrophies, degenerations and scarring.
2. **Tectonic** grafting may be carried out to restore or preserve corneal integrity in eyes with severe structural changes such as stromal thinning and descemetoceles.
3. **Therapeutic** corneal transplantation may afford removal of infected corneal tissue in eyes unresponsive to antimicrobial therapy.
4. **Cosmetic** grafting may rarely be performed to improve the appearance of the eye.

Donor tissue
Donor tissue should be removed within 24 hours of death. Corneas from infants are usually not used, being floppy and likely to result in high astigmatism. Corneas from donors over the age of 70 years may also be inappropriate due to low endothelial cell counts. Preoperative evaluation of donor tissue includes slit-lamp examination and specular microscopy. Donor corneas should not be utilized under the following circumstances.

- Death of unknown cause.
- Infectious diseases of the CNS (e.g. Creutzfeld–Jakob disease, systemic sclerosing panencephalitis, progressive multifocal leucoencephalopathy).
- Certain systemic infections (e.g. AIDS, viral hepatitis, syphilis, septicaemia).
- Leukaemia and lymphoma.
- Intrinsic eye disease (e.g. malignancy, active inflammation) or previous intraocular surgery.

Prognostic factors

The following factors may adversely affect the prognosis of a corneal graft and should therefore be addressed prior to surgery.

- Abnormalities of the eyelids such as blepharitis, ectropion, entropion and trichiasis should be corrected before surgery.
- Tear film dysfunction.
- Recurrent or progressive forms of conjunctival inflammation, such as atopic conjunctivitis and ocular cicatricial pemphigoid.

- Severe stromal vascularization, absence of corneal sensation, extreme thinning at the proposed host–graft junction and active corneal inflammation.
- Anterior synechiae.
- Uncontrolled glaucoma.
- Uveitis.

NB In general, the most favourable cases are localized scars, keratoconus and dystrophies.

Technique

1. **Determination of graft size** is done preoperatively with a variable slit beam and operatively, by trial placement of trephines with different diameters or measurement with a caliper. Grafts of diameter 8.5mm or more are prone to postoperative anterior synechiae formation, vascularization and increased intraocular pressure. An ideal size is 7.5mm; grafts smaller than this may give rise to high astigmatism.
2. **Excision of donor cornea** should always precede that of the host. Donor tissue is prepared by trephining a previously excised corneoscleral button, endothelial side up in a concave Teflon block. Alternatively, the donor may be trephined from the intact donor globe having first injected air or viscoelastic substance into the anterior chamber. The donor button is usually about 0.25mm larger in diameter than the planned diameter of the host opening, to facilitate watertight closure, minimize postoperative flattening and reduce the possibility of postoperative glaucoma.
3. **Excision of diseased host tissue** is then carried out taking care not to damage the iris and lens.
   a. Sutures are placed through the insertions of the superior and inferior rectus muscles.
   b. Partial-thickness trephination is performed (Fig. 10.1a).

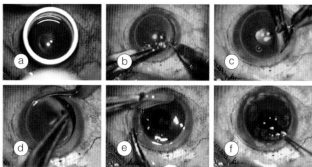

Fig. 10.1
Penetrating keratoplasty – excision of host tissue. **(a)** Partial-thickness trephination; **(b)** anterior chamber is entered with a knife; **(c)**, **(d)** and **(e)** excision is completed with scissors; **(f)** injection of viscoelastic (Courtesy of R Fogla)

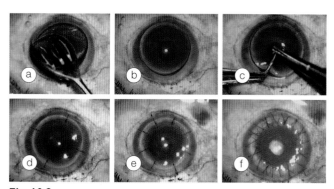

Fig. 10.2
Penetrating keratoplasty – fixation of donor button. **(a)** and **(b)** Donor button is placed onto the cornea; **(c)** initial cardinal suture is placed at 12 o'clock; **(d)** four interrupted cardinal sutures in place; **(e)** additional radial sutures; **(f)** continuous running suture (Courtesy of R Fogla)

   c. The anterior chamber is entered with a knife (Fig. 10.1b).
   d. Excision is completed with scissors (Fig. 10.1c, d and e).
   e. Viscoelastic is injected (Fig. 10.1f).
4. **Fixation of donor button** is usually with 10-0 monofilament nylon.
   a. The donor button is placed onto the cornea (Fig. 10.2a and b).
   b. Four interrupted radial 'cardinal' sutures are placed; the first at 12 o'clock (Fig. 10.2c), the second at 6 o'clock, the third at 3 o'clock and the last at 9 o'clock (Fig. 10.2d). The corneal 'bite' should be almost full-thickness to prevent wound gape.
   c. Further interrupted sutures are inserted (Fig. 10.2e).
   d. Closure is completed with a continuous running suture (Fig. 10.2f).
5. **Replacement of viscoelastic substance** with balanced salt solution.

Postoperative management

1. **Topical steroids** are used to reduce immunological graft rejection. After initial administration 2-hourly and then q.i.d. for a few weeks, the dose may be further tapered, depending on the condition of the eye. Steroids are usually continued at low doses such as once daily for a year or more.
2. **Mydriatics** b.d. for 2 weeks, or longer if uveitis persists.
3. **Oral aciclovir** may be used in the context of pre-existing herpes simplex keratitis to minimize the risk of recurrence.
4. **Removal of sutures** when the graft–host junction has healed is usually after 12–18 months, although in elderly patients it may take much longer.
5. **Rigid contact lenses** may be required to optimize visual acuity in eyes with astigmatism.

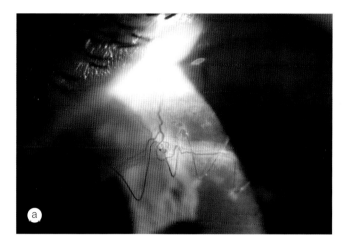

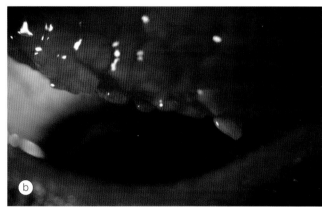

Fig. 10.3
(a) Protruding suture; **(b)** giant papillary conjunctivitis

Postoperative complications

1. **Early** complications include persistent epithelial defects, irritation by protruding sutures (Fig. 10.3a) which may give rise to papillary hypertrophy (Fig. 10.3b), wound leak, flat anterior chamber, iris prolapse, uveitis, elevation of intraocular pressure and infection. A rare complication is a fixed dilated pupil (Urrets–Zavalia syndrome).
2. **Late** complications include astigmatism, recurrence of initial disease process on the graft, late wound separation, retrocorneal membrane formation, glaucoma and cystoid macular oedema.

Corneal allograft rejection

Allograft rejection of any layer of the cornea can occur following penetrating keratoplasty and, less commonly, lamellar grafts. Endothelial rejection is the most common and most severe as it can lead to severe endothelial cell loss and

decompensation. Late graft failure through decompensation can also occur in the absence of further rejection episodes. Stromal rejection and epithelial rejection are less frequent and respond readily to topical steroid treatment with few long-term consequences. Elements of the different types of rejection can coexist.

1. **Pathogenesis.** The cornea is immunologically privileged and a normal cornea will usually not reject. However, if there is inflammation this privilege is lost and rejection may occur. Other important predisposition for rejection includes corneal vascularization, grafts over 8mm in diameter, eccentric grafts, infection, glaucoma and previous keratoplasty. If the host becomes sensitized to the major or minor histocompatibility antigens present in the donor, cornea type IV hypersensitivity can develop against the graft and rejection and graft failure may result. Antigen presenting cells in the donor cornea may initiate this process. HLA Class I matching has a small beneficial effect on graft survival.
2. **Symptoms** of graft rejection include blurred vision, photophobia and a dull periocular ache. However, many cases are asymptomatic until advanced rejection is established.
3. **Signs**
   - Ciliary injection and anterior uveitis is a pre-rejection manifestation (Fig. 10.4a).
   - Epithelial rejection may be accompanied by an elevated line of abnormal epithelium (Fig. 10.4b).
   - Stromal rejection is characterized by subepithelial infiltrates, reminiscent of adenoviral infection (Krachmer spots) on the donor cornea (Fig. 10.4c).
   - Endothelial rejection is characterized by linear pattern of keratic precipitates (Khodadoust endothelial rejection line) associated with an area of inflammation at the graft margin (Fig. 10.4d).
   - Stromal oedema is indicative of endothelial failure.
4. **Management.** Early treatment is essential as this greatly improves the chances of reversing the rejection episode.
   a. ***Topical steroids*** (dexamethasone phosphate 0.1% or prednisolone acetate 1%) hourly for 24 hours are the mainstay of therapy. The frequency is reduced gradually over several weeks but high risk patients should be maintained on the highest tolerated topical dose (e.g. prednisolone acetate 1% q.i.d).
   b. ***Systemic steroids*** (oral prednisolone 1mg/kg/day in divided doses, or a single intravenous dose of methylprednisolone 500mg) may help to reverse rejection and prevent further rejection episodes but only if given within 8 days of onset of rejection. Repeated intravenous methylprednisolone may be associated with loss of bone density and osteoporosis.
   c. ***Subconjunctival steroids*** (betamethasone 2mg) may be useful.
5. **Differential diagnosis** includes graft failure, reactivation of HSV, uveitis and epithelial down-growth.

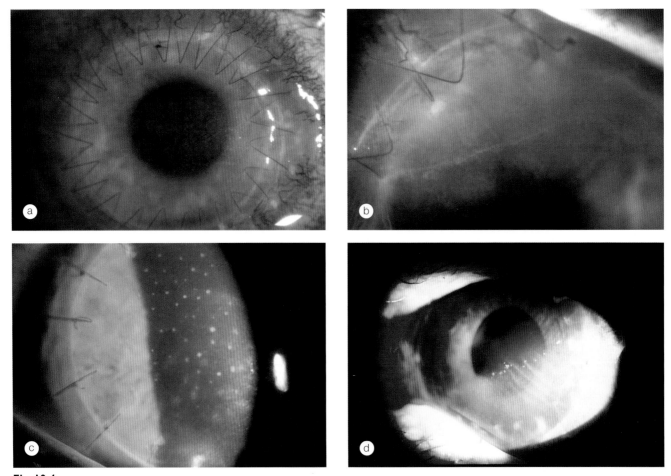

Fig. 10.4
Allograft rejection. **(a)** Ciliary injection in pre-rejection; **(b)** elevated epithelial line in epithelial rejection; **(c)** Krachmer spots in stromal rejection; **(d)** Khodadoust line in endothelial rejection (Courtesy of S Tuft – figs a, b and c; D Easty – fig. d)

Lamellar keratoplasty

Lamellar keratoplasty involves partial thickness excision of the corneal epithelium and stroma so that the endothelium and part of deep stroma are left behind.

1. Indications
- Opacification of the superficial one-third of the corneal stroma not caused by potentially recurrent disease.
- Marginal corneal thinning or infiltration as in recurrent pterygium, Terrien marginal degeneration and limbal dermoids or other tumours.
- Localized thinning or descemetocele formation.

2. Technique is similar to penetrating keratoplasty except that only a partial thickness of cornea is grafted.

Deep lamellar keratoplasty

Deep lamellar keratoplasty is a relatively new technique in which all opaque corneal tissue is removed almost to the level of Descemet membrane. The theoretical advantage is the decreased risk of rejection because the endothelium, a major target for rejection, is not transplanted.

1. Indications
- Disease involving the anterior 95% of corneal thickness with a normal endothelium and absence of breaks or scars in Descemet membrane.
- Chronic inflammatory disease such as atopic kerato-conjunctivitis which carries an increased risk of graft rejection.

2. Advantages

- No risk of endothelial rejection although epithelial rejection may occur.
- Less astigmatism and a structurally stronger globe as compared with penetrating keratoplasty.
- Increased availability of graft material since endothelial quality is irrelevant.

3. Disadvantages

- Difficult and time-consuming with a high risk of perforation in older patients.
- Interface haze may limit best final visual acuity.

NB The major difficulty lies in judging the depth of the corneal dissection as close as possible to Descemet membrane without perforating.

5. Postoperative management is similar to penetrating keratoplasty except that topical steroids are used less frequently and sutures can usually be removed after 6 months.

KERATOPROSTHESES

Keratoprostheses are artificial corneal implants (Fig. 10.5a) used in patients unsuitable for keratoplasty. The modern osteo-odonto-keratoprosthesis consists of the patient's own tooth root and alveolar bone which supports the central optical cylinder. This is usually covered with a buccal mucous membrane graft. Surgery is difficult and time consuming and is performed in two stages 2–4 months apart.

1. Indications

- Patients with bilateral blindness with visual acuity of hand movements or less but normal optic nerve and retinal function (i.e. accurate light projection, good pupillary responses if obtainable, normal electrophysiological tests and absence of retinal detachment on ultrasonography).
- Severe, debilitating but inactive anterior segment disease with no realistic chance of success from conventional keratoplasty (e.g. Stevens–Johnson syndrome, ocular cicatricial pemphigoid, chemical burns or trachoma).
- Multiple previous failed corneal grafts or other types of ocular surface reconstruction such as amniotic membrane or stem cell grafting.
- Normal intraocular pressure with or without medication.
- Absence of active ocular surface inflammation.
- Good patient motivation.

2. Complications include glaucoma, retroprosthesis membrane formation, tilting or extrusion of the cylinder (Fig. 10.5b), retinal detachment and endophthalmitis.

3. Results. Approximately 80% of patients experience visual improvement which varies from CF to 6/12 or even

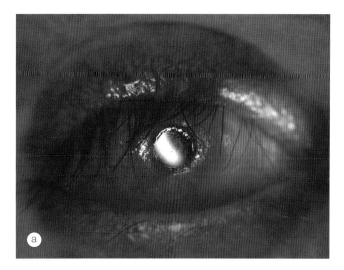

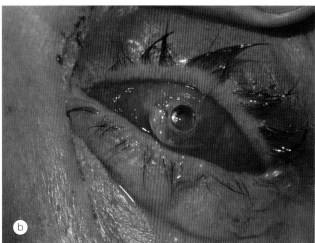

Fig. 10.5
(a) Keratoprosthesis; **(b)** extrusion (Courtesy of C Liu and G Facinelli – fig. a)

better. Poor visual outcome is often associated with pre-existing optic nerve or retinal dysfunction.

REFRACTIVE SURGERY

Introduction

Refractive surgery encompasses a range of procedures aimed at changing the refraction of the eye by altering the cornea and/or crystalline lens, which constitute the principal refracting components. Refractive errors corrected by such procedures include myopia, hypermetropia and astigmatism. The surgical correction of presbyopia by laser is still in its infancy. Lens extraction and the insertion of a multifocal/bifocal or accommodating implant can optically restore reading vision.

NB To settle any contact lens-induced corneal distortion, soft contact lenses should be discontinued 2 weeks before keratometry, and hard lenses for one week for each year of wear.

Correction of myopia

1. **Photorefractive keratectomy** (PRK – see below)
2. **Laser epithelial keratomileusis** (LASEK – see below).
3. **Laser in-situ keratomileusis** (LASIK – see below).
4. **Clear lens extraction** gives very good visual results but carries a small risk of retinal detachment.
5. **Iris clip (lobster claw)** implant is attached to the iris (Fig. 10.6a). Complications include subluxation and an oval pupil.
6. **Phakic posterior chamber implant** (implantable contact lens) is inserted behind the iris (Fig. 10.6b), in front of the crystalline lens and supported in the ciliary sulcus. The lens is composed of material derived from collagen with a power of −3D to −20.50D. Short term visual results are promising; however, this procedure should be used with caution because it may be associated with uveitis, glaucoma, endothelial cell loss and cataract formation.

Correction of hypermetropia

1. **PRK and LASEK** can correct low degrees of hypermetropia.
2. **LASIK** can correct up to 4D.
3. **Conductive keratoplasty** with a radiofrequency probe can correct low hypermetropia. Burns are placed in one or two rings in the corneal periphery. The resultant thermally induced stromal shrinkage is accompanied by increase in central corneal curvature. This change decays over time but the procedure can be repeated.
4. **Laser thermal keratoplasty** with a holmium laser can correct low hypermetropia. Laser burns are placed in one or two rings in the corneal periphery (Fig. 10.7a). The resultant thermally induced stromal shrinkage is accompanied by increase in central corneal curvature. This change decays over time but the procedure can be repeated.

Correction of astigmatism

1. **Limbal relaxing incisions/arcuate keratotomy** involves making paired arcuate incisions on opposite sides of the cornea in the axis of the correcting 'plus' cylinder (the steep meridian). The resultant flattening of the steep meridian coupled with a smaller steepening of the flat

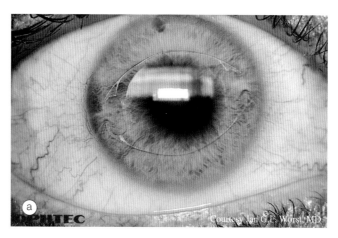

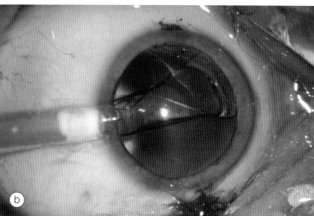

Fig. 10.6
Phakic intraocular implants for correction of myopia. **(a)** Anterior chamber 'lobster claw' implant; **(b)** posterior chamber implant is injected between the iris and anterior lens capsule (Courtesy of Krachmer, Mannis and Holland from *Cornea*, Mosby, 2005)

meridian at 90° to the incisions reduces astigmatism. The desired result can be controlled by varying the length and depth of the incisions and their distance from the optical centre of the cornea. Arcuate keratotomy may be combined with compression sutures placed in the perpendicular meridian, when treating large degrees of astigmatism such as may occur following penetrating keratoplasty.
2. **PRK and LASEK** can correct up to 3D.
3. **LASIK** can correct up to 5D.
4. **Lens surgery** involves using a toric intraocular implant at the time of cataract extraction. However, postoperative rotation of the implant away from the desired axis may occur.

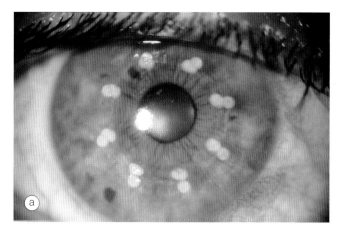

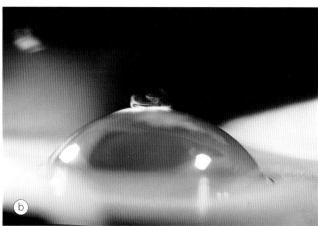

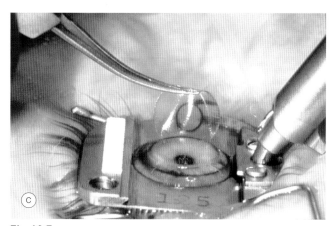

Fig. 10.7
Refractive laser procedures. **(a)** Thermal keratoplasty;
(b) photorefractive keratectomy; **(c)** laser *in-situ* keratomileusis
(Courtesy of H Nano Jr – fig. a; C Barry – fig. b; Eye Academy – fig. c)

Laser refractive procedures

Photorefractive keratectomy

Photorefractive keratectomy (PRK) is performed with the
excimer laser which can accurately ablate corneal tissue to

an exact depth with minimal disruption of surrounding
tissue. Myopia is treated by ablating the central anterior
corneal surface so that it becomes flatter; approximately
10μm of ablation corrects 1D of myopia. Hypermetropia is
treated by ablation of the periphery so that the centre
becomes steeper. PRK is able to correct myopia up to 6D,
astigmatism up to 3D and low hypermetropia.

1. **Technique**
   a. The visual axis is marked and the corneal epithelium
      removed
   b. The patient fixates on the aiming beam of the laser.
   c. The laser is applied to ablate only Bowman layer and
      anterior stroma (Fig. 10.7b). This usually takes 30–60
      seconds.

   The cornea usually heals within 48–72 hours aided by a
   bandage contact lens. A subepithelial haze invariably
   develops within 2 weeks and persists for 1–6 months. It rarely
   causes diminished visual acuity but may produce night glare.

2. **Complications** include slow-healing epithelial defects,
   corneal haze and haloes, poor night vision and regression
   of refractive correction. Uncommon problems include
   decentred ablations, scarring, abnormal epithelial healing,
   irregular astigmatism, hypoaesthesia, sterile infiltrates,
   infection and acute corneal necrosis.

Laser epithelial keratomileusis

Although LASEK is a relatively new procedure, its popularity
is on the increase. It is associated with less pain, less haze and
quicker visual recovery than PRK. LASEK works well with
low corrections and for patients who are unsuitable for
LASIK such as those with very thin corneas. The techniques
are as follows:

a. Alcohol 20% is applied for 30–40 seconds and an
   epithelial sheet is cleaved at the basement membrane.
b. Laser is applied.
c. The epithelial flap is re-positioned.

Functional vision is usually achieved within 4–7 days and
the procedure has a low risk of serious complications. The
main disadvantages compared with LASIK are the unpre-
dictability of postoperative pain and epithelial healing.

Laser in-situ keratomileusis

LASIK is currently the most frequently performed refractive
procedure. It is more versatile than PRK and can correct
hypermetropia of up to 4D, astigmatism of up to 5D and
myopia of up to 12D depending on corneal thickness. To
prevent corneal ectasia, a residual corneal base of 250μm
thickness must remain after the flap has been cut and tissue
ablated. The amount of tissue removed and the total
treatment is therefore limited by the original corneal
thickness (on pachymetry). The thickness of the flap can be
varied but thinner flaps are more difficult to handle and are
more prone to wrinkling.

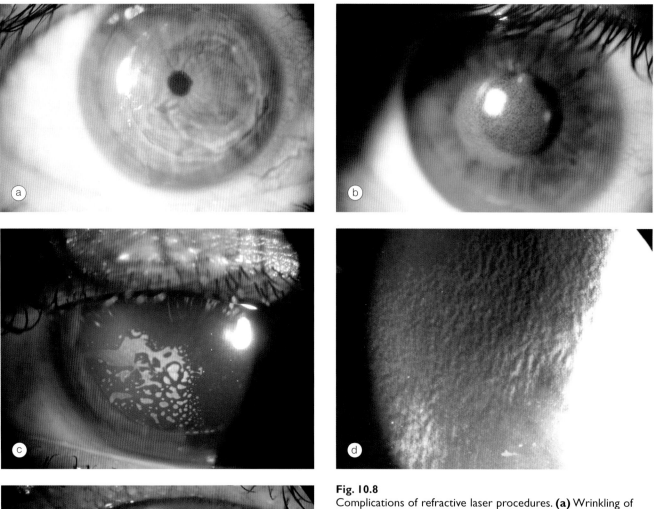

Fig. 10.8
Complications of refractive laser procedures. **(a)** Wrinkling of the flap; **(b)** subepithelial haze; **(c)** epithelial ingrowth; **(d)** diffuse lamellar keratitis; **(e)** bacterial keratitis (Courtesy of H Nano Jr – figs a and b; S Fogla – fig. c; S Tuft – figs d and e)

1. Technique

a. A suction ring is applied to the globe which raises the intraocular pressure to over 65mmHg. This may temporarily occlude the central retinal artery and extinguish vision.

b. The ring is centred on the cornea and provides a guide track into which an automated microkeratome is inserted.

c. The keratome is mechanically advanced across the cornea to create a very thin flap, which is reflected (Fig. 10.7c).

d. Suction is released and the bed is treated with the excimer laser as for PRK.

e. The flap is repositioned and allowed to settle undisturbed for 30 seconds.

Compared with LASEK, the procedure offers the advantages of minimal discomfort, faster visual rehabilitation, rapid stabilization of refraction and minimal stromal haze.

2. Complications

a. Operative complications include buttonholes, thin flaps, flap amputation, incomplete or irregular flaps, and rarely corneal perforation.

b. Postoperative

- Dry eyes are almost universal and may require treatment.

- Wrinkling (Fig. 10.8a), distortion or dislocation of the flap.
- Subepithelial haze that may cause glare at night (Fig. 10.8b).
- Epithelial defects that may predispose to epithelial ingrowth under the flap (Fig. 10.8c).
- Diffuse lamellar keratitis (sands of Sahara) may develop 1–7 days following LASIK. It is characterized by granular deposits at the flap interface (Fig. 10.8d). Treatment is with intensive topical antibiotics and steroids.
- Bacterial keratitis is rare (Fig. 10.8e).

EPISCLERA AND SCLERA

ANATOMY

The scleral stroma is composed of collagen bundles of varying size and shape that are not as uniformly orientated as in the cornea. The inner layer of the sclera (lamina fusca) blends with the suprachoroidal and supraciliary lamellae of the uveal tract. Anteriorly the episclera consists of a dense, vascular connective tissue which lies between the superficial scleral stroma and Tenon capsule. The three vascular layers that cover the anterior sclera are as follows:

1. **The conjunctival vessels** are the most superficial; arteries are tortuous and veins straight.
2. **The superficial episcleral plexus** vessels are straight with a radial configuration.
   - In episcleritis, maximal congestion occurs within this vascular plexus (Fig. 11.1a). Tenon capsule and the episclera are infiltrated with inflammatory cells, but the sclera itself is not swollen.
   - Instillation of topical phenylephrine will cause blanching of the conjunctival and to a certain extent

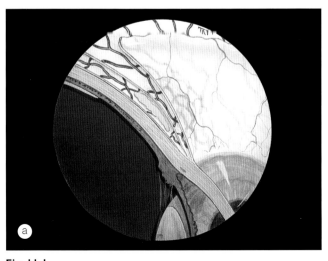
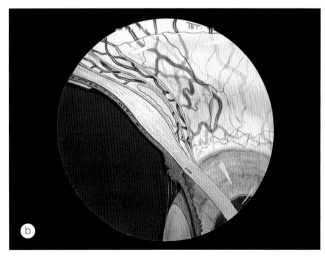

Fig. 11.1
(a) Episcleritis showing maximal vascular congestion of the superficial episcleral plexus; **(b)** scleritis showing scleral thickening and maximal vascular congestion of the deep vascular plexus

the superficial episcleral vessels, allowing visualization of the underlying sclera.

3. **The deep vascular plexus** lies in the superficial part of the sclera and shows maximal congestion in scleritis (Fig. 11.1b). There is also inevitably some engorgement of the superficial vessels, but this should be ignored. Examination in daylight is important to localize the level of maximal injection.

EPISCLERITIS

Simple episcleritis

Simple episcleritis accounts for three-quarters of all cases and predominantly affects females. It has a great tendency to recur either in the same eye, or sometimes both together. The attacks become less frequent and after many years disappear completely.

Diagnosis

1. **Presentation** is almost always sudden, the eye becoming red and uncomfortable within an hour of the start of an attack. The most common sensations described are hotness, pricking or generalized discomfort. Pain is unusual but if it occurs it is localized to the eye itself and does not radiate to the face or temple.
2. **Signs**
   - Redness may vary from a mild to a fiery red flush, and may be sectoral (Fig. 11.2a) or diffuse (Fig. 11.2b). Often it has an interpalpebral distribution in contrast with scleritis which most commonly starts in the upper temporal or upper nasal quadrants.
   - The attack reaches its peak within 12 hours and then gradually fades over the next 10–21 days.
   - The episcleritis usually flits from one eye to the other or may be bilateral. Some patients always have attacks in the same place.

Treatment

1. **First attack.** If the patient is seen within 48 hours of onset, topical steroids may be used half hourly during the day for 2 days, then q.i.d. for 1 day, b.d. for 1 day and daily for 2 days. The regressive phase requires no treatment other than cold artificial tears for symptomatic relief.
2. **Recurrent attacks,** if mild, require no treatment other than cold artificial tears. Treatment of extremely frequent or disabling attacks involves a systemic non-steroidal anti-inflammatory drug (NSAID) such as flurbiprofen 100mg t.i.d for 10 days. If recurrences occur thereafter, long-term treatment or a change of drug may be necessary.

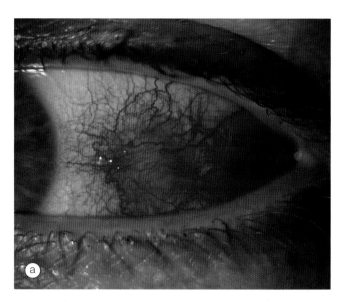

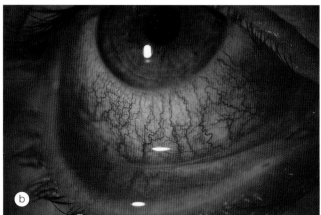

Fig. 11.2
Episcleritis. **(a)** Simple; **(b)** diffuse

Nodular episcleritis

Nodular episcleritis also tends to affect young females but has a less acute onset and a more prolonged course than simple episcleritis.

Diagnosis

1. **Presentation** is with a red eye typically first noted on waking.
   - Over the next 2–3 days the area of redness increases in size but remains in the same position.
   - During the same period the eye becomes more uncomfortable and by the time the disease is at its height is very tender.

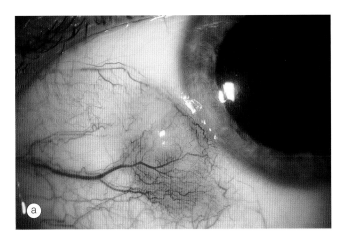

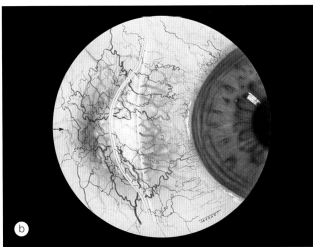

Fig. 11.3
(a) Nodular episcleritis; **(b)** slit-lamp examination of an episcleral nodule shows that the deep beam is not displaced above the scleral surface (Courtesy of P Watson)

2. Signs
- One or more tender nodules, almost always within the interpalpebral fissure (Fig. 11.3a).
- A thin slit-lamp section shows that the anterior scleral surface is flat, indicating absence of scleral involvement (Fig. 11.3b).
- Instillation of 10% phenylephrine drops will decongest the conjunctival and episcleral vessels allowing better visualization of underlying sclera.
- Each attack is self-limiting and usually clears without treatment, but lasts longer than simple episcleritis.
- After several attacks the vessels surrounding the inflamed area may become permanently dilated.

Treatment

1. **First attack.** Patients seen within 48 hours of onset should be treated with intensive topical steroids.
2. **Recurrent attacks** usually require no treatment but if necessary a NSAID can be used for 2–3 months.

> **NB** It is important to exclude a local cause for an episcleral nodule such as a foreign body or granuloma.

SCLERITIS

Scleritis is an uncommon condition characterized by oedema and cellular infiltration of the entire thickness of the sclera. It is much less common than episcleritis and covers a spectrum ranging in severity from trivial self-limiting episodes to a necrotizing disease that may involve adjacent tissues and threaten vision.

Anterior non-necrotizing scleritis

Diffuse

Diffuse disease is slightly more common in females and usually presents in the fifth decade of life.

1. **Presentation** is with ocular redness followed a few days later by aching and pain which may spread to the face and temple. The pain typically wakes the patient in the early hours of the morning and improves later in the day but responds poorly to common analgesics.
2. **Signs**
   - Vascular congestion and dilatation associated with oedema. If treatment is started early, which rarely happens, the disease can be completely inhibited.
   - The redness may be generalized (Fig. 11.4a) or localized to one quadrant. If confined to the areas under the upper eyelid the diagnosis may be missed if the eyelid is not elevated.
   - As the oedema resolves, the affected area often takes on a slight grey/blue appearance because of increased scleral translucency, due to rearrangement of scleral fibres rather than a decrease in scleral thickness (Fig. 11.4b).
   - Recurrences at the some location are common unless the underlying cause is eliminated.
   - The overall duration of disease is approximately 6 years and the frequency of recurrences decreases after the first 18 months. The long-term visual prognosis is very good.

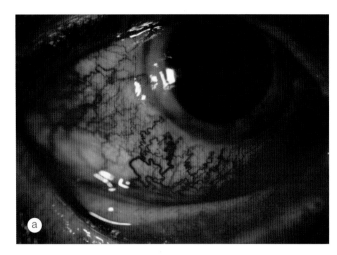

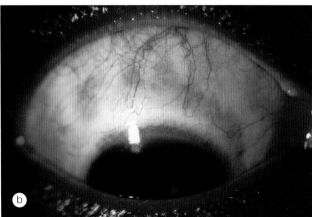

Fig. 11.4
Diffuse anterior non-necrotizing scleritis. **(a)** Intense episcleral inflammation with disruption of the limbal arcade; **(b)** scleral translucency following recurrent disease

Nodular

The incidence of nodular and diffuse anterior scleritis is the same but a disproportionately large number of those with nodular disease have had a previous attack of herpes zoster ophthalmicus. The age of onset is similar to that of diffuse scleritis.

1. **Presentation** is with an insidious onset of pain followed by increasing redness, tenderness of the globe and the appearance of a scleral nodule.
2. **Signs**
   • Scleral nodules may be single or multiple and most frequently develop in the interpalpebral region 3–4mm away from the limbus. They have a deeper blue-red colour than episcleral nodules and are immobile.

• Slit-lamp examination shows that the slit beam is displaced by the scleral nodule (Fig. 11.5a).
• Instillation of 10% phenylephrine drops will constrict the conjunctival and superficial episcleral vasculature but not the deep plexus over the nodule (Fig. 11.5b and c).
• Multiple nodules may coalesce, become confluent or expand – sometimes to an enormous size if treatment is delayed.
• As the inflammation in the nodule subsides, increased translucency of the sclera becomes apparent.
• The duration of the disease is similar to diffuse scleritis.

NB Over 10% of patients with nodular scleritis develop necrotizing disease but if treatment is instituted early superficial necrosis does not occur and the nodule heals from the centre leaving a small atrophic scar.

Necrotizing anterior scleritis with inflammation

Necrotizing disease is the aggressive form of scleritis. The age at onset is later than that of non-necrotizing scleritis with an average age of 60 years. The condition is bilateral in 60% of patients and unless appropriately treated, especially in its early stages, it may result in severe visual impairment and sometimes loss of the globe itself.

Diagnosis

1. **Presentation** is with gradual onset of pain which becomes severe and persistent, and radiates to the temple, brow or jaw; it frequently interferes with sleep and responds poorly to analgesia.
2. **Signs**
   • Nodular scleritis with deep vascular congestion (Fig. 11.6a).
   • Scleral thinning due to necrosis allows the blue choroid to show through the translucent hydrated scar tissue that has replaced normal sclera (Fig. 11.6b).
   • Progressive scleral thinning and extension of the necrotic process around the globe (Fig. 11.6c, d and e).
   • Healing is associated with reduction of vascular congestion, absorption of dead tissue leaving areas of dark choroid covered only by atrophic conjunctiva (Fig. 11.6f).

Specific types of necrotizing disease

1. **Vaso-occlusive** necrotizing scleritis is characterized by areas of congestion which coalesce and become avascular and necrotic (Fig. 11.7a).
2. **Granulomatous necrotizing scleritis** is often associated with Wegener granulomatosis and polyarteritis nodosa. The disease typically starts with injection adjacent

to the limbus and then extends posteriorly. Within 24 hours, the sclera, episclera, conjunctiva and adjacent cornea become irregularly raised and oedematous (Fig. 11.7b).

3. **Surgically-induced scleritis** typically starts within 3 weeks of the surgical procedure, but much longer intervals have been reported. Scleritis may be induced by any type of surgery including strabismus repair, trabeculectomy (Fig. 11.8a) and scleral buckling for retinal detachment (Fig.11.8b). The necrotizing process starts at the site of surgery and then extends outwards but, unlike other forms of necrotizing disease, it tends to remain localized to one segment.

Investigations

1. **Laboratory.** The commonest association of scleral inflammation is a connective tissue disease. Unfortunately there are few specific and reliable tests so the results should be employed as adjuncts to clinical signs. Specific tests include RF, ANA, cANCA and antiphospholipid antibodies.
2. **FA** can aid in deciding if necrotizing scleritis is present or is likely to occur. In most patients with necrotizing scleritis there is vascular non-perfusion (Fig. 11.9). However, in patients with a systemic vasculitis such as Wegener granulomatosis the pattern is primarily of transudation, localized areas of vasculitis and new vessel formation.

Corneal complications

1. **Acute infiltrative stromal keratitis** which may be localized or diffuse (Fig. 11.10a).
2. **Sclerosing keratitis** characterized by chronic thinning and opacification in which the peripheral cornea adjacent to the site of scleritis resembles sclera (Fig. 11.10b).
3. **Peripheral ulcerative keratitis** is characterized by progressive melting and ulceration which may eventually be more serious than the scleritis. In granulomatous scleritis the destruction extends directly from the sclera into the limbus and cornea (Fig. 11.10c). This characteristic pattern is seen in Wegener granulomatosis, polyarteritis nodosa and relapsing polychondritis.

NB Peripheral corneal ulceration can occur at any stage of a necrotizing scleritis and, in rare cases, may precede its onset.

Other complications

1. **Uveitis,** if severe, usually denotes aggressive disease.
2. **Uveal effusion** characterized by exudative retinal and choroidal detachments may occur in equatorial scleritis.

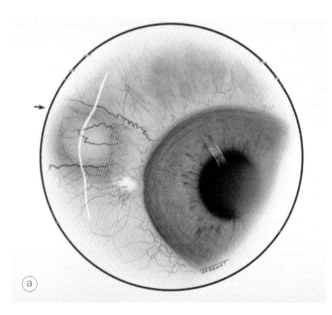
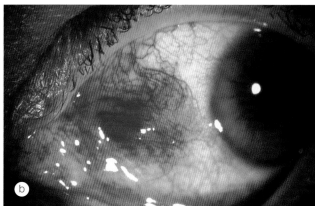
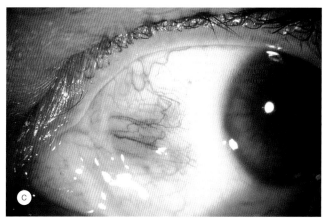

Fig. 11.5
Nodular anterior non-necrotizing scleritis. **(a)** Slit-lamp examination of scleral nodule shows displacement of the entire beam; **(b)** dilatation of conjunctival vessels, and the superficial episcleral and deep vascular plexus; **(c)** following instillation of 10% phenylephrine only the deep plexus over the nodule remains dilated (Courtesy of Dr Geux-Crosier in Watson, Hazelman, Pavesio and Green, from *The Sclera and Systemic Disorders,* Mosby, 2004)

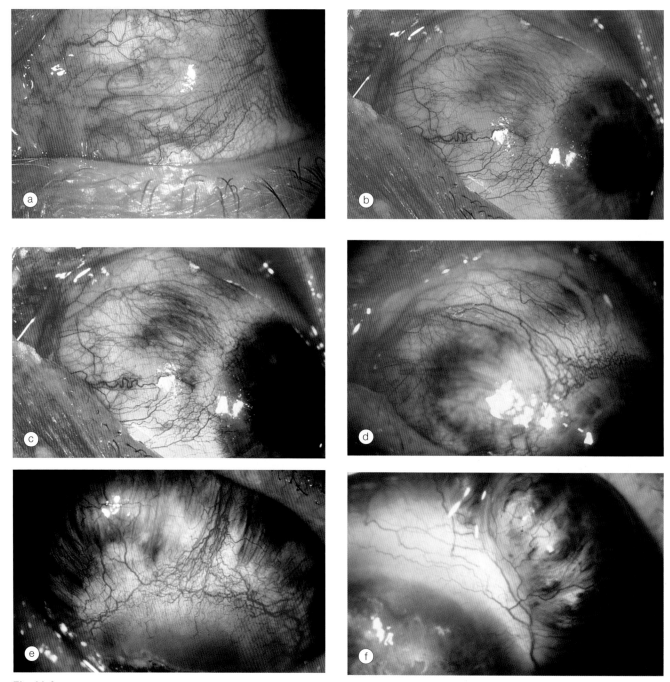

Fig. 11.6
Progression of anterior necrotizing scleritis. **(a)** Nodular scleritis; **(b)** early scleral thinning; **(c)**, **(d)** and **(e)** progressive scleral thinning; **(f)** the healed stage shows very severe scleral thinning and lack of vascular congestion (Courtesy of Watson, Hazelman, Pavesio and Green, from *The Sclera and Systemic Disorders*, Mosby, 2004)

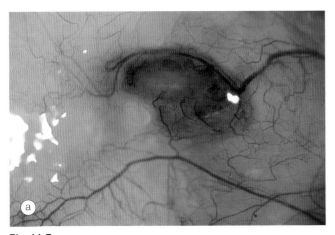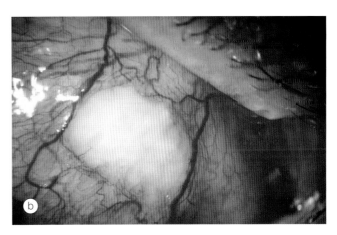

Fig. 11.7
Specific types of necrotizing scleritis. **(a)** Vaso-occlusive; **(b)** granulomatous

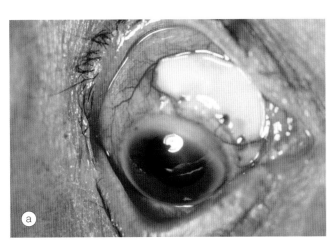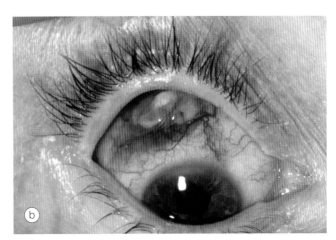

Fig. 11.8
Surgically-induced scleritis. **(a)** Following trabeculectomy; **(b)** following scleral buckling

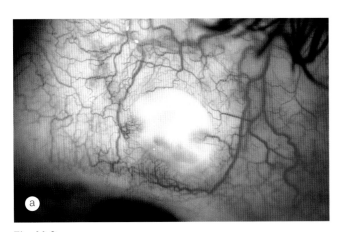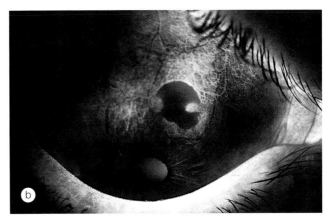

Fig. 11.9
(a) Patch of necrotizing scleritis; **(b)** fluorescein angiography shows complete lack of perfusion of the necrotic area (Courtesy of Watson, Hazelman, Pavesio and Green, from *The Sclera and Systemic Disorders*, Mosby, 2004)

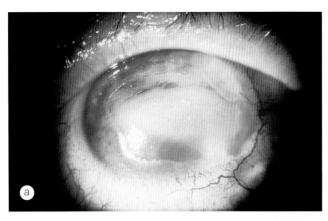

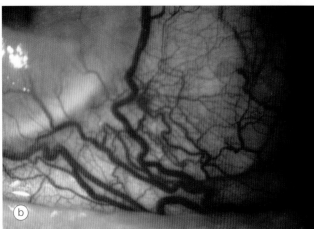

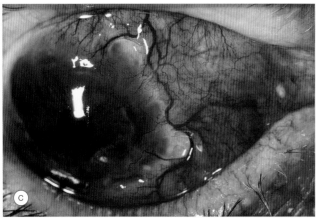

Fig. 11.10
Corneal complications of scleritis. **(a)** Acute diffuse stromal keratitis; **(b)** sclerosing keratitis; **(c)** peripheral ulcerative keratitis (Courtesy of Watson, Hazelman, Pavesio and Green, from *The Sclera and Systemic Diseases*, Mosby, 2004 – figs a and c)

3. **Glaucoma** is the most common cause of eventual loss of vision. The intraocular pressure is very difficult to control in the presence of active scleritis.
4. **Hypotony** may be the result of ciliary body detachment, inflammatory damage or ischaemia.

5. **Perforation** of the globe as a result of the inflammatory process alone is extremely rare.

Scleromalacia perforans

Scleromalacia perforans is a specific type of necrotizing scleritis without inflammation that typically affects elderly women with long-standing rheumatoid arthritis. The use of the word 'perforans' is unfortunate; perforation is extremely rare because the integrity of the globe is maintained by a thin, but complete, layer of fibrous tissue.

1. **Presentation** is with slight non-specific irritation and keratoconjunctivitis sicca may be suspected; pain is absent and vision unaffected.
2. **Signs**
   * Yellow scleral necrotic plaques near the limbus without vascular congestion (Fig. 11.11a).
   * Coalescence and enlargement of necrotic areas (Fig. 11.11b).
   * Very slow progression of scleral thinning and exposure of underlying uvea (Fig. 11.11 c and d).
3. **Treatment** may be effective in patients with very early disease but by the time most patients present, no treatment is either needed or effective. Repair of scleral perforation is very difficult but must be attempted otherwise phthisis bulbi ensues.

Posterior scleritis

Posterior scleritis is a serious, potentially blinding, condition, which is often misdiagnosed and treated very late. The age at onset is often under the age of 40 years. The disease is bilateral in 35% of cases. It is important to remember that the inflammatory changes seen in posterior and anterior scleral disease are identical and can arise in both segments simultaneously or separately. The presence of anterior scleritis is a great help if posterior scleritis is suspected but it only occurs in a minority of cases. Patients with posterior scleritis can go blind extremely rapidly, so correct, early diagnosis is crucial. Young patients are usually healthy but about a third of those over the age of 55 years have associated systemic disease.

Diagnosis

1. **Presentation** may be with discomfort or pain. Surprisingly pain does not correlate to the severity of inflammation but tends to be more severe in those with accompanying myositis. Tenderness to palpation is very common but photophobia is not a dominant feature.
2. **Signs**
   *a. **Exudative retinal detachment*** occurs in almost 25% of cases (Fig. 11.12a).

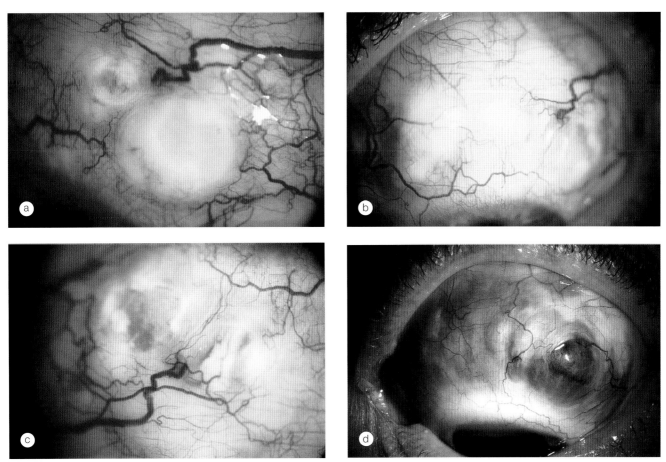

Fig. 11.11
Progression of scleromalacia perforans. **(a)** Scleral necrotic patches; **(b)** extension of scleral necrosis; **(c)** and **(d)** progressive scleral thinning and exposure of underlying sclera (Courtesy of Watson, Hazelman, Pavesio and Green, from *The Sclera and Systemic Diseases*, Mosby, 2004)

*b. **Uveal effusion*** characterized by exudative retinal detachment and choroidal detachment (Fig. 11.12b).

*c. **Choroidal folds*** represent an anterior displacement of the choroid and are usually confined to the posterior pole and run horizontally (Fig. 11.12c).

*d. **Subretinal mass*** characterized by a yellowish-brown elevation which may be mistaken for a choroidal tumour (Fig. 11.12d).

*e. **Disc oedema*** with an accompanying slight reduction of vision is common. It is caused by spread of the granulomatous process into the orbital tissue and sheaths of the optic nerve. Treatment must not be delayed in these patients as vision can be lost rapidly due to ischaemia.

*f. **Myositis*** is common and gives rise to diplopia, pain on eye movement, tenderness to touch and redness around a muscle insertion.

*g. **Proptosis*** is usually mild and frequently associated with ptosis.

*h. **Other features*** occasionally present include periorbital oedema, chemosis and conjunctival injection.

NB About 20% of the patients with definite ultrasonic evidence of posterior scleral disease have absolutely no clinical evidence of any abnormality in the posterior segment of the eye.

3. US is extremely useful in showing increased scleral thickness, scleral nodules and separation of Tenon capsule from the sclera. Fluid in Tenon space gives rise to the characteristic 'T' sign in which the stem of the T is formed by the optic nerve on its side and the cross bar by the gap containing fluid (Fig. 11.12e). Ultrasonography will also show disc oedema, choroidal folds or retinal detachment.

4. CT may show scleral thickening and proptosis (Fig. 11.12f).

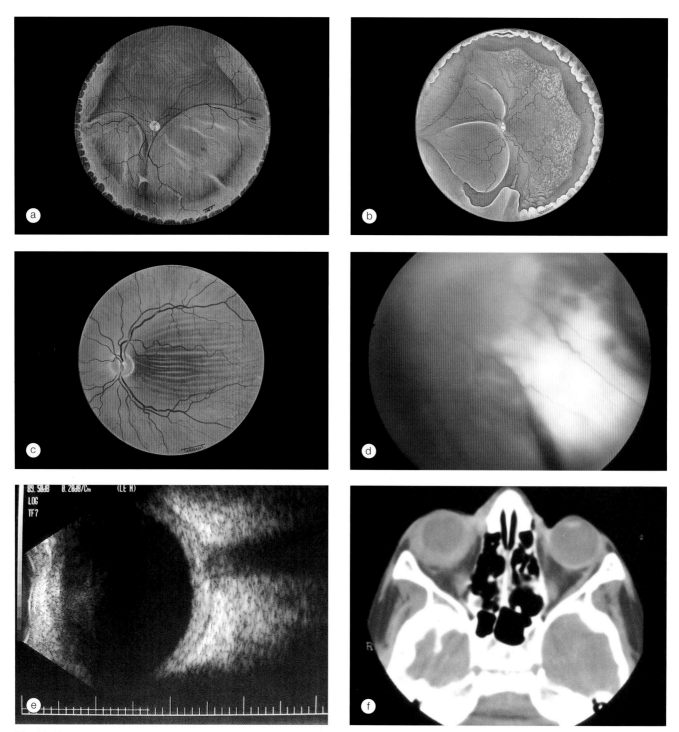

Fig. 11.12
Posterior scleritis. **(a)** Exudative retinal detachment; **(b)** uveal effusion; **(c)** choroidal folds; **(d)** subretinal mass; **(e)** ultrasonography showing scleral thickening and fluid in sub-Tenon space; **(f)** axial CT in right posterior scleritis shows scleral thickening and mild proptosis (Courtesy of Watson, Hazelman, Pavesio and Green, from *The Sclera and Systemic Disorders*, Mosby, 2004 – figs a and d)

Differential diagnosis

1. **Subretinal mass** must be differentiated from a granuloma associated with some other pathology, amelanotic choroidal melanoma, choroidal metastasis and choroidal haemangioma.
2. **Choroidal folds,** retinal striae and disc oedema may also occur in orbital tumours, orbital inflammatory disease, thyroid eye disease, papilloedema and hypotony.
3. **Exudative retinal detachment** also occurs in VKH syndrome and central serous retinopathy.
4. **Orbital cellulitis** may cause proptosis and periocular oedema but unlike posterior scleritis it is associated with pyrexia.

Systemic associations of scleritis

1. **Rheumatoid arthritis** (see Chapter 24) is by far the most common systemic association of scleritis. Patients with non-necrotizing scleritis usually have mild joint disease whereas necrotizing disease and scleromalacia perforans tend to affect patients with severe long-standing rheumatoid disease with extra-articular manifestations, most notably rheumatoid nodules.
2. **Wegener granulomatosis** is an idiopathic, multisystem granulomatous disorder characterized by generalized small vessel vasculitis affecting predominantly the respiratory tract and kidneys (see Chapter 24). The disease may be associated with rapidly progressive, necrotizing granulomatous scleritis. Because Wegener granulomatosis can be localized to the eye and the orbit, without any systemic involvement, orbital biopsy may be required for diagnosis.
3. **Relapsing polychondritis** is a rare idiopathic condition characterized by small vessel vasculitis involving cartilage resulting in recurrent, often progressive, inflammatory episodes involving multiple organ systems (see Chapter 24). It is a common cause of intractable scleritis which may be non-necrotizing or necrotizing.
4. **Polyarteritis nodosa (PAN)** is an idiopathic, potentially lethal, collagen vascular disease affecting medium-sized and small arteries, with frequent aneurysm formation (see Chapter 24). PAN may be associated with aggressive necrotizing disease although other types of scleritis may also occur. Ocular involvement may precede the systemic manifestations by several years.
5. **Systemic lupus erythematosus (SLE)** is an autoimmune, non-organ specific connective tissue disease (see Chapter 24). SLE may be associated with anterior diffuse or nodular scleritis. Necrotizing scleritis less common but is difficult to control if treatment is delayed.
6. **Other** uncommon associations include:
   a. *Spondyloarthropathies* are occasionally associated with mild diffuse scleritis and may antedate joint involvement.
   b. *Behçet syndrome* may rarely be associated with diffuse anterior scleritis which may occur in the absence of other ocular manifestations.
   c. *Sarcoidosis* may rarely manifest scleral nodules.
   d. *Gout* very rarely may be associated with diffuse episcleritis or scleritis.

Treatment of scleritis

1. **Topical steroids** do not affect the natural history of the scleral inflammation, but may relieve symptoms and oedema in non-necrotizing disease.
2. **Systemic NSAIDs** should be used only in non-necrotizing disease. There is little to choose between various agents in terms of relief of pain or regression of physical signs. It is unlikely that using them in combination will provide any more relief than using them singly. Because there is a large variation in individual responses to NSAIDs it is often necessary to try a number of different drugs before finding one that provides adequate relief of symptoms. Each drug should be given for 2 weeks to assess its efficacy. Guidelines for prescribing an NSAID:
   * Use a drug with which you are familiar
   * Prescribe cheaper, established drugs
   * Prescribe only one drug at a time, in adequate dosage
   * Prescribe for 2 weeks and review
3. **Periocular steroid injections** may be used in non-necrotizing and necrotizing disease but their effects are usually transient.
4. **Systemic steroids** are used when NSAIDs are inappropriate or ineffective (necrotizing disease). The dose of prednisolone is 1.0–1.5mg/kg daily. If a faster effect is required the drug should be administered intravenously at a dose of 0.5–1.0g (1–3mg/kg) daily.
5. **Cytotoxic agents** are usually necessary whenever disease activity is not completely controlled with steroids alone, or as a steroid-sparing measure in patients requiring very high doses. In patients with an underlying systemic vasculitis such as Wegener granulomatosis or PAN this form of therapy may also be life-saving. The most frequently used drugs are cyclophosphamide, which is the drug of choice in Wegener disease, azathioprine, mycophenolate mofetil and methotrexate.
6. **Immune modulators** such as ciclosporin and tacrolimus are less useful as long-term therapy but may be considered as a short-term measure in acute presentations before a cytotoxic agent is able to exert its action.

NB If pain and headache persist in spite of treatment then there is still active inflammation.

Scleral infection

1. **Herpes zoster** is the most common infective cause. Necrotizing scleritis is extremely resistant to treatment and may result in a punched-out area in the sclera, a very thin atrophic scar, or, very occasionally, staphyloma formation or perforation.
2. **Tuberculous scleritis** is rare and difficult to diagnose. The sclera may be infected by direct spread from a local conjunctiva or choroid lesion, or more commonly by haematogenous spread. Clinically involvement may be nodular (Fig. 11.13) or necrotizing.
3. **Leprosy.** Diffuse scleritis is associated with severe recurrent erythema nodosum leprosum reactions. Nodular scleritis may occur in lepromatous leprosy as a result of scleral infection or as part of an immune response.
4. **Syphilis.** Diffuse anterior scleritis may occur in secondary syphilis. Occasionally scleral nodules may be seen in tertiary syphilis.
5. **Lyme disease.** Scleritis is common but typically occurs long after initial infection.

NB Once the infective agent has been identified, specific therapy should be initiated. Topical and systemic steroids may also be used to reduce the inflammatory reaction.

SCLERAL DISCOLORATION

Focal

Focal discoloration may be caused by the following:
1. **Scleral hyaline plaques** are characterized by oval, dark-greyish areas located close to the insertion of the horizontal rectus muscles (Fig. 11.14). They typically affect elderly patients, are entirely innocuous and should not be confused with scleromalacia perforans.
2. **Alcaptonuria** is an inherited aminoacidopathy of phenylalanine/tyrosine metabolism due to absence of homogentistic acid oxidase. This results in accumulation of homogentisic acid in collagenous tissues such as cartilage (Fig. 11.15a) and tendon, especially in the ear and nose (ochronosis). Scleral involvement is characterized by brown-black discoloration at the insertions of horizontal recti (Fig. 11.15b and c).
3. **Haemochromatosis** causes rusty-brown discoloration.
4. **Systemic minocycline** may cause blue-grey paralimbal discoloration, usually denser in the interpalpebral area, possibly due to the photosensitizing properties of the drug.

This may be associated with pigmentation of skin, teeth, nails, mucosa, thyroid and bones.
5. **Metallic foreign body,** if long-standing, may produce rust staining.

Diffuse

1. **Yellow** discoloration is caused by jaundice.
2. **Blue** discoloration is caused by thinning and transparency of scleral collagen with visualization of the underlying uvea (Fig. 11.16). Important causes include osteogenesis imperfecta types 1 and 2, Ehlers–Danlos syndrome (usually type 6), pseudoxanthoma elasticum (dominant type 2) and Turner syndrome.

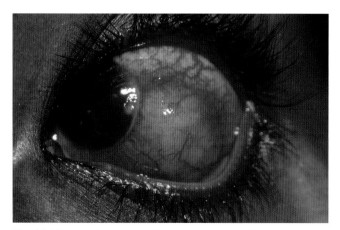

Fig. 11.13
Tuberculous scleritis (Courtesy of S Fogla)

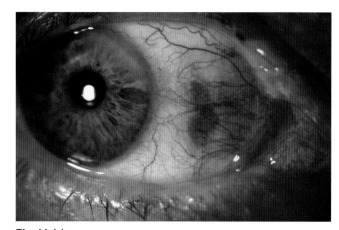

Fig. 11.14
Scleral hyaline plaques

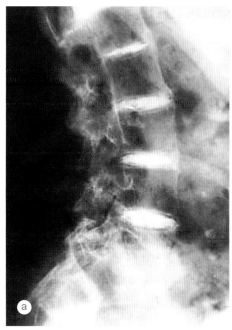

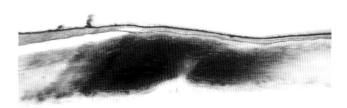

Fig. 11.15
Alcaptonuria. **(a)** Calcification of intervertebral discs; **(b)** scleral pigmentation; **(c)** histology shows brown-black pigmentation (Courtesy of J M H Moll – figs a and b; J Harry and G Misson, from *Clinical Ophthalmic Pathology*, Butterworth-Heinemann, 2001 – fig. c)

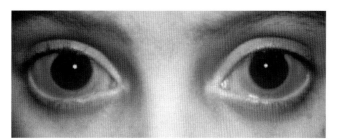

Fig. 11.16
Blue sclera

CHAPTER 12

LENS

INTRODUCTION

The crystalline lens is a biconvex, avascular, transparent structure enclosed by a capsule, which is a basement membrane secreted by the lens epithelium. The capsule, responsible for moulding the lens during accommodation, is thickest in the equatorial zone and thinnest at the posterior pole. A ring of zonular fibres, which insert in the equatorial region, suspends the lens from the ciliary body. A monolayer of epithelium lines only the anterior and equatorial lens capsule. Cells in the equatorial region exhibit mitotic activity. Newly formed epithelial cells elongate to form fibres, which lose their organelles, thus optimizing lens transparency. The lens may be conceptualized as consisting of the nucleus, the central compacted core, surrounded by the cortex. New lens fibres are continuously laid down under the capsule throughout life, resulting in older layers acquiring a progressively deeper location within the lens substance. The lens thus grows in both anteroposterior and equatorial dimensions throughout life. The normal lens is transparent; any congenital or acquired opacity in the lens capsule or substance, irrespective of the effect on vision, is a cataract.

ACQUIRED CATARACT

Age-related cataract

Subcapsular cataract

Anterior subcapsular cataract lies directly under the lens capsule and is associated with fibrous metaplasia of the lens epithelium. Posterior subcapsular opacity lies just in front of the posterior capsule and manifests a vacuolated, granular, or plaque-like appearance on oblique slit-lamp biomicroscopy (Fig. 12.1a) and appears black on retroillumination

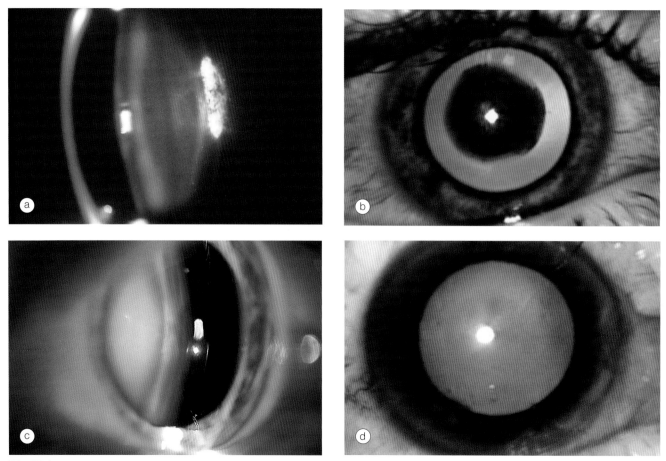

Fig. 12.1
Age-related cataract. **(a)** Posterior subcapsular; **(b)** posterior subcapsular seen on retroillumination; **(c)** nuclear; **(d)** early nuclear cannot be seen on retroillumination

(Fig. 12.1b). Due to its location at the nodal point of the eye, a posterior subcapsular opacity has a more profound effect on vision than a comparable nuclear or cortical cataract. Near vision is frequently impaired more than distance vision. Patients are particularly troubled under conditions of miosis, such as produced by headlights of oncoming cars and bright sunlight.

Nuclear cataract

Nuclear cataract starts as an exaggeration of the normal ageing changes involving the lens nucleus. It is often associated with myopia due to an increase in the refractive index of the nucleus and with increased spherical aberration. Some elderly patients may consequently be able to read again without spectacles ('second sight of the aged'). Nuclear sclerosis is characterized in its early stages by a yellowish hue

due to the deposition of urochrome pigment. This type of cataract is best assessed with oblique slit-lamp biomicroscopy (Fig. 12.1c) and not by retroillumination (Fig. 12.1d). When advanced, the nucleus appears brown (a brunescent cataract). Such cataracts are of hard consistency, which is surgically relevant.

Cortical cataract

Cortical cataract may involve the anterior, posterior or equatorial cortex. The opacities start as clefts (Fig. 12.2a) and vacuoles (Fig. 12.2b) between lens fibres due to hydration of the cortex. Subsequent opacification results in typical cuneiform (wedge-shaped) or radial spoke-like opacities (Fig. 12.2c and d) often initially in the inferonasal quadrant. Patients with cortical opacities frequently complain of glare due to light scattering.

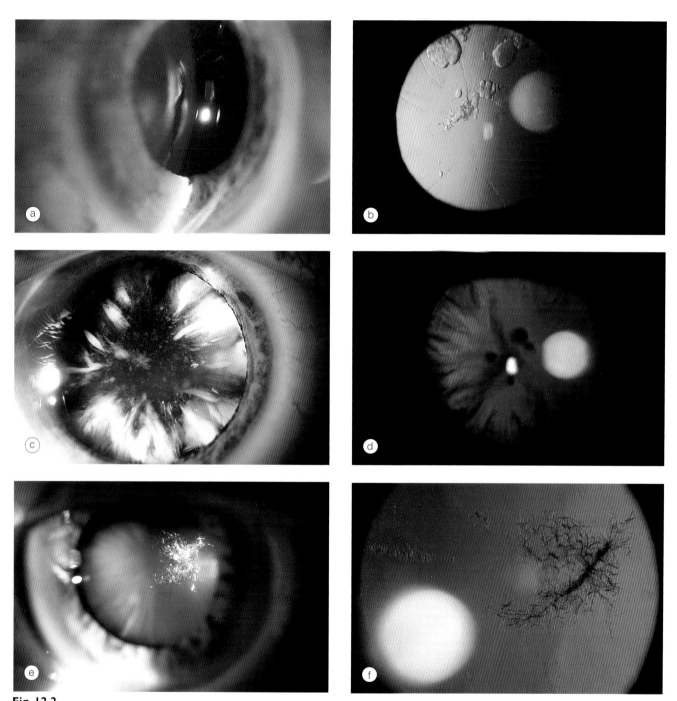

Fig. 12.2
Age-related cataract. **(a)** Cortical clefts; **(b)** cortical vacuoles seen on retroillumination; **(c)** wedge-shaped cuneiform; **(d)** cuneiform seen on retroillumination; **(e)** Christmas tree; **(f)** Christmas tree seen on retroillumination

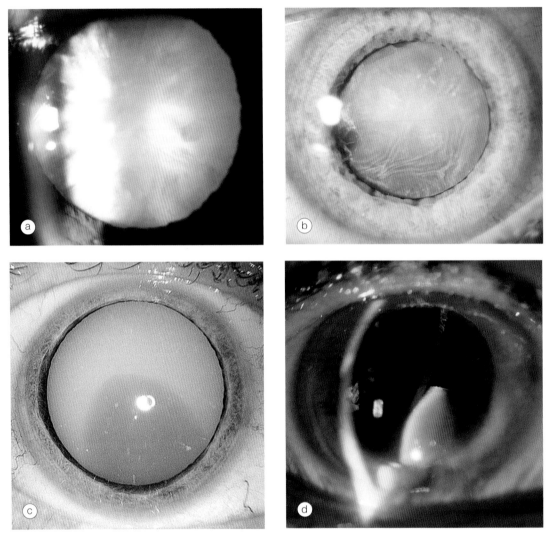

Fig. 12.3
Cataract maturity. **(a)** Mature; **(b)** hypermature with wrinkling of the anterior capsule; **(c)** morgagnian with liquefaction of the cortex and inferior sinking of the nucleus; **(d)** total liquefaction and absorption of the cortex with inferior sinking of the lens (Courtesy of P Gili – fig. d)

Christmas tree cataract

Christmas tree cataract, which is uncommon, is characterized by striking, polychromatic, needle-like deposits in the deep cortex and nucleus (Fig. 12.2e and f) which may be solitary or associated with other opacities.

Cataract maturity

1. **Immature** cataract is one in which the lens is partially opaque.
2. **Mature** cataract is one in which the lens is completely opaque (Fig. 12.3a).
3. **Hypermature** cataract has a shrunken and wrinkled anterior capsule due to leakage of water out of the lens (Fig. 12.3b).

4. **Morgagnian** cataract is a hypermature cataract in which liquefaction of the cortex has allowed the nucleus to sink inferiorly (Fig. 12.3c and d).

Cataract in systemic diseases

Diabetes mellitus

Diabetes mellitus (see Chapter 24), in addition to causing cataract, can affect the refractive index of the lens and also its amplitude of accommodation.

1. **Classical** diabetic cataract is rare. Hyperglycaemia is reflected in a high level of glucose in the aqueous humour, which diffuses into the lens. Here glucose is metabolized

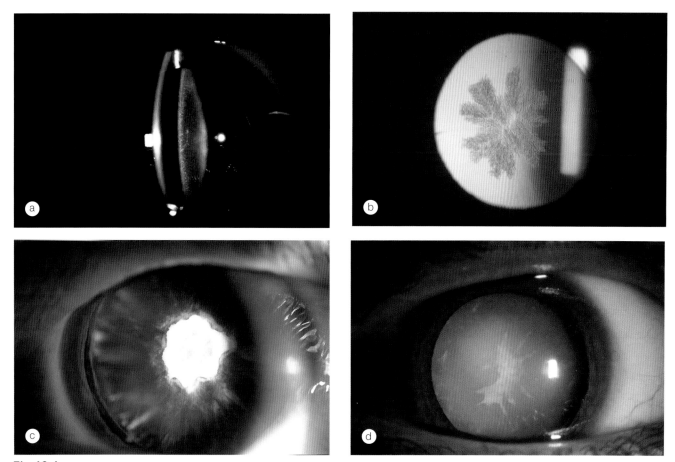

Fig. 12.4
Cataract in systemic disease. **(a)** Diabetic snowflake; **(b)** stellate posterior subcapsular in myotonic dystrophy seen on retroillumination; **(c)** shield-like anterior subcapsular in atopic dermatitis; **(d)** advanced in atopic dermatitis (Courtesy of A Fielder – fig. a; L Merin – fig. b; S Tuft – fig d)

by aldose reductase into sorbitol, which then accumulates within the lens, resulting in secondary osmotic over-hydration of the lens substance. In mild degree, this may affect the refractive index of the lens with consequent fluctuation of refraction pari-passu with the plasma glucose level (hyperglycaemia resulting in myopia). Cortical fluid vacuoles develop and later evolve into frank opacities. Classical diabetic cataract consists of snowflake cortical opacities (Fig. 12.4a) occurring in the young diabetic that may resolve spontaneously or mature within a few days.

2. Age-related cataract occurs earlier in diabetes mellitus. Nuclear opacities are common and tend to progress rapidly.

Myotonic dystrophy

About 90% of patients with myotonic dystrophy (see Chapter 24) develop visually innocuous, fine cortical iridescent opacities in the third decade. These evolve into a visually disabling stellate posterior subcapsular cataract by the fifth decade (Fig. 12.4b). Occasionally cataract may antedate myotonia.

Atopic dermatitis

About 10% of patients with severe atopic dermatitis (see Chapter 24) develop cataracts in the second to fourth decades. The opacities are often bilateral and may mature quickly. Shield-like dense anterior subcapsular plaque which wrinkles the anterior capsule is characteristic (Fig. 12.4c and d). Posterior subcapsular opacities resembling a complicated cataract may also occur.

Neurofibromatosis-2

Neurofibromatosis-2 (see Chapter 24) is associated with posterior subcapsular or posterior cortical opacities.

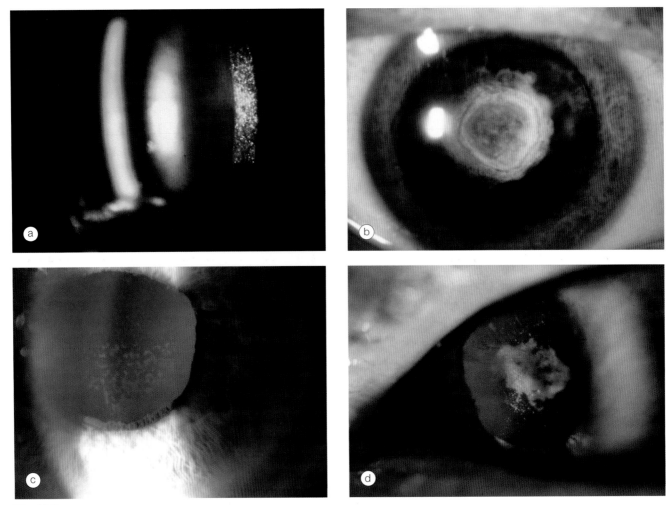

Fig. 12.5
Secondary cataract. **(a)** Posterior polychromatic; **(b)** dense posterior subcapsular plaque; **(c)** mild glaukomflecken; **(d)** severe glaukomflecken

Secondary cataract

A secondary (complicated) cataract develops as a result of some other primary ocular disease.

Chronic anterior uveitis

Chronic anterior uveitis is the most common cause of secondary cataract. The incidence is related to the duration and activity of intraocular inflammation that results in prolonged breakdown of the blood–aqueous or blood–vitreous barrier. The use of steroids, topically and systemically, is also important. The earliest finding is a polychromatic lustre at the posterior pole of the lens (Fig. 12.5a) which may not progress if the uveitis is arrested. If the inflammation persists, posterior (Fig. 12.5b) and anterior opacities develop and may progress to maturity. Lens opacities appear to progress more rapidly in the presence of posterior synechiae.

Acute congestive angle-closure

Acute congestive angle-closure may cause small, grey-white, anterior, subcapsular or capsular opacities within the pupillary area (glaukomflecken – Fig. 12.5c and d). They represent focal infarcts of the lens epithelium and are pathognomonic of past acute angle-closure glaucoma.

High myopia

High (pathological) myopia is associated with posterior subcapsular lens opacities and early-onset nuclear sclerosis, which may ironically increase the myopic refractive error.

Simple myopia, however, is not associated with such cataract formation.

Hereditary fundus dystrophies

Hereditary fundus dystrophies such as retinitis pigmentosa, Leber congenital amaurosis, gyrate atrophy and Stickler syndrome may be associated with posterior subcapsular lens opacities (see Chapter 18). Cataract surgery may occasionally improve visual acuity even in the presence of severe retinal changes.

MANAGEMENT OF AGE-RELATED CATARACT

Preoperative considerations

Indications for surgery

1. **Visual improvement** is by far the most common indication for cataract surgery, although requirements vary from person to person. Surgery is indicated only if and when cataract develops to a degree sufficient to cause difficulty in performing daily essential activities. If the patient desires to drive or continue a specific occupation, visual function below legally prescribed levels may necessitate surgery.
2. **Medical** indications are those in which a cataract is adversely affecting the health of the eye, for example, phacolytic glaucoma or phacomorphic glaucoma (see Chapter 13). Cataract surgery to improve the clarity of the ocular media may also be required in the context of fundal pathology (e.g. diabetic retinopathy) requiring monitoring or treatment.
3. **Cosmetic** indications are rare, such as when a mature cataract in an otherwise blind eye is removed to restore a black pupil.

Preoperative evaluation

Apart from a general medical examination, a patient due to undergo cataract surgery requires a detailed and pertinent ophthalmic examination.

1. **Visual acuity.** Although most patients will have visual acuity assessed using a Snellen chart, this is probably rather a crude approach as only high contrast vision is tested – usually in a darkened room. Contrast sensitivity charts and/or the use of LogMAR visual acuity measurement can give a better understanding of the quality of vision (see Chapter 1). Brightness acuity testing, when a chart is viewed through a glare source, also adds practical information about the patient's visual disability.
2. **Cover test.** A heterotropia may indicate amblyopia, which carries a guarded visual prognosis, or the possibility of diplopia if vision is improved.
3. **Pupillary responses.** Because a cataract never produces an afferent pupillary defect, its presence implies additional pathology, which may influence the final visual outcome.
4. **Ocular adnexa.** Dacryocystitis, blepharitis, chronic conjunctivitis, lagophthalmos, ectropion, entropion and tear film abnormalities may predispose to endophthalmitis and require effective preoperative treatment.
5. **Cornea.** A wide arcus senilis or stromal opacities may prejudice a good surgical view. Eyes with guttata and decreased endothelial cell counts are vulnerable to postoperative decompensation secondary to operative trauma. In these cases special precautions should be taken to protect the endothelium during surgery with viscoelastics (see below). Eyes with significant endothelial cell loss may be candidates for simultaneous penetrating keratoplasty. The amount of pre-existing corneal astigmatism should be measured, if freedom from at least distance glasses is envisaged following surgery. A decision as to whether astigmatism should be corrected can be made after discussion with the patient.
6. **Anterior segment.** A shallow anterior chamber can render cataract surgery difficult. Pseudoexfoliation indicates a weak zonule, with the possibility of problems during surgery. A poorly dilating pupil can make cataract surgery difficult. Recognition of this allows intensive preoperative mydriatic drops, planned stretching of the pupil prior to capsulorrhexis or intracameral injection of mydriatic. A poor red reflex compromises the performance of a good capsulorrhexis. This can be overcome by staining the capsule with a dye such as trypan blue.
7. **Lens.** The type of cataract is relevant. Nuclear cataracts tend to be harder and may require more phaco power, while cortical opacities tend to be softer. The colour of the nucleus depends on the age of the cataract and varies from transparent – grey – grey-yellow – amber – brown – black. The latter occupies most of the lens and is the hardest.
8. **Fundus** examination pathology such as age-related macular degeneration may affect the visual outcome. Ultrasonography may be required in eyes with very dense cataracts that preclude fundoscopy.

Biometry

Surgical removal of the crystalline lens subtracts approximately 20D from the refracting system of the eye. The aphakic eye is grossly hypermetropic; modern cataract surgery therefore involves the implantation of an intraocular lens (IOL), ideally in the same location as the surgically removed crystalline lens. Biometry affords calculation of the lens power likely to result in the desired postoperative refractive error.

In its simplest form, biometry involves two parameters: (a) keratometry – the curvature of the anterior corneal surface

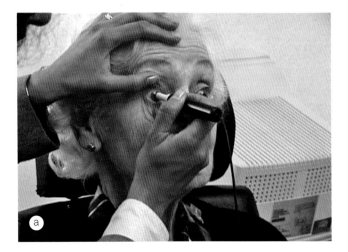
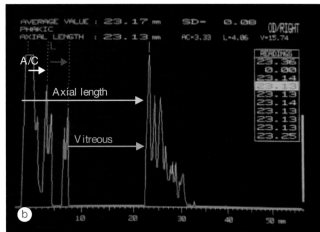
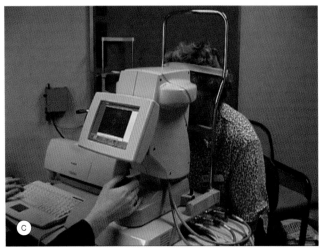
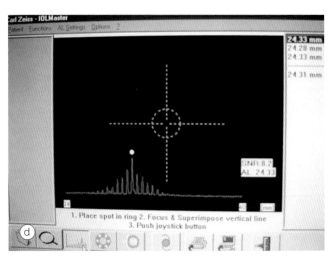

Fig. 12.6
Biometry **(a)** Technique of contact A-scan biometry; **(b)** ideal scan; **(c)** IOLMaster; **(d)** ideal scan (Courtesy of D Michalik and J Bolger)

(steepest and flattest meridians), expressed in dioptres or mm of radius of curvature and (b) axial length – the antero-posterior dimension of the eye in millimetres. There are two main methods used to measure axial length.

1. **A-scan ultrasonic biometry** in which an ultrasonic wave is passed through the eye and the time of its return after hitting intraocular structures produces a trace. Biometry can be either by direct contact (Fig. 12.6a) or more accurately, using a water bath. The display allows ocular structures to be identified and the distance from the front of the cornea to the retina determined. The sound beam must be aligned with the visual axis for maximal echo reflection. Each echo shows up as a spike on the oscilloscope screen (Fig. 12.6b). A certain amount of skill is required to obtain accurate measurements

2. **Zeiss IOLMaster** (Fig. 12.6c) is a non-contact method that utilizes two coaxial laser beams which are partially coherent and produce an interference pattern (partial

coherence inferometry). Measurements (Fig. 12.6d) have high reproducibility and generally require less skill than ultrasonic biometry. The IOLMaster is a complete biometry system which also performs keratometry, anterior chamber depth, corneal white to white and comes with formulae for calculating IOL power. Storage of data and validation of the A-constant is another useful feature. Aphakic, pseudophakic and silicone filled eyes can also be measured but eyes with dense posterior subcapsular opacities present a problem.

3. **IOL power calculation formulae.** Numerous formulae, incorporating additional parameters such as anterior chamber depth and individualized surgeon factors, have been developed to optimize the accuracy of preoperative prediction.

4. **Personalized A-constant** is the process of fine-tuning IOL calculation. It is done by back calculating the A-constant using at least 20 cases of average eyes. Most modern biometry machines have this facility already

programmed into them. If a constant error of say +1D is found in most cases, a new personalized A-constant can be used to ensure a better outcome.

Postoperative refraction

Emmetropia is often the ideal postoperative refraction, with spectacles needed only for close work (since an IOL cannot accommodate). In practice, most surgeons aim for a small degree of myopia (about 0.25D) to offset possible error in biometry. This is because a slight degree of myopia is acceptable in most patients, and may even be advantageous, while postoperative hypermetropia, which necessitates spectacles for clear vision at all distances, is poorly tolerated. The planning of postoperative refraction also needs to take account of the other eye. If the other eye has good vision with a significant refractive error and is unlikely to require surgery, then postoperative refraction should be targeted at within 2D of the other eye, to avoid problems with binocular coordination. Or else if the ametropia is extreme the patient can be offered refractive lens exchange in the fellow eye to target both at emmetropia. The idea of monovision, where the non-dominant eye is left −2.0D myopic to allow it to read whilst the dominant eye is left emmetropic, is attractive to some patients. There are now lens options available which allow degrees of multifocality as patients ask for more independence from spectacles following surgery. In order to achieve this, the question of correcting preoperative corneal astigmatism becomes important.

Intraocular lenses

Positioning

An IOL consists of the optic (the central refracting element) and the haptics, which sit in contact with the ocular structures (capsular bag, ciliary sulcus or anterior chamber angle) thus affording an optimal and stable position (centration) of the optic. Modern cataract surgery, with preservation of the capsular 'bag', affords positioning of the IOL in the ideal location – 'in the bag'. Complicated surgery with rupture of the posterior capsule may, however, necessitate alternative positioning of the IOL, in the posterior chamber, with haptics in the ciliary sulcus, or in the anterior chamber, with the haptics supported in the chamber angle. The latter is designated an AC-IOL in contrast to the former two, which are PC-IOLs.

Designs

Designs are numerous and continue to evolve.

1. **Rigid** IOL requires an incision larger than the diameter of the optic, often 5mm, for insertion. They are made entirely from PMMA and are now generally used only in developing countries where they are cheap and plentiful.

2. **Flexible** IOL may be folded with forceps, or loaded into an injector/delivery system and inserted through a much smaller incision.
   a. **Silicone** IOLs, both three-piece loop and one-piece plate haptics, are associated with lower rates of posterior capsular opacification (PCO) than PMMA lenses. They are more likely to be associated with contraction of the anterior capsule than soft acrylic IOLs.
   b. **Acrylic** IOLs, three-piece or one-piece, may be hydrophobic (water content < 1%) or hydrophilic (water content 18–35%). Hydrophobic acrylic IOLs with a sharp edge to the optic inhibit PCO. Hydrophobic materials have a much higher refractive index than hydrophilic lenses and are subsequently thinner.
   c. **Hydrogel** IOLs are similar to hydrophilic acrylic IOLs but have a high water content and tend to have a much higher incidence of PCO.

3. **Multifocal** IOLs are now available that allow clear vision at different distances. So called accommodative IOLs attempt to flex and change focal length but in practice the amplitude of accommodation is slight. Pseudo-accommodative IOLs achieve their purpose by refractive or diffractive means.

4. **Other features.** IOLs are now available that contain filters for blue light to counteract the possibility of damage to the retina by certain wavelengths of light. Aspheric optics to minimize spherical aberrations are also being introduced. Finally, a number of toric IOLs to correct pre-existing corneal astigmatism are available.

Anaesthesia

The vast majority of cataract surgery is performed under local anaesthesia (LA) although general anaesthesia is required for children, mentally handicapped patients and those with a head tremor.

1. **Peribulbar block** is the most commonly performed LA. It is given through the skin or conjunctiva with a 25mm needle (Fig. 12.7a and b).
2. **Sub-Tenon block** involves passing a blunt tipped cannula through an incision in the conjunctiva and Tenon capsule 5mm from the limbus, and along sub-Tenon space (Fig. 12.7c). The anaesthetic is injected beyond the equator of the globe (Fig. 12.7d). Although anaesthesia is good and complications minimal, akinesia is variable.
3. **Topical-intracameral anaesthesia** involves initial surface anaesthesia with drops or gel (proxymetacaine 0.5%, lidocaine 2%) which can be augmented with intracameral injection or infusion of diluted preservative-free lidocaine 1%, usually during hydrodissection. Although analgesia is adequate, patients need to be warned that there is not true anaesthesia as sensation is still intact. Despite the absence of akinesia most patients

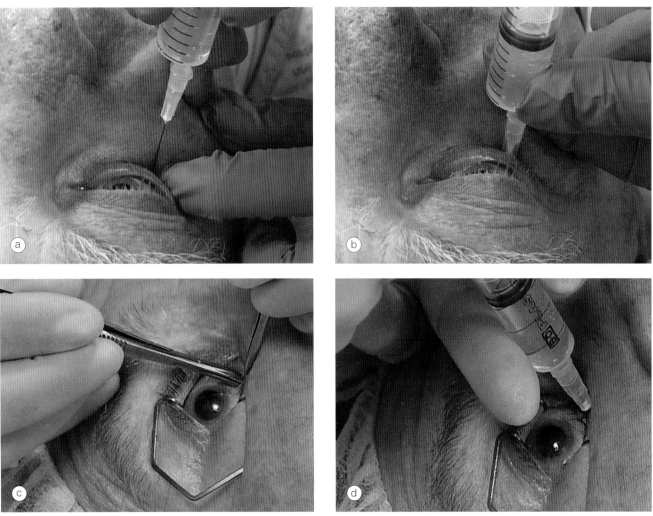

Fig. 12.7
Peribulbar anaesthesia. **(a)** Insertion of needle; **(b)** injection. Sub-Tenon anaesthesia. **(c)** Dissection; **(d)** injection

can cooperate sufficiently by fixing the microscope filament.

Extracapsular cataract extraction

When IOLs became more widely used in the 1980s the technique most surgeons used was extracapsular cataract extraction (ECCE) having changed from intracapsular extraction. Although ECCE requires a relatively large circumferential limbal incision (8–10mm) it was relatively simple and straightforward to learn without investment in new expensive equipment. After a 'can opener' capsulotomy was performed with a bent needle or cystitome the lens nucleus was expressed. Cortical matter was then aspirated, leaving behind an intact posterior capsule. This provided a satisfactory location for the insertion of the IOL into the

capsular bag. The incision was then sutured, sometimes inducing considerable corneal astigmatism. This slowed visual recovery as the stitches often required removal at about 3 months postoperatively and the astigmatism could change for some time thereafter.

Phacoemulsification

Introduction

Phacoemulsification (phaco) has become the preferred method over the last 15 years. The smaller incision of phacoemulsification compared to ECCE renders the operation safer, since decompression of the eye is avoided. In addition, the procedure is associated with little induced postoperative astigmatism and early stabilization of refraction (usually 3 weeks for 3mm incisions). Postoperative wound-related problems such as iris prolapse are almost eliminated. One disadvantage of phaco is that it requires complex machinery to break up the lens nucleus and remove it through a small incision. Considerable training is required to learn the techniques.

Phacodynamics

The surgeon must understand the machine dynamics and the interaction of fluidics in treating different forms of cataract. The various machines behave differently but the basic mechanism is similar. Choosing appropriate settings makes surgery easier and safer.

1. **Level of irrigating bottle** is measured from the level of the patient's eye. The purpose of having the bottle at a specific height is to maintain a stable eye at a reasonable intraocular pressure. The infusion flow is proportional to the height of the bottle and is dependent on gravity.
2. **Aspiration flow rate** (AFR) refers to the volume of fluid removed from the eye in ml/min. For a higher AFR the bottle must be elevated to compensate for increased fluid loss. High AFR results in attraction of lens material towards the phaco tip like a magnet with faster vacuum build up and swifter removal of lens matter but with less power.
3. **Vacuum** is measured in mmHg and is generated during occlusion when the pump is trying to aspirate fluid. Vacuum helps to hold nuclear material and provides the ability to manipulate lens fragments. High vacuum also decreases the need of the total power required to remove the lens.
4. **Surge.** When occlusion is broken pent up energy in the system results in surge. This may result in collapse of the anterior chamber and capsular rupture.

NB Once the concepts of AFR and vacuum are understood they can be modified as appropriate.

Pumps

1. **Flow peristaltic pumps** pull liquid and lens material into the phaco tip by milking fluid-filled tubing over rollers inside the cassette attached to the phaco machine. The speed at which this is performed is determined by the speed of turning of the rollers. However, in order for the pump to work effectively occlusion of the tip is required so that vacuum can build in the system. As vacuum builds to the preset level the pump slows down until it stops when the required vacuum is achieved.
2. **The Venturi** pump generates vacuum by creating a negative pressure in a vessel by passing compressed gas across its entrance. This means that there is no difference between vacuum and AFR. Depression of the foot pedal increases vacuum towards the preset level which is not dependent on occlusion. Tip vacuum is therefore always present in a machine with a Venturi pump.

Handpiece

The handpiece (Fig. 12.8a) contains a series of piezoelectric crystals which act as rapid switching devices to enable the tip to vibrate longitudinally at ultrasonic frequencies. The tip consists of a hollow titanium needle 1.1–0.7mm in diameter with a sleeve to protect the cornea from thermal and mechanical damage (Fig. 12.8b). Different shaped phaco needles have various characteristics in terms of emulsifying and holding nuclear material. Emulsification of the lens is the result of the following phenomena:

1. **Jackhammer** pneumatic drill effect is probably the most important.
2. **Cavitation** resulting from the swift movement of solid in a liquid. At the end of each oscillation backstroke, the tip retracts and creates a vacuum which causes cavitation bubbles. The bubbles implode and release large amounts of energy causing emulsification of the lens matter.
3. **Acoustic shock wave** generated by the excursion of the phaco tip.
4. **Impact of the fluid particle wave** as the tip impacts on aqueous. In softer cataracts it is possible to see this in action by removing tissue without direct contact.

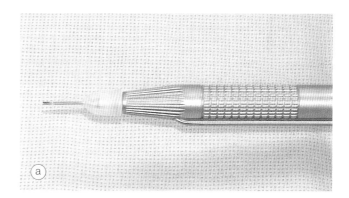

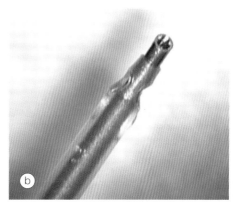

Fig. 12.8 (a) Phaco handpiece with tip; **(b)** phaco tip with sleeve

Viscoelastics

Viscoelastics are sophisticated biopolymers whose main constituents are glycosaminoglycans and hydroxypropyl-methylcellulose. The two main types are the following:

1. **Cohesive** (Healon, Healon 5, Healon GV and Provisc)
   - Long chains and high molecular weight.
   - Used to create and maintain intraocular spaces.
   - Cause raised intraocular pressure unless removed.
   - Easy to remove.
2. **Dispersive** (Viscoat)
   - Low molecular weight and a tendency to break up.
   - Used to coat and protect the endothelium.
   - Used to create and maintain space, forming compartments.
   - Do not cause raised intraocular pressure.
   - More difficult to remove than cohesive viscoelastics.
3. **Clinical uses**
   - Soft shell technique involves the injection of a dispersive and then a cohesive viscoelastic underneath. The former adheres to and protects the endothelium
   - If the capsulorrhexis is running out to the periphery, injecting a high molecular weight cohesive viscoelastic will flatten the anterior capsule and push the iris away.
   - In small pupils a high molecular weight cohesive viscoelastic will push the iris away from the lens and induce mydriasis.
   - In small posterior capsular tears a dispersive viscoelastic will push the vitreous back into the posterior chamber and plug the capsular defect.

Technique

It is beyond the scope of this book to describe the technique in detail. The following are the basic steps:

1. **Preparation**
   a. Topical anaesthetic is instilled into the conjunctival sac.
   b. Povidone-iodine 5% is instilled into the conjunctival sac (Fig. 12.9a) and is also used to paint the skin of the eyelids prior to draping (Fig. 12.9b).
   c. Careful draping is performed ensuring that the lashes and lid margins are isolated from the surgical field and a speculum is inserted (Fig. 12.9c).
2. **Incisions**
   a. Two side port stab incisions are made 180° apart, the first 30–60° to the left of the main incision.
   b. The corneal incision may be clear corneal or limbal (Fig. 12.10a); a temporal incision is preferred for topical anaesthesia.
   c. Viscoelastic is injected into the anterior chamber.
3. **Capsulorrhexis** should be continuous, central and curvilinear (Fig. 12.10b). It is performed either with a cystitome or bent needle and involves two movements:

   a. Shearing, in which a tangential vector force is applied along the direction of the tear.
   b. Ripping, in which a centripetal vector force strains and tears the capsule.
4. **Hydrodissection** is performed to separate the nucleus and cortex from the capsule so that the nucleus can be more easily and safely rotated.
   a. A 26-gauge blunt cannula with fluid is inserted just beneath the edge of the rhexis and fluid is injected under the capsule (Fig. 12.10c).
   b. A hydrodissection wave should be seen provided there is a good red reflex.
   c. The phaco probe is inserted and the superficial cortex and epinucleus are aspirated.
5. **Four quadrant** ('divide and conquer') technique for removal of the nucleus is well suited for the trainee surgeon because it is fairly easy to achieve consistency early in the learning process.
   a. 'Sculpting' is performed with the probe to create a groove (Fig. 12.10d).
   b. The nucleus is rotated and a second groove is made at right angle to the first.
   c. The probe and second instrument are engaged in opposite walls of the groove and the nucleus is cracked by applying force in opposite directions (Fig. 12.10e).
   d. The nucleus is rotated 90° and a crack made in the perpendicular groove in a similar manner.
   e. Each of the four quadrants is emulsified and aspirated in turn (Fig. 12.10f).
6. **Nuclear phaco chop** takes greater experience, but has the advantage of requiring much less expenditure of energy.
   a. In horizontal chopping a blunt-tipped chopper is placed horizontally underneath the capsule and then turned vertically as the equator is reached.
   b. Vertical chopping is performed with a pointed-tip chopper which does not need to pass beyond the capsulorrhexis.
   c. The nucleus is chopped into several pieces each of which is emulsified and aspirated.
7. **Cortical clean up.** The cortical fragments are engaged by vacuum, pulled centrally and aspirated (Fig. 12.11a).
8. **Insertion of IOL**
   a. The capsular bag is filled with viscoelastic (Fig. 12.11b).
   b. The corneal incision is enlarged (Fig. 12.11c).
   c. The IOL is folded and then inserted into the capsular bag (Fig. 12.11d); a special injector may be used to insert a pre-folded IOL.
   d. The IOL is centred by dialling (Fig. 12.11e).
9. **Completion**
   a. Viscoelastic is aspirated.
   b. The side port incisions are sealed with a jet of saline (Fig. 12.11f).
   c. A subconjunctival injection of steroid and antibiotic is given.

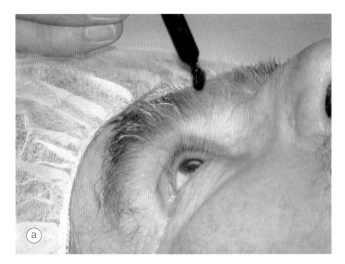

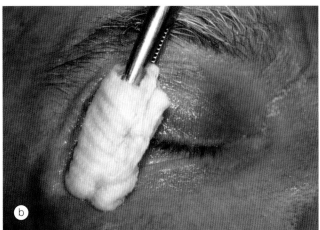

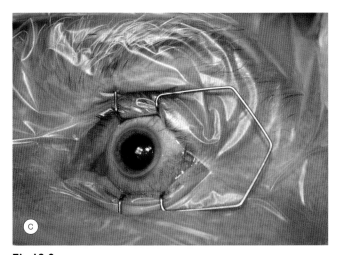

Fig.12.9
Preparation. **(a)** Povidone-iodine 5% is instilled; **(b)** skin is painted; **(c)** drapes isolate the eyelids from the operating field

Small incision manual cataract surgery

Small incision manual cataract surgery is a good alternative to phacoemulsification in countries where very high volume surgery with inexpensive instrumentation is required. The procedure is fast and has a low rate of complications, and can be performed on the dense cataract. The major disadvantage is that because round edge PMMA IOLs are used there is still a high incidence of PCO necessitating capsulotomy. The technique is as follows:

a. A self-sealing partial thickness scleral tunnel is dissected and the anterior chamber is entered (Fig. 12.12a).
b. Capsulorrhexis is performed (Fig. 12.12b).
c. Hydrodissection is performed and the nucleus partly prolapsed into the anterior chamber (Fig. 12.12c).
d. A small hook is inserted between the posterior capsule and nucleus, and the nucleus extracted (Fig. 12.12d). It is also possible to extract the nucleus with an irrigating vectis.
e. The epinucleus and residual cortex are aspirated with a Simcoe cannula (Fig. 12.12e).
f. The IOL is inserted (Fig. 12.12f).

Operative complications

Complications of cataract surgery can occur at any stage of the procedure. As this is not a textbook of cataract surgery all of the possible complications and their management will not be discussed.

Rupture of the posterior capsule

Capsular rupture is serious because it may be accompanied by vitreous loss, posterior migration of lens material and, rarely, expulsive haemorrhage. Long-term complications of vitreous loss, particularly if inappropriately managed, include up-drawn pupil, uveitis, vitreous touch, vitreous wick syndrome, endophthalmitis, glaucoma, posterior dislocation of the IOL, retinal detachment and chronic cystoid macular oedema.

1. **Signs**
   - Sudden deepening of the anterior chamber and momentary pupillary dilatation.
   - The nucleus falls away and will not come towards the phaco tip.
   - Vitreous may be aspirated into the phaco tip.
   - The torn capsule or vitreous may be directly visible.
2. **Management** depends on the magnitude of the tear and the presence or absence of vitreous prolapse. The main principles of management are as follows:
   a. Dispersive viscoelastic may be injected behind nuclear material with the purpose of expressing it into the anterior chamber and also preventing anterior herniation of vitreous.

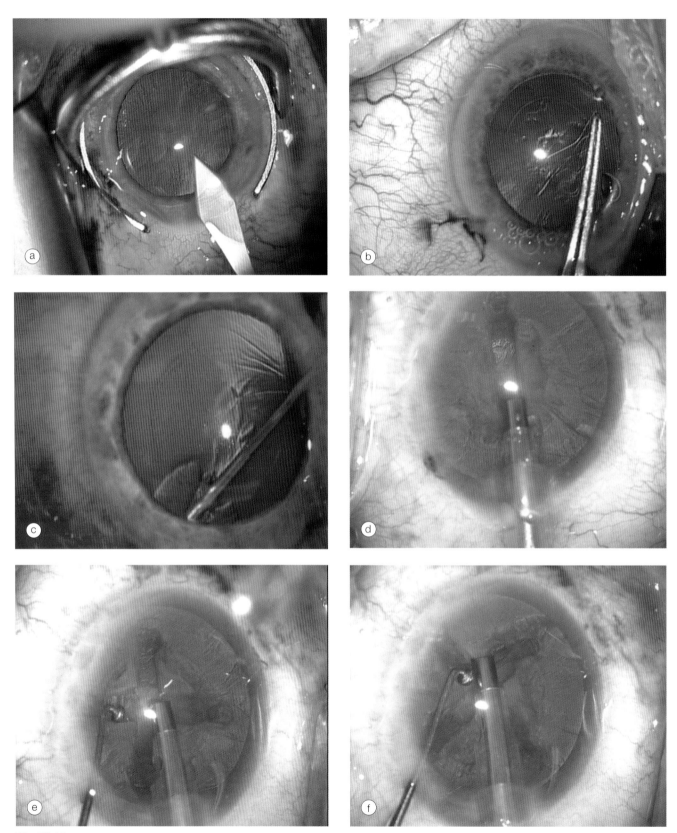

Fig. 12.10
Four quadrant ('divide and conquer') phacoemulsification. **(a)** Corneal incision; **(b)** capsulorrhexis; **(c)** hydrodissection; **(d)** nucleus is grooved; **(e)** nucleus is cracked; **(f)** each nuclear quadrant is emulsified and aspirated

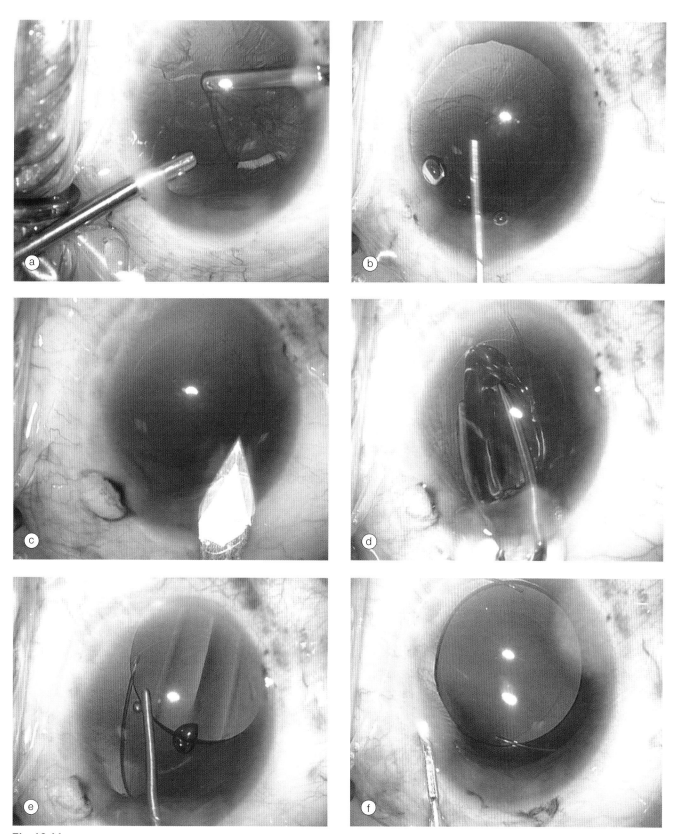

Fig. 12.11

Completion of phacoemulsification. **(a)** Cortical lens matter is pulled centrally and aspirated: **(b)** viscoelastic is injected into the capsular bag; **(c)** incision is enlarged; **(d)** IOL is inserted; **(e)** IOL is dialled; **(f)** sideports are hydrated

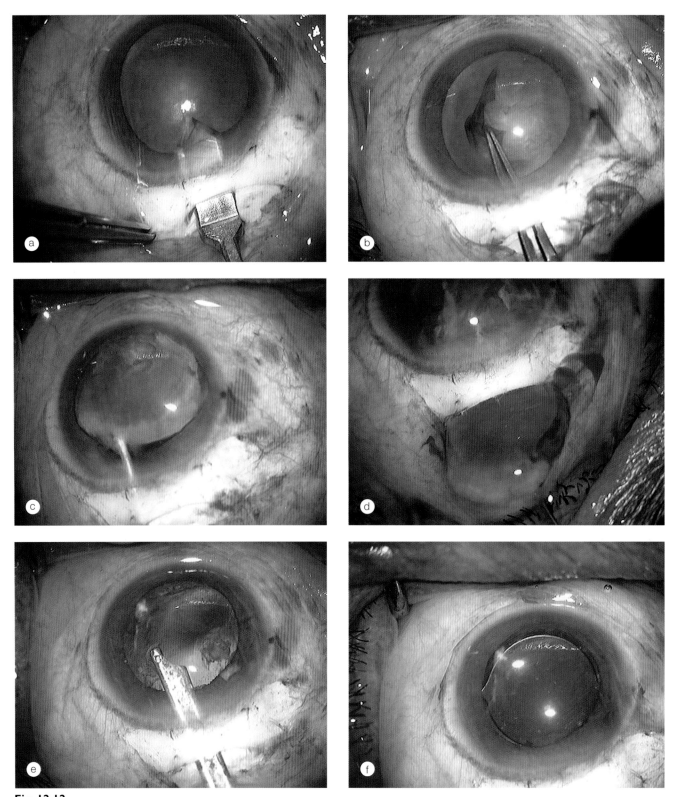

Fig. 12.12
Small incision manual cataract surgery. **(a)** Anterior chamber is entered; **(b)** capsulorrhexis; **(c)** partial prolapse of nucleus into anterior chamber; **(d)** extraction of nucleus with hook; **(e)** cortical cleanup; **(f)** IOL in place (Courtesy of A Hennig)

b. A lens glide is passed behind the lens fragments to cover the capsular defect (Fig. 12.13).

c. The lens fragments are removed by visco-expression or by phaco if it is desirable to maintain a small incision.

d. All vitreous is removed from the anterior chamber and the wound with a vitrector.

e. A small posterior capsular tear may allow careful in-the-bag implantation of a PC-IOL.

g. A large tear will usually allow ciliary sulcus fixation of a three piece PC-IOL with the optic captured in the capsular bag.

h. Insufficient capsular support may necessitate suturing the IOL to the sulcus or implanting an AC-IOL with the aid of a glide (Fig. 12.14). AC-IOLs are, however, associated with a higher risk of complications including bullous keratopathy, hyphaema, iris tuck and pupillary irregularities.

NB Conditions may not be favourable for correct positioning of an AC-IOL. It may then be safer not to proceed with implantation and to consider visual rehabilitation with a contact lens or secondary IOL implantation at a later date.

Posterior loss of lens fragments

Dislocation of fragments of lens material into the vitreous cavity after zonular dehiscence or posterior capsule rupture is rare but potentially serious because it may result in glaucoma, chronic uveitis, retinal detachment and chronic cystoid macular oedema. Initially, any uveitis or raised intraocular pressure must be treated. The patient should then be referred to a vitreoretinal surgeon for removal of nuclear fragments by pars plana vitrectomy.

Posterior dislocation of IOL

Dislocation of an IOL into the vitreous cavity (Fig. 12.15a) reflects inappropriate implantation and is rare. It is a serious complication, particularly if it is accompanied by posterior loss of nuclear material (Fig. 12.15b). If the IOL is left it may lead to vitreous haemorrhage, retinal detachment, uveitis and chronic cystoid macular oedema. Treatment involves pars plana vitrectomy with removal, repositioning or exchange of the IOL depending on the extent of capsular support.

Suprachoroidal haemorrhage

A suprachoroidal haemorrhage is a bleed into the suprachoroidal space which may result in extrusion of intraocular contents (expulsive haemorrhage) or apposition of retinal surfaces. It is a dreaded but rare complication and much less

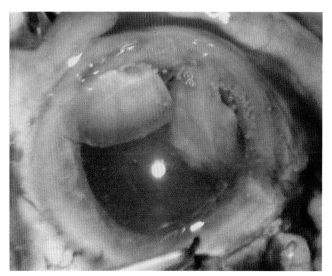

Fig. 12.13
Lens glide supporting nuclear fragments following rupture of the posterior capsule (Courtesy of R Packard)

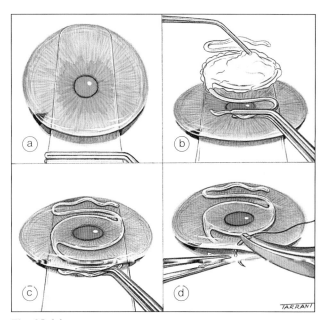

Fig. 12.14
Insertion of an anterior chamber IOL. **(a)** Glide is inserted; **(b)** IOL is coated with viscoelastic; **(c)** IOL is inserted; **(d)** incision is sutured

likely with phacoemulsification. The source of the bleeding is a ruptured long or short posterior ciliary artery. Although the exact cause is unknown, contributing factors include advanced age, glaucoma, increased axial length, systemic cardiovascular disease and vitreous loss.

1. **Signs** in chronological order
   a. Progressive shallowing of the anterior chamber, increased intraocular pressure and prolapse of the iris.
   b. Vitreous extrusion, loss of the red reflex and the appearance of a dark mound behind the pupil.
   c. In severe cases, all intraocular contents may be extruded through the incision.
2. **Immediate treatment** involves closure of the incision. Although posterior sclerotomy has been advocated, it may actually exacerbate the bleeding and result in a vicious circle with loss of the eye. Postoperatively, the patient should be treated with topical and systemic steroids to reduce intraocular inflammation.
3. **Subsequent management.** Ultrasonography may be used to assess severity. Surgery is performed 7–14 days later when the blood clot has liquefied. The blood is drained, and pars plana vitrectomy with air–fluid exchange performed. Although the visual prognosis is grave, useful vision may be salvaged in some cases.

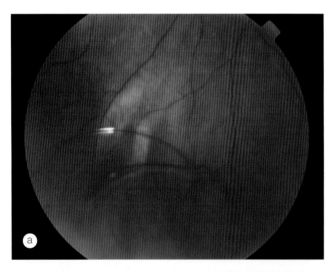

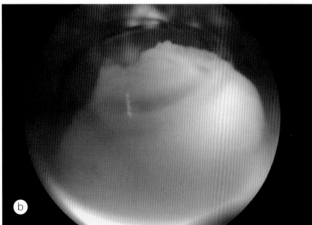

Fig. 12.15
(a) IOL on the retina; **(b)** IOL and large nuclear fragments in the vitreous (Courtesy of S Milewski)

Acute postoperative endophthalmitis

Pathogenesis

Acute endophthalmitis is a devastating complication of intraocular surgery. The estimated incidence following cataract surgery is approximately 0.15%. This has decreased over the last decade despite a great increase in the throughput of cataract surgery. Toxins produced by the infecting bacteria and the host inflammatory responses cause rapid and irreversible photoreceptor damage that can continue long after the ocular contents have been rendered sterile.

1. **Risk factors** include age over 80 years, diabetes, secondary lens implantation, posterior capsule rupture and cataract surgery combined with other procedures.
2. **Pathogens.** About 90% of isolates are Gram-positive and 10% Gram-negative. In order of frequency they include:
   - Coagulase-negative staphylococci (*S. epidermidis*).
   - Other Gram-positive organisms (*S. aureus* and *Streptococcus* spp.).
   - Gram-negative organisms (*Pseudomonas* spp. and *Proteus* spp.).
3. **The source of infection** usually cannot be identified with certainty. It is thought that the flora of the eyelids and conjunctiva are the most frequent source. Other potential sources of infection include contaminated solutions and instruments, the air in theatre, and the surgeon or operating room personnel.

Prophylaxis

Because of the low rate of endophthalmitis it is very difficult to prove that any method of prophylaxis is effective or superior to any other. Prophylaxis reduces the colony counts of organisms on the surface of the eye, but it cannot sterilize the surface. Apart from instilling povidone-iodine and careful draping the following measures may be beneficial:

1. **Treatment of pre-existing infections** such as blepharitis, conjunctivitis, chronic dacryocystitis and infection in the contralateral eye or socket.
2. **Prophylactic antibiotics**
   - Preoperative topical fluoroquinolone antibiotics given in regimen from 1 hour to 3 days before surgery.
   - Intracameral cefuroxime injected at the end of surgery.
   - Postoperative subconjunctival injection of antibiotics is commonly performed and can achieve bactericidal levels in the anterior chamber for 1–2 hours.

NB Intraoperative perfusion of the anterior chamber by adding vancomycin or gentamicin to the infusion fluid is unlikely to be effective as bactericidal levels are lost almost immediately after the end of surgery. This may also encourage emergence of vancomycin resistant strains of bacteria.

Clinical features

1. **Symptoms** are pain and visual loss.
2. **Signs** vary according to severity.
   - Chemosis, conjunctival injection and discharge.
   - Relative afferent pupil defect.
   - Corneal haze (Fig. 12.16a)
   - Fibrinous exudate and hypopyon (Fig. 12.16b).
   - Vitritis with impaired view of the fundus (Fig. 12.16c).
   - Severe vitreous inflammation and debris with loss of the red reflex (Fig. 12.16d).

Differential diagnosis

If there is any doubt about the diagnosis, treatment should be that of infectious endophthalmitis.

1. **Retained lens material** in the anterior chamber or vitreous may precipitate a severe uveitis, corneal oedema and raised intraocular pressure.
2. **Vitreous haemorrhage,** especially if blood in the vitreous is depigmented.
3. **Postoperative uveitis.** A confident diagnosis of infection can be difficult in patients with a prior history of uveitis. If signs of inflammation are mild a trial of topical steroid therapy and early review (< 6h) is appropriate. If there is not substantial improvement management should be that of endophthalmitis.
4. **Toxic reaction** to the use of inappropriate or contaminated irrigating fluid or viscoelastic. An intense fibrinous reaction with corneal oedema may develop although other signs of infectious endophthalmitis are absent. Treatment is with intensive topical steroids combined with cycloplegics.
5. **Complicated or prolonged surgery** may result in corneal oedema and uveitis.

Identification of pathogens

Samples for culture should be obtained from aqueous and vitreous to confirm the diagnosis. However, negative culture does not necessarily rule out infection and treatment should be continued. The samples can be taken in a minor procedures operating room as follows.

1. **Preparation**
   - Povidone-iodine 5% is instilled and the eye draped.
   - Topical and subconjunctival or peribulbar anaesthesia is administered.
2. **Aqueous samples**
   - 0.1–0.2ml of aqueous is aspirated via a limbal paracentesis using a 25G needle on a tuberculin syringe.
   - The syringe is capped and labelled.
3. **Vitreous samples** are more likely to yield a positive culture than aqueous.

- A 2ml syringe and a 23G needle may be used or a special disposable vitrector (Fig. 12.17a).
- The distance from the limbus for the scleral incision is measured with calipers and marked (Fig. 12.17b) – 4mm (phakic eye) or 3mm (aphakic eye).
- 0.2–0.4ml are aspirated from the mid-vitreous cavity (Fig. 12.17c).

Treatment

1. **Intravitreal antibiotics** are the key to management. They achieve levels above the minimum inhibitors concentration of most pathogens, and these are maintained for days. They should be administered immediately after culture specimens have been obtained. The two antibiotics used are ceftazidime, which will kill most Gram-negative organisms (including *P. aeruginosa*), and vancomycin, which will kill coagulase-negative and coagulase-positive cocci (including methicillin-resistant *S. aureus*).
   - The concentrations are ceftazidime (2mg in 0.1ml) and vancomycin (2mg in 0.1ml); amikacin (0.5mg in 0.1ml) can be used as an alternative to ceftazidime in patients allergic to penicillin but is more toxic to the retina.
   - The antibiotics are injected slowly into the mid-vitreous cavity using a 25 G needle (Fig. 12.17d).
   - After the first injection has been given, the syringe is disconnected but the needle is left inside the vitreous cavity so that the second injection can be given through the same needle. Alternatively, a second needle entry can be used.
2. **Periocular antibiotic injections** are often given but are of doubtful additional benefit if intravitreal antibiotics have been used. Suggested doses are vancomycin 50mg and ceftazidime 125mg (or amikacin 50mg).
3. **Topical antibiotics** are of limited benefit in the absence of associated infectious keratitis. Vancomycin 5% (50mg/ml) or ceftazidime 5% (50mg/ml) applied intensively may penetrate the cornea in therapeutic levels.
4. **Oral antibiotics** Fluoroquinolones penetrate the eye and moxifloxacin 400mg daily for 10 days is recommended; clarithromycin 500mg b.d. may be helpful for culture-negative infections.
5. **Oral steroids.** The rationale for the use of steroids is to limit the destructive complications of the inflammatory process. Prednisolone 60mg daily should be started in severe cases after 12 hours provided fungal infection has been excluded from examination of smears.
6. **Periocular steroids** dexamethasone (12mg) or triamcinolone (1.0mg) should be considered if systemic therapy is contraindicated.
7. **Topical dexamethasone** 0.1% q.i.d for anterior uveitis.
8. **Intravitreal steroids** (dexamethasone 400µm) is controversial. Although it reduces inflammation in the short term it does not influence the final visual outcome. Some

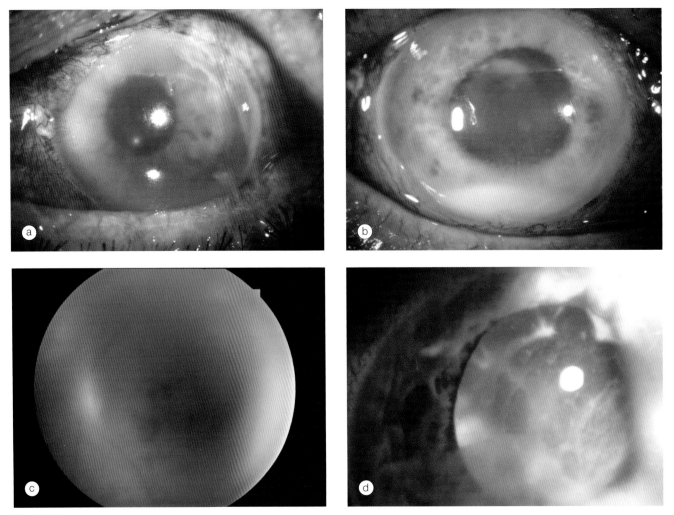

Fig. 12.16
Acute bacterial endophthalmitis. **(a)** Corneal haze; **(b)** fibrinous exudate and hypopyon; **(c)** vitreous haze and impaired fundus view; **(d)** severe vitritis (Courtesy of S Tuft – figs a, b and d)

studies even suggest a detrimental effect. Conversely, improvement in outcome in some bacterial sub-groups has been reported.

9. **Pars plana vitrectomy.** The Endophthalmitis Vitrectomy Study (EVS) showed a benefit from immediate pars plana vitrectomy in eyes with a visual acuity of perception of light (*not* hand movements vision or any better acuity level) at presentation, with a 50% reduction in severe visual loss.

   NB The conclusions of the EVS cannot be extrapolated to other forms of endophthalmitis that have a different microbiological spectrum.

Microbiology

The syringes should be sent directly to the laboratory during working hours even if they appear to be empty (do not send needles).

1. **Culture media**
   - Blood agar.
   - Cooked meat broth.
   - Brain–heart infusion.
   - Slide for Gram stain if sufficient sample is available.

   NB A standard blood culture bottle is an alternative if specific media are unavailable.

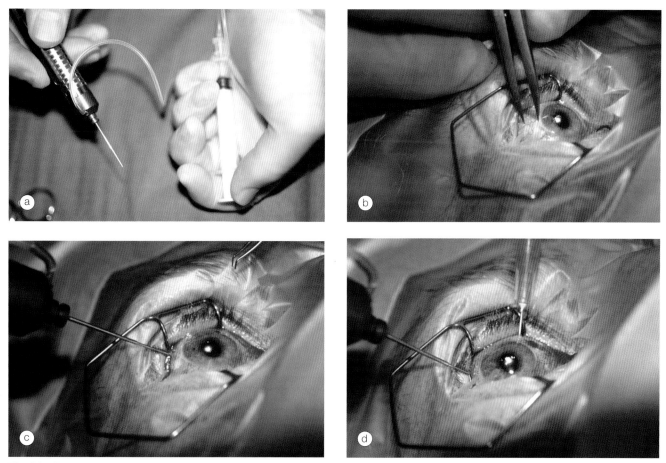

Fig. 12.17
Management of endophthalmitis. **(a)** Mini-vitrector for obtaining vitreous samples; **(b)** calipers measuring distance from limbus; **(c)** vitreous samples obtained with vitrector; **(d)** intravitreal antibiotic injection

2. **Polymerase chain reaction** (PCR) can be helpful in identifying unusual organisms, the cause of culture negative disease, and organisms after antibiotic treatment has been started. The great sensitivity means that contamination can lead to false positive results.

Subsequent management

Subsequent management is partly determined by culture results and clinical findings. Ultrasonography may be useful in assessing response to treatment.

1. **Signs of improvement** include contraction of fibrinous exudate, and reduction of anterior chamber cellular activity and hypopyon. In this situation treatment is not modified irrespective of culture results.
2. **If the clinical signs are worsening** after 48 hours antibiotic sensitivities should be reviewed and therapy modified accordingly. A vitrectomy should be considered if not previously performed. Intravitreal antibiotics can be repeated after 2 days.
3. **The outcome** is related to the duration of the infection prior to treatment and the virulence of organisms.
   • If visual acuity at presentation is light perception 30% of eyes achieve 6/12 following treatment. If visual acuity is better than light perception this increases to 60%.
   • Infection with *B. cereus* and streptococci has a poor visual outcome despite aggressive and appropriate therapy, probably due to early retinopathy from exotoxins released by the organisms.

Complications

Severe visual loss may occur in patients presenting with any level of visual acuity. The severity of endophthalmitis reflects the virulence of the offending organism. *Streptococcal* spp.,

S. aureus and *Enterococcus* spp. infections tend to be aggressive with a poor visual outcome despite early treatment. Endophthalmitis caused by *S. epidermidis* has a more gradual onset with milder disease. The main causes of visual loss are:
- Chronic uveitis, macular oedema and macular ischaemia.
- Secondary glaucoma.
- Retinal detachment.
- Phthisis.
- Panophthalmitis or perforation that requires evisceration.

Delayed-onset postoperative endophthalmitis

Pathogenesis

Delayed-onset endophthalmitis develops following cataract surgery when an organism of low virulence becomes trapped within the capsular bag. It has an onset ranging from 4 weeks to years (mean 9 months) postoperatively and typically follows uneventful surgery. It may rarely be precipitated by YAG-laser capsulotomy, which releases the sequestrated organism from the posterior capsule into the vitreous. The infection is caused most frequently by *P. acnes* and occasionally *S. epidermidis*, *Corynebacterium* spp. or *Candida parapsilosis*.

Diagnosis

1. **Presentation** is with painless mild progressive visual deterioration which may be associated with floaters.
2. **Signs**
   - Low-grade anterior uveitis, sometimes with mutton-fat keratic precipitates (Fig. 12.18a).
   - Vitritis is common but hypopyon infrequent.
   - An enlarging capsular plaque composed of organisms sequestrated in residual cortex within the peripheral capsular bag is characteristic (Fig. 12.18b).

   NB It is important to perform gonioscopy under mydriasis so as not to miss an equatorial plaque.

3. **Investigations.** The diagnosis should be confirmed by cultures of the aqueous and vitreous with growth of the organism. Anaerobic culture should be requested if *P. acnes* infection is suspected and isolates may take 10–14 days to grow. Detection rate of pathogens can be greatly improved with PCR.
4. **Clinical course.** Without antibiotic treatment the inflammation initially responds well to topical steroids (Fig. 12.18c), but recurs when treatment is stopped and eventually becomes steroid resistant (Fig. 12.18d).

Treatment

Because the sequestered organisms are isolated from host defences and antibiotics, antibiotic treatment alone is unlikely to be successful.

1. **Removal** of the capsular bag, residual cortex and IOL is recommended and requires pars plana vitrectomy. Secondary IOL implantation may be considered at a later date.
2. **Intravitreal vancomycin** (1mg in 0.1ml) is the antibiotic of choice although *P. acnes* is also sensitive to methicillin, cefazolin and clindamycin.

Posterior capsular opacification

Visually significant PCO is the most common late complication of uncomplicated cataract surgery. Apart from reducing visual acuity, it may impair contrast sensitivity, cause difficulties with glare or give rise to monocular diplopia. The incidence of PCO is reduced when the rhexis is in complete contact with the anterior surface of the IOL. Certain acrylic IOLs may be associated with lower rates of PCO than PMMA and silicone lenses. Implant design may also be relevant in this context; notably, a square 'edge' to the optic appears to inhibit PCO.

Signs

1. **Elschnig pearls** (bladder cells, Wedl cells) are caused by the proliferation and migration of residual equatorial epithelial cells along the posterior capsule at the site of apposition between the remnants of the anterior capsule and the posterior capsule. They impart a vacuolated appearance to the posterior capsule, best visualized on retroillumination (Fig. 12.19a). This is the most frequently seen type of opacification and is related to the patient's age. It is extremely common in children if a posterior capsulorrhexis is not performed at the time of surgery.
2. **Capsular fibrosis** (Fig. 12.19b), due to fibrous metaplasia of epithelial cells, is less common and usually appears earlier than Elschnig pearls.

Treatment

Treatment involves the creation of an opening in the posterior capsule, with the Nd:YAG laser.

1. **Indications** for capsulotomy include:
   - Diminished visual acuity.
   - Diplopia or glare, secondary to capsular wrinkling.
   - Inadequate fundus view impairing diagnosis, monitoring or treatment of retinal disease.

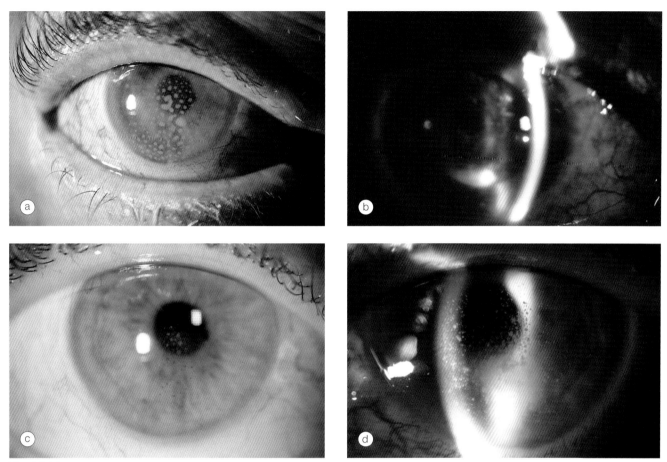

Fig. 12.18
Delayed-onset postoperative endophthalmitis. **(a)** Anterior uveitis with mutton-fat keratic precipitates; **(b)** white capsular plaque; **(c)** fewer keratic precipitates following topical steroid therapy; **(d)** severe recurrence 2 weeks following cessation of steroid therapy

2. **Technique.** Safe and successful laser capsulotomy involves accurate focusing and using the minimum energy required. Laser power is initially set 1mJ/pulse, and may be increased if necessary. A series of punctures are applied in a cruciate pattern, the first puncture aimed at the visual axis. An opening of about 3mm is usually adequate (Fig. 12.19c), but larger capsulotomies may be necessary for retinal examination or photocoagulation.

3. **Complications**
   - Damage to the IOL ('pitting') (Fig. 12.19d) may occur if the laser is poorly focused. Although undesirable, a few laser marks on the IOL do not alter visual function or impair ocular tolerance of the IOL.
   - Cystoid macular oedema is an occasional complication that may develop months after capsulotomy. It is less common when capsulotomy is delayed for 6 months or more after surgery.
   - Rhegmatogenous retinal detachment is rare, except in high myopes and may occur several months after capsulotomy.

   - Intraocular pressure elevation, which may be acute or chronic, is uncommon.
   - Posterior IOL subluxation or dislocation is rare but may occur, particularly with plate haptic silicone and hydrogel IOLs.
   - Chronic endophthalmitis due to release of sequestered organisms into the vitreous is very rare.

NB Most patients who develop complications have no identifiable risk factor. The number of laser pulses and the energy level are probably not related to their development.

Anterior capsular contraction

Since the advent of continuous curvilinear capsulorrhexis, contraction of the anterior capsular opening (capsulophimosis) has become one of the most common postoperative complications. It occurs several weeks after surgery and is

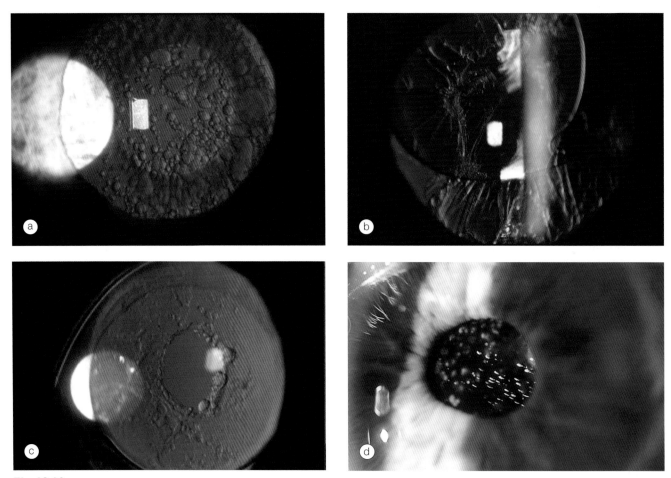

Fig. 12.19
Posterior capsular opacification. **(a)** Elschnig pearls; **(b)** capsular fibrosis; **(c)** appearance following laser capsulotomy; **(d)** laser pitting of the IOL (Courtesy of P Gili – figs a and b; R Packard – fig. c; R Curtis – fig. d)

accompanied by subcapsular fibrosis (Fig. 12.20). The contraction typically progresses for up to 3 months, and if severe, may require Nd:YAG laser capsulotomy. The severity of contraction is related to the optic material. The highest rate is with plate-haptic silicone IOLs and the lowest with three-piece acrylic optic-PMMA haptic IOLs. A small capsulorrhexis may also be of relevance.

Miscellaneous complications

Corneal oedema

Corneal oedema is usually transient and often caused by intraoperative trauma to the endothelium by contact with lens matter, instruments or IOL. Eyes with pre-existing Fuchs endothelial dystrophy are at increased risk. Other causes include excessive power during phacoemulsification,

complicated or prolonged surgery, and postoperative ocular hypertension. Use of appropriate viscoelastics to protect the corneal endothelium during surgery in at-risk eyes (Fuchs or hard nuclei) is prudent to minimize oedema.

Malposition of IOL

Although uncommon, malposition may be associated with both optical and structural problems. Annoying visual aberrations include glare, haloes, and monocular diplopia if the edge of the IOL becomes displaced into the pupil.

1. Causes

- Primary malposition occurs during initial surgery. This may be due to zonulodialysis, capsular rupture, or when, inadvertently, one haptic is inserted into the capsular bag and the other into the ciliary sulcus or rarely the angle (Fig. 12.21a).

- Postoperative causes include trauma, eye rubbing and capsular contraction.
2. **Treatment** with miotics may be successful in mild cases. Significant malposition may require replacement of the IOL (Fig. 12.21b).

Retinal detachment

Rhegmatogenous retinal detachment, although uncommon following uneventful ECCE or phaco, may be associated with the following risk factors:

1. **Preoperative**
   - Lattice degeneration or retinal breaks should be treated prophylactically prior to cataract surgery or laser capsulotomy if fundus view permits, or as soon as possible thereafter.
   - High myopia.
2. **Operative**
   - Disruption of the posterior capsule.
   - Vitreous loss, particularly if managed inappropriately, is associated with an approximate 7% risk of retinal detachment; myopia of over 6D increases the risk to 15%.
3. **Postoperative** laser capsulotomy, if performed within a year of cataract surgery.

Cystoid macular oedema

Cystoid macular oedema is quite common and may be demonstrated angiographically in eyes with good vision. Fortunately in most cases it is transient. It occurs more often after complicated surgery involving rupture of the posterior capsule and vitreous prolapse, sometimes with incarceration in the incision, although it may occur after uneventful surgery.

It usually presents 1–6 months after surgery. The clinical features and management are discussed in Chapter 17.

CONGENITAL CATARACT

Aetiology

Congenital cataracts occur in about 3:10,000 live births; two-thirds of cases are bilateral. The cause of cataract formation can be identified in about half of those with bilateral opacities. The most common cause is genetic mutation, usually autosomal dominant (AD). Other causes include chromosomal abnormalities such as Down syndrome, metabolic disorders such as galactosaemia and intrauterine insults such as rubella infection. Congenital cataract may also occur as part of a complex developmental disorder of the eye such as aniridia. The underlying factors of

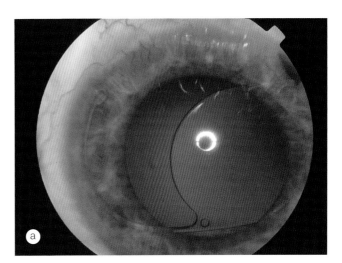

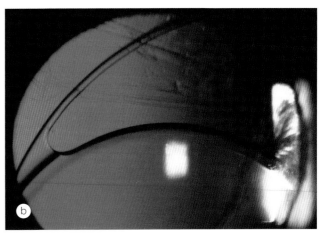

Fig. 12.21
(a) Decentred optic with one haptic in the angle and the other in the bag; **(b)** inferior subluxation of IOL (Courtesy of P Gili – fig. b)

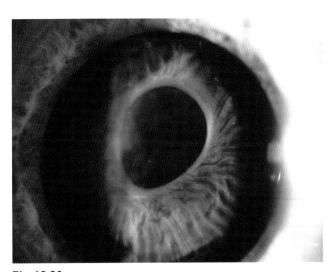

Fig. 12.20
Anterior capsular contraction and fibrosis

unilateral congenital cataracts remain less clear and the cause can be identified only in approximately 10% of cases. Unilateral cataracts are usually sporadic, without a family history or systemic disease, and affected infants are usually full-term and healthy. The most common association with unilateral cataracts is persistent anterior fetal vasculature.

Inheritance

Isolated hereditary cataracts account for about 25% of cases. The mode of inheritance is most frequently AD but may be autosomal recessive (AR) or X-linked (X-L). The morphology of the opacities and also frequently the need for surgery are usually similar in parent and offspring. About 10 loci for AD cataract have been mapped. Isolated inherited congenital cataracts carry a better visual prognosis than those with coexisting ocular and systemic abnormalities. This is because they are frequently partial at birth so that surgery may be delayed till the child is older, when there is a lower incidence of surgical complications and refractive correction is easier.

Morphology

The morphology of cataract is important because it may indicate a likely aetiology, mode of inheritance and effects on vision.

1. **Nuclear** opacities are confined to the embryonic or fetal nucleus of the lens. The cataract may be dense or composed of fine pulverulent (dust-like) opacities (Fig. 12.22a).
2. **Lamellar** opacities affect a particular lamella of the lens both anteriorly and posteriorly (Fig. 12.22b) and in some cases are associated with radial extensions (riders – Fig. 12.22c). Lamellar opacities may be AD and occur in isolation, as well as in infants with metabolic disorders and intrauterine infections.
3. **Coronary** (supranuclear) cataract, which lies in the deep cortex and surrounds the nucleus like a crown (Fig. 12.22d), is usually sporadic and only occasionally hereditary.
4. **Blue dot** opacities (cataracta punctata caerulea) (Fig. 12.22e) are common and innocuous, and may coexist with other types of lens opacities.
5. **Sutural,** in which the opacity follows the anterior or posterior Y suture, may occur in isolation or in association with other opacities (Fig. 12.22f).
6. **Anterior polar** cataract may be flat (Fig. 12.23a) or project as a conical opacity into the anterior chamber (pyramidal cataract – Fig. 12.23b). Flat anterior polar opacities are central, less than 3mm in diameter, bilateral in one-third of cases and visually insignificant. Pyramidal opacities are frequently surrounded by an area of cortical opacity and may affect vision. Occasional associations of anterior polar cataracts include persistent pupillary membrane (Fig. 12.23c), aniridia, Peters anomaly and anterior lenticonus.
7. **Posterior polar** cataract (Fig. 12.23d) may be occasionally associated with persistent hyaloid remnants (Mittendorf dots), posterior lenticonus and persistent anterior fetal vasculature.
8. **Central 'oil droplet'** opacities (Fig. 12.23e) are characteristic of galactosaemia.
9. **Membranous** cataract is rare and may be associated with Hallermann–Streiff–Francois syndrome. It occurs when the lenticular material partially or completely reabsorbs leaving behind residual chalky-white lens matter sandwiched between the anterior and posterior capsules (Fig. 12.23f).

Systemic associations

Many systemic paediatric conditions may be associated with congenital cataract. The vast majority are extremely rare and of interest only to paediatric ophthalmologists. The general ophthalmologist should, however, be aware of the following conditions.

Metabolic

1. **Galactosaemia** involves severe impairment of galactose utilization caused by absence of the enzyme galactose-1-phosphate uridyl transferase (GPUT). Inheritance is AR.
   a. **Systemic features**, which become manifest during infancy, include failure to thrive, lethargy, vomiting and diarrhoea. Reducing substance is found in the urine after drinking milk. Unless galactose, in the form of milk and milk products, is withheld from the diet, hepatosplenomegaly, renal disease, anaemia, deafness and mental handicap occur subsequently with ultimate death.
   b. **Cataract**, characterized by a central 'oil droplet' opacity (see Fig. 12.23e), develops within the first few days or weeks of life in a large percentage of patients. The exclusion of galactose from the diet prevents the progression of cataract and may reverse early lens changes.
2. **Lowe (oculocerebrorenal) syndrome** is a rare inborn error of amino acid metabolism which predominantly affects boys. Inheritance is X-L.
   a. **Systemic features** include mental handicap, Fanconi syndrome of the proximal renal tubules, muscular hypotonia, frontal prominence and sunken eyes. It is one of the few conditions in which congenital cataract and congenital glaucoma may coexist.
   b. **Cataract** is universal; the lens is also small, thin and disc-like (microphakia) and may show posterior lenticonus. Cataract may be capsular, lamellar, nuclear

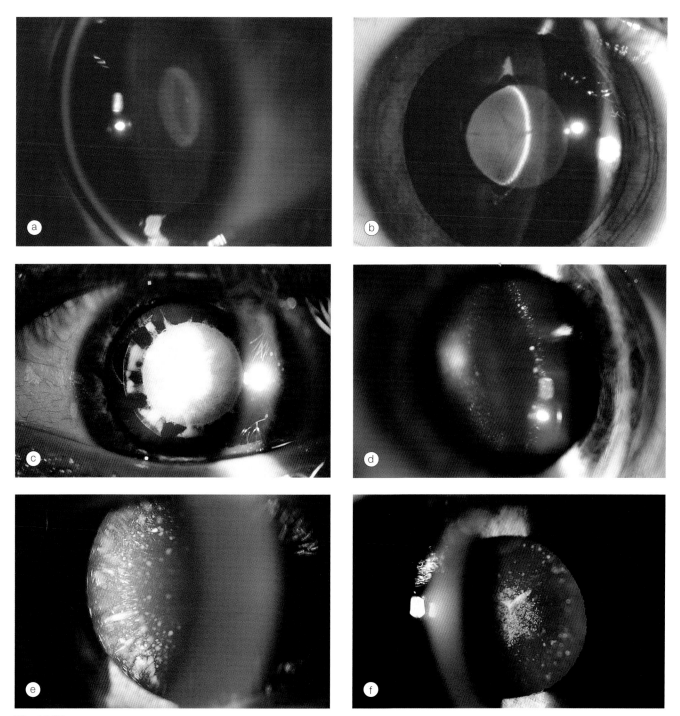

Fig. 12.22
Congenital cataract. **(a)** Nuclear pulverulent; **(b)** lamellar; **(c)** dense lamellar with riders; **(d)** coronary; **(e)** dense blue dot; **(f)** sutural and fine blue dot (Courtesy of R Curtis – fig. b; L Merin – fig. d)

or total. Female carriers manifest micropunctate cortical lens opacities, usually without visual impact.

c. *Congenital glaucoma* is present in 50% of cases.

3. **Other metabolic disorders** include hypoparathyroidism, pseudo-hypoparathyroidism, mannosidosis, Fabry disease, hypoglycaemia and hyperglycaemia.

Intrauterine infections

1. **Congenital rubella** is associated with cataract in about 15% of cases. After the gestational age of 6 weeks, the virus is incapable of crossing the lens capsule so that the lens is immune. Although the lens opacities (which may be

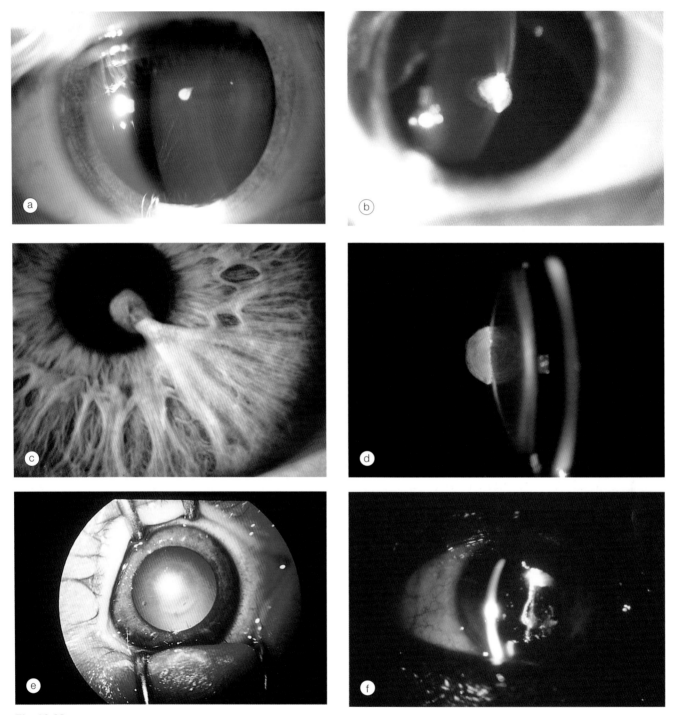

Fig. 12.23
Congenital cataract. **(a)** Flat anterior polar; **(b)** anterior pyramidal; **(c)** anterior polar with persistent pupillary membrane; **(d)** posterior polar; **(e)** 'oil droplet'; **(f)** membranous (Courtesy of K Nischal – fig. e)

unilateral or bilateral) are usually present at birth, they may occasionally develop several weeks or even months later. The opacity may involve the nucleus, with a dense pearly appearance, or may present as a more diffuse opacity involving most of the lens. The virus is capable of persisting within the lens for up to 3 years after birth.

2. **Other intrauterine infections** that may be associated with neonatal cataract are toxoplasmosis, cytomegalovirus, herpes simplex and varicella.

Chromosomal abnormalities

1. **Down syndrome (trisomy 21)**
   a. *Systemic features* include mental handicap, upward-slanting palpebral fissures, epicanthic folds, flat midface with relative prognathism, brachycephaly with flattening of the occiput, broad short hands and a protruding tongue.
   b. *Cataract* of varying morphology occurs in about 75% of patients. The opacities are usually symmetrical and often develop in late childhood.
2. **Other chromosomal abnormalities** associated with cataract include Patau (trisomy 13) and Edward (trisomy 18) syndromes.

Skeletal syndromes

1. **Hallermann–Streiff–François syndrome** is a sporadic disorder.
   a. *Systemic features* include frontal prominence, small beaked nose, baldness, progeria, micrognathia and pointed chin, short stature and hypodontia.
   b. *Cataract*, which may be membranous (see Fig. 12.23f), occurs in 90% of cases.
2. **Nance–Horan syndrome** is an X-L disorder.
   a. *Systemic features* include supernumerary incisors, prominent ears, anteverted pinnae and shortened metacarpals.
   b. *Cataract* may be dense and associated with mild microphthalmos. Female carriers may show mild sutural lens opacities.
   c. *Female carriers* may show a prominent Y suture or have Y suture opacities (see Fig. 12.22f).

Management

Ocular examination

Since a formal estimate of visual acuity cannot be obtained in the neonate, reliance is required on the density and morphology of the opacity, other ocular associated findings and visual behaviour of the child.

1. **Density** and potential impact on visual function is assessed on the basis of appearance of the red reflex and the quality of the fundus view on direct and indirect ophthalmoscopy. However, examination of a neonate has been made easier with the introduction of high quality portable slit-lamps. With assistance to restrain head movements, detailed anterior segment assessment should be possible. On ophthalmoscopy cataract density is graded as follows:
   - A very dense cataract occluding the pupil will preclude any view with either instrument and the decision to operate is straightforward.
   - A less dense cataract, which is still visually significant, will allow visualization of the retinal vasculature with the indirect but not with the direct ophthalmoscope. Other features of visually significant cataract are central or posterior opacities over 3mm in diameter.
   - A visually insignificant opacity will allow clear visualization of the retinal vasculature with both the indirect and direct ophthalmoscope. Other features of visually insignificant cataract are central opacities less than 3mm in diameter and peripheral, anterior or punctate opacities with intervening clear zones.
2. **Morphology** of the opacity can give important clues to aetiology, as described above.
3. **Associated ocular pathology** may involve the anterior segment (corneal clouding, microphthalmos, glaucoma, persistent anterior fetal vasculature) or the posterior segment (chorioretinitis, Leber amaurosis, rubella retinopathy, foveal or optic nerve hypoplasia). Examination under general anaesthesia may occasionally be required, as may repeat examinations, to document progression of cataract or associated disease. Ultrasonography using Doppler may be very useful to help diagnose persistent anterior fetal vasculature since blood flow may be seen in a persistent hyaloid artery.
4. **Other indicators of severe visual impairment** include absence of central fixation, nystagmus and strabismus. Nystagmus in particular signifies a poor visual prognosis.
5. **Special tests** such as forced choice preferential looking and visually evoked potentials also provide helpful information but should not be relied upon exclusively since they may be misleading.

Systemic investigations

Unless there is an established hereditary basis for the cataracts, the investigation of the infant with bilateral cataracts should include the following.

1. **Serology** for intrauterine infections (TORCH = toxoplasmosis, rubella, cytomegalovirus and herpes simplex). A history of maternal rash during pregnancy mandates the assay of varicella-zoster antibody titres.
2. **Urine.** Urinalysis for reducing substance after drinking milk (galactosaemia) and chromatography for amino acids (Lowe syndrome).
3. **Other investigations** include fasting blood glucose,

serum calcium and phosphorus, red blood cell GPUT and galactokinase levels.

4. **Referral to a paediatrician** may be warranted for dysmorphic features or suspicion of other systemic diseases. Chromosome analysis may be useful in this context.

Management

Timing is crucial and the main considerations are as follows.

1. **Bilateral dense** cataracts require early surgery when the child is 4–6 weeks of age to prevent the development of stimulus deprivation amblyopia. If the severity is asymmetrical, the eye with the denser cataract should be addressed first.
2. **Bilateral partial** cataracts may not require surgery until later, if at all. In cases of doubt it may be prudent to defer surgery, monitor lens opacities and visual function and intervene later if vision deteriorates.
3. **Unilateral dense** cataract merits urgent surgery (within days) followed by aggressive anti-amblyopia therapy, despite which the results are often poor. If the cataract is detected after 16 weeks of age then surgery is inadvisable because amblyopia is refractory.
4. **Partial unilateral** cataract can usually be observed or treated non-surgically with mydriasis and possibly part-time contralateral occlusion to prevent amblyopia.
5. **Surgery** involves anterior capsulorrhexis, aspiration of lens matter, capsulorrhexis of the posterior capsule, limited anterior vitrectomy and IOL implantation, if appropriate (see below).

> **NB** It is important to correct associated refractive errors.

Postoperative complications

Cataract surgery in children carries a higher incidence of complications than in adults.

1. **Posterior capsular opacification** is nearly universal if the posterior capsule is retained in a child under the age of 6 years. It is also of more significance in young children because of its amblyogenic effect. Opacification of the anterior hyaloid face may occur despite posterior capsulorrhexis if the anterior vitreous is left intact. The incidence of opacification is reduced when posterior capsulorrhexis is combined with vitrectomy.
2. **Secondary membranes** may form across the pupil, particularly in microphthalmic eyes or those with associated chronic uveitis. A fibrinous postoperative uveitis in an otherwise normal eye, unless vigorously treated, may also result in membrane formation. Thin membranes can be treated with laser capsulotomy although thick ones may require surgical excision.

Immediate postoperative fibrin may be removed by using intracameral recombinant TPA (tissue plasminogen activator)

3. **Proliferation of lens epithelium** is universal but usually visually inconsequential, since it does not involve the visual axis. It becomes encapsulated within the remnants of the anterior and posterior capsules and is referred to as a Soemmering ring.
4. **Glaucoma** eventually develops in about 20% of eyes.
   - Closed angle glaucoma may occur in the immediate postoperative period in microphthalmic eyes secondary to pupil block.
   - Secondary open-angle glaucoma may also develop years after the initial surgery. It is therefore important to monitor the intraocular pressure regularly for many years.
5. **Retinal detachment** is an uncommon and usually late complication.

Visual rehabilitation

Although the technical difficulties of performing cataract surgery in infants and young children have mostly been resolved, visual results continue to be disappointing because of severe and irreversible amblyopia. With regard to optical correction for the aphakic child, the two main considerations are age and laterality of aphakia.

1. **Spectacles** are useful for older children with bilateral aphakia, but not for unilateral aphakia because of associated anisometropia and aniseikonia. Even in infants with bilateral aphakia they may be inappropriate because of weight, unpleasant appearance, prismatic distortion and constriction of the visual field.
2. **Contact lenses** provide a superior optical solution for both unilateral and bilateral aphakia. Tolerance is usually reasonable until the age of about 2 years, although after this period, problems with compliance may start as the child becomes more active and independent. The contact lens may become dislodged or lost, leading to periods of visual deprivation with the risk of amblyopia. In bilateral aphakia, the solution is simply to prescribe spectacles, although in unilateral aphakia secondary IOL implantation may have to be considered.
3. **IOL implantation** is increasingly being performed in young children and even infants and appears to be effective and safe in selected cases. Awareness of the rate of myopic shift which occurs in the developing eye, combined with accurate biometry, allows the calculation of an IOL power targeted at initial hypermetropia (correctable with spectacles) which will ideally decay towards emmetropia later in life. However, final refraction is variable and emmetropia in adulthood cannot be guaranteed.
4. **Occlusion** to treat or prevent amblyopia is vital. Atropine penalization may also be considered.

ECTOPIA LENTIS

Ectopia lentis refers to a displacement of the lens from its normal position. The lens may be completely dislocated, rendering the pupil aphakic (luxated), or partially displaced, still remaining in the pupillary area (subluxated). Ectopia lentis may be hereditary or acquired. Acquired causes include trauma, a large eye (i.e. high myopia, buphthalmos), anterior uveal tumours and hypermature cataract. Only hereditary causes are discussed below.

Without systemic associations

1. **Familial ectopia lentis** is characterized by bilateral symmetrical superotemporal displacement. Inherited in an AD fashion, it may manifest congenitally or later in life.
2. **Ectopia lentis et pupillae** is a rare, congenital, bilateral, AR disorder characterized by displacement of the pupil and the lens in opposite directions. The pupils are small, slit like and dilate poorly (Fig. 12.24a). Other findings include iris transillumination, enlarged corneal diameter, glaucoma, cataract and microspherophakia.
3. **Aniridia** is occasionally associated with ectopia lentis (Fig. 12.24.b).

With systemic associations

Marfan syndrome

Marfan syndrome is a widespread AD disorder of connective tissue due to mutation of the fibrillin gene on chromosome 15q (see Chapter 24).

1. **Ectopia lentis,** bilateral and symmetrical, is present in 80% of cases. Subluxation is most frequently supero-temporal, but may be in any meridian. Because the zonule is frequently intact (Fig. 12.25a), accommodation is retained, although rarely the lens may dislocate into the anterior chamber or vitreous (Fig. 12.25b). The lens may also be microspherophakic.
2. **Angle anomaly** is present in 75% of eyes. It is charac-terized by dense iris processes and thickened trabecular sheets, and may be responsible for glaucoma.
3. **Retinal detachment** associated with lattice degeneration and high axial myopia is the most serious complication.
4. **Other features** include hypoplasia of dilator pupillae (rendering mydriasis difficult), peripheral iris transillu-mination, strabismus, flat cornea and blue sclera.

Homocystinuria

Homocystinuria is an AR inborn error of metabolism in which decreased hepatic activity of cystathionine beta-synthetase results in systemic accumulation of homocysteine and methionine.

1. **Systemic features** include skeletal anomalies with a Marfanoid habitus, fair hair and a tendency to thrombotic episodes.

   NB Giving a general anaesthetic without prior knowledge of the diagnosis of homocystinuria can be life-threatening.

2. **Ectopia lentis,** typically inferonasal (Fig. 12.25c), usually occurs by the age of 10 years. The zonule, which normally contains high levels of cysteine, often disintegrates so that accommodation is lost (Fig. 12.25d). Secondary angle-closure may occur as a result of pupil block caused by lens incarceration in the pupil, or a total dislocation into the anterior chamber.

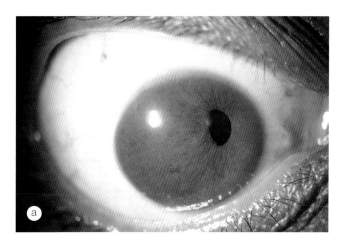

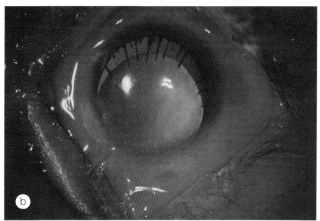

Fig. 12.24
Ectopia lentis without systemic association. **(a)** Ectopia lentis et pupillae; **(b)** inferior subluxation in aniridia (Courtesy of U Raina – fig. b)

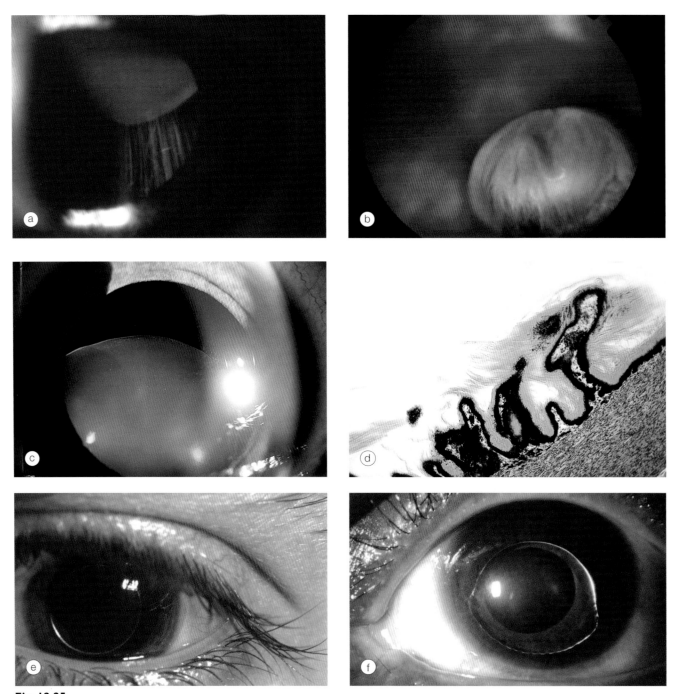

Fig. 12.25
Ectopia lentis in systemic disease. *1. Marfan syndrome.* **(a)** Superotemporal subluxation with intact zonule; **(b)** dislocation into the vitreous. *2. Homocystinuria.* **(c)** Inferior subluxation with zonular disintegration; **(d)** histology shows matted zonular fibres lying over the ciliary epithelium. *3. Weill–Marchesani syndrome.* **(e)** Microspherophakia; **(f)** dislocation into the anterior chamber (Courtesy of S Milewski – fig. b; J Harry and G Misson, from *Clinical Ophthalmic Pathology*, Butterworth-Heinemann, 2001 – fig. d; R Curtis – fig. f)

Weill–Marchesani syndrome

Weill–Marchesani syndrome is a rare systemic connective tissue disease, conceptually the converse of Marfan syndrome. Inheritance may be AD or AR.

1. **Systemic features** include short stature, brachydactyly with stiff joints and mental handicap.
2. **Ectopia lentis,** bilateral and inferior, occurs in about 50% of cases during the 'teens' or early twenties. Spherophakia is common (Fig. 12.25e) and the lens may be dislocated into the anterior chamber (Fig. 12.25f) causing pupil block angle-closure.
3. **Other features** include an angle anomaly, asymmetrical axial lengths and presenile vitreous liquefaction.

Miscellaneous conditions

1. **Hyperlysinaemia** is a very rare, AR, inborn error of metabolism caused by a deficiency in lysine alpha-ketoglutarate reductase. Systemic features include lax ligaments, hypotonic muscles, seizures and mental handicap. It is occasionally associated with ectopia lentis.
2. **Sulphite oxidase deficiency** is a very rare AR disorder of sulphur metabolism characterized by progressive muscular rigidity, decerebrate posture, mental handicap and demise usually before the age of 5 years. Ectopia lentis is universal.
3. **Stickler syndrome** is occasionally associated with ectopia lentis, retinal detachment being the most common problem (see Chapter 24).
4. **Ehlers–Danlos syndrome** (see Chapter 24) is occasionally associated with ectopia lentis.

Management

The main complications of ectopia lentis are (a) refractive error (lenticular myopia), (b) optical distortion due to astigmatism and/or lens edge effect, (c) glaucoma and, rarely, (d) lens-induced uveitis.

1. **Spectacle correction** may correct astigmatism induced by lens tilt or edge effect in eyes with mild subluxation. Aphakic correction may also afford good visual results if a significant portion of the visual axis is aphakic in the undilated state.
2. **Surgical removal** of the lens, using closed intraocular microsurgical techniques, is indicated for intractable ametropia, meridional amblyopia, cataract, lens-induced glaucoma, uveitis or endothelial touch.

CHAPTER 13

GLAUCOMA

BASIC SCIENCES

Aqueous secretion

Anatomy

The ciliary body extends from the root of the iris to the ora serrata. It is subdivided into two parts: an anterior pars plicata (2mm wide) and posterior pars plana (4mm wide). The pars plicata bears 70 radially orientated ciliary processes which project into the posterior chamber. Each ciliary process is lined by a pigmented epithelial layer continuous with the retinal pigment epithelium and a non-pigmented epithelial layer continuous with the neuroretina. Each process has a central arteriole ending in a rich capillary network. The capillaries of the stroma and those of individual ciliary processes are fenestrated, thus allowing easy passage of fluid and macromolecules. Tight junctions between adjacent non-pigmented epithelial cells constitute the blood–aqueous barrier.

Physiology

Aqueous humour is produced in two steps:
* Formation of a plasma filtrate within the stroma of the ciliary body.
* Formation of aqueous from this filtrate across the blood–aqueous barrier.

There are two mechanisms involved.

1. **Active secretion** by the non-pigmented ciliary epithelium accounts for the vast majority. It is the result of a metabolic process that depends on several enzyme systems, especially the $Na^+/K^+ATPase$ pump which secretes Na^+ ions into the posterior chamber. This creates an osmotic pressure difference across the ciliary epithelial cells so that water follows passively along the osmotic gradient. Cl^- secretion at the surface of the non-pigmented cells may be an important rate-limiting factor. Carbonic anhydrase also plays a role, but the precise mechanism is uncertain. Aqueous secretion is diminished by factors that inhibit active metabolism such as hypoxia and hypothermia but it is independent of the level of intraocular pressure (IOP).
2. **Passive secretion** by ultrafiltration and diffusion (which are dependent on the level of capillary hydrostatic pressure, the oncotic pressure and the level of IOP) is thought to play a minor role under normal conditions in the genesis of aqueous humour.

Conditions diminishing aqueous secretion

Aqueous secretion is diminished by the following:

1. **Drugs** such as beta-blockers, sympathomimetics and carbonic anhydrase inhibitors.

2. **Cyclodestructive procedures** such as cyclocryotherapy and laser ablation.
3. **Ciliary body shutdown** which may be caused by:
   * Detachment of the ciliary body.
   * Inflammation of the secretory ciliary epithelium associated with iridocyclitis.
   * Retinal detachment.

Aqueous outflow

Anatomy

1. **The trabecular meshwork** (trabeculum) is a sieve-like structure at the angle of the anterior chamber, through which 90% of the aqueous humour leaves the eye (Fig. 13.1). It consists of the following three portions (Fig. 13.2):
   a. The uveal meshwork is the innermost portion which consists of cord-like meshes that extend from the root of the iris to Schwalbe line. The intertrabecular spaces are relatively large and offer little resistance to the passage of aqueous.
   b. The corneoscleral meshwork forms the larger middle portion which extends from the scleral spur to Schwalbe line. The meshes are sheet-like and the intertrabecular spaces are smaller than in the uveal meshwork.
   c. The endothelial (juxtacanalicular) meshwork is the outer part of the trabeculum which links the corneoscleral meshwork with the endothelium of the inner wall of Schlemm canal. The juxtacanalicular tissue offers the major proportion of normal resistance to aqueous outflow.
2. **Schlemm canal** is a circumferential channel in the perilimbal sclera, bridged by septa. The inner wall of the canal is lined by irregular spindle-shaped endothelial cells

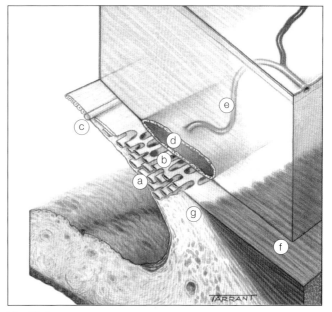

Fig. 13.2
Anatomy of outflow channels. **(a)** Uveal meshwork; **(b)** corneoscleral meshwork; **(c)** Schwalbe line; **(d)** Schlemm canal; **(e)** connector channels; **(f)** longitudinal muscle of the ciliary body; **(g)** scleral spur

which contain in-foldings (giant vacuoles). The outer wall of the canal is lined by smooth flat cells and contains the openings of the collector channels which leave at oblique angles and connect directly or indirectly with episcleral veins.

Physiology

Aqueous flows from the posterior chamber via the pupil into the anterior chamber, from where it exits the eye by two main routes (Fig. 13.3):

1. **Trabecular** (conventional) route accounts for approximately 90% of aqueous outflow. The aqueous flows through the trabeculum into Schlemm canal and is then drained by the episcleral veins. This is a bulk flow pressure-sensitive route so that increasing the pressure head will increase outflow. Trabecular outflow can be increased by drugs (miotics, sympathomimetics), laser trabeculoplasty and filtration surgery.
2. **Uveoscleral** (unconventional) route accounts for the remaining 10% of aqueous outflow. The aqueous passes across the face of the ciliary body into the suprachoroidal space and is drained by the venous circulation in the ciliary body, choroid and sclera. Uveoscleral outflow is decreased by miotics and increased by atropine, sympathomimetics and prostaglandins. Some aqueous also drains via the iris.

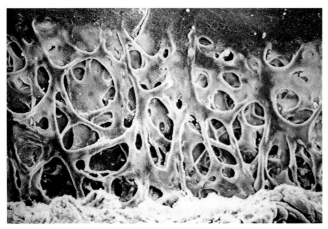

Fig. 13.1
Scanning electron micrograph of the trabecular meshwork

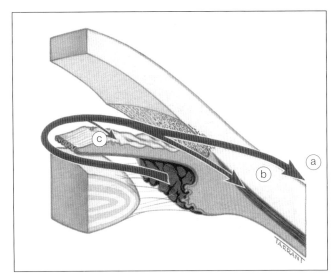

Fig. 13.3
Routes of aqueous outflow. **(a)** Trabecular; **(b)** uveoscleral;
(c) iris

Intraocular pressure

Determining factors

The IOP is determined by the rate of aqueous secretion and
rate of outflow. The latter is in turn related to the resistance
encountered in the outflow channels and the level of
episcleral venous pressure. The rate of aqueous outflow is
proportional to the difference between the intraocular and
episcleral venous pressure. The relationship between these
factors can be expressed as follows:

$$F = C (Po - Pe) \text{ where:}$$

F = rate of aqueous outflow (normal 2 μl/min)
C = facility of aqueous outflow (normal 0.2 μl/min/mmHg)
Po = IOP in mmHg
Pe = episcleral venous pressure (normal 10mmHg).
For example:

- If episcleral venous pressure is 20mmHg the IOP will be
  (2/0.2) + 20 = 30mmHg.
- If the facility of outflow is 0.05 the IOP will be (2/0.05) +
  10 = 50mmHg.

Distribution

The distribution of IOP within the general population has a
range of 11–21mmHg. Although there is no absolute cut-off
point, 21mmHg is considered the upper limit of normal and
levels above this are viewed with suspicion. However, in some
patients glaucomatous damage occurs with IOPs less than
21mmHg (normal-tension glaucoma) whilst others remain
unscathed with IOPs up to 30mmHg (ocular hypertension).
Although the actual level of IOP is important in the
development of glaucomatous damage, other factors also
play a part. The level of IOP is inherited so that first-degree
relatives of patients with primary open-angle glaucoma have
higher IOPs.

Fluctuation

Normal IOP varies with the time of day, heartbeat, blood
pressure level and respiration. The pattern of diurnal curves
of IOP varies, with a tendency to be higher in the morning
and lower in the afternoon and evening. Normal eyes
manifest a mean diurnal pressure variation of 5mmHg;
ocular hypertensive or glaucomatous eyes, however, exhibit
a wider fluctuation. In normal-tension glaucoma the
fluctuations are the same as in normals. A single normal
reading, particularly if taken during late afternoon, may
therefore be misleading and it may be necessary to take
several readings at different times of day (phasing). In clinical
practice phasing during the morning hours may be sufficient
because 80% of patients peak between 8am and 12am.

Definition

Glaucoma is a potentially blinding condition. Because the
pathophysiology, presentation and treatment of the different
types of glaucoma are so varied, there is no single definition
that adequately encompasses all forms. Understanding this
concept helps to explain, for example, why one patient
with 'glaucoma' may have no symptoms whilst another
experiences sudden pain and redness. In essence, glaucoma is
a disease which exhibits a characteristic optic neuropathy
which may result in progressive visual field loss. The most
important risk factor is raised IOP secondary to reduced
aqueous outflow through the filtration angle. On a molecular
level, glaucoma of diverse aetiology is linked by the presence
of endothelial leukocyte adhesion molecule 1 (ELAM-1), which
indicates activation of a stress response in the trabecular
meshwork cells of eyes with glaucoma.

Classification

Glaucoma may be (a) *congenital* (developmental) and (b)
acquired. Further sub-classification into open-angle and
angle-closure types is based on the mechanism by which
aqueous outflow is impaired. The glaucoma may also be
(a) *primary* or (b) *secondary* depending on the presence or
absence of associated factors contributing to the pressure
rise. In primary glaucoma the elevation of IOP is not
associated with any other ocular disorder whereas in
secondary glaucoma a recognizable ocular or non-ocular
disorder alters aqueous outflow which, in turn, results in
elevation of IOP. Secondary glaucoma may be acquired or
developmental and of the open-angle or angle-closure type.

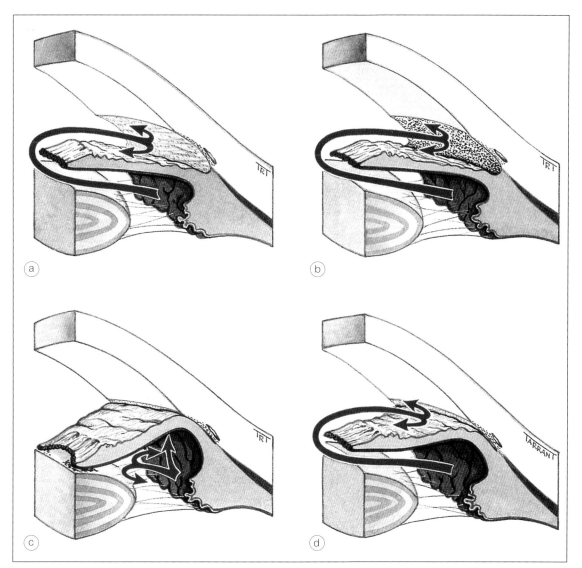

Fig. 13.4
Pathogenesis of secondary glaucoma. **(a)** Pre-trabecular obstruction; **(b)** trabecular obstruction by pigment granules; **(c)** angle closure with pupil block; **(d)** angle closure without pupil block

Secondary open-angle glaucoma

Secondary open-angle glaucoma can be subdivided on the basis of the site of aqueous outflow obstruction as follows:

1. **Pre-trabecular** glaucoma in which aqueous outflow is obstructed by a membrane covering the trabeculum (Fig. 13.4a), which may consist of:
   - Fibrovascular tissue (e.g. neovascular glaucoma).
   - Endothelial cells (e.g. iridocorneal endothelial syndrome).
   - Epithelial cells (e.g. epithelial ingrowth).

2. **Trabecular** glaucoma in which the obstruction occurs as a result of 'clogging up' of the meshwork by:
   - Pigment particles (e.g. pigmentary glaucoma – Fig. 13.4b).
   - Red blood cells (e.g. red cell glaucoma).
   - Degenerated red cells (e.g. ghost cell glaucoma).
   - Macrophages and lens proteins (e.g. phacolytic glaucoma).
   - Proteins (e.g. hypertensive uveitis.)
   - Pseudoexfoliative material (e.g. pseudoexfoliation glaucoma).

Trabecular glaucoma may also be caused by alteration of the trabecular fibres themselves by:

- Oedema (e.g. herpes zoster iritis).
- Scarring (e.g. post-traumatic angle recession glaucoma).

3. **Post-trabecular** glaucoma in which the trabeculum itself is normal but aqueous outflow is impaired as a result of elevated episcleral venous pressure due to:

- Carotid-cavernous fistula.
- Sturge–Weber syndrome.
- Obstruction of the superior vena cava.

Secondary angle-closure glaucoma

Secondary angle closure is caused by impairment of aqueous outflow secondary to apposition between the peripheral iris and the trabeculum by either posterior or anterior forces as follows:

1. **Posterior** forces push the peripheral iris against the trabeculum (e.g. iris bombé due to seclusio pupillae – Fig. 13.4c).
2. **Anterior** forces pull the iris over the trabeculum by contraction of inflammatory or fibrovascular membranes (e.g. late neovascular glaucoma – Fig. 13.4d).

OPTIC NERVE HEAD

Normal optic nerve head

Neuroretinal rim

The neuroretinal rim is the tissue between the outer edge of the cup and the disc margin. The normal healthy rim has an orange or pink colour and shows a characteristic con-figuration. The inferior rim is the broadest followed by superior, nasal and temporal (ISNT). A large physiological cup is due to a mismatch between the size of the scleral canal and the number of traversing nerve fibres which in health remains constant. Pathological cupping is caused by an irreversible decrease in the number of nerve fibres, glial cells and blood vessels.

Rim–disc ratio

The rim–disc ratio indicates the thickness of the rim in four quadrants expressed as a fraction of the diameter of the disc. It is useful in documenting progression of glaucomatous damage.

Cup

The optic cup may have one of three main appearances:
- A small dimple-like central cup (Fig. 13.5a).

- A punched-out deep central cup (Fig. 13.5b).
- A cup with a sloping temporal wall (Fig. 13.5c).

Cup–disc ratio

The cup–disc ratio which indicates the diameter of the cup expressed as a fraction of the diameter of the disc should be measured in both vertical and horizontal meridians (Fig. 13.6). This ratio is genetically determined and is also dependent on the area of the disc. The neuroretinal rim occupies a relatively similar area in different eyes; large discs therefore have large cups with high cup–disc ratios (Fig. 13.7). Most normal eyes have a vertical cup–disc ratio of 0.3 or less; only 2% have a ratio greater than 0.7. In any individual, asymmetry of 0.2 or more should also be regarded with suspicion until glaucoma has been excluded.

Blood vessels

The blood vessels from within the optic nerve enter the disc centrally and then course nasally following the edge of the cup. The central retinal artery is usually nasal to the vein.

Glaucomatous optic neuropathy

Glaucomatous damage results in characteristic signs involving (a) *retinal nerve fibre layer*, (b) *parapapillary area* and (c) *optic nerve head*.

Retinal nerve fibre layer

In glaucoma subtle retinal nerve fibre layer defects precede the development of detectable optic disc and visual field changes. Retinal nerve fibre drop-out may be diffuse or localized. Localized damage is characterized by slit defects in the retinal nerve fibre layer (Fig. 13.8a) which is best visualized with a green filter (Fig. 13.8b). As glaucomatous damage progresses the defects become larger.

Parapapillary changes

Chorioretinal atrophy surrounding the optic nerve head is conceptualized as consisting of two zones – an inner 'beta' zone, bordering the disc margin, which in turn is concentrically surrounded by an outer 'alpha' zone (Fig. 13.9a and b).

1. **The beta** zone exhibits chorioretinal atrophy with visibility of the sclera and large choroidal blood vessels.
2. **The alpha** zone displays variable irregular hyper- and hypopigmentation of the retinal pigment epithelium. Although the alpha zone is larger in patients with POAG, its frequency is similar in glaucomatous and normal subjects. However, the beta zone is not only larger but also occurs more frequently in patients with POAG than

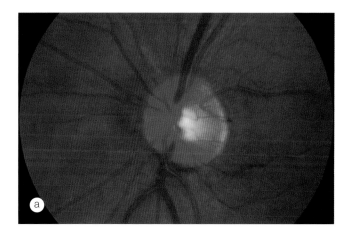

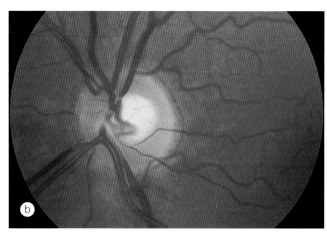

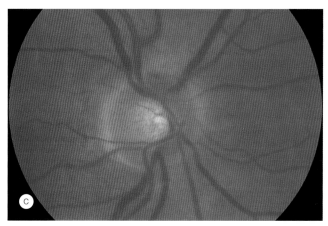

Fig. 13.5
Variations in appearance of a normal optic nerve head. **(a)** Small dimple-like cup; **(b)** deep punched-out cup; **(c)** cup with a sloping temporal wall

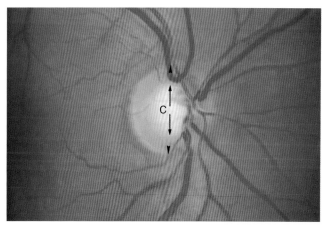

Fig. 13.6
Cup-disc ratio (C = cup; arrowheads = edge of optic disc)
(Courtesy of J Salmon)

damage. Approximately half of all ocular hypertensive eyes that convert to POAG exhibit progression of parapapillary atrophic changes.

Optic nerve head

Optic disc damage is superimposed upon physiological cupping present prior to the onset of raised IOP. If an eye with a small cup develops glaucoma, the cup will increase in size, but during the early stages its dimensions may still be smaller than that of a large physiological cup. An estimation of cup size alone is therefore of limited value in the diagnosis of early glaucoma, unless it is found to be increasing. Glaucomatous cups are usually larger than physiological cups, although a large cup is not necessarily pathological. Assessment of the thickness, symmetry and colour of the neuroretinal rim is, however, more important. The spectrum of disc damage in glaucoma ranges from highly localized tissue loss with notching of the neuroretinal rim to diffuse concentric enlargement of the cup as well as vascular changes.

Subtypes of glaucomatous damage

The appearance and pattern of disc damage may correlate with sub-types of glaucoma and provide clues as to the pathogenic mechanisms involved as follows:

1. **Focal ischaemic (type 1)** disc is characterized by focal tissue loss at the superior and/or inferior poles (polar notching) and an otherwise relatively intact neuroretinal rim (Fig. 13.10a). The notch may be associated with localized field defects near to fixation. Paradoxically, a large reduction in IOP may be beneficial. Type 1 discs tend to occur in females who may have vasospasm and migraine.

in normal individuals. In asymmetrical POAG, the changes are more advanced in the more severely affected eye (Fig. 13.9c). In ocular hypertension, the presence and size of parapapillary changes correlates with the subsequent development of optic disc and visual field

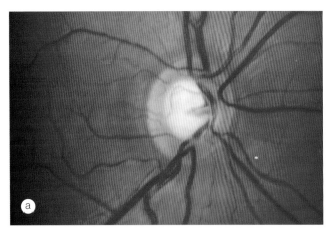
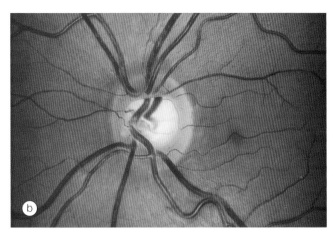

Fig. 13.7
Normal discs with large symmetrical physiological cups (Courtesy of J Salmon)

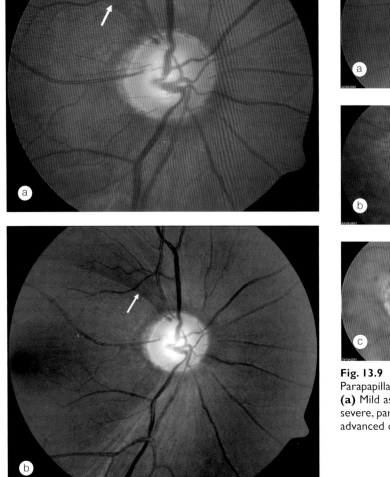

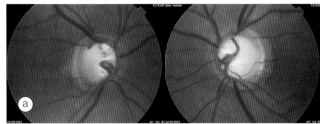
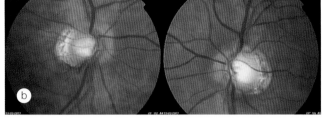
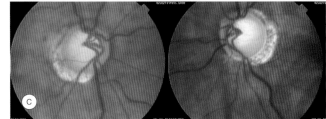

Fig. 13.9
Parapapillary changes associated with glaucomatous cupping.
(a) Mild asymmetrical; **(b)** more severe symmetrical; **(c)** very severe, particularly in the left eye which also shows more advanced cupping

Fig. 13.8
Retinal nerve fibre layer defects. **(a)** Superotemporal wedge-shaped defect; **(b)** same eye seen with a green filter (Courtesy of P Gili)

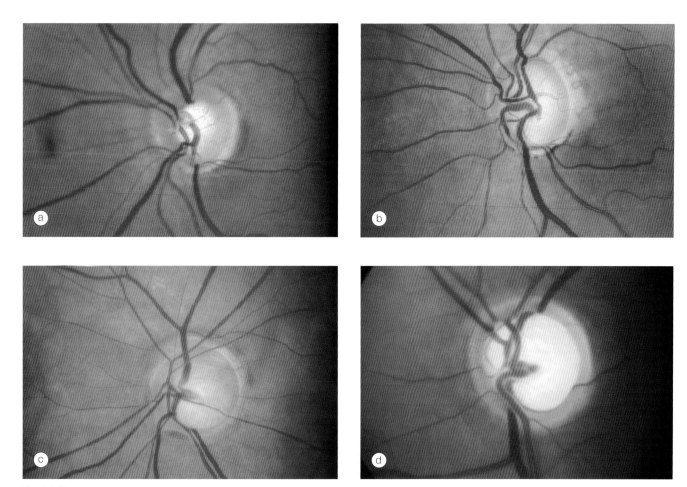

Fig. 13.10
Specific subtypes of glaucomatous damage. **(a)** Type 1 – focal ischaemic; **(b)** type 2 – myopic glaucomatous; **(c)** type 3 – senile sclerotic; **(d)** type 4 – concentrically enlarging

2. **Myopic glaucomatous (type 2)** disc is characterized by polar notching and a temporal crescent in the absence of degenerative myopia (Fig. 13.10b). It is associated with dense superior or inferior scotomas, which threaten fixation in 50% of cases. Progression of damage is frequent and may be rapid. Type 2 discs tend to occur in younger patients, particularly males.

3. **Senile sclerotic (type 3)** disc is characterized by a shallow, saucerized cup and a gently sloping neuroretinal rim, a 'moth-eaten appearance', variable parapapillary atrophy and peripheral visual field loss (Fig. 13.10c). It tends to affect older patients (both genders equally), and is associated with ischaemic heart disease and hypertension. Circulatory abnormalities have also been demonstrated in the retrobulbar vessels.

4. **Concentrically enlarging (type 4)** disc is caused by diffuse loss of nerve fibres involving the entire cross-section of the optic nerve head. It is characterized by thinning of the entire neuroretinal rim without notching (Fig. 13.10d) and is frequently associated with diffuse visual field loss. At presentation IOP is often significantly elevated. Type 4 discs tend to occur in younger patients and affect both genders equally.

5. **Mixed.** At least two-thirds of eyes have a mixed appearance, potentially the result of multiple pathogenic mechanisms.

Non-specific signs of glaucomatous damage

1. **Baring of circumlinear blood vessels** is a sign of early thinning of the superior or inferior neuroretinal rim. It is characterized by a space between a superficial blood vessel that runs from the superior or inferior aspects of the disc towards the macula, and the disc margin (Fig. 13.11a).

2. **Bayoneting** is characterized by double angulation of a blood vessel as it dives sharply backwards and then turns along the steep wall of the excavation before angling again onto the floor of the disc (Fig. 13.11b).

3. **The laminar dot sign** is caused by exposure of the lamina cribrosa due to loss of neuroretinal tissue

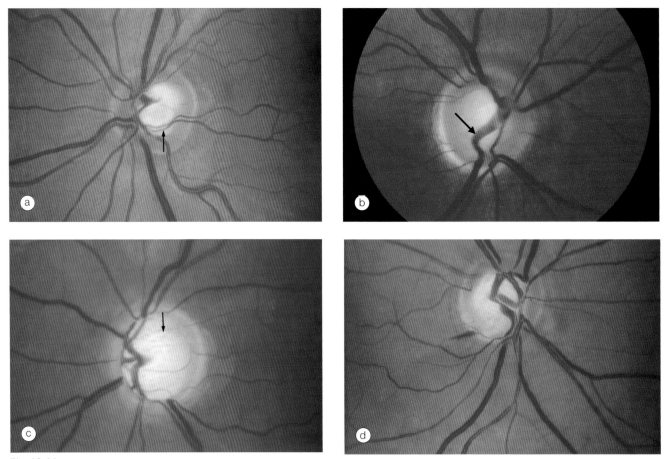

Fig. 13.11
Non-specific signs of glaucomatous damage. **(a)** Baring of circumlinear blood vessels; **(b)** bayoneting; **(c)** lamellar dot sign; **(d)** disc haemorrhage

(Fig. 13.11c). It is often seen in eyes with advanced glaucomatous damage but is not specific for glaucoma.

4. **Disc haemorrhages** are flame-shaped and extend onto the nerve fibre layer, most frequently infero-temporally (Fig. 13.11d). They are observed in glaucoma and occasionally in patients with hypertension, diabetes and the use of aspirin, and rarely in healthy individuals. In glaucoma their significance is as follows:
   • They occur more frequently in normal tension glaucoma.
   • They may precede a visual field defect, often by several months.

OCULAR HYPERTENSION

Definition

In the general population the mean IOP is 16mmHg; two standard deviations on either side of this gives a 'normal' IOP range of 11–21mmHg. The distribution is Gaussian with the curve skewed to the right (Fig. 13.12). In the elderly the mean IOP is higher, particularly in women, and the standard deviation greater than in younger individuals. This means that 'normal' IOP in elderly women may range up to 24mmHg and not 21mmHg. It is estimated that about 7% of the population over the age of 40 years have IOPs > 21mmHg without detectable glaucomatous damage on standard clinical tests. These individuals are referred to as ocular hypertensives or glaucoma suspects.

Risk factors for developing glaucoma

1. **Older age** is a risk factor because POAG is mainly a disease of old age although many elderly patients with ocular hypertension may not live long enough to develop POAG.
2. **Retinal nerve fibre defects** are an important risk factor because they precede changes in visual field (pre-perimetric glaucoma). It may therefore take several years before damage can be detected by conventional perimetry, which necessitates loss of 20% of the ganglion cell

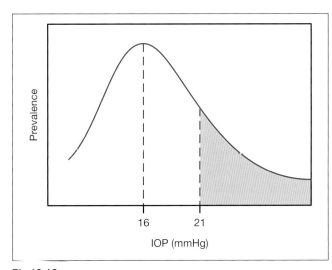

Fig.13.12
Distribution of intraocular pressure in the general population

Table 13.1   Relationship between prevalence of POAG and IOP

IOP (mmHg)	POAG (%)
16–21	1.5
22–29	8.0
30 or more	25.0

Table 13.2   Longitudinal risk of POAG in individuals with ocular hypertension

IOP (mmHg)	Developing visual field defects (%)	Relative risk
21–25	2.7	1.0
26–30	12.0	4.4
> 30	41.2	15.3

population. Objective measurement of retinal nerve fibre layer thickness may be helpful in patients with ocular hypertension.

3. **High vertical cup–disc ratio** is a risk factor on the premise that it represents an early glaucomatous change. It is also possible that an eye with a high cup–disc ratio unaltered by glaucoma may be at greater risk of developing POAG. Ideally, an objective method should be used to measure the cup–disc ratio such as a scanning laser ophthalmoscope (see Chapter 2).
4. **High IOP** is important because risk of damage increases as the IOP rises. The prevalence of POAG in relation to screening IOP is shown in Table 13.1 and the longitudinal risk of developing POAG in individuals with ocular hypertension is shown in Table 13.2
5. **Parapapillary changes** are present in over 50% of ocular hypertensive patients that convert to POAG.
6. **Thin central corneal thickness.** Eyes with a thin cornea have a true IOP that is greater than the measured IOP. Conversely, eyes with a thicker cornea have a true IOP that is lower than the measured IOP and they may be misdiagnosed as having ocular hypertension. Thus it is important to measure corneal thickness before instituting therapy in a patient with ocular hypertension.
7. **Family history** of POAG in a first degree relative is a moderate risk factor.
8. **High myopia** is a moderate risk factor because myopic discs are more susceptible to glaucomatous damage at a lower IOP than emmetropic discs.

Management

Untreated patients with ocular hypertension have a 9.5% cumulative risk of developing POAG after 5 years; treatment reduces this to 4.4%. However, only a subset of patients with POAG will lose functional vision during their lifetime. Most patients with ocular hypertension therefore do not require treatment and only those at high risk should be treated in order to delay or prevent the development of POAG. It should be remembered that once treatment is instituted, it is continued throughout the patient's lifetime and may have significant side-effects. Therapeutic decisions in individual patients are based on a combination of risk factors as follows:

1. **High risk**
   - Retinal nerve fibre layer defects.
   - Parapapillary changes.
   - IOP 30mmHg or more.
   - IOP 26mmHg or more and central corneal thickness < 555μm.
   - Vertical cup–disc ratio 0.4 or more and central corneal thickness < 555μm.

Most patients with high risk factors should be offered treatment because a reduction of IOP is effective in delaying or preventing the development of POAG in a significant proportion of cases. A change of IOP is more important than a specific level and it is reasonable to aim for a 20% reduction.

2. **Moderate risk**
   - IOP of 24–29mmHg without nerve fibre layer defects.
   - IOP of 22–25mmHg and central corneal thickness < 555μm.
   - Vertical cup–disc ratio 0.4 or more and central corneal thickness 555–588μm.
   - Family history of POAG in a first degree relative.
   - High myopia.

In these patients annual examination of the optic discs and perimetry is appropriate. Treatment is withheld until damage is documented.

3. Low risk
- IOP 22–23mmHg and a central corneal thickness >588µm.
- Vertical cup–disc ratio 0.4 or less and central corneal thickness >588µm.

In these patients examination every 2 years is adequate.

PRIMARY OPEN-ANGLE GLAUCOMA

Introduction

Definition

Glaucoma is a neurodegenerative disease of the optic nerve that presents to the practitioner at various stages of a continuum characterized by accelerated ganglion cell death, subsequent axonal loss and optic nerve damage, and eventual visual field loss. POAG, also referred to as chronic simple glaucoma, is a generally bilateral, but not always symmetrical disease, characterized by:
- Adult onset.
- An IOP >21mmHg.
- An open angle of normal appearance.
- Glaucomatous optic nerve head damage.
- Visual field loss.

Despite this definition it should be emphasized that approximately 16% of all patients with otherwise characteristic POAG will have IOPs consistently below 22mmHg. Moreover, the majority of individuals with IOP > 21mmHg do not have glaucoma. POAG is the most prevalent type of glaucoma, affecting approximately 1 in 100 of the general population over the age of 40 years. It affects both sexes equally and is responsible for about 12% of all cases of blind registration in the UK and the USA.

Risk factors and associations

1. **Age.** POAG is more common in older individuals, most cases presenting after the age of 65 years. It is unusual for this diagnosis to be made before the age of 40 years.
2. **Race.** POAG is significantly more common, develops earlier, and is more severe, in blacks than in whites.
3. **Family history** and inheritance. POAG is frequently inherited and is believed to have a genetic basis. The responsible genes are thought to show incomplete penetrance and variable expressivity in some families. IOP, facility of aqueous outflow and optic disc size are also genetically determined. First-degree relatives of patients with POAG are at increased risk of developing POAG; however, estimates of exact risk are lacking because the disease develops in older individuals and long-term follow-up is required for accurate figures. However, an approximate risk to siblings of 10% (i.e. three times the normal population) and to offspring of 4% (i.e. twice the normal population) has been suggested.
4. **Diabetes mellitus** – clinic-based studies and most prevalence studies show a correlation between diabetes and POAG.
5. **Reduction of perfusion pressure** (blood pressure minus IOP) is strongly associated with an increased prevalence of POAG. Visual field progression, despite well-controlled IOP, may occur in some cases because of a significant nocturnal dip in blood pressure.
6. **Myopia** is associated with an increased incidence of POAG and myopic eyes are also more susceptible to glaucomatous damage.
7. **Retinal disease.** Central retinal vein occlusion is associated with an increased incidence of POAG. Approximately 5% of patients with rhegmatogenous retinal detachment and 3% of those with retinitis pigmentosa have associated POAG.

Genetics

Linkage analysis in families with POAG has led to the detection of six different loci in the human genome associated with POAG designated GLC1A-F. Only two genes have been identified so far, the myocilin gene (MYOC) on chromosome 1q21-q31 and the optineurin gene in the GLC-1E interval on chromosome 10p. Myocilin is a 504 amino acid protein, formerly known as trabecular meshwork induced gluocorticoid response protein (TIGR). The specific mechanism whereby abnormal myocilin results in POAG is poorly understood. A number of different mutations of this gene have been described, including the Gln368 Stop mutation, which is associated with relatively late-onset POAG. A study of a group of unrelated POAG patients found myocilin mutations in at least 4% of the adult patients. However, if one family member develops POAG prior to age 35 years, the chances that the genetic defect is a mutation in the myocilin gene is up to 33%. In families with POAG where linkage to a proven locus or where a specific gene mutation has been demonstrated, it is possible to screen individuals members using molecular genetic techniques.

Steroid responsiveness

The normal population can be divided into three groups on the basis of their IOP response to a 6-week course of topical betamethasone.

1. **High** responders exhibit a marked elevation of IOP (> 30 mmHg).
2. **Moderate** responders display a moderate elevation of IOP (22–30mmHg).
3. **Non-responders** manifest virtually no change in IOP. The incidence of steroid responders is shown in Table 13.3. There is a marked increase in myocilin production by

Table 13.3   Incidence of steroid responsiveness

	High (%)	Moderate (%)	Non (%)
General population	5	35	60
Patients with POAG	90	10	0
Siblings of patients with POAG	30	50	20
Offspring of patients with POAG	25	70	5

the trabecular meshwork cells after treatment with dexamethasone but the exact mechanism whereby this results in a rise in IOP is unclear. It has been postulated that the response to topical steroids is determined genetically and so these drops should be used with caution in patients with POAG as well as in their siblings and offspring. However, in a high or intermediate steroid responder, the 'strong' steroids (dexamethasone, beta-methasone and prednisolone) are equipotent in their ability to raise IOP, while fluorometholone has a lesser propensity to raise IOP; fluorometholone raises IOP half as much as betamethasone.

NB Systemic steroids are much less prone to cause elevation of IOP, but more likely to induce cataract.

Pathogenesis of glaucomatous damage

Elevation of IOP in POAG is caused by increased resistance to aqueous outflow in the trabecular meshwork. Retinal ganglion cell death occurs predominantly through apoptosis (programmed cell death) rather than necrosis. The preterminal event is calcium ion influx into the cell body and an increase in intracellular nitric oxide. Glutamine metabolism has a profound effect on this process. The factors that influence the rate of cell death are multiple, but current opinion is polarized between ischaemic and mechanical aetiologies of damage.

1. **The ischaemic** theory postulates that compromise of the microvasculature with resultant ischaemia in the optic nerve head is responsible. The possible mechanisms include the following:
   - Loss of capillaries or alteration in capillary blood flow.
   - Interference with the delivery of nutrients or removal of metabolic products from axons.
   - Failure of blood flow regulation.
   - Delivery of hostile vasoactive substances to the blood vessels of the optic nerve head.
2. **The direct** mechanical theory suggests that raised IOP directly damages the retinal nerve fibres as they pass

through the lamina cribrosa. It is likely that the pressure gradient around the optic nerve head rather than the absolute IOP is relevant in this context.
3. **Optic nerve head remodelling** may be a primary or secondary response to local factors, such as elevation of IOP, ischaemia and axonal loss. Once the initial injury occurs, a cascade of events results in astrocyte and glial cell mediation, as well as alterations in the extracellular matrix of the lamina cribrosa, ultimately leading to collapse of the cribriform plates and loss of axonal support.

Screening

Population screening with tonometry alone is unsatisfactory, since it will label as 'normal' a significant number of cases with other features of POAG such as cupping and visual field loss. Even with the additional criterion of a vertical cup–disc ratio of >0.4, only 60% of potential POAG patients will be identified. Until more accurate methods of mass screening are available, screening should therefore include visual field examination, tonometry and ophthalmoscopy. Individuals with a family history of glaucoma in first-degree relatives should be screened from the age of 40 years. Provided initial assessment is normal, subsequent review should be at 2-yearly intervals until the age of 50 years and then annually thereafter.

Diagnosis

1. **Raised IOP.** This objective measurement has proved both a stumbling block and a great benefit in the diagnosis of POAG. Approximately 2% of the general population over the age of 40 years have IOPs >24mmHg and 7% have IOPs >21mmHg. However, only about 1% of these have glaucomatous visual field loss. This issue is further complicated by patients with 'normal' IOP (<22mmHg) who develop glaucomatous visual field loss and cupping.
2. **Diurnal fluctuations in IOP** of up to 5mmHg occur in approximately 30% of normals. In POAG this fluctuation is exaggerated and occurs in about 90% of cases. For this reason, a single pressure reading of 21mmHg or less does not necessarily exclude the diagnosis of POAG, nor should a single reading of >21mmHg do more than arouse suspicion. In order to detect fluctuations of IOP, it may be necessary to measure the IOP at different times during the day (phasing). Asymmetry in the IOP measurement between the two eyes of 5mmHg or more should arouse suspicion, since irrespective of the absolute value, the eye with the higher reading may be abnormal.
3. **Optic disc changes.** POAG is often diagnosed after finding suspicious optic or asymmetrical discs on routine examination (Fig. 13.13).
4. **Visual fields** show typical changes as described below.
5. **Gonioscopy** shows a normal open angle.

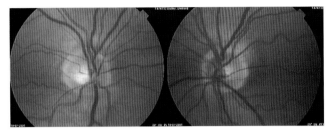

Fig. 13.13
Asymmetrical cupping

Visual field defects

Minimal criteria for glaucomatous damage

One of the following defects on Humphrey visual field testing (Anderson's criteria):

1. **Glaucoma hemifield test** outside normal limits on at least two consecutive occasions. This provides information concerning differences between the superior and inferior halves of the visual field by evaluating threshold at mirror image points above and below the horizontal meridian. This program also compares the overall height of the hill of vision with age-adjusted normal values.
2. **Cluster of three or more non-edge points** in a location typical for glaucoma, all of which are depressed on PSD at a $P < 5\%$ level and one of which is depressed at a $P < 1\%$ level, on two consecutive occasions (Fig. 13.14).
3. **CPSD** that occurs in less than 5% of normal individuals on two consecutive fields.

> **NB** Visual fields should not be interpreted in isolation but in conjunction with clinical findings such as the level of IOP, and the appearance of the optic disc and retinal nerve fibre layer.

Progression of glaucomatous damage

The characteristic defect in glaucoma is the retinal nerve fibre bundle defect that results from damage at the optic nerve head. The pattern of nerve fibres in the retinal area served by the damaged nerve fibre bundle will correspond to the specific defect in the visual field. The common names for the classical visual field defects are derived from their appearance when plotted on a kinetic visual field chart. In static perimetry, however, sample points are in a grid pattern which means that the representation of the visual field defect lacks the smooth contours suggested by such terms as 'arcuate'.

1. **Earliest** changes suggestive of glaucoma consist of increased variability of responses in areas that subsequently develop defects. Alternatively there may be slight asymmetry between the two eyes.

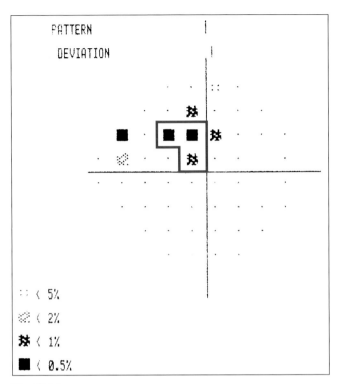

PATTERN
DEVIATION

:: < 5%

< 2%

< 1%

< 0.5%

Fig. 13.14
Minimal criterion for glaucoma showing a cluster of three non-edge points

2. **Paracentral,** small, relatively steep depressions, most commonly supero-nasally (Fig. 13.15a), constitute approximately 70% of all early glaucomatous field defects. Since the defects respect the distribution of the retinal nerve fibre layer they terminate at the horizontal midline. Defects above and below the horizontal therefore are not aligned with each other.
3. **Nasal (Roenne) step** represents a difference in sensitivity above and below the horizontal midline in the nasal field (Fig. 13.15b). It is a common finding usually associated with other defects. A temporal wedge is less common but has similar implications.
4. **Arcuate-shaped** defects develop as a result of coalescence of paracentral scotomas. They typically develop between 10° and 20° of fixation in areas that constitute downward or, more commonly, upward extensions from the blind spot around fixation (Bjerrum area). With time, they tend to elongate circumferentially along the distribution of arcuate nerve fibres (Seidel scotoma) and may eventually connect with the blind spot (arcuate scotoma) reaching to within 5° of fixation nasally (Fig. 13.15c)
5. **Enlargement** of scotomas due to damage to adjacent fibres (Fig. 13.15d).
6. **Deepening** of scotomas and development of fresh defects (Fig. 13.15e).

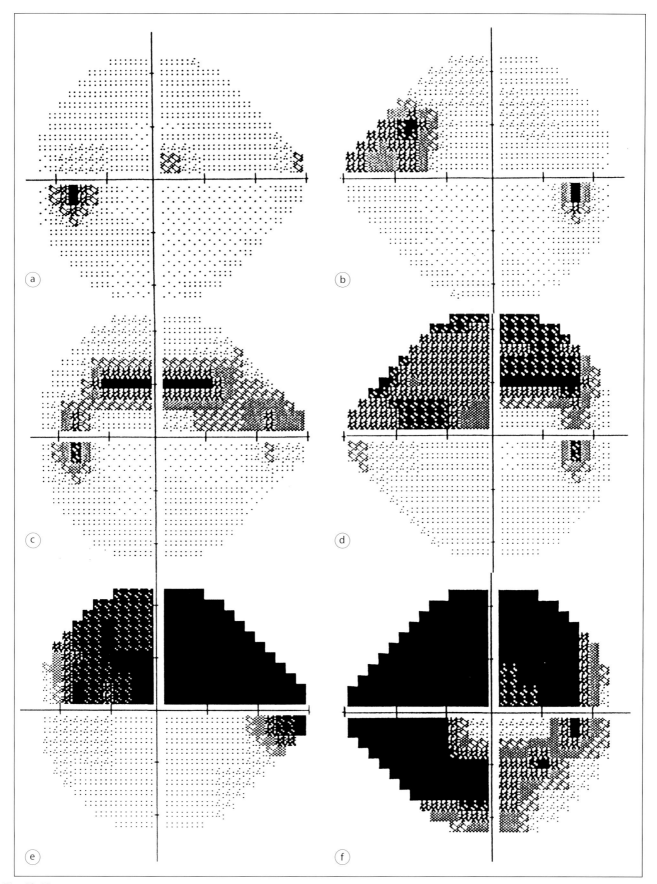

Fig. 13.15
Grey-scale display showing progression of glaucomatous visual field loss (see text)

7. **A ring scotoma** develops when arcuate defects in upper and lower halves of the visual field join (Fig. 13.15f). Misalignment between the two often preserves the nasal step.

8. **End-stage** changes are characterized by a small island of central vision and an accompanying temporal island. The temporal island is usually extinguished before the central.

NB Progression of damage can also be identified not only by progression of visual field defects but also by deterioration of total and pattern deviations and global indices (Fig. 13.16).

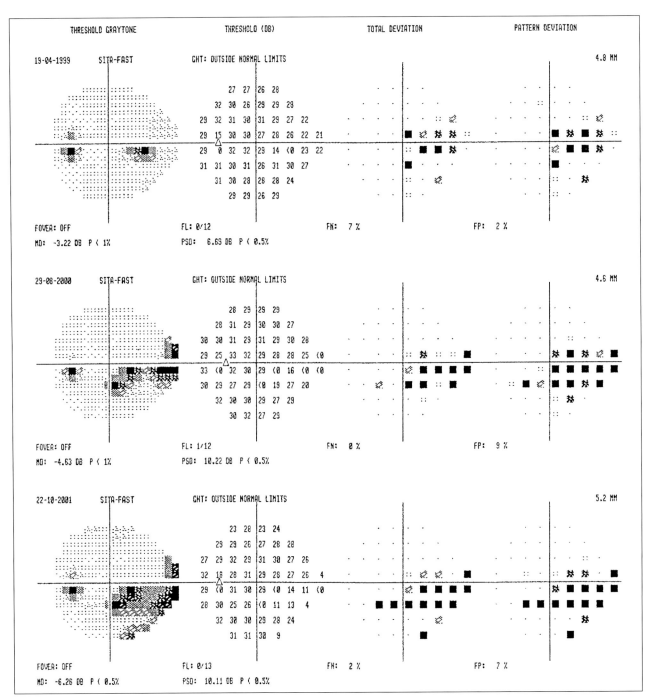

Fig. 13.16
Progression of visual field defects and deterioration of global indices over a period of 30 months

Management

The primary aim of treatment is to prevent functional impairment of vision within the patient's lifetime by slowing the rate of ganglion cell loss closer to that of the normal population (approximately 5000/year). Currently the best method of achieving this goal is the lowering of IOP. Other modalities aimed at inhibition of ganglion cell apoptosis are currently under evaluation.

Baseline evaluation

Clear and concise records of baseline parameters are essential to monitor future progress.

1. **Visual acuity and refractive state.**
2. **Slit-lamp biomicroscopy,** paying attention to signs of secondary glaucomas which may masquerade as POAG.
3. **Applanation tonometry,** noting the time of day.
4. **Gonioscopy,** if a coupling substance is required, should be delayed until the optic discs and visual fields have been assessed.
5. **Ophthalmoscopy** should be performed and the appearance of the disc documented by drawing and if possible also by photography.
6. **Perimetry.** The type of perimetry depends on the instrumentation available, the patient's age and visual acuity. In patients with significant lens opacities, perimetry should be performed with dilated pupils.

Patient instruction

A simple explanation should be offered concerning the nature of the disease and an explanatory booklet provided. The patient should be taught how to instil drops and the intervals between medications should be specified. At follow-up visits the patient's proficiency at instilling drops should be checked. In order to minimize systemic absorption the patient should be instructed either to perform lacrimal sac occlusion (by applying pressure at the medial canthus) or to close the eyes for about 3 minutes after instillation. Potential adverse effects should be explained and subsequently asked for at follow-up visits.

Grading of glaucomatous damage

1. **Mild** damage (grade 1) is characterized by minimal cupping (Fig. 13.17a), a nasal step or paracentral scotomas and a MD < −6dB (Fig. 13.17b).
2. **Moderate** damage (grade 2) is characterized by thinning of the neuroretinal rim (Fig. 13.18a), an arcuate scotoma and a MD < −12dB (Fig. 13.18b).
3. **Severe** damage (grade 3) is characterized by marked cupping (Fig. 13.19a), extensive visual field loss including defects within the central 5° and a MD > −12dB (Fig. 13.19b).

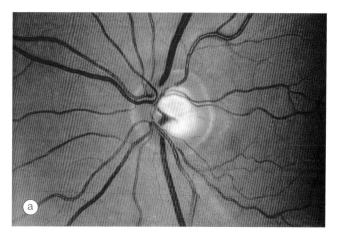

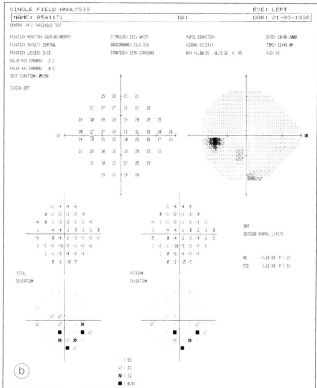

Fig. 13.17
Mild damage. **(a)** Minimal cupping; **(b)** small paracentral scotoma

4. **End-stage** damage (grade 4) is characterized by gross cupping (Fig. 13.20a) and a small residual field (Fig. 13.20b).

Treatment goals

1. **Target pressure.** It is assumed that the pre-treatment level of IOP has damaged the optic nerve and will continue to do so. An IOP level is identified below which further damage is considered unlikely (target pressure). The target

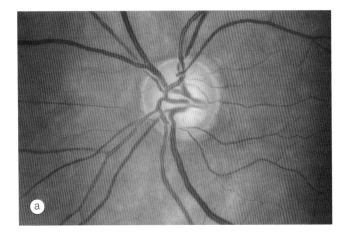

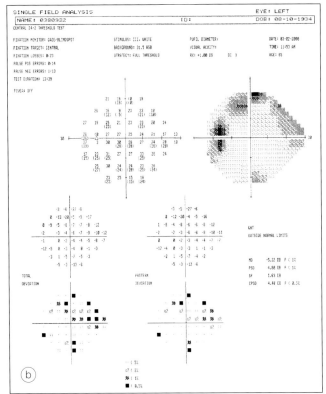

Fig. 13.18
Moderate damage. **(a)** Moderate cupping; **(b)** arcuate scotoma

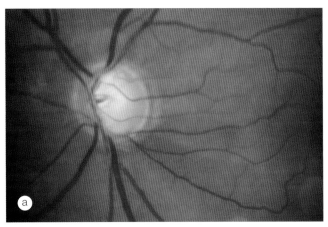

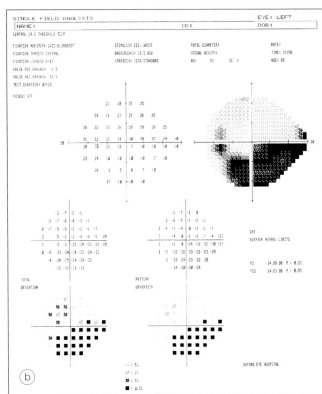

Fig. 13.19
Severe damage. **(a)** Marked cupping; **(b)** extensive visual field loss

pressure is identified taking into account the severity of existing damage, the level of IOP and the rapidity with which damage occurred (if that is known), as well as the age and general health of the patient. Therapy should maintain the IOP at or below the target level.

2. **Monitoring** is performed of the optic nerve and visual fields. In the event of further damage the target IOP is reset at a lower level. Although there is no 'safe' level, progression is uncommon if the IOP is < 16mmHg. As the disease progresses the degree of redundancy or 'reserve capacity' within the visual system diminishes and the loss of each remaining ganglion cell inflicts a greater impact on visual function. Low target pressures are therefore required in patients with advanced disease.

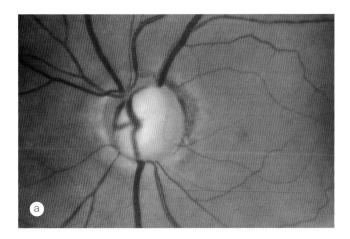

(a)

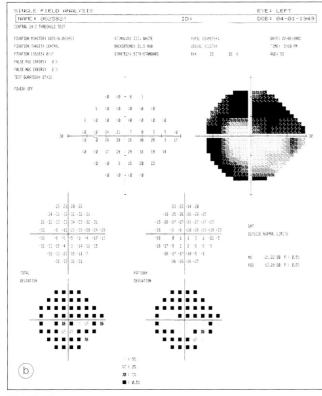

(b)

Fig. 13.20
End-stage damage; **(a)** Gross cupping; **(b)** very advanced visual field loss

Medical therapy

1. Principles
- Any chosen drug should be used in its lowest concentration and as infrequently as possible consistent with the desired therapeutic effect.
- Ideally the drug with the fewest potential side-effects should be used.

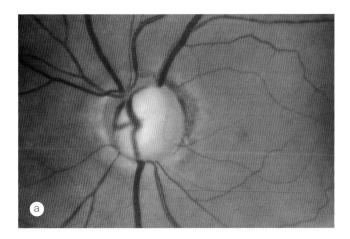

- Initial treatment is usually with one drug, usually a beta-blocker or prostaglandin analogue.

2. Follow-up after 4 weeks.
- A fall in IOP of >4mmHg is usually considered significant (i.e. caused by the drug as opposed to chance fluctuation).
- If both eyes require treatment it should not be assumed that the magnitude of response will be equal in both eyes.
- If the response is satisfactory subsequent assessment is after 2 months and at 3–4-monthly intervals thereafter.
- If the response is unsatisfactory the initial drug is withdrawn and another substituted.
- If the response is still unsatisfactory yet another drug is added or a combined preparation (e.g. timolol-dorzolamide) substituted. When two separate drugs are used the patient should be instructed to wait 5 minutes before instilling the second drug to prevent washout of the first drug.

3. Perimetry.
If control is good and the appearance of the optic disc stable, annual perimetry is sufficient.

4. Gonioscopy
should also be performed annually because the anterior chamber gradually shallows with age.

5. Causes of failure
- Inappropriate target pressure. If the IOP runs in the upper part of the statistically normal range, progressive field loss is relatively common.
- Non-compliance with therapy occurs in at least 25% of patients.
- Wide fluctuations in IOP frequently occur in patients treated medically.

Laser trabeculoplasty

In laser trabeculoplasty discrete argon or diode laser burns are applied to the trabeculum to enhance aqueous outflow and lower IOP. The therapeutic effect is often transient, lasting a few years, so that laser therapy may merely defer the need for filtration surgery. The following are the main indications:

1. Avoidance of polypharmacy,
usually with more than two preparations. In this situation laser therapy may be considered as a substitute for another drug.

2. Avoidance of surgery
- Elderly patients in whom laser therapy may defer the need for surgery to beyond life expectancy.
- In black patients in whom filtration surgery carries a poorer prognosis.

3. Primary therapy
in patients who are expected not to comply with medical therapy. Since IOP reduction with laser is seldom greater than 30%, an IOP >28mmHg is unlikely to be adequately controlled by laser alone.

Trabeculectomy

Trabeculectomy involves the creation of a fistula between the angle of the anterior chamber and the sub-Tenon space, which allows egress of aqueous from the anterior chamber into a 'drainage bleb'. Progressive damage is less likely after trabeculectomy than with medical therapy because the resultant IOP is often significantly lower and less likely to fluctuate. The timing of surgery depends on the amount of visual loss that has occurred, the rapidity of deterioration and life expectancy. The following are the main indications:

1. **Failed medical therapy and/or laser trabeculoplasty.**
2. **Unsuitability for laser therapy** due to poor patient cooperation or inadequate visualization of the trabeculum (narrow angle, corneal opacification).
3. **Advanced disease** requiring a very low target pressure may benefit from early surgery.

Prognosis

Most patients with POAG do not become blind in their lifetime. Fewer than 5% have the disease for longer than 15 years, and the average period from diagnosis to death is less than 13 years. Twenty-year follow-up of glaucoma-related blindness in one eye occurs in 25% of patients and in both eyes in only 10%.

NORMAL-TENSION GLAUCOMA

Definition

Normal-tension glaucoma (NTG), also referred to as low-tension glaucoma, is a variant of POAG. It is characterized by:
- A mean IOP ≤ 21 mmHg on diurnal testing.
- Glaucomatous optic disc damage and visual field loss.
- Open drainage angle on gonioscopy.
- Absence of secondary causes for glaucomatous optic disc damage.

> **NB** The classification of POAG into two types (i.e. normal-tension and high-tension) is based on an epidemiologically derived normal IOP. It is essentially an arbitrary division and may not have significant clinical value. The prevalence of NTG in individuals over the age of 40 years is 0.2% and the condition accounts for 16% of all cases of POAG.

Pathogenesis

The exact cause of NTG has not been conclusively determined although various mechanisms have been postulated such as vascular insufficiency, decreased optic disc resistance, IOP effects and optic nerve compression by normal carotid arteries.

Risk factors

1. **Age.** Patients with NTG tend to be significantly older than those with POAG.
2. **Gender.** Females are at greater risk than males by a 2:1 ratio.
3. **Race.** NTG occurs more frequently in Japan than in either Europe or North America.
4. **Family history.** The prevalence of POAG is greater in families of patients with NTG than in the normal population. A specific locus for NTG (*GLCIE*) has been assigned to 10p14-p15 (optineurin gene).

Diagnosis

1. **IOP** is usually in the high teens, but may rarely be lower. In asymmetrical disease the more damaged disc corresponds to the eye with the higher IOP.
2. **Optic nerve head**
   - Although the optic nerve head is larger in NTG than in POAG, glaucomatous cupping and parapapillary changes are identical.
   - Splinter haemorrhages at the disc margin (see Fig. 13.11d) and acquired optic disc pits characterized by localized excavations of the lamina cribrosa are more frequent in NTG than in POAG.
3. **Visual field defects** are essentially the same as in POAG although it has been suggested that in NTG they tend to be closer to fixation, deeper, steeper and more localized. In some patients, even without treatment, field changes are non-progressive. However, because of frequent delay in diagnosis, patients with NTG tend to present with more advanced damage than those with POAG. Patients with unilateral field defects have a 40% chance of developing field loss in the fellow eye within 5 years.
4. **Other characteristics** which are more common in NTG than in POAG are:
   - Peripheral vascular spasm on cooling (Raynaud phenomenon).
   - Migraine.
   - Nocturnal systemic hypotension.
   - Reduced blood flow velocity in the ophthalmic and posterior ciliary arteries. This can be demonstrated with colour Doppler imaging.
   - Paraproteinaemia and the presence of serum auto-antibodies.

Treatment

Perimetry should be performed at 4–6-monthly intervals to demonstrate progression, before specific medication is commenced. In some patients the visual field loss is non-progressive and treatment is not required. Without treatment 40% of patients do not deteriorate after 5 years of follow-up. With treatment that reduces IOP by 30% from baseline, 80% of patients are stable and 20% show progression of visual field defects after 5 years of follow-up. Risk factors for progression of visual field loss include presence of disc haemorrhages, female gender and migraine.

1. **Medical** treatment in progressive cases may include betaxolol because of its beneficial effects on optic nerve blood flow in addition to its IOP lowering properties. However, prostaglandin analogues tend to have a greater ocular hypotensive effect in eyes with normal IOP although they are ineffective in the long term in a significant proportion of patients.
2. **Trabeculectomy** should be considered, in at least one eye, if progressive field loss occurs despite IOP in the low teens.
3. **Monitoring of systemic blood pressure** for 24 hours. If a significant nocturnal drop is detected, it may be necessary to avoid anti-hypertensive medication (especially if taken prior to bed-time). Non-selective topical beta-blockers should not be used at bed-time, because they may cause a profound drop in systemic blood pressure in some individuals. The patient should also be encouraged to take normally salted food and increase physical activity (an afternoon walk may suffice).

Differential diagnosis

1. **POAG** presenting with normal IOP because of a wide diurnal fluctuation. This can be excluded by phasing over an 8-hour period in order to detect a pressure spike of > 21mmHg.
2. **Spontaneously resolved pigmentary glaucoma.**
3. **Previous episodes of raised IOP** as may occur as a result of ocular trauma, chronic anterior uveitis or topical steroid therapy.
4. **Progressive retinal nerve fibre defects not due to glaucoma** as may occur in myopic degeneration and optic disc drusen.
5. **Congenital disc anomalies** simulating glaucomatous cupping such as disc pits and colobomas.
6. **Neurological** lesions causing optic nerve or chiasmal compression may produce visual field defects, which may be misinterpreted as being glaucomatous. Neuroimaging should therefore be performed in patients who do not fit the profile of NTG.
7. **Previous anterior ischaemic optic neuropathy,** especially the arteritic form, may give rise to a disc appearance consistent with advanced glaucoma.
8. **Previous acute blood loss or shock** causing infarction of the optic nerve head is also relevant.

PRIMARY ANGLE-CLOSURE GLAUCOMA

Introduction

Definition

1. **Primary angle closure** occurs in anatomically predisposed eyes, without other pathology, in which vision is threatened by elevation of IOP as a consequence of obstruction of aqueous outflow by occlusion of the trabecular meshwork by the peripheral iris. The condition may manifest as an ophthalmic emergency or may remain asymptomatic until visual loss occurs. Unlike POAG, the diagnosis depends largely on examination of the anterior segment and careful gonioscopy. Management requires an understanding of the underlying pathophysiological mechanisms.
2. **Primary angle-closure glaucoma** (PACG) is a term that should be used only when primary angle closure has resulted in optic nerve damage and visual field loss. It is important to note that until recently PACG was not defined by optic nerve damage, in distinction to the contemporary definition. This inconsistency in use of the word glaucoma has a historical rather than a scientific basis and can be a source of confusion when reviewing previous publications.

Risk factors

1. **Age.** The average age at presentation is about 60 years; prevalence increases thereafter.
2. **Gender.** Females are more commonly affected than males by a ratio of 4:1.
3. **Race.** In Caucasians the condition accounts for about 6% of all glaucomas and it affects approximately 1:1000 individuals over the age of 40 years. PACG is more common in South-East Asians, Chinese and Eskimos but is uncommon in blacks.
4. **Family history.** First degree relatives are at increased risk because predisposing anatomical factors are often inherited (see below).

Anatomical predisposing factors

- Relatively anterior location of the iris-lens diaphragm secondary to short axial length.
- Shallow anterior chamber.
- Narrow entrance to the chamber angle.

The proximity of the peripheral iris to the cornea facilitates angle closure. The following three interrelated factors are responsible for these characteristics.

1. **Lens size.** The lens is the only ocular structure which continues to increase in size throughout life. Axial

(anteroposterior) growth brings its anterior surface closer to the cornea, while equatorial growth slackens the suspensory ligament, allowing the iris-lens diaphragm to move anteriorly. Both these factors cause gradual and progressive shallowing of the anterior chamber. Eyes with PACG have shallower anterior chambers (1.8mm) than normal eyes (2.8mm), and women have shallower anterior chambers than men.

2. **Corneal diameter.** Anterior chamber depth and angle width are related to the corneal diameter. Eyes with PACG have corneal diameters 0.25mm smaller than normal.

3. **Axial length.** The position of the lens and the corneal diameter are related to the axial length of the globe. A short eye, which is also frequently hypermetropic, has a small corneal diameter and a relatively anteriorly located lens.

Pathogenesis

The pathogenesis of acute PACG is incompletely understood. Normally the pressure in the posterior chamber exceeds that in the anterior chamber due to a physiological degree of resistance at the pupil, since the iris rests posteriorly on the anterior lens capsule.

1. **The dilator muscle theory** postulates that contraction of the dilator pupillae exerts a posterior vector force. This increases the amount of apposition between the iris and the anteriorly located lens, enhancing the degree of physiological pupil block (Fig. 13.21a). Simultaneous dilatation of the pupil renders the peripheral iris more flaccid. The pupil block causes the pressure in the posterior chamber to increase and the peripheral iris bows anteriorly (iris bombé – Fig. 13.21b). Eventually the iris touches the posterior corneal surface, obstructing the angle, and the IOP rises (Fig. 13.21c).

2. **The sphincter muscle theory** postulates that the sphincter pupillae is the prime culprit in precipitating angle closure. The pupillary blocking force of the sphincter is greatest when the diameter of the pupil is approximately 4mm.

Classification

Although primary angle closure can be divided into five overlapping stages, the condition does not necessarily progress from one stage to the next in an orderly sequence. In practice, a combination of these clinical stages is often seen.

1. **Angle closure suspect.**
2. **Intermittent (subacute) angle closure.**
3. **Acute angle closure:** congestive and post-congestive.
4. **Chronic angle closure:** without and with glaucomatous damage.
5. **Absolute angle closure** is the end-stage of acute congestive PACG in which the eye is completely blind and will not be discussed further.

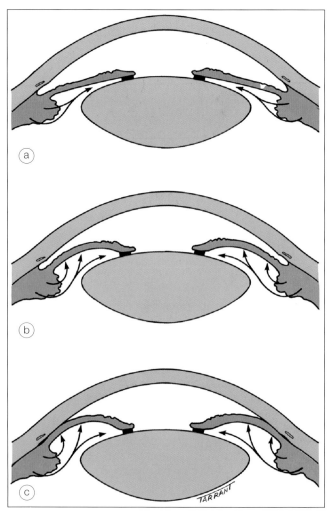

Fig. 13.21
Mechanism of angle closure. **(a)** Relative pupil block; **(b)** iris bombé; **(c)** iridocorneal contact

Angle closure suspect

Diagnosis

Angle closure suspect is a retrospective diagnosis, only made with any degree of certainty in one eye during an attack of acute congestive angle closure in the other. Essentially, the term implies an anatomically predisposed eye.

1. **Symptoms** are absent.
2. **Slit-lamp biomicroscopy**
   - Axial anterior chamber depth is less than normal and the iris-lens diaphragm is convex (Fig. 13.22a).
   - Close proximity of the iris to the cornea (Fig. 13.22b).
3. **Gonioscopy** shows an 'occludable' angle in which the pigmented trabecular meshwork is not visible (Shaffer

grade 1 or 0) without indentation or manipulation in at least three quadrants (Fig. 13.22c).

4. **The clinical course** without treatment may be as follows:
   - IOP may remain normal.
   - Acute or subacute angle closure may ensue.
   - Chronic angle closure may develop, without passing through subacute or acute stages.

Treatment

The need to treat is based on the following criteria:
- If one eye has had acute or subacute angle closure, the fellow eye should undergo prophylactic peripheral laser iridotomy because, without treatment, the risk of an acute pressure rise during the next five years is about 50%.
- If both eyes have occludable angles, there is no parameter or provocative test that is sufficiently sensitive or accurate to determine whether acute angle closure will later develop. However, since the risks of laser iridotomy are small, if carefully undertaken, laser treatment may be considered.

NB Although prophylactic laser iridotomy will prevent an acute attack, 15% of eyes develop a late rise in IOP.

Intermittent angle closure

Intermittent (subacute) angle closure occurs in a predisposed eye with an occludable angle in association with intermittent pupillary block. Rapid closure of the angle results in sudden increase in IOP. The pupillary block is then spontaneously relieved, the angle opens and the IOP returns to normal. Attacks may be precipitated by physiological mydriasis (watching television in a dark room), or by physiological shallowing of the anterior chamber when the patient assumes a prone or semi-prone position (when sewing or reading). Emotional stress may occasionally be a precipitating factor.

1. **Diagnosis** is based on a characteristic history of transient blurring of vision associated with haloes around lights due to corneal epithelial oedema (the blue end of the spectrum being nearer the source). There may also be associated ocular discomfort or frontal headache. The attacks are recurrent and are usually broken after 1–2 hours by physiological miosis (exposure to bright sunlight or sleep). During an attack the eye is usually white and in between attacks looks normal although the angle is narrow.

2. **The clinical course without treatment** is variable. Some eyes develop an acute attack and others may develop chronic angle closure.

3. **Treatment** is with prophylactic peripheral laser iridotomy.

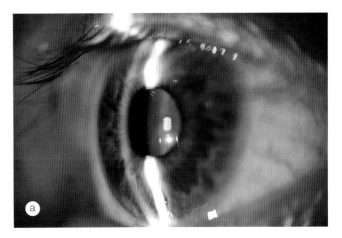

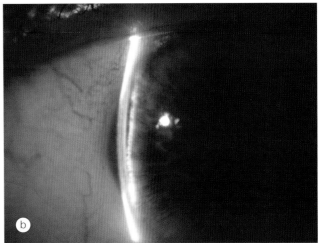

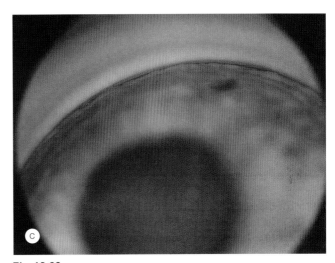

Fig. 13.22
Angle closure suspect. **(a)** Shallow anterior chamber and convex shaped iris-lens diaphragm; **(b)** close proximity of the iris to the peripheral cornea; **(c)** very narrow angle (Courtesy of L MacKeen – fig. c)

Acute congestive angle closure

Acute congestive angle closure ('acute glaucoma') is a sight-threatening emergency, manifesting with painful loss of vision due to sudden and total closure of the angle.

Diagnosis

1. **Presentation** in classical cases there is rapidly progressive unilateral visual loss associated with periocular pain and congestion. Nausea and vomiting may occur in severe cases. It is, however, important to be aware of the variability of symptoms. Some patients, particularly blacks in whom the condition is uncommon, have remarkably little pain and no congestion despite very high IOPs, the only symptom being impairment of vision.

2. **Slit-lamp biomicroscopy**
   * 'Ciliary' flush due to injection of the limbal and conjunctival blood vessels.
   * Shallow anterior chamber and corneal oedema with epithelial vesicles and stromal thickening (Fig. 13.23a).
   * Shallow anterior chamber with peripheral iridocorneal contact.
   * Aqueous flare and cells may be seen once the corneal oedema has resolved.
   * The pupil is vertically oval, fixed in the semi-dilated position and unreactive to both light and accommodation (Fig. 13.23b).
   * The iris blood vessels are dilated.
   * IOP is severely elevated (50–100mmHg).

3. **Gonioscopy** may need to be deferred until the corneal oedema has resolved, either with ocular hypotensive medication or topical glycerine. It is, however, vital to perform this examination on the fellow eye, which usually exhibits characteristics of latent angle closure. The affected eye shows complete peripheral iridocorneal contact (Shaffer grade 0 – Fig. 13.23c).

NB The diagnosis should be questioned if the fellow eye does not show a narrow angle on gonioscopy.

Medical treatment

1. **Immediate.** The patient should be positioned supine to allow the lens to shift posteriorly.
   a. Acetazolamide 500mg intravenously and 500mg orally (not slow-release) provided there is no vomiting.

   NB Check for sulphonamide allergy.

   b. Topical
   – Predsol or dexamethasone q.i.d.
   – Timolol 0.5% if there is no contraindication.
   c. Analgesia and anti-emetics as required.

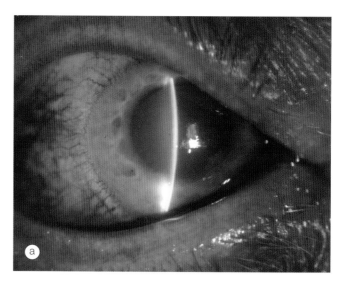

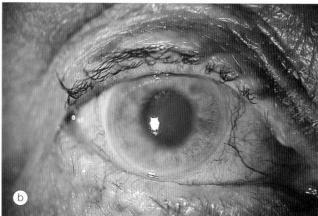

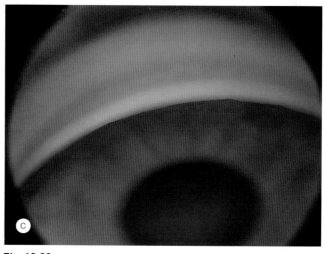

Fig. 13.23
Acute congestive angle closure. **(a)** Shallow anterior chamber and corneal oedema; **(b)** fixed oval dilated pupil; **(c)** complete angle closure (Courtesy of L MacKeen – fig. c)

NB Laser iridotomy may also be effective in relatively mild cases.

2. **After one hour** pilocarpine 2% q.i.d should be started half to one hour after commencement of treatment, by which time reduction of iris ischaemia and lowering of IOP allows the sphincter pupillae to respond to the drug. There is no place for 'intensive' miotic therapy. The fellow eye is also treated prophylactically with pilocarpine 1% q.i.d until prophylactic laser iridotomy is performed.
3. **After a further 30 minutes**
   - Re-check IOP.
   - If the IOP has not fallen to below 35mmHg give oral 50% glycerol 1g/kg (with caution in diabetics) and limit fluid intake for maximum effect.
   - If the patient is vomiting or is unable to tolerate oral glycerol give 20% mannitol (1–2g/kg) intravenously over 45 minutes.

NB A high IOP unresponsive to ocular hypotensive medication may sometimes respond to axial corneal indentation with a squint hook or a Zeiss goniolens. If angle closure is appositional, this allows aqueous humour to force its way between the iris and cornea to the angle, thus opening it and gaining access to the trabecular meshwork.

Nd:YAG laser iridotomy

1. **Purpose** of peripheral laser iridotomy is to re-establish communication between the posterior and anterior chambers by making an opening in the peripheral iris.
2. **Timing** varies with the severity of the attack and the rapidity of corneal clearing. Iridotomy has been advocated as initial treatment to break pupil block but may be difficult until the corneal thickening and iris congestion have settled (usually 48 hours). After an explanation has been given, it may be appropriate to perform a prophylactic laser iridotomy on the fellow eye in the interim period. Laser iridotomy is effective in about 75% of eyes with acute angle-closure glaucoma. Unresponsive cases may require trabeculectomy.

NB It is important to confirm that the angle is open after peripheral iridotomy even if the IOP is normal.

3. **Favourable prognostic factors** for laser iridotomy include:
   - Good response to medical therapy with early miosis indicating that a sufficient portion of the angle is open.
   - More than 50% of the angle without peripheral anterior synechiae.
   - Absence of glaucomatous damage.

Differential diagnosis

Although the diagnosis is usually straightforward the following conditions should be considered in differential diagnosis:

1. **Secondary acute angle closure** due to an intumescent (swollen) or dislocated lens.
2. **Neovascular glaucoma** may occasionally cause a sudden onset of pain and congestion.
3. **Glaucomatocyclitic crisis** may cause severe elevation of IOP with pain and haloes.
4. **Pigment dispersion** with sudden elevation of IOP.
5. **Pseudoexfoliation** with sudden elevation of IOP.
6. **Other causes of headache** around the eye such as migraine or migrainous neuralgia (cluster headache).

Post-congestive angle closure

Clinical settings

Post-congestive angle closure refers to the aftermath of an attack of acute angle closure. It may be seen in the following three clinical settings:

1. **Postsurgical** in which the IOP is normalized by successful peripheral iridotomy. Occasionally, even after peripheral iridotomy, with the angle open 180° or more, IOP may still be elevated due to associated trabecular damage. Medical therapy or trabeculectomy may be needed to control the IOP.
2. **Spontaneous angle re-opening** without treatment may occur in a few cases; management is as for intermittent angle closure.
3. **Ciliary body shutdown** involves temporary cessation of aqueous secretion due to ischaemic damage to the ciliary epithelium. Subsequent recovery of ciliary function may lead to chronic elevation of IOP with cupping and field loss.

Diagnosis

1. **Slit-lamp biomicroscopy**
   - Folds in Descemet membrane, if the IOP has been reduced rapidly (Fig. 13.24a).
   - Fine pigment granules on the corneal endothelium.
   - Aqueous flare and cells.
   - Glaukomflecken characterized by small, grey-white, anterior subcapsular or capsular lens opacities in the pupillary zone is diagnostic of a previous congestive attack (Fig. 13.24b). It represents focal necrosis of the lens epithelium.
   - Stromal iris atrophy with a spiral-like configuration (Fig. 13.24c).

- Fixed and semi-dilated pupil due to a combination of paralysis of the sphincter and posterior synechiae (Fig. 13.24c).
- IOP may be normal, subnormal or elevated.

2. **Gonioscopy** shows a narrow angle which may be open or partly closed. If open, trabecular hyperpigmentation may be present. A straight line of pigment may be seen anterior to Schwalbe line at the site of previous iridocorneal contact.

3. **Ophthalmoscopy** may reveal congestion of the optic disc and choroidal folds if the IOP is very low. The disc may be atrophic as a result of infarction.

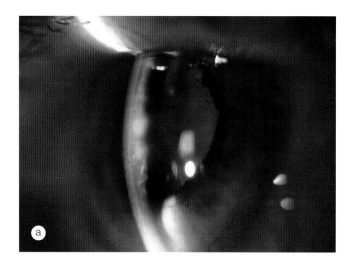

Chronic angle closure

Pathogenesis

1. **Type 1** (creeping) is caused by gradual and progressive synechial angle closure which always starts superiorly and spreads circumferentially. This may be caused by anteriorly situated ciliary processes; many eyes have a plateau iris configuration (see below).

2. **Type 2** is caused by synechial angle closure as a result of intermittent (subacute) attacks secondary to pupillary block.

3. **Type 3** (mixed) is caused by a combination of POAG with narrow angles usually associated with the long-term use of miotics.

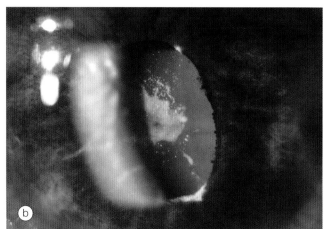

Diagnosis

1. **Gonioscopy** shows a variable amount of angle closure, although permanent peripheral anterior synechiae do not usually develop until late. The diagnosis will be missed unless routine gonioscopy is performed on all glaucomatous eyes.

2. **Ophthalmoscopy** shows optic disc changes similar to those in POAG except when infarction of the optic nerve head has caused pallor and shallow temporal shelving.

Treatment

1. **Type 1** (creeping) is initially treated by laser iridotomy to eradicate any element of pupil block. Any residual elevation of IOP is then treated medically. If this fails, trabeculectomy should be required.

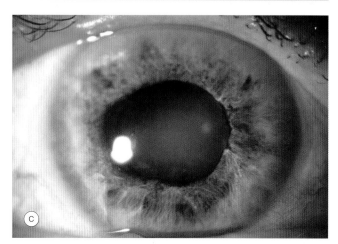

2. **Type 2** will already have undergone iridotomy. Medical therapy should be added as necessary.

3. **Type 3** (mixed) will already be on medical therapy for POAG and should be treated by laser iridotomy.

Fig. 13.24
Post-congestive angle closure. **(a)** Stromal corneal oedema and folds in Descemet membrane; **(b)** glaukomflecken; **(c)** spiral-shaped atrophic iris, dilated pupil and posterior synechiae

NB Treatment of associated cataract may be beneficial in controlling IOP provided no more than two quadrants of synechial angle closure are present.

Plateau iris configuration and syndrome

Diagnosis

1. **Plateau iris configuration** is characterized by a narrow anterior chamber angle in association with a flat iris plane and a normal depth central anterior chamber. An anterior position of the ciliary processes results in an abnormal configuration of the peripheral iris (Fig. 13.25a). Although this mechanism of angle closure is rare in whites, it is not uncommon in South-East Asians.
2. **Plateau iris syndrome** describes acute angle closure which occurs either spontaneously or after pupillary dilatation, despite a patent iridotomy. The syndrome tends to occur at a younger age than angle closure with pupillary block. When the pupil dilates, the peripheral iris becomes 'bunched up' and occludes the trabeculum (Fig. 13.25b). All the features of acute congestive angle closure are present except that the axial anterior chamber depth is normal and the iris plane is flat rather than convex.

Treatment

1. **Medical** treatment is with pilocarpine 1% drops after laser peripheral iridotomy has been performed.
2. **Peripheral iridoplasty** involves applying argon laser burns to the iris in order to flatten the 'hump' by contracting iris tissue. The initial settings are 200µm, 0.2sec and 400mW. Approximately 10 burns are placed in each quadrant. If iris contraction is inadequate further applications may be required.

PSEUDOEXFOLIATION

Pseudoexfoliation syndrome

Introduction

The pseudoexfoliation (PEX) syndrome is a relatively common but easily overlooked cause of chronic open-angle glaucoma. When an eye with PEX develops secondary trabecular block glaucoma the condition is referred to as PEX glaucoma, which is also sometimes referred to as glaucoma capsulare. PEX is more common in females but males appear to be at higher risk of developing glaucoma. Although no clear hereditary pattern has been established the condition is particularly common in Scandinavia and is associated with a gene locus at 2p16. PEX should be differentiated from true exfoliation, which is very rare and involves lamellar splitting of the lens capsule secondary to infra-red damage.

Pathogenesis

PEX (Fig. 13.26a) is a grey-white, fibrillogranular, extra-cellular, matrix material composed of a protein core surrounded by glycosaminoglycans. It is produced by abnormal basement membranes of ageing epithelial cells in the trabeculum, equatorial lens capsule, iris and ciliary body, and then deposited on the anterior lens capsule, zonules, ciliary body, iris, trabeculum, anterior vitreous face and conjunctiva.

NB In addition to its occurrence within the eye, exfoliative fibrillopathy has been reported in skin and visceral organs, suggesting that PEX may be an ocular manifestation of a systemic disorder.

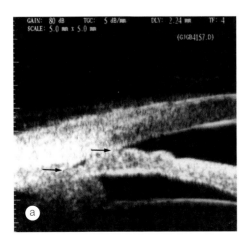
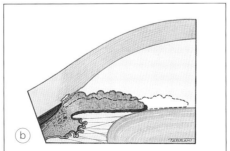

Fig. 13.25
(a) High-resolution ultrasonography in plateau iris configuration shows anteriorly rotated ciliary processes and a slit-like angle (arrows); **(b)** angle closure in plateau iris syndrome (Courtesy of J Salmon – fig. a)

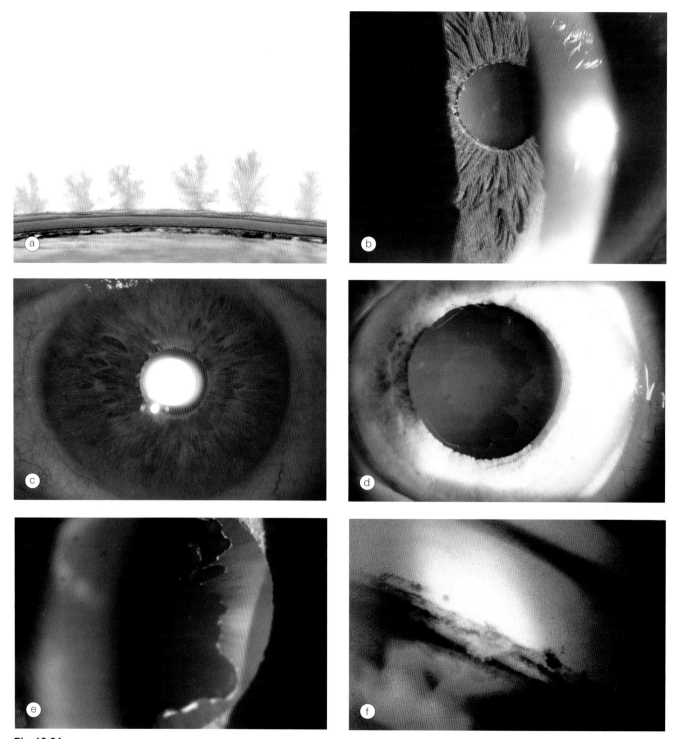

Fig. 13.26

Pseudoexfoliation syndrome. **(a)** Christmas-tree like deposits of pseudoexfoliative material (PEX) on the lens capsule; **(b)** PEX on the pupillary margin; **(c)** transillumination defect corresponding to sphincter iris atrophy; **(d)** central disc of PEX; **(e)** peripheral band of PEX; **(f)** gonioscopy shows patchy trabecular hyperpigmentation and deposits of PEX (Courtesy of J Harry and G Misson, from *Clinical Ophthalmic Pathology*, Butterworth-Heinemann, 2001– fig a; E Michael Van Buskirk, from *Clinical Atlas of Glaucoma*, W B Saunders, 1986 – fig. f)

Diagnosis

1. **Cornea** occasionally shows PEX on the endothelium as well as pigment deposition which is usually diffuse, although occasionally it may take the form of a Krukenberg spindle (Fig. 13.28a).
2. **Mild aqueous flare** due to breakdown of the iris blood–aqueous barrier.
3. **Iris** shows PEX on the pupillary margin (Fig. 13.26b) and sphincter atrophy characterized by 'moth-eaten' transillumination defects, most evident in eyes with pupillary ruff defects (Fig. 13.26c).
4. **PEX on the anterior lens surface**
   - The constant rubbing of the pupil scrapes the material off the mid-zone of the lens giving rise to a central disc and a peripheral band of PEX, with a clear zone in between.
   - The central disc is translucent, well demarcated and its edges may contain rolled-up fragments (Fig. 13.26d).
   - The peripheral band is granular and has a well-delineated inner border with multiple radial striations (Fig. 13.26e). It can be detected only after the pupil has been dilated.
5. **Gonioscopy**
   - Trabecular hyperpigmentation is common and is usually most marked inferiorly. It may antedate the appearance of PEX by several years. The pigment lies on the surface of the trabeculum and has a patchy distribution (Fig. 13.26f). A scalloped band of pigment running on to or anterior to Schwalbe line (Sampaolesi line) is also frequently seen.
   - PEX deposits in the trabeculum give rise to a 'dandruff-like' appearance (Fig. 13.26f).
   - Narrow angles are present in some cases; even in eyes with wide open angles, the IOP may become elevated when the pupil is dilated.

NB Cataract surgery may be more hazardous due to a combination of poorly dilating pupil, increased risk of zonulodialysis and vitreous loss. There is also an increased incidence of postoperative capsular opacification and contraction, and spontaneous decentration or dislocation of the IOL. Other problems that may occur include prolonged intraocular inflammation and corneal decompensation that may occur with only moderate rises in IOP.

Pseudoexfoliation glaucoma

Pathogenesis

Many unresolved questions exist concerning the relationship between PEX and glaucoma. Potential causes of elevation of IOP include secondary trabecular blockage due to a combination of 'clogging up' of the trabeculum by PEX and/or pigment released from the iris, as well as trabecular endothelial cell dysfunction.

Risk factors

- The cumulative risk of glaucoma in eyes with PEX is 5% at 5 years and 15% at 10 years. Individuals with PEX should be informed of this risk and advised to undergo annual ocular examination.
- A patient with unilateral PEX glaucoma and only PEX in the fellow eye is at high risk (50% in 5 years) of developing glaucoma in the fellow eye.
- A patient with unilateral PEX glaucoma who does not have PEX in the fellow eye is at very small risk of developing glaucoma in the normal eye.

Diagnosis

1. **Presentation** is usually in the seventh decade, which is later than POAG.
2. **Signs.** The majority of patients have a chronic open-angle glaucoma which is usually unilateral. Occasionally the IOP may rise acutely despite a wide-open angle; this may be confused with primary angle-closure. There is no apparent association between angle characteristics and the severity of glaucoma.

Treatment

1. **Medical** treatment is the same as for POAG. However, despite initial success in most cases, there is a high incidence of late failure and patients are likely to require laser therapy or surgery.
2. **Laser trabeculoplasty** is particularly effective, possibly because of trabecular hyperpigmentation. However, after an initial good response a gradual late rise of IOP occurs so that after 4 years the results are the same as in POAG.
3. **Early trabeculectomy** may be advantageous and has the same success rate as in POAG with no unusual complications.
4. **Bimanual trabecular aspiration** is a recently described procedure with early results comparable to trabeculectomy but fewer complications.

Prognosis

The prognosis is less good than in POAG because the IOP is often significantly elevated and may also exhibit great fluctuation so that severe damage may develop rapidly. It is therefore important to monitor patients closely until the IOP is brought under control.

PIGMENT DISPERSION

Pigment dispersion syndrome

Introduction

Pigment dispersion syndrome (PDS) is a usually bilateral condition characterized by the liberation of pigment granules from the iris pigment epithelium and their deposition throughout the anterior segment. PDS primarily affects whites and may be inherited as AD with variable penetrance. There is a significant linkage between the disease phenotype and genetic markers located on 7q35-36 named GLC1F. Myopia predisposes to the phenotypical manifestations and the development of a secondary open-angle 'pigmentary' glaucoma. However, some manifestations of PDS may be extremely subtle and go undetected.

Pathogenesis

Pigment shedding is caused by the mechanical rubbing of the posterior pigment layer of the iris against packets of lens zonules as a result of excessive posterior bowing of the mid-peripheral portion of the iris. It is postulated that an increase in anterior chamber pressure (relative to the posterior chamber) occurs due to 'reverse pupil block', with resultant posterior bowing of the iris and irido-zonular touch (Fig. 13.27a). This is supported by the observation that neutralization of reverse pupil block with peripheral iridotomy flattens the iris and decreases irido-zonular contact (Fig. 13.27b). The pigment epithelium itself may be abnormally susceptible to shedding; in some patients strenuous exercise may precipitate episodes of pigment dispersion associated with a rise in IOP. The pigment granules are released into the aqueous humour, dispersed by aqueous currents and deposited on all anterior chamber structures, including the zonular fibres and ciliary body.

Diagnosis

1. **Cornea** shows pigment deposition on the endothelium, in a vertical spindle-shaped distribution (Krukenberg spindle) (Fig. 13.28a). This sign, although common, is neither universal nor pathognomonic of PDS, and in long-standing cases, may be more difficult to detect because it tends to become smaller and lighter in colour.
2. **Anterior chamber** is very deep (see Fig. 13.27a) and melanin granules may be seen floating in the aqueous.
3. **Iris**
   - Fine surface pigment granules that may extend onto the lens (Fig. 13.28b).
   - Pigment epithelial atrophy due to shedding of pigment from the mid-periphery gives rise to characteristic radial slit-like transillumination defects (Fig. 13.28c). If asymmetrical, the eye with more iris atrophy may exhibit a slightly larger pupil.

   - Partial loss of the pupillary ruff (frill) is common (see Fig. 13.28b).
4. **Gonioscopy**
   - Wide open angle with characteristic mid-peripheral iris concavity that may increase with accommodation.
   - Trabecular hyperpigmentation is most marked over the posterior trabeculum (Fig. 13.28d).

   NB The pigment is finer than in PEX and appears to lie both on and within the trabecular meshwork. It also has a more homogeneous appearance and forms a dense band involving the entire circumference of the meshwork uniformly. Pigment may also be seen on or anterior to Schwalbe line.

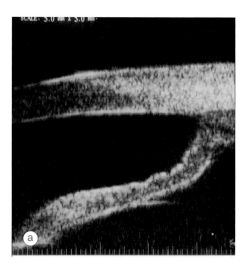

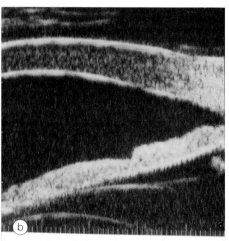

Fig. 13.27
High-frequency ultrasonography in pigment dispersion syndrome. **(a)** Very deep anterior chamber and posterior bowing of the peripheral iris; **(b)** flattening of the peripheral iris following laser iridotomy (Courtesy of J Salmon)

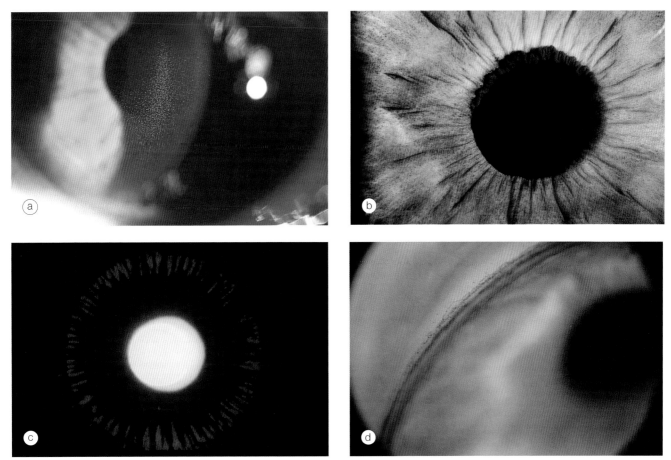

Fig. 13.28
Pigment dispersion syndrome. **(a)** Krukenberg spindle; **(b)** pigment granules on the surface of the iris and partial loss of the pupillary ruff; **(c)** radial slit-like transillumination defects; **(d)** homogeneous trabecular hyperpigmentation (Courtesy of L Merin – fig. c; L MacKeen – fig. d)

Pigmentary glaucoma

Pathogenesis

Elevation of IOP appears to be caused by pigmentary obstruction of the intertrabecular spaces and damage to the trabeculum secondary to denudation, collapse and sclerosis.

Risk factors

About a third of patients with PDS eventually develop ocular hypertension or chronic open-angle glaucoma after 15 years. Men are affected twice as frequently as women. The optic disc is more susceptible to the effects of elevated IOP because of the underlying myopia. It is therefore important to regularly follow patients with the condition, particularly myopic males with Krukenberg spindles. However, initial IOP, cup–disc ratio and degree of trabecular hyperpigmentation are not helpful in identifying those who will eventually develop glaucoma. Patients with pigmentary glaucoma have an increased incidence of steroid responsiveness. Although PDS is rare in black patients they are at increased risk of developing glaucoma which is of a more severe form than that in whites.

Diagnosis

1. **Presentation** is usually with chronic glaucoma, most commonly in the third and fourth decades, although in women it tends to develop 10 years later. Occasionally, the sudden release of pigment granules, following vigorous movement of the pupil or strenuous physical exercise, may precipitate an acute rise in IOP, with corneal oedema and haloes.

2. **IOP** may initially be very unstable, so that a single normal reading does not exclude glaucoma. Some patients exhibit higher levels and wider fluctuations of IOP than in POAG, and at the time of diagnosis it is common to find advanced disease in one eye and relatively mild damage in the other.

Treatment

1. **Medical** treatment is similar to that of POAG. Miotics may, theoretically, be of particular benefit because they decrease irido-zonular contact in addition to facilitating aqueous outflow. They, however, carry the disadvantage of exacerbating myopia. Topical carbonic anhydrase inhibitors, brimonidine and prostaglandin analogues are also effective.
2. **Laser trabeculoplasty** is often initially effective and younger patients appear to respond better. It is important not to over-treat eyes with heavily pigmented angles and to start at a relatively low power laser setting. At least one-third of patients will require trabeculectomy within 5 years of laser trabeculoplasty.
3. **Laser iridotomy** may be effective in preventing further pigment deposition by reversing iris concavity and eliminating irido-zonular contact (see Fig. 13.27). It appears to work best in patients under the age of 40 years but its long-term efficacy is not known.
4. **Trabeculectomy** is required in patients unresponsive to medical therapy and laser trabeculoplasty although the results are less predictable in younger patients. The use of adjunctive antimetabolites may improve surgical outcome. A higher percentage of patients with pigmentary glaucoma require surgery as compared with POAG and men require it earlier.

Prognosis

Prognosis is relatively good and over time the control of IOP becomes easier. Occasionally the IOP may spontaneously revert to normal. This may or may not be associated with a decrease in trabecular pigmentation. Patients with undetected previous pigmentary glaucoma may later be erroneously diagnosed as having normal-tension glaucoma.

Differential diagnosis

1. **POAG** may be associated with a hyperpigmented trabeculum. However, the pigment tends to be concentrated in the inferior sector of the angle, unlike in PDS. Patients with POAG are also usually older and lack Krukenberg spindles and iris transillumination defects.
2. **PEX glaucoma** may exhibit trabecular hyperpigmentation and pigment dispersion. However, transillumination defects are evident at the margin of the pupil rather than in the periphery. In contrast with pigmentary glaucoma, PEX glaucoma usually affects patients over the age of 60

years, is unilateral in 50% of cases and has no predilection for a myopic refractive error.
3. **Pseudophakic pigmentary glaucoma** occurs in the context of rubbing of the haptics and optics of a posterior chamber intraocular lens against the posterior surface of the iris, with resultant pigment dispersion and outflow obstruction.
4. **Anterior uveitis** may result in trabecular hyperpigmentation and iris atrophy. Clustered small old pigmented keratic precipitates may be mistaken for a Krukenberg spindle on cursory examination.
5. **Subacute angle-closure glaucoma** may be associated with a heavily pigmented trabeculum where the iris root has been in contact with the angle.

NEOVASCULAR GLAUCOMA

Introduction

Pathogenesis

Neovascular glaucoma (NVG) is a relatively common and serious condition which occurs as a result of iris neovascularization (rubeosis iridis). The common aetiological factor is severe, diffuse and chronic retinal ischaemia. It is postulated that hypoxic retinal tissue produces heparin-binding growth factors in an attempt to revascularize hypoxic areas. The most important of these is vascular endothelial growth factor (VEGF). Apart from inducing retinal neovascularization (proliferative retinopathy) such factors also diffuse into the anterior segment and initiate rubeosis iridis and neovascularization in the angle of the anterior chamber. The latter initially impairs aqueous outflow in the presence of an open angle and later contracts to produce a secondary angle-closure glaucoma which is usually severe and relentless (Fig. 13.29a). NVG can often be prevented by timely treatment of ischaemic retina by laser photocoagulation.

Causes of rubeosis iridis

1. **Ischaemic central retinal vein occlusion** accounts for 36% of cases. Approximately 50% of eyes develop NVG following ischaemic central retinal vein occlusion. Extensive peripheral retinal capillary non-perfusion on fluorescein angiography is the most valuable predictor of the risk of subsequent NVG, although in some patients non-ischaemic occlusion may subsequently become ischaemic. Glaucoma typically occurs 3 months after the occlusion ('100-day glaucoma') but intervals from 4 weeks to 2 years have been documented.
2. **Diabetes mellitus** accounts for 32% of cases. Patients with long-standing diabetes (10 years or more) with proliferative retinopathy are at particular risk. The risk of

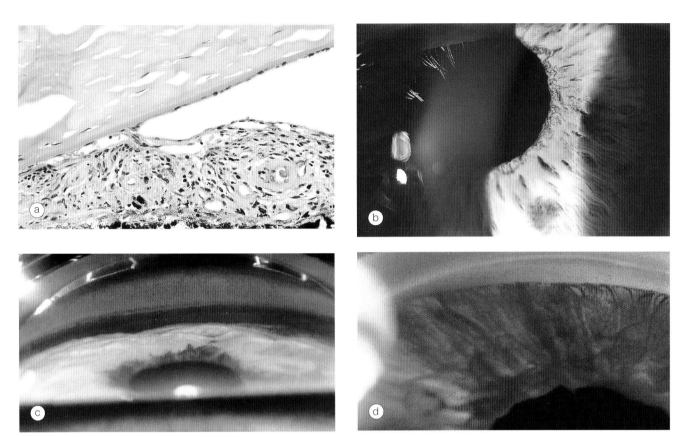

Fig. 13.29
Neovascular glaucoma. **(a)** Rubeosis iridis and angle closure; **(b)** tiny capillary tufts on the pupil margin; **(c)** invasion of angle structures by new vessels; **(d)** progressive synechial angle closure (Courtesy of J Harry and G Misson, from *Clinical Ophthalmic Pathology*, Butterworth-Heinemann, 2001 – fig. a)

glaucoma is decreased by appropriate panretinal photocoagulation and increased by cataract extraction, particularly if the posterior capsule is breached. Frequent review is therefore essential during the first four postoperative weeks, which represent the crucial period for the development of rubeosis iridis. Pars plana vitrectomy may also precipitate rubeosis iridis if inadequate laser therapy is applied or tractional retinal detachment persists.

3. **Miscellaneous** causes include central retinal artery occlusion, carotid obstructive disease, intraocular tumours, long-standing retinal detachment and chronic intraocular inflammation.

Classification

Despite a degree of overlap it is convenient to divide NVG into the following three stages: (a) *rubeosis iridis*, (b) *secondary open-angle glaucoma* and (c) *secondary synechial angle-closure glaucoma*.

Rubeosis iridis

Diagnosis

In chronological order rubeosis develops as follows:
- Tiny dilated capillary tufts or red spots develop at the pupillary margin and may be missed unless the iris is examined carefully under high magnification (Fig. 13.29b).
- The new vessels grow radially over the surface of the iris towards the angle, sometimes joining dilated blood vessels at the collarette. At this stage the IOP may still be normal; and the new vessels may regress either spontaneously or with treatment.

NB Angle neovascularization in the absence of pupillary involvement may occur after an ischaemic central retinal vein occlusion. It is therefore important to perform careful gonioscopy in eyes at high risk even when the pupillary border is uninvolved.

Treatment

1. **Panretinal photocoagulation,** if performed early, is often effective in inducing regression of the new vessels and preventing subsequent progression to glaucoma.
2. **Retinal surgery.** If rubeosis develops or persists following vitrectomy in a diabetic patient with residual retinal detachment, reattachment should be attempted since, if successful, the rubeosis will frequently regress. Additional panretinal photocoagulation will also be beneficial.

Secondary open-angle glaucoma

Diagnosis

The new blood vessels continue to grow across the iris surface towards the iris root. The neovascular tissue then proliferates across the face of the ciliary body and scleral spur to invade the angle (Fig. 13.29c). Here the new blood vessels arborize and form a fibrovascular membrane, which blocks the trabeculum and gives rise to secondary open-angle glaucoma.

Treatment

1. **Medical** treatment is as for POAG.
2. **Panretinal photocoagulation** should still be performed even if the IOP is adequately controlled medically, although this will not influence the fibrous component of the fibrovascular membrane.

Secondary angle-closure glaucoma

Diagnosis

If the rubeosis iridis continues to progress the angle becomes progressively closed by contraction of fibrovascular tissue with pulling of the peripheral iris over the trabeculum (Fig. 13.29d). The angle thus closes circumferentially in a zipper-like fashion resulting in very high IOP, severe visual impairment, congestion of the globe and pain.

Treatment

The main aim is to relieve pain, as the prognosis for maintaining visual function is extremely poor.

1. **Medical** treatment is initially with topical beta-blockers and systemic acetazolamide. Topical atropine and steroids may decrease inflammation and make the eye more comfortable and less congested, even if the IOP remains high.
2. **Retinal ablation** is performed with laser if the fundus can be adequately visualized. Eyes with opaque media are treated by trans-scleral diode laser photocoagulation or cryotherapy.
3. **Filtration surgery** may be considered if vision is hand movements or better. The two options are trabeculectomy with adjunctive mitomycin C or artificial filtering shunts.
4. **Cyclodestruction** by trans-scleral diode laser may effectively control IOP and render the eye more comfortable, particularly in conjunction with medical therapy.
5. **Retrobulbar alcohol injection** is useful in relieving pain but it may cause permanent ptosis and does not relieve congestion.
6. **Enucleation** may be considered if all else fails.

Differential diagnosis

1. **Primary congestive angle-closure glaucoma.** NVG may occasionally present with sudden onset of pain, congestion and corneal oedema. Gonioscopy after clearing the cornea with ocular hypotensive agents and/or topical glycerine is useful to differentiate the two. Moreover the fellow eye manifests a normal angle.
2. **Postvitrectomy inflammation** in diabetic patients may be associated with congested and prominent iris vasculature and a transient rise in IOP, which may be mistaken for NVG. However, these features usually resolve following the intensive administration of topical steroids.

INFLAMMATORY GLAUCOMA

Introduction

Elevation of IOP secondary to intraocular inflammation frequently presents a diagnostic and therapeutic challenge. The elevation of IOP may be transient and innocuous, or persistent and severely damaging. The prevalence of secondary glaucoma increases with chronicity and severity of disease. Secondary glaucoma is particularly common in Fuchs uveitis syndrome and chronic anterior uveitis associated with juvenile idiopathic arthritis.

NB A common cause of raised IOP in individuals with ocular inflammation is the use of topical steroids.

Classification

1. **Angle-closure with pupil block**
2. **Angle-closure without pupil block**
3. **Open angle**
4. **Posner–Schlossman syndrome**

Diagnostic dilemmas

1. **IOP fluctuation** may be dramatic in uveitic glaucoma

and phasing may be helpful in patients with borderline IOP.

2. **Ciliary body shutdown** caused by acute exacerbation of chronic anterior uveitis is frequently associated with lowering of IOP that may mask the underlying tendency to glaucoma. Even eyes with considerably elevated IOP (30–35mmHg) may become hypotonous during acute exacerbations of uveitis. Return of ciliary body function with subsidence of uveitis may be associated with a rise in IOP in the presence of permanently compromised outflow facility.

> **NB** It is important to perform gonioscopy in eyes with anterior uveitis and to continue monitoring the IOP as the inflammation resolves.

3. **Pathogenesis** of elevation of IOP may be uncertain; multiple mechanisms may be involved. Steroid-responders often represent a therapeutic challenge.
4. **Assessment of glaucomatous damage** may be hampered by a miotic pupil or opacities in the media. Poor visual acuity may also compromise accurate perimetry.

Angle-closure glaucoma with pupil block

Pathogenesis

Secondary angle closure is caused by posterior synechiae extending for 360° (seclusio pupillae) which obstruct aqueous flow from the posterior to the anterior chamber (Fig.13.30a). The resultant increased pressure in the posterior chamber produces anterior bowing of the peripheral iris (iris bombé – Fig. 13.30b) resulting in shallowing of the anterior chamber and apposition of the peripheral iris to the trabeculum and peripheral cornea (Fig. 13.30c). Such an inflamed iris easily sticks to the trabeculum; and the iridocorneal contact becomes permanent with the development of peripheral anterior synechiae (PAS).

> **NB** Angle-closure glaucoma with pupil block is uncommon; most eyes with seclusio pupillae exhibit a normal or subnormal IOP due to concomitant chronic ciliary body shutdown. In some cases the IOP may subsequently become elevated as ciliary body function returns.

Diagnosis

1. **Slit-lamp biomicroscopy** shows seclusio pupillae, iris bombé and a shallow anterior chamber.
2. **Gonioscopy** shows angle closure from iridotrabecular contact. Indentation gonioscopy with a Zeiss four-mirror goniolens, or equivalent, may be used to assess the extent of appositional as opposed to synechial angle closure.

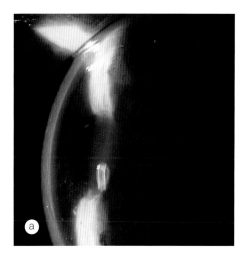

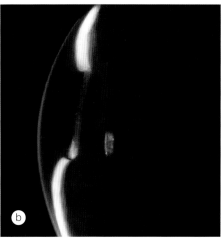

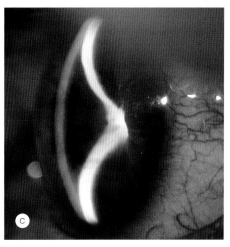

Fig. 13.30
Secondary angle closure with pupil block. **(a)** Seclusio pupillae; **(b)** iris bombé; **(c)** iridocorneal contact

Angle-closure glaucoma without pupil block

1. **Pathogenesis.** Chronic anterior uveitis causes the deposition of inflammatory cells and debris in the angle (Fig. 13.31a and b), subsequent organization and contraction of which pulls the peripheral iris over the trabeculum (Fig. 13.31c), thereby causing gradual and progressive synechial angle closure with eventual elevation of IOP (Fig. 13.31d). The eye with a pre-existing narrow angle may be at higher risk, as may one with granulomatous inflammation with inflammatory nodules in the angle.
2. **Diagnosis.** The anterior chamber is deep but gonioscopy shows extensive angle closure by PAS.

Open-angle glaucoma

In acute anterior uveitis

In acute anterior uveitis the IOP is usually normal or subnormal due to concomitant ciliary shutdown. Occasionally, however, secondary open-angle glaucoma develops due to obstruction of aqueous outflow, most commonly as the acute inflammation is subsiding and ciliary body function is returning. This effect, which is often transient and innocuous, may be steroid-induced or caused by a combination of the following mechanisms:

1. **Trabecular obstruction** by inflammatory cells and debris which may be associated with increased aqueous

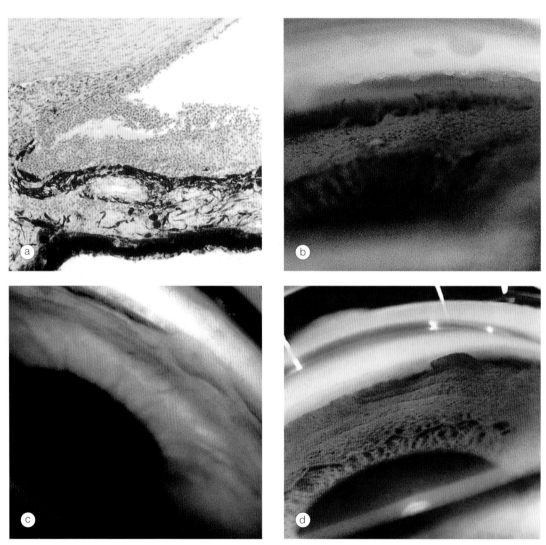

Fig. 13.31
Secondary angle closure without pupil block. **(a)** Deposition of inflammatory cells in the angle; **(b)** gonioscopy shows an open angle containing inflammatory debris; **(c)** peripheral anterior synechiae; **(d)** progressive synechial angle closure (Courtesy of J Harry and G Misson, from *Clinical Ophthalmic Pathology*, Butterworth-Heinemann, 2001 – fig. a)

viscosity due to leakage of proteins from the inflamed iris blood vessels.

2. **Acute trabeculitis,** involving inflammation and oedema of the trabecular meshwork with secondary diminution of intertrabecular porosity, may result in a reduction in outflow facility. It is thought that this is relevant in anterior uveitis associated with herpes zoster and herpes simplex.

In chronic anterior uveitis

In chronic anterior uveitis the main mechanism for reduced outflow facility is thought to be trabecular scarring and/or sclerosis secondary to chronic trabeculitis. The exact incidence and importance of this mechanism is, however, difficult to determine as most eyes also have some degree of synechial angle closure. Because of the variable appearance of the angle on gonioscopy, definitive diagnosis of trabecular damage is difficult. Theoretically, the angle should be open and, in some eyes, a gelatinous exudate resembling 'mashed potatoes' is seen on the trabeculum.

Treatment

Medical

- Medical control of IOP is more likely to be achieved if the angle is completely open, and there are no PAS or pigment deposits.
- The aim of therapy in terms of IOP level to be attained depends on the health of the optic nerve head; eyes with advanced damage require a low target IOP to prevent further damage.
- In steroid-reactors it is important not to sacrifice control of inflammation for fear of steroid-induced IOP elevation. Long-acting depot preparations should be used with great caution in patients with a history of a steroid response.
- The IOP-lowering effect of ocular hypotensive drugs is less predictable in uveitis and some cases may be unexpectedly sensitive to topical carbonic anhydrase inhibitors (CAI).
- The use of prostaglandin analogues as first-line agents in uveitic glaucoma is tempered by the small risk of precipitating a uveitic episode or CMO.
- A topical beta-blocker is therefore usually the first drug of choice.
- The choice of a second line agent often depends on the IOP level. If the IOP is very high, a systemic CAI (e.g. acetazolamide) may be required in the short-term. On the other hand if elevation of IOP is moderate (e.g. less than 35mmHg on a beta-blocker) in the absence of significant glaucomatous damage, an alpha-adrenergic agonist (e.g. brimonidine), a topical CAI (e.g. dorzolamide) or prostaglandin analogue might be appropriate.

NB Miotics are contraindicated because they increase vascular permeability and may induce inflammation, and miosis enhances the formation of posterior synechiae.

Laser iridotomy

- Laser iridotomy is performed to re-establish communication between the posterior and anterior chambers in eyes with pupil-block angle closure. The resulting hole is usually quite small and likely to become occluded in the presence of an active uveitis.
- It is important to bear in mind that correction of pupil block may not control the IOP if there is insufficient open angle for drainage. In cases of progressive angle closure, iridotomy may, nevertheless, prevent further PAS formation.
- Intensive topical steroid therapy should be used to minimize post-laser inflammation.

Surgery

As in any type of glaucoma, the decision to operate is based on the level of the IOP, the response to medication and the health of the optic nerve head.

1. **Preoperative preparation**
   - Control of uveitis for a minimum of 3 months before surgery is ideal but often impractical as glaucoma surgery is rarely an elective procedure.
   - Preoperative topical steroids should be used, not only as prophylaxis against recurrent inflammation, but also to reduce the conjunctival inflammatory cell population and enhance the success rate of a filtration procedure.
   - In patients with particularly labile inflammatory disease systemic steroids should be considered.
2. **Trabeculectomy** is the procedure of choice.
   - Combined cataract and glaucoma surgery is not appropriate. Ideally cataract surgery should be performed about 6 months after trabeculectomy because the results are better.
   - Adjunctive antimetabolites, particularly mitomycin C, are required since these eyes carry a high risk of failure.
   - Postoperative hypotony is a risk where a delicate balance may exist between reduced aqueous production and severely restricted aqueous outflow. If production drops in the early postoperative period, any filtration may be excessive. It is therefore imperative to perform tight scleral suturing in order to prevent early hypotony.
   - After trabeculectomy steroids are tapered according to the level of inflammation and the appearance of the filtering bleb, and usually discontinued after 2–3 months, although earlier tapering may be necessary in cases of over-filtration.

3. **Glaucoma drainage devices (GDD)** should be considered in cases where trabeculectomy, even with adjunctive antimetabolites, has a poor success rate. This includes aphakic eyes, children with chronic anterior uveitis, or a previously failed trabeculectomy.
   - While their exact role of GDD has yet to be clearly defined, it is widely accepted that the threshold for using these devices is lower in uveitic glaucoma than other types.
   - GDD implantation generally produces better IOP control in uveitic eyes than in other glaucomas, probably because it also reduces aqueous secretion. For this reason, implants with smaller surface areas for drainage, such as the Ahmed valve, single plate Molteno and 250 Baerveldt, are preferred.
   - Postoperative hypotony is a problem with these devices and a two-step procedure is recommended, using a suture fed inside the tube, which is later removed.

4. **Cyclodestructive** procedures should be used with caution because they may not only exacerbate the intraocular inflammation but also result in profound hypotony which may proceed to phthisis bulbi. Even eyes with seemingly intractable uveitic glaucoma may paradoxically develop ciliary body insufficiency in the longer term.

5. **Angle procedures** include trabeculodialysis, and goniotomy may be successful in children. The former procedure involves making an incision along Schwalbe line in order to establish communication between the anterior chamber and Schlemm canal.

Posner–Schlossman syndrome

Posner–Schlossman syndrome (glaucomatocyclitic crisis) is characterized by recurrent attacks of unilateral, acute secondary open-angle glaucoma associated with mild anterior uveitis. The cause of the raised IOP is presumed to be acute trabeculitis. There is some evidence that the herpes simplex virus may play a pathogenetic role. Posner–Schlossman syndrome is a rare condition typically affecting young adults, 40% of whom are positive for HLA-Bw54. Males are affected more frequently than females. The IOP is elevated for a few hours to several days. The attacks are unilateral, although 50% of patients have bilateral involvement at different times. The intervals between attacks vary and, with time, usually become longer. Patients should be followed, even after the attacks have completely subsided, because a significant percentage will develop chronic elevation of IOP.

Diagnosis

1. **Presentation** is with mild discomfort, haloes around lights and slight blurring of vision.

2. **Slit-lamp biomicroscopy** shows corneal epithelial oedema due to a high IOP (40–80mmHg), a few aqueous cells and fine white central keratic precipitates.

3. **Gonioscopy** shows an open angle. Unless it is performed the condition may be confused with acute primary angle-closure glaucoma. The absence of PAS helps in the differentiation from other inflammatory glaucomas.

Treatment

Topical steroids are used to control the inflammation and aqueous suppressants for the raised IOP. Oral non-steroidal anti-inflammatory agents may also be beneficial.

LENS-RELATED GLAUCOMA

Phacolytic glaucoma

Pathogenesis

Phacolytic glaucoma (lens protein glaucoma) is open-angle glaucoma occurring in association with a hypermature cataract. It is more common in underdeveloped countries where patients with cataract often present late. Trabecular obstruction is caused by high molecular weight lens proteins which have leaked through the intact capsule into the aqueous humour. Lens protein containing macrophages may also contribute to trabecular blockage (Fig. 13.32a and b).

> **NB** Phacolytic glaucoma should not be confused with phacoanaphylactic (phacoantigenic) uveitis which is an autoimmune granulomatous reaction to lens proteins occurring in an eye with a ruptured capsule.

Diagnosis

1. **Presentation** is with pain. Vision is already poor due to cataract.

2. **Slit-lamp biomicroscopy** shows corneal oedema, a hypermature cataract and a deep anterior chamber. The aqueous may manifest floating white particles (Fig. 13.32c), which may form a pseudohypopyon if very dense (Fig. 13.32d).

3. **Gonioscopy** shows an open angle.

Treatment

Once the IOP is controlled medically, the proteinaceous material is flushed out and the cataract removed. Care should be taken not to rupture the zonules when performing anterior capsulotomy.

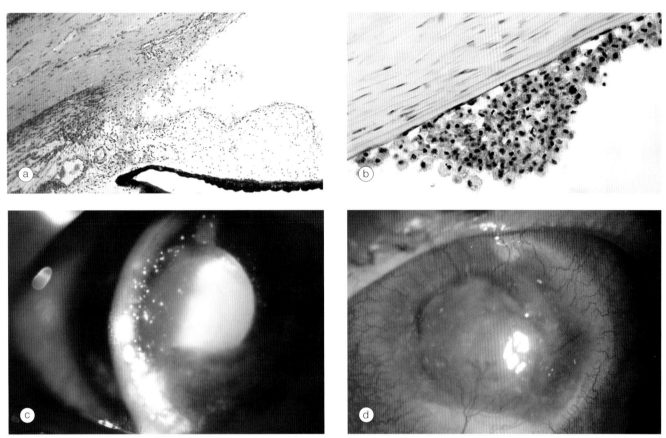

Fig. 13.32
Phacolytic glaucoma. **(a)** Lens-protein containing macrophages in the angle; **(b)** lens-protein containing macrophages on the corneal endothelium similar to keratic precipitates; **(c)** hypermature cataract and lens-protein containing macrophages floating in the aqueous; **(d)** neglected end-stage glaucoma with corneal vascularization and a small pseudo-hypopyon (Courtesy of J Harry – figs a and b)

Phacomorphic glaucoma

Pathogenesis

Phacomorphic glaucoma is an acute secondary angle-closure glaucoma precipitated by an intumescent cataractous lens. A history of gradual impairment of vision or an increase in myopia may be obtained. The crystalline lens continues to grow throughout life. Equatorial growth (which slackens the suspensory ligament, thus allowing the lens to move anteriorly) combines with anteroposterior growth to increase iridolenticular contact and potentiate pupillary block and iris bombé. Phacomorphic glaucoma and primary angle closure therefore conceptually overlap, and it may be difficult to distinguish the two in a clinical setting.

Diagnosis

1. **Presentation** is similar to acute primary angle closure with a shallow anterior chamber and dilated pupil. Cataract is usually evident (Fig. 13.33).
2. **Examination** of the fellow eye may demonstrate a deep anterior chamber and an open angle, thus excluding the diagnosis of primary angle closure. Axial length measurement and records of the refraction may also be helpful in distinguishing between the two conditions.

Treatment

Treatment is initially similar to acute primary angle closure. Laser iridotomy is performed once the IOP is controlled, although it has been suggested that laser iridotomy is safe

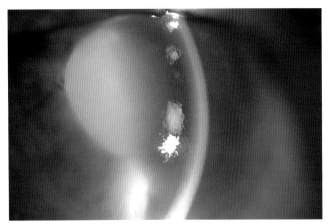

Fig. 13.33
Intumescent cataract, shallow anterior chamber, dilated pupil and corneal oedema in phacomorphic glaucoma

and effective as first-line therapy without initial medical treatment. Cataract surgery is performed once the eye is quiet but is associated with an increased risk of capsular rupture and vitreous loss. A surgical iridectomy should always be performed.

Dislocated lens into the anterior chamber

Causes

1. **Blunt ocular trauma,** even if relatively trivial, may result in lens dislocation in eyes with weak zonules (e.g. buphthalmos, homocystinuria – Fig. 13.34a).
2. **Small lenses** (microspherophakia) as in Weill–Marchesani syndrome.

Diagnosis

The dislocated lens causes acute pupil block and a sudden and severe elevation of IOP with associated visual impairment. This constitutes an acute emergency because lenticulocorneal contact may cause permanent endothelial damage.

Treatment

The IOP is initially reduced with osmotic agents. Subsequent management is dependent on the absence or presence of some remaining zonular attachments and the hardness of the lens as follows:

1. **Some remaining attachments.** The patient is placed into the supine position and the pupil dilated in an attempt to reposition the lens into the posterior chamber.

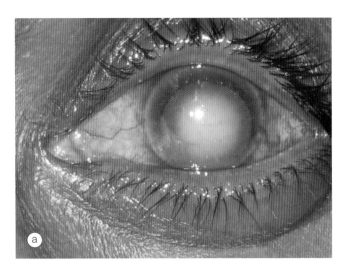

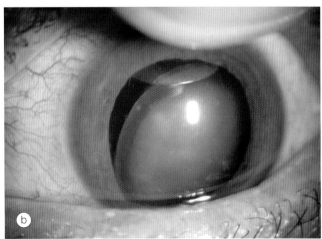

Fig. 13.34
Lens-induced pupil-block glaucoma. **(a)** Lens dislocation into the anterior chamber; **(b)** lens incarceration in the pupil (Courtesy of S Kumar Puri – fig. a)

2. **Soft lens without zonular attachments.** A lensectomy is performed through a limbal incision. Lenses in patients over the age of 35 years are usually too hard to be removed by this technique.
3. **Hard lens without zonular attachments** is managed by intracapsular extraction.

Incarcerated lens in the pupil

1. **Pathogenesis.** The rise in IOP is caused by pupil block by a microspherical lens in which only part of the zonule has been disrupted so that the intact zonule acts as a hinge (Fig. 13.34b).
2. **Treatment** involves relieving pupil block with mydriatics or laser iridotomy. Miotics are contraindicated because they will worsen pupil block. The fellow eye should undergo prophylactic laser iridotomy.

TRAUMATIC GLAUCOMA

Red cell glaucoma

Pathogenesis

A traumatic hyphaema may be associated with IOP elevation due to trabecular blockage by red blood cells. Pupillary occlusion by a blood clot may superimpose an angle closure component. Secondary haemorrhage, often more severe than the primary bleed, may develop within 3–5 days of the initial injury, particularly in black patients. Patients with sickle-cell haemoglobinopathies are at increased risk of developing complications associated with traumatic hyphaema.

Risk of glaucoma

Although most traumatic hyphaemas are relatively innocuous and transient, occasionally severe and prolonged elevation of IOP may damage the optic nerve and cause blood staining of the cornea. The latter can progress very rapidly and may take years to clear. The optic nerve is endangered by IOP > 50mmHg for 2 days. The size of a hyphaema is a useful indicator of visual prognosis and risk of complications:

- Hyphaema involving less than half the anterior chamber (Fig. 13.35a) is associated with a 4% incidence of raised IOP, a 22% incidence of complications and a final visual acuity of > 6/18 in 78% of eyes.
- Hyphaema involving more than half the anterior chamber (Fig. 13.35b) is associated with an 85% incidence of raised IOP, 78% incidence of complications and a final visual acuity of > 6/18 in only 28% of eyes.

Treatment

Hospital admission is required for large hyphaemas.

1. **Medical**
   - Topical and/or systemic aqueous suppressants, depending on the IOP. Miotics should be avoided as they may increase pupil block.
   - Topical steroids should always be used since they reduce the risk of secondary haemorrhage and reduce ocular inflammation.
   - Mydriatics are useful. It is preferable to achieve constant mydriasis rather than a mobile pupil in order to minimize the chances of secondary haemorrhage from the iris or ciliary body.
2. **Surgical evacuation** of the blood with or without trabeculectomy is indicated in the following circumstances:
   - IOP of > 50mmHg for 2 days or > 35mmHg for 7 days.
   - Early corneal blood staining because it can progress to a dense opacity within a few hours.
   - Total hyphaema for more than 5 days to prevent the development of PAS and chronic elevation of IOL.

Angle recession glaucoma

Pathogenesis

Angle recession involves rupture of the face of the ciliary body (the portion that lies between the iris root and the scleral spur) due to blunt trauma. Although a large percentage of eyes with traumatic hyphaema exhibit some degree of angle recession, only 6–9% develop glaucoma after

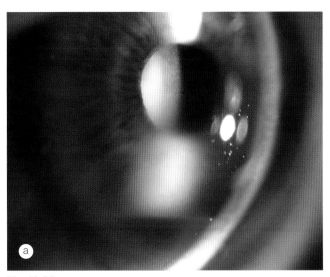

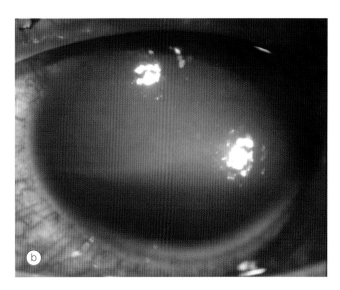

Fig. 13.35
(a) Small hyphaema; (b) total hyphaema

10 years. It is thought that the rise in IOP is secondary to trabecular damage rather than from angle recession itself. However, the risk of glaucoma is directly related to the extent of angle recession. Since glaucoma may not develop until months or even years after the initial injury, angle recession mandates periodic review.

Diagnosis

1. **Presentation** is with unilateral chronic glaucoma. The diagnosis may be easily missed unless a careful past history is taken and gonioscopy performed.
2. **Slit-lamp biomicroscopy** often shows signs of previous blunt trauma, which may be mild, such as a small sphincter rupture.
3. **Gonioscopy** may show irregular widening of the ciliary body which may be associated with scarring and pigment within the recess (Fig. 13.36a). In long-standing cases, the cleft may be obscured by fibrosis. On cursory examination, hyperpigmentation in the angle (Fig. 13.36b) may be mistaken for pigmentary glaucoma, particularly if the corneal endothelium is also covered by pigment granules.

NB It is important to compare the angle appearance in the two eyes and also to compare different sectors of the angle in the same eye.

Treatment

1. **Medical** treatment is as for other types of secondary open-angle glaucoma but is frequently unsatisfactory (laser trabeculoplasty is ineffective).
2. **Trabeculectomy** with adjunctive antimetabolites is the most effective surgical procedure.
3. **An artificial filtering shunt** should be considered if trabeculectomy fails.

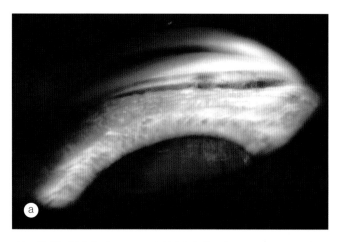

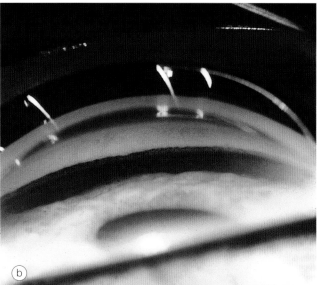

Fig. 13.36
(a) Angle recession; **(b)** old angle recession with hyperpigmentation (Courtesy of R Curtis – fig. a)

IRIDOCORNEAL
ENDOTHELIAL SYNDROME

Classification

The iridocorneal endothelial (ICE) syndrome typically affects one eye of a middle-aged woman. It consists of the following three very rare and frequently overlapping disorders: (a) *progressive iris atrophy*, (b) *iris naevus* (Cogan–Reese) syndrome and (c) *Chandler syndrome*.

Pathogenesis

The common link between the three variants of the ICE syndrome is an abnormal corneal endothelial cell layer which has the capacity to proliferate and migrate across the angle and onto the surface of the iris. The term 'proliferative endotheliopathy' has therefore been suggested to describe this disorder. The ICE syndrome may progress to glaucoma, corneal decompensation or both. Glaucoma is due to synechial angle closure secondary to contraction of this abnormal tissue. Polymerase chain reaction shows the presence of herpes simplex virus DNA in a substantial percentage of ICE syndrome corneal specimens, suggesting that the condition may be of viral origin.

General features

1. **Slit-lamp biomicroscopy**
   - Corectopia (malposition of the pupil – Fig. 13.37a).

- Pseudopolycoria (supernumerary false pupils) in a previously normal iris (Fig. 13.37b).
- Iris atrophy of varying severity (Fig. 13.37c and d).

2. **Gonioscopy** shows broad-based PAS that often extend anterior to Schwalbe line (Fig. 13.38).
3. **Glaucoma** is present in about 50% of cases.

Specific features

In their purest form, the three conditions are easily distinguished from each other. However, there is frequently considerable overlap and clear differentiation may be difficult. Occasionally, during follow-up one condition can be observed to change into another. The differentiation depends primarily on the iris.

1. **Progressive iris atrophy** is characterized by severe iris changes (see Fig. 13.37).
2. **The iris naevus (Cogan–Reese) syndrome** is characterized by either a diffuse naevus which covers the anterior iris (Fig. 13.39a) or iris nodules (Fig. 13.39b). Iris atrophy is absent in 50% of cases and in the remainder it is usually mild to moderate, although corectopia may be severe.

NB It is important not to misdiagnose a diffuse iris melanoma as the iris naevus syndrome.

3. **Chandler syndrome** is characterized by 'hammered-silver' corneal endothelial abnormalities (Fig. 13.40a) and frequently presents with blurred vision and haloes due to corneal oedema (Fig. 13.40b). Stromal atrophy is absent in about 60% of cases and in the remainder is variable in its severity; corectopia is mild to moderate. Glaucoma is usually less severe than in the other two syndromes, and at presentation the IOP may be normal.

Treatment of glaucoma

1. **Medical** treatment may be tried but is often ineffective.
2. **Trabeculectomy,** even when combined with adjunctive antimetabolites, is frequently unsuccessful because of late-onset bleb failure.
3. **Artificial filtering shunts** are eventually required in many cases.

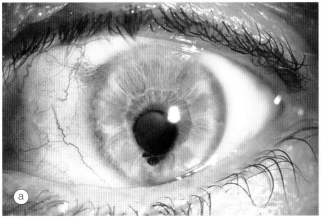
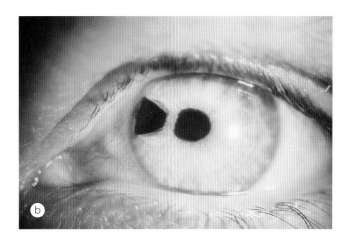
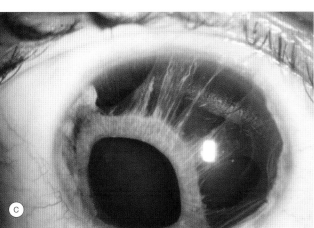
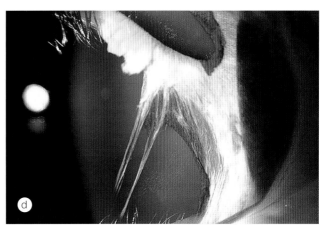

Fig. 13.37
Progressive iris atrophy. **(a)** Corectopia; **(b)** pseudopolycoria; **(c)** iris atrophy; **(d)** very severe iris atrophy

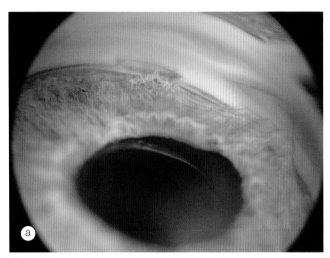
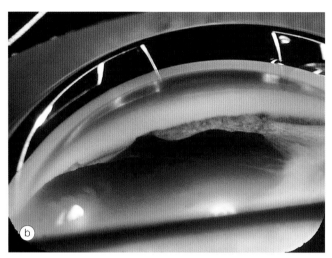

Fig. 13.38
Synechial angle closure in iridocorneal endothelial syndrome. **(a)** Early; **(b)** late (Courtesy of L MacKeen – fig. a)

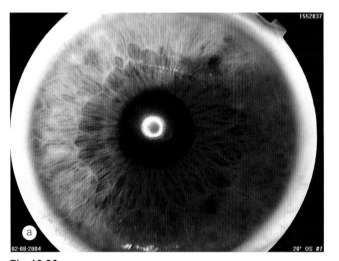
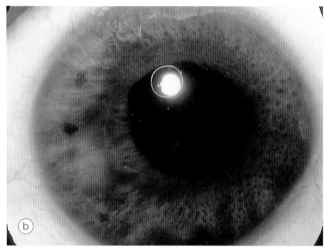

Fig. 13.39
Cogan–Reese iris naevus syndrome. **(a)** Diffuse iris naevus; **(b)** multiple iris nodules

GLAUCOMA IN INTRAOCULAR TUMOURS

Approximately 5% of eyes with intraocular tumours develop a secondary elevation of IOP. Depending on the location of the tumour one or more of the following mechanisms may be responsible:

Trabecular block

Trabecular block may be the result of one of the following:

1. **Angle invasion** by a solid iris melanoma (Fig. 13.41a).
2. **Trabecular infiltration** by neoplastic cells originating from an iris melanoma (Fig. 13.41b). Rarely tumour seeding from a retinoblastoma may also invade the trabeculum.
3. **Melanomalytic** glaucoma may occur in some eyes with iris melanoma; and is due to trabecular blockage by macrophages which have ingested pigment and tumour cells similar to phacolytic glaucoma (Fig. 13.41c).

Secondary angle closure

Secondary angle closure may be the result of one of the following:

or diffuse manner. The latter is characterized by the proliferation of sheets of epithelial cells over the posterior cornea, trabeculum, iris and ciliary body (Fig. 13.42a), and is more commonly associated with secondary glaucoma than the cystic variety. Elevation of IOP is caused by a combination of often pre-existing PAS, destruction of the trabeculum by the epithelial membrane, and/or obstruction of the trabeculum by desquamated epithelial cells and associated inflammatory cells.

Diagnosis

- Persistent postoperative anterior uveitis.
- Diffuse epithelialization is characterized by a translucent membrane with scalloped border involving the posterior corneal surface (Fig. 13.42) and anterior vitreous face in the sector of the incision.
- Pupillary distortion.

Treatment

The aim of treatment is to eradicate the invading epithelium to avoid recurrence or the conversion of epithelial cysts into diffuse epithelialization with consequent intractable glaucoma.

1. **Block excision** involves simultaneous excision of adjacent iris, pars plicata of the ciliary body, together with all layers of the sclera and cornea in contact with the lesion. The resultant defect is covered with a tectonic corneoscleral graft. The area of iris involvement may be identified by applying argon laser burns which will cause whitening of the affected area.
2. **Cryotherapy** may be applied trans-sclerally to devitalize the epithelium remaining on the posterior surface of the cornea, in the angle and on the ciliary body. Intraocular air is used to insulate other tissues from the effects of the cryotherapy.
3. **Artificial filtering shunts** are of value for medically uncontrolled glaucoma associated with extensive epithelial ingrowth unsuitable for surgical excision.

GLAUCOMA IN IRIDOSCHISIS

Iridoschisis is a rare condition which typically affects the elderly and is often bilateral. It is associated with underlying angle closure glaucoma in 90% of cases. It is thought that acute or intermittent angle-closure results in iris atrophy because of high IOP.

1. **Slit-lamp biomicroscopy**
   - Shallow anterior chamber (Fig. 13.43a).

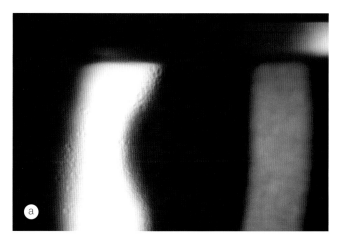
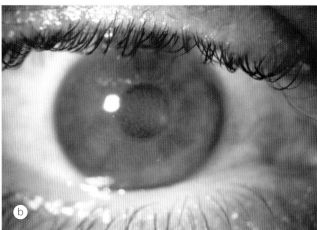

Fig. 13.40
Chandler syndrome. **(a)** Hammered-silver endothelial changes; **(b)** corneal oedema due to endothelial decompensation (Courtesy of J McAllister – fig. b)

1. **Neovascular glaucoma** is the most common mechanism in eyes with choroidal melanoma or retinoblastoma.
2. **Anterior displacement of iris-lens diaphragm** may occur in an eye with a ciliary body melanoma (Fig. 13.41d) or a large tumour of the posterior segment.

GLAUCOMA IN EPITHELIAL INGROWTH

Pathogenesis

Epithelial ingrowth is a rare and potentially blinding complication of anterior segment surgery or trauma. Conjunctival or corneal epithelial cells migrate through the wound and proliferate in the anterior segment, in a cystic

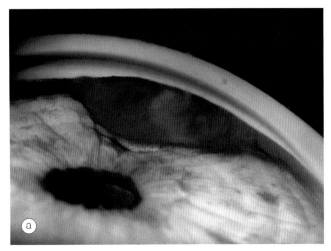
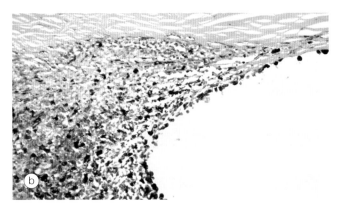
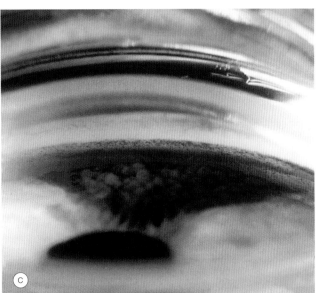
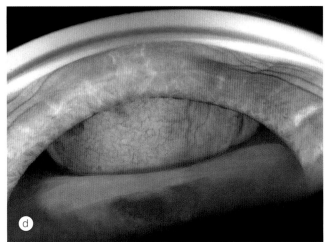

Fig. 13.41
Glaucoma in intraocular tumours. **(a)** Angle invasion by a solid iris melanoma; **(b)** melanoma cells infiltrating the trabeculum; **(c)** melanomalytic glaucoma; **(d)** angle closure by a large ciliary body melanoma (Courtesy of R Curtis – figs a and c; J Harry – fig. b)

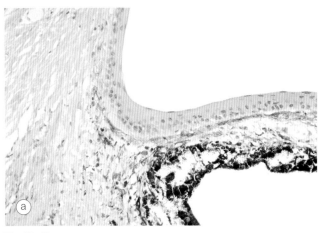
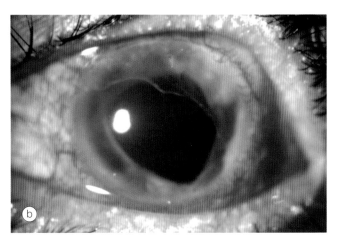

Fig.13.42
Diffuse epithelial ingrowth. **(a)** Stratified squamous epithelium lining the anterior iris surface and filtration angle; **(b)** translucent membrane with a scalloped border involving the posterior corneal surface (Courtesy of J Harry and G Misson, from *Clinical Ophthalmic Pathology*, Butterworth-Heinemann, 2001 – fig. a)

- Iridoschisis usually involves the inferior iris.
- The severity ranges from intrastromal atrophy (Fig. 13.43b) to extensive splitting of the anterior leaf (Fig. 13.43c) and disintegrated iris fibrils (Fig. 13.43d).
2. **Gonioscopy** shows a narrow occludable angle which may be associated with PAS.
3. **Treatment** initially involves peripheral laser iridotomy. Subsequent treatment is aimed at limiting glaucomatous damage.

PRIMARY CONGENITAL GLAUCOMA

Introduction

Genetics

Most cases of primary congenital glaucoma (PCG) are sporadic. In approximately 10% inheritance is AR with incomplete penetrance. Gene loci have been designated GLC3. The first gene to be identified (GLC3A) is a mutation of the cytochrome P4501B1 gene (*CYP1B1*) on the 2p21 region which participates in the metabolism of a molecule important for normal development and function of the anterior segment. The GLC3B locus resides on chromosome 1p36.

Pathogenesis

Impaired aqueous outflow in PCG is caused by maldevelopment of the angle of the anterior chamber, unassociated with any other major ocular anomalies (isolated trabeculodysgenesis). Clinically, trabeculodysgenesis is characterized by absence of the ciliary body band due to translucent amorphous material that obscures the trabeculum (Fig. 13.44).

Classification

1. **True** congenital glaucoma (40%) in which IOP becomes elevated during intrauterine life.

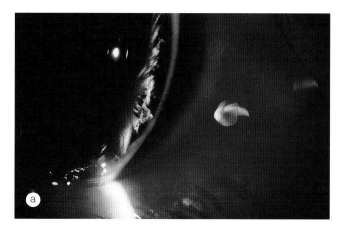
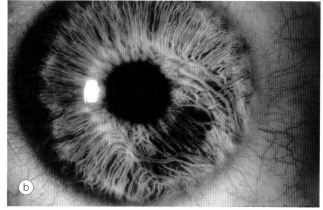
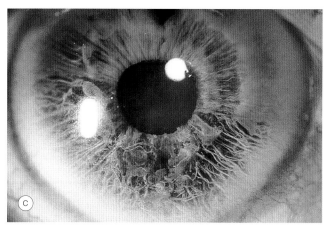
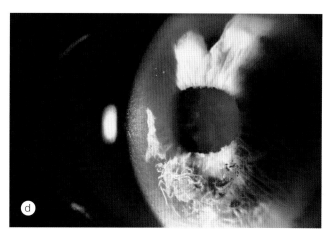

Fig. 13.43
Iridoschisis. **(a)** Shallow anterior chamber; **(b)** mild; **(c)** severe; **(d)** very severe – note peripheral iridectomy (Courtesy of R Curtis – fig. b)

2. **Infantile** glaucoma (55% of cases) which manifests prior to the third birthday.
3. **Juvenile** glaucoma, the least common, in which the pressure rise develops after the third birthday but before the age of 16 years. Gonioscopy is normal or reveals trabeculodysgenesis.

Diagnosis

Although PCG is the most common of the congenital glaucomas it is still a very rare condition, affecting 1:10,000 births; 65% are boys. The clinical features depend on the age of onset and the level of IOP. Both eyes are affected in 75% of cases although involvement is frequently asymmetrical.

1. **Corneal haze** is often the first sign noticed by the parents (Fig. 13.45a). It is caused by epithelial and stromal oedema secondary to raised IOP and may be associated with lacrimation, photophobia and blepharospasm (Fig. 13.45b).
2. **Buphthalmos** is a large eye as a result of stretching due to elevated IOP prior to the age of 3 years (Fig. 13.45c). It is not usually reported by the parents unless unilateral and advanced. As the sclera stretches it becomes thinner and translucent; the eye then takes on a blue appearance due to enhanced visualization of the underlying uvea (Fig. 13.45d). As ocular enlargement continues the anterior chamber deepens, and in advanced cases, the zonular fibres stretch and the lens may rarely subluxate. The increased axial length also causes axial myopia, which may give rise to anisometropic amblyopia.

3. **Breaks in Descemet membrane** secondary to corneal stretching may be associated with a sudden influx of aqueous into the corneal stroma. Haab striae represent healed breaks in Descemet membrane and appear as horizontal curvilinear lines (Fig. 13.45e). Chronic stromal oedema may lead to permanent scarring and vascularization (Fig. 3.45f).
4. **Optic disc cupping** in infants may regress once the IOP is normalized. Most normal infants exhibit no apparent cup and very few have a cup–disc ratio greater than 0.3, unlike a high percentage of infants with PCG. In contrast to the adult eye, the scleral canal in the infant eye enlarges as part of the generalized enlargement of the globe and the lamina cribrosa may bow posteriorly, in response to elevated IOP. Cup size may therefore be increased from neuronal loss, enlargement of the scleral canal, or both.

Management

Initial evaluation

The initial evaluation should be performed under general anaesthesia with intravenous ketamine, since other agents may lower IOP. Examination of the optic discs should be undertaken first, followed by measurement of IOP and corneal diameters, and finally gonioscopy.

1. **IOP** is measured with the Perkins tonometer (see Fig. 1.15c) or TonoPen (see Fig. 1.16a).
2. **Corneal diameter** is measured in both vertical and

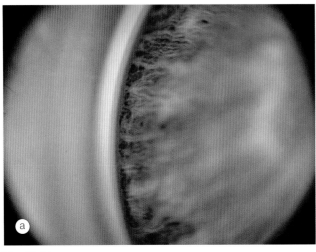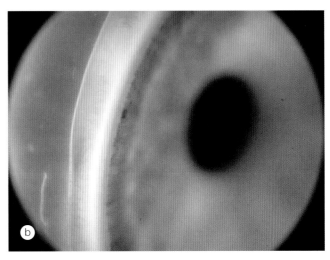

Fig. 13.44
Gonioscopy. **(a)** Normal infant angle shows iris root, prominent ciliary body band and trabeculum but no discernible scleral spur; **(b)** angle in congenital glaucoma shows the iris root but not the ciliary body band due to translucent amorphous tissue that obscures the trabeculum (Courtesy of K Nischal)

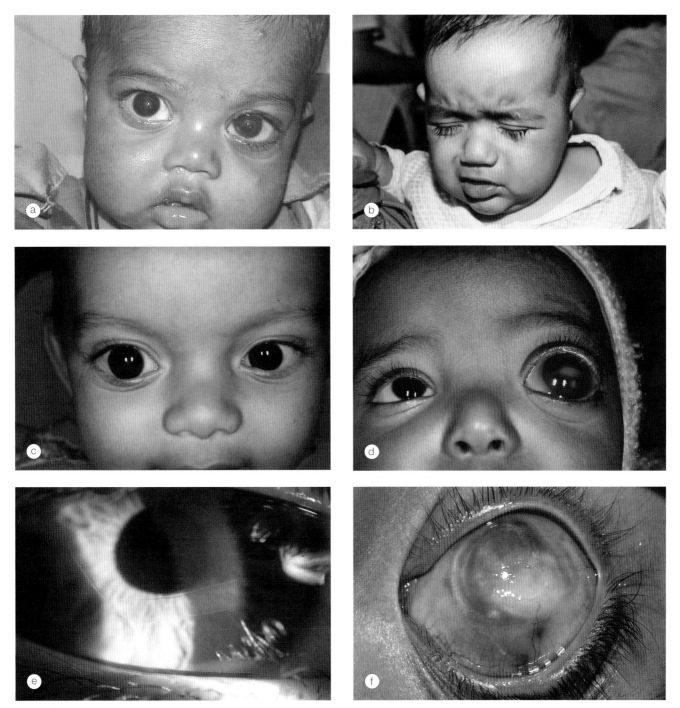

Fig. 13.45
Congenital glaucoma. **(a)** Corneal haze; **(b)** photophobia and blepharospasm; **(c)** buphthalmos; **(d)** severe buphthalmos and scleral thinning; **(e)** Haab striae; **(f)** corneal scarring and vascularization (Courtesy of M Parulekar – fig. a; U Raina – figs b, c and d; K Nischal – fig. e; L MacKeen – fig. f)

horizontal meridians with calipers. A diameter >11mm prior to the age of one year or >13mm at any age should be viewed with suspicion. Diameters of 14mm are typical of advanced buphthalmos.

3. **Gonioscopy** is performed with a Koeppe lens (see Fig. 1.19c) or a direct goniolens.

Surgery

1. **Goniotomy** is performed at the initial examination if the diagnosis is confirmed, provided there is sufficient corneal clarity and the angle can be visualized. The procedure involves making a horizontal incision at the midpoint of

the superficial layers of the trabecular meshwork (Fig. 13.46). Although goniotomy may need to be repeated, the eventual success rate is about 85%. However, the results are poor if the corneal diameter is 14mm or more because in such eyes the canal of Schlemm is obliterated.

2. **Trabeculotomy** may be necessary if corneal clouding prevents visualization of the angle or when repeated goniotomy has failed. In this procedure a partial thickness scleral flap is fashioned (Fig. 13.47a and b), Schlemm canal is found (Fig. 13.47c) and a trabeculotome is inserted into Schlemm canal and then rotated into the anterior chamber (Fig. 13.47d). However, the technique is highly demanding and requires previous experience and good anatomical landmarks to achieve predictable results. In addition, Schlemm canal may be difficult to canalize because of hypoplasia or angle anomaly.

3. **Trabeculectomy** is often successful, particularly when combined with adjunctive antimetabolites.

4. **Combined** trabeculectomy and trabeculotomy has been used but it is debatable if it is superior to trabeculectomy alone.

Follow-up

The patient should be reviewed one month after initial surgery. The IOP and corneal diameters should be monitored at regular intervals because progressive enlargement of the corneal diameter is as important a sign of uncontrolled congenital glaucoma as progressive visual field loss is in adult glaucoma. Cycloplegic refraction should be performed at 6-monthly intervals. About 50% of patients suffer visual loss from optic nerve damage, anisometropic amblyopia, corneal scarring, cataract and lens subluxation. A buphthalmic eye is also susceptible to traumatic damage.

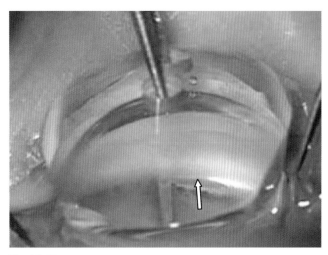

Fig. 13.46
Goniotomy – arrow shows the cleft (Courtesy of K Nischal)

Differential diagnosis

1. **Cloudy cornea at birth**
   - Birth trauma, which gives rise to corneal oedema due to breaks in Descemet membrane.
   - Intrauterine rubella, which results in a cloudy cornea due to keratitis.

   NB 10% of infants with the rubella syndrome also have congenital glaucoma due to an angle anomaly similar to that in PCG. This may be missed because the eye may not appear significantly enlarged, due to pre-existing microphthalmos.

   - Metabolic disorders such as mucopolysaccharidoses and mucolipidoses.
   - Congenital hereditary endothelial dystrophy.
2. **Large cornea** due to megalocornea or very high myopia.
3. **Lacrimation** resulting from delayed canalization of the nasolacrimal duct.
4. **Secondary infantile glaucoma**
   - Tumours such as retinoblastoma and juvenile xanthogranuloma.
   - Persistent anterior fetal vasculature.
   - Retinopathy of prematurity.
   - Intraocular inflammation.
   - Trauma.
   - Ectopia lentis.

PHACOMATOSES

Sturge–Weber syndrome

The systemic features are described in Chapter 24.

Pathogenesis

Glaucoma develops in about 30% of patients ipsilateral to the facial haemangioma, especially if the lesion affects the upper eyelid (Fig. 13.48a). Elevation of IOP occurs within the first 2 years of life in 60% of patients and may result in buphthalmos. In the remainder glaucoma may develop at any time from infancy to adulthood. The pathogenesis is controversial and often obscure.
- Isolated trabeculodysgenesis may be instrumental in infants.
- Raised episcleral venous pressure (associated with an arteriovenous communication in an episcleral haemangioma) (Fig. 13.48b) may be responsible in older patients.

Treatment

1. **Medical** treatment with topical prostaglandin analogues may be successful.

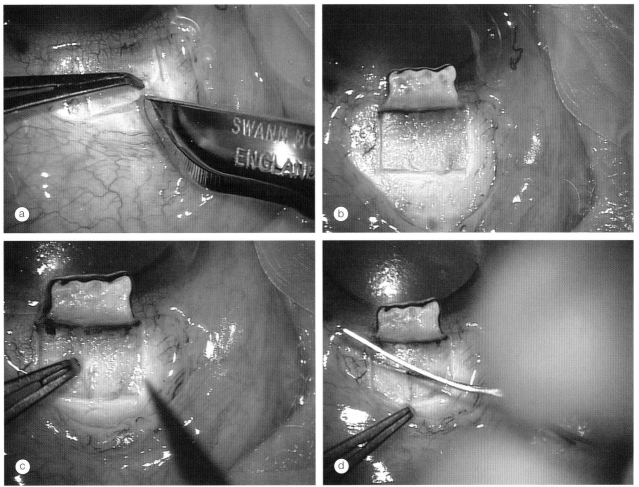

Fig. 13.47
Trabeculotomy. (**a** and **b**) A partial thickness flap is fashioned; (**c**) Schlemm canal is identified; (**d**) trabeculotome is inserted (Courtesy of K Nischal)

2. **Goniotomy** may be successful in eyes with angle anomalies.
3. **Combined** trabeculotomy-trabeculectomy gives good results in early-onset cases. The rationale is that trabeculotomy addresses the barrier to aqueous outflow posed by a congenital angle anomaly, while trabeculectomy bypasses the episcleral veins.

NB Surgery carries a high risk of choroidal effusion and suprachoroidal haemorrhage.

Neurofibromatosis-1

The systemic features are described in Chapter 24. Glaucoma is uncommon, usually unilateral and congenital. About 50% of patients with glaucoma have an ipsilateral plexiform neurofibroma of the upper eyelid (Fig. 13.49a) or exhibit facial hemiatrophy. One or more of the following may be responsible for glaucoma:

• Obstruction of aqueous outflow by neurofibromatous tissue in the angle (Fig. 13.49b).
• Developmental angle anomaly which may be associated with congenital ectropion uveae (Fig. 13.49c).
• Secondary angle-closure caused by forward displacement of the peripheral iris associated with neurofibromatous thickening of the ciliary body.
• Secondary synechial angle closure caused by contraction of a fibrovascular membrane.

GLAUCOMA MEDICATIONS

Most glaucoma medications are administered topically. As a general rule, treatment is indicated whenever glaucomatous damage is deemed likely to occur. The decision on which

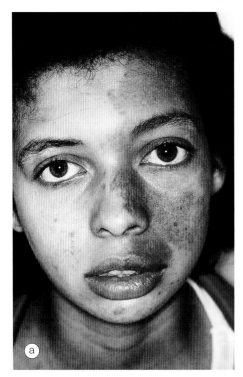

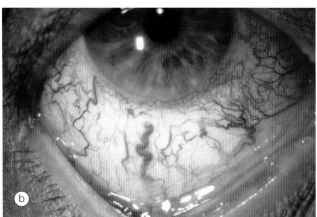

Fig. 13.48
Glaucoma in Sturge–Weber syndrome. **(a)** Left naevus flammeus and mild buphthalmos; **(b)** episcleral haemangioma (Courtesy of J Salmon – fig. a)

medication to prescribe depends not only on the type of glaucoma, but also on the patient's medical history (e.g. presence of asthma or bradycardia). This requires a detailed knowledge of the potential side-effects. To improve compliance, patients should be fully informed not only about their disease but also the medications used, how to administer the drug, and what side-effects to expect. The efficacy of therapy should be regularly evaluated and the regimen altered to improve efficacy, if appropriate, or to reduce adverse effects.

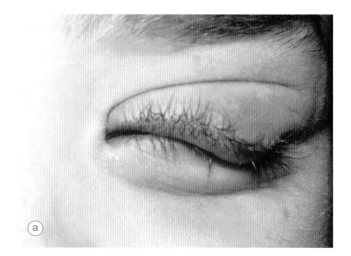

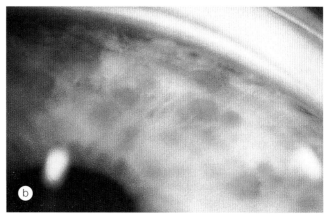

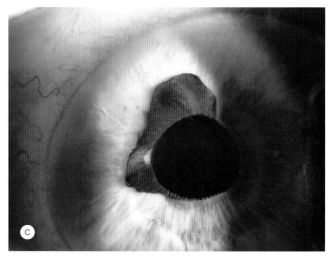

Fig. 13.49
Glaucoma in neurofibromatosis-1. **(a)** Ipsilateral eyelid plexiform neurofibroma; **(b)** neurofibromatous tissue in the angle and Lisch nodules on the iris; **(c)** congenital ectropion uveae (Courtesy of E M Van Buskirk, from *Clinical Atlas of Glaucoma*, W B Saunders, 1986 – fig. b)

Beta-blockers

Pharmacology

Adrenergic neurones secrete noradrenaline at sympathetic post-ganglionic nerve endings. Adrenergic receptors are of the following four main types:

1. **Alpha-1** receptors are located in the arterioles, dilator pupillae and Müller muscle. Stimulation gives rise to hypertension, mydriasis and lid retraction.
2. **Alpha-2** inhibitory receptors are located in the ciliary epithelium. Stimulation results in increase in the facility of aqueous outflow.
3. **Beta-1** receptors are located in the myocardium and give rise to tachycardia and increased cardiac output when stimulated.
4. **Beta-2** receptors are located in the bronchi and ciliary epithelium. Stimulation causes bronchodilatation and increased aqueous production.

Beta-blockers are drugs that antagonize the effects of catecholamines at beta receptors. Non-selective beta blockers are equipotent at beta-1 and beta-2 receptors, while cardioselective are more potent at beta-1 receptors. The advantage, at least in theory, is that the bronchoconstrictive effect of beta-2 blockade is minimized. Betaxolol is the only cardioselective agent currently available for the treatment of glaucoma.

Mode of action

Beta-blockers reduce IOP by decreasing aqueous secretion and are therefore useful in all types of glaucoma, irrespective of the state of the angle. The exact pharmacological basis for this is unclear. However, in approximately 10% of cases the pressure response decreases with time. This may occur within a few days of starting treatment ('short-term escape') or within a few months ('long-term drift'). As a general rule, no additional effect is obtained if a topical beta-blocker is used in a patient who is already on a systemic beta-blocker. During sleep, aqueous flow is normally less than half the daytime flow and therefore beta-blockers have little effect. When a beta-blocker is used in combination with brimonidine or a topical carbonic anhydrase inhibitor, an additional 15% reduction in IOP may be achieved. When combined with a prostaglandin analogue, the reduction is even greater (20%).

Side-effects

1. **Ocular** side-effects include occasional allergy, corneal punctate epithelial erosions and reduced aqueous tear secretion.
2. **Systemic** side-effects tend to occur during the first week of administration. Although uncommon they may be serious.
   - Bradycardia and hypotension can result from beta-1

blockade. The patient's pulse must be palpated before prescribing a beta-blocker.
   - Bronchospasm may be induced by beta-2 blockade and may be fatal in pre-existing asthma or severe chronic pulmonary obstruction.
   - Miscellaneous side effects include sleep disorders, hallucinations, confusion, depression, fatigue, headache, nausea, dizziness, decreased libido and possible reduction of plasma high-density lipoprotein level.
3. **Reduction of systemic absorption** may be achieved by:
   - Lacrimal occlusion following instillation, by closing the eyes and applying digital pressure over the lacrimal sac area for about 3 minutes. Apart from obstructing lacrimal drainage and reducing systemic absorption this also prolongs eye–drug contact and increases therapeutic efficacy.
   - Merely closing the eyes for 3 minutes will reduce systemic absorption by about 50%.
4. **Contraindications** to beta-blockers include congestive cardiac failure, 2nd or 3rd degree heart block, bradycardia, asthma and obstructive airways disease. Beta-blockers should not be used at bed-time because they may cause a profound drop in blood pressure while the individual is asleep, thus reducing optic disc perfusion and potentially causing visual deterioration.

Preparations

1. **Timolol** is available in three forms:
   - Timoptol 0.25%, 0.5% b.d.
   - Timoptol-LA 0.25%, 0.5% once daily.
   - Nyogel 0.1% once daily.
2. **Betaxolol** (Betoptic) 0.5% b.d. Although the ocular hypotensive effect is less than timolol, the effect on preservation of the visual field appears to be superior. Betaxolol may increase optic disc flow, probably because of a calcium-channel blocking effect on the microcirculation of the disc.
3. **Levobunolol** (Betagan) 0.5% daily or b.d. is similar to timolol.
4. **Carteolol** (Teoptic) 1%, 2% b.d. is similar to timolol and also exhibits intrinsic sympathomimetic activity. It has a more selective action on the eye than on the cardiopulmonary system and may therefore induce less bradycardia than timolol.
5. **Metipranolol** 0.1%, 0.3% b.d. is similar to timolol but may occasionally cause a granulomatous anterior uveitis. It is available only in preservative-free units and is therefore useful in patients allergic to preservatives or wearing soft contact lenses (in whom benzalkonium chloride should be avoided).

Alpha-2 agonists

Alpha-2 agonists decrease IOP by both decreasing aqueous secretion and enhancing uveoscleral outflow. Because the drugs cross the blood–brain barrier they should not be used in children.

1. **Brimonidine** (Alphagan) 0.2% b.d. is a highly selective alpha-2 agonist which also has a neuroprotective effect. Its efficacy is less than timolol but better than betaxolol. It exhibits additivity with beta-blockers. The major ocular side-effect is allergic conjunctivitis that may be delayed for up to a year after commencement of therapy (Fig. 13.50a). Acute granulomatous anterior uveitis has been reported. Systemic side-effects include xerostomia, drowsiness and fatigue.
2. **Apraclonidine** (Iopidine) 0.5%, 1% is mainly used after laser surgery on the anterior segment to offset an acute rise in IOP. It is not suitable for long-term use because of tachyphylaxis (loss of therapeutic effect over time) and a high incidence of local side-effects.

Prostaglandin and prostamide analogues

This group of agents have a sustained IOP-lowering effect during the nocturnal period.

Pharmacology

1. **Latanoprost and travoprost** are F2-alpha analogues that act as selective FP prostanoid receptor agonists; both enhance aqueous humour outflow through the uveoscleral route.
2. **Bimatoprost** is a synthetic prostamide analogue structurally similar to prostaglandins that selectively mimics naturally occurring prostamide. This agent appears to have a range of affinities from high to low for the FP receptor and promotes outflow through both uveoscleral and trabecular routes.

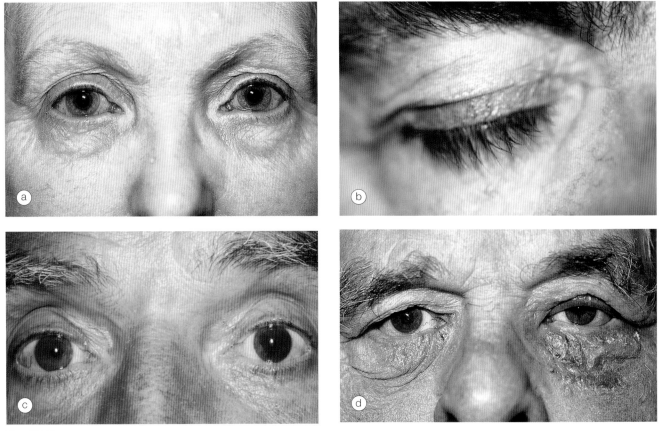

Fig. 13.50
Side-effects of topical medication. **(a)** Allergic conjunctivitis due to brimonidine; **(b)** lengthening and hyperpigmentation of lashes due to a prostaglandin analogue; **(c)** darkening of irides due to a prostaglandin analogue; **(d)** blepharoconjunctivitis due to a topical carbonic anhydrase inhibitor (Courtesy of J Salmon – fig. a; P Watson – fig. c)

3. **Unoprostone isopropyl** is a structural analogue of prostaglandin F2-alpha (a docosanoid) that has no affinity for prostaglandin receptors. It appears to promote aqueous outflow primarily through the trabecular meshwork.

Preparations

1. **Latanoprost** (Xalatan) 0.005% used once daily in the evening. Its pressure lowering effect is superior to timolol although a proportion of patients show no response. Latanoprost produces an additive reduction of IOP of 14–28% when combined with timolol but not with pilocarpine.
2. **Travoprost** (Travatan) 0.004% once daily is similar to latanoprost except in black patients where it appears to be more effective. Conjunctival hyperaemia occurs in up to 50% of patients but tends to subside with time.
3. **Bimatoprost** (Lumigan) 0.03% once daily is similar to latanoprost but may cause more conjunctival hyperaemia but fewer headaches and perhaps also less iris hyperpigmentation.
4. **Unoprostone isopropyl** (Rescula) 0.15% b.d is not as effective as latanoprost in lowering IOP and is perhaps unsuited for monotherapy.

Side-effects

1. **Ocular**
   - Conjunctival hyperaemia and a foreign body sensation are common.
   - Eyelash lengthening, thickening, hyperpigmentation and occasionally increase in number (Fig. 13.50b).
   - Iris hyperpigmentation, which is irreversible, occurs in 11–23% of patients after 6 months (Fig. 13.50c). The highest incidence is in green-brown irides, less in yellow-brown irides and least in blue-grey/brown irides. Hyperpigmentation is caused by an increase in the number of pigmented granules within the superficial stroma rather than an increase in the number of melanocytes. Iris naevi and freckles are, however, not affected.
   - Hyperpigmentation of periorbital skin is uncommon.
   - Cystoid macular oedema may occur in eyes that have independent risk factors for the development of cystoid macular oedema such as capsular rupture and vitreous loss at the time of cataract surgery.
   - Anterior uveitis is very rare and usually responsive to steroid therapy. The drug should therefore be used with caution in uveitic glaucoma.
   - Increase in severity and recurrence of herpetic keratitis is also rare.
   - Conjunctival hyperpigmentation has also been reported.
2. **Systemic** side-effects include occasional headache, precipitation of migraine in susceptible individuals, skin rash and mild upper respiratory tract symptoms. These preparations should not be used in pregnancy because animal studies have shown potential teratogenic effects.

Topical carbonic anhydrase inhibitors

The carbonic anhydrase inhibitors (CAIs) are chemically related to the sulphonamides. They lower IOP by inhibiting aqueous secretion.

1. **Dorzolamide** (Trusopt) 2% t.i.d. as monotherapy or b.d. as adjunctive treatment is similar in efficacy to betaxolol but inferior to timolol. The main side-effects are allergic blepharoconjunctivitis (Fig. 13.50d) and a transient bitter taste. The drug should be used with caution in patients with corneal endothelial dysfunction as it may precipitate decompensation.
2. **Brinzolamide** (Azopt) 1% b.d. or t.i.d. is similar to dorzolamide, but with a lower incidence of stinging and local allergy.

Miotics

Pharmacology

Miotics are parasympathomimetic drugs that act by stimulating muscarinic receptors in the sphincter pupillae and ciliary body.

1. **In POAG** miotics reduce IOP by contraction of the ciliary muscle, which increases the facility of aqueous outflow through the trabecular meshwork.
2. **In PACG** contraction of the sphincter pupillae and the resultant miosis pulls the peripheral iris away from the trabeculum, thus opening the angle. It is often necessary to reduce IOP with systemic medication before miotics can take effect.

Ocular side-effects include miosis, brow ache, myopic shift and exacerbation of symptoms of cataract. Visual field defects appear denser and larger.

Preparations

1. **Pilocarpine** is equal in efficacy to beta-blockers. It is available in the following forms:
   - Pilocarpine drops 1%, 2%, 3%, 4% is used q.i.d. as monotherapy. When used in combination with a beta-blocker, b.d. administration is adequate.
   - Pilocarpine gel (Pilogel) consists of pilocarpine adsorbed on to a plastic gel, instilled once daily at bedtime so that the induced myopia and miosis last only during sleep. The main disadvantage is the development of a diffuse superficial corneal haze in 20% of users, although this rarely affects visual acuity.

2. **Carbachol** 3% t.i.d. is a good alternative to pilocarpine in resistant or intolerant cases.

Combined preparations

Combined preparations with similar ocular hypotensive effects to the sum of the individual components improve convenience and patient compliance. They are also more cost effective. Examples include:

1. **Cosopt** (timolol + dorzolamide) b.d.
2. **Xalacom** (timolol + latanoprost) once daily.
3. **TimPilo** (timolol + pilocarpine) b.d.
4. **Combigan** (timolol + brimonidine) b.d.
5. **Duotrav** (timolol + travoprost) once daily.
6. **Ganfort** (timolol + bimatoprost) once daily.

Systemic carbonic anhydrase inhibitors

Preparations

1. **Acetazolamide** is available in the following forms:
   - Tablets 250mg. The dose is 250–1000mg in divided doses. The onset of action is within 1 hour, with a peak at 4 hours and duration up to 12 hours.
   - Sustained-release capsules 250mg. The dose is 250–500mg daily with duration of up to 24 hours.
   - Powder 500mg vials for injection. The onset of action is almost immediate, with a peak at 30 minutes and duration up to 4 hours. This is the only CAI preparation available for injection and is useful in acute angle-closure glaucoma.
2. **Dichlorphenamide** tablets 50mg. The dose is 50–100mg (2–3 times daily). The onset of action is within 1 hour, with a peak at 3 hours and duration up to 12 hours.
3. **Methazolamide** tablets 50mg. The dose is 50–100mg (2–3 times daily). The onset of action is within 3 hours, with a peak at 6 hours and duration up to 10–18 hours. This is a useful alternative to acetazolamide with a longer duration of action but is currently not available in the United Kingdom.

Systemic side-effects

Systemically administered CAIs may be useful as short-term treatment, particularly in patients with acute glaucoma. Because of their systemic side-effects long-term use is reserved for patients at high risk of visual loss. The patient should always be warned of potential side-effects as this decreases anxiety and improves compliance.

1. **Paraesthesia** characterized by tingling of the fingers, toes, hands or feet, and occasionally at the mucocutaneous junctions, is a universal finding and usually innocuous. Compliance is suspect if the patient denies this symptom.
2. **Malaise complex** is characterized by a combination of malaise, fatigue, depression, weight loss and decreased libido. A supplemental 2-week course of sodium acetate may often be helpful.
3. **Gastrointestinal complex** is characterized by gastric irritation, abdominal cramps, diarrhoea and nausea. This can occur independently of the malaise syndrome and is unrelated to any specific changes in blood chemistry.
4. **Renal stone formation** is uncommon.
5. **Stevens–Johnson syndrome** may rarely occur since CAIs are sulphonamide derivatives (see Chapter 24).
6. **Blood dyscrasias** are extremely rare and may be of two types:
   - Dose-related bone marrow suppression, which usually recovers when treatment is stopped.
   - Idiosyncratic aplastic anaemia, which is not dose-related and has a mortality of 50%. It may occur after only one dose but usually does so during the first 2–3 months and very rarely after 6 months' administration.

Osmotic agents

Physiological principles

Osmotic pressure is dependent on the number rather than on the size of solute particles in a solution. Lower molecular weight solutes therefore exert a greater osmotic effect per gram. Osmotic agents remain intravascular, thus increasing blood osmolality. They lower IOP by creating an osmotic gradient between blood and vitreous so that water is 'drawn out' from the vitreous. The higher the gradient the greater the reduction of IOP. To be effective in the eye, an osmotic agent must therefore be unable to penetrate the blood–aqueous barrier. If penetration occurs, an osmotic equilibrium is set up and any further effect is lost. Osmotic agents are therefore of limited value in the treatment of inflammatory glaucomas in which the integrity of the blood–aqueous barrier is compromised.

Clinical uses

When a temporary drop in IOP is required that cannot be obtained by other means.
- In acute angle-closure glaucoma.
- Prior to intraocular surgery when the IOP is very high, as may occur from dislocation of the lens into the anterior chamber.

   NB These preparations should be given fairly rapidly and the patient should not subsequently be given fluids to quench thirst.

Side-effects

1. **Cardiovascular overload** may occur as a result of increased extracellular volume. Osmotic agents should therefore be used with great caution in patients with cardiac or renal disease.
2. **Urinary retention** may occur in elderly men following intravenous administration. Catheterization may be necessary in those with prostatism.
3. **Miscellaneous** side-effects include headache, backache, nausea and mental confusion.

Preparations

1. **Glycerol** is an oral agent with a sweet and sickly taste. Pure lemon (not orange) juice often needs to be added to avoid nausea. The dose is 1g/kg body weight or 2ml/kg body weight (50% solution). Peak action is within 1 hour, with duration up to 3 hours. Although glycerol is metabolized to glucose, it may be given to well controlled diabetics.
2. **Isosorbide** is an oral agent with a minty taste. Metabolically inert, it may be given to diabetics without insulin cover. The dose is the same as for glycerol.
3. **Mannitol** is the most widely used intravenous osmotic agent. The dose is 1g/kg body weight or 5ml/kg body weight (20% solution in water). Peak of action is achieved within 30 minutes, with duration up to 6 hours.

LASER THERAPY

Argon laser trabeculoplasty

Argon laser trabeculoplasty (ALT) involves the application of discrete laser burns to the trabecular meshwork. This enhances aqueous outflow and lowers IOP. ALT is performed in open angle glaucomas, usually as an adjunct to medical therapy. It is believed that the procedure causes increased outflow facility by the following mechanisms: (a) mechanical tightening of the trabecular meshwork and opening of adjacent, untreated trabecular spaces, and/or (b) inducing cell division and migration of macrophages to clear the trabecular meshwork of debris.

Technique

a. A drop of apraclonidine 1% or brimonidine 0.2% is instilled to prevent early post-laser rise in IOP.
b. Two drops of a topical anaesthetic are instilled.
c. A goniolens is inserted with the mirror at the 12 o'clock position to visualize the inferior angle (usually the easiest part to see).
d. The scleral spur, Schwalbe line (which may be pigmented) and the three-dimensional ground-glass appearance of the trabecular meshwork are identified.
e. The aiming beam is focused at the junction of the pigmented and non-pigmented trabecular meshwork ensuring that the spot is round and has a clear edge (Fig. 13.51a). An oval spot with an indistinct outline (Fig. 13.51b) means that the aiming beam is not perpendicular to the trabecular surface.
f. Initial laser settings are commonly: 50μm spot size, 0.1sec duration and 700mW power.
g. The laser is fired; the ideal reaction is a transient blanching (Fig. 13.52a) or appearance of a minute gas bubble (Fig. 13.52b) at the point of incidence. A large gas bubble (Fig. 13.52c) is excessive.
h. If the reaction is inadequate, the power is increased by 200mW. In a heavily pigmented meshwork, a power setting of 400mW may suffice, whereas a non-pigmented meshwork may require up to 1200mW (the average is about 900mW).
i. 25 burns are applied at regularly spaced intervals from one end of the mirror to the other.
j. The goniolens is rotated clockwise by 90° and a further 25 burns applied, making a total of 50 over 180° of the angle. It is important to be familiar with the rotational pattern of the mirror so that adjacent quadrants are treated systematically. With practice it is possible to perform ALT by continuously rotating the goniolens and applying each burn through the centre of the mirror. Some ophthalmologists initially treat 180° and later treat the other 180° if the response is unsatisfactory. Others, however, treat the entire circumference with 100 burns at the initial sitting.
k. Iopidine 1% or brimonidine 0.2% is instilled.
l. Topical fluorometholone q.i.d. for a week is prescribed; glaucoma medical therapy is continued.

Follow-up

Four to six weeks should be allowed for the treatment to take effect. If the IOP is reduced significantly by 6 weeks, gradual

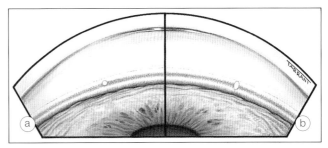

Fig. 13.51
Laser trabeculoplasty. **(a)** Correct focus of aiming beam; **(b)** incorrect focus

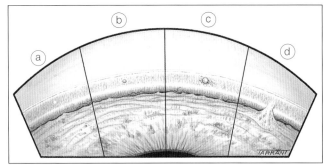

Fig. 13.52
Laser trabeculoplasty. **(a)** Blanching of trabecular meshwork – appropriate; **(b)** small bubble – also appropriate; **(c)** large bubble – excessive; **(d)** peripheral anterior synechiae due to poor technique

withdrawal of medication may be attempted, although total withdrawal is seldom possible. The main aim of ALT is to obtain a safe IOP; the reduction of medication is usually a secondary consideration. If IOP remains high and only 180° has been treated, the remaining 180° is treated. Following 360° ALT, re-treatment is unlikely to be beneficial and filtration surgery merits consideration.

Complications

1. **Peripheral anterior synechiae** (Fig. 13.52d) may develop if the burns are applied too posteriorly or if the energy level is high. In the majority of cases this does not compromise aqueous outflow.
2. **Small haemorrhages** may develop if the blood vessels on the peripheral iris or ciliary body are inadvertently treated. Such bleeding is easily stopped by applying pressure on the globe with the goniolens.
3. **Acute elevation of IOP** may occur if prophylactic apraclonidine or brimonidine is not used.
4. **Anterior uveitis** is fairly common but usually mild, transient and innocuous.
5. **Adverse effect on subsequent filtration surgery.** The incidence of encapsulated blebs following filtration surgery is up to three times higher in eyes previously treated by ALT.

Results

1. **In POAG** the initial success rate is 75–85%. The average reduction in IOP is about 30% – eyes with initially high IOPs therefore manifest a greater reduction of IOP. Up to 50% of eyes are still controlled after 5 years and about 33% after 10 years. Failure occurs most frequently in the first year; therefore if the IOP is still controlled at one year, the probability of control after 5 years is 65% and after 10 years 40%. If ALT is used as primary treatment, 50% of cases require additional medical therapy within 2 years.

Following initially successful ALT, re-treatment carries a low success rate (30% after one year and only 15% after 2 years). In general, the results are less good in patients under the age of 50 years. Black patients respond as well as whites initially, but tend to have a more rapid loss of effect.
2. **In normal-tension glaucoma** 50–70% of patients have a good response, but the absolute reduction in IOP is less than in POAG.
3. **In pigmentary glaucoma** results are generally good, although less so in older patients.
4. **In pseudoexfoliation glaucoma** initial results are excellent, although failure may occur earlier than in POAG and subsequent rise may be rapid.

NB ALT is ineffective in paediatric and most secondary glaucomas.

Selective laser trabeculoplasty

Selective laser trabeculoplasty (SLT) is a relatively new procedure which uses a 532nm frequency-doubled, Q-switched Nd:YAG laser which selectively targets melanin pigment in the trabecular meshwork cells, leaving non-pigmented cells and structures unscathed. It may therefore be safer than ALT as there is no thermal or structural damage to non-targeted tissue. Initial results show that it is probably as effective as ALT, although its exact place in the treatment of open angle glaucoma is yet to be defined.

Nd:YAG laser iridotomy

Indications

- PACG – acute, intermittent and chronic.
- Fellow eye of a patient with acute angle closure.
- Narrow 'occludable' angles.
- Secondary angle closure with pupil block.
- POAG with narrow angles and combined mechanism glaucoma.

Technique

a. A drop of apraclonidine 1% or brimonidine 0.2% is instilled.
b. The pupil should be miosed with topical pilocarpine, although this may not be possible following acute glaucoma.
c. A topical anaesthetic is instilled.
d. A special contact lens such as the Abraham iridotomy lens is inserted.
e. A site is selected, preferably in the superior iris, so that it is covered by the eyelid, thus preventing monocular diplopia.

The iridotomy should also be as peripheral as possible to minimize damage to the crystalline lens, although an arcus senilis may render this difficult. Finding an iris crypt is beneficial but not essential.

f. The beam is angled so that it is non-perpendicular and aimed towards the peripheral retina to avoid the remote possibility of a macular burn.

g. Laser settings vary with different machines. Most iridotomies are made with settings of 4–8millijoules (mJ). For a thin blue iris the required energy level is 1–4mJ per shot, with 2–3 shots per burst. Thick, velvety smooth, brown irides necessitate higher energy levels, which may be achieved with higher power or more shots per burst. Although such higher energy levels and more shots per burst render penetration of the iris easier, they carry an increased risk of intraocular damage. As a general guideline three bursts of 3–6mJ are usually effective.

h. The beam is focused precisely and the laser fired. Successful penetration is characterized by a gush of pigment debris. On average seven shots are required to produce an adequate iridotomy (Fig. 13.53a) although with practice this can be reduced to one or two.

i. A drop of apraclonidine 1% or brimonidine 0.2% is instilled.

j. A strong topical steroid (e.g. dexamethasone) is prescribed every 10 minutes for 30 minutes and thereafter q.i.d. for one week.

Technical problems

1. **Initial failure** is managed by re-treating the same site or moving to a different site and increasing the energy level. The decision to re-treat the same site depends in part on the degree of pigment dispersion and haemorrhage caused by the previous partial treatment. In thick brown irides, incomplete treatment may result in a thick cloud of dispersed iris pigment which impairs visualization and accurate focusing on the base of the crater. Further applications applied into the cloud often merely increase the pigment and haemorrhage, without producing an opening. In this situation it is best to wait for the cloud to disperse and then re-treat the same site, or to increase the energy level and try a different site. Alternatively a potential site may be pre-treated with an argon laser.

2. **Opening too small** (Fig. 13.53b). It is sometimes easier to create an additional opening at a different site rather than to try to enlarge the opening. The ideal diameter is 150–200μm.

Complications

1. **Bleeding** occurs in about 50% of cases. It is usually slight and stops after several seconds. Persistent bleeding can be terminated by pressing the contact lens against the cornea.

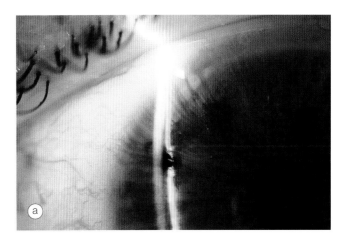
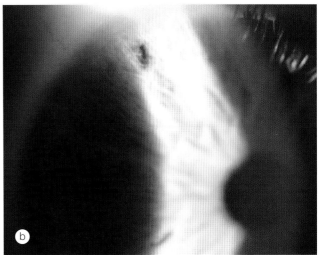
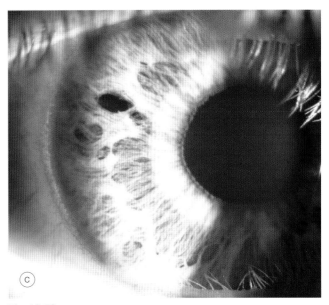

Fig. 13.53
Nd:YAG iridotomy. **(a)** Appropriate size; **(b)** too small; **(c)** not covered by the eyelid and perhaps not sufficiently peripheral

2. IOP elevation within one hour of treatment is common. It is mild and transient because dangerous spikes are avoided by pre-treatment with apraclonidine or brimonidine.

3. Iritis is common and usually mild. Severe iritis, which may result in the formation of posterior synechiae, is invariably caused by over-treatment and inadequate post-laser steroid therapy.

4. Corneal burns may occur if a contact lens is not used or if the anterior chamber is shallow.

5. Lens opacities which are localized and non-progressive occasionally develop at the treatment site.

6. Glare and diplopia may rarely occur if the iridotomy is not sited under the upper eyelid (Fig. 13.53c).

Diode laser cycloablation

Cycloablation lowers IOP by destroying part of the secretory ciliary epithelium, thereby reducing aqueous secretion. In the past it was used mainly in uncontrolled end-stage secondary glaucoma with minimal visual potential, mainly to control pain. However, it is now apparent that it can also be used in eyes with reasonably good vision which may be retained provided control of IOP is adequate.

Technique

a. A sub-Tenon or peribulbar anaesthetic is administered.
b. Laser settings are 1.5–2sec and 1500–2000mW.
c. The power is adjusted until a 'popping' sound is heard and then reduced to just below that level.
d. Approximately 2–40 burns are placed 1.2mm posteriorly to the limbus over 180° but avoiding the posterior ciliary nerves at 3 and 9 o'clock (Fig. 13.54).
e. A strong topical steroid is prescribed hourly on the day of treatment and then q.i.d. for 2 weeks.
f. Oral non-steroidal anti-inflammatory agents are prescribed for 2 days.

> **NB** Frequently more than one treatment session is required for adequate pressure control.

Complications

Mild pain and anterior segment inflammation are common. Serious complications are rare and include chronic hypotony, phthisis bulbi, scleral thinning, corneal decompensation and retinal or choroidal detachment. However, since the aim of the procedure is usually to relieve pain, vision-threatening complications do not have the same significance as those following conventional filtering procedures.

Results

The success rate is dependent on the type of glaucoma;

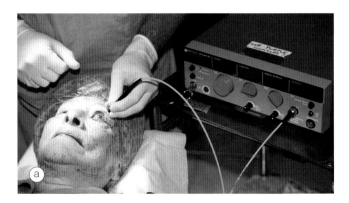

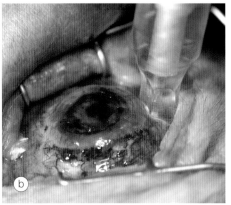

Fig. 13.54
(a) Diode laser cycloablation; **(b)** close up of the probe (Courtesy of J Salmon – fig. a; Krachmer, Mannis and Holland, from *Cornea*, Mosby, 2005 – fig. b)

frequently the procedure has to be repeated. Pain relief is generally good, but does not appear to be solely related to pressure control.

TRABECULECTOMY

Trabeculectomy lowers IOP by creating a fistula, which allows aqueous outflow from the anterior chamber to the sub-Tenon space. The fistula is protected or 'guarded' by a superficial scleral flap (Fig. 13.55). The procedure is usually performed when medical therapy has failed to achieve adequate control of IOP.

Technique

a. The pupil should be miosed.
b. A bridle suture is inserted either into peripheral clear cornea superiorly or into the superior rectus muscle.
c. A limbal or fornix-based flap of conjunctiva and Tenon capsule is fashioned superiorly.
d. Episcleral tissue is cleared. An outline of the proposed superficial scleral flap is made with wet-field cautery.

e. Incisions are made along the cautery marks through two-thirds of scleral thickness, to create a 'trapdoor' lamellar scleral flap (Fig. 13.56a). This flap may be rectangular (3mm × 4mm) or triangular, according to preference.

f. The superficial flap is dissected forwards until clear cornea has been reached (Fig. 13.56b).

g. A paracentesis is made in superotemporal peripheral clear cornea.

h. The anterior chamber is entered along the entire width of the trapdoor flap.

i. A block of deep sclera (1.5mm × 2 mm) is outlined (Fig. 13.56c) and excised with a knife and scissors (Fig. 13.56d) or a special punch (Fig. 13.56e).

j. A peripheral iridectomy is performed in order to prevent blockage of the internal opening (Fig. 13.56f).

k. The superficial scleral flap is sutured at its posterior corners so that it is lightly apposed to the underlying bed.

l. Alternatively, the flap may be sutured tightly with releasable sutures to reduce the risk of postoperative scleral flap leakage and shallow anterior chamber.

m. Balanced salt solution is injected into the anterior chamber through the paracentesis. This tests the patency of the fistula and facilitates the detection of any holes or leaks in the flap.

n. Conjunctiva/Tenon capsule flap is sutured. Irrigation through the paracentesis is repeated to produce a bleb, which is then checked for leakage.

o. A drop of atropine 1% is instilled.

p. A steroid and an antibiotic are injected under the inferior conjunctiva.

q. Steroid-antibiotic drops are used q.i.d. for 1–2 weeks and then changed to prednisolone acetate 1% for a further 4–8 weeks.

Shallow anterior chamber

A shallow anterior chamber may be due to (a) *pupillary block*, (b) *overfiltration* or (c) *malignant glaucoma* (aqueous misdirection). Severe and sustained shallowing is uncommon (Fig. 13.57a and b), the chamber re-forming spontaneously in most cases. However, those that do not may develop severe complications such as peripheral anterior synechiae, corneal endothelial damage (Fig.13.57c) and cataract (Fig. 13.57d).

Pupil block

Pupil block is caused by a non-patent peripheral iridectomy.

1. **Signs**
   • High IOP and flat bleb.
   • Negative Seidel test.
   • Iris bombé with a non-patent iridectomy.
2. **Treatment** involves YAG laser to the pigment epithelium at the iridectomy site if the anterior iris stroma appears to have been largely penetrated, or a new laser iridotomy is performed.

Overfiltration

Overfiltration may be caused by a scleral flap leakage due to insufficient resistance to outflow by the lamellar scleral flap or bleb leakage through an inadvertent buttonhole. Inadequate closure of the conjunctiva and Tenon capsule is perhaps the most common cause.

1. **Signs**
   • Low IOP, a well formed bleb in a scleral flap leak and flat in a bleb leak.
   • Seidel test is negative in a scleral flap leak and positive in a bleb leak (Fig. 13.58a).

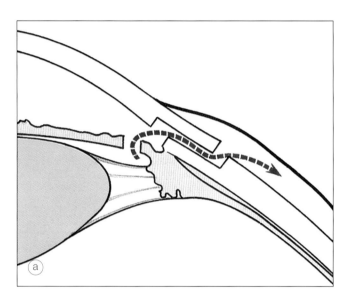

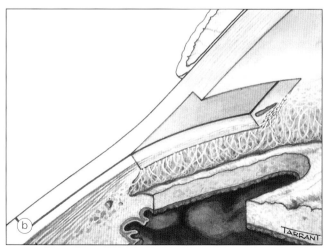

Fig. 13.55
Trabeculectomy principles. **(a)** Pathway of aqueous egress following trabeculectomy; **(b)** appearance from inside the eye following completion

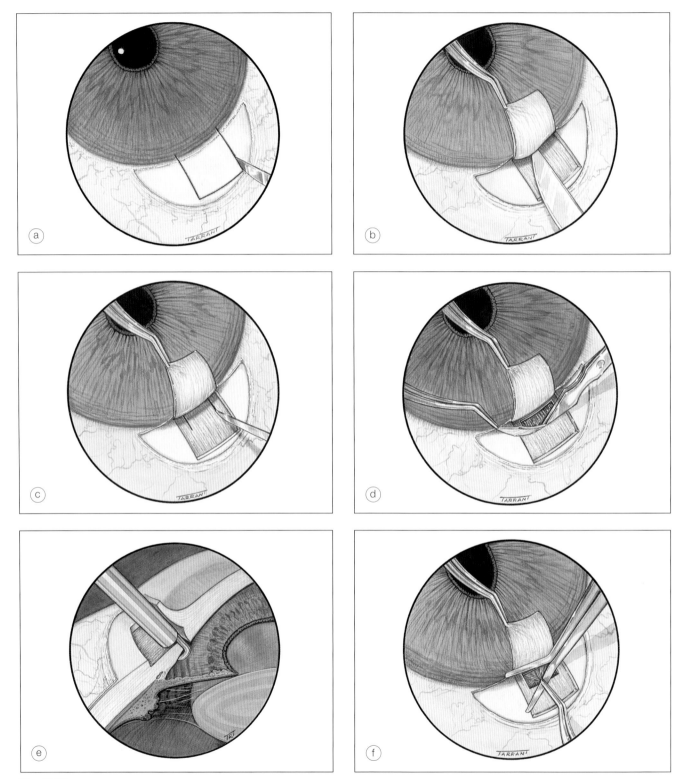

Fig. 13.56
Trabeculectomy. **(a)** Outline of superficial scleral flap; **(b)** dissection of superficial scleral flap; **(c)** incision for deep sclerectomy; **(d)** excision of deep scleral flap with Vannas scissors; **(e)** excision of deep scleral tissue with a punch (alternative); **(f)** peripheral iridectomy

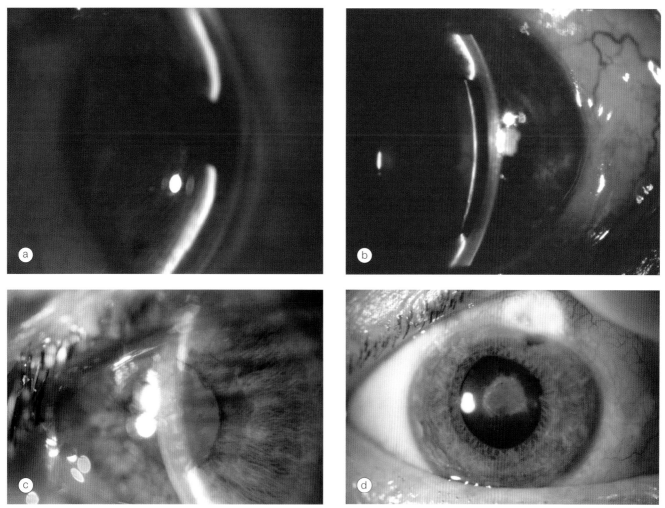

Fig. 13.57
Shallow anterior chamber. **(a)** Peripheral iris-corneal apposition; **(b)** pupillary border-corneal apposition; **(c)** lenticulo-corneal apposition resulting in corneal oedema; **(d)** cataract following inappropriate management

- The cornea may manifest signs of hypotony such as folds in Descemet membrane.
- Choroidal detachment may be present (Fig. 13.58b).
2. **Treatment** depends on the cause and degree of shallowing.
   a. Initial conservative treatment in eyes without lens-corneal touch is with atropine to prevent pupil block and aqueous suppressants (topical beta-blockers or oral acetazolamide) to promote spontaneous healing by temporarily reducing aqueous flow through the fistula.
   b. Subsequent treatment, if the above measures are ineffective, involves temporary tamponade of the conjunctiva to enhance spontaneous healing by simple pressure patching, a large diameter soft bandage contact lens, a collagen shield or a Simmons shell designed for the purpose.
   c. Definitive treatment for progressive shallowing and imminent or established lens-corneal touch involves

reformation of the anterior chamber with air, sodium hyaluronate or sulphur hexafluoride (SF6) and drainage of choroidal detachments if they are very deep and in danger of touching (kissing choroidals). The scleral flap and conjunctiva are re-sutured.

Malignant glaucoma

Malignant (ciliary-block) glaucoma (aqueous misdirection) is rare but serious. It is caused by blockage of aqueous flow at the pars plicata of the ciliary body, so that the aqueous is forced backwards into the vitreous.

1. **Signs**
   - High IOP and absent bleb.
   - Negative Seidel test.
2. **Treatment**
   a. Initial treatment is with mydriatics (atropine 1% and

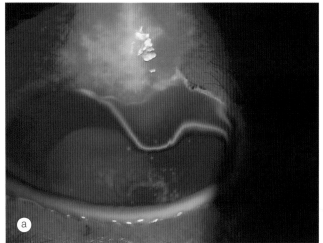
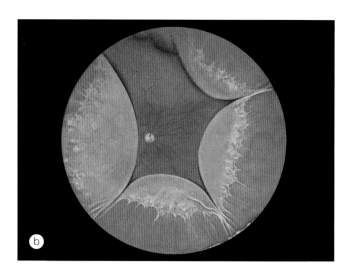

Fig. 13.58
(a) Positive Seidel test; (b) choroidal detachment

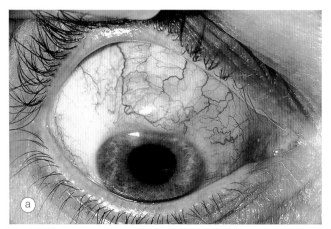

Fig. 13.59
Poorly filtering blebs. (a) Flat and vascularized; (b) encapsulated – Tenon cyst

phenylephrine 10%) to dilate the ciliary ring and increase the distance between the ciliary processes and the equator of the lens, thereby tightening the zonule and pulling the lens posteriorly into its normal position. Intravenous mannitol may be used if mydriatics are ineffective in order to shrink the vitreous gel and allow the lens to move posteriorly.

b. *Subsequent* treatment, if medical therapy fails, is with Nd:YAG laser fired through the iridectomy in order to disrupt the anterior hyaloid face and break the ciliary block. In pseudophakic eyes posterior capsulotomy and disruption of the anterior hyaloid face should be performed. Pars plana vitrectomy is performed if laser therapy fails. Sufficient vitreous gel is excised to allow free flow of aqueous to the anterior chamber.

Failure of filtration

Diagnosis

Poor filtration is indicated by increasing IOP and a bleb with one of the following appearances:

1. **Vascularized** bleb due to episcleral fibrosis (Fig. 13.59a).
2. **Encapsulated** bleb (Tenon cyst) which typically develops 2–8 weeks postoperatively. It is characterized by a localized, highly elevated, dome-shaped, firm, fluid-filled cavity of hypertrophied Tenon capsule with engorged surface blood vessels (Fig. 13.59b).

Causes

Causes of failure can be classified according to the site of blockage:

1. **Extraocular** causes include (a) subconjunctival and episcleral fibrosis and (b) occasionally bleb encapsulation.
2. **Scleral** causes include (a) an over-tight suturing of the scleral flap and (b) gradual scarring in the scleral bed may lead to obstruction of the fistula at that level.
3. **Intraocular** causes are uncommon and include (a) blockage of the sclerostomy by vitreous, blood or uveal tissue and (b) obstruction of the internal opening by a variety of thin membranes derived from surrounding cornea or sclera.

Management

Management of filtration failure depends on the cause and may involve one or more of the following:

1. **Ocular compression** in an effort to force outflow through the surgical fistula may be performed by (a) digital compression through the lower lid with the eyes closed and the patient looking straight ahead or (b) at the slit-lamp with a moistened sterile cotton bud at the edge of the scleral flap in an attempt to promote outflow.
2. **Suture manipulation** may be considered 7–14 days postoperatively if the eye has high IOP, a flat bleb and a deep anterior chamber. Releasable sutures can be cut or released according to the technique of initial placement. Argon laser suture lysis is useful if releasable sutures have not been used. It may be performed through a Hoskins (suture lysis lens) or a Zeiss four-mirror goniolens.
3. **Needling** of an encysted bleb may be performed at the slit-lamp or operating microscope under topical anaesthesia. It can be augmented with 5-fluorouracil to enhance the success rate.
4. **Subconjunctival injection of 5-fluorouracil** may be used in the first 7–14 days to suppress episcleral fibrosis; 5mg (0.1ml of 50mg/ml solution) is injected approximately 10mm away from the bleb.

Late bleb leakage

1. **Cause** is dissolution of conjunctiva overlying the sclerostomy, following previous operative application of antimetabolites, particularly mitomycin C. Necrosis of the surface epithelium results in transconjunctival drainage of aqueous.
2. **Complications** of untreated leaks include corneal decompensation, PAS, choroidal haemorrhage, infection, hypotony and maculopathy (see Chapter 17).
3. **Signs**

- Low IOP and an avascular cystic bleb.
- Seidel testing is initially negative; and only multiple punctate breaks in staining areas (sweating) are seen. Later the formation of a hole results in gross leakage with a positive test.
- Shallow anterior chamber and choroidal detachment may be present in severe cases.
4. **Treatment** is difficult. The following are some of the methods used, none of which are universally successful.
   a. **Initial** treatment is as for early postoperative over-filtration but is seldom successful.
   b. **Subsequent** treatment depends on the whether the leakage involves merely 'sweating' or is due to a hole.
   – Sweating blebs may be treated by injection of autologous blood into the bleb and compression sutures.
   – Full thickness holes usually require revisional surgery, such as conjunctival advancement to hood the existing bleb, free conjunctival patch autografts with removal of the existing bleb and scleral grafts to limit flow through the sclerostomy.

Bleb-associated bacterial infection and endophthalmitis

Glaucoma filtration-associated infection is classified as limited to the bleb (blebitis) or endophthalmitis, although there is some overlap. The incidence of blebitis following trabeculectomy with mitomycin is estimated to be 5% per year and endophthalmitis about 1% per year.

Pathogenesis

Adjunctive antifibrotic agents (mitomycin C, 5-fluorouracil) are frequently used to increase the success of glaucoma filtration surgery. The use of these agents can lead to a very thin walled drainage bleb (Fig. 13.60a) that significantly increases the risk of late-onset infection. The infection presumably gains access directly through the thin and avascular wall of the drainage bleb. All patients with such blebs should be warned of the possibility of late infection and strongly advised to report immediately should they develop a red and sticky eye, or blurred vision (RSVP – red, sticky, visual loss, pain).

1. **Risk factors** include blepharitis, long-term topical antibiotic use, an inferior or nasally placed bleb, and bleb leak. Late bleb leaks should be treated aggressively to reduce the risk of infection.
2. **Pathogens.** The most frequent are *H. influenzae*, *Streptococcus* spp., and *Staphylococcus* spp. The often poor visual prognosis is related to the virulence of these organisms.

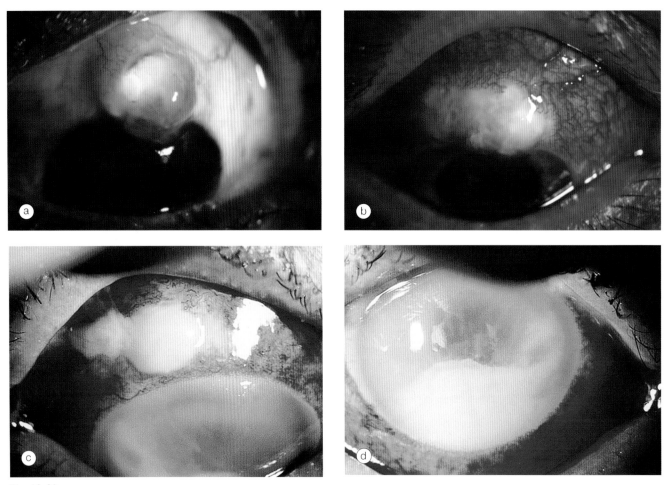

Fig. 13.60
(a) Thin-walled bleb; **(b)** blebitis; **(c)** purulent bleb and endophthalmitis; **(d)** endophthalmitis with hypopyon

Blebitis

Blebitis describes infection without vitreous involvement.

1. **Presentation** is with mild discomfort and redness.
2. **Signs**
   - A white bleb that appears to contain inflammatory material (Fig. 13.60b).
   - Anterior uveitis is absent.
   - The red reflex is normal.
3. **Investigation.** A conjunctival swab should be taken.

   NB Do not try to aspirate a sample from within the bleb.

4. **Treatment**
   - Topical ofloxacin and cefuroxime (or vancomycin 50mg/ml) hourly.
   - Oral augmentin 625mg t.d.s. and ciprofloxacin 750mg

b.d. for 5 days; azithromycin 500mg daily 5 days is an alternative to augmentin.

Endophthalmitis

1. **Presentation** is with a short history of rapidly worsening vision, pain and redness.
2. **Signs**
   - White milky bleb containing pus (Fig. 13.60c).
   - Severe anterior uveitis that may be associated with hypopyon (Fig. 13.60d).
   - Vitritis and impairment of the red reflex.
3. **Treatment** involves topical and systemic therapy as for blebitis and intravitreal antibiotics as for acute postoperative endophthalmitis following cataract extraction (see Chapter 12).

   NB Successfully treated eyes remain at risk of recurrent infection.

NON-PENETRATING SURGERY

Introduction

In non-penetrating filtration surgery the anterior chamber is not entered and the internal trabecular meshwork preserved, thus reducing the incidence of postoperative overfiltration and hypotony and its potential sequelae. Two lamellar scleral flaps are fashioned and the deep flap excised, leaving behind a thin membrane consisting of trabeculum/Descemet membrane through which aqueous diffuses from the anterior chamber to the subconjunctival space. Non-penetrating surgery is easier to perform in blacks than whites because the trabecular meshwork is easily visible as a consequence of the increased pigmentation. The surgery is technically challenging and requires meticulous dissection of a deep scleral flap without entering the delicate anterior trabecular meshwork.

Indications

The main indication for non-penetrating surgery is POAG. In general the IOP reduction is less than that achieved by trabeculectomy so that topical medication often needs to be recommenced. Conventional filtration is therefore still the procedure of choice when the target IOP is in the low teens.

Technique

The two currently used procedures are:

1. **Deep sclerectomy** in which a Descemet window is created that allows aqueous seepage from the anterior chamber (Fig. 13.61). Subsequent egress is subconjunctival resulting in a shallow filtration bleb, as well as along deeper suprachoroidal routes. The long-term results can be enhanced by using a collagen implant at the time of surgery and postoperative application of Nd:YAG laser to the meshwork at the surgical site using a gonioscope (goniopuncture).

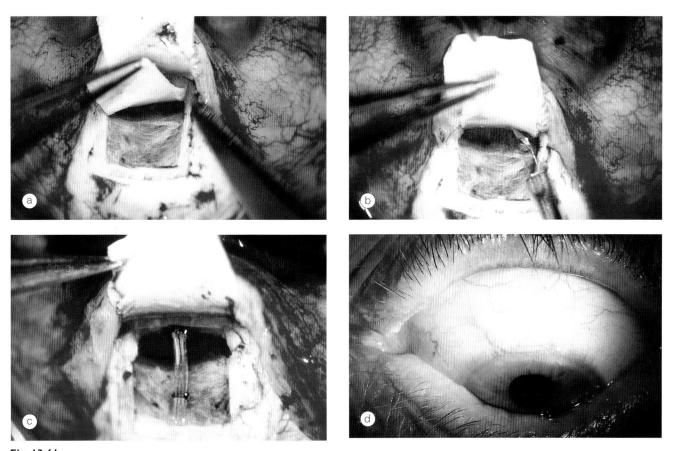

Fig. 13.61
Non-penetrating filtration surgery. **(a)** Dissection of scleral flap; **(b)** dissection into clear cornea exposing Schlemm canal; **(c)** collagen implant; **(d)** shallow diffuse avascular bleb (Courtesy of A Mermoud)

2. **Viscocanalostomy** involves the creation of a filtering window and identification and dilatation of Schlemm canal with high density viscoelastic. The superficial scleral flap is sutured tightly so that subconjunctival fluid outflow and bleb formation are minimized. The procedure probably causes inadvertent microscopic ruptures in the juxtacanalicular tissue and meshwork.

ANTIMETABOLITES IN FILTRATION SURGERY

Indications

Adjunctive antimetabolites inhibit the natural healing response that may preclude successful filtration surgery. They should, however, be used with caution because of the serious nature of potential complications; and primarily considered in the context of known risk factors for failure of trabeculectomy.

1. **High risk factors**
   * Neovascular glaucoma.
   * Previous failed trabeculectomy or artificial filtering devices.
   * Certain secondary glaucomas (e.g. inflammatory, post-traumatic angle recession and iridocorneal endothelial syndrome).
2. **Intermediate risk factors**
   * Patients on topical antiglaucoma medication (particularly sympathomimetics) for over 3 years.
   * Previous conjunctival surgery.
   * Previous cataract surgery.
3. **Low risk factors**
   * Black patients.
   * Patients under the age of 40 years.

   NB In uncomplicated glaucoma the use of low-dose antimetabolites may improve long-term control of IOP but this benefit should be weighed against possible complications such as corneal epithelial defects, chronic hypotony and late-onset bleb leakage.

5-Fluorouracil

5-fluorouracil (5-FU) inhibits DNA synthesis and is active on the 'S' phase (synthesis phase) of the cell cycle. Fibroblastic proliferation is inhibited, but fibroblastic attachment and migration are unaffected. It is the antimetabolite of choice in elderly patients who have risk factors for failure. The drug can be used in the following two ways:

1. **Subconjunctival** injection of 5mg daily for 5–7days as follows:
   * The eye is anaesthetized with a cotton pledget soaked in amethocaine.
   * 0.5ml of 5-FU (50mg/ml) is drawn up into a tuberculin syringe.
   * The 27-gauge needle is exchanged for a 30-gauge needle.
   * The bubbles are shaken to the top of the syringe.
   * 0.4ml of 5-FU is expressed so that only 0.1ml remains in the syringe.
   * The contents of the syringe are injected sub-conjunctivally 180° away from the filtration site.
   * Any reflux is caught on a dry cotton-tipped applicator or irrigated out.
2. **Operative** application is as follows:
   * The conjunctival flap is dissected.
   * A cellulose sponge measuring 4.5mm × 4.5mm is soaked in a 50mg/ml solution of 5-FU.
   * The sponge is placed under the dissected flap of Tenon capsule at the site of filtration making sure that the edges of the conjunctival incision are not exposed to the drug.
   * The sponge is removed after 5 minutes.
   * The space between the conjunctiva and episclera is thoroughly irrigated with balanced salt solution.
   * The trabeculectomy is completed.

Mitomycin C

Mitomycin C (MMC) is an alkylating agent rather than an antimetabolite, which selectively inhibits DNA replication, mitosis and protein synthesis. The drug inhibits proliferation of fibroblasts, suppresses vascular ingrowth and is much more potent than 5-FU. Optimum concentration and exposure times are not known and vary between 0.2–0.5mg/ml and 1–5 minutes. In general, low or intermediate risk indicates use of a low concentration (0.2mg/ml), whilst high risk implies the need for a higher concentration (0.4–0.5mg/ml). Higher concentrations and extended exposure times are associated with an increased risk of complications. The technique of intraoperative application is the same as for 5-FU and great care should be taken to prevent contamination of the anterior chamber. MMC can also be applied externally to the bleb with a sponge in the postoperative period.

Complications

1. **Corneal epithelial defects** and postoperative wound leaks occur mainly after the use of 5-FU.
2. **Cystic thin-walled blebs** may occur following the use of both 5-FU and mitomycin C and may predispose to chronic hypotony, late-onset bleb leak and endophthalmitis.

DRAINAGE IMPLANTS

Principles

Artificial drainage shunts are plastic devices which create a communication between the anterior chamber and sub-Tenon space. All such shunts consist of a tube attached to a posterior episcleral explant. Some contain pressure-sensitive valves for regulation of aqueous flow. Reduction of IOP is due to passive, pressure-dependent flow of aqueous across the capsular wall.

1. **Molteno** implant consists of a silicone tube connected to one or two polypropylene plates 13mm in diameter (Fig. 13.62).

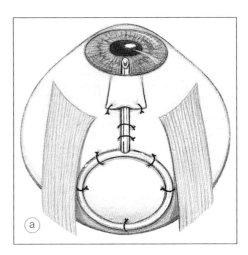

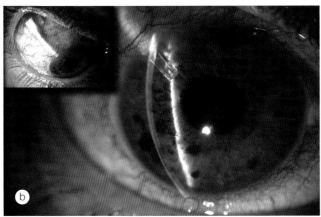

Fig. 13.62
(a) Molteno implant; **(b)** postoperative appearance (Courtesy of P Gili – fig. b)

2. **Baerveldt** implant consists of a silicone tube connected to a large area silicone plate impregnated with barium.
3. **Ahmed** implant consists of a silicone tube connected to a silicone sheet valve held in a polypropylene body. The valve mechanism consists of two thin silicone elastomer membranes which create a Venturi-shaped chamber.

Indications

- Uncontrolled glaucoma despite previous trabeculectomy with adjunctive antimetabolite therapy.
- Secondary glaucoma where routine trabeculectomy, with or without adjunctive antimetabolites, is unlikely to be successful. Examples include neovascular glaucoma and glaucoma following traumatic anterior segment disruption.
- Eyes with severe conjunctival scarring precluding accurate dissection of the conjunctiva.
- Certain congenital glaucomas where conventional procedures have failed (i.e. goniotomy, trabeculotomy and trabeculectomy).

Complications

Because shunts are used in severely compromised eyes, the complication rate tends to be greater than following trabeculectomy.

1. **Excessive drainage** may occur due to leakage around or down the tube if the occluding suture is loose and result in hypotony and a shallow anterior chamber (Fig. 13.63a).
2. **Malposition** may result in endothelial or lenticular touch (Fig. 13.63b).
3. **Tube erosion** through the sclera and conjunctiva (Fig. 13.63c).
4. **Drainage failure** may occur as a result of blockage of the end of the tube by vitreous, blood or iris tissue.
5. **Bleb encapsulation** over the footplate may result in poor drainage (Fig. 13.63d). This occurs in about 10% of cases and is the most significant late complication.

Results

The results depend on the type of glaucoma. In general, an IOP < 21mmHg is achieved in 50–70% of cases but topical medication is often required to maintain the IOP at this level. Less than 33% of cases achieve adequate control of IOP without additional medical therapy. The long-term success rate in neovascular glaucoma is particularly disappointing because of progressive retinal disease with loss of vision and late development of phthisis bulbi. Adjunctive mitomycin C may enhance the success rate of drainage shunt surgery but is associated with a higher complication rate.

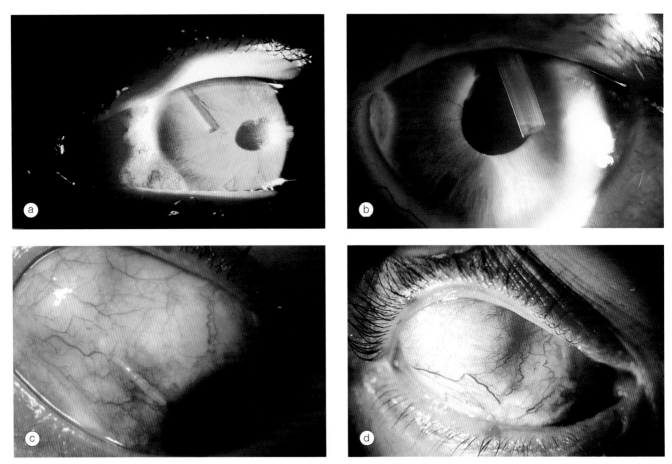

Fig. 13.63
Complications of drainage implants. **(a)** Flat anterior chamber due to excessive drainage; **(b)** malposition; **(c)** tube erosion; **(d)** bleb encapsulation over the footplate (Courtesy of J Salmon)

UVEITIS

INTRODUCTION

Anatomical classification

The uvea is the intermediate vascular coat of the eye which comprises the iris, ciliary body and choroid (Fig. 14.1).

1. **Uveitis,** by strict definition implies an inflammation of the uveal tract. However, the term is now used to describe many forms of intraocular inflammation involving not only the uveal tract but also the retina and its vessels.
2. **Anterior uveitis** may be subdivided into:
   - Iritis in which the inflammation primarily involves the iris.
   - Iridocyclitis in which both the iris and ciliary body are involved.
3. **Intermediate** uveitis is defined as inflammation predominantly involving the vitreous.
4. **Posterior uveitis** involves the fundus posterior to the vitreous base.
   - Retinitis with the primary focus in the retina.
   - Choroiditis with the primary focus in the choroid.
   - Vasculitis which may involve veins, arteries or both.
5. **Panuveitis (diffuse)** implies involvement of the entire uveal tract without a predominant site of inflammation.

6. **Endophthalmitis** implies inflammation, often purulent, involving all intraocular tissues except the sclera.
7. **Panophthalmitis** involves the entire globe, often with orbital extension.

   NB Anterior uveitis is the most common, followed by posterior, intermediate and panuveitis.

Definitions

1. **Onset** of uveitis may be either *sudden* or *insidious*.
2. **Duration** of an attack may be either *limited*, if it is 3 months or less in duration, or *persistent*, if it is longer.
3. **Course**
   a. Acute uveitis describes the course of a specific uveitis syndrome characterized by sudden onset and limited duration.
   b. Recurrent uveitis is characterized by repeated episodes of uveitis separated by periods of inactivity without treatment lasting at least 3 months.
   c. Chronic uveitis describes persistent inflammation characterized by prompt relapse (in less than 3 months) after discontinuation of therapy.
   d. Remission refers to inactive disease for at least 3 months after discontinuation of treatment.

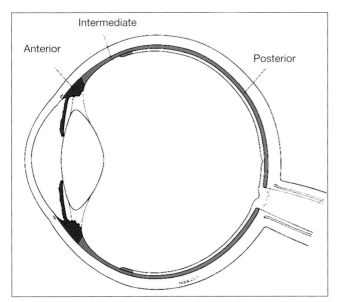

Fig. 14.1
Anatomical classification of uveitis

History

Establishing the aetiological diagnosis in uveitis is based on obtaining an accurate ocular and medical history as well as performing a detailed examination. Laboratory tests may be helpful, but very few conclusively establish the diagnosis.

1. **Age** at presentation is very important because certain types of uveitis are confined to patients within a specific age group whilst others may occur at any age. For example:
   - Uveitis associated with juvenile idiopathic arthritis (JIA) and ocular toxocariasis typically affects children.
   - Birdshot chorioretinopathy and serpiginous choroiditis are more prevalent in the fifth to seventh decades of life.
   - HLA-B27-associated uveitis and Behçet syndrome usually affect young adults.
   - Acute retinal necrosis and toxoplasmosis may affect individuals of any age group.

   NB It is less common for primary uveitis to first manifest in old age; suspect a masquerade syndrome, especially intraocular lymphoma.

2. **Race** is especially important in conditions such as Behçet syndrome (Mediterranean, Middle Eastern and Asian), sarcoidosis (blacks) and VKH (Chinese, Asians, and in the USA those with native Indian ancestry).
3. **Geographic location** may be of importance because infectious uveitis (e.g. Lyme disease and presumed ocular histoplasmosis) may be endemic in certain locations.

4. **Past ocular history** may occasionally be helpful. For example, recurrent attacks of unilateral acute anterior uveitis would be suggestive of HLA-B27-related disease whereas a history of previous trauma or surgery would point to the diagnosis of sympathetic ophthalmitis or lens-induced uveitis.
5. **Past medical history** is of paramount importance, particularly in identifying exposure to infectious agents, such as tuberculosis and syphilis as well as supporting the diagnosis of Behçet syndrome (oral and genital ulcers). Certain medications such as rifabutin and cidofovir may occasionally cause uveitis.
6. **Hygiene and dietary habits** are important when considering infectious diseases such as toxocariasis (history of pica), toxoplasmosis (undercooked meat – ingestion of water in rural areas seems to be a more important factor) and cysticercosis (ingestion of pork in endemic areas).
7. **History of sexual practices** are especially important for the diagnosis of syphilis and HIV infection.
8. **Recreational drugs** are a risk factor for HIV infection and fungal endophthalmitis.
9. **Pets.** Cats are linked to the transmission of toxoplasmosis and cat-scratch disease, while exposure to puppies is associated with toxocariasis.

SPECIAL INVESTIGATIONS

Indications

1. **Not necessary**
   - Single attack of mild unilateral acute anterior uveitis without suggestion of a possible underlying disease.
   - A specific uveitis entity such as sympathetic ophthalmitis and Fuchs uveitis syndrome.
   - When a systemic diagnosis compatible with the uveitis is already apparent such as Behçet syndrome or sarcoidosis.
2. **Indications**
   - Recurrent granulomatous anterior uveitis.
   - Bilateral disease.
   - Systemic manifestations without a specific diagnosis.
   - Confirmation of a suspected ocular picture, which depends on the test result as part of the criteria for diagnosis such as HLA-A29 testing for birdshot chorioretinopathy.

Skin tests

1. **Tuberculin skin tests (Mantoux and Heaf)** involve the intradermal injection of purified protein derivative of *M. tuberculosis.*

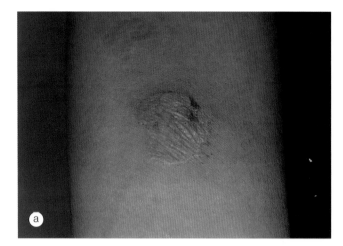

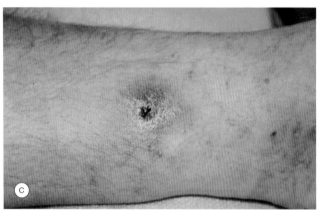

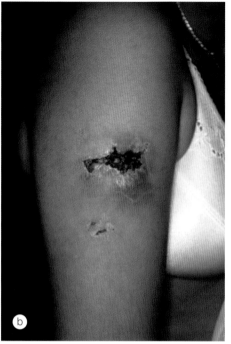

Fig. 14.2
Skin tests in the investigation of uveitis. **(a)** Positive tuberculin skin reaction; **(b)** strongly positive tuberculin skin reaction; **(c)** positive pathergy test in Behçet syndrome (Courtesy of U Raina – fig. a; B Noble – fig. c)

a. Positive result is characterized by the development of an induration of 5–14mm within 48 hours (Fig. 14.2a).

b. Negative result usually excludes TB, but may also occur in patients with advanced consumptive disease.

c. Weakly positive result does not necessarily distinguish between previous exposure and active disease. This is because most individuals have already received BCG (Bacille Calmette-Guérin) vaccination and will therefore exhibit a hypersensitivity response.

d. Strongly positive result (induration >15mm) is usually indicative of active disease since this level of response is not expected after long exposure to the vaccine (Fig. 14.2b).

2. **Pathergy** test (increased dermal sensitivity to needle trauma) is a criterion for the diagnosis of Behçet syndrome, but the results vary and it is only rarely positive in the absence of systemic activity. A positive response is the formation of a pustule following pricking of the skin with a needle (Fig. 14.2c).

Serology

Syphilis

Because of the variable presentation serology should be performed in all patients with uveitis who require investigation. Serological tests rely on detection of non-specific antibodies (cardiolipin) or specific treponemal antibodies.

1. **Non-treponema tests** such as rapid plasma regain (RPR) or Venereal Disease Research Laboratory (VDRL) are best used to diagnose primary infection, monitor disease activity or response to therapy based on titre. The patient's serum is mixed with commercially prepared carbon-like cardiolipin antigen (Fig. 14.3a). The results may be negative in up to 30% of patients with documented syphilitic uveitis. They also tend to become negative 6–18 months after therapy.

2. **Treponema antibody tests** are highly sensitive and specific and more useful to prove past infection, or secondary or tertiary forms of clinical infection. The

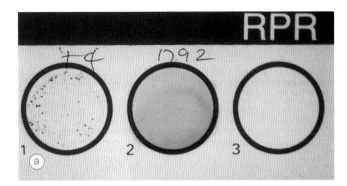

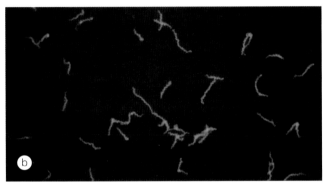

Fig. 14.3
Serological tests for syphilis. **(a)** Rapid plasma reagin (RPR)
showing clumping of the antigenic particles (left) after 4 minutes;
(b) positive fluorescent treponema antibody test (FTA-ABS)
(Courtesy of Mims, Dockrell, Goering, Roitt, Wakelin and Zuckerman,
from *Medical Microbiology*, Mosby, 2004)

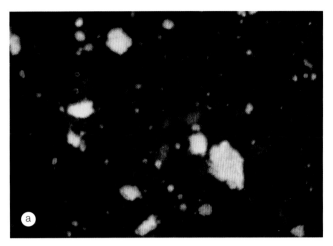

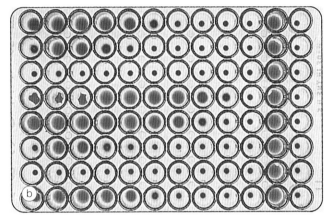

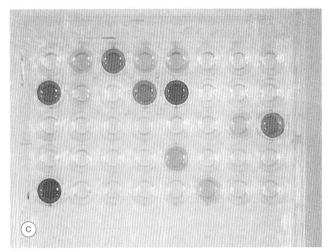

Fig. 14.4
Serological tests for toxoplasmosis. **(a)** Positive immunofluorescent
antibody test; **(b)** haemagglutination test; **(c)** ELISA test showing
positive (yellow-brown) and negative wells

fluorescent treponemal antibody absorption test (FTA-ABS) and the more specific microhaemagglutination treponema pallidum test (MHA-TP) are most commonly used. The antibody in the patient's serum binds to bacteria and is visualized by a fluorescent dye (Fig. 14.3b). The result cannot be titrated and is either positive (reactive) or negative (non-reactive). A positive result always remains positive (serological scar).

Toxoplasmosis

1. **Dye test (Sabin–Feldman)** utilizes live organisms which are exposed to the patient's serum complement. The cell membranes of the organisms are lysed in the presence of the specific anti-Toxoplasma IgG, and as a consequence the organisms fail to stain with methylene-blue dye. This test remains as the gold standard for the diagnosis of toxoplasmosis.
2. **Immunofluorescent antibody** tests utilize dead organisms exposed to the patient's serum and antihuman globulin labeled with fluorescein. The results are read using a fluorescent microscope (Fig. 14.4a).

3. **Haemagglutination** tests involve coating of lysed organisms on to red blood cells which are then exposed to the patient's serum; positive sera cause the red cells to agglutinate (Fig. 14.4b).

4. **Enzyme-linked immunosorbent assay (ELISA)** involves binding of the patient's antibodies to an excess of solid phase antigen (Fig. 14.4c). This complex is then incubated with an enzyme-linked second antibody. Assessment of enzyme activity provides measurement of specific antibody concentration. The test can also be used to detect antibodies in the aqueous which are more specific than those in the serum. The test is also useful in other conditions such as cat-scratch fever and toxocariasis.

NB Any positive titre, even in undiluted serum, is significant in the presence of a fundus lesion compatible with toxoplasmic retinitis. Reactivation of ocular disease alone will have no impact on the titre.

Antinuclear antibody

Antinuclear antibody (ANA) is mainly used to identify children with JIA who are at high risk of developing anterior uveitis and therefore require closer follow-up.

NB Rheumatoid factor is relevant only when investigating aetiology of scleritis. It should not be ordered in the work-up of patients with uveitis only.

Enzyme assay

1. **Angiotensin-converting enzyme (ACE)** is a non-specific test which indicates the presence of a granulomatous disease such as sarcoidosis, tuberculosis or leprosy. Elevations occur in up to 80% of patients with sarcoidosis, and it is more likely to be elevated in acute disease. It is normally elevated in children and therefore of less diagnostic value.

2. **Lysozyme** has good sensitivity but less specificity than ACE for the diagnosis of sarcoidosis but using both tests seems to increase sensitivity and specificity.

HLA tissue typing

See Table 14.1 for details of HLA types and related systemic diseases.

Imaging

1. **Fluorescein angiography (FA)** is useful in the following conditions:

Table 14.1   HLA type and systemic disease

HLA type	Associated disease
B27	Spondyloarthropathies, particularly ankylosing spondylitis
A29	Birdshot chorioretinopathy
B51	Behçet syndrome
HLA-B7 and HLA-DR2	POHS and APMPPE

- Diagnosis and assessment of severity of retinal vasculitis.
- Diagnosis of cystoid macular oedema (CMO).
- Demonstrating macular ischaemia as the cause of visual loss rather than CMO.
- Differentiation between inflammatory and ischaemic cause of retinal neovascularization.
- Diagnosis and monitoring of choroidal neovascularization (CNV).

NB FA is less appropriate in choroiditis because deep lesions will be hidden by the choroidal flush. For this reason more lesions are seen clinically than angiographically in birdshot chorioretinopathy.

2. **Indocyanine green angiography (ICG)** is better suited for choroidal disease because the dye does not readily leak out of choroid vessels, which are better visualized through the RPE. ICG is able to detect non-perfusion of the choriocapillaris and provide information regarding inflammation affecting the stroma.

3. **Ultrasonography (US)** is of particular value when opaque media hamper adequate fundus examination, especially in excluding a retinal detachment or an intraocular mass.

4. **Optical coherence tomography (OCT)** is as effective as FA in detecting CMO. It can also identify vitreoretinal traction as the mechanism of CMO.

Biopsy

Histopathology still remains the gold standard for definitive diagnosis of many conditions. Biopsies of the skin or other organs may establish the diagnosis of a systemic disorder associated with the ocular manifestations, such as in sarcoidosis. However, intraocular structures are relatively inaccessible to this procedure without running the risk of significant morbidity.

1. **Conjunctiva and lacrimal gland** biopsy may be useful for the diagnosis of sarcoidosis but only in the presence of clinically apparent disease.

2. **Aqueous samples** for polymerase chain reaction (PCR) may occasionally be useful in the diagnosis of viral retinitis.

3. **Vitreous biopsy,** apart from its already well established role in infectious endophthalmitis, can also be used for the diagnosis of other infectious conditions by obtaining samples for culture and PCR. It is also used for diagnosis of intraocular lymphoma.
4. **Retinal and choroidal biopsies** may be useful in the following conditions:
   • Diagnosis not established.
   • No response to therapy.
   • Further deterioration despite therapy.
   • To exclude possibility of malignancy or infection.

Radiology

1. **Chest radiographs** are to exclude tuberculosis and sarcoidosis.
2. **Sacro-iliac joint x-ray** is helpful in the diagnosis of a spondyloarthropathy in the presence of symptoms of low back pain and uveitis.
3. **CT and MR** of the brain and thorax may be appropriate in the investigation of sarcoidosis, multiple sclerosis and primary intraocular lymphoma. A thorax CT scan may clarify any doubts regarding the presence of hilar adenopathy.

CLINICAL FEATURES

Acute anterior uveitis

Anterior uveitis is the most common form of uveitis. Acute anterior uveitis (AAU) is the most common form of anterior uveitis, accounting for three-quarters of cases. It is characterized by sudden onset and duration of 3 months or less. It is easily recognized due to the severity of symptoms which will force the patient to seek medical attention.

Symptoms

Presentation is typically with sudden onset of unilateral, pain, photophobia and redness, which may be associated with lacrimation.

NB Patients may notice mild ocular discomfort a few days before the acute attack when clinical signs are absent.

Signs

1. **Visual acuity** is usually good at presentation except in very severe cases with hypopyon.
2. **Ciliary (circumcorneal) injection** has a violaceous hue (Fig. 14.5a).

3. **Miosis** due to sphincter spasm may predispose to the formation of posterior synechiae unless the pupil is dilated (Fig. 14.5b).
4. **Endothelial dusting** by a myriad of cells is present early and gives rise to a 'dirty' appearance (Fig. 14.5c); true keratic precipitates usually appear only after a few days and are usually non-granulomatous (see below).
5. **Aqueous cells** indicate disease activity and their number reflects disease severity (Fig. 14.5d). Grading of cells is performed with a 2mm long and 1mm wide slit beam with maximal light intensity and magnification. The findings are recorded in the notes as shown in Table 14.2.

Table 14.2 Grading anterior chamber cells

Grade	Cells in field
0	< 1
0.5+	1–5
1+	6–15
2+	16–25
3+	26–50
4+	> 50

NB *Improvement* of inflammation is defined as either a two-step decrease in the level of activity or a decrease to 'inactive', and *worsening* is defined as either a two-step increase in the level of activity or an increase to the maximum grade.

6. **Anterior vitreous cells** indicate iridocyclitis.
7. **Aqueous flare** reflects the presence of protein due to a breakdown of the blood–aqueous barrier (see Fig. 14.5d). Flare may be graded by laser interferometry using a flare meter or clinically by observing the degree of interference in the visualization of iris using the same settings as for cells (Table 14.3).

Table 14.3 Grading or anterior chamber flare

Grade	Description
0	Nil
1+	Faint
2+	Moderate (iris and lens details clear)
3+	Marked (iris and lens details hazy)
4+	Intense (fibrinous exudate)

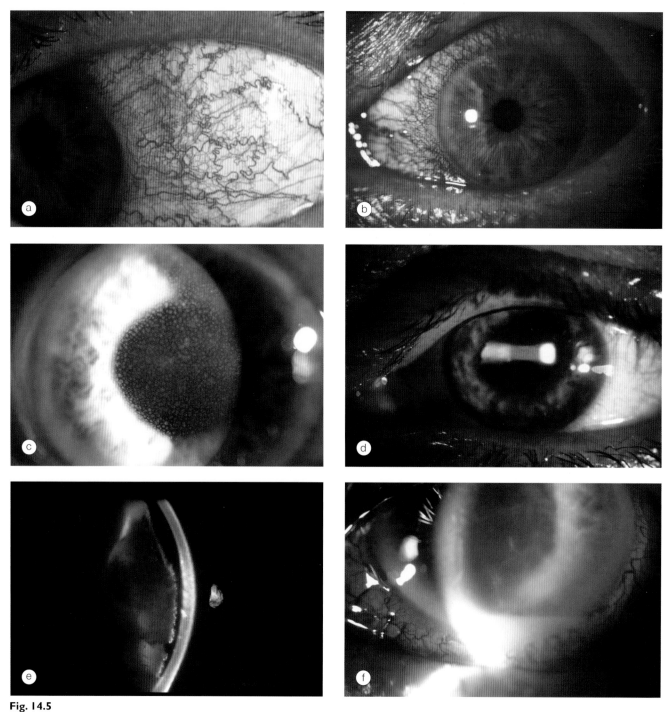

Fig. 14.5
Signs of acute anterior uveitis. (a) Ciliary injection; (b) miosis; (c) endothelial dusting by cells; (d) aqueous flare and cells; (e) fibrinous exudate; (f) fibrinous exudate and hypopyon

8. **Aqueous fibrinous exudate** typically occurs in HLA-B27-associated AAU (Fig. 14.5e).
9. **Hypopyon** is a feature of intense inflammation in which cells settle in the inferior part of the anterior chamber and form a horizontal level (Fig. 14.5f).
   • In AAU associated with the HLA-B27 the hypopyon

has a high fibrin content which makes it dense, immobile and slow to absorb.
• In patients with Behçet syndrome the hypopyon has minimal fibrin and therefore shifts according to the patient's head position and may disappear quickly.

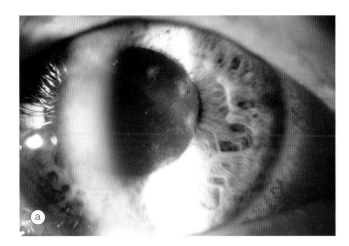

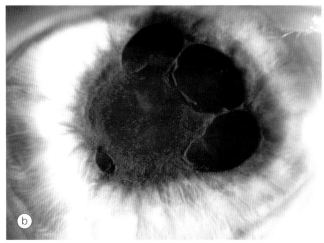

Fig. 14.6
Posterior synechiae. **(a)** Early synechiae formation in active acute anterior uveitis; **(b)** extensive synechiae and pigment on the lens following a severe attack of acute anterior uveitis

- Hypopyon associated with blood occurs in herpetic infection and in eyes with associated rubeosis iridis.
10. **Posterior synechiae** may develop quite quickly (Fig. 14.6a) and must be broken down before they become permanent (Fig. 14.6b).
11. **Low intraocular pressure** is the rule as a result of reduced secretion of aqueous by the ciliary epithelium. Occasionally the intraocular pressure may be elevated (hypertensive uveitis) in herpetic uveitis and Posner–Schlossman syndrome.

NB Although fundus examination is usually normal, it should always be performed to exclude 'spillover' anterior uveitis associated with a posterior focus, most notably toxoplasmosis.

Course and prognosis

With appropriate therapy the inflammation tends to completely resolve within 5–6 weeks, with an excellent visual prognosis. Complications and poor visual prognosis are related to delayed or inadequate management. Steroid-induced hypertension may occur but glaucomatous damage is uncommon.

Chronic anterior uveitis

Chronic anterior uveitis (CAU) is less common than the acute type and is characterized by persistent inflammation that promptly relapses, in less than 3 months, after discontinuation of treatment. The inflammation may be granulomatous or non-granulomatous. Simultaneous bilateral involvement is more common than in AAU.

Symptoms

Presentation is insidious and many patients are asymptomatic until the development of complications such as cataract or band keratopathy.

NB Because of the lack of symptoms patients at risk of developing CAU should be routinely screened; this applies particularly in patients with JIA.

Signs

1. **External.** The eye is usually white or occasionally pink during periods of exacerbation of inflammatory activity.
2. **Aqueous cells** vary in number according to disease activity but even patients with numerous cells may have no symptoms.
3. **Aqueous flare** may be more marked than cells in eyes with prolonged activity and its severity may act as an indicator of disease activity (contrary to previous teaching).
4. **Keratic precipitates** (KP) are clusters of cellular deposits on the corneal endothelium composed of epithelioid cells, lymphocytes and polymorphs (Fig. 14.7a). Their characteristics and distribution may indicate the probable type of uveitis.
   - Large KP in granulomatous disease have a greasy ('mutton-fat') appearance. They are often more numerous inferiorly and may form in a triangular pattern with the apex pointing up (Fig. 14.7b) as the result of gravity and normal convection flow of aqueous.
   - Resolved 'mutton-fat' KP leave behind a ground-glass appearance (ghost KP) which is evidence of previous granulomatous inflammation (Fig. 14.7c).

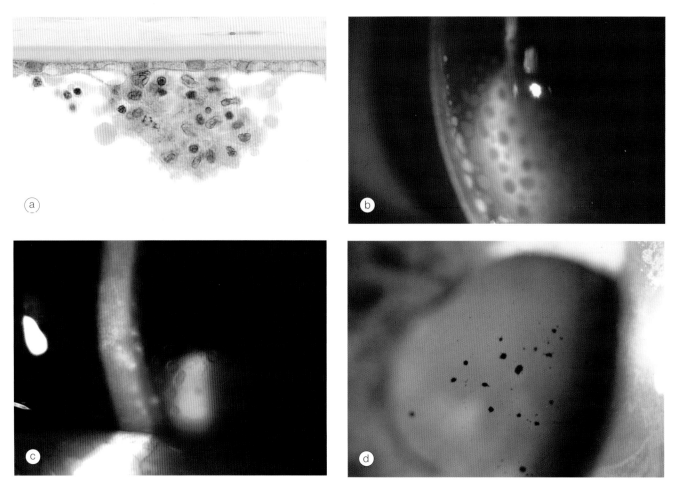

Fig. 14.7
Keratic precipitates. **(a)** Aggregate of inflammatory cells on the corneal endothelium; **(b)** large 'mutton-fat' keratic precipitates; **(c)** 'ghost' keratic precipitates; **(d)** old pigmented keratic precipitates (Courtesy of J Harry and G Misson, from *Clinical Ophthalmic Pathology*, Butterworth-Heinemann, 2001 – fig. a)

- Long-standing non-granulomatous KP may become pigmented (Fig. 14.7d).
5. Iris nodules typically occur in granulomatous disease.
  - Koeppe nodules are small and situated at the pupillary border (Fig. 14.8a).
  - Busacca nodules are stromal (Fig. 14.8b).
  - Large pink nodules are characteristic of sarcoid uveitis (Fig. 14.8c).

Course and prognosis

The inflammation persists for longer than 3 months and in some cases even years. Remissions and exacerbations of inflammatory activity are common and it is difficult to determine when the natural course of the disease has come to an end. Because of the chronicity of the disease, delay in presentation and prolonged therapy, the prognosis is guarded and complications such as cataract and glaucoma are common.

Posterior uveitis

Posterior uveitis encompasses retinitis, choroiditis and retinal vasculitis. Some lesions may originate primarily in the retina or choroid but often there is involvement of both (retinochoroiditis and chorioretinitis).

Symptoms

Presenting symptoms vary according to the location of the inflammatory focus and the presence of vitritis. For example, a patient with a peripheral lesion may complain of floaters whereas a patient with a lesion involving the macula will predominantly complain of impaired central vision.

Signs

1. Retinitis may be focal (solitary) or multifocal. Active lesions are characterized by whitish retinal opacities

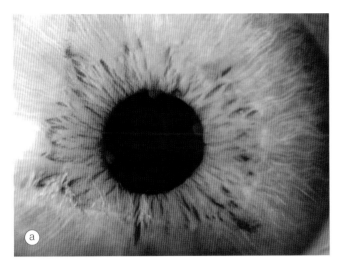

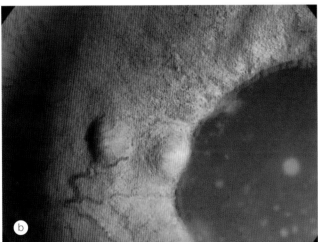

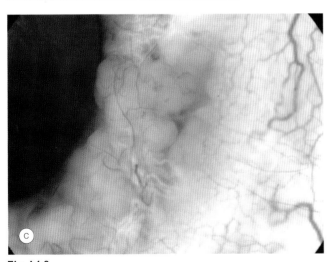

Fig. 14.8
Iris nodules in granulomatous anterior uveitis. **(a)** Koeppe nodules; **(b)** Busacca nodules; **(c)** very large nodules in sarcoid uveitis (Courtesy of C Pavesio – figs b and c)

with indistinct borders due to surrounding oedema (Fig. 14.9a). As the lesion resolves, the borders become better defined.

2. **Choroiditis** may also be focal, multifocal or geographic. It does not usually induce vitritis in the absence of concomitant retinal involvement. Active choroiditis is characterized by a round, yellow nodule (Fig. 14.9b).

3. **Vasculitis** may occur as a primary condition or as a secondary phenomenon adjacent to a focus of retinitis. Both arteries (periarteritis) and veins (periphlebitis) may be affected, although venous involvement is more common. Active vasculitis is characterized by yellowish or grey-white, patchy, perivascular cuffing (Fig. 14.9c). Quiescent vasculitis may leave perivascular scarring, which should not be mistaken for active disease (Fig. 14.9d).

TREATMENT

Treatment of immune-mediated uveitis involves predominantly the use of anti-inflammatory and immunosuppressive agents. Antibiotic therapy for infectious diseases will be discussed in the specific sections. It is important to keep in mind that nearly all drugs used to treat uveitis are capable of producing side-effects, and this should always be weighted against the decision to treat. Also, it must be emphasized that the use of systemic therapy should be carried out in conjunction with a physician who is competent to deal with complications associated with the underlying disease or therapy.

Mydriatics

Preparations

1. **Short-acting**
   a. *Tropicamide* (0.5% and 1%) has duration of 6 hours.
   b. *Cyclopentolate* (0.5% and 1%) has duration of 24 hours.
   c. *Phenylephrine* (2.5% and 10%) has duration of 3 hours but no cycloplegic effects.
2. **Long-acting**
   a. *Homatropine 2%* has duration of up to 2 days.
   b. *Atropine 1%* is the most powerful cycloplegic and mydriatic with duration of up to 2 weeks.

Indications

1. **To promote comfort** by relieving spasm of the ciliary muscle and pupillary sphincter, with atropine or homatropine, although it is usually unnecessary to use these agents for more than 1–2 weeks. Once the inflammation shows signs of subsiding a short-acting preparation can be used.

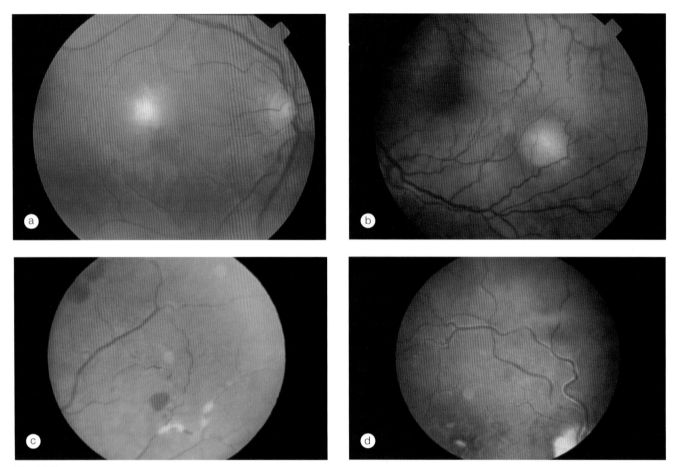

Fig. 14.9
Signs of posterior uveitis. **(a)** Retinitis; **(b)** choroiditis; **(c)** active vasculitis; **(d)** old vasculitis

2. **To break down recently formed posterior synechiae** with intensive topical mydriatics (atropine, phenylephrine) or subconjunctival injections of mydricaine (adrenaline, atropine and procaine) in eyes that do not respond to drops. A subconjunctival injection (0.5ml) of mydricaine is divided into the four quadrants for maximal effect by pulling from all directions. A good alternative to injections is to insert cotton pledget soaked in Mydricaine into the superior and inferior fornices for 5 minutes.

   NB Tissue plasminogen activator (12.5µg in 0.05ml) injected into the anterior chamber (intracamerally) with a 25-gauge needle will dissolve fibrinous exudate and help break down persistent posterior synechiae.

3. **To prevent formation of posterior synechiae** following control of acute inflammation by using a short-acting mydriatic that allows some mobility of the pupil and prevents synechiae in the dilated position. In mild chronic anterior uveitis, the mydriatic can be instilled once at bedtime to prevent difficulties with accommodation during the day. Moreover, the pupil should not be kept constantly dilated because posterior synechiae can still form in the dilated position. In young children, constant uniocular atropinization may induce amblyopia.

NB Subconjunctival Mydricaine may induce tachycardia and hypertension and should be used with caution in patients with cardiovascular disease.

Topical steroids

Topical steroids are useful only for anterior uveitis because therapeutic levels are not reached behind the lens. A solution penetrates the cornea better than a suspension or ointment. Because ointment causes blurring of vision it is usually instilled at bedtime. The frequency of instillation of drops depends on the severity of inflammation.

NB If a suspension is used (e.g. Pred Forte) the patient must be instructed to shake the bottle vigorously before use since the active component of the preparation will settle at the bottom of the bottle and exert no effect.

Indications

1. **Treatment of AAU** is relatively straightforward and depends on the severity of inflammation.
   - Initial intensive therapy involves instillation either hourly or every minute for the first 5 minutes of every hour.
   - Once the inflammation is well controlled the frequency should be carefully tapered to 2-hourly, followed by 3-hourly, then four times a day and eventually reduced by one drop a week. The drops are usually discontinued altogether by 5–6 weeks.
2. **Treatment of CAU** is more difficult because the inflammation may last for months and even years so that long-term steroids are often required with the risk of complications such as cataract and steroid-induced elevation of intraocular pressure.
   - Weak steroid preparations, such as rimexolone or loteprednol etabonate, may be attempted, particularly in steroid-reactors, as they have much lesser propensity for elevation of intraocular pressure, but they are less effective in controlling the inflammation.
   - It may be difficult to discontinue therapy since exacerbations are common.
   - Exacerbations are initially treated in the same way as AAU. If the inflammation is controlled with no more than +1 aqueous cells, the rate of instillation can be gradually further reduced by one drop/month.
   - The classic teaching that only cellular reaction in the anterior chamber represents active inflammation has been challenged. Flare is caused by chronic breakdown of the blood–aqueous barrier, but the intensity of the flare can also indicate an active process, which may respond to therapy. In this regard, the use of the Kowa Flare Meter represents an improvement in the monitoring of these patients. The measurement of the flare gives a direct quantification of the integrity of the blood–aqueous barrier. Unfortunately this machine is not available in most centres so that monitoring is based on clinical assessment of cells and flare.

NB Following cessation of treatment, the patient should be re-examined within a short time to ensure that the uveitis has not recurred.

Complications

1. **Elevation of intraocular pressure** (IOP) is common in susceptible individuals (steroid-reactors), but long-term exposure to topical steroids may eventually result in ocular hypertension in many patients.
2. **Cataract** can be induced by both systemic and, less frequently, topical steroid administration. The risk increases with dose and duration of therapy.
3. **Corneal** complications, which are uncommon, include secondary infection with bacteria and fungi, recrudescence of herpes simplex keratitis, and corneal melting, which may be enhanced by inhibition of collagen synthesis.
4. **Systemic** side-effects are rare, but may occasionally occur following prolonged administration, particularly in children.

Periocular steroids

1. **Advantages over topical administration**
   - Therapeutic concentrations behind the lens may be achieved.
   - Water soluble drugs, incapable of penetrating the cornea when given topically, can enter the eye transsclerally when given by periocular injection.
   - A prolonged effect can be achieved with long-acting preparations such as triamcinolone acetonide (Kenalog) or depot steroids such as methylprednisolone acetate (Depomedrone).
2. **Indications**
   - In unilateral or asymmetrical intermediate or posterior uveitis, periocular injections should be considered as first-line therapy to control inflammation and CMO.
   - In bilateral posterior uveitis either to supplement systemic therapy or when systemic steroids are contraindicated.
   - Poor compliance with topical or systemic medication.
   - At the time of surgery in eyes with uveitis.
3. **Complications**
   - Globe penetration.
   - Elevation of IOP.
   - Ptosis.
   - Subdermal fat atrophy.
   - Extraocular muscle paresis.
   - Optic nerve injury.
   - Retinal and choroidal vascular occlusion.
   - Cutaneous hypopigmentation.
4. **Technique**
   a. Conjunctival anaesthesia
   - A topical anaesthetic such as amethocaine is instilled.
   - A small cotton pledget impregnated with amethocaine (or equivalent) is placed into the superior fornix at the site of injection for 2 minutes.
   b. Posterior sub-Tenon injection
   - The vial containing the steroid is shaken.
   - 1.5ml steroid is drawn up into a 2-ml syringe and the drawing-up needle replaced with a 25-gauge 5/8 inch (16mm).

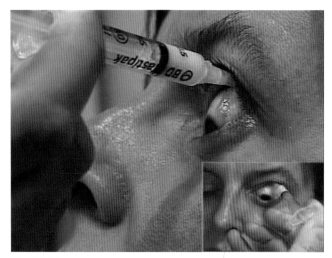

Fig. 14.10
Posterior sub-Tenon steroid injection (Courtesy of C Pavesio)

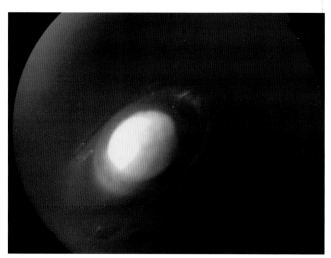

Fig. 14.11
Slow-release steroid implant (Courtesy of C Pavesio)

- The patient is asked to look away from the site of injection; most frequently inferiorly when the injection is being given supero-temporally.
- The bulbar conjunctiva is penetrated with the tip of the needle, bevel towards the globe, slightly on the bulbar side of the fornix.
- The needle is slowly inserted posteriorly, following the contour of the globe, keeping it as close to the globe as possible. In order not to penetrate the globe accidentally, wide side-to-side motions are made as the needle is being inserted and the limbus watched; movement of the limbus means that the sclera has been engaged!
- When the needle has been advanced to the hub and cannot be inserted any further (Fig. 14.10), the plunger is slightly withdrawn and, if no blood has entered the syringe, 1ml is injected. If the needle is too far away from the globe, adequate trans-scleral absorption of steroid will not occur.

Intraocular steroids

1. Injection
- Triamcinolone acetonide (4mg in 0.1ml) is an option in the treatment of uveitis and CMO unresponsive to other forms of therapy.
- It produces fast resolution of CMO lasting about 4 months and may be used to determine reversibility of visual loss due to CMO.
- Injections may be used following surgery on eyes with uveitis when other forms of prophylaxis are not appropriate.
- Repeated injections should be considered with caution due to significant risk of complications, especially high IOP.

- Other complications include cataract, endophthalmitis (sterile or infectious), hemorrhage and retinal detachment.

2. Slow-release implants appear to be useful in patients with posterior uveitis who do not respond to or are intolerant to conventional treatment.
- The implant, containing an insoluble steroid (fluocinolone acetonide), is implanted via a pars plana incision and sutured to the sclera (Fig. 14.11).
- The steroid is continuously released for 3 years and this may obviate the use of long-term systemic steroids.
- Complications are similar to those of intravitreal triamcinolone injection.

Systemic steroids

1. Preparations
   a. Oral prednisolone 5mg or 25mg tablets are the main preparations.
   b. Intravenous injection methylprednisolone 1g/day, repeated for 2–3 days is an option in severe bilateral disease but does not seem to offer any major advantages over high-dose oral therapy.

2. Indications
- Intermediate uveitis unresponsive to posterior sub-Tenon injections.
- Sight-threatening posterior or panuveitis, particularly with bilateral involvement.
- Rarely, anterior uveitis resistant to topical therapy.

3. Contraindications
- Poorly controlled diabetes is a relative contraindication.
- Peptic ulceration.
- Osteoporosis.
- Active systemic infection.
- Psychosis on previous exposure to steroids.

4. General rules of administration

- Start with a large dose and then reduce.
- The starting dose of prednisolone is 1–2mg/kg/day given in a single morning dose, after breakfast.
- A high level is maintained until a clinical effect is seen, followed by a slow taper over several weeks to avoid reactivation.
- Doses of 40mg or less for 3 weeks or less do not require gradual reduction.
- Doses of more than 15mg/day are unacceptable long-term so that the use of a steroid-sparing agent has to be considered.

NB A common cause of failure of treatment is suboptimal dosage.

5. Side-effects depend on the duration and dose of administration.

- *a.* **Short-term** therapy may cause dyspepsia, mental changes, electrolyte imbalance, aseptic necrosis of the head of the femur and, very rarely, hyperosmolar hyperglycaemic non-ketotic coma.
- *b.* **Long-term** therapy may cause a Cushingoid state, osteoporosis, limitation of growth in children, reactivation of infections such as TB, cataract and exacerbation of pre-existing conditions such as diabetes and myopathy.

NB Occasionally systemic steroids may cause severe ocular hypertension in children, even when administered only for several days.

Antimetabolites

Indications

1. **Sight-threatening uveitis,** which is usually bilateral, non-infectious, reversible and has failed to respond to adequate steroid therapy.
2. **Steroid-sparing therapy** in patients with intolerable side-effects from systemic steroids. Once a patient has been started on an immunosuppressive drug and the appropriate dose ascertained, treatment should continue for 6–24 months, after which gradual tapering and discontinuation of medication should be attempted over the next 3–12 months. However, some patients may require long-term therapy for control of disease activity.

Azathioprine

1. **Indications.** Onset of action takes several weeks but its effects persist after treatment has been discontinued. It is therefore a good option for long-term use in chronic diseases, particularly Behçet syndrome, but not for acute disease.

2. Regimen

- Starting dose is 1mg/kg/day (50mg tablets) administered once daily or in divided doses.
- After 1–2 weeks the dose is doubled.
- If appropriate control of inflammation is achieved the dose of other drugs (e.g. steroids, ciclosporin and tacrolimus) can be tapered.
- Azathioprine is stopped only after the disease has been inactive for over 1 year, ciclosporin or tacrolimus has been withdrawn and the daily steroid dose is under 7.5mg.
3. **Side-effects.** Bone marrow suppression and gastrointestinal upset and hepatotoxicity are the most important. They can be reversed by dose reduction or temporary withdrawal of the drug.
4. **Monitoring** involves a complete blood count, initially weekly and then every 4–6 weeks, and liver function tests every 12 weeks.

Methotrexate

1. **Indications** are mainly as a steroid-sparing agent in patients with uveitis associated with sarcoidosis and JIA.
2. **Regimen**
- Adult dose is 10–15mg/week.
- Children require a higher dose (up to 30mg/week) since the clearance of the drug is increased.
- Folic acid 2.5–5.0mg/day is administered to reduce bone marrow toxicity.
3. **Side-effects.** Bone marrow suppression, hepatotoxicity, acute pneumonitis (hypersensitivity reaction) are the most serious, but rarely occur with low-dose therapy.

NB Patients must be warned to abstain from alcohol.

4. **Monitoring** involves a full blood count and liver function tests every 1–2 months. Occasionally liver biopsies may be required in patients on long-term therapy.

Mycophenolate mofetil

1. **Indications.** A good alternative to azathioprine in unresponsive or intolerant patients but it is not recommended in children.
2. **Dose** is 1g b.d. which may be increased to 4g daily.
3. **Side-effects** include gastrointestinal disturbance and bone marrow suppression.
4. **Monitoring** involves a full blood count initially weekly for 4 weeks and then monthly.

Immune modulators

Ciclosporin

1. **Indications.** It is the drug of choice for Behçet syndrome, and may also be used in intermediate uveitis, birdshot

retinochoroidopathy, Vogt–Koyanagi–Harada syndrome, sympathetic ophthalmitis and idiopathic retinal vasculitis.

2. **Regimen**
   - Initial dose is 5mg/kg/day either as a single daily dose or in two divided doses to avoid serum spikes and renal toxicity.
   - Following control of the inflammation the dose should be tapered to 2–3mg/kg/day.
   - Ciclosporin should not be stopped abruptly because rebound of inflammation may occur.
3. **Side-effects** include nephrotoxicity, hyperlipidaemia, hepatotoxicity, hypertension, hirsutism and gingival hyperplasia. Poorly controlled hypertension and renal disease are relative contraindications. The drug should also be used with caution in patients over 55 years of age because of less renal reserve.
4. **Monitoring** involves blood pressure, and renal and liver function tests every 6 weeks. Serum creatinine level should not be permitted to rise 30% over baseline.

Tacrolimus

1. **Indications.** An alternative to ciclosporin in intolerant or unresponsive patients.
2. **Dose.** Maximal is 0.1–0.15mg/kg which should be introduced gradually.
3. **Side-effects** include hyperglycaemia, neurotoxicity and nephrotoxicity which are more common than with ciclosporin.
4. **Monitoring** involves blood pressure, renal function tests and blood glucose, initially weekly and then less frequently.

Biological blockers

Biological blockers are used principally for organ transplantation. They have not been licensed for the treatment of ocular inflammatory conditions but clinical trials are currently in progress.

1. **IL-2 receptor antagonists.** Daclizumab (Zenapax) may be useful to treat uveitis.
2. **Anti-tumour necrosis factor (TNF) alpha therapy**
   a. **Infliximab** (Remicade) shows promise in patients with predominant retinal vasculitis and vitritis, as in Behçet syndrome, especially when resistant to conventional treatment. It is given as intravenous infusions every 8 weeks in a maintenance phase.
   b. **Adalimumab** is similar to infliximab but is administered subcutaneously weekly or every other week.

NB The clinical experience with these agents is very limited and there is concern regarding aggravating tuberculosis and induction of demyelinating disease. The cost is still very high and the long-term effects on the immune system unknown.

INTERMEDIATE UVEITIS

Intermediate uveitis (IU) is an insidious, chronic, relapsing disease in which the vitreous is the major site of the inflammation. The condition may be idiopathic or associated with a systemic disease (see below). Pars planitis (PP) is a subset of idiopathic IU in which there is snowbanking or snowball formation. It occurs more commonly in children while other forms of IU occur in an older age group (25–35 years), reflecting an increase in systemic associations. Disease starting before the age of 10 years tends to be more aggressive, whilst that starting later in life tends to be less severe. IU accounts for up to 15% of all uveitis cases and about 20% of paediatric uveitis. The diagnosis is essentially clinical, and investigations are carried out to exclude a systemic association, especially in the presence of suggestive findings and in older individuals.

NB The exact age of onset of IU may be difficult to determine, since a long time may go by before patients become symptomatic.

Symptoms

Presentation is with an insidious onset of blurred vision often accompanied by vitreous floaters. The initial symptoms are usually unilateral, but the condition is typically bilateral and often asymmetrical, so that only careful examination of the apparently normal eye may reveal minor abnormalities of the peripheral retina, such as vascular sheathing or localized vitreous condensations.

Signs

1. **Anterior uveitis**
   - In PP anterior uveitis is mild with small scattered KP which occasionally have a linear distribution in the inferior cornea and are associated with epithelial oedema (endotheliopathy).
   - In the other forms of IU, anterior uveitis can be severe, especially in patients with MS, sarcoidosis and Lyme disease.
2. **Vitreous**
   - Vitreous cells with anterior predominance are universal (Fig. 14.12a).
   - Vitreous condensation (Fig. 14.12b).
   - 'Snowballs' often most numerous inferiorly (Fig. 14.12c).
3. **Posterior segment**
   - Peripheral periphlebitis and perivascular sheathing are common, particularly in patients with MS (Fig. 14.13a).
   - 'Snowbanking' is characterized by a grey-white fibrovascular plaque which may occur in all quadrants, but is most frequently found inferiorly (Fig. 14.13b).

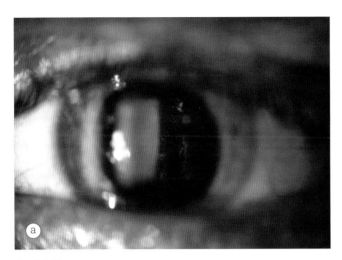
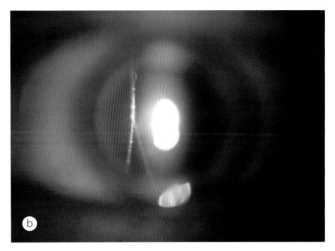

Fig. 14.12
Vitreous signs of intermediate uveitis. **(a)** Mild vitritis; **(b)** vitreous condensations; **(c)** severe vitritis and 'snowballs'

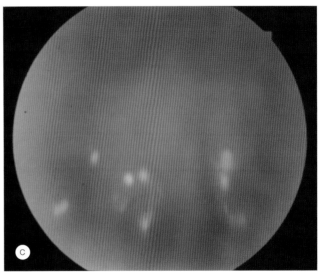

- Neovascularization may occur on the snowbank (Fig. 14.13c) or the optic nerve head; the latter usually resolves when inflammatory activity is controlled.
- Subtle disc oedema may be seen in young patients.

Course

- A minority of patients have a benign course, which may not require treatment, with spontaneous resolution within several years.
- In other patients the disease is more severe and prolonged with episodes of exacerbations that tend to become progressively worse. 'Snowbanking' is a common finding which is associated with CMO and visual loss.
- IU associated with systemic diseases has a variable course depending on the disease and its severity.
- The inflammation may last as long as 15 years and preservation of vision will depend on control of macular disease. In short follow-up of up to 4 years up to 75% of the patients have a visual acuity of 6/12 or better.

Complications

- CMO occurs in 30% of cases and is the major cause of impaired visual acuity.
- Macular epiretinal formation is common.
- Cataract and glaucoma may occur in eyes with prolonged inflammation, particularly if requiring long-term steroid therapy.
- Peripheral retinal vasoproliferative tumours are uncommon.
- Retinal detachment is uncommon, but may occur in advanced cases. The detachment may be tractional (Fig. 14.13c), rhegmatogenous and occasionally exudative; retinoschisis has also been described.

- Vitreous haemorrhage may occur from the snowbank or disc new vessels, particularly in children.

Treatment

1. **Medical therapy.** The most common reason to initiate therapy is reduction of vision due to CMO. Initial treatment involves posterior sub-Tenon injections of triamcinolone. Further options in unresponsive cases include systemic steroids and immunosuppressive agents. IU associated with multiple sclerosis (see below) may benefit from treatment with interferon beta.
2. **Vitrectomy** may be beneficial for CMO as well as the inflammatory process itself. It may therefore be considered following failure of systemic steroids to control CMO but prior to the use of immunosuppressive agents. Other indications for vitrectomy include tractional retinal detachment, severe vitreous opacification, non-resolving vitreous haemorrhage and epiretinal membranes.

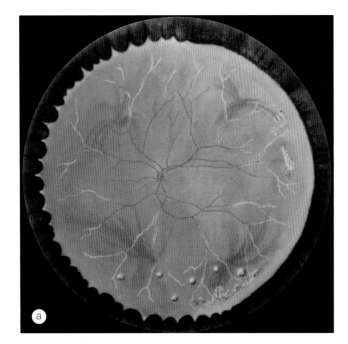

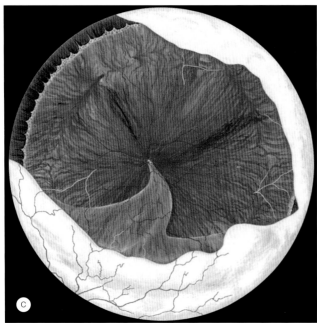

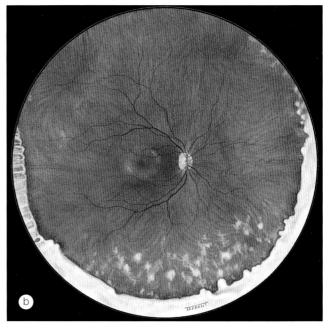

Fig. 14.13
Posterior segment signs in intermediate uveitis. **(a)** Peripheral periphlebitis and a few snowballs inferiorly; **(b)** inferior snowbanking and snowballs; **(c)** severe snowbanking, neovascularization and inferior retinal detachment (Courtesy of C L Schepens, M E Hartnett and T Hirose, from *Schepens' Retinal Detachment and Allied Diseases*, Butterworth-Heinemann, 2000 – figs a and c)

Systemic associations

1. **Multiple sclerosis** associated IU may precede or antedate the diagnosis demyelination. MS should be suspected in females in the third to fifth decades, especially if they are carriers of HLA-DR15 (a suballele of HLA-DR2).

   NB Other causes of neurological concomitants of uveitis include: Vogt–Koyanagi–Harada syndrome, sarcoidosis, Behçet syndrome, AIDS, primary central nervous system lymphoma, herpes virus infections, syphilis, acute posterior multifocal placoid pigment epitheliopathy and Whipple disease.

2. **Sarcoidosis** associated IU is relatively uncommon and may antedate the onset of systemic disease. The presence of associated granulomatous anterior uveitis should arouse suspicion.

3. **Lyme disease** associated IU also often manifests severe anterior uveitis. Visits to endemic areas and a history of a tick bite should be elicited, and confirmed by serology.

3. **Cryotherapy** is currently seldom used but may be considered for peripheral exudative retinal detachments associated with telangiectatic vessels and vasoproliferative tumours.

4. **Laser photocoagulation** of the peripheral retina is useful in eyes with neovascularization of the vitreous base.

4. **HTLV-I infection** associated may be associated with extensive periphlebitis but CMO is rare.

Differential diagnosis

Chronic conditions which produce vitritis, or peripheral retinal changes mimicking IU include the following:

1. **Fuchs uveitis syndrome** may be associated with severe vitreous inflammation but it is usually unilateral, not associated with CMO and manifests characteristic anterior segment findings.
2. **Primary intraocular lymphoma** may also present with vitritis but the infiltrate is more homogeneous and snowballs are absent.
3. **A peripheral toxocara granuloma** may resemble snowbanking and be associated with mild vitritis but is invariably unilateral.
4. **Other conditions**
   - Amyloidosis may produce vitritis without vasculitis or CMO.
   - Whipple disease may be associated with vitritis without snowballs.

UVEITIS IN SPONDYLOARTHROPATHIES

HLA-B27 and spondyloarthropathies

The prevalence of HLA B-27 is as follows:
- 6–8% of the Caucasian population of the USA.
- 50% of patients with AAU who are otherwise fit and well.
- 90% of patients with AAU who have an associated spondyloarthropathy.

The AAU associated with HLA-B27 is typically unilateral, severe, recurrent and associated with a higher incidence of posterior synechiae. A fibrinous exudate in the anterior chamber is common. Patients who do not carry HLA-B27 tend to have a more benign course with fewer recurrences.

Ankylosing spondylitis

Ankylosing spondylitis (AS) is characterized by inflammation, calcification and finally ossification of ligaments and capsules of joints with resultant bony ankylosis of the axial skeleton. It typically affects males, of whom about 95% are HLA-B27 positive (see Chapter 24).

1. **AAU** occurs in about 25% of patients with AS; conversely, 25% of males with AAU will have AS. Either eye is frequently affected at different times but bilateral simultaneous involvement is rare. There is no correlation between the severity and activity of eye and joint involvement. In a few patients with many recurrent attacks the inflammation may eventually become chronic.
2. **Other** uncommon manifestations include scleritis and conjunctivitis.

Reiter syndrome

Reiter syndrome (RS), also referred to as reactive arthritis, is characterized by the triad of non-specific (non-gonococcal) urethritis, conjunctivitis and arthritis. About 85% of patients with RS are positive for HLA-B27 but the diagnosis is clinical and based on the presence of arthritis and other characteristic manifestations (see Chapter 24).

1. **AAU** occurs in up to 12% of patients. The prevalence is, however, higher in carriers of HLA-B27.
2. **Conjunctivitis** is very common and usually follows the urethritis by about 2 weeks and precedes the arthritis. The inflammation is usually mild, bilateral and mucopurulent with a papillary or follicular reaction. Spontaneous resolution occurs within 7–10 days and treatment is not required. Cultures for bacteria are usually negative.
3. **Other** uncommon manifestations include nummular keratitis, scleritis, episcleritis, intermediate uveitis, papillitis, retinal oedema and retinal vasculitis.

Psoriatic arthritis

About 7% of patients with psoriasis develop arthritis. Psoriatic arthritis affects both sexes equally and is associated with an increased prevalence of HLA-B27 and HLA-B17 (see Chapter 24).

1. **AAU** occurs in approximately 7% of patients and it has also been suggested that patients with psoriasis alone may be predisposed to anterior uveitis.
2. **Other** manifestations include conjunctivitis, keratitis in the form of raised, marginal, corneal infiltrates, and secondary Sjögren syndrome.

UVEITIS IN JUVENILE ARTHRITIS

Juvenile idiopathic arthritis

JIA is an inflammatory arthritis of at least 6 week's duration occurring before the age of 16 years (see Chapter 24). It is by far the most common disease associated with childhood anterior uveitis.

Classification

Classification of JIA is based on the onset and the extent of joint involvement during the first 6 months as follows:

1. **Pauciarticular onset** JIA affects four or fewer joints, commonly the knees (Fig. 14.14), and accounts for about 60% of cases. Uveitis affects about 20% of children. Risk factors for uveitis are early-onset of JIA, and positive findings for ANA and HLA-DR5.
2. **Polyarticular onset** JIA affects five or more joints and accounts for a further 20% of cases. Uveitis occurs in about 5% of cases.
3. **Systemic onset** JIA accounts for about 20% of cases but is not associated with uveitis.

   NB The term 'Still disease' is reserved for patients with systemic onset disease.

Anterior uveitis

In the vast majority of patients arthritis antedates the diagnosis of uveitis, although rarely ocular involvement may precede joint disease by several years. The intraocular inflammation is chronic, non-granulomatous, and bilateral in 70% of cases. It is unusual for unilateral uveitis to become bilateral after more than a year. When bilateral, the severity of inflammation is usually symmetrical.

NB There is no correlation between the activity of joint and eye inflammation.

1. **Presentation** is invariably asymptomatic; the uveitis is frequently detected on routine slit-lamp examination. Even during acute exacerbations with +4 aqueous cells, it is rare for patients to complain, although a few report an increase in vitreous floaters.

   NB Often uveitis may not be suspected until the parents recognize complications such as strabismus, or an abnormal appearance of the eye due to band keratopathy or cataract.

2. **Signs**
   - Uninjected eye even in the presence of severe uveitis.
   - Small to medium size KP.
   - During acute exacerbations, the entire endothelium shows 'dusting' by many hundreds of cells, but hypopyon is absent.
   - Posterior synechiae are common in long-standing undetected uveitis.

   NB Not all children with chronic anterior uveitis have or will develop JIA.

3. **Prognosis**
   - In about 10% of cases the uveitis is mild, with never more than +1 aqueous cells and persists for less than 12 months.
   - About 15% of patients have one attack, which lasts less than 4 months, the severity of inflammation varying from +2 to +4 aqueous cells.
   - In 50% of cases, the uveitis is moderate to severe and persists for more than 4 months.
   - In 25% of cases, the uveitis is very severe, lasts for several years and responds poorly to treatment. In this subgroup, band keratopathy (Fig. 14.15) occurs in 40% of patients, cataract in 30% and secondary glaucoma in 15%.

   NB The presence of complications at initial examination appears to be an important risk factor for a poor prognosis, regardless of therapy.

4. **Treatment** with topical steroids is usually effective; acute exacerbations require very frequent instillations. Poor responders to topical administration may benefit

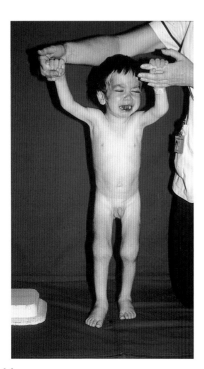

Fig. 14.14
Involvement of the knees in pauciarticular onset juvenile idiopathic arthritis

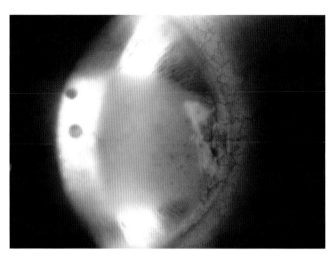

Fig. 14.15
Band keratopathy in chronic anterior uveitis associated with juvenile idiopathic arthritis

from periocular injections. Low-dose methotrexate is useful for steroid resistance.

5. **Screening.** Because the onset of intraocular inflammation is invariably asymptomatic, it is extremely important to regularly screen children at risk for at least 7 years from the onset of arthritis or until the age of 12 years. The frequency of slit-lamp examination is governed by the following risk factors:
   - Systemic onset = not required.
   - Polyarticular onset = every 9 months
   - Polyarticular onset + ANA = every 6 months
   - Pauciarticular onset = every 3 months
   - Pauciarticular onset + ANA = every 2 months.

Differential diagnosis

1. **Idiopathic juvenile chronic iridocyclitis.** Whilst JIA is the most common systemic association of CAU in children, many patients with juvenile CAU are otherwise healthy. The majority of patients are female. As the onset of intraocular inflammation is frequently insidious and asymptomatic, most cases are not diagnosed until visual acuity is reduced from complicated cataract or the parents notice a white patch on the cornea caused by band keratopathy. In a small number of cases the uveitis is detected by chance.
2. **Other types of juvenile arthritis and uveitis**
   a. *Juvenile ankylosing spondylitis* is uncommon and typically affects boys around the age of 10 years. Early diagnosis may be difficult, because in children the disease frequently presents with peripheral lower limb arthritis and radiological evaluation of the sacro-iliac

joints is usually not helpful during the early stages. Just like adults, some children develop AAU.
   b. *Juvenile Reiter syndrome* is very rare and is invariably post-dysenteric. A few cases of AAU have been reported.
   c. *Juvenile psoriatic arthritis* is relatively uncommon and is characterized by asymmetrical involvement of both large and small joints in association with skin lesions and nail pitting. Chronic anterior uveitis is uncommon.
   d. *Juvenile bowel-associated arthritis* is rare. Joint involvement is usually mild and affects large joints in association with either ulcerative colitis or Crohn disease. Anterior uveitis, which may be acute or chronic, has been reported in a few patients.
3. **Juvenile sarcoidosis** is rare and less frequently associated with pulmonary involvement than in adults, and typically manifests with skin, joint and eye disease. Chest radiographs are therefore of less diagnostic value in children with sarcoidosis. Serum angiotensin-converting enzyme may also be misleading because children have higher normal values than adults. When uveitis is confined to the anterior segment it can be confused with JIA-associated uveitis. Unlike JIA-associated uveitis, however, it may also be granulomatous and also involve the posterior segment.
4. **Lyme disease** usually presents with intermediate uveitis with significant anterior uveitis, in contrast with pars planitis where anterior uveitis is insignificant.
5. **Neonatal-onset multisystem inflammatory disease** is a rare, idiopathic, chronic relapsing disease that predominantly involves the skin, joints and the central nervous system. About 50% of children develop recurrent anterior uveitis. The absence of posterior synechiae and no tendency to glaucoma and cataract formation are characteristic.

Familial juvenile systemic granulomatosis syndrome

Familial juvenile systemic granulomatosis (Blau syndrome, Jabs disease), is a rare AD disorder characterized by childhood onset of granulomatous disease of skin, eyes and joints. It is associated with CARD15/Nod2 mutation.

1. **Systemic features,** which develop in the first decade of life, include painful cystic joint swelling which may progress to flexion contractures (camptodactyly), and an intermittent perioral rash.
2. **Ocular manifestations** include panuveitis and multifocal choroiditis. Complications include cataract, band keratopathy and CMO.
3. **Differential diagnosis** includes sarcoidosis and JIA.

UVEITIS IN BOWEL DISEASE

Ulcerative colitis

Ulcerative colitis is an idiopathic, chronic, relapsing inflammatory disease, involving the rectum and extending proximally to involve part or all of the large intestine (see Chapter 24).

1. **AAU** occurs in about 5% of patients and may synchronize with exacerbation of colitis. As expected, uveitis is commoner in patients with associated AS.
2. **Other** manifestations include peripheral corneal infiltrates, conjunctivitis, episcleritis, scleritis and rarely posterior segment involvement in the form of papillitis, multifocal choroiditis and retinal vasculitis.

Crohn disease

Crohn disease (regional ileitis) is an idiopathic, chronic, relapsing disease characterized by multifocal, full-thickness, non-caseating granulomatous inflammation of the intestinal wall (see Chapter 24).

1. **AAU** occurs in about 3% of patients.
2. **Other** manifestations include conjunctivitis, episcleritis, peripheral corneal infiltrates and retinal periphlebitis.

Whipple disease

Whipple disease (intestinal lipodystrophy) is a rare, chronic, relapsing, bacterial infection with Gram-positive *Tropheryma whippelii* that primarily involves the gastrointestinal tract and its lymphatic drainage. It occurs mostly in white middle-aged men and is fatal if untreated. Extraintestinal manifestations may involve the CNS, lungs, heart, joints and eyes. Long-term antibiotic therapy is necessary (see Chapter 24).

1. **Secondary to CNS involvement** includes gaze palsy, nystagmus, ophthalmoplegia, papilloedema and optic atrophy.
2. **Intraocular inflammation** in the form of vitritis, retinitis, retinal haemorrhages and cotton-wool spots, and multifocal choroiditis may occur with or without concomitant CNS disease.

UVEITIS IN RENAL DISEASE

Tubulointerstitial nephritis

Tubulointerstitial nephritis and uveitis (TINU) is an uncommon oculo-renal disorder of immune origin characterized by a combination of idiopathic acute tubulointerstitial nephritis and uveitis. It typically occurs in adolescent girls. Renal disease usually precedes uveitis.

1. **Presentation** is with constitutional symptoms, proteinuria, anaemia, hypertension and renal failure. The response to systemic steroid therapy is good and the condition resolves within a few months.
2. **Uveitis** is usually anterior, bilateral, non-granulomatous and responds well to steroids. Some cases become chronic and relapsing and may require immunosuppressive therapy. Intermediate uveitis, posterior uveitis and disc oedema may also occur.

IgA glomerulonephritis

IgA glomerulonephritis is a common disease in which IgA is found in the glomerular mesangium.

1. **Presentation** is usually in the third to fifth decades with recurrent macroscopic haematuria which may be associated with upper respiratory tract infection.
2. **Ocular manifestations,** which are uncommon, include anterior uveitis, keratoconjunctivitis and scleritis.

SARCOIDOSIS

Sarcoidosis is a T-lymphocyte-mediated non-caseating granulomatous inflammatory disorder of unknown cause. The clinical spectrum of disease varies from mild single-organ involvement to potentially fatal multisystem disease which can affect almost any tissue (see Chapter 24).

Signs

1. **AAU** typically affects patients with acute-onset sarcoid and responds well to topical steroids.
2. **Granulomatous CAU** (Fig. 14.16) tends to affect older patients with chronic pulmonary disease. Treatment is more difficult than for acute anterior uveitis; periocular and systemic steroids may be required.
3. **Intermediate uveitis** is uncommon and may antedate the onset of systemic disease. The presence of associated granulomatous anterior uveitis should arouse suspicion.
4. **Periphlebitis**
   - Yellowish or grey-white perivenous sheathing (Fig. 14.17a).
   - Occlusive periphlebitis is uncommon (Fig. 14.17b).
   - Perivenous exudates referred to as 'candle wax drippings' (*en taches de bougie*) are typical of severe involvement (Fig. 14.17c).
5. **Choroidal infiltrates** are uncommon and vary in appearance:

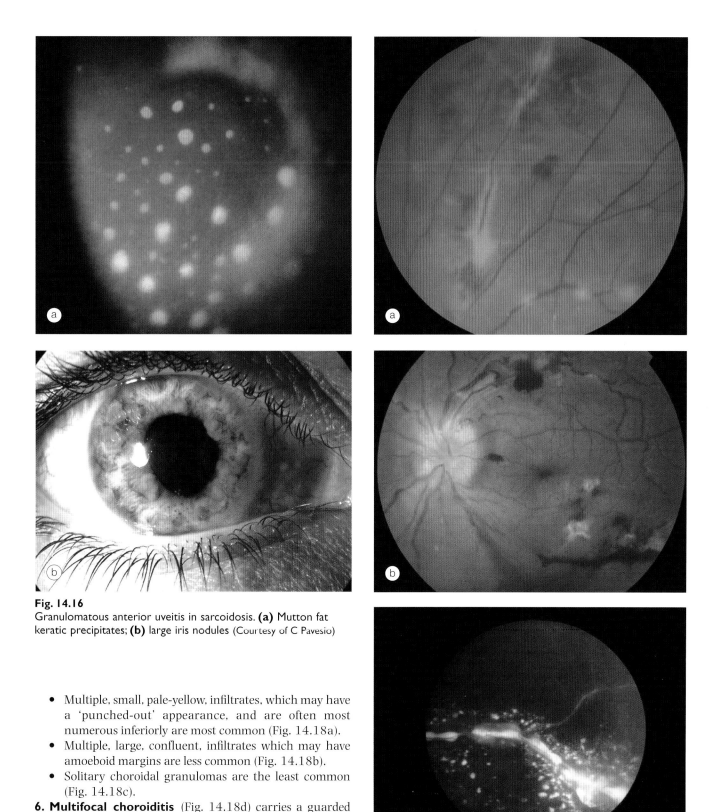

Fig. 14.16
Granulomatous anterior uveitis in sarcoidosis. **(a)** Mutton fat keratic precipitates; **(b)** large iris nodules (Courtesy of C Pavesio)

- Multiple, small, pale-yellow, infiltrates, which may have a 'punched-out' appearance, and are often most numerous inferiorly are most common (Fig. 14.18a).
- Multiple, large, confluent, infiltrates which may have amoeboid margins are less common (Fig. 14.18b).
- Solitary choroidal granulomas are the least common (Fig. 14.18c).

6. **Multifocal choroiditis** (Fig. 14.18d) carries a guarded visual prognosis because it may cause loss of central vision as a result of secondary CNV, which may be peripapillary or associated with a chorioretinal scar.

7. **Retinal granulomas** are small, discrete, yellow lesions (Fig. 14.18e).

Fig. 14.17
Periphlebitis in sarcoidosis. **(a)** Mild; **(b)** occlusive with disc oedema; **(c)** 'candle wax drippings' (Courtesy of C Barry – fig. a; C Pavesio – fig. b; P Morse – fig. c)

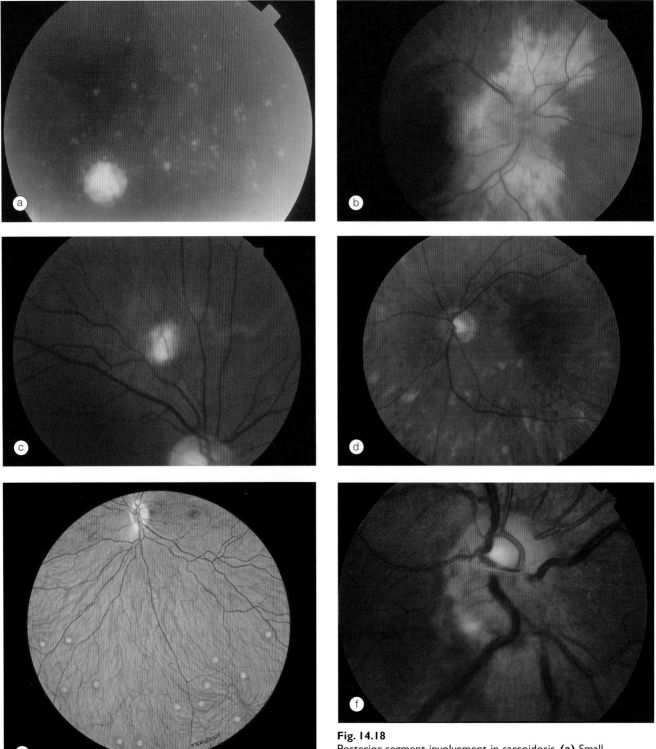

Fig. 14.18
Posterior segment involvement in sarcoidosis. **(a)** Small peripheral choroidal granulomas; **(b)** confluent choroidal infiltrates; **(c)** solitary choroidal granuloma; **(d)** multifocal choroiditis; **(e)** multiple small retinal granulomas; **(f)** disc granuloma

8. **Peripheral retinal neovascularization** may develop secondary to retinal capillary dropout. In black patients it may be mistaken for proliferative sickle-cell retinopathy.
9. **Optic nerve** involvement may take the following forms:
   - Focal granulomas, which do not usually affect vision (Fig. 14.18f).
   - Papilloedema due to CNS involvement may occur in the absence of other ocular manifestations.
   - Persistent disc oedema is a frequent finding in patients with retinal or vitreous involvement.

Treatment

Treatment of vision-threatening posterior segment disease may be with posterior sub-Tenon steroid injections or systemic steroids. Rarely ciclosporin or methotrexate is required.

Differential diagnosis of posterior segment sarcoid

1. **Small choroidal lesions**
   - Multifocal choroiditis with panuveitis.
   - Birdshot chorioretinopathy.
   - Tuberculosis.
2. **Large choroidal infiltrates**
   - Metastatic tumour.
   - Large cell lymphoma.
   - Harada disease.
   - Serpiginous choroidopathy.
3. **Periphlebitis**
   - Tuberculosis.
   - Behçet syndrome.
   - Cytomegalovirus retinitis.

BEHÇET SYNDROME

Behçet syndrome (BS) is an idiopathic, multisystem disease characterized by recurrent episodes of orogenital ulceration and vasculitis which may involve small, medium and large veins and arteries (see Chapter 24). Ocular complications occur in up to 95% of men and 70% of women. Eye disease typically occurs within 2 years of oral ulceration, but rarely the delay may be as long as 14 years. Conversely, intraocular inflammation is the presenting manifestation in about 10% of cases. It is unusual for the systemic and ocular manifestations to develop simultaneously. Ocular disease is usually bilateral and only in 6% does it remain uniocular.

Special tests

Pathergy test (increased dermal sensitivity to needle trauma) is a criterion for the diagnosis of BS, but the results vary and it is only rarely positive in the absence of systemic activity.

A positive response is the formation of a pustule following pricking of the skin with a needle (see Fig. 14.2c).

Signs

1. **Recurrent AAU,** which may be simultaneously bilateral and frequently associated with a transient mobile hypopyon in a relatively white eye (Fig. 14.19a), is often a mild manifestation when compared to posterior segment involvement and usually responds well to topical steroids.
2. **Retinal infiltrates** are white, superficial, necrotic, cellular lesions, which may be seen during the acute stage of the systemic disease (Fig. 14.19b); they heal without scarring.
3. **Retinal vasculitis** may involve both veins and arteries and result in occlusion (Fig. 14.19c).
4. **Vascular leakage** may give rise to diffuse retinal oedema, CMO and disc oedema.
5. **Vitritis,** which may be severe and persistent, is universal in eyes with active disease.
6. **Other manifestations,** which are uncommon, include conjunctivitis, conjunctival ulcers, episcleritis, scleritis, and ophthalmoplegia from neurological involvement.

Treatment of posterior uveitis

1. **Systemic steroids** may shorten the duration of an inflammatory episode but are not effective long-term so that an additional agent is usually required.
2. **Azathioprine** does not act fast enough in acute disease but is suitable for long-term therapy.
3. **Ciclosporin** is effective and rapidly acting but is associated with nephrotoxicity, particularly at doses higher than 5mg/kg/day; relapses after cessation often limit its use.
4. **Subcutaneous interferon alfa-2a** (6 million units daily) is very effective for mucocutaneous lesions and may also be used to treat ocular disease resistant to high-dose steroids. Side-effects are dose-dependent and include flu-like symptoms, hair loss, itching and depression.
5. **Biological agents** such as infliximab (Remicade) are currently undergoing clinical trials and show promise in treating retinal vasculitis.

Prognosis

The prognosis is guarded and about 20% of eyes become blind despite treatment. The end stage of posterior segment involvement is characterized by optic atrophy, vascular attenuation, chronic sheathing and variable chorioretinal scarring (Fig. 14.19d).

Differential diagnosis

In patients with suggestive ocular findings but lack of classical systemic manifestations the diagnosis becomes uncertain,

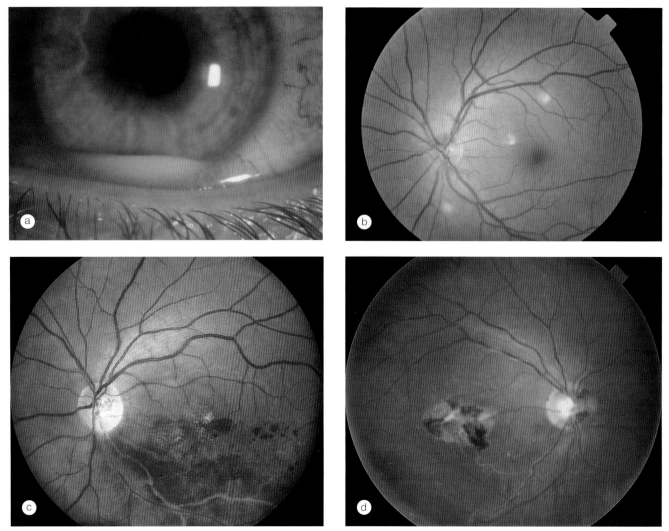

Fig. 14.19
Behçet syndrome. **(a)** Hypopyon in a white eye; **(b)** retinal infiltrates; **(c)** occlusive vasculitis; **(d)** end-stage (Courtesy of A Curi – fig. a; S Milewski – fig. b; A Dick – fig d.)

especially due to the lack of definitive laboratory tests. It is therefore important to consider the following conditions:

1. **Recurrent anterior uveitis with hypopyon** may occur in spondyloarthropathies. However, the uveitis is not usually simultaneously bilateral and the hypopyon is not mobile because it is frequently associated with a fibrinous exudate. In BS uveitis is frequently simultaneously bilateral and the hypopyon shifts with gravity as the patient changes head position.
2. **Retinal vasculitis** may be associated with sarcoidosis. However, sarcoid vasculitis involves only veins in a segmental manner and is rarely occlusive. In contrast, BS may affect both arteries and veins, is diffuse, frequently occlusive and is associated with vitritis, which is uncommon in sarcoid-related vasculitis.

3. **Retinal infiltrates** similar to those in BS may be seen in viral retinitis such as the acute retinal necrosis syndrome. However, in viral retinitis the infiltrates eventually coalesce. Multiple retinal infiltrates also occur in idiopathic acute multifocal retinitis.

VOGT–KOYANAGI–HARADA SYNDROME

Vogt–Koyanagi–Harada syndrome (V-K-H) is an idiopathic, multisystem, autoimmune disease against melanocytes causing inflammation of melanocyte-containing tissues such as the uvea, ears, skin and meninges (see Chapter 24).

Signs

1. **Anterior uveitis** is usually non-granulomatous during the acute phase but shows granulomatous features during recurrences which involve only the anterior segment.
2. **Posterior uveitis** occurs in patients with Harada disease and is frequently bilateral. In chronological order the findings are as follows:
   - Diffuse choroidal infiltration.
   - Multifocal detachments of the sensory retina and disc oedema (Fig. 14.20a).
   - Exudative retinal detachment.
   - The chronic phase is characterized by diffuse RPE atrophy (sunset-glow fundus) which may be associated with small, peripheral, discrete atrophic spots, often labeled Dalen–Fuchs nodules (Fig. 14.21a).
   - CNV and subretinal fibrosis (Fig. 14.21b) may be responsible for significant visual loss.

Investigations

1. **CSF analysis** shows pleocytosis with predominant small lymphocytes in about 80% of patients within 1 week and 97% within 3 weeks of disease onset.
2. **FA** shows multifocal hyperfluorescent dots at the level of the RPE and the accumulation of dye in the subretinal space (see Fig. 14.20b and c). The chronic phase shows areas of hyperfluorescence due to RPE window defects.
3. **ICG** demonstrates hypofluorescent dark spots which probably represent choroidal granulomas, delayed or patchy filling, indistinct choroidal vessels in the early phase and hyperfluorescence over the posterior pole in the late phase. ICG is useful in monitoring the evolution of the choroidal inflammation and the effect of therapy.
4. **US** may be helpful in cases of poor visualization of the fundus, and may show diffuse thickening of the posterior choroid, serous retinal detachment and vitreous opacities.

Treatment

Posterior segment involvement is treated with intravenous or high-dose oral steroids. Steroid-resistant patients may require ciclosporin. Eyes with subfoveal CNV may benefit from surgical excision or PDT.

NB The prognosis depends on early recognition and aggressive control of the early stages of the disease. Late diagnosis or incorrect initial therapy is more likely to be associated with a guarded prognosis with only 50% of patients having a final visual acuity better than 6/12.

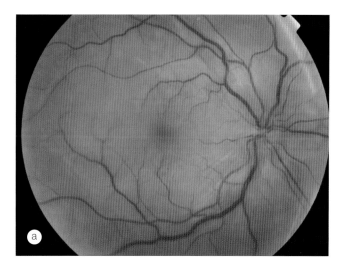
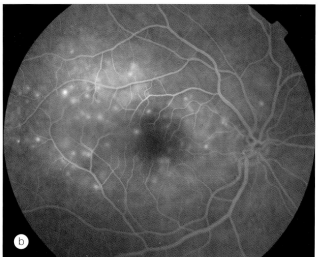
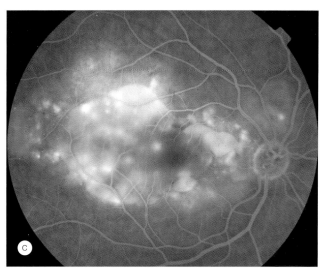

Fig. 14.20
Active Harada disease. **(a)** Multifocal serous retinal detachments; **(b)** FA venous shows multiple hyperfluorescent spots; **(c)** late phase shows extensive areas of hyperfluorescence due to pooling of dye under the serous detachments (Courtesy of Moorfields Eye Hospital)

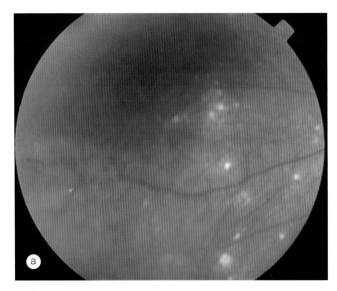

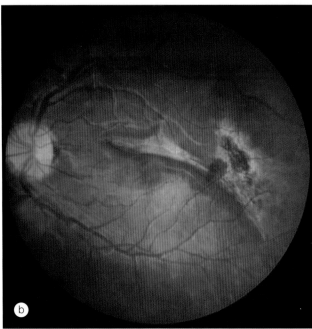

Fig. 14.21
Sequelae of Harada disease. **(a)** 'Sunset-glow' fundus with scattered depigmented spots; **(b)** subretinal fibrosis (Courtesy of C Pavesio)

Differential diagnosis of bilateral exudative retinal detachments

- Carcinoma metastatic to the choroid.
- Uveal effusion syndrome.
- Posterior scleritis.
- Eclampsia.
- Central serous retinopathy.

PARASITIC UVEITIS

Toxoplasma retinitis

Pathogenesis

Toxoplasma gondii, an obligate intracellular protozoan (see Chapter 24), is the most frequent cause of infectious retinitis in immunocompetent individuals. Although some cases may occur as a result of reactivation of prenatal infestation the vast majority are acquired postnatally. Recurrent episodes of inflammation are common and occur when the cysts rupture and release hundreds of tachyzoites into normal retinal cells. Recurrences usually take place between the ages of 10 and 35 years (average age 25 years). The scars from which recurrences arise may be the residua of previous congenital infestation or, more frequently, remote acquired involvement.

Diagnosis

The diagnosis of toxoplasma retinitis is based on a compatible fundus lesion and positive serology for toxoplasma antibodies. Any antibody titre is significant because in recurrent ocular toxoplasmosis no correlation exists between the titre and the activity of retinitis.

1. **Presentation** is with unilateral, sudden onset of floaters, visual loss and photophobia.
2. **Signs**
   - 'Spill-over' anterior uveitis, which may be granulomatous, is common.
   - Solitary inflammatory focus near an old pigmented scar ('satellite lesion' – Fig. 14.22a and b).
   - Multiple foci are uncommon (Fig. 14.22c).
   - Severe vitritis may greatly impair visualization of the fundus, although the inflammatory focus may still be discernible ('headlight in the fog' appearance) (Fig. 14.22d).
3. **Atypical features** that may occur in immunocompromised individuals are:
   - Extensive confluent areas of retinitis, which may be difficult to distinguish from a viral retinitis (Fig. 14.23a).
   - Inflammatory focus not associated with a pre-existing scar (Fig. 14.23b) implying that the infestation has been newly acquired and disseminated to the eye from extraocular sites.

Course

The rate of healing is dependent on the virulence of the organism, the competence of the host's immune system and especially the size of the lesion. In uncompromised hosts healing occurs within 6–8 weeks (Fig. 14.24a–c) although vitreous opacities take longer to resolve. The inflammatory focus is replaced by a sharply demarcated atrophic scar with

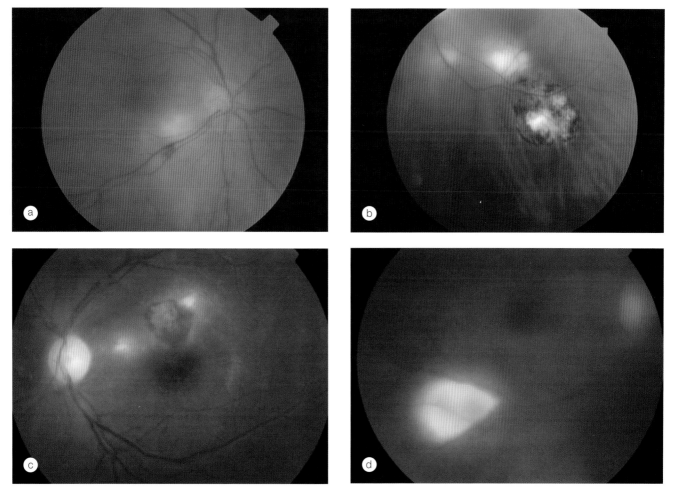

Fig. 14.22
Toxoplasma retinitis. **(a)** Small solitary focus; **(b)** larger solitary focus; **(c)** two small foci; **(d)** severe vitreous haze and 'headlight in the fog' appearance (Courtesy of C Pavesio – figs c and d)

a hyperpigmented border. Resolution of anterior uveitis is a reliable sign of posterior segment healing. After the first attack, the mean recurrence rate within 3 years is about 50% and the average number of recurrent attacks per patient is 2.7.

NB In elderly patients the course may be progressive and should be differentiated from viral retinitis and lymphoma.

Complications

Nearly 25% of eyes develop serious visual loss as a result of the following:
- Involvement of the macula (Fig. 14.25a).
- Secondary optic nerve head involvement due to juxtapapillary lesion (Fig. 14.25b).

- Primary optic nerve head involvement is rare and may mimic anterior ischaemic optic neuropathy (Fig. 14.25c).
- Occlusion of a major blood vessel by the inflammatory focus (Fig. 14.25d).

Treatment

1. Aims
- To reduce the duration and severity of acute inflammation.
- To lessen the risk of permanent visual loss by reducing the size of the eventual retinochoroidal scar.
- To reduce the risk of recurrences.

2. Indications. Unfortunately, there is lack of evidence that treatment with antibiotics achieves any of the above aims although adjunctive corticosteroids may diminish the duration and severity of inflammation. Despite these

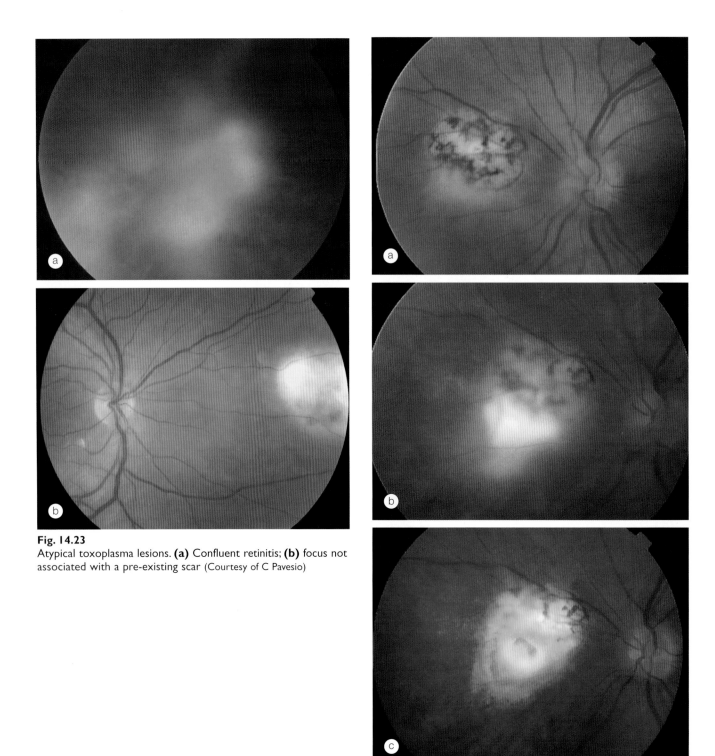

Fig. 14.23
Atypical toxoplasma lesions. **(a)** Confluent retinitis; **(b)** focus not associated with a pre-existing scar (Courtesy of C Pavesio)

Fig. 14.24
Progression of toxoplasma retinitis. **(a)** Mild fluffy haze adjacent to an old scar at presentation; **(b)** after 2 weeks the area of retinitis is larger and denser; **(c)** after 7 weeks the retinitis has nearly resolved

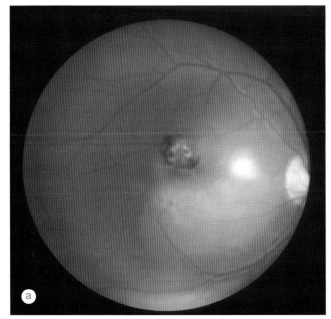

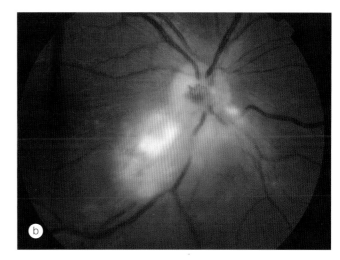

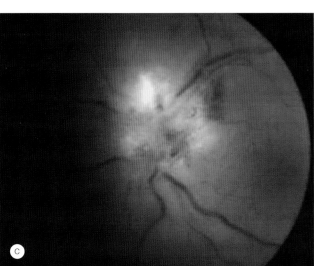

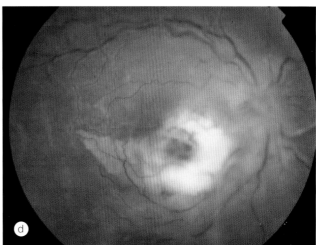

Fig. 14.25
Complications of toxoplasma retinitis. **(a)** Scar at the fovea and a fresh lesion involving the papillomacular bundle; **(b)** juxtapapillary lesion involving the optic nerve head; **(c)** primary optic nerve head involvement; **(d)** periarteritis resulting in branch retinal artery occlusion (Courtesy of C de A Garcia – fig. c; C Pavesio – fig. d)

reservations treatment may be considered for the following vision-threatening lesions:

- A lesion involving the macula, papillomacular bundle, optic nerve head or a major blood vessel.
- Very severe vitritis because of the risk of vitreous fibrosis and tractional retinal detachment.
- In immunocompromised patients all lesions should be treated irrespective of location or severity.

3. Regimen. There is no universally agreed therapeutic regimen and no evidence to support the specific form of treatment. Systemic prednisolone (1mg/kg) is given initially and tapered according to clinical response, but should always be used in conjunction with one or more of the following agents:

a. Clindamycin 300mg q.i.d. for 3–4 weeks. However, if used alone it may rarely cause a pseudomembranous colitis secondary to clostridial overgrowth. The risk of colitis is reduced when clindamycin is used together with a sulphonamide that inhibits clostridial overgrowth. Treatment of colitis is with oral vancomycin 500mg 6-hourly for 10 days.

b. Sulfadiazine 1g q.i.d. for 3–4 weeks is usually given in combination with pyrimethamine. Side-effects of sulphonamides include renal stones, allergic reactions and Stevens–Johnson syndrome.

c. Pyrimethamine (Daraprim) is administered as a loading dose of 50mg followed by 25–50mg daily for 4 weeks in combination with oral folinic acid 5mg (mixed with orange juice) three times a week to prevent thrombocytopenia, leucopenia and folate deficiency. Weekly blood counts should be performed. In AIDS pyrimethamine is avoided because of possible pre-existing bone marrow suppression and the antagonistic effect of zidovudine when the drugs are combined.

  d. Co-trimoxazole (Septrin) 960mg b.d. for 4–6 weeks may be used as monotherapy or in combination with clindamycin. Side-effects are similar to those of the sulphonamides.

  e. Atovaquone 750mg t.i.d. has been used mainly in the treatment of systemic pneumocystosis and toxoplasmosis in AIDS but it is also effective for toxoplasma retinitis in immunocompetent individuals. The drug is relatively free of serious side-effects but is expensive.

  f. Azithromycin 500mg daily is a good alternative to sulfadiazine and is as effective but less toxic.

Toxocariasis

Toxocariasis is caused by an infestation with a common intestinal ascarid (roundworm) of dogs called *Toxocara canis* (see Chapter 24). ELISA can be used to determine the level of serum antibodies to *T. canis*. When ocular toxocariasis is suspected, exact ELISA titres should be requested, including testing of undiluted serum. Any positive titre is consistent with, but not necessarily diagnostic of, toxocariasis. It must therefore be interpreted in conjunction with the clinical findings. A positive titre does not therefore exclude the possibility of some other condition such as retinoblastoma.

Chronic endophthalmitis

1. **Presentation** is between the ages of 2 and 9 years with leukocoria (Fig. 14.26a), strabismus or unilateral visual loss.
2. **Signs**
   - Anterior uveitis and vitritis.
   - In some cases, there may be a peripheral granuloma.
   - The peripheral retina and pars plana may be covered by a dense greyish-white exudate, similar to the 'snowbanking' seen in pars planitis (Fig. 14.26b).
3. **Ultrasonography** may be useful in establishing the diagnosis in eyes with hazy media and excluding other causes of leukocoria (Fig. 14.26c).
4. **Treatment** with steroids, either periocular or systemic, may be used to reduce the inflammatory activity.
5. **Prognosis** in most cases is very poor and some eyes eventually require enucleation. The main causes of visual loss are tractional retinal detachment, hypotony and phthisis bulbi caused by separation of the ciliary body from the sclera by contraction of a cyclitic membrane (Fig. 14.26d).

Posterior pole granuloma

1. **Presentation** is typically with unilateral visual impairment between the ages of 6 and 14 years.
2. **Signs**
   - Absence of intraocular inflammation.
   - Round, yellow-white, solid granuloma which varies between one to two disc-diameters in diameter in the posterior fundus (Fig. 14.27a and b).
   - Associated findings include vitreoretinal traction bands (Fig. 14.27b) and localized tractional retinal detachment (Fig. 14.27d).

Peripheral granuloma

1. **Presentation** is usually in adolescence or adult life with visual impairment from distortion of the macula or retinal detachment. In uncomplicated cases, the lesion may remain undetected throughout life.
2. **Signs**
   - Absence of intraocular inflammation.
   - A white hemispherical peripheral granuloma in any quadrant of the fundus (Fig. 14.28a).
   - Vitreous bands may extend from the lesion to the posterior fundus and result in 'dragging' of the disc and macula (Fig. 14.28b).

Onchocerciasis

Onchocerciasis is caused by the filarial parasite *Onchocerca volvulus* which is transmitted by the bite of a blackfly (Simulium) and results in the migration of millions of tiny worms (microfilariae) throughout the body (see Chapter 24).

Diagnosis

1. **Aqueous** may show live floating microfilariae after the patient has bent face down for a few minutes and is then immediately examined on the slit lamp.
2. **Anterior uveitis** may result in pear-shaped pupillary distortion.
3. **Chorioretinitis** is usually bilateral and predominantly involves the posterior fundus. The severity varies from atrophy and clumping of the RPE which may resemble choroidal 'sclerosis' (Fig. 14.29a) to widespread chorioretinal atrophy (Fig. 14.29b).
4. **Other** manifestations include punctate keratitis and sclerosing keratitis.

Treatment

Treatment is aimed at eradicating the source of the microfilariae with ivermectin. Anterior uveitis responds to steroids but the chorioretinal lesions are irreversible.

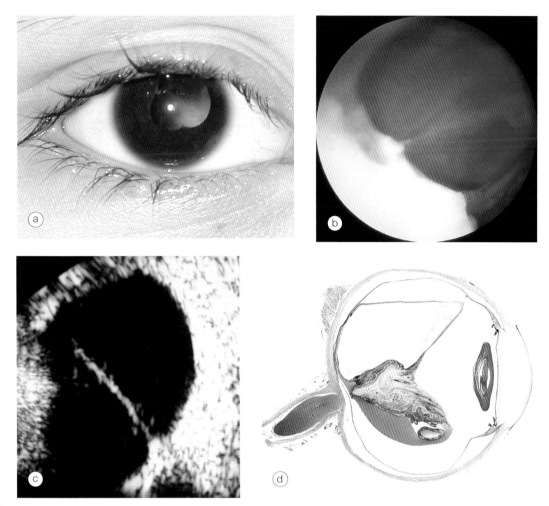

Fig. 14.26
Chronic toxocara endophthalmitis. **(a)** Leukocoria; **(b)** peripheral exudation and vitreoretinal traction bands; **(c)** ultrasonography shows a vitreoretinal traction band; **(d)** inflammatory mass and total retinal detachment (Courtesy of N Rogers – figs a and c; S Lightman – fig. b; J Harry and G Misson, from *Clinical Ophthalmic Pathology*, Butterworth-Heinemann, 2001 – fig. d)

Cysticercosis

Cysticercosis refers to a parasitic infestation by *Cysticercus cellulosae*, the larval form of the pork tapeworm *Taenia solium* (see Chapter 24).

1. **Subconjunctival** cysts are commonly seen in Asian patients.
2. **Anterior chamber** shows a free-floating cyst (Fig. 14.30a).
3. **Subretinal cyst with retinal detachment** (Fig. 14.30b). The larvae enter the subretinal space and can pass into the vitreous where released toxins incite an intense inflammatory reaction which may ultimately lead to blindness.
4. **Treatment** involves surgical removal of the larvae. Subretinal cysts may be removed trans-sclerally and intravitreal cysts transvitreally. Medical therapy with albendazole is not indicated for ocular disease, since dead parasite may induce intense inflammation.

Diffuse unilateral subacute neuroretinitis

Diffuse unilateral subacute neuroretinitis (DUSN) is characterized by a motile subretinal nematode that typically causes monocular visual loss in an otherwise healthy individual. *Baylisascaris procyonis*, the raccoon roundworm, as well as *Ancylostoma caninum*, the dog hookworm, have been implicated but it is possible that different worms are capable of producing the same clinical picture.

1. **Presentation** is with insidious, usually severe loss of peripheral and central vision.
2. **Signs**
   - Papillitis, retinal vasculitis and recurrent crops of evanescent grey-white outer retinal lesions (Fig. 14.31a).
   - Vitritis.

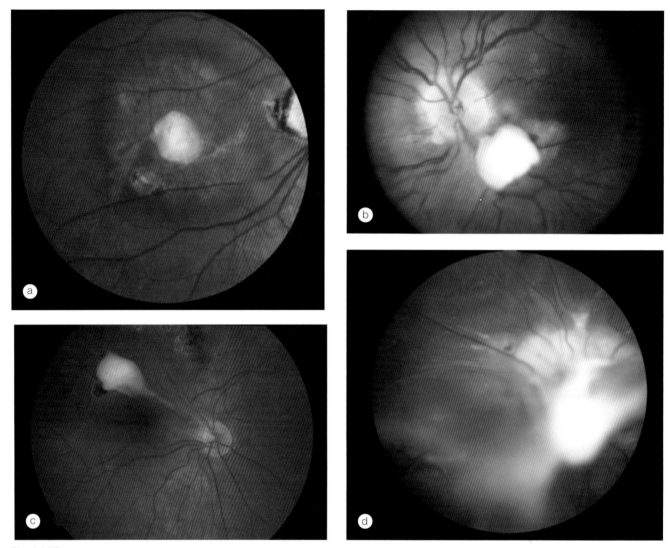

Fig. 14.27
Posterior toxocara granuloma. **(a)** Granuloma at the macula; **(b)** juxtapapillary granuloma: **(c)** granuloma with vitreoretinal bands to the disc; **(d)** granuloma associated with a localized tractional retinal detachment

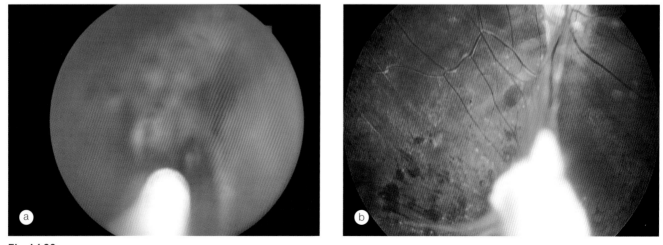

Fig. 14.28
Peripheral toxocara granuloma. **(a)** Inferior granuloma; **(b)** vitreous band extending between the disc and the granuloma

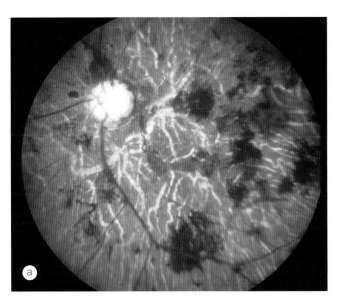
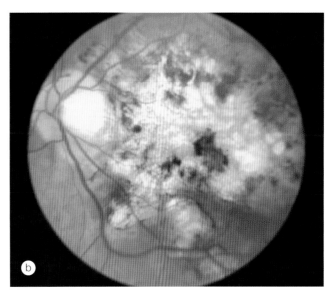

Fig. 14.29
Onchocerciasis. **(a)** Choroidal 'sclerosis' and pigmentary changes; **(b)** severe chorioretinal atrophy

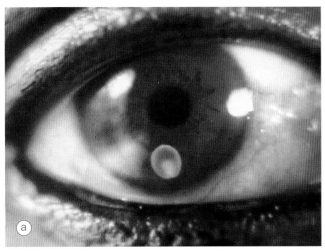
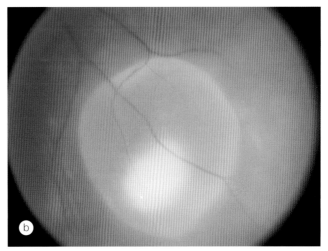

Fig. 14.30
Cysticercosis. **(a)** Anterior chamber cyst; **(b)** subretinal cysticercus cyst with overlying retinal detachment (Courtesy of A Pearson)

- Optic atrophy, retinal vascular attenuation and diffuse RPE degeneration (Fig. 14.31b).
- Subretinal scarring (Fig. 14.31c).

3. ERG is subnormal.

4. Treatment involves direct laser photocoagulation of the subretinal nematode by first surrounding it with a ring of burns, which restrict its movement, and then applying heavy burns to the entire area. Systemic albendazole also may be beneficial.

Choroidal pneumocystosis

Pneumocystis carinii, an opportunistic protozoan parasite, is a major cause of morbidity and mortality in AIDS. The presence of choroidal involvement can be an important sign of extrapulmonary systemic dissemination. Most patients with choroiditis have received inhaled pentamidine as prophylaxis against *Pneumocystis carinii* pneumonia. In contrast with systemic prophylaxis this protects only the lungs, allowing the organisms to disseminate throughout the body.

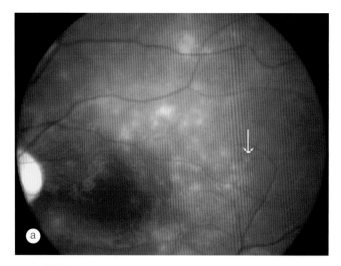

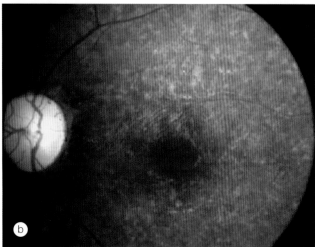

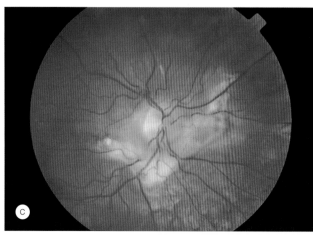

Fig. 14.31
Diffuse unilateral subacute neuroretinitis. **(a)** Active retinal
lesions; **(b)** optic atrophy, vascular attenuation and diffuse RPE
degeneration; **(c)** subretinal scarring (Courtesy of C de A Garcia –
figs a and b; R Curtis – fig. c)

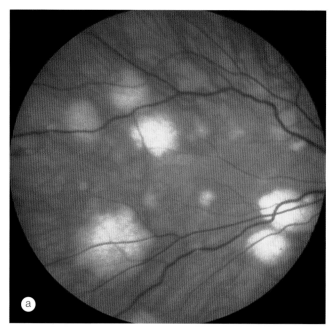

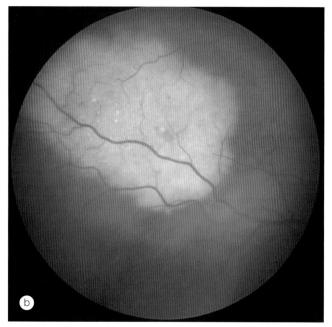

Fig. 14.32
Choroidal pneumocystosis. **(a)** Multifocal choroidal lesions;
(b) large coalescent lesion (Courtesy of S Mitchell – fig. a)

I. Signs

- Flat, yellow, round, choroidal lesions, scattered
  throughout the posterior pole, which are frequently
  bilateral and not associated with vitritis (Fig. 14.32a).
- The lesions may coalesce and produce large geographic
  patches (Fig. 14.32b).
- Even when the fovea is involved there is little visual
  impairment.

2. Treatment involves intravenous trimethoprim and sulfamethoxazole or parenteral pentamidine.

VIRAL UVEITIS

Human immunodeficiency virus uveitis

HIV microangiopathy

Retinal microangiopathy is the most frequent retinopathy in patients with AIDS, developing in up to 70% of patients and is associated with a declining CD4+ count. Postulated causes include immune complex deposition, HIV infection of the retinal vascular endothelium, haemorheological abnormalities and abnormal retinal haemodynamics.

1. **Signs.** Cotton-wool spots which may be associated with retinal haemorrhages and capillary abnormalities (Fig. 14.33a).
2. **Differential diagnosis.** The lesions may be mistaken for early CMV retinitis. However, in contrast to CMV retinitis, lesions are usually asymptomatic and almost invariably disappear spontaneously after several weeks.

HIV retinitis

1. **Signs**
   - Anterior uveitis and vitritis.
   - Small, irregular, grey-white or yellow lesions located in the midperipheral and anterior fundus (Fig. 14.33b) that may slowly enlarge or remain static.
2. **Treatment** is with anti-retroviral therapy – but not aciclovir or ganciclovir. The prognosis is good.

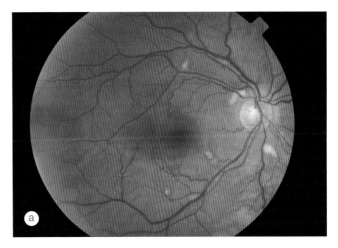

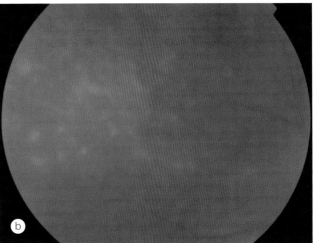

Fig. 14.33
HIV infection. **(a)** Microangiopathy; **(b)** retinitis (Courtesy of C Barry – fig. a; C Pavesio – fig. b)

Cytomegalovirus retinitis

Cytomegalovirus (CMV) retinitis is the most common ocular opportunistic infection among patients with AIDS (see Chapter 24). Since the advent of HAART its incidence has declined and its rate of progression reduced, even in patients with low CD4+ T-cell counts. It also appears that the rates of second eye involvement and retinal detachment are less than in the pre-HAART era.

Diagnosis

1. **Indolent retinitis** frequently starts in the periphery and progresses slowly. It is characterized by a mild granular opacification which may be associated with a few punctate haemorrhages but vasculitis is absent (Fig. 14.34).
2. **Fulminating retinitis**
   - Mild vitritis.

- Vasculitis with perivascular sheathing and retinal opacification (14.35a).
- Dense, white, well-demarcated, geographical area of confluent opacification often associated with retinal haemorrhages (Fig. 14.35b).
- Slow but relentless 'brushfire-like' extension along the course of the retinal vascular arcades that may involve the optic nerve head (Fig. 14.35c).
- Without treatment the entire retina becomes involved within a few months (Fig. 14.35d).
- Regression is characterized by fewer haemorrhages, less opacification, followed by diffuse atrophic and mild pigmentary changes (Fig. 14.35e).
- Retinal detachment associated with large posterior breaks may occur in uncontrolled disease (Fig. 14.35f) and require vitreoretinal surgery and the use of silicone oil tamponade.

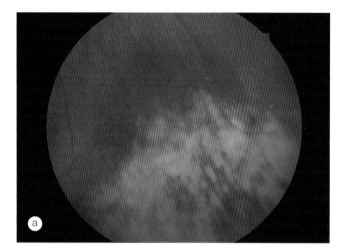

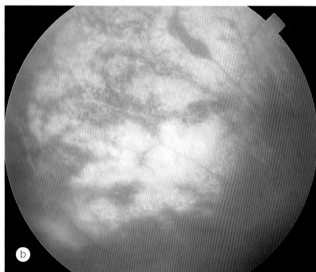

Fig. 14.34
Indolent cytomegalovirus retinitis. **(a)** Early involvement;
(b) more advanced disease (Courtesy of C Pavesio)

Systemic treatment

1. **Ganciclovir** is initially given intravenously (induction) 5mg/kg every 12 hours for 2–3 weeks, then 5mg/kg every 24 hours. Patients with stable retinitis may be treated with oral ganciclovir 300–450mg daily for prophylaxis and maintenance. Ganciclovir is effective in 80% of patients but 50% subsequently relapse and require re-induction of therapy. The drug carries a high risk of bone marrow suppression which often forces interruption of treatment.
2. **Valganciclovir** is a pro-drug of ganciclovir that has better gastrointestinal absorption and is as effective as intravenous ganciclovir itself for treatment and prophylaxis. The induction dose is 900mg b.d. and maintenance is 900mg daily.

3. **Intravenous foscarnet,** unlike ganciclovir, may also improve life expectancy. The initial dose is 60mg/kg every 8 hours for 2–3 weeks and then 90–120mg every 24 hours. Side-effects include nephrotoxicity, electrolyte disturbances and seizures. Foscarnet can also be given intravitreally (2.4mg in 0.1ml).
4. **Intravenous cidofovir,** 5mg/kg once weekly for 2 weeks and then every 2 weeks, may be used where other agents are unsuitable. It must be administered in combination with probenecid. Side-effects include nephrotoxicity, neutropenia and anterior uveitis.

Intravitreal treatment

1. **Ganciclovir slow-release device** (Vitrasert) is as effective as intravenous therapy (Fig. 14.36). The duration of efficacy is 8 months, which is superior to intravenous therapy with either ganciclovir or foscarnet (average 60 days). However, it does not prevent involvement of the fellow eye. Complications include cataract, vitreous haemorrhage, retinal detachment and endophthalmitis.
2. **Intravitreal injections**
   a. **Ganciclovir** may be injected prior to implantation of a slow-release implant to determine the likely response to the drug.
   b. **Fomivirsen** has a different mechanism of action from other agents. Adverse effects include anterior uveitis, vitritis, cataract and rarely retinopathy.
   c. **Cidofovir** may occasionally cause severe inflammation which may result in hypotony and even phthisis bulbi.

Prognosis

Initially 95% of cases respond to treatment. Unfortunately, all relapse within 2 weeks when treatment is discontinued and there is a 50% relapse rate within 6 months in patients on maintenance therapy. Since the introduction of HAART the incidence of CNV retinitis has decreased and many patients have had their treatment of retinitis stopped after immune recovery (CD4 >100–150). Unfortunately, many patients with HAART-induced immune recovery develop intraocular inflammation which may cause macular edema and epiretinal membrane formation.

Progressive outer retinal necrosis

Although progressive outer retinal necrosis (PORN) occurs predominantly in AIDS, it may also occur in patients with drug-induced immunosuppression. It is a rare but devastating necrotizing retinitis caused by varicella zoster virus, which behaves aggressively probably as a consequence of the profound immunosuppression of the host. The name is actually not appropriate since it is only in the early stages that the infection is limited to the outer retina and there is rapid progression to a full thickness retinal necrosis.

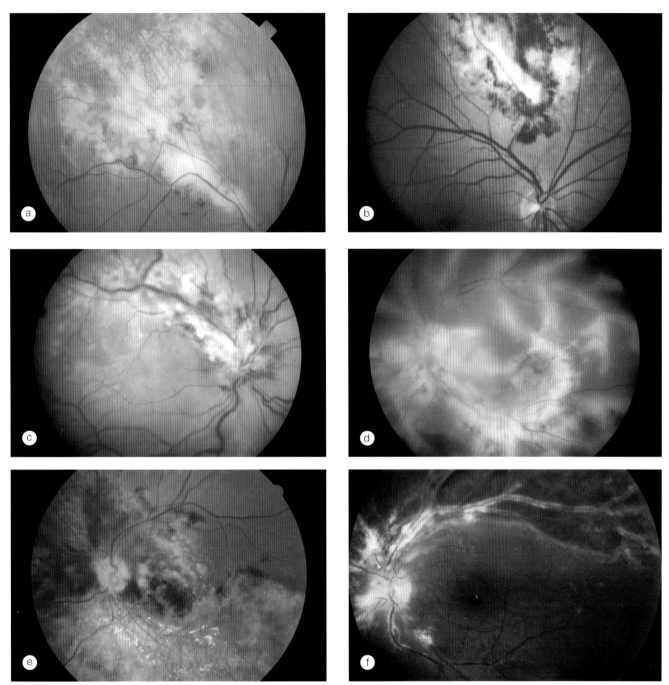

Fig. 14.35
Fulminating cytomegalovirus retinitis. **(a–d)** Progression of disease process; **(e)** regression following treatment; **(f)** large posterior retinal tear and localised retinal detachment (Courtesy of L Merin – figs d and e; C Barry – fig. f)

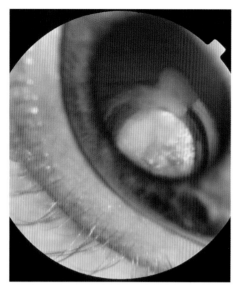

Fig. 14.36
Slow-release intravitreal implant containing ganciclovir (Courtesy of S Milewski)

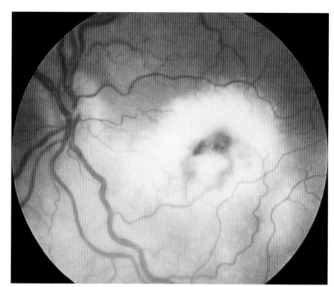

Fig. 14.37
Progressive outer retinal necrosis involving the macula (Courtesy of S Mitchell)

1. **Presentation** is with rapidly progressive visual loss which is initially unilateral in 75% of cases.
2. **Signs** in chronological order:
   • Minimal anterior uveitis.
   • Multifocal, yellow-white, retinal infiltrates with minimal vitritis.
   • Early macular involvement (Fig. 14.37).
   • Rapid confluence and full-thickness retinal necrosis.

   NB Vitreous inflammation is usually late and reflects extensive retinal necrosis.

3. **Investigations.** Specific PCR-based diagnostic assay for varicella zoster virus DNA may be performed on vitreous samples.
4. **Treatment** with intravenous ganciclovir alone or in combination with foscarnet, or intravitreal foscarnet is often disappointing and most patients become blind in both eyes within a few weeks as a result of macular necrosis or retinal detachment. In addition, 50% of patients are dead 5 months after diagnosis. Vitreoretinal surgery for retinal detachment often also yields poor results.

Acute retinal necrosis

Acute retinal necrosis (ARN) is a rare but devastating necrotizing retinitis which typically affects otherwise healthy individuals of all ages. Males are more frequently affected than females by a 2:1 ratio. ARN is a biphasic disease which tends to be caused by HSV in younger patients and VZV in older individuals. Some patients have a past history of HSV encephalitis, many years before developing ARN, and occasionally encephalitis and ARN develop simultaneously.

1. **Presentation** is initially unilateral and varies according to severity. Some patients develop severe visual impairment over a few days associated with pain whereas others have an insidious onset with mild visual symptoms such as floaters.
2. **Signs**
   • Anterior granulomatous uveitis and vitritis are universal.
   • Peripheral periarteritis associated with multifocal, deep, yellow-white, retinal infiltrates that gradually coalesce and progress (Fig. 14.38a and b).
   • Progressive full-thickness retinal necrosis (Fig. 14.38c).
   • The posterior pole is usually spared so that visual acuity may remain fairly good despite severe necrosis of the surrounding retina (Fig. 14.38d).
   • The acute lesions resolve within 6–12 weeks, leaving behind a transparent necrotic retina with hyper-pigmented borders.

   NB Unless the patient receives appropriate treatment the second eye becomes involved in 30% of patients, usually within 2 months, although in some patients the interval may be much longer.

3. **Treatment** is with aciclovir, initially intravenously (10mg/kg every 8 hours) for 10–14 days and then orally

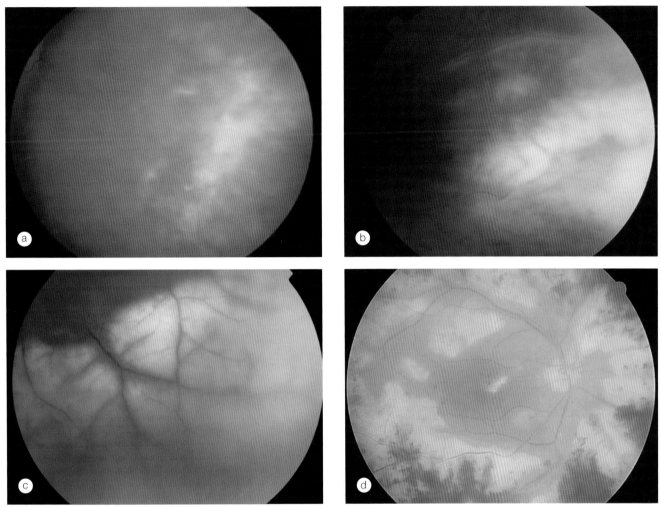

Fig. 14.38
Acute retinal necrosis. **(a)** and **(b)** Progression of peripheral retinal infiltration; **(c)** full-thickness necrosis; **(d)** advanced disease with relative macular sparing (Courtesy of C Pavesio – figs c and d)

800mg five times daily for 6–12 weeks. This may hasten resolution of the acute retinal lesions and reduce the risk of second eye involvement, but it does not prevent retinal detachment. Recurrences may occur in some patients and long-term therapy may be required. Systemic steroids may be started 24 hours after initiation of antiviral therapy and is usually indicated in severe cases, especially showing optic nerve involvement.

NB Prophylactic laser photocoagulation, aimed at limiting posterior spread of retinitis, has been largely abandoned.

4. Prognosis is relatively poor with 60% of patients having a final visual acuity of less than 6/60 as a result of the retinal detachment, ischaemic optic neuropathy and occlusive periphlebitis.

Herpes simplex anterior uveitis

1. **Granulomatous CAU,** which may be associated with trabeculitis and high IOP (hypertensive uveitis), may occur with or without active corneal disease. Iris atrophy which is often patchy and occasionally sectoral is common (Fig. 14.39). Spontaneous hyphema may also occur but is uncommon.
2. **Treatment** involves topical steroids (in the absence of active epithelial disease) and oral aciclovir (400mg five times a day).

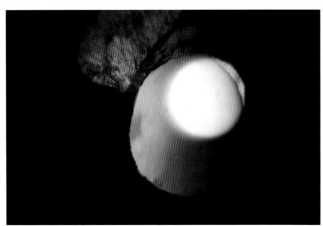

Fig. 14.39
Iris atrophy in herpes simplex anterior uveitis

Varicella zoster anterior uveitis

1. **Granulomatous CAU** affects nearly 50% of the patients with herpes zoster ophthalmicus (HZO), particularly when the rash involves the side of the nose (Hutchinson sign) (Fig. 14.40). The inflammation is often mild and asymptomatic although rarely it may be severe with fibrinous exudation and hypopyon or hyphaema. Residual sectoral iris atrophy is seen in 25% of cases and is thought to be due to occlusive vasculitis.
2. **Treatment** is with topical steroids although systemic steroids are occasionally required.

NB All patients with HZO must be examined regularly for 6 weeks from the onset of the rash to detect anterior uveitis because it is often asymptomatic.

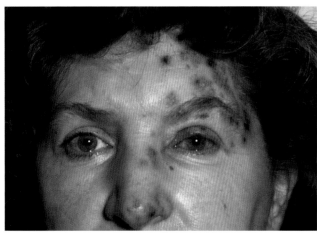

Fig. 14.40
Hutchinson sign in herpes zoster ophthalmicus

Congenital rubella

Rubella (German measles) is usually a benign febrile exanthema. Congenital rubella results from transplacental transmission of virus to the fetus from an infected mother, usually during the first trimester of pregnancy (see Chapter 24).

1. **Anterior uveitis** may result in iris atrophy.
2. **Retinopathy** is a common manifestation, but the exact incidence is unknown because cataracts frequently impair visualization of the fundus.
   - 'Salt and pepper' pigmentary disturbance involving the periphery (Fig. 14.41a) and posterior pole (Fig. 14.41b).
   - Prognosis is usually good although a small percentage of eyes may later develop CNV.
3. **Other** manifestations include cataract, microphthalmos, glaucoma, keratitis and extreme refractive errors.

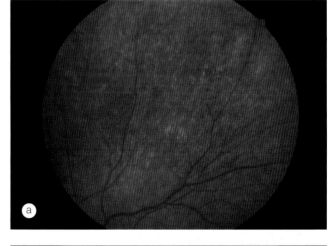

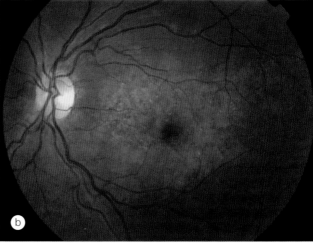

Fig. 14.41
Rubella retinopathy. **(a)** Peripheral involvement; **(b)** macular involvement (Courtesy of A Moore – fig. b)

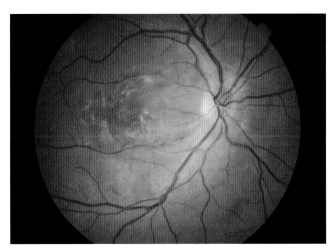

Fig. 14.42
Retinal involvement in subacute sclerosing panencephalitis
(Courtesy of Z Bashshur)

Subacute sclerosing panencephalitis

Subacute sclerosing panencephalitis is a chronic, progressive neurodegenerative and usually fatal disease of children caused by the measles virus.

1. **Systemic features** include insidious personality change followed by progressive psychomotor deterioration, myoclonus and seizures. Death ensues within years.
2. **Posterior uveitis** is characterized by papillitis, macular oedema, whitish retinal infiltrates and choroiditis (Fig. 14.42).

FUNGAL UVEITIS

Presumed ocular histoplasmosis syndrome

Pathogenesis

Histoplasmosis is caused by *Histoplasma capsulatum* acquired by inhalation of infective mycelia fragments and/or spores with dust particles. The organisms then pass via the bloodstream to the spleen, liver and, on occasion, the choroid, setting up multiple foci of granulomatous inflammation. Although ocular histoplasmosis has never been reported in patients with active, systemic histoplasmosis, eye disease has an increased prevalence in areas where histoplasmosis is endemic, such as the Mississippi–Missouri river valley. It is thought that presumed ocular histoplasmosis syndrome (POHS) represents an immunologic mediated

response in individuals previously exposed to the fungus. Patients with POHS show an increased prevalence of HLA-B7 and HLA-DR2.

General signs

POHS is asymptomatic unless it causes a maculopathy. The following types of fundus lesion are seen, which are bilateral in 60% of cases.

1. **Absence of intraocular inflammation.**
2. **Acute stage** may manifest localized swelling of the choroid, which may also lead to changes in the overlying RPE.
3. **Atrophic 'histo'** spots consist of roundish, slightly irregular, yellowish-white lesions about 200μm in diameter, often associated with pigment clumps within or at the margins of the scars. They are scattered in the mid-retinal periphery and posterior fundus (Fig. 14.43a and b).
4. **Peripapillary atrophy** may be diffuse (Fig. 14.43c) or focal or a combination of both.

Exudative maculopathy

1. **Exudative (wet) maculopathy** associated with CNV is a late manifestation which usually develops between the ages of 20 and 45 years in about 5% of eyes. In most cases, CNV is associated with an old macular 'histo spot', although occasionally it develops within a peripapillary lesion. Very rarely, the CNV occurs in the absence of a pre-existing scar.
2. **Clinical course** of maculopathy may show the following patterns:
   - Leakage from CNV causes serous macular elevation which may be associated with an underlying focal yellow-white or grey lesion. In 12% of eyes the subretinal fluid absorbs spontaneously and visual symptoms regress.
   - A dark green-black ring frequently develops on the surface of the yellow-white lesion and bleeding occurs into the sub-sensory retinal space, causing a marked drop in visual acuity (Fig. 14.43d). In a few eyes, the subretinal haemorrhage resolves and visual acuity improves.
   - The initial CNV may remain active for about 2 years, giving rise to recurrent haemorrhages and subsequently disciform scarring with permanent loss of central vision.

NB Patients with maculopathy in one eye and an asymptomatic atrophic macular scar in the other are likely to develop CNV in the second eye. They should therefore test themselves every day with an Amsler grid to detect early metamorphopsia because without treatment 60% of eyes with CNV have a final visual acuity of less than 6/60.

3. **Treatment of CNV** may involve argon laser photocoagulation for extrafoveal CNV and photodynamic

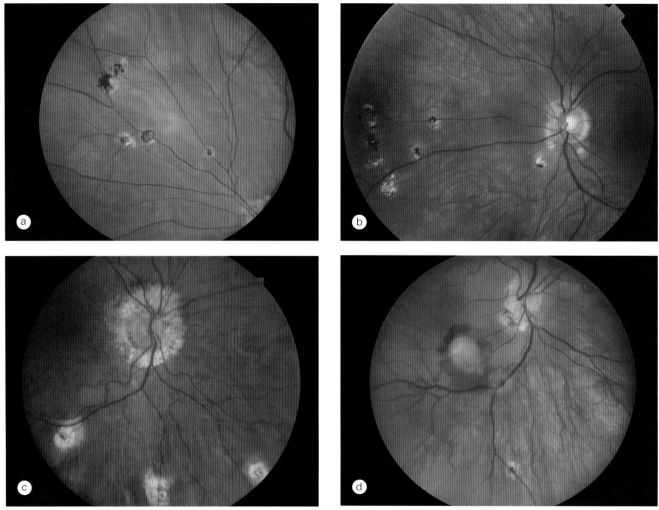

Fig. 14.43
Presumed ocular histoplasmosis syndrome. **(a)** Peripheral 'histo' spots; **(b)** peripheral and juxtapapillary 'histo' spots; **(c)** circumferential peripapillary atrophy and 'histo' spots; **(d)** subretinal haemorrhage from choroidal neovascularization

therapy (PDT) for subfoveal membranes. Intravitreal triamcinolone acetonide may be effective for both extrafoveal and subfoveal CNV but the effect is transient. Surgical removal may be feasible in selected cases. Systemic steroids may halt progression of CNV and prevent recurrence after subfoveal surgery.

Cryptococcosis

Soil contaminated with pigeon droppings contains an encapsulated yeast, *Cryptococcus neoformans*, which enters the body through inhalation (see Chapter 24). Cryptococcal infection is usually limited to patients with cell-mediated immune dysfunction and occurs in 5–10% of patients with

AIDS. Ocular involvement is present in approximately 6% of patients with cryptococcal meningitis. The most likely route of infection is via direct extension from the optic nerve or by haematogenous spread to the choroid and retina.

1. **Signs**
   - Meningitis-associated manifestations are the most common and include papilloedema, ophthalmoplegia, ptosis, optic neuropathy and sixth nerve palsy.
   - Multifocal choroiditis (Fig. 14.44).
   - Iris infiltration, keratitis and conjunctival granuloma have been reported.
2. **Treatment** of sight-threatening lesions is with intravenous amphotericin, oral fluconazole and itraconazole.

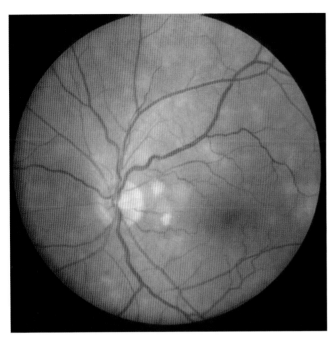

Fig. 14.44
Multifocal cryptococcal choroiditis (Courtesy of A Curi)

Endogenous fungal endophthalmitis

Pathogenesis

The major source of fungal infection within the eye is metastatic spread from a septic focus associated with catheters, intravenous drug abuse, parenteral nutrition and chronic lung disease such as cystic fibrosis. Neutropenia following immunosuppression and AIDS are also major risk factors. Approximately 75% of isolates are *Candida* spp.; other pathogens include *Cryptococcus* spp., *Sporothrix schenckii* and *Blastomyces* spp.

Diagnosis

1. **Presentation** is dependent on the location of the inflammatory focus. Peripheral lesions may cause few or no visual symptoms while central lesions or those resulting in severe vitritis will manifest earlier. The progression is, however, much slower than in bacterial endophthalmitis and bilateral involvement is common.
2. **Signs**
   • Anterior uveitis is uncommon in the early stages but may become prominent later.
   • Creamy white chorioretinal lesions with overlying vitritis (Fig. 14.45a).
   • Extension into the vitreous (Fig. 14.45b).
   • Vitritis and floating 'cotton-ball' colonies (Fig. 14.45c).
   • Chronic endophthalmitis characterized by severe vitreous infiltration and abscess formation (Fig. 14.45d).

3. **Course** is relatively chronic and may result in the development of retinal necrosis and retinal detachment associated with severe proliferative vitreoretinopathy.
4. **Investigations** involving vitreous biopsy and smears and cultures may be required to confirm the diagnosis and test sensitivity of the organisms to antifungal agents.

Treatment

1. **Medical** treatment is indicated for systemic disease and ocular disease without vitreous involvement.
   • Intravenous amphotericin 5% dextrose; the initial dose is 5mg and after a few days can be increased to 20mg.
   • Oral fluconazole 100–200mg/day (400–800mg for disseminated disease) for 3–6 weeks. It can be used in conjunction with flucytosine (100mg/kg/day).
   • Oral voriconazole to treat cases resistant to fluconazole.

   NB Systemic steroids are contraindicated in fungal infections.

2. **Pars plana vitrectomy** combined with intravitreal injection of amphotericin 5–10µg in 0.1ml is indicated in the presence of vitreous involvement.

BACTERIAL UVEITIS

Tuberculosis

Tuberculosis (TB) is a chronic granulomatous infection caused by the tubercle bacillus which is of the genus Mycobacterium (see Chapter 24). TB uveitis is rare in the developed world and may be difficult to diagnose because it may occur in patients without systemic manifestations of TB. The diagnosis is therefore often presumptive, based on indirect evidence, such as intractable uveitis unresponsive to steroid therapy, a positive history of contact, a positive skin test and negative findings for other causes of uveitis.

Diagnosis

1. **CAU**, usually granulomatous, but occasionally non-granulomatous, is the most frequent feature.
2. **Choroiditis** is caused by direct infection.
   • Unilateral focal or less frequently multifocal.
   • Extensive diffuse choroiditis may occur in patients with AIDS (Fig. 14.46a).
   • Choroiditis may occasionally resemble serpiginous choroidopathy (Fig. 14.46b).
3. **Large solitary choroidal granulomas** are uncommon.
4. **Periphlebitis** is often bilateral and represents a manifestation of hypersensitivity to the bacillus. It may be mild and innocuous or occlusive, resulting in severe

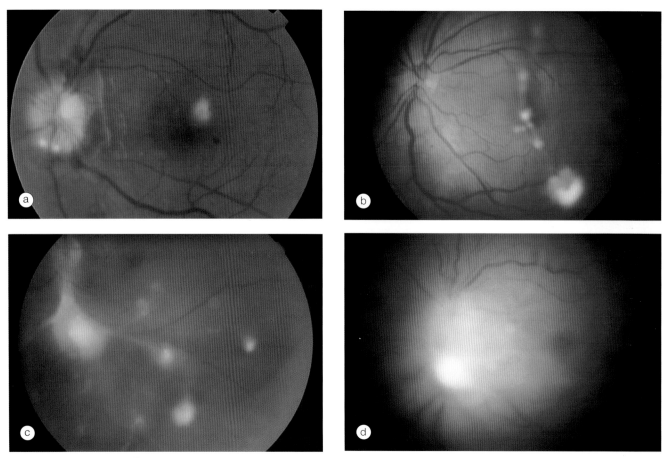

Fig. 14.45
Fungal endophthalmitis. **(a)** Focal retinitis; **(b)** multifocal retinitis with early vitreous extension; **(c)** vitritis and 'cotton ball' colonies; **(d)** vitreous abscess (Courtesy of A Curi – fig. c)

retinal ischaemia and secondary retinal neovascularization (Fig. 14.47).

Treatment

Treatment is initially with at least three drugs (isoniazid, rifampicin, pyrazinamide or ethambutol) and then with isoniazid and rifampicin. Quadruple therapy is sometimes necessary in resistant cases, more frequently seen in highly endemic areas such as India. Concomitant systemic steroid therapy is also frequently necessary. The steroid dose needs to be adjusted when given with rifampicin.

Syphilis

Syphilis is sexually-transmitted disease caused by the spirochaete *Treponema pallidum* (see Chapter 24). Ocular syphilis is uncommon and there are no pathognomonic signs. Eye involvement typically occurs during the secondary and tertiary stages, although occasionally it may be seen during primary syphilis. The disease must therefore be suspected in any case of intraocular inflammation resistant to conventional therapy. Because of variable presentation serology should be performed in all patients with uveitis who require investigation. Serological tests rely on detection of non-specific antibodies (cardiolipin) or specific treponemal antibodies.

Anterior uveitis

Iridocyclitis occurs in about 4% of patients with secondary syphilis and is bilateral in 50%. The inflammation is usually acute and unless appropriately treated becomes chronic. In some cases, iritis is first associated with dilated iris capillaries (roseolae) (Fig. 14.48) which may develop into more localized papules and subsequently into larger yellowish nodules. Various types of post-inflammatory iris atrophy may ensue.

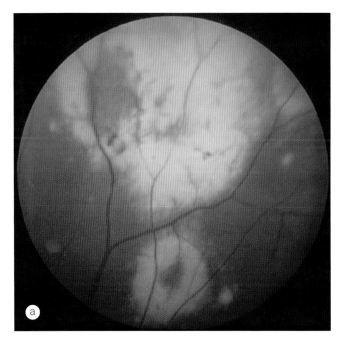

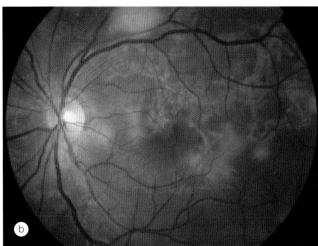

Fig. 14.46
Tuberculous choroiditis. **(a)** Diffuse involvement in a patient with AIDS; **(b)** resembling serpiginous choroidopathy (Courtesy of C de A Garcia – fig. a; C Pavesio – fig. b)

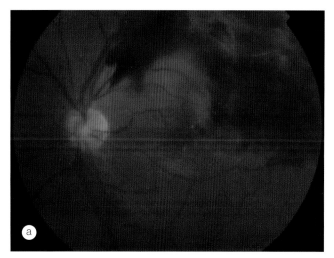

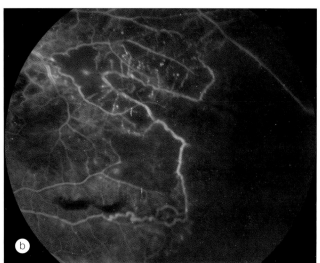

Fig. 14.47
Occlusive tuberculous periphlebitis. **(a)** Superior retinal branch occlusion; **(b)** fluorescein angiography shows extensive hypofluorescence due to capillary non-perfusion (Courtesy of C Pavesio)

Posterior uveitis

The absence of pathognomonic signs and the ability of syphilis to mimic any ocular and systemic inflammatory disease often leads to misdiagnosis and delay in appropriate treatment.

1. Chorioretinitis
- Multifocal disease is frequently bilateral (Fig. 14.49a).
- Acute posterior placoid chorioretinitis is characterized by bilateral, large, solitary, placoid, pale-yellowish subretinal lesions (Fig. 14.49b).

2. **Neuroretinitis,** unless treated, gives rise to secondary optic atrophy and replacement of retinal vessels by white strands.
3. **Periphlebitis** may be occlusive.

Syphilis in HIV-positive patients

Syphilis is an uncommon cause of uveitis in HIV-infected patients. Because syphilis may pursue a more aggressive course in HIV patients and respond less well to conventional therapy it seems reasonable to test all patients with ocular syphilis for HIV and vice-versa.

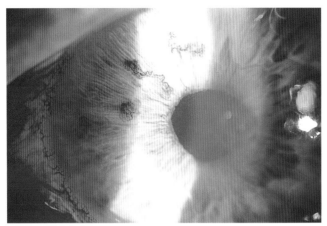

Fig. 14.48
Dilated iris vessels (roseolae) in syphilitic anterior uveitis

Treatment

Conventional doses of penicillin are inadequate; the therapeutic regimen is the same as for neurosyphilis (which should be ruled out by lumbar puncture). One of the following regimens may be used:

1. **Intravenous aqueous penicillin G** 12–24MU (mega units) daily for 10–15 days.
2. **Intramuscular procaine penicillin** 2.4MU daily, supplemented with oral probenecid (2g daily), for 10–15 days.
3. **Oral amoxicillin** 3g b.d. for 28 days.

   NB Penicillin-allergic patients can be treated with oral tetracycline or erythromycin 500mg q.i.d. for 30 days.

Lyme disease

Lyme disease (borreliosis) is an infection caused by a flagellated spirochaete, *Borrelia burgdorferi*, transmitted through the bite of a hard-shelled tick of the genus *Ixodes* which feeds on a variety of large mammals, particularly deer (see Chapter 24).

1. **Uveitis** is uncommon and may take the following forms: anterior, intermediate, peripheral multifocal choroiditis, retinal periphlebitis and neuroretinitis.
2. **Other** manifestations include follicular conjunctivitis, episcleritis, keratitis, scleritis, orbital myositis, optic neuritis, ocular motor nerve palsies and reversible Horner syndrome.
3. **Treatment** of uveitis is with steroids.

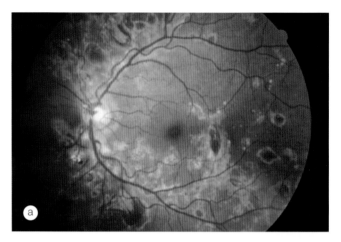

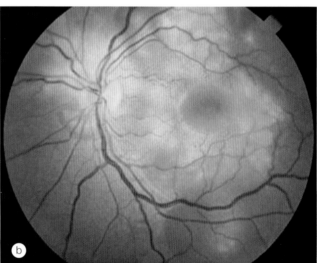

Fig. 14.49
Syphilitic chorioretinitis. **(a)** Old multifocal chorioretinitis: **(b)** acute posterior placoid chorioretinitis (Courtesy of J Salmon – fig. a; C de A Garcia – fig. b)

Brucellosis

Zoonoses are human diseases caused by a pathogen that has an animal reservoir. Brucellosis is a zoonotic disease caused by the Gram-negative bacteria *Brucella melitensis* or *Brucella abortus*. It is transmitted from animals to man through the ingestion of unpasteurised milk products or uncooked meat.

1. **Systemic features** include fever, arthralgia, myalgia, anorexia, sweating, headache and malaise. The onset of symptoms may be acute or insidious, generally beginning within 2–4 weeks after inoculation.

2. **Treatment** involves tetracycline for 6 weeks and streptomycin for 2 weeks. Doxycycline and rifampicin are alternatives.

3. **Ocular involvement** usually develops after the acute phase and may be characterized by CAU, multifocal choroiditis and, rarely, endogenous endophthalmitis. Other manifestations include dacryoadenitis, episcleritis, nummular keratitis and optic neuritis.

Endogenous bacterial endophthalmitis

Pathogenesis

Endogenous (metastatic) endophthalmitis occurs when organisms enter the eye through the blood–eye barrier from the bloodstream. However, no ocular infection occurs in the vast majority of cases of bacteraemia, although Roth spots develop in about 1% of cases. Both eyes are involved in about 12% of cases.

1. **Risk factors** are diabetes, cardiac disease and malignancy. Other risks include indwelling catheters, intravenous drug abuse, liver abscess, pneumonia, endocarditis, cellulitis, urinary tract infection (*E. coli*), meningitis, septic arthritis and abdominal surgery.

2. **Pathogens.** The most common is *Klebsiella* spp. although a wide variety of organisms may be responsible.

Clinical features

Misdiagnosis as uveitis, conjunctivitis or acute glaucoma is common, and this may delay treatment. Diagnosis and management may be difficult if the patient is immobile or moribund.

1. **Symptoms**
   - Pain, blurred vision, floaters, photophobia and headache.
   - The patient is usually systemically unwell with fever and rigors.
2. **Anterior segment**
   - Proptosis, chemosis, swollen lids and corneal oedema.
   - Discrete iris nodules or plaques, anterior fibrinous uveitis and hypopyon in severe cases (Fig. 14.50a).
3. **Posterior segment**
   - White or yellow retinal infiltrates (Fig.14.50b).
   - Vitreous haze or abscess.
   - Retinal necrosis in severe cases.
   - Spread to the orbit may occur.

Investigations

1. **Systemic**
   - Search for septic foci (skin, joints); collaboration with physician or intensive care specialist is essential.
   - Blood and urine cultures in all patients.
   - Appropriate cultures from other sites depending on the clinical features (e.g. catheter tips, cerebrospinal fluid, skin wounds, abscesses and joints.
   - Investigations for endocarditis (chest x-ray, ECG and echocardiography).
   - Abdominal ultrasound.

NB Exclude meningitis in children using PCR on blood for *N. meningitidis*.

2. **Ocular.**
   - Aqueous and vitreous samples should be taken.

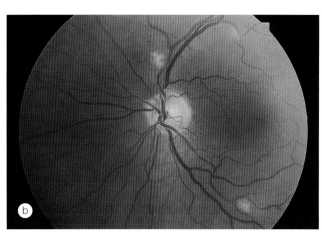

Fig. 14.50
Endogenous bacterial endophthalmitis. **(a)** Fibrinous anterior uveitis; **(b)** retinal infiltrates

Table 14.4   Comparison of postoperative and endogenous endophthalmitis

	Postoperative	*Endogenous*
Ocular cultures	Always	Always
Blood cultures	No	Always
Systemic investigations	No	Always
Topical antibiotics	Yes	Yes
Systemic antibiotics	Oral fluoroquinolone	Intravenous (various)
Intravitreal antibiotics	Always	Always
Steroids	Yes	No proven value
Visual outcome	70% > 6/60	70% < count fingers
Mortality	None	10%

- Fine needle biopsy of a focal abscess should be considered.

Treatment

1. **Systemic infection** is treated with intravenous antibiotics. The choice is based on culture and sensitivity results and should continue for 2–3 weeks, or longer if there is endocarditis. Patients without an evident source of infection should be treated with a combination of ceftazidime 1g every 12 hours and vancomycin 1g every 12 hours. If an organism is identified specialist micro-biological advice should be obtained.
2. **Endophthalmitis** is treated with oral ciprofloxacin and intravitreal antibiotics although the benefits of the latter are less clear than for acute postoperative bacterial endophthalmitis, which presents much earlier.

Prognosis

The prognosis is poor with 70% of eyes reduced to light perception – probably as a result of delay in presentation and the virulence of the organism. Phthisis or evisceration occurs in 25%. Table 14.4 is a comparison of postoperative and endogenous endophthalmitis.

NB There is a mortality of 5–10% from associated systemic disease.

Cat-scratch disease

Cat-scratch disease (benign lymphoreticulosis) is a subacute infection caused by *Bartonella henselae*, a Gram-negative rod. The infection is transmitted by the scratch or bite of an apparently healthy cat (see Chapter 24). Neuroretinitis is the most common manifestation and is characterized by the following:

1. **Presentation** is with unilateral, painless, visual impairment which starts gradually and then becomes most marked after about a week.
2. **Signs** in chronological order:
   - VA is impaired to a variable degree.
   - Papillitis associated with peripapillary and macular oedema. In severe cases venous engorgement and splinter-shaped haemorrhages may be present (Fig. 14.51a).
   - A macular star figure composed of hard exudates subsequently ensues (Fig. 14.51b).
   - After several months visual acuity improves, with first resolution of papillitis and then hard exudates, although initially the exudates may increase as disc swelling is resolving (Fig. 14.51c).
   - The fellow eye occasionally becomes involved but recurrences in the same eye are uncommon.
3. **Other less common manifestations** include Parinaud oculoglandular syndrome, focal choroiditis, intermediate uveitis, exudative maculopathy, retinal vascular occlusion and panuveitis.
4. **Treatment** is with oral doxycycline or erythromycin, with or without rifampicin.

Leprosy

Lepromatous leprosy (see Chapter 24) may result in chronic anterior uveitis as the result of direct invasion of the iris by bacilli.

1. **Signs**
   - Low-grade inflammation associated with the formation of synechiae.
   - A pathognomonic sign is the presence of iris pearls formed from dead bacteria (Fig. 14.52a). They slowly enlarge and coalesce, become pedunculated and drop into the anterior chamber, from which they eventually disappear.
   - The pupil becomes miosed (Fig. 14.52b) and the iris atrophic (Fig. 14.52c) as a result of damage to the sympathetic innervation to the dilator pupillae.
2. **Treatment** involves systemic antibiotics and topical steroids.

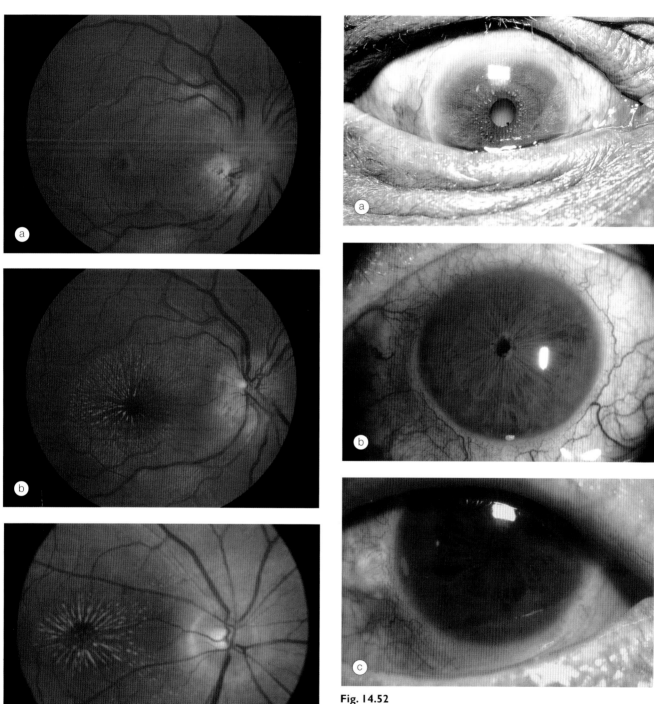

Fig. 14.51
Neuroretinitis. **(a)** Papillitis; **(b)** macular star and resolving papillitis; **(c)** increase in macular star and nearly resolved papillitis (Courtesy of P Saine – figs a and b)

Fig. 14.52
Lepromatous chronic anterior uveitis. **(a)** Iris pearls; **(b)** miosis; **(c)** iris atrophy (Courtesy of M Hogeweg, from P G Watson, B L Hazelman, C E Pavesio and W R Green, *The Sclera and Systemic Disorders*, Butterworth-Heinemann, 2004 – fig. a; P Gili – fig. b; T ffytche – fig. c)

PRIMARY IDIOPATHIC INFLAMMATORY CHORIOCAPILLAROPATHIES (WHITE DOT SYNDROMES)

Acute posterior multifocal placoid pigment epitheliopathy

Acute posterior multifocal placoid pigment epitheliopathy (APMPPE) is an uncommon, idiopathic, usually bilateral condition, which typically affects individuals in the third to sixth decades. It affects both sexes equally and is associated with HLA-B7 and HLA-DR2. In about one-third of patients APMPPE follows a flu-like illness and occasionally it may be the initial manifestation of a CNS angiitis. APMPPE has been described in association with a variety of systemic conditions including tuberculosis, anti-hepatitis B vaccination, mumps, Wegener granulomatosis, polyarteritis nodosa, ulcerative colitis, sarcoidosis and Lyme disease.

Diagnosis

1. **Presentation** is with subacute visual impairment associated with central and paracentral scotomas and often photopsia. Within a few days to several weeks the fellow eye becomes affected.
2. **Signs**
   - Mild vitritis.
   - Multiple, large, cream-coloured or greyish-white, placoid lesions at the level of the RPE which typically begin at the posterior pole and then extend to the post-equatorial fundus (Fig. 14.53a).
   - After a few days the lesions begin to fade centrally but this is not accompanied by immediate improvement of vision.
   - Within 2 weeks the majority of acute lesions are replaced by RPE changes of varying severity.
   - New lesions may appear so that different stages of evolution may be seen.
   - Within several months visual acuity recovers although occasionally paracentral scotomas may persist.
3. **FA** of active lesions shows early dense hypofluorescence associated with non-perfusion of the choriocapillaris (Fig. 14.53b) and late hyperfluorescence due to staining (Fig. 14.53c).
4. **ICG** is superior to FA in demonstrating non-perfusion of the choriocapillaris (Fig. 14.53d).
5. **EOG** may be subnormal.

Differential diagnosis

1. **Early serpiginous choroidopathy** may occasionally be confused with APMPPE but it tends to affect an older age group, runs a recurrent course and has a poor prognosis.
2. **Multiple evanescent white dot syndrome** can also cause acute visual loss in healthy young adults. However, the lesions are smaller, unilateral and at the level of outer retina and RPE. FA shows early hypofluorescence and late staining of the lesions which are much more numerous than clinically observed. The ERG is usually abnormal.
3. **Harada disease** is characterized by diffuse choroidal infiltrates during acute stage and similar residual RPE changes to APMPPE. However, it typically affects specific ethnic groups and is characterized by exudative retinal detachment.
4. **Other causes** of multifocal deep lesions include diffuse unilateral subacute neuroretinitis (DUSN), multifocal choroiditis with panuveitis, sarcoidosis, secondary syphilis, sympathetic ophthalmitis and metastatic choroidal infiltrates.

Birdshot retinochoroidopathy

Birdshot retinochoroidopathy is an uncommon, idiopathic, chronic, recurrent, bilateral disease which typically affects individuals in the fifth to seventh decades of life, predominantly females. Over 95% of patients are positive for HLA-A29.

Diagnosis

1. **Presentation** is with insidious impairment of central vision associated with photopsia and floaters, or night blindness and impairment of colour vision. The severity of visual disturbance is frequently out of proportion to the measured visual acuity, indicating diffuse retinal dysfunction.
2. **Signs** are usually bilateral but may be asymmetrical.
   - Moderate vitritis without snowballs or snowbanking.
   - Retinal vasculitis involving large and small vessels.
   - Multiple, small, ill-defined, cream-coloured, choroidal spots in the posterior pole and mid-periphery (Fig. 14.54a).
   - Over several years new spots may appear and old lesions may enlarge.
   - Inactive lesions consist of well delineated, atrophic spots, which show no tendency to become hyperpigmented (Fig. 14.54b).

NB Occasionally the fundus spots appear several years after the onset of vitritis, vasculitis and CMO, resulting in misdiagnosis.

3. **FA** shows early hypofluorescence and late mild hyper-fluorescence. The disc may show hyperfluorescence due to leakage, and CMO may be present (Fig. 14.54c). Fewer lesions are seen on FA than clinically because they dis-

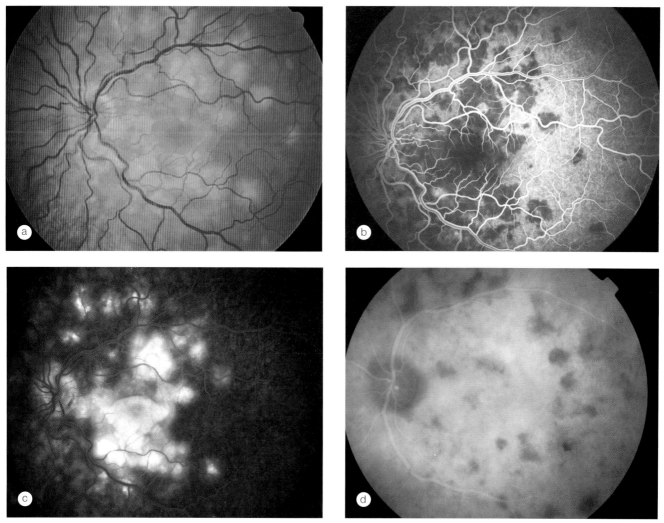

Fig. 14.53
(a) Active posterior multifocal placoid pigment epitheliopathy; **(b)** FA early venous phase shows dense foci of hypofluorescence; **(c)** late phase shows hyperfluorescence; **(d)** ICG shows focal hypofluorescence (Courtesy of C Barry)

appear after the choroidal flush and only become apparent when the RPE is involved.

4. **ICG** reveals well defined hypofluorescent spots in the early phases (Fig. 14.54d), becoming hyperfluorescent later. Many more spots can be seen by ICG than either clinically or on FA.

5. **ERG** is normal in early disease but with time the b-wave amplitude and then oscillatory potential become decreased. A delay in implicit time of the 30Hz flicker ERG is the most sensitive change. ERG findings seem to reflect intraretinal oedema and for this reason correlate well with the severity of retinal vasculopathy rather than choroidal involvement.

Treatment

The decision to start treatment is based on ERG abnormalities, which can be reversed by early treatment (i.e. before reduction of visual acuity). Although good response may be achieved with systemic steroids optimal treatment may involve a steroid-sparing agent such as azathioprine or mycophenolate mofetil. Discontinuation of therapy should not be attempted while ERG abnormalities are still present as this will lead to deterioration. Periocular steroids are useful for treatment of CMO but do not seem to offer the same level of benefit for global retinal function.

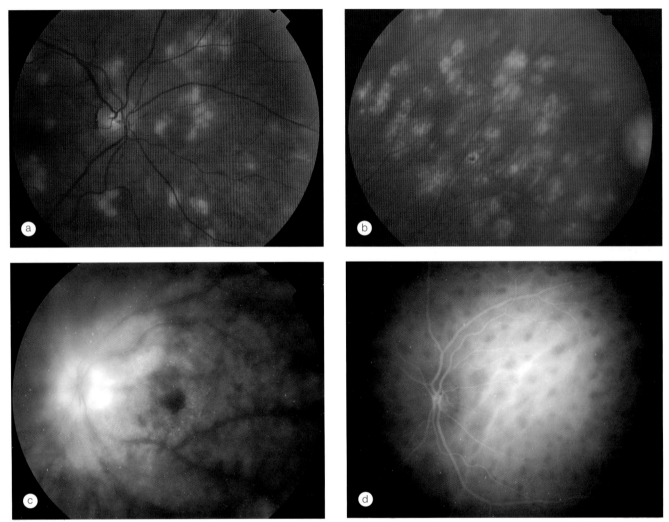

Fig. 14.54
Birdshot chorioretinopathy. **(a)** Active stage; **(b)** inactive lesions; **(c)** late phase fluorescein angiogram shows disc hyperfluorescence and cystoid macular oedema; **(d)** early phase indocyanine green angiogram shows numerous hypofluorescent lesions (Courtesy of C Pavesio – fig. c; P Gilli – fig. d)

Prognosis

The prognosis is guarded. About 20% of patients have a self limited course and maintain normal visual acuity at least in one eye. The remainder has variable impairment of visual acuity in one or both eyes, with approximately 40% reaching levels of 6/60 after 10 years of follow-up as a result of maculopathy (CMO, pucker, CNV) or progressive retinal degeneration.

NB The introduction of early therapy based on ERG findings may significantly impact on the prognosis of this condition.

Punctate inner choroidopathy

Punctate inner choroidopathy (PIC) is an uncommon idiopathic disease which typically affects young myopic women. Both eyes are frequently involved but not simultaneously.

Diagnosis

1. **Presentation** is with blurring of central vision or paracentral scotomas which may be associated with photopsia.
2. **Signs**
   - Absent or minimal intraocular inflammation.

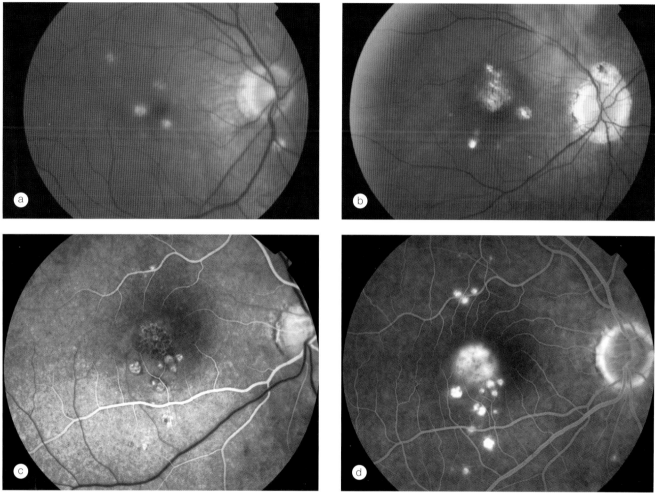

Fig. 14.55
Punctate inner choroidopathy. **(a)** Active stage; **(b)** inactive disease; **(c)** FA arterial phase shows several hyperfluorescent spots with hypofluorescent edges inferior to the fovea and mild lacy hyperfluorescence at the fovea due to choroidal neovascularization; **(d)** late phase shows more hyperfluorescent spots and intense hyperfluorescence at the fovea due to leakage from choroidal neovascularization (Courtesy of M Westcott – figs c and d)

- Multiple, small, yellow-white spots with fuzzy borders at the level of the inner choroid. The lesions are all of the same age and principally involve the posterior pole (Fig. 14.55a).
- Plentiful lesions occasionally may be associated with an overlying serous sensory retinal detachment which often resolves spontaneously.
- Large visual field defects probably caused by acute damage to retinal receptors.
- After a few weeks the acute lesions resolve leaving sharply demarcated atrophic scars which may subsequently become pigmented (Fig. 14.55b).
- CNV (type 2 – under the sensory retina) develops in up to 40% of patients.

- After a variable period of time the fellow eye frequently becomes similarly involved.
3. **FA** of PIC lesions shows early hyperfluorescence and late staining. It is of particular value in detecting CNV (Fig. 14.55c and d).
4. **ERG** is normal.

Treatment of CNV

1. **Argon laser photocoagulation,** usually under steroid cover, for extrafoveal CNV – particularly if there is evidence of progression towards the fovea.
2. **Systemic steroids** may be used for subfoveal CNV in order to reduce subretinal vascular leakage but the

response is unpredictable for CNV larger than 200μm in diameter.

3. **Photodynamic therapy** (PDT), also under steroid cover, may be considered in cases that have failed to respond to oral steroids.

4. **Surgical excision** of subfoveal CNV may be appropriate in selected cases, taking into account the timing of surgery and location of the membrane. Surgery is usually not indicated for CNV of less than 3 months duration, especially in the presence of good visual acuity, since spontaneous resolution may occur. However, if treatment is delayed too long, fibrosis will develop and surgery will not be beneficial. Unfortunately, recurrences are common, restricting long-term visual outcome.

Prognosis

The prognosis is guarded because central vision may become compromised by either foveal involvement by a lesion or CNV, which usually occurs within the first year of presentation. Subfoveal CNV may undergo spontaneous involution, with or without recovery of central vision. Small, well-defined subfoveal areas of CNV carry a reasonable prognosis and many patients retain a visual acuity of 6/18 or better.

Differential diagnosis

1. **Multifocal choroiditis and panuveitis** is characterized by similar lesions when they affect the posterior pole and in contrast to PIC is associated with intraocular inflammation and involvement of the peripheral fundus.

2. **POHS** is characterized by punched-out chorioretinal scars, CNV and absence of intraocular inflammation. However, there is also peripapillary atrophy as well as linear peripheral streaks and peripheral lesions.

3. **Myopic maculopathy** may have similar macular changes, CNV and absence of intraocular inflammation. However, the severity of myopic changes may be greater with the presence of more extensive degenerative changes. Axial length of the eye and refraction will establish the diagnosis.

Serpiginous choroidopathy

Serpiginous choroidopathy (SC) is an uncommon, chronic, recurrent disease which is usually bilateral but the extent of involvement is frequently asymmetrical. It affects individuals in the fourth to sixth decades of life. It affects men more than women and is associated with HLA-B7. SC has a chronic, recurrent evolution, which is variable between individuals and may remain inactive for months or years.

1. **Presentation** is with unilateral blurring of central vision, scotoma or metamorphopsia as a result of macular involvement. After a variable period of time the fellow eye is also affected, although it is not uncommon to find evidence of inactive asymptomatic disease in one eye at presentation.

2. **Signs**
   - Mild vitritis is present in up to 50% of eyes and mild anterior uveitis may occur.
   - Active lesions are grey-white to yellow in appearance located at the level of the RPE or inner choroid (Fig. 14.56a).
   - They develop first around the optic disc and then gradually spread in a serpentine manner towards the macula and peripheral fundus.
   - The course lasts many years in an episodic and recurrent fashion, and disease activity may recur after several months of remission.
   - Recurrences are characterized by yellow-grey extensions, contiguous or as satellites to existing areas of chorioretinal atrophy.
   - Inactive lesions are characterized by scalloped, atrophic, 'punched-out' areas of choroidal and RPE atrophy (Fig. 14.56b).
   - Uncommon complications include subretinal fibrosis and CNV.

3. **FA** of active lesions shows early hypofluorescence due to non-perfusion of the choriocapillaris (Fig. 14.56c) and late hyperfluorescence due to staining (Fig. 14.56d).

4. **ICG** of active lesions reveals marked hypofluorescence throughout all phases of the angiogram. It may also show localized areas of hyperfluorescence outside these areas that do not correspond to clinically visible changes, which might represent areas of subclinical involvement.

5. **ERG** may be abnormal in eyes with extensive retinal damage.

6. **Treatment.** Currently there is no definitive treatment strategy although long-term immunosuppression may prolong remission. Options include triple therapy with systemic steroids, azathioprine and ciclosporin, although early monotherapy with ciclosporin may be adequate.

7. **Prognosis** is poor and 50–75% of patients will eventually develop visual loss in one or both eyes despite treatment. Loss of vision can be caused by either macular involvement by the disease or secondary CNV. The latter develops in about 25% of cases and may be amenable to argon laser photocoagulation, PDT or intravitreal injection of triamcinolone.

Multifocal choroiditis with panuveitis

Multifocal choroiditis with panuveitis (MCP) is an uncommon, usually bilateral, chronic recurrent, frequently asymmetrical disease. The disease typically affects individuals in the third and fourth decades of life; predominantly myopic females.

1. **Presentation** is usually with blurring of central vision which may be associated with floaters and photopsia.

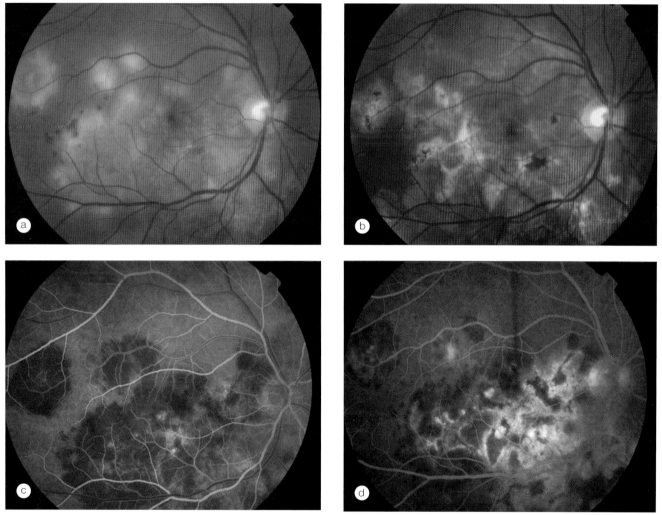

Fig. 14.56
Serpiginous choroidopathy. **(a)** Active stage; **(b)** inactive disease; **(c)** FA early venous phase in active disease shows hypofluorescence of the spots and lacy hyperfluorescence at the fovea due to choroidal neovascularization; **(d)** late phase shows hyperfluorescence at the fovea due to leakage from choroidal neovascularization (Courtesy of C Pavesio)

2. Signs
- Vitritis of variable intensity is universal and anterior uveitis is present in 50% of cases.
- Bilateral, multiple, discrete, round or ovoid, yellowish-gray lesions located at the level of the RPE and choriocapillaris.
- The lesions involve the posterior pole and/or periphery and may be arranged in clumps or linear streaks (Schlagel lines) (Fig. 14.57a).
- Occasionally, in older patients, the lesions are confined to the periphery.
- Peripapillary atrophy may be present.
- Mild disc oedema and blind spot enlargement may be present.
- CMO affects more than 40% of patients with prolonged disease.

- Inactive lesions have sharp 'punched-out' margins and pigmented borders resembling POHS (Fig. 14.57b).
- The course is prolonged with the development of new lesions and recurrent inflammatory episodes.
- Subretinal fibrosis is uncommon.

3. FA of active lesions shows early hypofluorescence due to blockage and late hyperfluorescence due to staining. Old inactive lesions show RPE window defects.

4. ICG shows hypofluorescent acute lesions which may not be clinically apparent. Old lesions remain hypofluorescent throughout and correspond to atrophic chorioretinal scars seen on fundus examination.

5. ERG remains normal until there is advanced retinal atrophy and substantial mid-peripheral field loss, at which time visual loss may be irreversible. Multifocal ERG shows moderate to severe depression of retinal function.

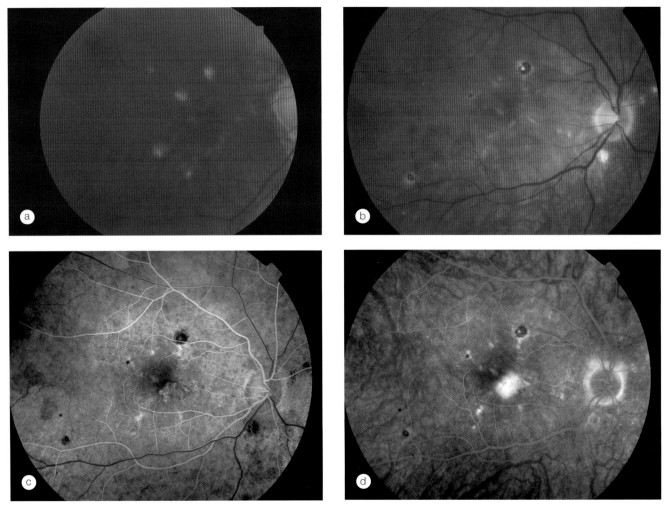

Fig. 14.57
Multifocal choroiditis with uveitis. **(a)** Active disease in which some small lesions form a linear streak (Schlagel line); **(b)** inactive lesions; **(c)** early venous phase fluorescein angiogram shows variable hypo- and hyperfluorescence of the lesions and lacy hyperfluorescence at the fovea associated with choroidal neovascularization; **(d)** late phase shows hyperfluorescence at the fovea due to leakage from choroidal neovascularization (Courtesy of Moorfields Eye Hospital)

6. **Large visual field defects** may appear acutely and are not explained on the basis of fundus abnormalities.
7. **Treatment** with systemic and periocular steroids is effective when administered early. Steroid-resistant patients require immunosuppressive therapy. Eyes with CNV (Fig. 14.57c and d) may require argon laser photocoagulation or PDT, preferably under steroid cover.
8. **Prognosis** is variable because the disease has a wide spectrum varying between those with few lesions and short periods of activity to patients with progressive scarring and visual loss due to maculopathy or diffuse subretinal fibrosis.
9. **Differential diagnosis**
   a. Sarcoidosis may also present as multifocal choroiditis

and panuveitis. However, the lesions are usually more numerous in the inferior fundus and CNV is less common.
   b. PIC is also characterized by multifocal choroidal lesions affecting the posterior pole and CNV. However, there is absence of intraocular inflammation.

Progressive subretinal fibrosis and uveitis syndrome

Progressive subretinal fibrosis and uveitis syndrome is a rare, idiopathic, chronic, bilateral condition which typically affects healthy young women who are frequently myopic.

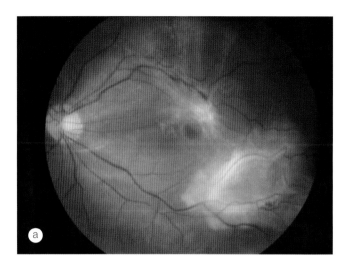

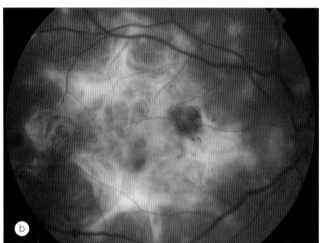

Fig. 14.58
Subretinal fibrosis. **(a)** Early involvement; **(b)** advanced disease

1. **Presentation** is with gradual unilateral blurring of vision although both eyes are usually eventually involved.
2. **Signs**
   • Mild anterior uveitis and vitritis.
   • Yellow, indistinct subretinal lesions which coalesce into dirty-yellow mounds at the posterior pole and midperiphery (Fig. 14.58a).
   • Eventually large areas of subretinal fibrosis develop (Fig. 14.58b).
3. **FA** reveals normal retinal and choroidal filling, early mottled hyperfluorescence and window defects with late hyperfluorescence along the edges of the lesions.
4. **ERG** may be decreased.
5. **Treatment** with non-steroidal immunosuppressive agents may be beneficial. Systemic steroids are usually not effective once the fibrotic process is established but may be useful in the treatment of recurrences, CNV and CMO.
6. **Prognosis.** The course is prolonged and recurrences common, with poor visual prognosis.

7. **Differential diagnosis.** The late stage has similar appearance to serpiginous choroidopathy and disciform age-related macular degeneration.

Multiple evanescent white dot syndrome

Multiple evanescent white dot syndrome (MEWDS) is an uncommon, idiopathic, usually unilateral, self-limiting disease which typically affects individuals between the ages of 20 and 40 years, particularly females. About one-third of patients have a preceding viral-like illness. MEWDS may form part of a spectrum of disease that includes acute idiopathic blind spot enlargement, acute zonal occult outer retinopathy and acute macular neuroretinopathy (see below).

NB Although uncommon, it is important to be aware of MEWDS because the subtle signs may be overlooked and a misdiagnosis made of a more serious disorder such as retrobulbar neuritis.

1. **Presentation** is with sudden onset decreased vision or paracentral scotomas which may be associated with photopsia, typically affecting the temporal visual field.
2. **Signs**
   • Mild afferent pupillary defect.
   • Mild vitritis.
   • Numerous, very small, ill-defined, white dots at the level of the outer retina and inner choroid involving the posterior pole and mid-periphery (Fig. 14.59a).
   • The macula is spared but has a granular appearance which renders the foveal reflex abnormal or absent.
   • Optic disc oedema and enlargement of the physiological blind spot.
   • Over several weeks to months the dots and disc oedema fade and central vision returns to normal or near normal levels. However, the foveal granularity may remain (Fig. 14.59b) and blind spot enlargement may take much longer to diminish in size.
3. **FA** shows subtle punctate hyperfluorescence, some of which may form a cluster or 'wreath-shaped' pattern (Fig. 14.59c).
4. **ICG** shows more numerous hypofluorescent spots than are apparent clinically or on FA (Fig. 14.59d). Peripapillary non-perfusion, as demonstrated by fluorescein and ICG angiography, explains the enlarged blind spot.
5. **ERG** shows a decrease in a-wave amplitude which returns to a normal pattern within a few weeks.
6. **Prognosis** is excellent and treatment not appropriate. The course is short with resolution of visual symptoms over several weeks, although occasionally photopsia may persist. Relapses occur in about 10% of cases and a very small minority of eyes develops chorioretinal scarring or CNV.

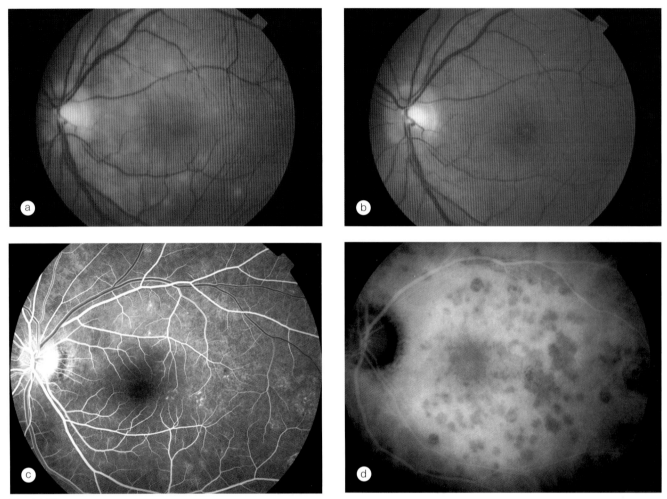

Fig. 14.59
Multiple evanescent white dot syndrome. **(a)** Active lesions; **(b)** residual foveal granularity; **(c)** FA arteriovenous phase of active lesions shows subtle hyperfluorescent spots; **(d)** ICG shows hypofluorescent spots which are more numerous than on FA (Courtesy of S Milewski – figs a and b; Moorfields Eye Hospital – figs c and d)

Acute idiopathic blind spot enlargement syndrome

Acute idiopathic blind spot enlargement syndrome is a rare condition which seems to exclusively affect women between the third and sixth decades of life. It shares common features with MEWDS and perhaps represents a different form of the same disease. It was first described as a neuro-ophthalmological condition in young patients, with enlarged blind spots and photopsia. However, further studies suggested a retinal origin for the enlarged blind spots.

1. **Presentation** is with photopsia and decreased vision, which may be misdiagnosed as migraine or optic neuritis.

Occasionally photopsia may precede visual loss by several weeks.

2. **Signs**
   - Visual acuity may be normal or reduced.
   - Afferent pupillary defect may be present.
   - Blind spot enlargement with steep margins but variable size is universal showing a clustering of lesions around the optic nerve.
   - Mild disc swelling or hyperaemia with peripapillary subretinal pigmentary changes in 50% of cases.

3. **FA** may show late staining of the optic nerve head.

4. **Prognosis** is good. Visual acuity improves spontaneously but blind spot enlargement may persist. Recurrence may occur in the same or fellow eye.

MISCELLANEOUS ANTERIOR UVEITIS

Fuchs uveitis syndrome

Fuchs uveitis syndrome (FUS) or Fuchs heterochromic cyclitis is a chronic, non-granulomatous, anterior uveitis of insidious onset. It typically affects one eye of a young adult, although it can also occur during childhood. Bilateral simultaneous involvement occurs in about 5% of cases. Although FUS accounts for about 4% of all cases of uveitis, it is frequently misdiagnosed and over-treated. The heterochromia (difference in iris colour) may be absent or difficult to detect, particularly in brown-eyed individuals.

Diagnosis

The diagnosis is based on ocular signs, which in early cases may be subtle and easily overlooked.

1. **Presentation**
   - Chronic, annoying vitreous floaters is often the presenting symptom.
   - Gradual blurring of vision secondary to cataract formation is common.
   - Colour difference between the two eyes.
   - Incidental detection.
2. **General signs**
   - Absence of posterior synechiae, except following cataract surgery.
   - The keratic precipitates are characteristically small, round or stellate, grey-white in colour and scattered throughout the corneal endothelium and frequently associated with feathery fibrin filaments (Fig. 14.60a and b); they may come and go but never become confluent or pigmented.
   - Small, transparent nodules at the pupillary border (Fig. 14.60c) and stroma (Fig. 14.60d) are seen in 30% of cases.
   - Aqueous humour shows a faint flare and mild cellular reaction.
   - Vitritis and stringy opacities may be dense enough to reduce vision.
3. **Diffuse iris atrophy**
   - The earliest finding is loss of iris crypts.
   - Advanced stromal atrophy makes the affected iris appear dull with loss of detail giving rise to a washed-out appearance, particularly in the pupillary zone (see Fig. 14.60c). The normal radial iris blood vessels appear prominent due to lack of stromal support.
   - Posterior pigment layer iris atrophy is best detected by retroillumination (Fig. 14.60e).
   - Mydriasis resulting from atrophy of the pupillary sphincter may be present.

4. **Heterochromia iridis** is an important and common sign.
   - Most frequently the affected eye is hypochromic (Fig. 14.61).
   - It is easily seen in green eyes, but if the iris is blue or deep brown, heterochromia will be difficult to detect.
   - The nature of heterochromia is determined by the relative degrees of atrophy of the stroma and posterior pigment epithelium, as well as the patient's natural iris colour.
   - In blue eyes, predominant stromal atrophy allows the posterior pigmented layer to show through and become the dominant pigmentation, so that the eye may become hyperchromic (reverse heterochromia).
5. **Gonioscopy** may be normal or may show one of the following:
   - Fine radial twig-like vessels in the angle (see Fig. 14.60f) which are responsible for the filiform haemorrhages which develop on anterior chamber paracentesis (Amsler sign).
   - A membrane obscuring angle details.
   - Small, non-confluent, irregular, peripheral anterior synechiae.
6. **Systemic association.** Parry–Romberg syndrome (hemifacial atrophy) is found in a small minority of cases.

Complications

FUS runs a chronic course lasting many years with periods of increased activity. The two main complications are cataract and glaucoma, both of which may be enhanced by the inadvertent use of topical steroids.

1. **Cataract** is extremely common and is often the presenting feature (see Figs 14.60d and 14.61). It does not differ from that associated with other types of anterior uveitis. The results of surgery with posterior chamber intraocular lens implantation are good.
2. **Glaucoma** is a late manifestation which typically develops only after several years of follow-up. It is usually well controlled on topical therapy, but some patients may require trabeculectomy.

Treatment

1. **Posterior sub-Tenon** injections of a long-acting steroid preparation such as triamcinolone acetonide may be beneficial for troublesome vitreous floaters, although improvement is usually temporary.
2. **Vitrectomy** may be considered for severe vitreous opacification that is reducing vision or is very disturbing.

NB Topical steroids are ineffective and mydriatics unnecessary because of lack of posterior synechiae.

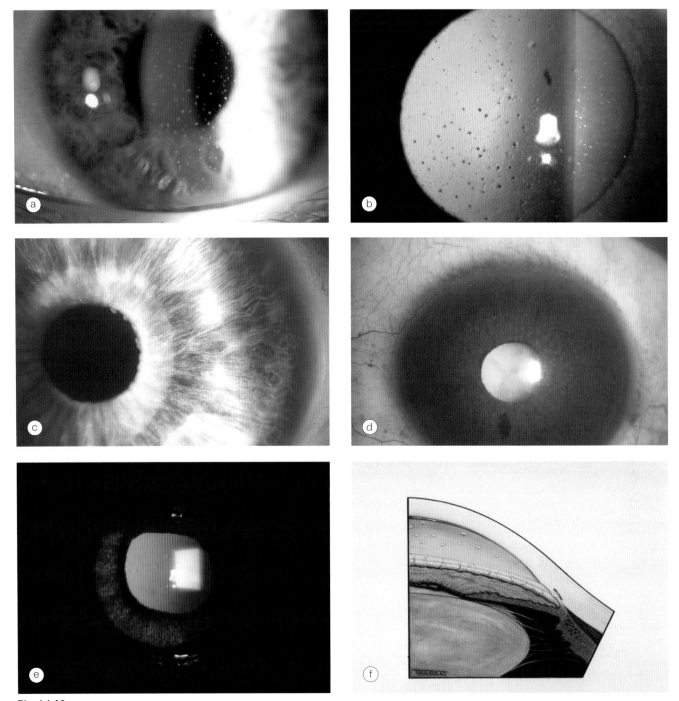

Fig. 14.60
Fuchs uveitis syndrome. **(a)** and **(b)** Keratic precipitates; **(c)** stromal iris atrophy rendering the sphincter pupillae prominent and small pupillary nodules; **(d)** stromal nodules and mature cataract; **(e)** posterior pigment layer atrophy seen on retroillumination; **(f)** angle vessels (Courtesy of C Pavesio – figs b and d)

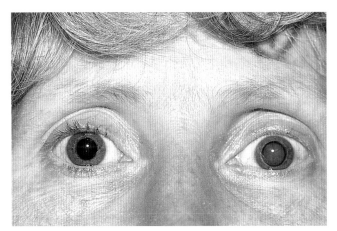

Fig. 14.61
Heterochromia iridis and mature left cataract in Fuchs uveitis syndrome

Other causes of heterochromia iridis

1. **Hypochromic**
   - Congenital.
   - Horner syndrome, particularly if congenital.
2. **Hyperchromic**
   - Oculodermal melanocytosis (naevus of Ota).
   - Ocular siderosis.
   - Diffuse iris naevus or melanoma.
   - Unilateral use of a topical prostaglandin analogue for glaucoma.
   - Sturge–Weber syndrome (rare).

Lens-induced uveitis

Lens-induced uveitis is triggered by an immune response to lens proteins following rupture of the lens capsule which may be due to trauma or incomplete cataract extraction (Fig. 14.62).

Phacoanaphylactic endophthalmitis

1. **Presentation** is with abrupt reduction in visual acuity and pain, which is less severe than in bacterial endophthalmitis, days to weeks after rupture of the lens capsule.
2. **Signs**
   - Anterior uveitis is granulomatous and of variable severity.
   - The IOP is frequently high.
   - The posterior segment is not involved.
3. **Differential diagnosis** is bacterial endophthalmitis; in doubtful cases vitreous taps may be required.

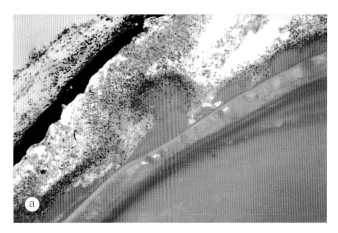

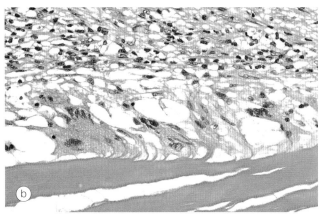

Fig. 14.62
Lens-induced uveitis. **(a)** Escaping lens material producing an inflammatory reaction; **(b)** giant cells in relation to extracapsular material (Courtesy of J Harry and G Misson, from *Clinical Ophthalmic Pathology*, Butterworth-Heinemann, 2001)

4. **Treatment** involves removal of all lens material in conjunction with intensive steroid therapy.

Phacogenic non-granulomatous uveitis

1. **Signs.** Anterior uveitis is less severe and more chronic than in phacoanaphylactic endophthalmitis, and develops within 2–3 weeks after lens capsule rupture.
2. **Differential diagnosis** includes low-grade bacterial and fungal endophthalmitis, sympathetic ophthalmitis and IOL-induced inflammation.
3. **Treatment** of mild cases is with topical steroids but periocular and systemic therapy will be necessary for more intense inflammation. Removal of remaining lens material may also be necessary.

MISCELLANEOUS POSTERIOR UVEITIS

Acute retinal pigment epitheliitis

Acute retinal pigment epitheliitis is a rare, idiopathic, self-limiting inflammatory condition of the macular RPE. It typically affects young adults and although there is no treatment the visual prognosis is excellent. The condition is unilateral in 75% of cases.

1. **Presentation** is with sudden onset impairment of central vision which may be associated with metamorphopsia.
2. **Signs**
   - Absence of intraocular inflammation.
   - The fovea shows a blunted reflex with discrete clusters of a few, subtle, small and brown or grey spots at the level of the RPE which may be surrounded by hypopigmented yellow halos (Fig. 14.63a).
   - These lesions tend to appear 1–2 weeks after the onset of symptoms. The loss of visual function is out of proportion to clinical signs.
   - After 6–12 weeks the acute fundus lesions resolve and visual acuity returns to normal, although innocuous residual pigment clumping at the fovea may remain. Recurrences are uncommon.
3. **FA** may be normal or show small hyperfluorescent dots with hypofluorescent centres ('honeycomb' appearance) without leakage (Fig. 14.63b).
4. **EOG** is subnormal.

Acute macular neuroretinopathy

Acute macular neuroretinopathy is a rare, self-limiting condition that typically affects healthy females between the second and fourth decades of life. The disease may affect one or both eyes and may be preceded by a flu-like illness. Occasionally it may be associated with MEWDS and idiopathic blind spot enlargement syndrome, as well as the use intravenous iodine contrast agents, oral contraceptives and trauma.

1. **Presentation** is with sudden decrease of visual acuity and paracentral scotomas.
2. **Signs**
   - Absence of intraocular inflammation.
   - Darkish, brown-red, wedge-shaped lesions in a flower petal arrangement around the centre of the macula (Fig. 14.64).
   - Amsler grid and perimetry reveal remarkable correspondence of the lesions with the shape and location of the scotoma.
   - Within several months visual symptoms gradually improve and the lesions fade but do not completely resolve for many years. Recurrences are uncommon.

Acute idiopathic maculopathy

Acute idiopathic maculopathy is a very rare, self-limiting condition which typically affects young adults. It is most frequently unilateral and may be preceded by a flu-like illness.

1. **Presentation** is with a unilateral sudden and severe loss of vision with the presence of a central scotoma.

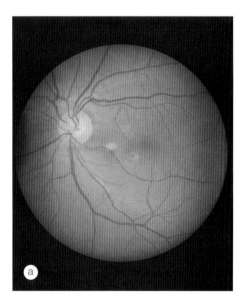
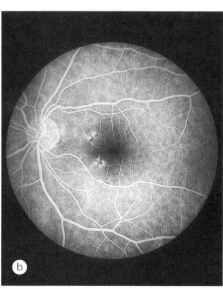

Fig. 14.63
(a) Acute retinal pigment epitheliitis;
(b) FA venous phase shows corresponding focal hyperfluorescence
(Courtesy of M Prost)

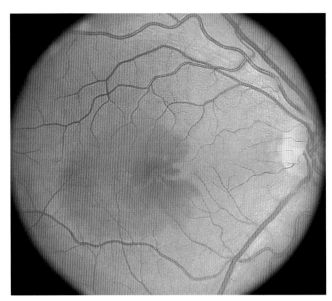

Fig. 14.64
Acute macular neuroretinopathy (Courtesy of J Donald M Gass from *Stereoscopic Atlas of Macular Disease*, Mosby, 1997)

2. Signs
- Detachment of the sensory retina at the macula with an irregular outline (Fig. 14.65a).
- Smaller, greyish subretinal thickening at the level of the RPE beneath the detachment is frequently present.
- Iritis, papillitis and mild vitritis may be present.
- Within a few weeks the exudative changes resolve with nearly complete recovery of vision. Innocuous residual RPE atrophic changes which may have a 'bull's eye' pattern remain.

3. FA
- Early phase shows minimal subretinal hypo-fluorescence and hyperfluorescence beneath the sensory retinal detachment (Fig. 14.65b).
- The mid-venous phases show two levels of hyper-fluorescence, one from staining of the subretinal thickening at the level of the RPE, and the second from pooling of dye within the subretinal space (Fig. 14.65c).
- The late phase shows complete staining of the overlying sensory retinal detachment (Fig. 14.65d).

Acute multifocal retinitis

Acute multifocal retinitis is a very rare, frequently bilateral, self-limiting condition that typically affects healthy, young-to-middle aged adults. It may be preceded by a flu-like illness, usually 1–2 weeks before the onset of the visual symptoms. It has been postulated by some that acute multifocal retinitis may be an unusual presentation of cat-scratch disease.

1. Presentation is with sudden onset of mild visual loss.
2. Signs
- Bilateral, multiple areas of retinitis posterior to the equator (Fig. 14.66).
- Mild vitritis and disc oedema are frequent.
- A macular star is present in a few cases.
- Small retinal branch artery occlusions occur in a minority.
- After 2–4 months the fundus lesions resolve and vision recovers.

Solitary idiopathic choroiditis

Solitary idiopathic choroiditis is a distinct clinical entity that may give rise to diagnostic problems as it may simulate other pathology.

1. Presentation is with mild visual loss and floaters.
2. Signs
- Vitritis is present during active disease.
- Discrete, post-equatorial, dull-yellow, choroidal elevation with ill-defined margins.
- Associated findings include adjacent subretinal fluid and a macular star figure.
- As the inflammation resolves the lesion develops a better defined margin with resolution of subretinal fluid and exudation (Fig. 14.67).
- Occasional features include retinal vascular dilatation and focal retinal haemorrhages.

NB The lesions tend to be small so ultrasonography is of little diagnostic value.

3. Treatment of active, vision-threatening lesions is with systemic steroids. Most inactive lesions either remain stable or resolve without treatment.
4. Differential diagnosis includes inflammatory lesions (sarcoidosis, tuberculosis, nodular posterior scleritis and syphilis) and amelanotic tumours (amelanotic melanoma, metastasis and circumscribed choroidal haemangioma).

Frosted branch angiitis

Frosted branch angiitis (FBA) describes a characteristic fundus picture, usually bilateral, which may represent a specific syndrome (primary form) or a common immune pathway in response to multiple infective agents. Secondary FBA may be associated with infectious retinitis, most notably cytomegalovirus retinitis, but it may also occur in association with other conditions such as glomerulonephritis and central retinal vein occlusion. Primary FBA is rare and typically affects children and young adults.

1. Presentation is with a subacute bilateral visual loss, floaters or photopsia.

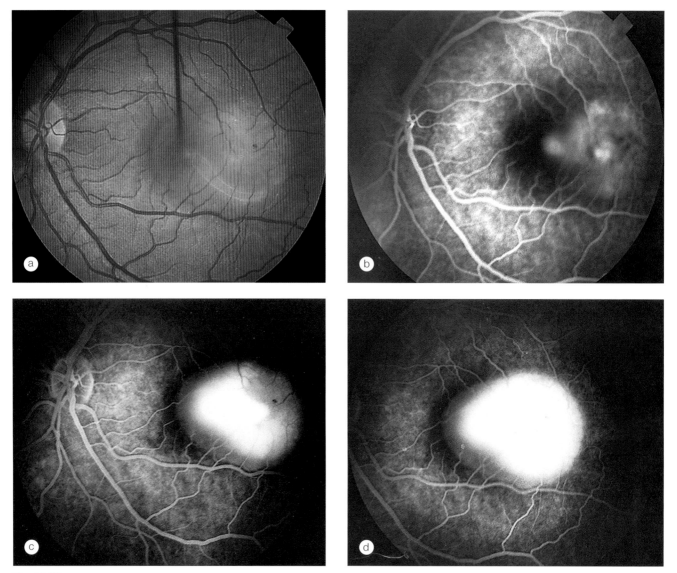

Fig. 14.65
Acute idiopathic maculopathy. **(a)** Detachment of the sensory retina at the macula with an irregular outline; **(b)** FA early phase shows minimal subretinal hypofluorescence and hyperfluorescence; **(c)** mid-venous phases show two levels of hyperfluorescence; **(d)** late phase shows complete staining of the overlying sensory retinal detachment (Courtesy of S Milewski)

2. Signs
- Visual acuity is usually very poor.
- Florid translucent retinal perivascular sheathing of both arterioles and venules (Fig. 14.68a).
- Anterior uveitis, vitritis and retinal oedema are common.
- Uncommon findings include papillitis, hard exudates, retinal haemorrhages and venous occlusion (Fig. 14.68b).

3. Treatment is with systemic and topical steroids, but the optimal regimen has not been established. The primary form has a good visual prognosis but significant visual loss may result in secondary forms.

Acute zonal occult outer retinopathy (AZOOR)

The acute zonal outer retinopathies (AZOR) are a group of very rare, idiopathic syndromes characterized by acute onset of loss of one or more zones of visual field caused by damage to the retinal receptor elements. Although AZOR is a rare condition it is important to be aware of its existence to save the patient inappropriate and unrewarding medical and neurological investigations.

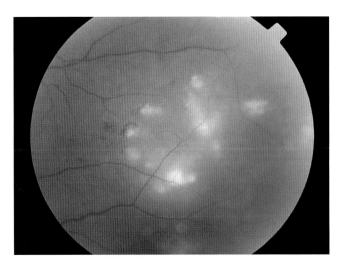

Fig. 14.66
Acute multifocal retinitis (Courtesy of S Milewski)

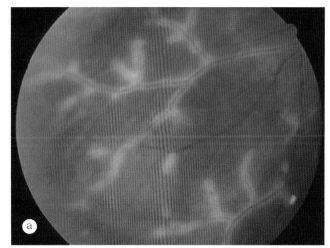

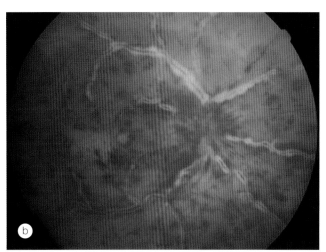

Fig. 14.68
Frosted branch angiitis. **(a)** Perivascular sheathing; **(b)** secondary venous occlusion (Courtesy of C Barry – fig. b)

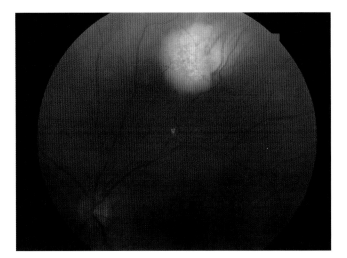

Fig. 14.67
Solitary idiopathic choroiditis

AZOOR is the most common of the AZOR syndromes. It typically affects healthy, young, frequently myopic women, some of whom have an antecedent viral-like illness. Although autoimmunity has been implicated, there are several factors that suggest that AZOOR is probably not primarily an autoimmune disease – asymmetric nature of retinal involvement, lack of improvement with steroids and difficulty in detecting circulating retinal antibodies.

1. **Presentation** is with acute loss affecting one or more zones of the visual field, which is frequently associated with photopsia. The temporal field is frequently involved but the central field is usually spared; bilateral involvement occurs in 50% of patients.
2. **Signs** in chronological order.
   - Normal fundus.

- After several weeks there may be mild vitritis, attenuation of retinal vessels in the affected zone and occasionally periphlebitis, particularly in patients with large visual field defects.
- The zones may enlarge, or less frequently they remain the same or improve.
- In 50% of cases visual field loss stabilizes within 4–6 months.
- Late findings are characterized by RPE clumping and arteriolar narrowing in the involved area (Fig. 14.69) although if the retinal cells survive the fundus remains normal.

3. **Perimetry** should include both peripheral and central visual fields because large peripheral zones of visual field loss may go undetected if only central fields are tested. Visual field loss does not correlate with retinal findings.

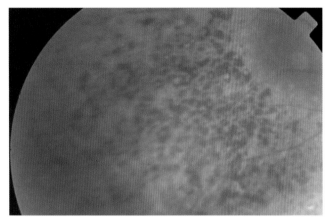

Fig. 14.69
Retinal pigment epithelial changes in acute zonal occult outer retinopathy (Courtesy of C Pavesio)

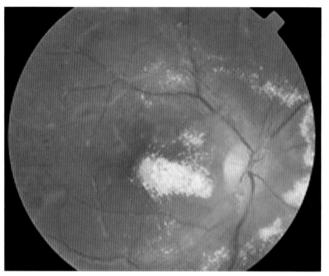

Fig. 14.70
Idiopathic retinal vasculitis, aneurysms and neuroretinitis syndrome (Courtesy of A Abu El-Asrar)

4. **ERG** characteristically shows a-wave and b-wave amplitude reduction and delayed 30Hz flicker.
5. **EOG** shows absence or severe reduction of the light rise.
6. **Prognosis** is good with a final visual acuity of 6/12 in at least one eye in 85% of cases. A recurrence rate of 25% to the affected eye and delayed involvement of the fellow eye may occur.

Idiopathic retinal vasculitis, aneurysms and neuroretinitis syndrome

Idiopathic retinal vasculitis, aneurysms and neuroretinitis syndrome is a rare entity that most frequently affects healthy young women.

1. **Signs**
   - Multiple, leaking, tied-knot-like aneurysmal dilatations along the retinal arteriolar tree that give rise to exudation and macular oedema (Fig. 14.70).
   - Neuroretinitis.
   - Extensive peripheral capillary non-perfusion.
   - The aneurysms may increase in number and leak and then some may spontaneously regress.
2. **Treatment** by laser photocoagulation may be beneficial in eyes with extensive peripheral ischaemia and retinal neovascularization.

15

OCULAR TUMOURS AND RELATED CONDITIONS

BENIGN CONJUNCTIVAL TUMOURS

Naevus

A conjunctival naevus is a relatively uncommon, benign, usually unilateral lesion.

1. **Histology** is similar to cutaneous naevi except that there is no dermis so that subepithelial or stromal replaces dermal in the nomenclature.
   a. *Junctional naevi* are characterized by nests of naevus cells at the epithelial–subepithelial junction (Fig. 15.1a).
   b. *Compound* naevi are characterized by naevus cells at the epithelial–subepithelial junction and within the subepithelial stroma, with downward proliferation of surface epithelium containing goblet cells (Fig. 15.1b). They are more common than junctional naevi.
2. **Presentation** is usually during the first two decades of life with either ocular irritation or a pigmented lesion.
3. **Signs**
   - Solitary, sharply demarcated, flat or slightly elevated, pigmented, intraepithelial bulbar lesion, most frequently in the juxtalimbal area (Fig. 15.1c).
   - The extent of pigmentation is variable and some may be virtually non-pigmented (Fig. 15.1d).
   - Cystic spaces within the naevus are frequent (Fig. 15.1e).
   - The second most common location is the plica and caruncle (Fig. 15.1f).
   - In children and adolescents, a conjunctival naevus may appear inflamed, with dilated feeder vessels.
   - Around puberty the naevus may enlarge and become more pigmented.
4. **Signs of potential malignancy**
   - An unusual site such as palpebral or forniceal conjunctiva.
   - Extension onto the cornea.
   - Sudden increase in pigmentation or growth.
   - Development of vascularity except in a child.
5. **Treatment** is by excision and is indicated mainly for cosmetic reasons. Less common indications include irritation and suspicion of malignant transformation.

Papilloma

Pedunculated

Pedunculated papillomas are caused by infection with human papillomavirus which may occur by mother-to-infant transmission at birth through an infected vagina.

1. **Histology** shows a fibrovascular core covered by irregular proliferation of non-keratinized, stratified squamous epithelium containing goblet cells (Fig. 15.2a).
2. **Presentation** may be at any age.
3. **Signs.** The papillomas, which may be multiple and occasionally bilateral, are most frequently located in the juxtalimbal area (Fig. 15.2b), caruncle (Fig. 15.2c) or fornix (Fig. 15.2d).
4. **Treatment** of small lesions may not be required because they often resolve spontaneously. Large lesions are treated by excision biopsy or cryotherapy. Treatment options for recurrences include subconjunctival alpha-interferon, topical mitomycin C or oral cimetidine (Tagamet).

Sessile papilloma

Sessile (neoplastic) papilloma is not infectious.

1. **Presentation** is usually in middle-age.
2. **Signs.** The lesion is unilateral and most frequent on the bulbar (Fig. 15.2e) and juxtalimbal area (Fig. 15.2f).
3. **Treatment** is by excision.

Epibulbar choristoma

A choristoma is a congenital overgrowth of normal tissue in an abnormal location. There are two main types: (a) *solid dermoid* and (b) *dermolipoma*.

Solid dermoid

1. **Histology** shows a mass of collagen containing dermal elements covered by stratified squamous epithelium.
2. **Presentation** is in early childhood.
3. **Signs**
   - Smooth, soft, yellowish, subconjunctival masses most frequently located at the infero-temporal limbus (Fig. 15.3a).
   - Occasionally the lesions are large and may virtually encircle the limbus (complex choristoma – Fig. 15.3b).
4. **Treatment** is indicated for cosmetic reasons, chronic irritation, dellen formation and involvement of the visual axis. Small lesions can be excised although the removal of large lesions may require lamellar corneal or scleral grafting.
5. **Systemic associations** include Goldenhar syndrome (Fig. 15.3c), and less commonly Treacher Collins syndrome and naevus sebaceus of Jadassohn.

Dermolipoma

Dermolipomas are similar to solid dermoids but contain fatty tissue.

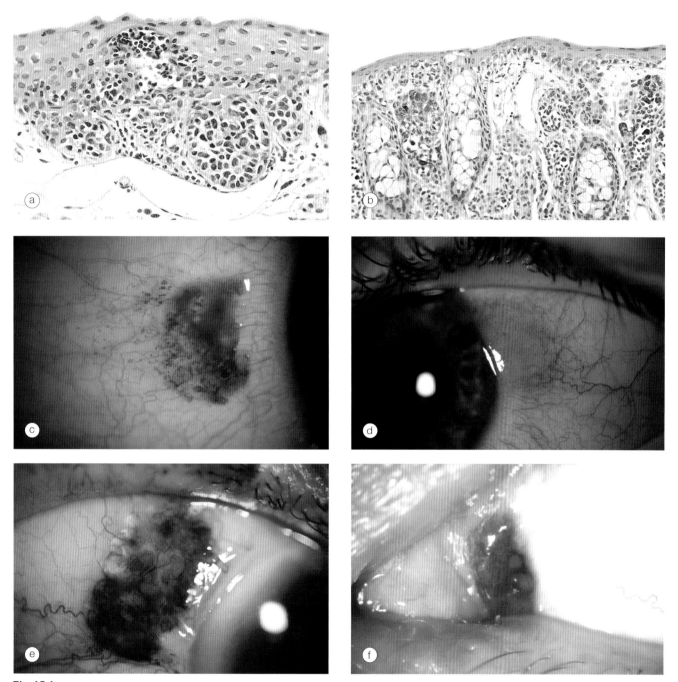

Fig. 15.1
Conjunctival naevus. **(a)** Histology of a junctional naevus shows nests of naevus cells at the epithelial–subepithelial junction; **(b)** histology of a compound naevus shows naevus cells at the epithelial–subepithelial junction and within the stroma, and downward proliferation of surface epithelium containing goblet cells (evident as clear spaces); **(c)** pigmented naevus; **(d)** non-pigmented naevus; **(e)** large naevus with cystic spaces; **(f)** naevus involving the plica (Courtesy of J Harry and G Misson, from *Clinical Ophthalmic Pathology*, Butterworth-Heinemann, 2001 – figs a and b; R Fogla – fig. c; B Damato – fig. f)

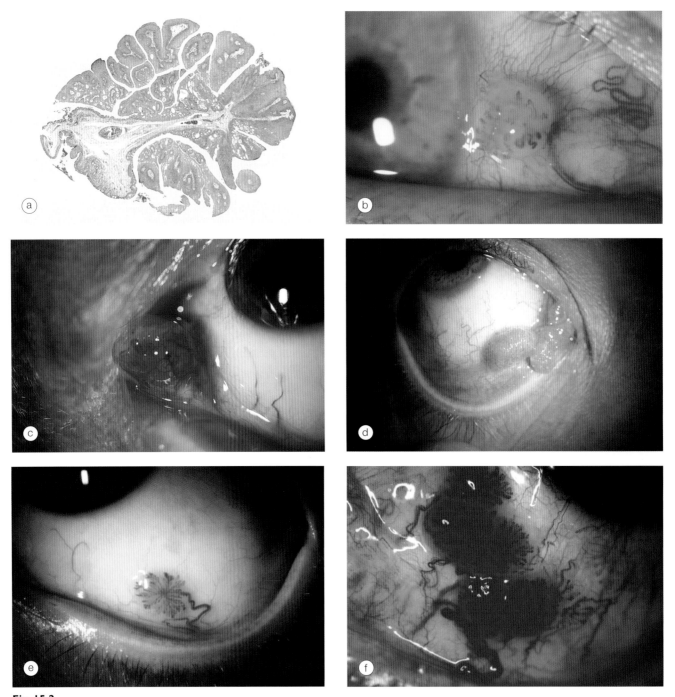

Fig. 15.2
Conjunctival papilloma. **(a)** Histology shows irregular proliferation of stratified squamous epithelium containing goblet cells overlying a fibrovascular core; **(b)** pedunculated papilloma at the limbus; **(c)** pedunculated papilloma at the caruncle; **(d)** multiple pedunculated papillomas; **(e)** small sessile papilloma; **(f)** multiple sessile papillomas (Courtesy of J Harry – fig. a; B Damato – fig. b)

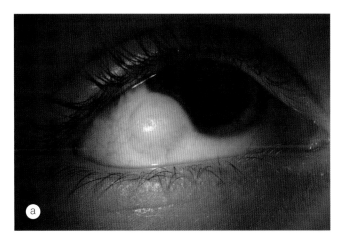

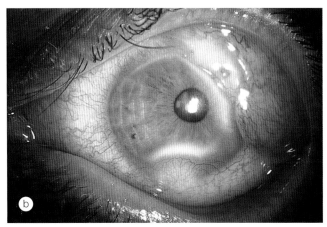

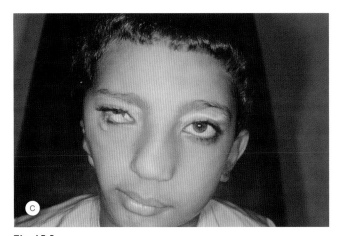

Fig. 15.3
Limbal dermoid. **(a)** Typical dermoid; **(b)** complex choristoma; **(c)** dermoids in a patient with Goldenhar syndrome (Courtesy of A Pearson – fig. a; U Raina – fig. c)

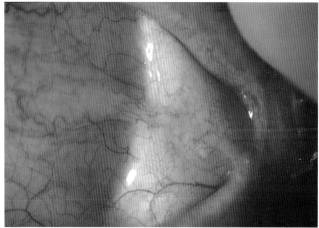

Fig. 15.4
Dermolipoma

1. **Presentation** is in adult life.
2. **Signs.** Soft, movable, subconjunctival mass most commonly located at the outer canthus (Fig. 15.4).
3. **Treatment** should be avoided because surgery may be complicated by scarring, ptosis, dry eye and ocular motility problems. However, if they are particularly unsightly, then debulking the anterior portion may improve cosmesis without compromising ocular motility.

Pyogenic granuloma

A pyogenic granuloma is a proliferation of granulation tissue that develops after procedures that involve conjunctival incisions such as pterygium excision, chalazia, placement of hydroxyapatite implant motility pegs and eye muscle surgery. Patients undergoing repeated surgery do not seem to be at increased risk for pyogenic granuloma formation, and the occurrence of a pyogenic granuloma does not increase the risk of developing pyogenic granulomas in future surgeries.

1. **Histology** is similar to that of cutaneous pyogenic granuloma (see Fig. 4.15a).
2. **Presentation** is frequently a few weeks after conjunctival surgery.
3. **Signs.** A fast growing, pink, fleshy, vascularized conjunctival mass near the conjunctival wound (Fig. 15.5).
4. **Treatment** with topical steroids is usually successful. Resistant cases require excision.
5. **Differential diagnosis** includes suture granuloma, Tenon granuloma or cyst, and a vascular tumour.

NB The term 'pyogenic granuloma' is a misnomer because the lesion is neither pyogenic nor granulomatous.

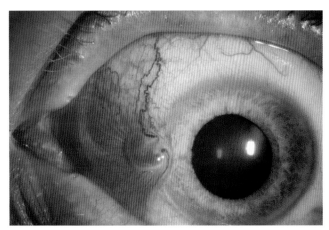

Fig. 15.5
Pyogenic granuloma (Courtesy of R Curtis)

MALIGNANT CONJUNCTIVAL TUMOURS

Primary acquired melanosis

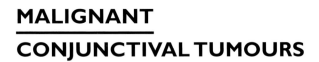

Primary acquired melanosis (PAM) is an uncommon unilateral condition which typically affects middle-aged Caucasians. The term primary acquired 'melanosis' is inaccurate because the lesion is characterized by proliferation of conjunctival epithelial melanocytes and not deposition of pigment – a more appropriate term is conjunctival melanocytic intraepithelial neoplasia.

Classification

There are two histological types:
1. **PAM without melanocytic cellular atypia** is a benign intraepithelial proliferation of epithelial melanocytes (Fig. 15.6a).
2. **PAM with melanocytic cellular atypia** has a 50% chance of developing infiltrating malignancy within 5 years. Intraepithelial melanocytes increase in number and exhibit pleomorphism. PAM with atypia, if severe, can be regarded as melanoma *in situ*.

Diagnosis

1. **Presentation** of PAM without atypia can be at any age, but PAM with atypia is usually seen after the age of 45 years.
2. **Signs**
   - Irregular, unifocal or multifocal areas of flat, brown pigmentation which may involve any part of the conjunctiva (Fig. 15.6b).

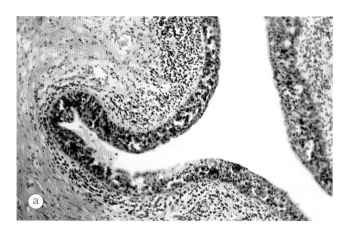

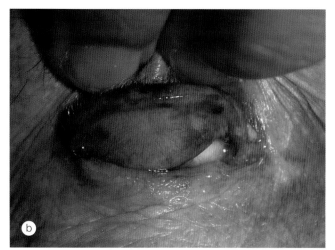

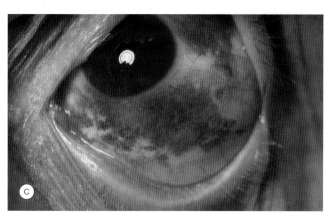

Fig. 15.6
Primary acquired melanosis (PAM). **(a)** Histology shows intraepithelial proliferation of conjunctival epithelial melanocytes; **(b)** small area of PAM associated with lentigo maligna of the lid margin; **(c)** large area of PAM (Courtesy of J Harry – fig. a; D Selva – fig. b; B Jay – fig. c)

- The lesions involve the epithelium and can therefore be moved over the surface of the globe.
- PAM may expand (Fig. 15.6c), shrink or remain stable for long periods of time. It may also lighten or darken focally.

NB Multiple biopsies assisted by immunohistochemistry are required for diagnosis because the clinical features of PAM with and without atypia are the same. A sign of malignant transformation of PAM to melanoma is the sudden appearance of one or more nodules in otherwise flat lesions (see Fig. 15.7b).

Treatment

1. **PAM without atypia** does not require treatment.
2. **PAM with atypia**
   • Small areas are treated by excision.
   • Larger areas that cannot be excised may be treated with cryotherapy or by topical application of mitomycin C.

Melanoma

Conjunctival melanoma accounts for about 2% of all ocular malignancies.

Histology

The histological features are similar to cutaneous melanoma and show sheets of melanoma cells within the subepithelial stroma (Fig. 15.7a).

Classification

1. **Melanoma arising from PAM with atypia** accounts for 75% of cases. It is characterized by the development of areas of thickening and nodularity (Fig. 15.7b).
2. **Melanoma arising from a pre-existing naevus** (junctional or compound) accounts for 20%.
3. **Primary melanoma** is the least common and will be considered below.

Diagnosis

1. **Presentation** is in the sixth decade except in patients with the rare dysplastic naevus syndrome, who develop multiple melanomas earlier.

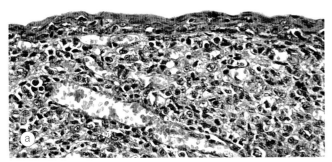
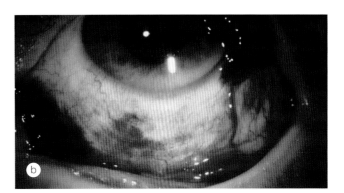
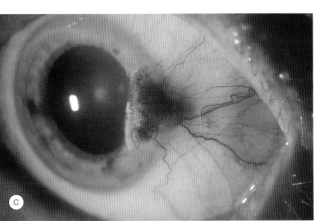
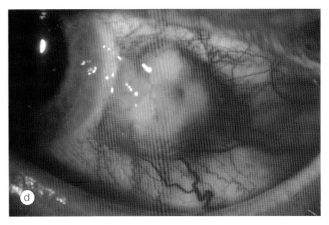

Fig. 15.7
Conjunctival melanoma. **(a)** Histology shows melanoma cells within the epithelium and subepithelial stroma; **(b)** multifocal melanoma arising from PAM; **(c)** pigmented melanoma; **(d)** amelanotic melanoma (Courtesy of J Harry – fig. a; B Damato – figs c and d)

2. Signs
- A common site is the limbus although the tumour may arise anywhere in the conjunctiva.
- A black or grey nodule containing dilated feeder vessels which may become fixed to the episclera (Fig. 15.7c).
- Amelanotic tumours are pink and have a characteristic, smooth, fish-flesh appearance (Fig. 15.7d).

Treatment

1. Circumscribed melanoma
- Surgical excision with a wide clearance and cryotherapy to prevent recurrence. It is vitally important not to touch normal conjunctiva with any instruments and swabs that have come into contact with the tumour, to avoid seeding.
- If histology reveals tumour extension to the deep surface of the specimen, adjunctive radiotherapy can be administered once the conjunctiva has healed. This usually consists of beta irradiation with a strontium applicator or ruthenium plaque. Proton beam radiotherapy can be useful for caruncular tumours. If there is diffuse superficial spread, adjunctive topical chemotherapy can be prescribed, once the conjunctival wound has healed.
- Re-examination of the patient is at 6–12-monthly intervals for life. At each visit the entire conjunctival surface is examined and any suspicious areas examined histologically by means of biopsy or impression cytology.

2. Diffuse melanoma
associated with PAM is treated by excision of localized nodules and cryotherapy or mitomycin C to the diffuse component.

3. Orbital recurrences
(Fig. 15.8) are treated by local resection and radiotherapy. Exenteration does not improve the survival rate and is therefore reserved for patients with extensive and aggressive disease that cannot be controlled by other methods.

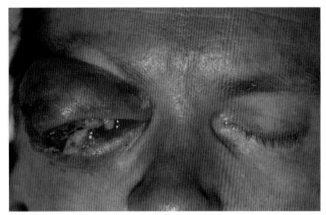

Fig. 15.8
Orbital recurrent melanoma

4. Lymph node involvement
is treated by surgical excision and radiotherapy.

5. Palliation
for metastatic disease is with chemotherapy or radiotherapy.

Prognosis

The overall mortality is about 12% at 5 years and 25% at 10 years. The main sites for metastases are regional lymph nodes, lung, brain and liver. Poor prognostic indicators include:
- Multifocal tumours.
- Extralimbal tumours involving the caruncle, fornix or palpebral conjunctiva.
- Tumour thickness of 2mm or more.
- Recurrence.
- Lymphatic or orbital spread.

Differential diagnosis

1. **Large naevus** growing during puberty but unlike melanoma it does not involve the cornea.
2. **Ciliary body melanoma** with extraocular extension.
3. **Melanocytoma** is a rare, congenital, black, slowly-growing lesion which cannot be moved freely over the globe.
4. **Pigmented conjunctival carcinoma** in a dark-skinned individual.

Conjunctival intraepithelial neoplasia

Conjunctival intraepithelial neoplasia (CIN) is an uncommon, slowly progressive unilateral disease. Risk factors include ultraviolet light exposure, human papilloma virus (type 16) infection, AIDS and xeroderma pigmentosum.

Histology

The spectrum includes:
1. **Conjunctival epithelial dysplasia,** with dysplastic cells in the basal layers of the epithelium.
2. **Carcinoma *in situ*,** with dysplastic cells involving the full thickness of the epithelium (Fig. 15.9a).
3. **Squamous cell carcinoma** is rare and is characterized by invasion of the underlying stroma (Fig. 15.9b).

NB Clinical differentiation between these three conditions is unreliable.

Diagnosis

1. **Presentation** is usually in late adult life with ocular irritation or a mass.
2. **Papillomatous** lesions are discrete and have surface corkscrew-like blood vessels (Fig. 15.9c).

3. Nodular squamous cell carcinoma is a fleshy, pink papillomatous mass with feeder vessels often at the limbus but may be anywhere. Well-differentiated lesions grow slowly and may have a leukoplakia appearance (Fig. 15.9d). Corneal involvement may occur (Fig. 15.9e). Metastasis can rarely occur to regional lymph nodes and systemically.

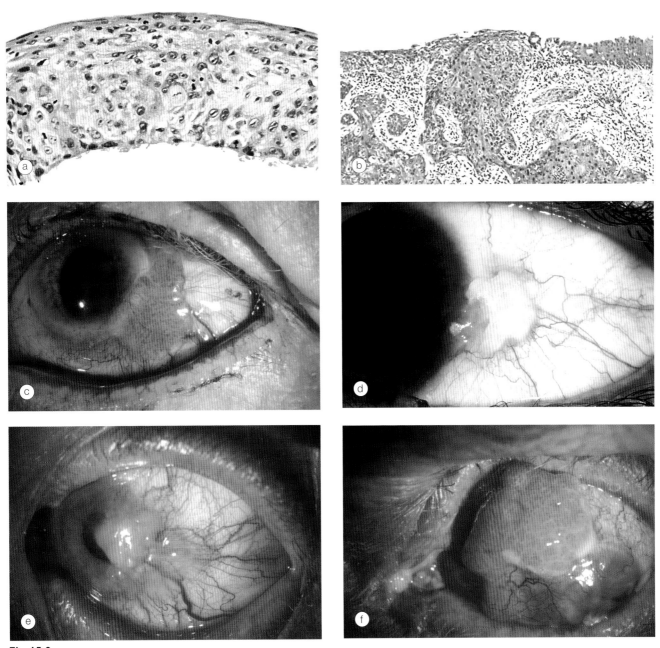

Fig. 15.9
Conjunctival intraepithelial neoplasia. **(a)** Histology of carcinoma *in situ* shows dysplastic changes throughout the thickened epithelium; **(b)** histology of squamous cell carcinoma shows downward proliferation of irregular, dysplastic, squamous epithelium with infiltration of subepithelial tissue; **(c)** papillomatous lesion; **(d)** well-differentiated carcinoma with leukoplakia; **(e)** carcinoma with corneal involvement; **(f)** very extensive carcinoma (Courtesy of J Harry – figs a and b; L Merin – fig. c; B Damato – figs e and f)

NB All varieties may be associated with grey-white hyperplastic epithelium that extends onto the cornea. Impression cytology may be useful in diagnosis.

Treatment

1. **Localized** lesions are treated by excision, possibly with autologous conjunctival or limbal transplantation or amniotic membrane graft. Measures for reducing the incidence of local recurrence include 2–3mm safety margins, assessment of surgical clearance with frozen sections, as well as adjunctive cryotherapy, brachytherapy or topical chemotherapy.
2. **Diffuse** disease is more difficult to treat because the poorly defined borders render involved tissue clinically indistinguishable from healthy tissue. This frequently results in incomplete excision and a high rate of recurrence. Other treatment modalities have therefore been introduced, either as alternatives or as adjuncts to surgery. These include topical mitomycin C, 5-fluorouracil and interferon alpha-2b.
3. **Enucleation** is usually necessary in very large tumours (Fig. 15.9f) particularly with intraocular invasion.
4. **Exenteration** for advanced cases with orbital involvement.

Differential diagnosis

1. **Atypical conjunctival papilloma.**
2. **Pterygium** which is also associated with exposure to ultraviolet radiation.
3. **Pseudo-epitheliomatous hyperplasia** which is a rapidly-growing, white, hyperkeratotic, juxtalimbal nodule which develops secondary to irritation.
4. **Amelanotic melanoma.**

Lymphoproliferative lesions

Most conjunctival lymphoproliferative lesions are reactive lymphoid hyperplasia, a proliferation of B and T cells with germinal follicle formation (Fig. 15.10a). Conjunctival lymphoma may arise in three clinical settings: (a) *de novo*, (b) extension from orbital lymphoma and (c) occasionally associated with systemic involvement. Sometimes reactive lymphoid hyperplasia undergoes transformation to lymphoma. Most conjunctival lymphomas are B cell lymphomas and arise from MALT (mucosa-associated lymphoid tissue).

1. **Presentation** is usually in late adult life with irritation or painless swelling which may be bilateral.
2. **Signs**
   - Slowly growing, mobile, salmon-pink or flesh-coloured infiltrate in the fornices (Fig. 15.10b) or epibulbar surface (Fig. 15.10c).

- Rarely a diffuse lesion (Fig. 15.10d) may mimic chronic conjunctivitis.
3. **Treatment** is most frequently with radiotherapy. Other options include chemotherapy, excision, cryotherapy and local injection of interferon alpha-2b.

Kaposi sarcoma

Kaposi sarcoma is a slow-growing tumour which occurs in patients with AIDS.

1. **Histology** shows proliferation of spindle-shaped cells, vascular channels and inflammatory cells (Fig. 15.11a).
2. **Presentation** is in adult life with irritation or painless discolouration.
3. **Signs.** A flat bright-red lesion (Fig. 15.11b) that may mimic a subconjunctival haemorrhage.
4. **Treatment** is required for cosmetic reasons, bleeding or infection. Options include focal radiotherapy and excision, with or without adjunctive cryotherapy.

IRIS TUMOURS

Iris naevus

1. **Histology** shows proliferation of melanocytes in the superficial iris stroma – predominantly spindle cells but dendritic and balloon cells may also be seen (Fig. 15.12a).
2. **A typical naevus** is a pigmented, flat or slightly elevated tumour, usually less than 3mm in diameter. It disrupts the normal iris architecture and may occasionally cause mild distortion of the pupil and ectropion uveae (Fig. 15.12b).
3. **A diffuse naevus** is flat and has indistinct margins (Fig. 15.12c). It may occur in patients with the iris-naevus syndrome, also known as Cogan–Reese syndrome (see Chapter 13), and may be associated with numerous, small, pedunculated nodules resembling mammillations (see Fig. 13.39b).

Iris melanoma

General predispositions to uveal melanoma

Uveal melanomas are extremely rare in blacks and there is no sexual predominance. Conditions associated with or predisposing to uveal melanomas are: (a) *fair skin*, (b) *light iris colour*, (c) *numerous cutaneous naevi*, (d) *congenital ocular melanocytosis*, (e) *oculodermal melanocytosis* (i.e. *naevus of Ota*), (f) *uveal melanocytoma*, (g) *dysplastic cutaneous naevi*, (h) *familial cutaneous melanoma* and (i) *neurofibromatosis 1*.

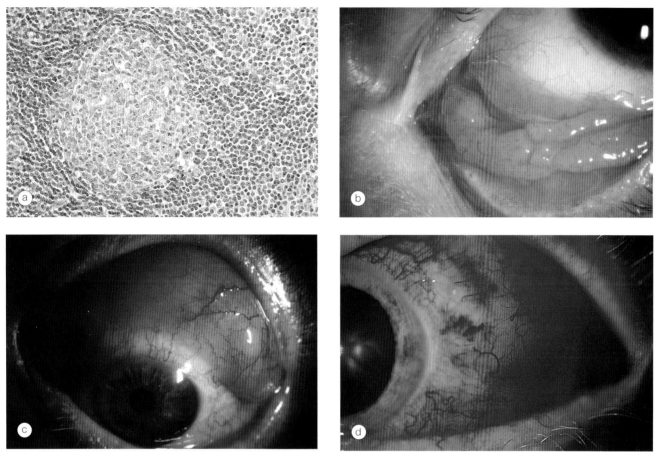

Fig. 15.10
Conjunctival lymphoproliferative lesions. **(a)** Histology of reactive lymphoid hyperplasia shows a germinal lymphoid follicle consisting of immature lymphoid cells at the centre and mature cells at the periphery; **(b)** forniceal; **(c)** epibulbar; **(d)** diffuse (Courtesy of J Harry and G Misson, from *Clinical Ophthalmic Pathology*, Butterworth-Heinemann, 2001 – fig. a; R Curtis – fig. b; P Gili – fig. c)

Histology

The majority are composed of spindle cells and are of low grade malignancy (Fig. 15.13a). A minority contain an epithelioid cell component and can be aggressive.

Diagnosis

About 3% of uveal melanomas arise in the iris. The prognosis is very good and only about 5% of patients develop metastases within 10 years of treatment.

1. **Presentation** is in the fifth to sixth decades, earlier than ciliary body and choroidal melanoma, usually with enlargement of a pre-existing iris lesion.
2. **Typical**
   - A pigmented or non-pigmented nodule at least 3mm in diameter and 1mm thick, usually located in the inferior half of the iris and often associated with surface blood vessels (Fig. 15.13b and c).

- Pupillary distortion, ectropion uveae and occasionally localized cataract may be seen, although these can also occur with large naevi.
- The tumour usually grows very slowly along the iris surface and may invade the angle (Fig. 15.13d) and anterior ciliary body.
- Features associated with malignancy include prominent vascularity, rapid growth, diffuse spread and seeding.

3. **Rare variants**
   - Diffusely growing intrastromal melanoma may give rise to ipsilateral hyperchromic heterochromia (Fig. 15.13e).
   - 'Tapioca melanoma' is characterized by multiple surface nodules (Fig. 15.13f).

Treatment

1. **Observation** of suspicious lesions involves documentation by slit-lamp examination, gonioscopy and photo-

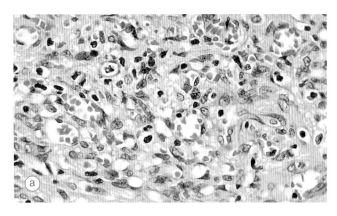

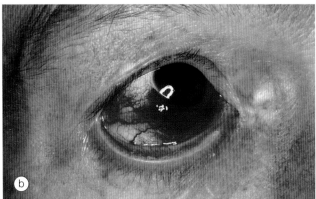

Fig. 15.11
Conjunctival Kaposi sarcoma. **(a)** Histology shows proliferation of vascular endothelial cells, occasional mitotic figures, vascular channels and chronic inflammatory cells; **(b)** clinical appearance (Courtesy of J Harry – fig. a)

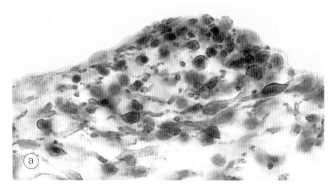

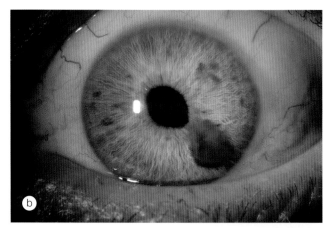

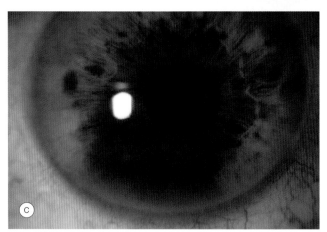

Fig. 15.12
Iris naevus. **(a)** Histology shows localized proliferation of melanocytes on the anterior iris stroma; **(b)** multiple iris freckles and a large naevus causing mild ectropion uveae; **(c)** diffuse naevus (Courtesy of J Harry – fig. a; P Saine – fig. b)

graphy. Follow-up should be life-long because growth may occur after several years of apparent inactivity. Initially the patient is reviewed after 3–6 months, then 6–9 months and later annually.

2. **Iridectomy** for small tumours with iris reconstruction to reduce postoperative photophobia.
3. **Iridocyclectomy** for tumours invading the angle.
4. **Radiotherapy** with a radioactive plaque (brachytherapy) or external irradiation with a proton beam.
5. **Enucleation** may be required for diffusely growing tumours, if radiotherapy is not possible.

Differential diagnosis

1. **Large iris naevus.**
2. **Ciliary body melanoma** with extension through the iris root and usually associated with sentinel episcleral vessels
3. **Adenoma of the iris pigment epithelium** is a rare benign tumour characterized by a dark grey-black nodule with a smooth or multinodular surface, most frequently in the peripheral iris. The lesion causes anterior displace-ment and thinning of the iris stroma, which eventually erodes, disclosing the tumour on slit-lamp biomicroscopy.
4. **Leiomyoma** is an extremely rare benign tumour which arises from smooth muscle. The appearance is similar to that of an amelanotic melanoma except that it is not necessarily confined to the inferior half of the iris. Often the diagnosis can be established only histologically.

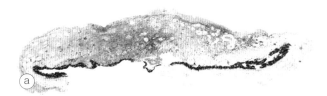

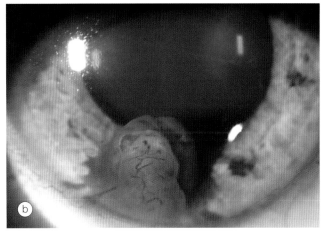

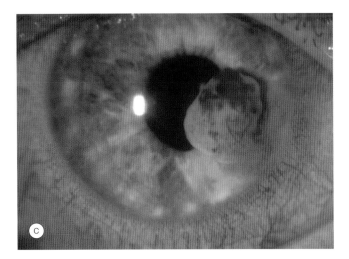

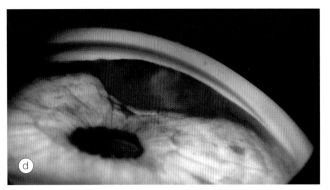

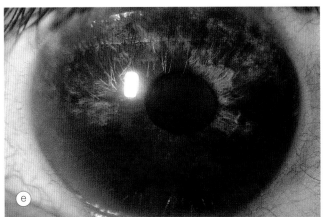

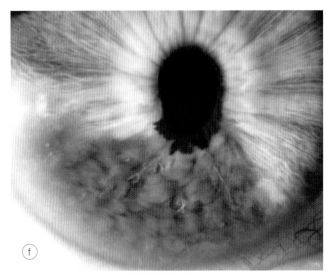

Fig. 15.13
Iris melanoma. **(a)** Histology shows infiltration of the entire thickness of the stroma; **(b)** highly pigmented tumour; **(c)** amelanotic tumour; **(d)** invasion of the angle; **(e)** extensive diffusely growing tumour; **(f)** 'tapioca' melanoma (Courtesy of J Harry and G Misson, from *Clinical Ophthalmic Pathology*, Butterworth-Heinemann, 2001 – fig. a; C Barry – fig. b; B Damato – figs c and f; R Curtis – fig. d)

5. **Melanocytoma** is a deeply-pigmented nodular mass with a mossy, granular surface and no intrinsic vessels. It can undergo spontaneous necrosis resulting in seeding of the iris stroma and chamber angle. Dispersion of melanophages may result in elevation of intraocular pressure.

Iris metastasis

Metastasis to the iris is rare and is characterized by a white, pink or yellow, fast-growing mass (Fig. 15.14a) which may be associated with anterior uveitis and occasionally hyphaema (Fig. 15.14b). Small, multiple deposits may also be seen (Fig. 15.14c).

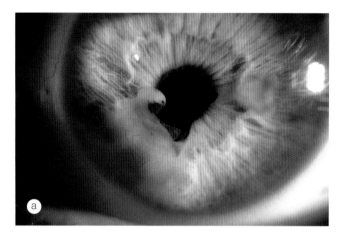

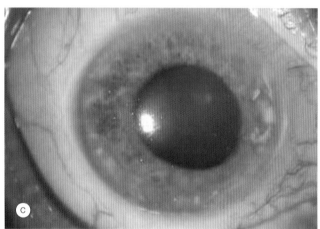

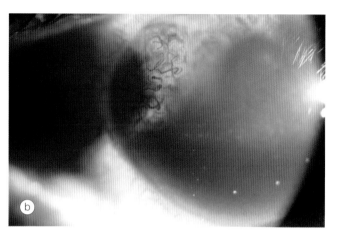

Fig. 15.14
Iris metastasis. **(a)** Solitary fast-growing mass; **(b)** vascularized deposit with hyphaema; **(c)** multiple small deposits (Courtesy of P Saine – fig. a; B Damato – fig. c)

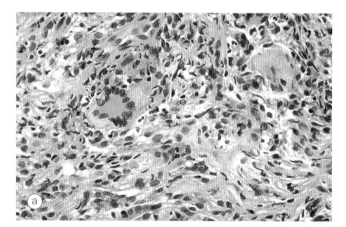

Iris xanthogranuloma

Juvenile xanthogranuloma is a rare, idiopathic granulo-matous disease of early childhood involving proliferation of non-Langerhans histiocytes (Fig. 15.15a).

1. **Cutaneous** involvement is characterized by yellowish papules that have a tendency for spontaneous regression.
2. **Iris** involvement is characterized by localized or diffuse yellow lesions that may be associated with spontaneous hyphaema, or less commonly anterior uveitis and glaucoma (Fig. 15.15b).
3. **Treatment** is with topical steroids.

Small multiple benign lesions

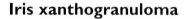

1. **Freckles** are smaller than naevi and never distort the iris architecture (Fig. 15.16a).
2. **Brushfield spots** are pale lesions in the peripheral stroma that may be found in some normal individuals as well as in the majority of patients with Down syndrome (Fig. 15.16b).

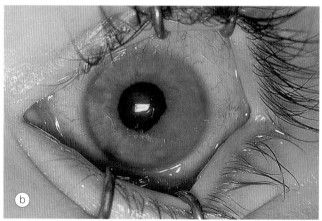

Fig. 15.15
Juvenile xanthogranuloma. **(a)** Histology shows histiocytes and a multinucleated Touton giant cell centrally; **(b)** iris xanthogranuloma (Courtesy of J Harry and G Misson, from *Clinical Ophthalmic Pathology*, Butterworth-Heinemann, 2001 – fig. a)

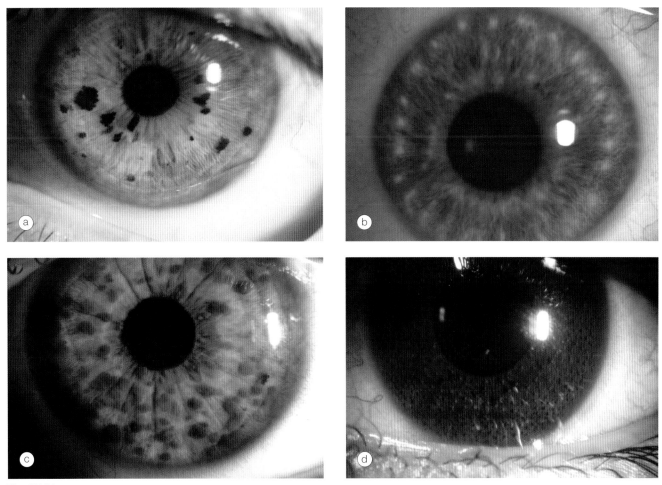

Fig. 15.16
Multiple small benign iris lesions. **(a)** Freckles; **(b)** Brushfield spots; **(c)** Lisch nodules; **(d)** mammillations (Courtesy of P Gili – fig. c)

3. **Lisch nodules** are, small, bilateral, iris naevi found after the age of 16 years in virtually all patients with neuro-fibromatosis-1 (Fig. 15.16c).
4. **Mammillations** are tiny, villiform lesions that are uncommon in normal individuals but occur with increased frequency in patients with congenital ocular melanocytosis, neurofibromatosis-1, Axenfeld-Rieger anomaly and Peters anomaly (Fig. 15.16d).

IRIS CYSTS

Primary cysts

Primary iris cysts are rare curiosities arising from the iris epithelium or, rarely, the stroma. Epithelial cysts lie between the two layers of the pigment epithelium (Fig. 15.17a).

1. **Epithelial**
   - They are unilateral or bilateral, solitary or multiple, globular structures which may be brown or transparent, depending on whether they arise in the iris epithelium or iridociliary epithelium respectively.
   - The cysts may be located at the pupillary border (Fig. 15.17b), in the midzone or the iris root.
   - Occasionally they become dislodged and float freely in the anterior chamber (Fig. 15.17c).
   - The vast majority are asymptomatic and innocuous. Rarely large cysts may obstruct vision and require treatment with argon laser photocoagulation.
2. **Stromal** cysts present in the first years of life.
   - They are solitary, unilateral, have a smooth, translucent anterior wall and contain fluid.
   - The cyst may remain dormant for many years or suddenly enlarge and cause secondary glaucoma, corneal decompensation and show a fluid-debris level reminiscent of a pseudo-hypopyon (Fig. 15.17d).

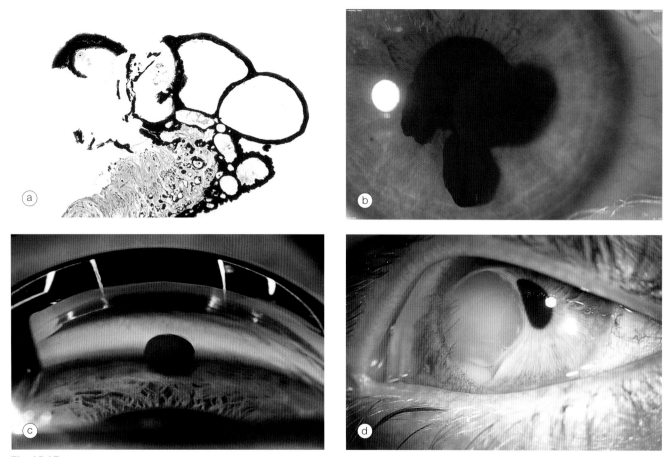

Fig. 15.17
Primary iris cysts. **(a)** Histology of epithelial cysts shows that they lie between the two layers of the pigment epithelium; **(b)** epithelial pupil margin cysts; **(c)** dislodged epithelial cyst in the angle; **(d)** stromal cyst with a fluid-debris level reminiscent of a pseudohypopyon (Courtesy of J Harry and G Misson, from *Clinical Ophthalmic Pathology*, Butterworth-Heinemann, 2001 – fig. a)

- Although spontaneous regression can occur, most require treatment by needle aspiration or excision. Injection of ethanol into the cyst for one minute may avoid the need for excision of a recalcitrant cyst.

Secondary cysts

Secondary iris cysts develop as a result of the following:

1. **Implantation** cysts are the most common. They originate by deposition of surface epithelial cells from the conjunctiva or cornea after penetrating or surgical trauma.
   a. *Pearl* cysts are small, white, solid lesions with opaque walls located in the stroma and are not connected to the wound (Fig. 15.18a).
   b. *Serous* cysts are translucent, filled with fluid and may be connected to the wound (Fig. 15.18b). They frequently enlarge, leading to corneal oedema, anterior uveitis and glaucoma. Ultrasound biomicroscopy may show the location and extent of the lesions when surgical excision is contemplated.
2. **Prolonged use of long-acting miotics** may be associated with usually bilateral, small, multiple cysts located along the pupillary border (Fig. 15.18c). Their development can be prevented by the use of topical phenylephrine 2.5%.
3. **Parasitic** cysts are very rare (Fig. 15.18d).

CILIARY BODY TUMOURS

Ciliary body melanoma

Ciliary body melanomas comprise 5% of uveal melanomas.

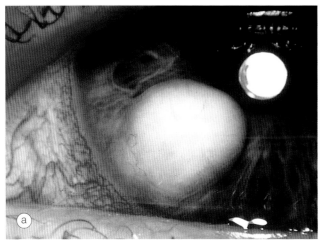
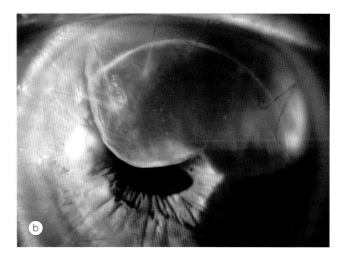
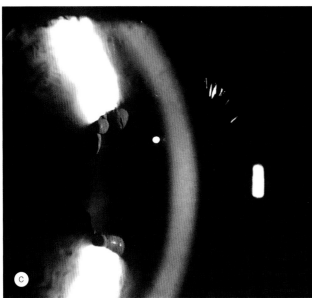
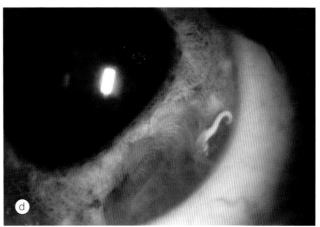

Fig. 15.18
Secondary iris cysts. **(a)** Pearl cyst; **(b)** large serous cyst following penetrating keratoplasty; **(c)** small pupil border cysts due to miotics; **(d)** parasitic cyst

Clinical features

1. **Presentation** is in the sixth decade with visual symptoms but occasionally the tumour may be discovered incidentally.
2. **Signs** depend on the size and location of the tumour.
   - Small tumours cannot usually be visualized without pupillary dilatation and gonioscopy.
   - A large tumour may be visualized on fundoscopy following dilatation of the pupil (Fig. 15.19a).
   - Dilated episcleral blood vessels in the same quadrant as the tumour (sentinel vessels – Fig. 15.19b).
   - Erosion through the iris root that may mimic an iris melanoma (Fig. 15.19c).
   - Pressure on the lens may give rise to astigmatism, subluxation or cataract formation (Fig. 15.19d).
   - Extraocular extension through the scleral emissary vessels may produce a dark epibulbar mass (Fig. 15.19e) which may be mistaken for a conjunctival melanoma.
   - Exudative retinal detachment may be caused by posterior extension (Fig. 15.19f).
   - Anterior uveitis, caused by tumour necrosis, is uncommon.
   - Circumferential (annular) growth for 360° carries the worst prognosis because early diagnosis is difficult.

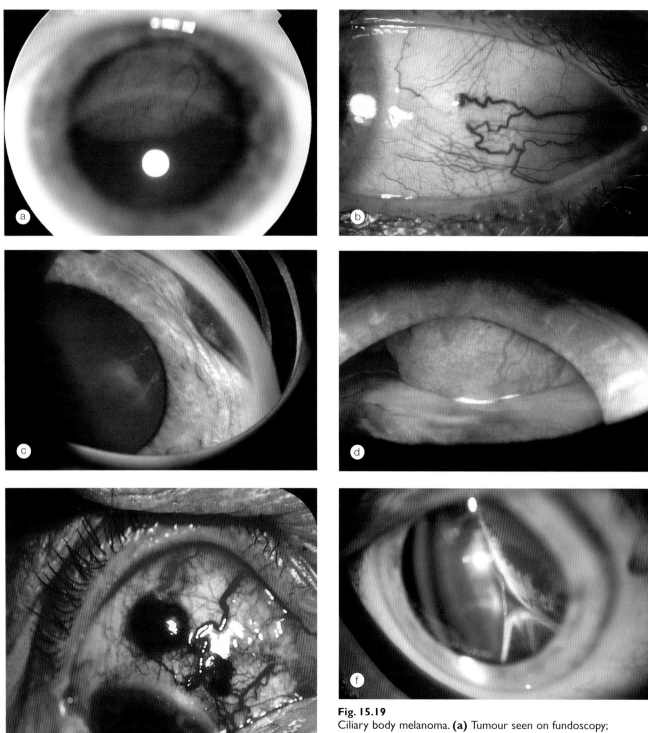

Fig. 15.19
Ciliary body melanoma. **(a)** Tumour seen on fundoscopy;
(b) sentinel vessels in the same quadrant as the tumour;
(c) erosion of the tumour through the iris root; **(d)** pressure on
the lens; **(e)** extraocular extension; **(f)** displacement of the lens
and inferior retinal detachment (Courtesy of R Curtis – figs c and d;
B Damato – fig. e)

Investigations

1. **Triple-mirror contact lens** examination through a well-dilated pupil is essential and is particularly useful in detecting forward erosion through the iris root into the angle.
2. **Transillumination** may give an approximate indication of tumour extent but is of little diagnostic value because an amelanotic melanoma may transilluminate.
3. **Ultrasonography (US)** is very useful in showing the dimensions and extent of the tumour.
4. **Biopsy** involving excisional, incisional or fine-needle aspiration techniques may be helpful in selected cases.

Treatment

1. **General considerations** (see choroidal melanoma below).
2. **Iridocyclectomy** for small or medium-sized tumours involving no more than one-third of the angle. Complications are iris coloboma, vitreous haemorrhage, cataract, lens subluxation, hypotony and incomplete resection.
3. **Radiotherapy** by brachytherapy or proton beam irradiation.
4. **Enucleation** for large tumours and those causing secondary glaucoma, resulting from extensive invasion of Schlemm canal.

Differential diagnosis

1. **Uveal effusion syndrome** may resemble circumferential ciliary body melanoma. However, the effusion is lobulated, transilluminates brightly and appears cystic on US.
2. **Congenital epithelial iridociliary cysts** may displace the lens but can be readily differentiated from melanomas by US.
3. **Other ciliary body tumours,** which are extremely rare, include melanocytoma, medulloepithelioma, metastases, adenocarcinoma, adenoma neurolemmoma and leiomyoma. In most of these the correct diagnosis can be made only histologically.

Medulloepithelioma

Medulloepithelioma (previously known as diktyoma) is a rare embryonal neoplasm that arises from the inner layer of the optic cup which can be benign or malignant. The latter may be fatal as a result of intracranial spread or metastatic disease.

1. **Histology**
   - Teratoid tumours contain heterotopic elements or tissue such as brain, cartilage and skeletal muscle (Fig. 15.20a).
   - Non-teratoid tumours lack these elements.
   - Both types may be benign or malignant.
2. **Presentation** is usually in the first decade with visual loss, pain, photophobia or leukocoria.
3. **Signs**
   - Unilateral, white, pink, yellow or brown cystic ciliary body mass that may be solid or polycystic (Fig. 15.20b).
   - An anterior chamber mass that may contain grey-white opacities consisting of cartilage (Fig. 15.20c).
   - A sheet-like tumour growing behind the lens may resemble a cyclitic membrane.
4. **Complications include** glaucoma, cataract and retinal detachment.
5. **Treatment** is difficult and most patients require enucleation.

TUMOURS OF THE CHOROID

Choroidal naevus

Choroidal naevi are present in about 5–10% of Caucasians but are very rare in dark-skinned races. They can be associated with neurofibromatosis-1 and the dysplastic naevus syndrome. Although they are probably present at birth, growth occurs mainly during the pre-pubertal years and is extremely rare in adulthood. For this reason clinically detectable growth should arouse suspicion of malignancy.

Histology

The tumour is composed of proliferation of spindle cell melanocytes in the choroid but sparing of the choriocapillaris (Fig. 15.21a).

Diagnosis

1. **Presentation.** The vast majority of naevi are asymptomatic and detected by routine examination. Rarely symptoms may be caused by involvement of the fovea by the tumour itself or by secondary serous retinal detachment.
2. **Signs**
   - Usually post-equatorial, oval or circular, slate-blue or grey lesion with detectable but not sharp borders (Fig. 15.21b).
   - Dimensions are < 5mm in basal diameter (i.e. three disc diameters) and < 1mm thickness.
   - Surface drusen may be present, particularly in the central area of a larger lesion (Fig. 15.21c).
   - Secondary choroidal neovascularization is uncommon.
3. **Fluorescein angiography (FA)** findings depend on the amount of pigmentation within the naevus and associated

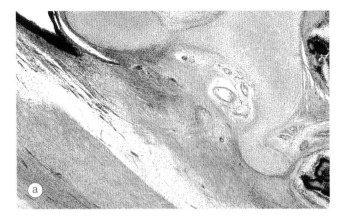

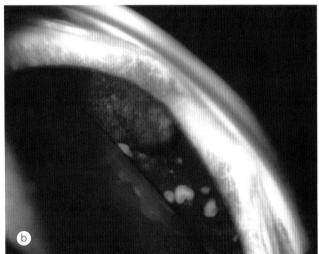

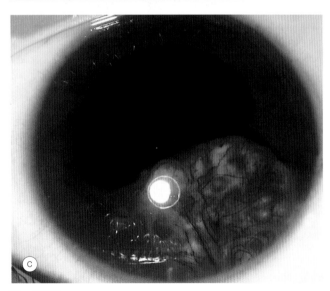

Fig. 15.20
Medulloepithelioma. **(a)** Histology of the teratoid type containing cartilage; **(b)** brown cystic ciliary body mass; **(c)** anterior segment mass (Courtesy of J Harry – fig. a; R Curtis – fig. b)

changes in the overlying retinal pigment epithelium (RPE). Most naevi are avascular and pigmented, giving rise to hypofluorescence caused by blockage of background choroidal fluorescence. Association with surface drusen will result in areas of hyperfluorescence (Fig. 15.21d).

NB FA is not helpful in distinguishing a small melanoma from a naevus although multiple pinpoint areas of hyperfluorescence may predict future growth.

4. **Indocyanine green angiography (ICG)** shows hypofluorescence relative to the surrounding choroid (Fig. 15.21e).
5. **US** shows a localized flat or slightly elevated lesion with high internal acoustic reflectivity (Fig. 15.21f); a low internal reflectivity on A-scan is suggestive of malignancy.
6. **Atypical naevus**
   - An amelanotic naevus (Fig. 15.22a).
   - A 'halo' naevus which is surrounded by a pale zone resembling choroidal atrophy (Fig. 15.22b).

Suspicious naevus

The following features may suggest that a melanocytic lesion is not a naevus but a small melanoma.
- Symptoms such as blurred vision, metamorphopsia, field loss and photopsia.
- Dimensions > 5mm in diameter and > 1mm in thickness.
- Traces of surface orange (lipofuscin) pigment.
- Absence of surface drusen on a relatively thick lesion.
- Margin of the lesion at or near the optic disc.
- Serous retinal detachment either over the surface of the lesion or inferiorly.

NB The greater the number of these features, the higher the chance that the lesion is a melanoma.

Management

1. **Typical naevi** do not require special follow-up because the risk of malignant transformation is extremely low.
2. **Suspicious naevi** require baseline fundus photography and US, and then indefinite follow-up. Subsequently the ophthalmoscopic appearance is compared with the baseline photograph, using landmarks such as retinal blood vessels. It is difficult to detect small changes in thickness by US, because of measurement variation of +0.5mm. Once growth has been documented, the lesion should be reclassified as a melanoma and managed accordingly.

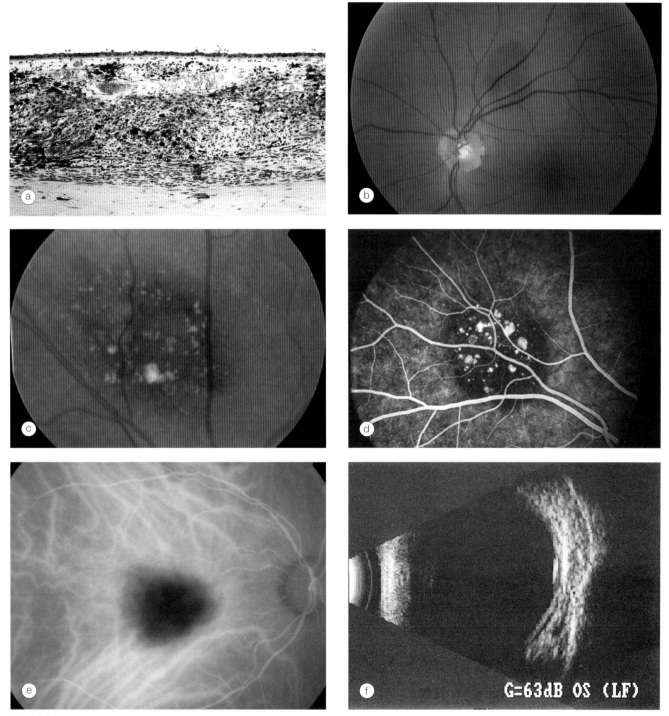

Fig. 15.21
Choroidal naevus. **(a)** Histology shows proliferation of melanocytes in the choroid but sparing of the choriocapillaris; **(b)** typical naevus; **(c)** naevus with surface drusen; **(d)** FA shows hypofluorescence of the naevus and hyperfluorescence of drusen; **(e)** ICG shows hypofluorescence relative to the surrounding choroid; **(f)** US shows slight elevation with internal acoustic reflectivity (Courtesy of J Harry – fig. a; M Karolczak-Kulesza – fig. f)

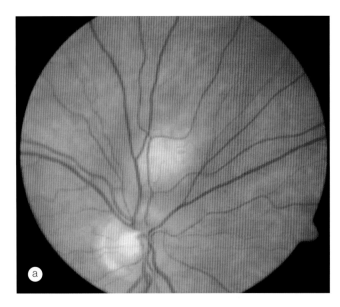

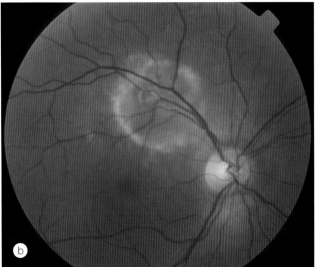

Fig. 15.22
Atypical choroidal naevi. **(a)** Presumed amelanotic naevus;
(b) 'halo' naevus (Courtesy of B Damato – fig. a)

NB It is not known at what stage melanomas begin to metastasize. Lethal systemic spread may start when they are indistinguishable from large, atypical naevi so that once a definitive clinical diagnosis of malignancy is made it may be too late to prevent metastasis. There is therefore a trend towards biopsy as well as earlier treatment, especially if these are unlikely to cause significant visual loss.

Differential diagnosis

1. **Congenital hypertrophy of the RPE** is dark and flat, with a well defined outline.

2. **Melanocytoma of the choroid** is clinically indistinguishable from a large naevus.
3. **Small melanoma** is usually associated with serous retinal detachment and clumps of orange lipofuscin pigment.

Choroidal melanoma

Choroidal melanoma has an overall incidence of about 5 per million per year with no significant gender difference. It is the most common primary intraocular malignancy in adults and accounts for 90% of all uveal melanomas.

Cell type

1. **Spindle** cells are arranged in tight bundles, their cell membranes are indistinct and the cytoplasm is fibrillary or finely granular. Nuclei vary from slender to plump and nucleoli may or may not be distinct (Fig. 15.23a).
2. **Epithelioid** cells are larger and more pleomorphic than spindle cells, often appearing polyhedral with abundant eosinophilic cytoplasm. The cell membranes are distinct and an extracellular space often separates adjacent cells. The nuclei are large with a coarse chromatin pattern and prominent nucleoli. Mitotic figures are more frequent than in spindle cells (Fig. 15.23b).

Classification of uveal melanomas

The classification of uveal melanomas is that issued by the Armed Forces Institute of Pathology (AFIP), Washington DC. It is a modification of the Callender classification. Two types are recognised:

1. **Spindle cell** melanomas formed exclusively by spindle cells.
2. **Mixed cell melanomas** in which there is a mixture of spindle and epithelioid cells.

Other histological features

1. **Fascicular pattern** of cell growth which may be vasocentric in which the cells are arranged perpendicular to a central vessel or ribbon-like (Fig. 15.23c).
2. **Necrosis** where the cell type may not be recognizable (Fig. 15.23d).

Pattern of tumour spread

- Penetration of Bruch membrane and RPE, with herniation into the subretinal space, often with the development of a 'collar-stud' shape (Fig. 15.23e).
- Invasion of scleral channels for blood vessels and nerves resulting in orbital spread (Fig. 15.23f).
- Invasion of vortex veins.

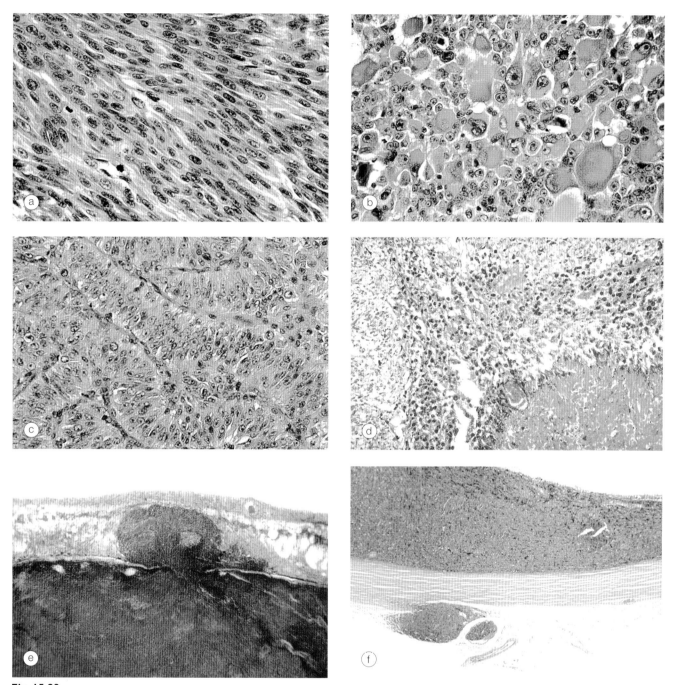

Fig. 15.23
Histology of choroidal melanoma. **(a)** Spindle cells – tightly arranged fusiform cells with indistinct cell membranes and slender or plump oval nuclei; **(b)** epithelioid cells – large pleomorphic cells with distinct cell membranes, large vesicular nuclei with prominent nucleoli, and abundant cytoplasm; **(c)** fascicular pattern – ribbon-like; **(d)** necrotic tumour – cell type cannot be determined; **(e)** penetration of Bruch membrane in a 'collar-stud' fashion; **(f)** extraocular extension and an embolus of neoplastic cells within a blood vessel (Courtesy of J Harry – figs a and b; J Harry and G Misson, from *Clinical Ophthalmic Pathology*, Butterworth-Heinemann, 2001 – figs c, d, e and f)

- Metastatic haematogenous spread primarily to the liver and occasionally to the lungs, bone, skin and brain.
- Optic invasion is very rare, the tumour tending to surround the disc.

Adverse prognostic factors

1. **Histological features** implying an adverse prognosis include large numbers of epithelioid cells, long and wide nuclei, long and multiple nucleoli, closed vascular loops within the tumour and lymphocytic infiltration.
2. **Chromosomal abnormalities** within the melanoma cells, particularly loss in chromosome 3 and gains in chromosome 8, are associated with poor prognosis. Gains in the short arm of chromosome 6 carry a favourable prognosis.
3. **Size:** large tumours have a worse prognosis than small tumours because of lead time bias (i.e. the tumour and any metastases being present for a longer time), and because they show aggressive histological and cytogenetic features.
4. **Extrascleral extension,** because the tumour is advanced and aggressive.
5. **Location:** anterior tumours involving ciliary body have a worse prognosis, most likely because they have grown relatively large by the time of presentation.
6. **Local tumour recurrence** after conservative treatment is associated with poor survival probably because the recurrence is an indication that the original tumour was aggressive.

Clinical features

1. **Presentation** peaks at around the age of 60 years and occurs in one of the following ways:
   - An asymptomatic tumour detected by chance on routine fundus examination performed for other reasons.
   - A symptomatic tumour causing decreased visual acuity, metamorphopsia, visual field loss, floaters, or photopsia, consisting of a brief 'ball of light' travelling across the visual field 2–3 times a day, most apparent in subdued lighting.
2. **Signs**
   - An elevated, subretinal, dome-shaped mass, which may be pigmented (Fig. 15.24a) or amelanotic (Fig. 15.24b).
   - Clumps of orange pigment (lipofuscin) are frequently seen in the RPE overlying the tumour (Fig. 15.24c).
   - If the tumour breaks through Bruch membrane it acquires a 'collar-stud' appearance, with visible blood vessels if the tumour is amelanotic (Fig. 15.24d).
   - A diffuse tumour is rare and is characterized by extensive flat, grey or brown, irregular discolouration (Fig. 15.24e). Extraocular extension is common because this type of tumour tends to be aggressive.
   - Exudative retinal detachment, which is initially confined to the surface of the tumour and which later shifts inferiorly and becomes bullous (Fig. 15.24f).
   - Choroidal folds, haemorrhage, rubeosis, secondary glaucoma, cataract and uveitis may occur.

NB Unlike rhegmatogenous retinal detachment, the subretinal fluid shifts with ocular movement and gravity ('shifting fluid'). In addition, the retina does not show the fine, silvery rippling that occurs in the presence of a tear.

Ocular investigations

1. **FA** is of limited diagnostic value because there is no pathognomonic pattern. Most dome-shaped melanomas show a mottled fluorescence during the arteriovenous phase and progressive leakage and staining. Collar-stud tumours show a 'dual circulation' consisting of tumour vessels and retinal vessels (Fig. 15.25a).
2. **US** is useful in detecting tumours when the media are opaque and also identifies any extraocular extension. The characteristic findings are acoustic hollowness, choroidal excavation and orbital shadowing (Fig. 15.25b). A collar-stud configuration is almost pathognomonic (Fig. 15.25c). Ultrasonography is also useful for measuring tumour dimensions.
3. **ICG** provides more information about the extent of the tumour, because there is less interference caused by RPE changes.
4. **MR,** particularly when combined with surface coils and fat suppression sequences, shows hyperintensity in T1-weighted images (Fig. 15.25d) and hypointensity in T2-weighted images, but these features are not pathognomonic. Enhancement with gadolinium improves image quality, demonstrating optic nerve and orbital invasion and facilitating differentiation from other tumours.
5. **Colour-coded Doppler imaging** may differentiate pigmented tumours from intraocular haemorrhage, particularly in eyes with opaque media.
6. **Biopsy** is useful when the diagnosis cannot be established by less invasive methods. It may be performed either with a fine needle or using the 25-gauge vitrectomy system, which provides a larger sample.

NB Binocular indirect ophthalmoscopy combined with indirect slit-lamp biomicroscopy is sufficient for diagnosis in the vast majority of cases.

Systemic investigations

Systemic investigation is aimed at the following:

1. **Excluding a metastasis to the choroid,** if there is uncertainty about whether the ocular tumour is a melanoma

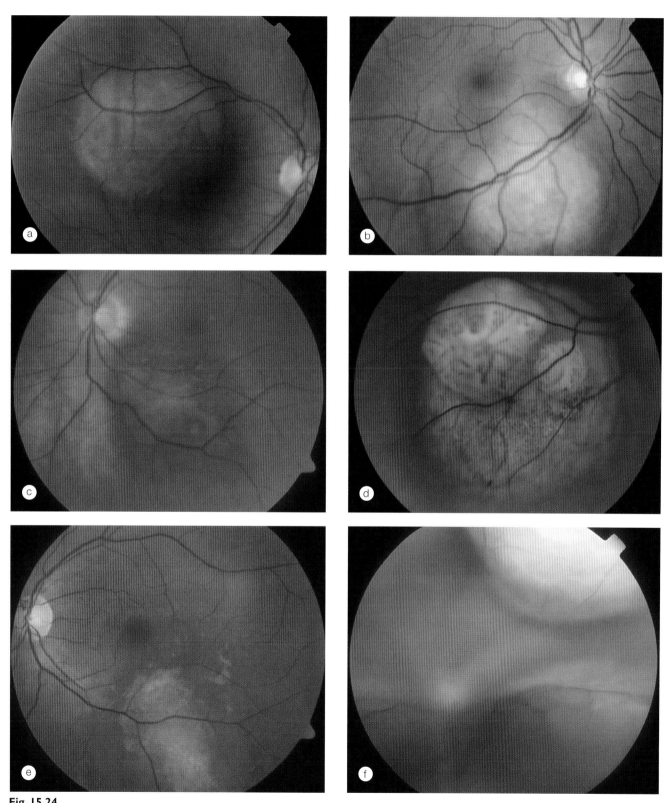

Fig. 15.24
Choroidal melanoma. **(a)** Pigmented melanoma; **(b)** amelanotic melanoma; **(c)** pigmented melanoma with surface orange pigment; **(d)** amelanotic 'collar-stud' melanoma with intrinsic vessels; **(e)** diffuse melanoma; **(f)** superior amelanotic melanoma with inferior bullous retinal detachment (Courtesy C Barry – fig. b; B Damato – figs c, e and f; Moorfields Eye Hospital – fig. d)

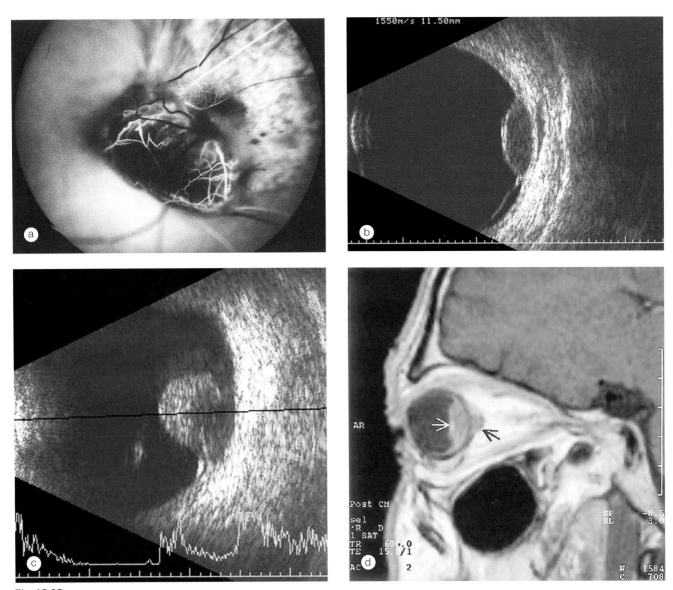

Fig. 15.25
Imaging in choroidal melanoma. **(a)** FA early phase of a 'collar-stud' tumour shows a 'dual circulation'; **(b)** US of a dome-shaped tumour shows choroidal excavation; **(c)** US of a 'collar-stud' tumour; **(d)** T1-weighted sagittal MR shows a choroidal melanoma (white arrow) and extraocular extension (black arrow) (Courtesy of B Damato – figs a and b; S Milewski – fig. c; M Karolczak-Kulesza – fig. d)

or a metastasis. Ocular secondaries arise most frequently from the lung in both sexes and from the breast in women. Occasionally, the primary site is the kidney or gastro-intestinal tract. If metastasis is suspected, initial invest-igations should include chest radiography, rectal examination, serum PSA and CEA, and mammography in females.

2. **Detecting metastatic spread from the choroid** if there is suspicion of metastatic disease because of large tumour size (i.e. basal diameter > 16mm), symptoms such as dyspepsia, abdominal pain, weight loss, palpable enlargement of the liver, or abnormal liver function tests. Hepatic involvement can be detected by US and elevated lactate dehydrogenase, gamma-glutamyl transpeptidase and alkaline phosphatase levels. Whole body positron emission tomography (PET) is a sensitive tool for the detection and localization of metastases. Chest radiography rarely shows lung secondaries in the absence of liver metastases. Only about 1–2% of patients have detectable metastases at the time of presentation.

Principles of treatment

Treatment is performed to avoid the development of a painful and unsightly eye, preferably conserving as much useful vision as possible. Since it is not known when metastatic spread occurs it is uncertain as to whether or not ocular treatment influences survival. Theoretically the smaller the tumour the greater the opportunity for preventing metastasis and therefore the more urgent is the need for treatment. Management should be tailored to the individual patient taking the following factors into consideration:

- Size, location and extent of the tumour together with effects on vision.
- State of the fellow eye.
- General health and age of the patient.
- The patient's wishes and fears.

Treatment not required

- If the tumour is slow-growing and present in the only seeing eye of a very elderly or chronically ill patient.
- If it is not possible to determine clinically whether a tumour is a small melanoma or a large naevus. In this case the lesion is observed and treatment is administered only if growth is documented by sequential US or photography.

The risks involved in delaying treatment are uncertain so that it is essential to confirm and document in writing that the patient understands the situation fully.

Brachytherapy

Brachytherapy with ruthenium-106 or iodine-125 applicator (Fig. 15.26a) is usually the treatment of first choice because it is relatively straightforward and effective.

1. **Indications** are tumours <20mm in basal diameter in which there is a reasonable chance of salvaging vision. It is possible to treat tumours up to 5mm thick with a ruthenium plaque and up to 10mm thick with an iodine plaque. Supplemental transpupillary thermotherapy may be required to sterilize the tumour or to reduce exudation.
2. **Technique**
   a. The tumour is localized by transillumination or binocular indirect ophthalmoscopy.
   b. A template consisting of a transparent plastic dummy or metal ring with eyelets is sutured to the sclera with a releasable bow.
   c. Once it has been established that the template is correctly positioned, the sutures are loosened and used to secure the radioactive plaque.
   d. The plaque is removed once the appropriate dose has been delivered, usually within 3–7 days. At least 80Gy need to be delivered to the tumour apex. Tumour regression starts about 1–2 months after treatment and continues for several years, leaving a flat or dome-shaped pigmented scar.

3. **Tumour response** is usually gradual. Amelanotic tumours tend to become more pigmented as they regress (Fig. 15.26b and c).
4. **Complications** depend on the size of the tumour and its distance from optic nerve and fovea. Morbidity from excessive irradiation of lens, optic nerve and macula includes cataract, papillopathy (with or without disc neovascularization) and maculopathy respectively. The irradiated tumour can cause macular oedema, retinal hard exudates, serous retinal detachment, rubeosis and neovascular glaucoma (i.e. 'toxic tumour syndrome'). Complications are more severe in diabetic patients. Macular oedema after radiotherapy does not usually respond to grid laser photocoagulation but can regress for several months after intravitreal injection of triamcinolone.
5. **Survival** is similar to that following enucleation of comparable tumours.

Charged particle irradiation

Irradiation with charged particles such as protons achieves a high dose in the tumour with a relatively small dose in the superficial tissues.

1. **Indications** are tumours unsuitable for brachytherapy either because of large size or posterior location, which might make positioning of a plaque unreliable.
2. **Technique**
   a. Radio-opaque tantalum markers are sutured to the sclera and used to locate the tumour radiographically.
   b. The patient is seated in a mechanized chair with the head immobilized.
   c. The eyes look at an adjustable fixation target.
   d. Four fractions of radiotherapy are delivered over four consecutive days.
3. **Tumour regression** is slower than with brachytherapy and choroidal atrophy around the base of the tumour takes longer to develop.
4. **Complications** involving intraocular structures are similar to brachytherapy. Extraocular complications include loss of lashes, eyelid depigmentation, canaliculitis with epiphora, conjunctival keratinization and keratitis. Local tumour recurrence is rare.
5. **Survival results** are similar to those following brachytherapy or enucleation.

Stereotactic radiotherapy

Radiation is focussed on the tumour by aiming multiple, highly collimated beams from different directions, either concurrently or sequentially, so that only the tumour receives a high dose of radiation. This is still a new technique, which is gaining in popularity in centres where proton beam radiotherapy is not available.

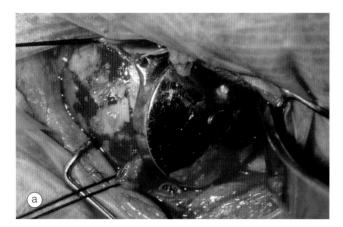

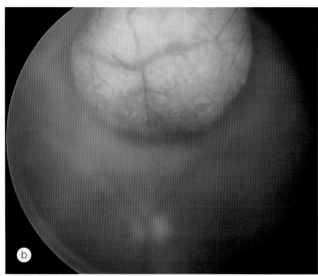

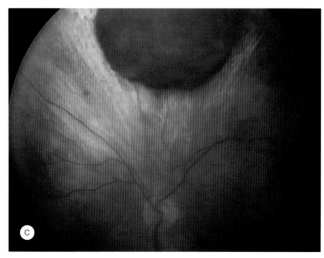

Fig. 15.26
Brachytherapy for choroidal melanoma. **(a)** Placement of plaque;
(b) amelanotic tumour prior to treatment; **(c)** increase in
pigmentation following treatment (Courtesy of C Barry)

Transpupillary thermotherapy

Transpupillary thermotherapy (TTT) uses an infrared laser
beam to induce tumour cell death by hyperthermia but not
coagulation. It is an outpatient procedure requiring retrobulbar or peribulbar anaesthesia.

1. **Indications**
   - Small, pigmented choroidal tumour when differentia-
     tion between naevus and melanoma is not possible and
     when radiotherapy is considered unsuitable.
   - Small choroidal melanoma when radiotherapy is
     inappropriate because of poor general health or
     reduced life-expectancy.
   - After radiotherapy, as a treatment for exudation
     threatening vision.
2. **Technique**
   a. Overlapping one-minute applications of a 3mm diode
      laser beam are applied all over the tumour surface,
      adjusting the power so that retinal blanching does not
      develop before 45 seconds.
   b. A 2mm rim of surrounding choroid is treated to pre-
      vent marginal recurrence.
   c. Adjunctive plaque radiotherapy is administered, if
      possible, to prevent recurrence from deep intrascleral
      deposits.
   d. The treatment is repeated after 6 months if there is
      residual tumour.
3. **Tumour response** is gradual, with the lesion first becoming darker and flatter, eventually disappearing to leave
   bare sclera.
4. **Complications** include retinal traction, rhegmatogenous
   detachment, vascular occlusion, neovascularization, iris
   burns and lens opacities. Local recurrence is common,
   especially if the tumour is thick, amelanotic or involving
   the disc margin.

NB TTT a useful adjunct to radiotherapy, reducing
oedema and preventing local recurrence.

Trans-scleral choroidectomy

Choroidectomy is a difficult procedure and is therefore not
performed widely.

1. **Indications**
   - Carefully selected tumours that are too thick for radio-
     therapy and usually less than 16mm in diameter.
   - Severe exudative retinal detachment and/or neo-
     vascular glaucoma after radiotherapy.
2. **Technique**
   - The tumour is localized by transillumination.
   - The eye is decompressed by limited vitrectomy.

- A partial-thickness scleral flap is created over the tumour (Fig. 15.27a).
- The tumour is resected together with the deep scleral lamella, if possible leaving the retina intact (Fig. 15.27b).
- After scleral closure (Fig. 15.27c), the eye is filled with balanced salt solution.
- Adjunctive brachytherapy is administered, either immediately (Fig. 15.27d) or after healing has occurred.

3. **Complications** include retinal detachment, hypotony, wound dehiscence and local tumour recurrence.

Enucleation

1. **Indications** for excision of the globe are large tumour size, optic disc invasion, extensive involvement of the ciliary body or angle, irreversible loss of useful vision, and poor motivation to keep the eye.
2. **Technique** is the same as for other conditions, using the surgeon's preferred orbital implant. It is essential to perform ophthalmoscopy and to do this *after* draping the patient to ensure that the correct eye is treated.
3. **Complications** are the same as with enucleation for other conditions. Orbital recurrence is rare if there is no extraocular tumour spread or if any such extension is completely excised.

Exenteration

Removal of the globe and orbital contents is indicated when orbital disease cannot be controlled by lumpectomy and radiotherapy.

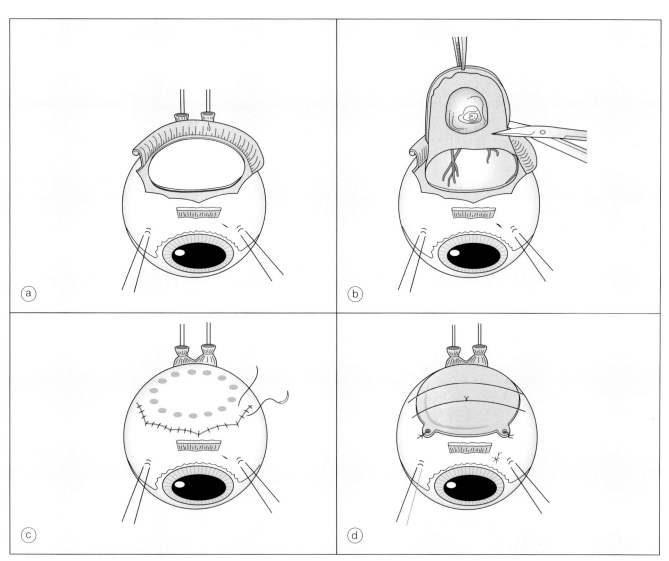

Fig. 15.27
Trans-scleral choroidectomy. **(a)** Scleral flap; **(b)** tumour excision; **(c)** closure of flap; **(d)** insertion of plaque (Courtesy of B Damato)

Treatment of metastatic disease

1. **Systemic** chemotherapy and/or immunotherapy rarely induce responses but remission has been reported with intra-hepatic chemotherapy.
2. **Partial hepatectomy** for removal of small metastatic deposits can prolong life significantly.

Differential diagnosis

Although the diagnosis is usually straightforward, the following conditions should be considered in the differential diagnosis of atypical cases:

1. **Pigmented lesions**
   - Large naevus, which usually shows numerous surface drusen, without serous retinal detachment and little if any orange pigment.
   - Melanocytoma, which is deeply pigmented and usually located at the optic disc.
   - Congenital hypertrophy of the RPE, which is flat and has a discrete margin.
   - Haemorrhage in the subretinal space or suprachoroidal space such as from choroidal neovascularization or retinal artery macroaneurysm.
   - Metastatic cutaneous melanoma, which has a smooth surface, a light brown colour, indistinct margins, extensive retinal detachment and often a past history of malignancy.
2. **Non-pigmented lesions**
   - Circumscribed choroidal haemangioma, which is typically posterior, pink, dome-shaped, and has a smooth surface.
   - Metastasis, which is often associated with exudative retinal detachment.
   - Solitary choroidal granulomas associated with sarcoidosis or tuberculosis.
   - Posterior scleritis, which can present with a large elevated lesion, but unlike melanoma, pain is a common feature.
   - Large elevated disciform lesion, which can be macular or eccentrically located, usually in the temporal preequatorial region. These neovascular lesions are usually associated with hard exudates and fresh haemorrhages, both of which rarely accompany a melanoma.
   - Prominent vortex vein ampulla is characterized by a small, smooth, brown, dome-shaped lesion, which disappears on exerting pressure on the eye.

Circumscribed choroidal haemangioma

Histology

The tumour is composed of varying-sized vascular channels that form a mass within the choroid (Fig. 15.28a).

Diagnosis

The lesion is not usually associated with systemic disease. It may be dormant throughout life or may give rise to symptoms, usually in adulthood as a result of exudative retinal detachment. Slight progressive enlargement can occur over many years.

1. **Presentation** is in the fourth to fifth decades in one of the following ways:
   - Unilateral blurring of central vision, visual field defect or metamorphopsia.
   - Hypermetropia may occur if the retina is elevated by tumour or fluid.
   - Some patients are asymptomatic with normal visual acuity.
2. **Signs**
   - An oval mass with indistinct margins, which has the same orange-red colour as the surrounding choroid (Fig. 15.28b).
   - It is located usually posterior to the equator and in the peripapillary area.
   - The median base diameter of the lesion is 6mm and median thickness 3mm.
3. **FA** reveals rapid, spotty hyperfluorescence in the pre-arterial or early arterial phase (Fig. 15.28c) and diffuse intense late hyperfluorescence.
4. **ICG** shows hyperfluorescence in the early frames by 1 minute (Fig. 15.28d) and hypofluorescence ('washout') at 20 minutes.
5. **US** shows an acoustically solid lesion with a sharp anterior surface and high internal reflectivity but without choroidal excavation and orbital shadowing (Fig. 15.28e).
6. **MR** shows that the tumour is iso- or hyperintense to the vitreous in T1-weighted images and isointense in T2-weighted images, with marked enhancement with gadolinium.

Complications

- Fibrous metaplasia over the tumour (Fig. 15.28f).
- Retinal oedema and accumulation of subretinal fluid over the tumour, maybe result in cystoid retinal degeneration.
- Exudation may lead to extensive retinal detachment and neovascular glaucoma.
- RPE degeneration, and rarely macular atrophy and choroidal neovascularization.

Treatment

Treatment of asymptomatic lesions is unnecessary. Treatment of vision-threatening haemangiomas is as follows:

1. **Photodynamic therapy** using the same method as for choroidal neovascular membranes. The treatment may

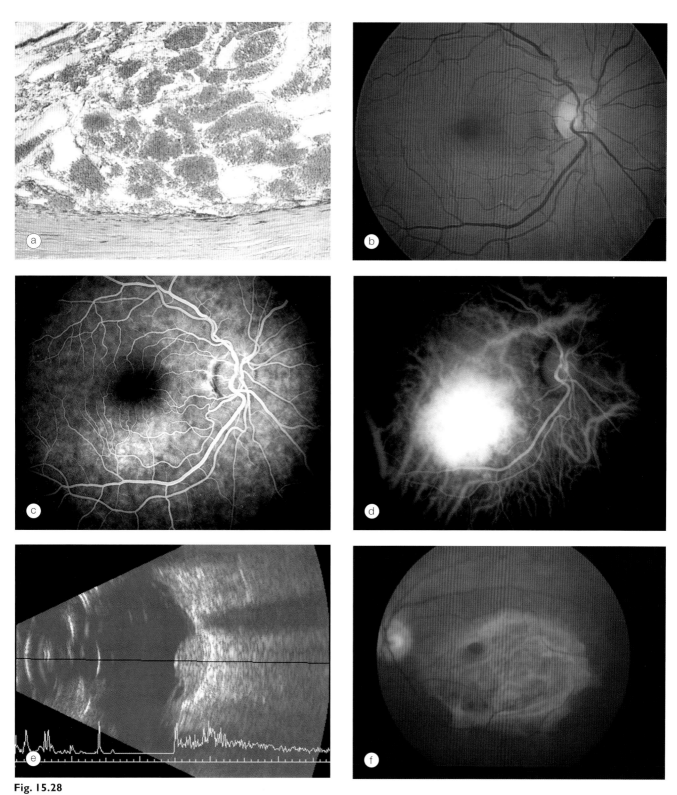

Fig. 15.28

Circumscribed choroidal haemangioma. **(a)** Histology shows varying-sized congested vascular channels forming a mass within the choroid; **(b)** clinical appearance; **(c)** FA early phase shows hyperfluorescence; **(d)** ICG shows early hyperfluorescence; **(e)** US shows an acoustically solid lesion with a sharp anterior surface and high internal reflectivity but without choroidal excavation and orbital shadowing; **(f)** surface fibrous metaplasia (Courtesy of J Harry – fig. a; P Gili – figs b, c and d; B Damato – figs e and f)

need to be repeated after a few months if subretinal fluid persists.

2. **TTT** for lesions not involving the macula – but this causes peripheral visual field loss.

3. **Radiotherapy** may involve lens-sparing external beam irradiation, proton beam radiotherapy or plaque brachytherapy. Only a low dose of radiotherapy is needed, but even this can cause collateral damage to normal tissues.

Differential diagnosis

1. **Amelanotic choroidal melanoma** has a yellow tan colour, often with subtle intrinsic pigment.
2. **Choroidal metastasis** is creamy yellow and may be multifocal. However, metastatic deposits from carcinoid tumour, renal cell carcinoma and thyroid carcinoma may appear orange, similar to a haemangioma.
3. **RPE detachment** is acoustically hollow and shows different staining on FA.
4. **Posterior scleritis** is associated with pain and shows scleral thickening and episcleral oedema on US.

Diffuse choroidal haemangioma

Diffuse choroidal haemangioma usually affects over half of the choroid and enlarges very slowly. It occurs almost exclusively in patients with the Sturge–Weber syndrome ipsilateral to the naevus flammeus (see Chapter 24).

1. **Signs.** The fundus has a deep-red 'tomato ketchup' colour that is most marked at the posterior pole (Fig. 15.29a).
2. **US** shows diffuse choroidal thickening (Fig. 15.29b).
3. **Complications** include secondary cystoid retinal degeneration and exudative retinal detachment. Neovascular glaucoma can result if exudative retinal detachment is not treated.
4. **Treatment** involves external beam radiotherapy, if necessary.

Melanocytoma

Melanocytoma (magnocellular naevus) is a rare, distinctive, heavily pigmented tumour which is seen most frequently in the optic nerve head but which can rarely arise anywhere in the uvea. In contrast with choroidal melanoma, melanocytomas are relatively more common in dark-skinned individuals, particularly females. In most cases the tumour is stationary with little tendency to change.

1. **Histology** shows, large, deeply pigmented polyhedral or spindle cells with small nuclei (Fig. 15.30a).

2. **Signs**
   - A dark brown or black lesion with feathery edges within the retinal nerve fibre layer that extends over the edge of the disc (Fig. 15.30b).
   - Occasionally the tumour is elevated and occupies most of the disc surface (Fig. 15.30c).
   - An afferent pupillary conduction defect may be present, even if visual acuity is good.

3. **FA** shows hypofluorescence of deep vessels due to blockage (Fig. 15.30d).

4. **Complications,** which are rare, include malignant transformation, spontaneous tumour necrosis, optic nerve compression and retinal vein obstruction.

5. **Treatment** is not required except in the very rare event of malignant transformation.

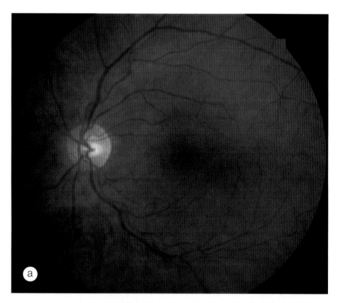

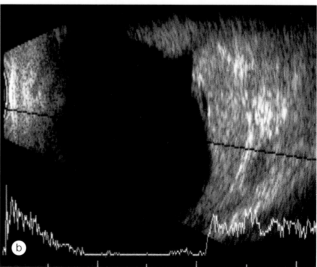

Fig. 15.29
(a) Diffuse choroidal haemangioma; **(b)** US shows diffuse choroidal thickening (Courtesy of B Damato – fig. b)

Osseous choristoma

Osseous choristoma (choroidal osteoma) is a very rare, benign, slow-growing, ossifying tumour which is more common in women. Familial cases have been reported. Both eyes are affected in about 25% of cases but not usually simultaneously. Histology shows mature, cancellous bone, which causes overlying RPE atrophy.

Diagnosis

1. **Presentation** is in the second to third decades with gradual visual impairment if the macula is involved by the tumour itself or by secondary choroidal neovascularization.
2. **Signs**

- An orange-yellow lesion with well-defined, scalloped borders near the disc or at the posterior pole (Fig. 15.31a).
- Slow growth can occur over several years and long-standing cases may show overlying RPE changes (Fig. 15.31b).
- Spontaneous decalcification can occur, with visual loss if the macula is involved.

3. **FA** manifests irregular, diffuse mottled hyperfluorescence during the early and late phases (Fig. 15.31c); choroidal neovascularization may be evident.
4. **ICG** shows early hypofluorescence (Fig. 15.31d) and late staining.
5. **US** shows a highly reflective anterior surface which causes orbital shadowing (Fig. 15.31e).
6. **CT** demonstrates bone-like features (15.31f).

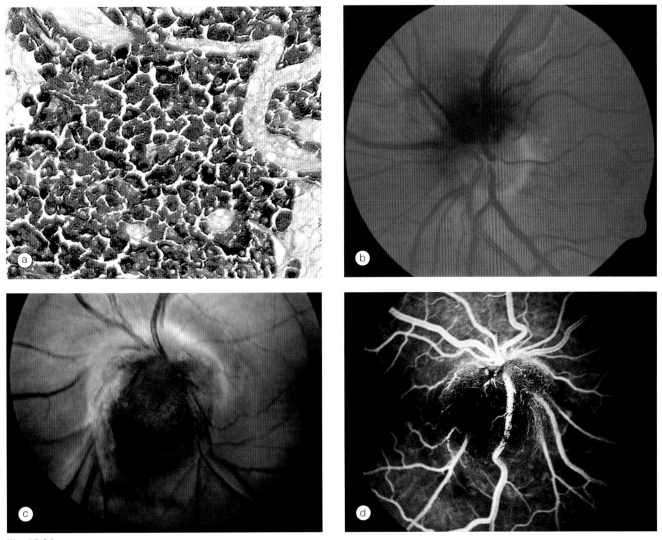

Fig. 15.30
Melanocytoma. **(a)** Histology shows heavily pigmented polyhedral cells; **(b)** relatively flat tumour; **(c)** large elevated tumour; **(d)** FA shows hypofluorescence of deeper disc vessels due to blockage (Courtesy of B Damato – fig. a; P Gili – fig. b)

Treatment

Treatment is confined to secondary choroidal neovascularization using photodynamic therapy if the macula is not involved. Conventional laser photocoagulation has limited effect because of lack of pigment in the tumour and atrophy of the overlying RPE. Laser treatment has been reported to induce decalcification, and recent evidence suggests that this may arrest growth towards the fovea.

Differential diagnosis

1. **Choroidal metastasis,** which may also be bilateral, but typically affects an older age group.
2. **Amelanotic choroidal naevus or melanoma** does not cause such extensive orbital shadowing.
3. **Osseous metaplasia,** which may occur in association with choroidal haemangiomas.
4. **Sclerochoroidal calcification** is an uncommon condition characterized by multifocal, geographic, yellow-white fundus lesions which are usually found in both eyes of older adults.

Metastatic choroidal tumours

The choroid is by far the most common site for uveal metastases accounting for about 90%, followed by the iris and ciliary body. Retinal metastases are very rare. Metastatic tumours to the choroid are more common than primary malignancies but are usually undetected or overshadowed by the patient's general illness. The most frequent primary site is the breast in women and the bronchus in men. A choroidal secondary may be the initial presentation of a bronchial carcinoma, whereas a past history of breast cancer is the rule in patients with breast secondaries. Other less common primary sites include the gastrointestinal tract, kidney and skin melanoma. The prostate is, however, an extremely rare primary site. Patient survival is generally poor, with a median of 8–12 months for all patients; 8–15 months for breast carcinoma and 3–5 months for bronchial carcinoma. In patients with breast carcinoma risk factors for choroidal metastases include dissemination of disease in more than one organ and the presence of lung and brain metastases.

Diagnosis

1. **Presentation** is usually with visual impairment although metastases may be asymptomatic if located away from the macula.
2. **Signs**
   - A fast-growing, creamy-white, placoid lesion most frequently located at the posterior pole (Fig. 15.32a).
   - The deposits are multifocal in about 30% of patients and both eyes are involved in 10–30% of cases.
   - Secondary exudative retinal detachment is frequent

and may occur in eyes with relatively small deposits (Fig. 15.32b).
   - Occasionally the deposits assume a globular shape and may mimic an amelanotic melanoma (Fig. 15.32c).
3. **US** of a placoid tumour shows diffuse choroidal thickening. A dome-shaped lesion shows moderately high internal acoustic reflectivity throughout the tumour which is suggestive but not pathognomonic (Fig. 15.32d).
4. **FA** shows early hypofluorescence and diffuse late staining (Fig. 15.32e) but in contrast with choroidal melanomas a 'dual circulation' is not seen.
5. **ICG** shows usually shows hypofluorescence (Fig. 15.32f) through the study and may show subtle deposits not evident on FA.
6. **Biopsy** by fine needle aspiration or using a 25-gauge vitrectomy system may be appropriate when the primary site is unknown.

Treatment

1. **Observation,** if the patient is asymptomatic or receiving systemic chemotherapy.
2. **Radiotherapy,** either external beam or brachytherapy.
3. **TTT** is useful for small tumours with minimal subretinal fluid.
4. **Systemic therapy** for the primary tumour may be beneficial for choroidal metastases.
5. **Enucleation** may be required for a painful blind eye.

TUMOURS OF THE RETINA

Retinoblastoma

Retinoblastoma is the most common primary, intraocular malignancy of childhood and accounts for about 3% of all childhood cancers. Even so, it is rare, occurring in about 1:17,000 live births.

Histology

The tumour is composed of small basophilic cells (retinoblasts) with large hyperchromatic nuclei and scanty cytoplasm. Many retinoblastomas are undifferentiated (Fig. 15.33a) but varying degrees of differentiation are characterized by the formation of rosettes, of which there are three types:

1. **Flexner–Wintersteiner** rosettes consist of a central lumen surrounded by tall columnar cells. The nuclei of these cells lie away from the lumen (Fig. 15.33b).
2. **Homer–Wright** rosettes have no lumen and the cells form around a tangled mass of eosinophilic processes.
3. **Fleurettes** are foci of tumour cells, which exhibit photoreceptor differentiation. Clusters of cells with long

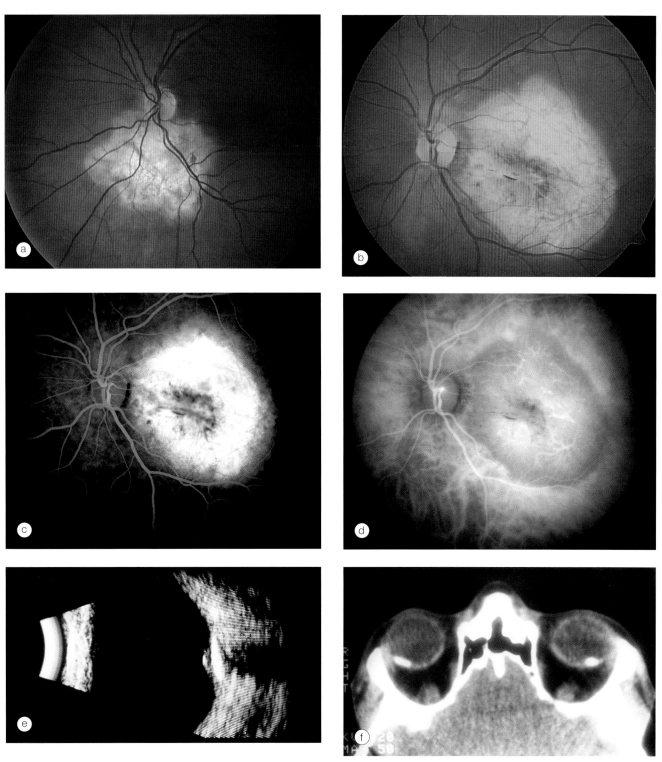

Fig. 15.31
Osseous choristoma. (a) Early juxtapapillary lesion; (b) longstanding tumour with overlying RPE changes; (c) FA late phase shows mottled hyperfluorescence; (d) ICG early phase shows hypofluorescence; (e) US shows a highly reflective anterior surface and orbital shadowing; (f) axial CT demonstrates bilateral lesions that have the same consistency as bone (Courtesy of C Barry – fig. a; P Gili – figs b, c and d)

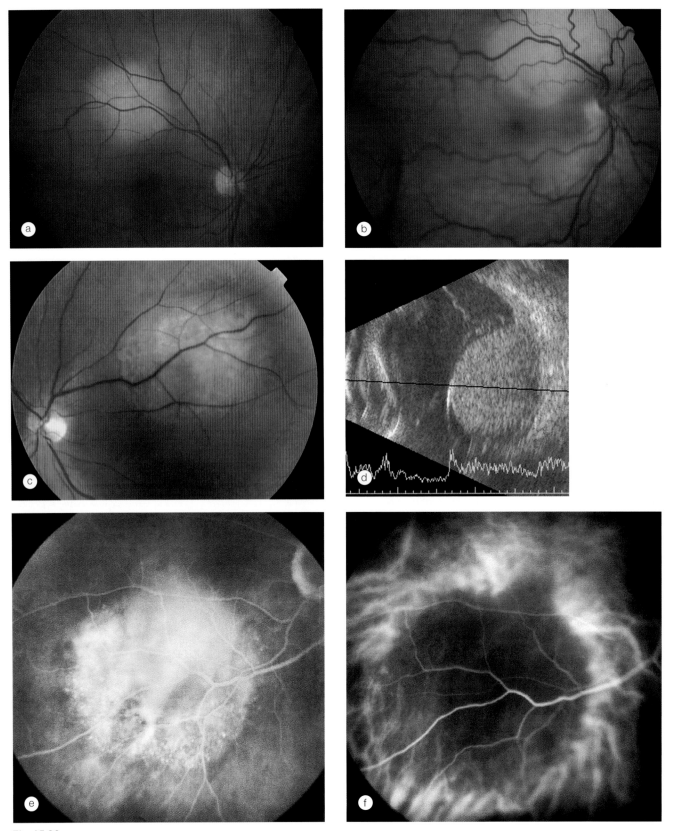

Fig. 15.32
Choroidal metastasis. **(a)** Small placoid deposit; **(b)** deposit above the disc associated with shallow exudative retinal detachment; **(c)** elevated deposit; **(d)** US shows a dome-shaped lesion with moderately high internal acoustic reflectivity throughout; **(e)** FA late phase shows diffuse hyperfluorescence; **(f)** ICG early phase shows hypofluorescence (Courtesy of C Barry – fig. a; B Damato – figs b and d; S Milewski – figs e and f)

cytoplasmic processes project through a fenestrated membrane and the appearance resembles a bouquet of flowers (Fig. 15.33c).

Patterns of tumour spread

1. **Growth pattern** may be endophytic (into the vitreous), with seeding of tumour cells throughout the eye or exophytic (into the subretinal space), causing retinal detachment (Fig. 15.33d).
2. **Optic nerve invasion,** with spread of tumour along the subarachnoid space to the brain (Fig. 15.33e).
3. **Diffuse infiltration** of the retina, without exophytic or endophytic growth.
4. **Metastatic spread,** which is to regional nodes, lung, brain and bone.

> **NB** In both heritable and non-heritable retinoblastoma, the risk of metastatic disease is greater if the tumour is advanced, retrolaminar optic nerve invasion, massive choroidal invasion, anterior chamber involvement and orbital spread. Repeated recurrences after conservative treatment also indicate an increased risk of metastasis.

Genetics

Retinoblastoma results from malignant transformation of primitive retinal cells before final differentiation. Because these cells disappear within the first few years of life, the tumour is seldom seen after 3 years of age. Retinoblastoma may be heritable or non-heritable. The predisposing gene (*RB1*) is at 13q14.

1. **Heritable** (germ line) retinoblastoma accounts for 40%. An association with advanced paternal age suggests that in some patients the mutation has occurred in the father's sperm. In heritable retinoblastoma one allele of the *RB1* (a tumour suppressor gene) is mutated in all body cells. When a further mutagenic event ('second hit') affects the second allele, the cell undergoes malignant transformation. Because all the retinal precursor cells contain the initial mutation, these children develop bilateral and multifocal tumours. Heritable retinoblastoma patients also have a predisposition to non-ocular cancers; most notably pineal or suprasellar primitive neuroectodermal tumour (PNET) (also known as pinealoblastoma and trilateral retinoblastoma), which occurs in about 3%. Second malignant neoplasms include osteosarcoma, melanoma, and malignancies of the brain and lung. The risk of second malignancy is about 6% but this increases five-fold if external beam irradiation has been used to treat the original tumour, the second tumour tending to arise within the irradiated field.
   - The mutation is transmitted in 50% but because of incomplete penetrance only 40% of offspring will be affected.

- If a child has heritable retinoblastoma, the risk to siblings is 2% if the parents are healthy, and 40% if a parent is affected.
- About 15% of patients with hereditary retinoblastoma manifest unilateral involvement.
2. **Non-heritable** (somatic) retinoblastoma accounts for 60% of cases. The tumour is unilateral, not transmissible and does not predispose the patient to second non-ocular cancers. If a patient has a solitary retinoblastoma and no positive family history, this is probably but not definitely non-heritable so that the risk in each sibling and offspring is about 1%.

> **NB** Siblings at risk of retinoblastoma should be screened by prenatal US and by ophthalmoscopy soon after birth and then regularly until the age of 5 years.

Presentation

Presentation is within the first year of life in bilateral cases and around 2 years of age if the tumour is unilateral.
- Leukocoria (white pupillary reflex) is the commonest (60%) and may be first noticed in family photographs (Fig. 15.34a).
- Strabismus is the second most common (20%); fundus examination is therefore mandatory in all cases of childhood strabismus.
- Secondary glaucoma, which is occasionally associated with buphthalmos (Fig. 15.34b).
- Diffuse retinoblastoma invading the anterior segment tends to present in older children. It may cause a red eye due to tumour-induced uveitis (Fig. 15.34c), and iris nodules which may be associated with pseudo-hypopyon (Fig. 15.34d).

> **NB** It is important to consider retinoblastoma in the differential diagnosis of unusual chronic uveitis in children.

- Orbital inflammation (Fig. 15.34e) mimicking orbital or preseptal cellulitis may occur with necrotic tumours. It does not necessarily imply extraocular extension and the exact mechanism is not known.
- Orbital invasion with proptosis and bone invasion may occur in neglected cases (Fig. 15.34f).
- Metastatic disease involving regional lymph nodes and brain before the detection of ocular involvement is rare.
- Raised intracranial pressure due to 'trilateral retinoblastoma' before the diagnosis of ocular involvement is very rare.
- Routine examination of a patient known to be at risk.

Signs

Indirect ophthalmoscopy with scleral indentation must be performed on both eyes after full mydriasis. This is because without indentation pre-equatorial tumours may be missed

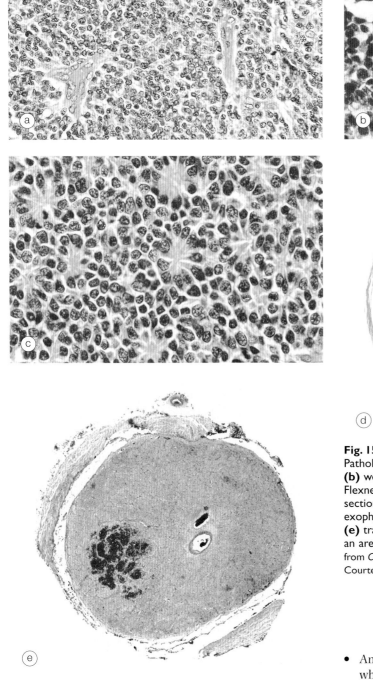

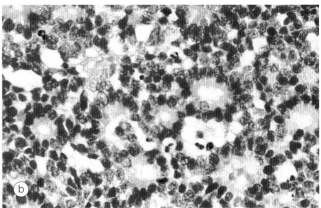

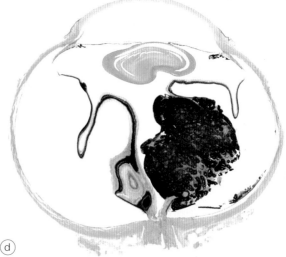

Fig. 15.33
Pathology of retinoblastoma: **(a)** Undifferentiated tumour; **(b)** well-differentiated tumour shows abundant Flexner–Wintersteiner rosettes; **(c)** fleurettes; **(d)** whole eye section shows a mixed endophytic (into the vitreous) and exophytic (into the subretinal space) growth pattern; **(e)** transverse section of the cut end of the optic nerve with an area of tumour infiltration (Courtesy of J Harry and G Misson, from *Clinical Ophthalmic Pathology*, Butterworth-Heinemann, 2001 – fig. a; Courtesy of J Harry – figs b, c, d and e)

(Fig. 15.35a) and one eye may harbour multiple tumours. The clinical signs depend on tumour size and growth pattern.

- An intraretinal tumour is a homogeneous, dome-shaped white lesion which becomes irregular, often with white flecks of calcification (Fig. 15.35b).
- An endophytic tumour projects into the vitreous as a white mass (Fig. 15.35c) that may seed into the vitreous.
- An exophytic tumour forms subretinal, multilobulated white masses, with overlying retinal detachment (15.35d).

Investigations

1. US is used mainly to assess tumour size. It also detects calcification within the tumour (Fig. 15.36a) and is helpful in the diagnosis of simulating lesions such as Coats disease.

2. **CT** also detects calcification (Fig. 15.36b) but entails a significant dose of radiation and is performed only if US has not detected calcification.

3. **MR** cannot detect calcification but it is superior to CT for optic nerve evaluation and detection of extraocular extension or a pinealoblastoma (Fig. 15.36c), especially with contrast and fat suppression. MR may also be useful to differentiate retinoblastoma from simulating conditions.

4. **Systemic** investigations include physical examination and MR scans of the orbit and skull, as a minimum in high-risk cases. If these indicate the presence of metastatic disease, then bone scans, bone marrow aspiration and lumbar puncture are also performed.

5. **Genetic** studies require fresh tumour tissue from the enucleated eye and a blood sample for DNA analysis. Blood samples from the patient's relatives and a sperm sample from the father may also be useful.

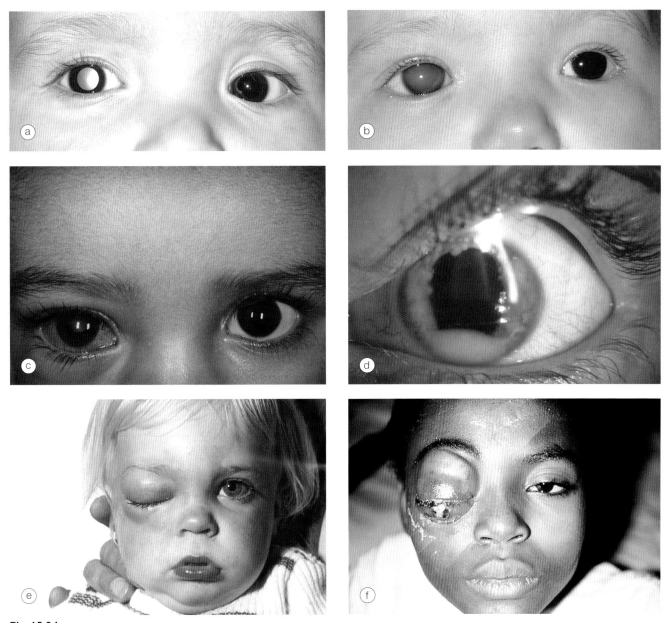

Fig. 15.34
Presentation of retinoblastoma. **(a)** Unilateral leukocoria; **(b)** secondary glaucoma and buphthalmos; **(c)** red eye due to uveitis; **(d)** iris nodules and pseudo-hypopyon; **(e)** orbital inflammation; **(f)** orbital invasion (Courtesy of N Rogers – figs a and b; U Raina – fig. c)

Treatment of small tumours

Small tumours, no more than 3mm diameter and 2mm thickness, may be treated as follows:

1. **Photocoagulation** using a low-energy 532nm argon or 810nm diode laser achieves focal consolidation after chemotherapy. At least three treatment sessions are needed but excessive laser energy can cause vitreous seeding.
2. **Cryotherapy** using the triple freeze-thaw technique is useful for pre-equatorial tumours without either deep invasion or vitreous seeding. Repeated treatment may be necessary. Complications include vitreous haemorrhage, retinal detachment and scleral thinning.

3. **Chemotherapy** without other treatment can be attempted for a macular tumour, to conserve as much vision as possible, but there is an increased risk of tumour recurrence.

Treatment of medium-sized tumours

Medium sized tumours, up to 12mm diameter and 6mm thickness, may be treated as follows:

1. **Brachytherapy** using iodine-125 or ruthenium-106 is indicated for an anterior tumour if there is no vitreous seeding.
2. **Primary chemotherapy** with intravenous carboplatin, etoposide and vincristine (CEV) is given in three to six

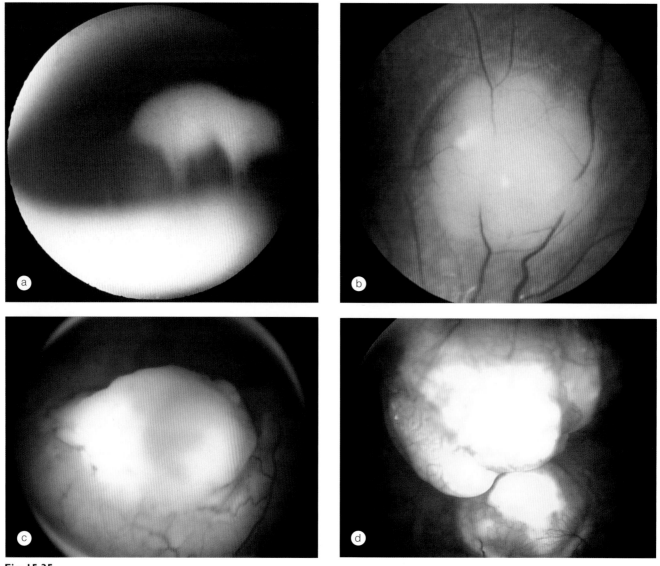

Fig. 15.35
Signs of retinoblastoma. **(a)** Small peripheral tumour; **(b)** intraretinal tumour; **(c)** endophytic tumour; **(d)** exophytic tumour (Courtesy of L Merin – fig. c; L MacKeen – fig. d)

cycles according to the grade of retinoblastoma. Single agent chemoreduction with carboplatin alone has recently been found to give similar results to multi-agent therapy. Systemic treatment can be supplemented with sub-Tenon carboplatin injections. This may be followed by local treatment with cryotherapy or TTT to consolidate tumour control.

3. **External beam radiotherapy** is avoided, if possible, in patients with heritable retinoblastoma because of the risk of inducing a second malignancy such as osteosarcoma. Hypoplasia of the bony orbit can occur, especially if radiotherapy is administered in the first 6 months of life. Early radiotherapy can also cause growth hormone deficiency and neurocognitive defects. In some centres, the risks of external beam radiotherapy can be minimized by methods such as proton beam and stereotactic radiotherapy.

Treatment of large tumours

1. **Chemotherapy** to shrink the tumour (chemoreduction), facilitating subsequent local treatment, thereby avoiding enucleation or external beam radiotherapy. Chemotherapy also will have a beneficial effect if a smaller tumour is present in the fellow eye or if there is a pinealoblastoma.
2. **Enucleation** is indicated if there is rubeosis, vitreous haemorrhage or optic nerve invasion. It is also performed if chemoreduction fails or a normal fellow eye makes aggressive chemotherapy inappropriate. It is also useful for diffuse retinoblastoma because of poor visual prognosis and high risk of risk of recurrence with other therapeutic modalities. Enucleation should be performed with minimal manipulation and it is imperative to obtain a long piece of optic nerve (12–15mm). Inadvertent scleral perforation greatly increases the chances of orbital recurrence and metastatic disease. The orbital implant should be as large as possible. Tenon capsule and conjunctiva should be closed separately. Any postoperative chemotherapy should be delayed for at least a week, to allow healing. A fresh tumour specimen should be taken by an experienced surgeon or pathologist together with a blood sample for *RB1* gene testing.

Treatment of extraocular extension

1. **Adjuvant chemotherapy** consisting of a 6-month course of CEV may be given after enucleation if there is retrolaminar or massive choroidal spread.
2. **External beam radiotherapy** is indicated when there is tumour extension to the cut end of the optic nerve at enucleation, or extension through the sclera.

Treatment of metastatic disease

Metastatic disease is treated according to its extent using various techniques, which include high dose chemotherapy,

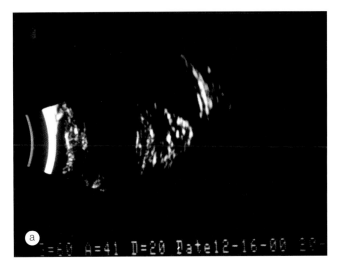

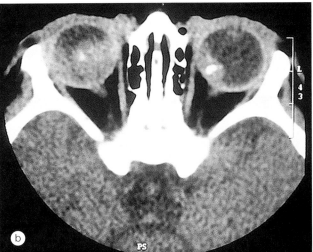

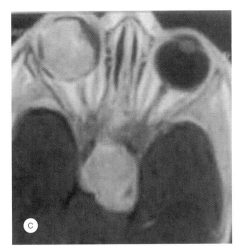

Fig. 15.36
Imaging of retinoblastoma. **(a)** US with low gain shows echoes from calcification; **(b)** axial CT shows bilateral tumours and calcification; **(c)** axial T1-weighted MR shows a very large retinoblastoma in the right eye and a pinealoblastoma (Courtesy of H Atta – fig. a; K Nischal – fig. b; J Pe'er – fig. c)

intrathecal chemotherapy, myeloablative therapy with bone marrow rescue, focal, cranio-spinal or total body radiotherapy. Patients with malignant cells in the cerebrospinal fluid may require intrathecal methotrexate.

Follow-up

- After radiotherapy or chemotherapy, tumours regress to a 'cottage-cheese' calcified mass (Fig. 15.37a), a translucent

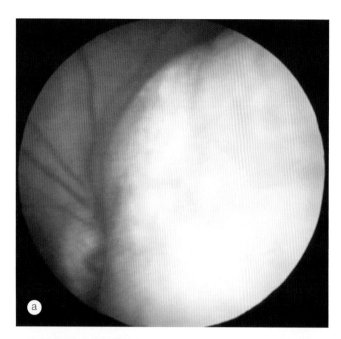

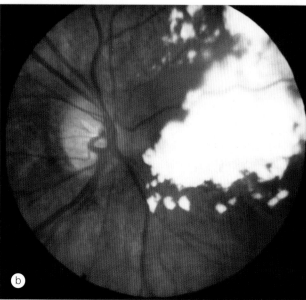

Fig. 15.37
Brachytherapy for retinoblastoma. **(a)** Before treatment; **(b)** 'cottage-cheese' appearance after treatment (Courtesy of N Bornfeld)

'fish-flesh' mass, a mixture of both, or a flat atrophic scar.
- New tumours can develop in patients with heritable retinoblastoma, especially those treated at a very young age. These tend to be anterior and are not prevented by chemotherapy because they have no blood supply. Local tumour recurrences usually occur within 6 months of treatment.
- If retinoblastoma has been treated conservatively examination without anaesthesia is necessary every 2–8 weeks until the age of 3 years, after which time examination without anaesthesia is performed every 6 months until the age of about 5 years, then annually until the age of 10 years.
- Orbital MR is indicated in high risk cases for about 18 months. If the child has any risk of developing a second malignant neoplasm, the parents should be educated to be alert to features of pain, tenderness and swelling and to seek medical attention if there is no improvement within a week.

Differential diagnosis

1. **Congenital cataract** giving rise to leukocoria.
2. **Persistent anterior fetal vasculature** is an important cause of congenital leukocoria (see Chapter 3).
3. **Coats disease** is unilateral, more common in boys and tends to present later than retinoblastoma (see Chapter 16).
4. **Retinopathy of prematurity,** if advanced, may cause retinal detachment and leukocoria. Diagnosis is usually straightforward because of the history of prematurity and low birth weight (see Chapter 16).
5. **Toxocariasis.** Chronic toxocara endophthalmitis may cause a cyclitic membrane and a white pupil. A granuloma at the posterior pole may resemble an endophytic retinoblastoma (see Chapter 14).
6. **Uveitis** may mimic the diffuse infiltrating type of retinoblastoma seen in older children. Conversely, retinoblastoma may be mistaken for uveitis, endophthalmitis or orbital cellulitis.
7. **Retinal dysplasia** is characterized by a congenital pink or white retrolental membrane in a microphthalmic eye, with a shallow anterior chamber and elongated ciliary processes (see Chapter 3).
8. **Incontinentia pigmenti** (Bloch–Sulzberger syndrome) is a rare X-linked dominant disorder affecting girls (see Chapter 3). About one-third of children develop cicatricial retinal detachment in the first year of life which may cause leukocoria.
9. **Retinoma** (retinocytoma) is a benign variant of retinoblastoma. It is characterized by a smooth, dome-shaped mass, which slowly involutes spontaneously to a calcified mass associated with RPE alteration and chorioretinal atrophy. The final appearance is remarkably similar to that of a retinoblastoma following irradia-

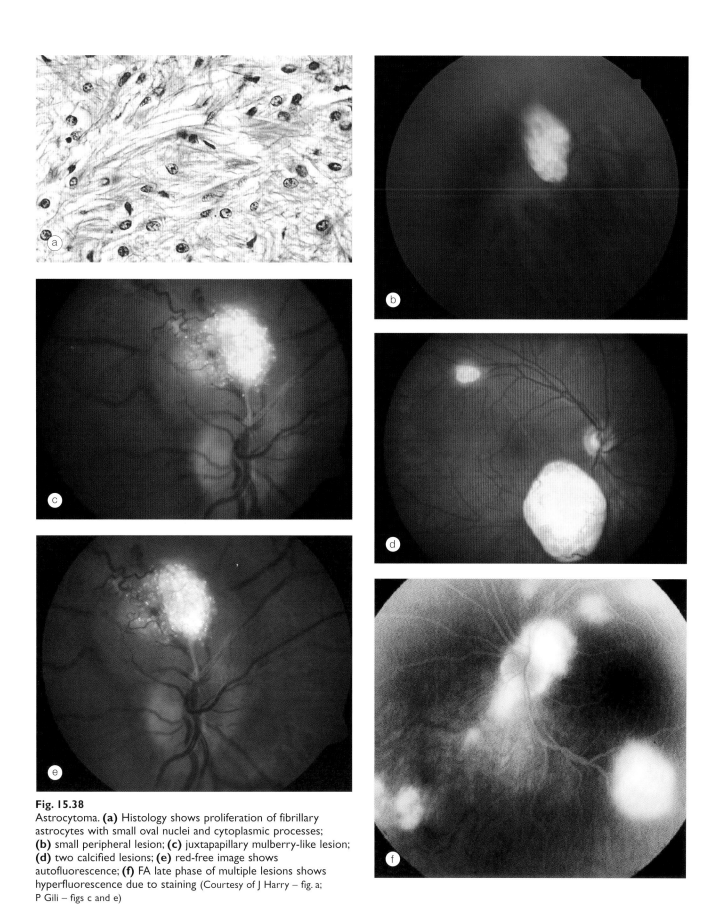

Fig. 15.38
Astrocytoma. **(a)** Histology shows proliferation of fibrillary astrocytes with small oval nuclei and cytoplasmic processes; **(b)** small peripheral lesion; **(c)** juxtapapillary mulberry-like lesion; **(d)** two calcified lesions; **(e)** red-free image shows autofluorescence; **(f)** FA late phase of multiple lesions shows hyperfluorescence due to staining (Courtesy of J Harry – fig. a; P Gili – figs c and e)

tion. Rarely, a retinoma can transform into a rapidly growing retinoblastoma.

10. **Retinal astrocytoma,** which may be multifocal and bilateral.

Astrocytoma

Astrocytoma of the retina or optic nerve head is a rare benign tumour which does not threaten vision. Most are endophytic, protruding into the vitreous, but exophytic subretinal tumours can occur. Astrocytomas may occasionally be encountered as an incidental solitary lesion in normal individuals but are most frequently seen in tuberous sclerosis (see Chapter 24). About 50% of patients with tuberous sclerosis have fundus astrocytomas which may be multiple and bilateral.

1. **Histology** shows fibrillary astrocytes with small oval nuclei and cytoplasmic processes (Fig. 15.38a).
2. **Signs**
   - Peripheral, yellowish plaque or nodule (Fig. 15.38b).
   - A peripapillary mulberry-like lesion (Fig. 15.38c).
   - Most tumours are static but long-standing lesions may become calcified (Fig. 15.38d).
3. **Autofluorescence** is characteristic (Fig. 15.38e).
4. **FA** shows hyperfluorescence due to staining without leakage (Fig. 15.38f).
5. **Treatment** is not required.
6. **Differential diagnosis**
   a. *Large optic disc drusen* lying deep in the disc.
   b. *Myelinated nerve fibres* may resemble a small, flat astrocytoma.
   c. *Retinoblastoma*, endophytic or regressed, may mimic a mulberry astrocytoma.

Retinal haemangioblastoma

Retinal haemangioblastoma is a rare sight-threatening tumour that may occasionally occur in isolation although about 50% of patients with solitary lesions and virtually all patients with multiple lesions have von Hippel–Lindau disease (VHL – see Chapter 24). The prevalence of retinal tumours in VHL is approximately 60%. Vascular endothelial growth factor (VEGF) is important in the development of retinal tumours.

Histology

The tumour is composed of capillary-like vascular channels between large foamy cells that possibly represent histiocytes, endothelial cells or astrocytes (Fig. 15.39a). The tumour is usually endophytic but occasionally it may be exophytic arising from the outer retina.

Endophytic tumour

1. **Presentation.** The median age at diagnosis in patients with VHL is earlier (median 18 years) than in those without VHL (median 31 years). The tumour may be detected by screening of those at risk or because of symptoms due to macular exudates or retinal detachment.
2. **Signs**
   - A small, well-defined oval red lesion within the capillary bed between an arteriole and venule (Fig. 15.39b).
   - A round orange-red mass with dilatation and tortuosity of the supplying artery and draining vein (Fig. 15.39c and 15.39d).
   - The tumour may involve the optic nerve head (Fig. 15.39f).
   - Fibrotic tumours, which have regressed spontaneously, are white and without feeder vessels.
3. **FA** shows early hyperfluorescence (Fig. 15.39e) and late leakage.
4. **Complications**
   - Exudate formation in the area surrounding the tumour and/or at the macula (Fig. 15.39f).
   - Bleeding and leakage resulting in macular oedema and exudative retinal detachment.
   - Fibrotic bands, which can cause tractional or rhegmatogenous retinal detachment.
   - Vitreous haemorrhage, secondary glaucoma and phthisis bulbi.

Exophytic tumour

1. **Presentation** is with visual loss due to exudation or bleeding.
2. **Signs**
   - A sessile, ill-defined, placoid, juxtapapillary lesion with dilated blood vessels.
   - Associated retinal oedema, serous elevation, hard exudates (Fig. 15.40a) and haemorrhage are common (Fig. 15.40b).
3. **FA** shows hyperfluorescence of the tumour and masking by blood or exudate (Fig. 15.40c).

Treatment

1. **No treatment** is advised for asymptomatic juxtapapillary haemangiomas without exudation, because these may remain inactive for many years and because of the high risk of iatrogenic visual loss.
2. **Laser photocoagulation** of small lesions. After closing the feeder vessels, the tumour is treated with low-energy, long duration burns. Multiple sessions may be needed.
3. **Cryotherapy** for larger peripheral lesions or those with exudative retinal detachment. Vigorous treatment of a large lesion may cause a temporary but extensive exudative retinal detachment.

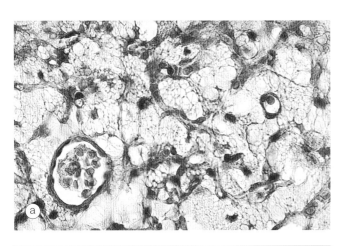

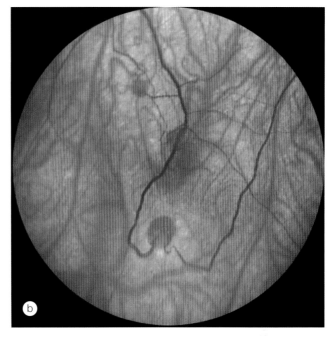

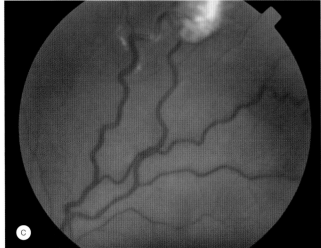

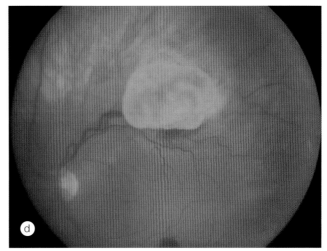

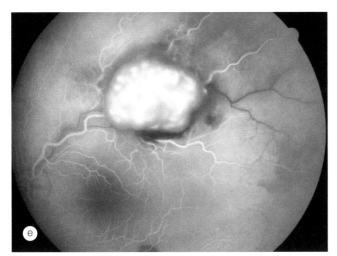

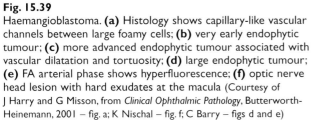

Fig. 15.39

Haemangioblastoma. **(a)** Histology shows capillary-like vascular channels between large foamy cells; **(b)** very early endophytic tumour; **(c)** more advanced endophytic tumour associated with vascular dilatation and tortuosity; **(d)** large endophytic tumour; **(e)** FA arterial phase shows hyperfluorescence; **(f)** optic nerve head lesion with hard exudates at the macula (Courtesy of J Harry and G Misson, from *Clinical Ophthalmic Pathology*, Butterworth-Heinemann, 2001 – fig. a; K Nischal – fig. f; C Barry – figs d and e)

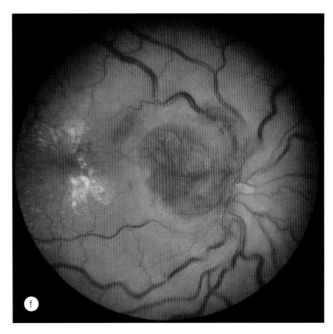

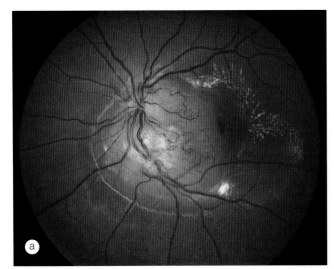

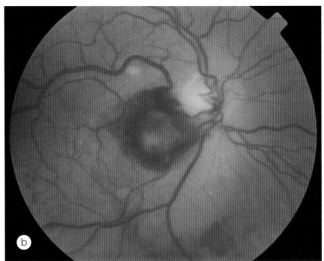

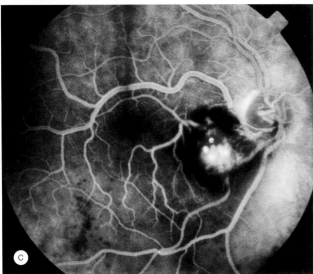

Fig. 15.40
Exophytic haemangioblastoma. **(a)** Diffuse juxtapapillary lesion associated with shallow serous retinal elevation and peripheral hard exudates; **(b)** tumour associated with haemorrhage; **(c)** FA arteriovenous phase shows hyperfluorescence of the tumour and hypofluorescence corresponding to blockage by blood (Courtesy of P Saine – fig. a; S Milewski – figs b and c)

skin and CNS ('neuro-oculo-cutaneous phacomatosis' or 'cavernoma multiplex').

1. **Presentation** may be in the second to third decades with vitreous haemorrhage or, more frequently, as a chance finding.
2. **Signs**
   - Sessile clusters of saccular aneurysms resembling a 'bunch of grapes' on the peripheral retina (Fig. 15.41a and c).
   - Because of sluggish flow of blood, the red cells may sediment and separate from plasma, giving rise to 'menisci', or fluid levels within the lesion, best seen on fluorescein angiography (Fig. 15.41b).
   - The lesion may also affect the optic nerve (Fig. 15.41d).
3. **Complications,** which are uncommon, include haemorrhage (Fig. 15.41e) and epiretinal membrane formation.
4. **Treatment.** Photocoagulation should be avoided as it may result in haemorrhage or tumour enlargement. Rarely vitrectomy may be necessary for non-absorbing vitreous haemorrhage. MR of the CNS is indicated in patients and close relatives as local excision or proton beam radiotherapy may avoid intracranial haemorrhage.

4. **Brachytherapy** for lesions too large for cryotherapy.
5. **Vitreoretinal surgery** may be required for non-absorbing vitreous haemorrhage, epiretinal fibrosis or tractional retinal detachment. If appropriate, the tumour may be destroyed by endolaser photocoagulation or excised.
6. **Other modalities** include photodynamic therapy, which avoids damage to adjacent tissues, and anti-vascular endothelial growth factor (VEGF) agents. These are worth considering with juxtapapillary tumours, which are otherwise virtually untreatable without visual loss.

Cavernous haemangioma

Cavernous haemangioma of the retina or optic nerve head is a rare, congenital, unilateral, vascular hamartoma. It is usually sporadic but occasionally can be inherited as AD with incomplete penetrance, in combination with lesions of the

Racemose haemangioma

Racemose haemangioma (also known as arteriovenous malformation) of the retina and optic nerve head is a rare,

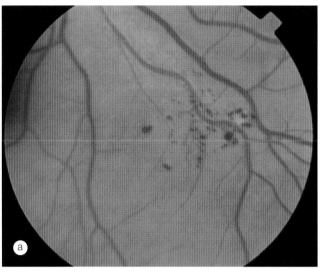

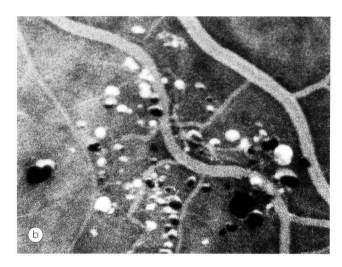

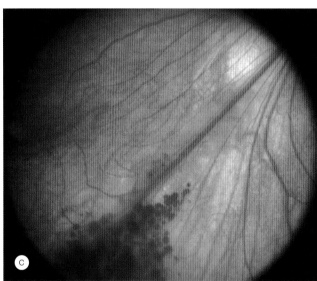

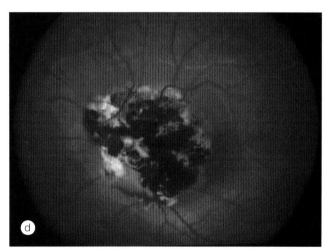

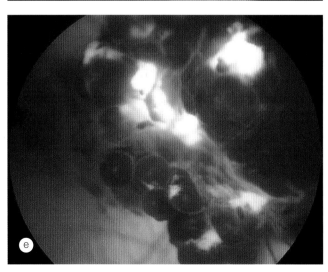

Fig. 15.41
Cavernous haemangioma. **(a)** Very small peripheral lesion; **(b)** FA shows fluid levels due to separation of red cells (hypofluorescent) and plasma (hyperfluorescent); **(c)** larger peripheral lesion; **(d)** optic nerve lesion; **(e)** very large lesion with haemorrhage (Courtesy of S Milewski – figs a and b; A Singh – fig. c; P Lommatzsch – fig. d; T Link – fig. e)

sporadic, usually unilateral, congenital malformation involving direct communication between the arteries and veins without an intervening capillary bed. Some patients have similar ipsilateral lesions involving the midbrain, basofrontal region and posterior fossa (an association referred to as the Wyburn–Mason syndrome). Brain involvement may lead to spontaneous haemorrhage or epilepsy. Occasionally, malformations may involve the maxilla and mandible, predisposing the patient to haemorrhage after dental treatment. Facial skin lesions have also been reported.

1. **Presentation** is usually as a chance finding.
2. **Signs**
   - Enlarged, tortuous blood vessels which are often more numerous than normal with the vein and artery appearing similar (Fig. 15.42a).
   - With time the vessels become more dilated and tortuous, and may become sclerotic (Fig. 15.42b).
3. **FA** shows hyperfluorescence but absence of leakage (Fig. 15.42c).
4. **Treatment** is not required.

Vasoproliferative tumour

Retinal vasoproliferative tumour is a rare gliovascular lesion which can be primary or secondary to conditions such as intermediate uveitis, ocular trauma and retinitis pigmentosa. Secondary lesions may be multiple and occasionally bilateral depending on the underlying aetiology.

1. **Presentation** is usually in the fifth to sixth decades with blurring of vision due to macular exudation.
2. **Signs**
   - A reddish-yellow, retinal or subretinal mass containing telangiectatic vessels, most frequently located in the inferotemporal periphery (Fig. 15.43).
   - Rarely the lesion may be diffuse and involve large areas of the fundus.
3. **Complications** include visual loss from maculopathy caused by hard exudates, oedema, exudative retinal detachment and epiretinal membrane. Untreated, this tumour causes severe vitreous haemorrhage, exudative retinal detachment, rubeosis and neovascular glaucoma.
4. **Treatment** with cryotherapy or brachytherapy induces regression of the tumour and exudation but the visual prognosis is guarded if there is maculopathy.

Primary intraocular lymphoma

Primary intraocular lymphoma (PIOL) represents a subset of primary central nervous system lymphoma (PCNSL), which is a variant of extranodal non-Hodgkin lymphoma.

The lymphoma cells are large, pleomorphic B lymphocytes with large multilobular nuclei, prominent nucleoli and scanty cytoplasm (Fig. 15.44a). The tumour arises from within the brain (Fig. 15.44b), spinal cord and leptomeninges, and has a very poor prognosis. Onset is in the sixth and seventh decades. About 20% of patients with PCNSL have ocular manifestations, which can precede or follow neurological involvement. Most patients with PIOL develop CNS symptoms after a mean delay of 29 months.

Ocular features

1. **Presentation** is with unilateral floaters, blurred vision, red eye or photophobia, which frequently becomes bilateral after a variable interval.
2. **Signs**
   - Mild anterior uveitis with cells, flare and keratic precipitates.
   - Vitritis is very common and may impede visualization of the fundus (Fig. 15.44c).
   - Multifocal, large, yellowish, solid sub-RPE infiltrates that progress to involve the choroid are common (Fig. 15.44d).
   - Occasionally coalescence of sub-RPE deposits may form a ring encircling the equator (Fig. 15.44e).
   - Diffuse retinal or subretinal infiltration (Fig. 15.44f).
   - Other features include retinal vasculitis, vascular occlusion, exudative retinal detachment and optic atrophy.

> **NB** Lack of CMO is an important diagnostic clue, since in true uveitis significant vitritis is almost always accompanied by CMO.

Neurological features

1. **Presentation**
   - An intracranial mass may cause headache, nausea, personality change, focal deficit and seizures.
   - Leptomeningeal disease may cause neuropathy.
   - Spinal cord involvement may cause bilateral motor and sensory deficits.
2. **Signs** are elicited with:
   - Abnormal clinical neurological examination, such as cranial nerve palsies, hemiparesis and ataxia.
   - MR of head and spine, with gadolinium, which can detect one or more intracranial tumours, diffuse meningeal or periventricular lesions, and/or localized intradural spinal masses.
   - Lumbar puncture, which can demonstrate malignant cells in CSF in a minority of patients with abnormal MR; a positive result avoids the need for brain or ocular biopsy.

Treatment

1. **Radiotherapy** is first-line treatment for PIOL, but recurrence is common.
2. **Intravitreal** methotrexate is useful for recurrent disease, but close monitoring is needed to detect ocular complications and any recurrence.
3. **Systemic chemotherapy** with a variety of regimens including methotrexate can prolong survival in patients with CNS disease. This can be given in combination with whole brain irradiation but neurotoxicity is a problem. Systemic treatment is usually effective for eye disease and this is preferred to ocular radiotherapy because in addition to avoiding radiation-induced complications it may improve survival.

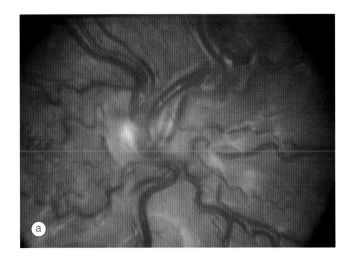
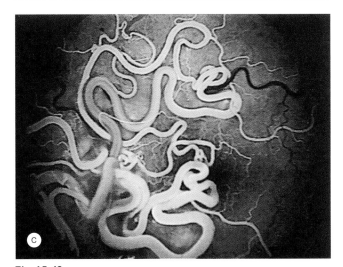
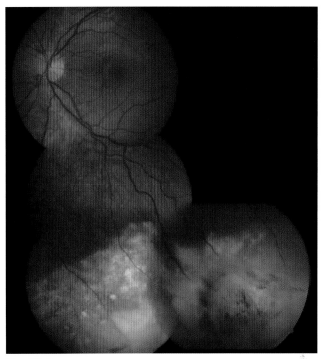

Fig. 15.42
Racemose haemangioma. **(a)** Vascular dilatation and tortuosity; **(b)** more severe lesion in which some vessels show sclerosis; **(c)** FA shows hyperfluorescence but absence of leakage (Courtesy of S Milewski – figs b and c)

Fig. 15.43
Vasoproliferative tumour (Courtesy of C Mosci-Genova)

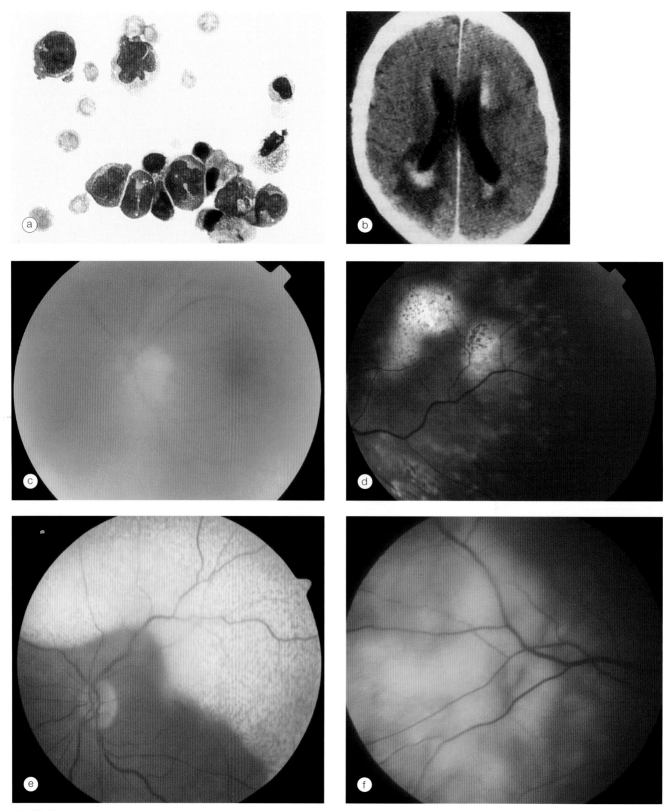

Fig. 15.44
Primary intraocular lymphoma. **(a)** Vitreous biopsy shows cells with irregular large nuclei and scanty cytoplasm; **(b)** axial CT shows cerebral lymphoma; **(c)** vitreous haze due to vitritis; **(d)** multifocal subretinal infiltrates; **(e)** coalescent subretinal infiltrates; **(f)** diffuse involvement (Courtesy of P Smith – fig. a; A Singh – figs b and f; B Damato – fig. e)

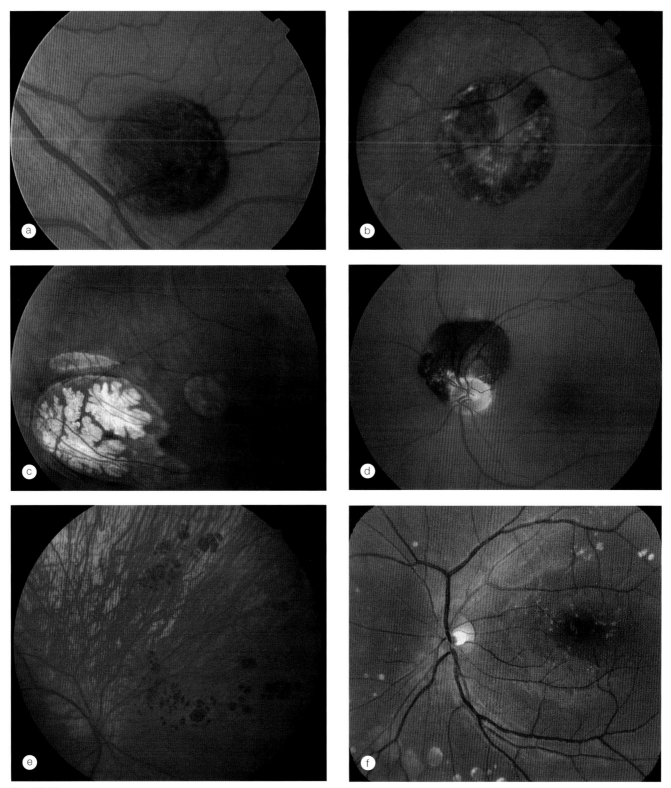

Fig. 15.45
Typical congenital hypertrophy of the retinal pigment epithelium. **(a)** Completely pigmented lesion; **(b)** partly depigmented lesion; **(c)** largely depigmented lesion; **(d)** juxtapapillary lesion; **(e)** 'bear-track' lesions; **(f)** 'polar bear-track' lesions (Courtesy of J Donald M Gass, from *Stereoscopic Atlas of Macular Diseases*, Mosby, 1997 – fig. f)

TUMOURS OF THE RETINAL PIGMENT EPITHELIUM

Typical congenital hypertrophy of the RPE

Congenital hypertrophy of the retinal pigment epithelium (CHRPE) is a common benign lesion which may be: (a) *typical*, either solitary or grouped, or (b) *atypical*. It is important to differentiate the two types because the latter may have important systemic implications (see below).

1. **Solitary CHRPE**
   - A flat, dark-grey or black, round or oval lesion with discrete margins usually located near the equator (Fig. 15.45a).
   - Depigmented lacunae are common (Fig. 15.45b).
   - Some lesions are depigmented apart from a thin rim (Fig. 15.45c).
   - Juxtapapillary lesions are uncommon (Fig. 15.45d).
2. **Grouped CHRPE**
   - Multiple lesions organized in a pattern simulating animal footprints (bear-track pigmentation) often confined to one sector or quadrant of the fundus with the smaller spots usually located more centrally (Fig. 15.45e).
   - Rarely the lesions may be completely depigmented (polar bear tracks) (Fig. 15.45f).

Atypical congenital hypertrophy of the RPE

Signs

Multiple, bilateral, widely separated, frequently oval or spindle-shaped lesions of variable size associated with hypopigmentation at one margin (Fig. 15.46a and b). The lesions have a haphazard distribution and may be pigmented, depigmented or heterogeneous.

Systemic associations

1. **Familial adenomatous polyposis (FAP)** is an AD condition characterized by adenomatous polyps throughout the rectum and colon which usually start to develop in adolescence (Fig. 15.46c). If untreated, virtually all patients with FAP develop carcinoma of the colorectal region by the age of 50 years. From the age of 10 years, persons at risk should undergo regular endoscopic examinations and a prophylactic total colectomy should be performed early in adult life in all affected persons. As a result of the dominant inheritance pattern, intensive survey of family members is imperative. The APC (Adenomatous Polyposis Coli) gene has been identified on chromosome 5(5q21-q22). Thus, molecular genetic analysis may identify carriers of the disease in selected cases. Over 80% of patients with FAP have atypical CHRPE lesions, which are present at birth. A positive criterion for FAP is the presence of at least four lesions whatever their size, or at least two lesions – one of which must be large. Such fundus lesions in a family member should therefore arouse suspicion of FAP but their absence does not exclude FAP.
2. **Gardner syndrome** is characterized by FAP, osteomas of the skull, mandible and long bones, and cutaneous soft tissue tumours such as epidermoid cysts, lipomas and fibromas.
3. **Turcot syndrome** is characterized by FAP and tumours of the CNS, particularly medulloblastoma (Fig. 15.46d) and glioma. Inheritance can be AD or AR.

Combined hamartoma of the retina and RPE

Combined hamartoma of the retina and RPE is a rare, usually unilateral congenital malformation that predominantly affects males. It usually occurs sporadically in normal individuals and occasionally in patients with neurofibromatosis 2, Gorlin syndrome and incontinentia pigmenti. The lesion is composed of RPE, sensory retina, retinal blood vessels and vitreoretinal membranes to varying degrees. Occasional optic disc associations include disc pit, drusen and coloboma.

1. **Presentation** is in late childhood or early adulthood with strabismus, blurred vision or metamorphopsia.
2. **Signs**
   - Deep greyish pigmentation with superficial whitish gliosis resulting in retinal wrinkling and vascular tortuosity.
   - The lesion is usually juxtapapillary (Fig. 15.47a), peripapillary (Fig. 15.47b) or at the posterior pole (Fig. 15.47c).
   - Peripheral lesions are uncommon (Fig. 15.47d).
   - Large lesions may cause 'dragging' of the disc (see Fig. 15.47c) or macula.
   - Uncommon associated findings include hard exudate formation (see Fig. 15.47b) and occasionally choroidal neovascularization at the margins of the lesion.
3. **FA** shows early hyperfluorescence of the vascular abnormalities and blockage by pigment (Fig. 15.47e); late phase shows intense hyperfluorescence due to leakage (Fig. 15.47f).
4. **Treatment** is not indicated.

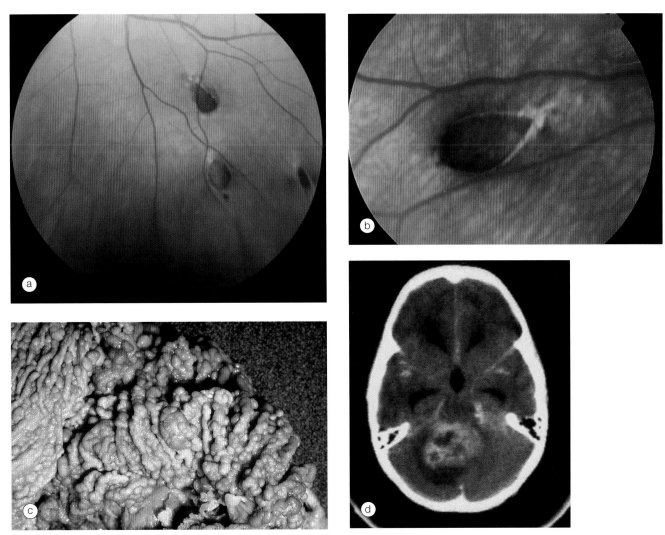

Fig. 15.46
(a) Atypical congenital hypertrophy of the retinal pigment epithelium; **(b)** magnification shows characteristic depigmentation at one margin; **(c)** adenomatous polyposis; **(d)** axial CT showing a medulloblastoma in Turcot syndrome (Courtesy of P Trend, M Swash and C Kennard, from *Colour Guide Neurology*, Churchill Livingstone, 1992 – fig. d)

Congenital hamartoma of the RPE

Congenital hamartoma of the RPE is a rare entity, usually incidentally diagnosed in asymptomatic children and young adults.

1. Signs
- Small, jet-black, nodular lesion, with well-defined margins, which usually appears to involve the full thickness of the retina and to spill onto the inner retinal surface in a mushroom configuration.
- The lesion is typically located immediately adjacent to the foveola and is 1.5mm or less in diameter (Fig. 15.48).
- Visual acuity is usually normal, but may occasionally be impaired as a result of surrounding foveal traction or central foveal involvement.

2. Treatment is not appropriate.

PARANEOPLASTIC SYNDROMES

Paraneoplastic syndromes are rare diseases that might be missed or misdiagnosed by the unwary observer. Many patients present with visual symptoms before the primary malignancy is diagnosed. It is therefore important for clinicians to be familiar with these syndromes so as to detect the underlying malignancy as early as possible.

Bilateral diffuse uveal melanocytic proliferation

Bilateral diffuse uveal melanocytic proliferation (BDUMP) is a very rare paraneoplastic syndrome occurring usually in

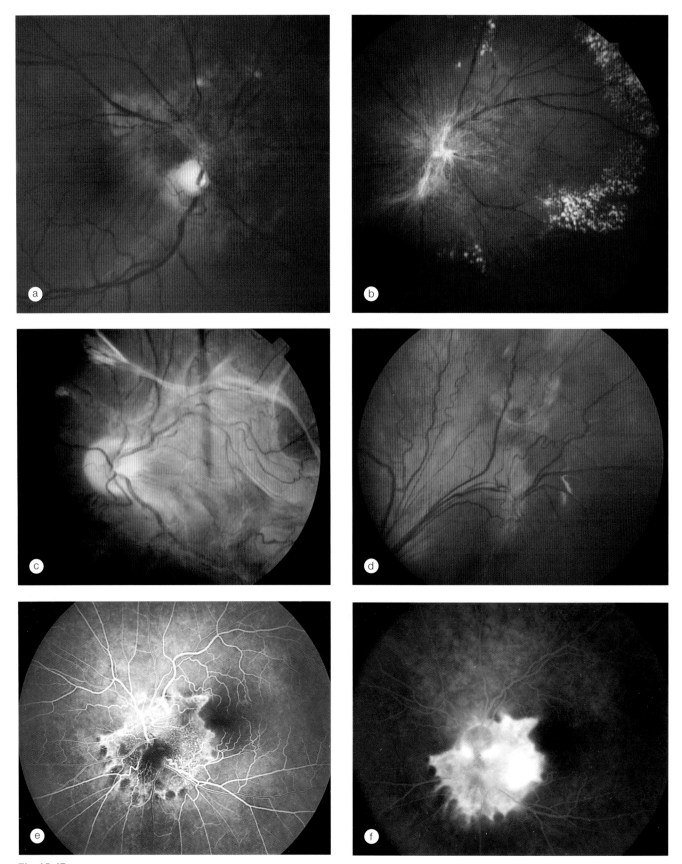

Fig. 15.47
Combined hamartoma of the retina and retinal pigment epithelium. **(a)** Small juxtapapillary lesion; **(b)** large peripapillary lesion with peripheral hard exudates; **(c)** large posterior pole lesion with 'dragging' of the disc; **(d)** peripheral lesion; **(e)** FA early venous phase shows hyperfluorescence of the vascular abnormality and blockage by pigment; **(f)** late phase shows intense hyperfluorescence due to leakage (Courtesy of B Damato – fig. a; S Milewski–fig. c; C Barry – figs e and f)

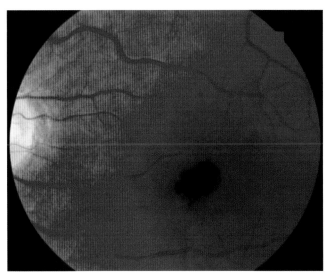

Fig. 15.48
Congenital hamartoma of the retinal pigment epithelium

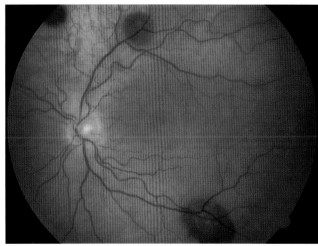

Fig. 15.49
Naevus-like lesions in diffuse uveal melanocytic proliferation
(Courtesy of A Leys)

patients with systemic, often occult, malignancy. It is characterized by proliferation of benign melanocytes in the outer choroid.

1. **Signs**
   - Multiple naevus-like choroidal lesions (Fig. 15.49).
   - Multiple red-grey subretinal patches which may have a reticular pattern.
   - Exudative retinal detachment.
   - Rapidly developing cataracts.
   - Vitreous and anterior chamber cells.
   - Episcleral nodules, and anterior uveal cysts and tumours.
2. **US** shows diffuse choroidal thickening and multiple tumours.
3. **ERG** is often reduced.
4. **Treatment** of BDUMP itself is not possible but successful treatment of the underlying primary tumour may be followed by regression of BDUMP but without improvement in vision.

Cancer-associated retinopathy

Cancer-associated retinopathy (CAR) is most frequently associated with small cell bronchial carcinoma, followed by gynecological and breast cancer.

1. **Symptoms**
   - Subacute bilateral visual loss over 6–18 months.
   - Visual symptoms precede the diagnosis of malignancy in half the cases, usually by several months.
   - Positive visual phenomenon of shimmering or flickering lights.

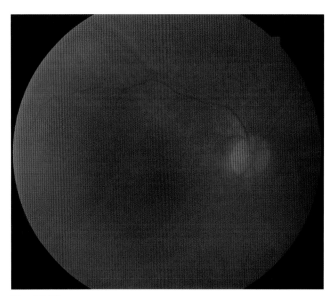

Fig. 15.50
Arteriolar attenuation in cancer-associated retinopathy

   - Progressive reduction of visual acuity and colour vision, glare, photosensitivity and central scotoma attributed to cone dysfunction.
   - Night blindness, impaired dark adaptation, ring scotoma and peripheral field loss due to rod dysfunction in advanced cases.
2. **Signs**
   - Fundus often appears normal on presentation.
   - Attenuated arterioles, optic disc pallor and mild RPE changes develop as the disease progresses (Fig. 15.50).

3. **Investigations**
   a. ***ERG*** is severely attenuated under photopic and scotopic conditions; dark adaptation is abnormal.
   b. ***Lumbar puncture*** may show elevated cerebral spinal fluid protein and lymphocytosis.
   c. ***Search for an underlying malignancy.***
4. **Prognosis** for both vision and life is poor.

Melanoma-associated retinopathy

Melanoma-associated retinopathy (MAR) differs from CAR because the visual symptoms usually arise after the diagnosis of cutaneous melanoma. There may be concurrent vitiligo. The specific antigen responsible has not been identified, but autoantibodies from MAR sera react against bipolar cells in human retina. Clinical and electrophysiological data also implicate the bipolar cells as the primary abnormality.

1. **Symptoms** are shimmering or flickering lights and nyctalopia.
2. **Signs**
   • Central visual loss, which is sudden.
   • Fundus appears normal initially, but optic disc pallor, retinal vascular attenuation and vitreous cells can develop.
3. **ERG** shows marked reduction of dark adapted and light adapted b-wave and preservation of a-wave (normal photoreceptor function). Both the amplitude and implicit time of the b-wave are abnormal. There is also a 'negative ERG', similar to the pattern seen in congenital stationary night blindness.
4. **Prognosis** for vision is good.

CHAPTER 16

RETINAL VASCULAR DISEASE

RETINAL CIRCULATION

Arterial system

1. **The central retinal artery** is an end artery that enters the optic nerve approximately 1 cm behind the globe. Like other arteries in the body it is composed of the following anatomical layers:
   a. *The intima*, the innermost, is composed of a single layer of endothelium resting on a collagenous zone.
   b. *The internal elastic lamina* separates the intima from the media.
   c. *The media* consists mainly of smooth muscle.
   d. *The adventitia* is the outermost and is composed of loose connective tissue.
2. **Retinal arterioles** arise from the central retinal artery. They contain smooth muscle within their walls but unlike arteries their internal elastic lamina is discontinuous.

Capillaries

Retinal capillaries supply the inner two-thirds of the retina, the outer third being supplied by the choriocapillaris. The inner capillary network is located in the ganglion cell layer and the outer in the inner nuclear layer. Capillary-free zones are present around arterioles (periarteriolar capillary-free zone – Fig. 16.1a) and at the fovea (foveal avascular zone). Retinal capillaries are devoid of smooth muscle and elastic tissue and their walls consist of the following (Fig. 16.1b):

1. **Endothelial cells** form a single layer on a basement membrane and are linked by tight junctions that form the inner blood–retinal barrier.

2. **Pericytes** lie external to endothelial cells and have multiple pseudopodial processes that envelop the capillary. They have contractile properties and are thought to participate in autoregulation of the microvascular circulation.

Venous system

Retinal venules and veins drain blood from the capillaries.

1. **Small venules** are larger than capillaries but have a similar structure.
2. **Larger venules** contain smooth muscle and gradually merge to form veins.
3. **Veins** contain a small amount of smooth muscle and elastic tissue in their walls and are relatively distensible. They gradually expand in diameter as they pass posteriorly towards the central retinal vein.

DIABETIC RETINOPATHY

Introduction

Risk factors

Diabetic retinopathy (DR) is commoner in type 1 (40%) than in type 2 (20%), and is the most prevalent cause of legal blindness between the ages of 20 and 65 years.

1. **Duration of diabetes** is the most important risk factor. In patients diagnosed before the age of 30 years, the incidence of DR after 10 years is 50% and after 30 years 90%. DR rarely develops within 5 years of the onset of diabetes or before puberty, but about 5% of type 2 diabetics

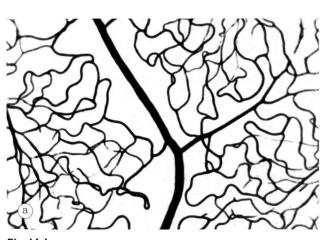
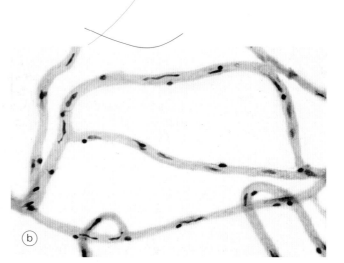

Fig. 16.1
Normal retinal capillary bed. **(a)** Periarteriolar capillary-free zone – flat preparation of Indian ink injected retina; **(b)** endothelial cells with elongated nuclei and pericytes with rounded nuclei – trypsin digest preparation (Courtesy of J Harry and G Misson, from *Clinical Ophthalmic Pathology*, Butterworth-Heinemann, 2001)

have DR at presentation. It appears that duration of diabetes is a strong predictor for maculopathy and proliferative disease, but relatively more important for the latter.

2. **Poor metabolic control** is less important than duration, but is nevertheless relevant to the development and progression of DR. It has been shown that tight blood glucose control, particularly when instituted early, can prevent or delay the development or progression of DR. It is, however, associated with an increased risk of hypoglycaemic events. Type 1 diabetic patients appear to obtain greater benefit from tight control than those with type 2. Unfortunately, perfect glycaemic control remains elusive in many patients. Raised HbA1c is associated with an increased risk of proliferative disease.

3. **Pregnancy** is occasionally associated with rapid progression of DR. Predicating factors include poor pre-pregnancy control of diabetes, too rapid control during the early stages of pregnancy, and the development of pre-eclampsia and fluid imbalance.

4. **Hypertension,** which is very common in patients with type 2 diabetes, should be rigorously controlled (< 140/80mmHg). Tight control appears to be particularly beneficial in type 2 diabetics with maculopathy.

5. **Nephropathy,** if severe, is associated with worsening of DR. Conversely, treatment of renal disease (e.g. renal transplantation) may be associated with improvement of retinopathy and a better response to photocoagulation.

6. **Other risk factors** include obesity, particularly increased body mass and a high waist-to-hip ratio, hyperlipidaemia and anaemia.

Pathogenesis

DR is a microangiopathy the exhibits features of both microvascular occlusion and leakage. Hyperglycaemia appears to initiate the following downstream vascular events:

1. **Capillaropathy** involves degeneration and loss of pericytes (Fig. 16.2b), proliferation of endothelial cells, thickening of the basement membrane and occlusion.

2. **Haematological changes** that predispose to decreased capillary blood flow:
   - Deformation of erythrocytes and rouleaux formation.
   - Activation and reduced deformability of white cells.
   - Increased platelet stickiness and aggregation.
   - Increased plasma viscosity.

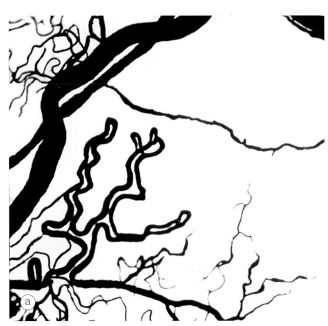

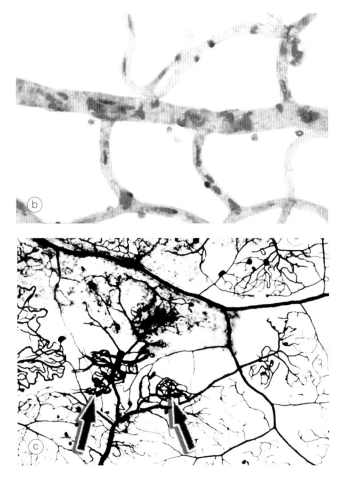

Fig. 16.2
Diabetic capillary bed. **(a)** Capillary closure with adjacent dilated and elongated capillaries – flat preparation of Indian ink injected retina; **(b)** degenerate pericytes which are eosinophilic – trypsin digest preparation; **(c)** new capillaries (arrows) on the inner retinal surface growing from vessels in relation to non-perfused areas – flat preparation of Indian ink injected retina (Courtesy of J Harry)

3. **Microvascular occlusion** results in capillary non-perfusion (Fig. 16.2a) and retinal hypoxia which may cause the following:

   a. *Arteriovenous shunts* that run from arterioles to venules are associated with significant capillary occlusion ('drop-out') and are referred to as intraretinal microvascular abnormalities (IRMA).

   b. *Neovascularization* which is thought to be caused by angiogenic growth factors and results in new vessel formation on the retina (Fig. 16.2c) and optic disc (proliferative retinopathy), and occasionally on the iris (rubeosis iridis).

Background diabetic retinopathy

Diagnosis

Figure 16.3 shows the lesions in background diabetic retinopathy (BDR) and their location.

1. **Microaneurysms** are localized saccular outpouchings of the capillary wall that may be formed by either focal dilatation of the capillary wall where pericytes are absent or fusion of two arms of a capillary loop (Fig. 16.4a). They are frequently seen in relation to areas of capillary non-perfusion (Fig. 16.4b). Loss of pericytes may also lead to endothelial cell proliferation with the formation of cellular microaneurysms (Fig. 16.4c). Microaneurysms may leak plasma constituents into the retina as a result of breakdown in the blood–retinal barrier or become thrombosed (Fig. 16.4d).

   a. *Signs*. Tiny, red dots, initially temporal to the fovea are the earliest signs of DR (Fig. 16.4e). When coated with blood they may be indistinguishable from dot haemorrhages.

   b. *FA.* Early frames show tiny hyperfluorescent dots (Fig. 16.4f), representing non-thrombosed microaneurysms,

typically more numerous than visible clinically. Late frames show diffuse hyperfluorescence due to leakage.

2. **Retinal haemorrhages** (Fig. 16.5a)

   a. *Retinal nerve fibre layer haemorrhages* arise from the larger superficial pre-capillary arterioles and, because of the architecture of the retinal nerve fibres, are flame-shaped (Fig. 16.5b).

   b. *Intraretinal haemorrhages* arise from the venous end of capillaries and are located in the compact middle layers of the retina with a resultant red, 'dot-blot' configuration (Fig. 16.5c).

3. **Macular oedema.** Diffuse oedema is caused by extensive capillary leakage. Localized retinal oedema is caused by focal leakage from microaneurysms and dilated capillary segments. The fluid is initially located between the outer plexiform and inner nuclear layers. Later it may also involve the inner plexiform and nerve fibre layers, until eventually the entire thickness of the retina becomes oedematous. With further accumulation of fluid the fovea assumes a cystoid appearance (cystoid macular oedema – CMO).

   a. *Signs*. Retinal thickening, which is best detected by indirect slit-lamp biomicroscopy.

   b. *FA* shows diffuse late hyperfluorescence due to retinal capillary leakage that may have a flower-petal pattern if CMO is present (Fig. 16.6a).

   c. *OCT* (optical coherence tomography) shows retinal thickening and, if present, cystoid spaces (Fig. 16.6b). It may be used to assess response to treatment.

4. **Hard exudates** are caused by chronic localized retinal oedema. They develop at the junction of normal and oedematous retina and are composed of lipoprotein and lipid-filled macrophages located mainly within the outer plexiform layer (Fig. 16.7a).

   a. *Signs*
   - Waxy, yellow lesions with relatively distinct margins often arranged in clumps and/or rings at the posterior pole that typically surround leaking microaneurysms (Fig. 16.7b and c).
   - With time number and size tends to increase, and the fovea may be threatened or involved (Fig. 16.7d and e).
   - When leakage ceases, they absorb spontaneously over a period of months or years, either into the healthy surrounding capillaries or by phagocytosis of their lipid content.
   - Chronic leakage leads to enlargement of the exudates and the deposition of cholesterol (Fig. 16.7f).

   b. *FA* shows hypofluorescence due to blockage of background choroidal fluorescence.

Management

Patients with mild BDR require no treatment but should be reviewed annually. Apart from optimal control of diabetes, associated factors such as hypertension, anaemia or renal failure should also be addressed. Patients with more severe

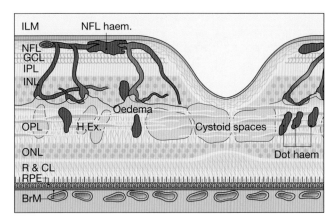

Fig. 16.3
Location of lesions in background diabetic retinopathy

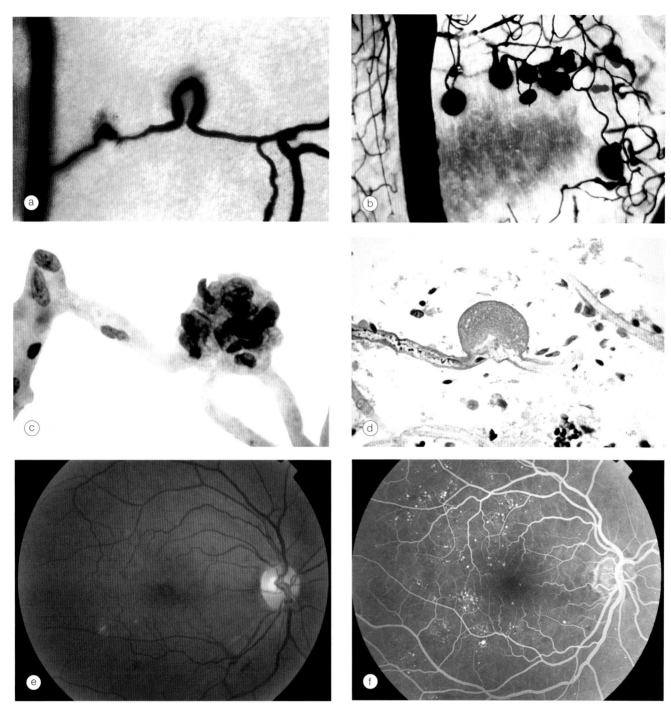

Fig. 16.4

Retinal microaneurysm. **(a)** Two arms of a capillary loop are not yet fused to become a microaneurysm – flat preparation of Indian ink injected retina; **(b)** an area of capillary non-perfusion and adjacent microaneurysms – flat preparation of Indian ink injected retina; **(c)** microaneurysm with endothelial cell proliferation (cellular microaneurysm) – trypsin digest preparation; **(d)** thrombosed microaneurysm – PAS and haematoxylin stain; **(e)** microaneurysms at the posterior pole; **(f)** FA shows scattered hyperfluorescent spots in the posterior fundus (Courtesy of J Harry and G Misson, from *Clinical Ophthalmic Pathology*, Butterworth-Heinemann, 2001 – fig. a; J Harry – figs b, c and d)

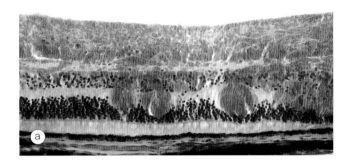

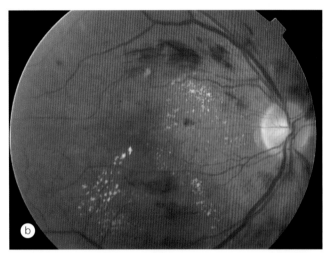

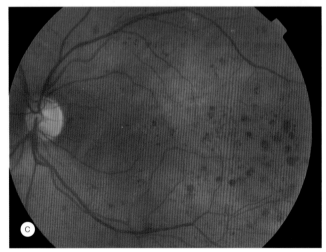

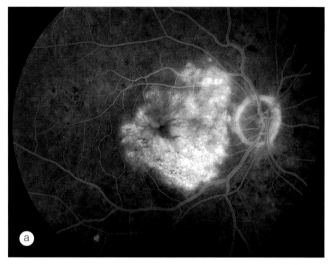

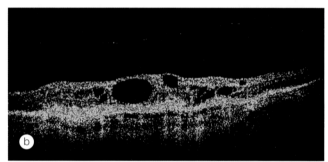

Fig. 16.6
Diffuse macular oedema. **(a)** FA shows diffuse hyperfluorescence with a central flower-petal configuration due to CMO; **(b)** OCT shows retinal thickening and cystoid spaces (Courtesy of Moorfields Eye Hospital – fig. a; Oxford Eye Hospital – fig. b)

Fig. 16.5
Retinal haemorrhages. **(a)** Histology shows blood lying diffusely in the retinal nerve fibre and ganglion cell layers and as globules in the outer layers; **(b)** retinal nerve fibre layer haemorrhages; **(c)** deep 'dot-blot' haemorrhages (Courtesy of J Harry and G Misson, from *Clinical Ophthalmic Pathology*, Butterworth-Heinemann, 2001 – fig. a; Moorfields Eye Hospital – fig. c)

disease should be carefully assessed to determine whether they have clinically significant macular oedema (see below).

Differential diagnosis

The diagnosis of BDR is usually straightforward, but occasionally the following conditions may give rise to diagnostic problems:

1. **Macular drusen** are bilateral, focal yellow spots which may be mistaken for hard exudates. However, they are not arranged in clumps or rings and are not associated with retinal microvascular changes.
2. **Hypertensive retinopathy** is characterized by bilateral retinal oedema, hard exudates and flame-shaped haemorrhages and may coexist with BDR. However, in hypertension the hard exudates typically form a macular star figure and are not arranged in clumps or rings.
3. **Old branch retinal vein occlusion** is characterized by hard exudates, retinal oedema and microvascular

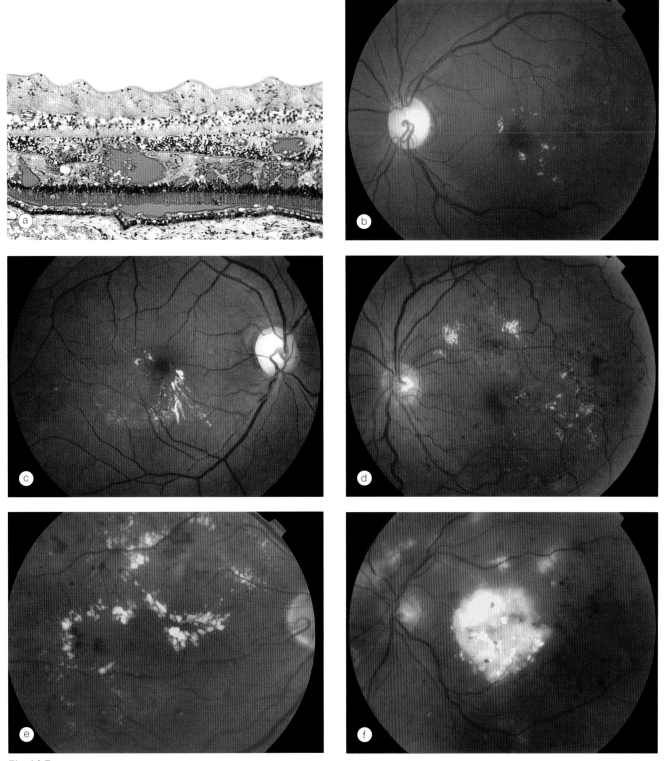

Fig. 16.7

Hard exudates. **(a)** Histology shows irregular eosinophilic deposits mainly in the outer plexiform layer; **(b)** a few small hard exudates and microaneurysms; **(c)** incomplete ring of hard exudates and a few microaneurysms; **(d)** diffusely scattered hard exudates, microaneurysms and small dot haemorrhages; **(e)** extensive involvement of the posterior pole by hard exudates and blot haemorrhages; **(f)** plaque of hard exudates at the macula associated with cholesterol deposition (Courtesy of J Harry – fig. a; Moorfields Eye Hospital – figs b–f)

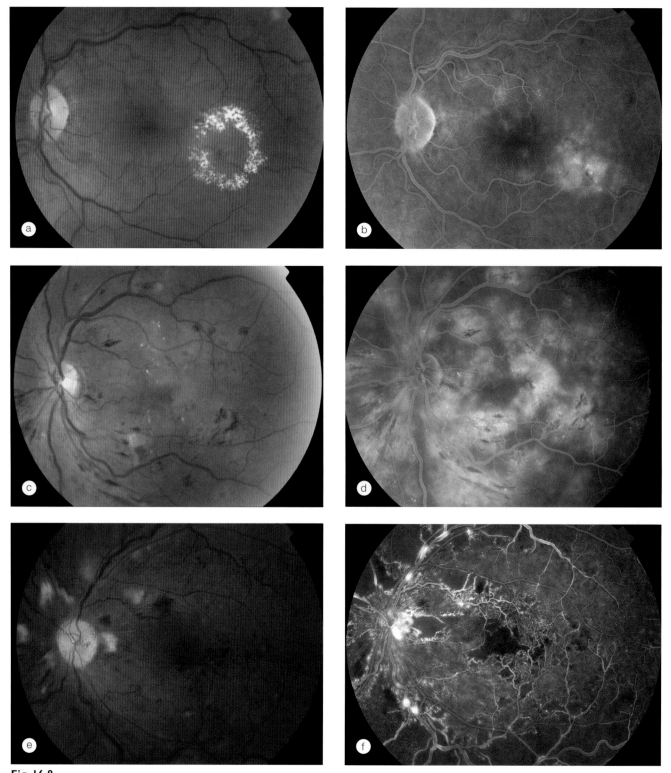

Fig. 16.8
Diabetic maculopathy. *1. Focal.* **(a)** A ring of hard exudates temporal to the macula; **(b)** FA late phase shows focal area of
hyperfluorescence due to leakage corresponding to the centre of the exudate ring. *2. Diffuse.* **(c)** Dot and blot haemorrhages;
(d) FA late phase shows extensive hyperfluorescence at the posterior pole due to leakage. *3. Ischaemic.* **(e)** Dot and blot haemorrhages
and cotton-wool spots; **(f)** FA venous phase shows hypofluorescence due to capillary non-perfusion at the macula and elsewhere
(Courtesy of Moorfields Eye Hospital)

changes. However, the condition is usually unilateral, confined to one quadrant and associated with collaterals.

4. **Retinal artery macroaneurysm** is characterized by retinal oedema, hard exudates and haemorrhage. However, it is usually unilateral and the retinal changes are more localized.

5. **Idiopathic juxtafoveolar retinal telangiectasis group I** is characterized by hard exudates and other microvascular anomalies which may resemble microaneurysms. However, the condition is unilateral and the changes are confined to the fovea.

Diabetic maculopathy

Diagnosis

Involvement of the fovea by oedema, hard exudates or ischaemia (diabetic maculopathy) is the most common cause of visual impairment in diabetic patients, particularly those with type 2 diabetes.

1. **Focal maculopathy** is characterized by well-circumscribed retinal thickening associated with complete or incomplete rings of hard exudates (Fig. 16.8a). FA shows late, focal hyperfluorescence due to leakage and good macular perfusion (Fig. 16.8b).
2. **Diffuse maculopathy** is characterized by diffuse retinal thickening, which may be associated with cystoid changes. Landmarks are obliterated by severe oedema which may render localization of the fovea impossible (Fig. 16.8c). FA shows late diffuse hyperfluorescence which may assume a central flower-petal if CMO is present (Fig. 16.8d).
3. **Ischaemic maculopathy.** The signs are variable and the macula may look relatively normal despite reduced visual acuity. In other cases preproliferative diabetic retinopathy (PPDR – see below) may be present (Fig. 16.8e). FA shows capillary non-perfusion at the fovea and frequently other areas of capillary non-perfusion at the posterior pole and periphery (Fig. 16.8f).
4. **Clinically significant macular oedema** (CSMO) is defined as follows (Fig. 16.9):
   - Retinal oedema within 500μm of the centre of the macula (upper left).
   - Hard exudates within 500μm of the centre of the macula, if associated with retinal thickening (which may be outside the 500μm – upper right).
   - Retinal oedema one disc area (1500μm) or larger, any part of which is within one disc diameter of the centre of the macula (lower centre).

Argon laser photocoagulation

1. **Indications**
   - All eyes with CSMO should be considered for laser photocoagulation irrespective of the level of visual acuity because treatment reduces the risk of visual loss by 50%.
   - Pre-treatment FA is useful to delineate the area and extent of leakage and also to detect ischaemic maculopathy which carries a poor prognosis and, if severe, is a contraindication to treatment.
2. **Focal treatment**
   - Burns are applied to microaneurysms and microvascular lesions in the centre of rings of hard exudates located 500–3000μm from the centre of the macula (Fig. 16.10a).
   - The spot size is 50–100μm and exposure time 0.1 sec with sufficient power to obtain gentle whitening or darkening of the lesions.
   - Treatment up to 300μm from the centre of the macula may be considered if CSMO persists despite previous treatment and visual acuity is less than 6/12. In these cases a shorter exposure time of 0.05sec is recommended.
3. **Grid treatment**
   - Burns are applied to areas of diffuse retinal thickening more than 500μm from the centre of the macula and 500μm from the temporal margin of the optic disc.
   - The spot size is 100μm and exposure time is 0.1sec giving a very light intensity burn (Fig. 16.10b).
4. **Results.** Approximately 70% of eyes achieve stable visual acuity, 15% show improvement and 15% subsequently deteriorate. Since it may take up to 4 months for the oedema to resolve, re-treatment should not be considered prematurely.
5. **Poor ocular prognostic factors**
   - Hard exudates involving the centre of the macula.

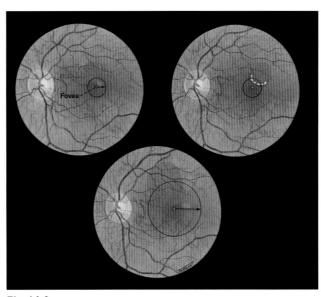

Fig. 16.9
Clinically significant macular oedema

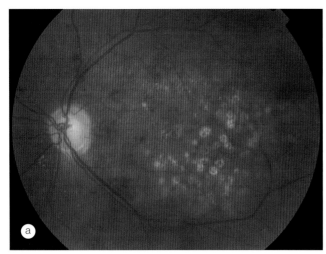
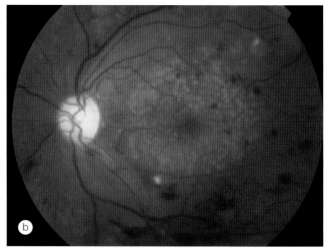

Fig. 16.10
Laser photocoagulation for clinically significant macular oedema. **(a)** Appearance several weeks following focal laser photocoagulation shows laser scars and absence of hard exudates; **(b)** appearance immediately following grid laser photocoagulation (Courtesy of Moorfields Eye Hospital)

- Diffuse macular oedema.
- CMO.
- Mixed exudative-ischaemic maculopathy.
- Severe retinopathy at presentation.
6. **Poor systemic prognostic factors**
   - Uncontrolled hypertension.
   - Renal disease.
   - Elevated glycosylated haemoglobin levels.

Other forms of laser therapy

1. **Low energy treatment** with a Nd:YAG (532nm – frequency doubled) green laser in which the energy employed is the lowest capable of producing barely visible burns at the level of the RPE is a promising new technique that is less destructive to the retina than conventional methods.
2. **Subthreshold micropulse diode laser** (810nm) therapy is also a promising new technique in which short duration (microseconds) burns are applied to the RPE without significantly affecting the outer retina and choriocapillaris.

Other forms of treatment

1. **Pars plana vitrectomy** may be indicated when macular oedema is associated with tangential traction from a thickened and taut posterior hyaloid. In these cases laser therapy is of limited benefit but surgical release of traction may be beneficial. Clinically, a taut thickened posterior hyaloid is characterized by an increased glistening of the pre-macular vitreous face. Typically FA shows diffuse leakage and prominent CMO. It has also been suggested that some eyes without a taut posterior hyaloid may benefit from vitrectomy although this has not been shown to be the case in randomized trials. OCT is invaluable in demonstrating eyes with marked vitreo-macular traction that may benefit most from surgery.

2. **Intravitreal triamcinolone acetonide** is a promising new therapy for the treatment of diffuse macular oedema that fails to respond to conventional laser photo-coagulation although it is also being used as primary treatment. Complications include endophthalmitis, intra-ocular haemorrhage, retinal detachment and raised intraocular pressure. The therapeutic effect fades after 6 months and macular oedema frequently returns. Studies are ongoing to produce a longer lasting steroid implant.

3. **Posterior sub-Tenon triamcinolone acetonide injection** may improve visual outcome in diffuse maculopathy when combined with laser photocoagulation but long-term results are lacking.

4. **Oral atorvastatin** in patients with type 2 diabetes with dyslipidaemia has been shown to reduce the severity of hard exudates and subfoveal lipid migration in eyes with CSMO and may become an important therapeutic adjunct.

Preproliferative diabetic retinopathy

Diagnosis

BDR that exhibits signs of imminent proliferative disease is termed preproliferative diabetic retinopathy (PPDR). The clinical signs of PPDR (Fig. 16.11a) indicate progressive retinal ischaemia, seen on FA as extensive hypofluorescent

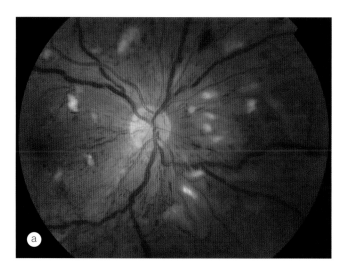

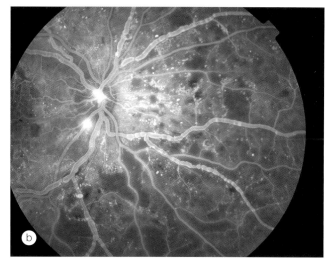

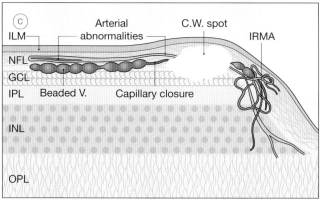

Fig. 16.11
Pre-proliferative diabetic retinopathy. **(a)** Cotton-wool spots, IRMA and venous changes; **(b)** FA shows extensive areas of hypofluorescence due to capillary non-perfusion, and venous beading; **(c)** location of lesions (Courtesy of Moorfields Eye Hospital – figs a and b)

areas representing retinal non-perfusion (capillary dropout – Fig. 16.11b). Figure 16.11c shows the lesions and their location. The risk of progression to proliferative disease appears proportional to the number of lesions. Some patients may have PDR in one eye and PPDR in the other.

1. **Cotton-wool spots** are composed of accumulations of neuronal debris within the nerve fibre layer. They result from disruption of nerve axons, the swollen ends of which are known as cytoid bodies, seen on light microscopy as globular structures in the nerve fibre layer (Fig. 16.12a). As cotton-wool spots heal, debris is removed by autolysis and phagocytosis.
   a. *Signs*. Small, whitish, fluffy superficial lesions which obscure underlying blood vessels that are clinically evident only in the post-equatorial retina, where the nerve fibre layer is of sufficient thickness to render them visible (Fig. 16.12b).
   b. *FA* shows focal hypofluorescence due to blockage of background choroidal fluorescence frequently associated with adjacent capillary non-perfusion.
2. **Intraretinal microvascular abnormalities** (IRMA) are arteriolar-venular shunts that run from retinal arterioles

to venules, thus by passing the capillary bed, and are therefore often seen adjacent to areas of capillary closure (Fig. 16.12c).
   a. *Signs*. Fine, irregular, red lines that run from arterioles to venules (Fig. 16.12d).
   b. *FA* shows focal hyperfluorescence associated with adjacent areas of capillary closure (dropout).

NB The main distinguishing features of IRMA are intraretinal location, failure to cross major retinal blood vessels and absence of leakage on FA.

3. **Other features**
   a. *Venous changes* consist of dilatation and tortuosity, looping (Fig. 16.13a), beading and 'sausage-like' segmentation (Fig. 16.13b).
   b. *Arterial changes* include peripheral narrowing, silver-wiring and obliteration (Fig. 16.13c), resembling a branch retinal artery occlusion.
   c. *Dark blot haemorrhages* represent haemorrhagic retinal infarcts and are located within the middle retinal layers (Fig. 16.13d).

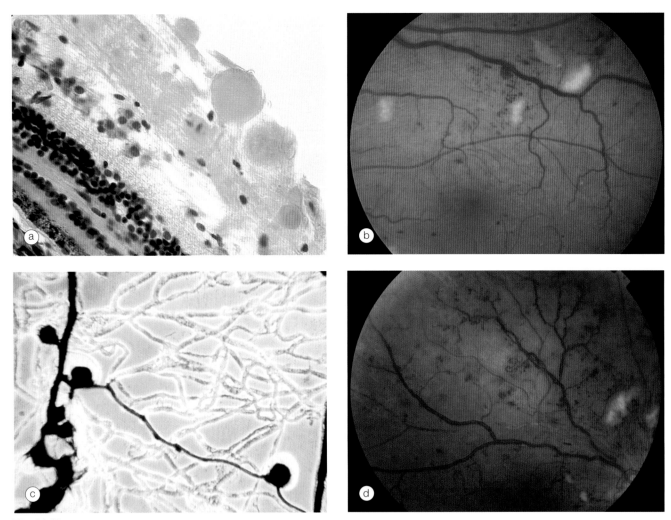

Fig. 16.12
Preproliferative diabetic retinopathy. **(a)** Histology shows cytoid bodies in the nerve fibre layer; **(b)** three cotton-wool spots, microaneurysms, flame-shaped haemorrhages and mild venous tortuosity; **(c)** arteriolar-venular shunt and a few microaneurysms within a poorly perfused capillary bed – flat preparation of Indian ink injected retina; phase contrast microscopy; **(d)** IRMA, venous changes and cotton-wool spots (Courtesy of J Harry – figs a and c; Moorfields Eye Hospital – fig. d)

Management

Patients with PPDR should be watched closely because of the risk of proliferative diabetic retinopathy (PDR – Fig. 16.14). Laser treatment is usually not appropriate unless regular follow-up is not possible, or vision in the fellow eye has been already lost due to proliferative disease. Every effort should be made to encourage maximal diabetic control and reduction of other systemic risk factors.

Proliferative diabetic retinopathy

PDR affects 5–10% of the diabetic population. Type 1 diabetics are at particular risk with an incidence of about

60% after 30 years. Protective factors include posterior vitreous separation, high myopia and optic atrophy.

Pathogenesis

The primary feature of PDR is neovascularization which is caused by angiogenic growth factors elaborated by hypoxic retinal tissue in an attempt to re-vascularize hypoxic retina. These substances promote neovascularization on the retina and optic nerve head and occasionally on the iris. Many angiogenic stimulators have been identified: vascular endothelial growth factor (VEGF) appears to be of particular importance, others include placental growth factor and pigment epithelium-derived factor. Similarly, several

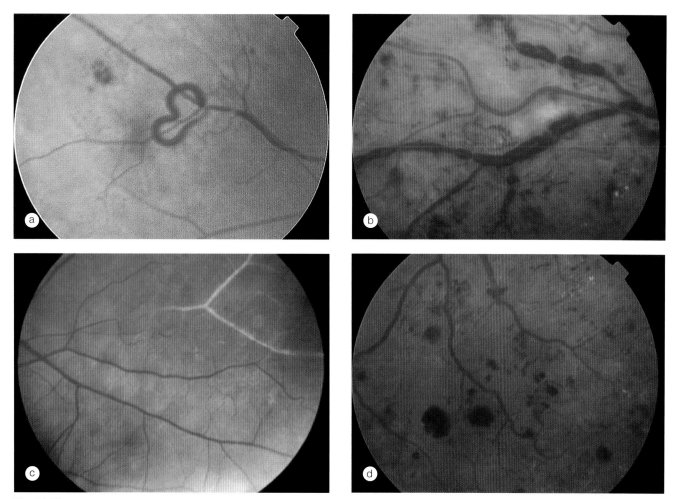

Fig. 16.13
Preproliferative diabetic retinopathy. **(a)** Venous loop; **(b)** venous beading and sausage-like segmentation; **(c)** peripheral arteriolar occlusion; **(d)** dark blot haemorrhages

endogenous inhibitors of angiogenesis have also been reported such as endostatin, platelet factor 4 and angiostatin. It has been hypothesised that the net balance between VEGF and endostatin is associated with the activity of retinopathy. It has been estimated that over one-quarter of the retina has to be non-perfused before PDR develops.

Diagnosis

1. **New vessels at disc** (NVD) describes neovascularization on or within one disc diameter of the optic nerve head (Fig. 16.15a).
2. **New vessels elsewhere** (NVE) describes neovascularization further away from the disc.
3. **FA,** although not required to make the diagnosis, high-

lights the neovascularization during the early phases of the angiogram (Fig. 16.15b and c) and shows hyperfluorescence during the later stages due to intense leakage of dye from neovascular tissue (Fig. 16.15d).

Clinical assessment

1. **Severity** of PDR is determined by the area covered with new vessels in comparison with the area of the disc as follows:
   - NVD is mild when less than one-third disc area in extent (Fig. 16.16a) and severe when more than this (Fig. 16.16b).
   - NVE is mild if less than half disc area in extent (Fig. 16.16c) and severe if more than this (Fig. 16.16d).

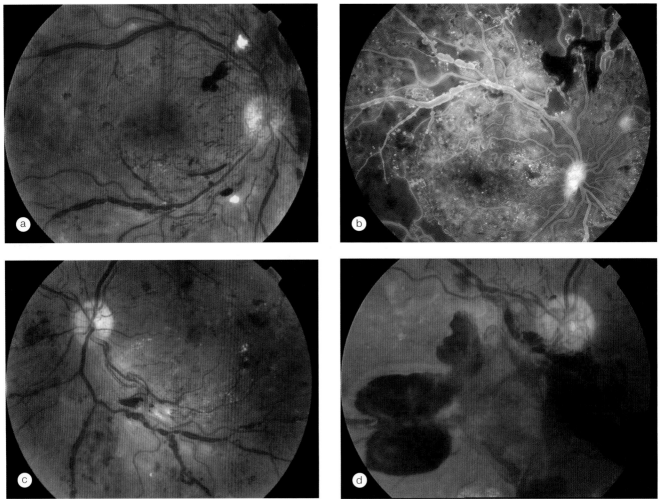

Fig. 16.14
Proliferative and preproliferative retinopathy. **(a)** Right eye shows severe proliferative retinopathy; **(b)** FA shows extensive areas of hypofluorescence due to capillary non-perfusion and hyperfluorescence at the disc due to leakage; **(c)** left eye shows pre-proliferative disease; **(d)** 4 months later the left eye has developed severe proliferative retinopathy and haemorrhage

2. **Elevated new vessels** are less responsive to laser therapy than flat.
3. **Fibrosis** associated with neovascularization (Fig. 16.16e) is important, since significant fibrous proliferation (Fig. 16.16f) carries an increased risk of tractional retinal detachment (see Chapter 19).
4. **High risk characteristics.** The following signify a high risk of severe visual loss within 2 years, if untreated:
   - Mild NVD with haemorrhage carries a 26% risk of visual loss, which is reduced to 4% with treatment.
   - Severe NVD without haemorrhage carries a 26% risk of visual loss, which is reduced to 9% with treatment.
   - Severe NVD with haemorrhage carries a 37% risk of visual loss, which is reduced to 20% with treatment.
   - Severe NVE with haemorrhage carries a 30% risk of visual loss, which is reduced to 7% with treatment.

Treatment

Laser therapy is aimed at inducing involution of new vessels and preventing visual loss.

1. **Laser settings**
   a. **Spot size** depends on the contact lens used.
   - With the Goldmann lens, spot size is set at 200–500µm, but with a panfundoscopic type lens it is set at 100–300µm because of induced magnification (varies with exact lens used).
   - In the beginner's hands, a panfundoscopic lens is perhaps safer than the Goldmann, since it is relatively easy to inadvertently photocoagulate the posterior pole through the latter, with disastrous consequences.
   b. **Duration** of the burn is 0.1–0.2sec.
   c. **Power** should be sufficient to produce only a light

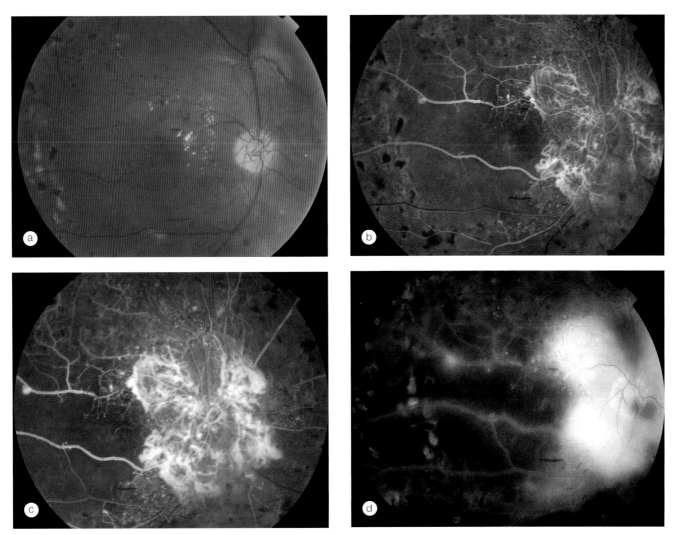

Fig. 16.15
Proliferative diabetic retinopathy. **(a)** Disc new vessels and laser scars; **(b)** FA arteriovenous phase highlights the vessels and shows extensive hypofluorescence at the macula due to capillary non-perfusion; **(c)** venous phase shows filling of the vessels; **(d)** late phase shows extensive hyperfluorescence due to leakage (Courtesy of Moorfields Eye Hospital)

intensity burn (Fig. 16.17), with the intention of stimulating the RPE rather than ablating the retina.

NB The main effect is related to surface area treated rather than the number of burns; a small variation in the size of the laser burn therefore has a profound effect on area treated (area = πr^2).

2. **Initial treatment** involves 1000–2000 burns in a scatter pattern extending from the posterior fundus to cover the peripheral retina in one or more sessions. PRP completed in a single session carries a slightly higher risk

of complications. The amount of treatment during any one session is governed by the patient's pain threshold and ability to maintain concentration. Topical anaesthesia is adequate in most patients, although peribulbar or sub-Tenon anaesthesia may be necessary. The sequence is as follows:

a. Step 1. Close to the disc (Fig. 16.18a); below the inferior temporal arcades (Fig. 16.18b and c).

b. Step 2. Protective barrier around the macula (Fig. 16.19a) to prevent inadvertent treatment of the fovea; above the superotemporal arcade (Fig. 16.19b and c).

c. Step 3. Nasal to the disc (Fig. 16.20a and b); completion of posterior pole treatment (Fig. 16.20c).

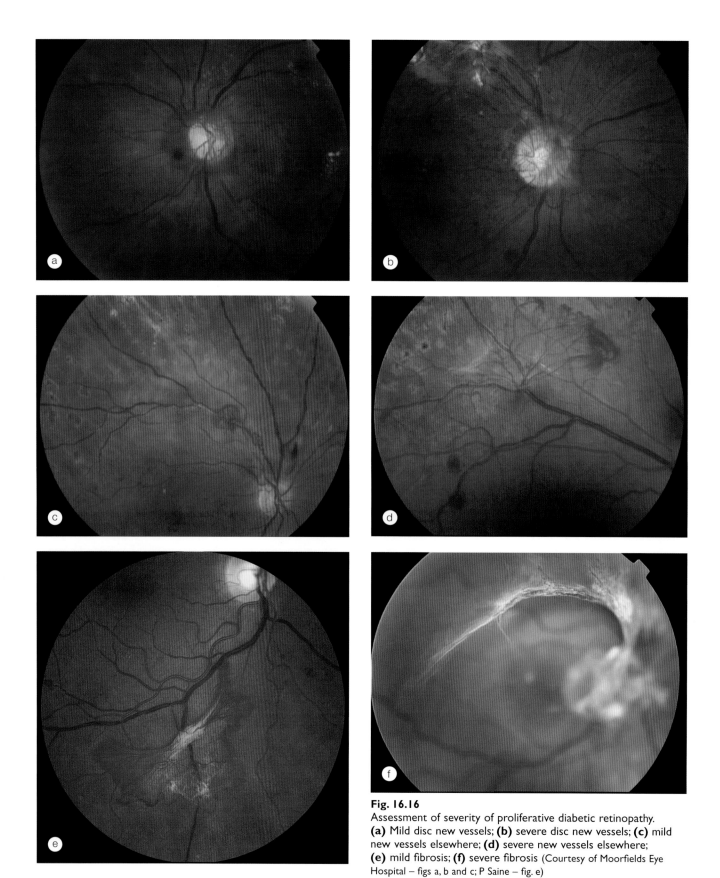

Fig. 16.16
Assessment of severity of proliferative diabetic retinopathy.
(a) Mild disc new vessels; **(b)** severe disc new vessels; **(c)** mild new vessels elsewhere; **(d)** severe new vessels elsewhere; **(e)** mild fibrosis; **(f)** severe fibrosis (Courtesy of Moorfields Eye Hospital – figs a, b and c; P Saine – fig. e)

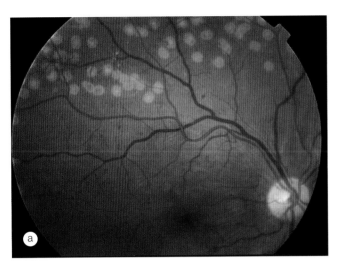 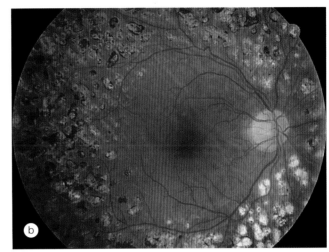

Fig. 16.17
(a) Appropriate laser burns; **(b)** appearance several weeks after completion of treatment (Courtesy of C Barry – fig. b)

d. Step 4. Peripheral treatment (Fig.16.21a and b) until completion (Fig. 16.21c).

NB In very severe PDR is advisable to treat the inferior fundus first, since any vitreous haemorrhage will gravitate inferiorly and obscure this area, precluding further treatment.

3. Follow-up is after 4–6 weeks. In eyes with severe NVD, several treatment sessions involving 5000 or even more

burns may be required. Occasionally complete elimination of NVD may be difficult but once the tips of the vessels start to fibrose and become inactive they pose much less threat to vision. Such fibrosed vessels can be observed although it should be remembered that the commonest cause of visual loss is inadequate treatment to persistently active neovascular proliferation.

4. Signs of involution are regression of neovascularization leaving 'ghost' vessels or fibrous tissue (Fig. 16.22), decrease in venous changes, absorption of retinal haemor-

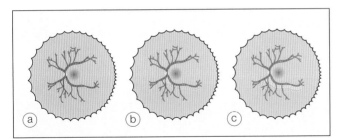

Fig. 16.18
PRP technique – step 1

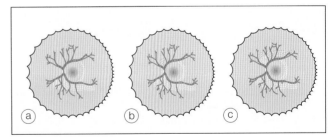

Fig. 16.19
PRP technique – step 2

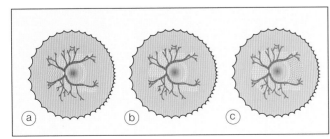

Fig. 16.20
PRP technique – step 3

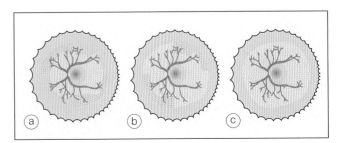

Fig. 16.21
PRP technique – step 4

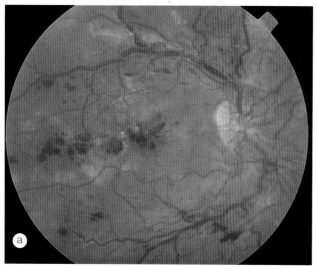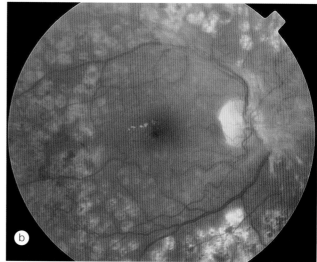

Fig. 16.22
Treatment of proliferative diabetic retinopathy. **(a)** Severe proliferative disease; **(b)** 3 months later new vessels have regressed and there is residual fibrosis at the disc (Courtesy of S Milewski)

rhages and disc pallor. In most eyes, once the retinopathy is quiescent, stable vision is maintained. In a few eyes, recurrences of PDR occur despite an initial satisfactory response; it is therefore necessary to re-examine the patient at intervals of approximately 6–12 months.

NB PRP influences only the vascular component of the fibrovascular process. Eyes in which new vessels have regressed leaving only fibrous tissue should not be re-treated.

5. **Treatment of recurrences** may involve:
   a. *Further laser photocoagulation*, filling in any gaps between previous laser scars or utilizing indirect laser to treat very peripheral retina.
   b. *Cryotherapy* to the peripheral retina is occasionally useful when further photocoagulation is impossible as a result of inadequate visualization of the fundus caused by opaque media.

NB It should be explained to patients that PRP may result in visual field defects of sufficient severity to legally preclude driving a motor vehicle.

Advanced diabetic eye disease

Serious vision-threatening complications of DR (advanced diabetic eye disease) occur in patients who have not had laser therapy or in whom laser photocoagulation has been unsuccessful or inadequate. One or more of the following complications may occur.

Diagnosis

1. **Haemorrhage** may be preretinal (retrohyaloid), intragel or both. A preretinal haemorrhage often has a crescentic shape which demarcates the level of posterior vitreous detachment (Fig. 16.23a). Intragel haemorrhages usually take longer to clear than preretinal haemorrhages because the former are usually the result of a more extensive bleed. In some eyes, altered blood becomes compacted on the posterior vitreous face to form an 'ochre membrane'. Patients should be warned that bleeding may be precipitated by severe physical exertion or straining, hypoglycaemia and direct ocular trauma. Ultrasonography is used in eyes with dense vitreous haemorrhage to detect the possibility of associated retinal detachment (Fig. 16.23b).

2. **Tractional retinal detachment** is caused by progressive contraction of fibrovascular membranes over areas of vitreoretinal attachment. Posterior vitreous detachment in eyes with PDR is often incomplete due to the strong adhesions between cortical vitreous and areas of fibrovascular proliferation (see Chapter 19).

3. **Tractional retinoschisis** with or without retinal detachment may also occur. Differentiation between retinoschisis and tractional retinal detachment is clinically difficult but very important, because recovery of central vision after macular reattachment is better in eyes with tractional detachment than in retinoschisis. In this respect OCT may be useful in the differentiation between these two conditions preoperatively

4. **Rubeosis iridis** may occur in eyes with PDR, and if severe may lead to neovascular glaucoma (see Chapter 13). Rubeosis is particularly common in eyes with severe

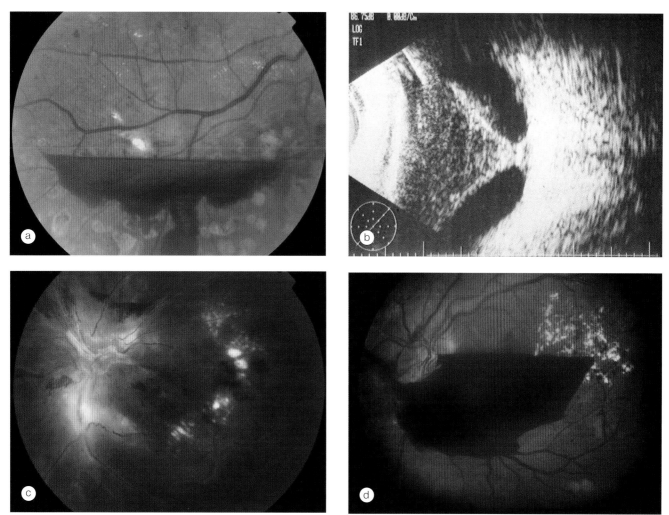

Fig. 16.23
Advanced diabetic eye disease. **(a)** Preretinal haemorrhage; **(b)** ultrasound shows tabletop tractional retinal detachment and dense intragel haemorrhage; **(c)** tractional retinal detachment involving the macula; **(d)** dense premacular subhyaloid haemorrhage (Courtesy Moorfields Eye Hospital – figs a and c; M Hamza – fig. b)

retinal ischaemia or persistent retinal detachment following unsuccessful pars plana vitrectomy.

Treatment

Pars plana vitrectomy is the main method of treating severe complications of PDR.

1. Indications

    a. Severe persistent vitreous haemorrhage is the most common indication. In these cases the density of the haemorrhage precludes adequate PRP. In the absence of rubeosis iridis, vitrectomy is traditionally considered within 3 months of the initial vitreous haemorrhage in type 1 diabetics and at about 6 months in type 2 diabetics. However, vitrectomy is frequently offered earlier regardless of diabetic type and certainly in any case with bilateral haemorrhage.

    b. Progressive tractional RD threatening or involving the macula must be treated without delay (Fig. 16.23c). However, extramacular tractional detachments may be observed, since they often remain stationary for prolonged periods of time.

    c. Combined tractional and rhegmatogenous RD should be treated urgently, even if the macula is not involved, because subretinal fluid is likely to spread quickly to involve the macula.

    d. Premacular subhyaloid haemorrhage, if dense (Fig. 16.23d) and persistent should be considered for vitrectomy because, if untreated, the internal limiting membrane or posterior hyaloid face may serve as a scaffold for subsequent fibrovascular proliferation and consequent tractional macular detachment or macular epiretinal membrane formation.

2. **Visual results** depend on the specific indications for surgery and the complexity of pre-existing vitreoretinal abnormalities. In general, about 70% of cases achieve visual improvement, about 10% are made worse and the rest are unchanged. It appears that the first few post-operative months are vital. If an eye is doing well after 6 months, then the long-term outlook is good because the incidence of subsequent vision-threatening complications is low. Favourable prognostic factors are:
- Good preoperative visual function.
- Age of 40 years or less.
- Absence of preoperative rubeosis iridis and glaucoma.
- Previous PRP of at least one-quarter of the fundus.

NB Intravitreal injection of bovine hyaluronidase has recently been shown to promote the absorption of vitreous haemorrhage.

Screening for diabetic retinopathy

All diabetic patients aged over 12 years and/or entering puberty should be screened, and those with risk factors for visual loss referred to an ophthalmologist. Screening involves measurement of visual acuity and fundus examination following pupillary dilatation.

General screening

1. **Annual review**
   - Normal fundus.
   - Mild BDR with small haemorrhages and/or small hard exudates more than one disc diameter from the fovea.
2. **Routine referral**
   - BDR with large exudates within the major temporal arcades but not threatening the fovea.
   - BDR without maculopathy but with reduced visual acuity, in order to determine the cause of visual impairment.
3. **Early referral**
   - BDR with hard exudates and/or haemorrhages within one disc diameter from the fovea.
   - PPDR.
4. **Urgent referral**
   - PDR.
   - Preretinal or vitreous haemorrhage.
   - Rubeosis iridis.
   - Retinal detachment.

Screening in pregnancy

Diabetic retinopathy can significantly worsen during preg-

nancy. The risk of progression is related to the severity of DR in the first trimester as follows:
1. **No retinopathy** 10% risk to progression to mild BDR.
2. **Mild BDR** 20% risk of developing moderate BDR or worse.
3. **Moderate to severe BDR** 25% risk of PDR, so monthly screening should be performed.
4. **Diabetic macular oedema** usually resolves spontaneously after pregnancy and need not be treated if it develops in late pregnancy.

RETINAL VENOUS OCCLUSIVE DISEASE

Pathogenesis

Arteriolosclerosis is an important causative factor for branch retinal vein occlusion (BRVO). Because a retinal arteriole and its corresponding vein share a common adventitial sheath, thickening of the arteriole appears to compress the vein. This causes secondary changes, including venous endothelial cell loss, thrombus formation and potential occlusion. Similarly, the central retinal vein and artery share a common adventitial sheath at arteriovenous crossings posterior to the lamina cribrosa so that atherosclerotic changes of the artery may compress the vein and precipitate central retinal vein occlusion (CRVO). It therefore appears that both arterial and venous disease contribute to retinal vein occlusion. Venous occlusion causes elevation of venous and capillary pressure with stagnation of blood flow. This results in hypoxia of the retina drained by the obstructed vein, which in turn results in damage to the capillary endothelial cells and extravasation of blood constituents. The tissue pressure is increased, causing further stagnation of the circulation and hypoxia, so that a vicious cycle is established.

Predisposing factors

Common

1. **Advancing age** is the most important factor; over 50% of cases occur in patients over the age of 65 years.
2. **Hypertension** is present in up to 64% patients over the age of 50 years and in 25% of younger patients with retinal vein occlusion. It is most prevalent in patients with BRVO, particularly when the site of obstruction is at an arteriovenous crossing. Inadequate control of hypertension may also predispose to recurrence of RVO in the same eye or fellow eye involvement.
3. **Hyperlipidaemia** (cholesterol >6.5mmol/l) is present in 35% of patients, irrespective of age.

4. **Diabetes mellitus** is present in about 10% of cases over the age of 50 years but is uncommon in younger patients. This may be due to an increase of other cardiovascular risk factors such as hypertension, which is present in 70% of type 2 diabetics.
5. **Raised intraocular pressure** increases the risk of CRVO, particularly when the site of obstruction is at the edge of the optic cup.

Uncommon

Uncommon predispositions (listed below) may assume more importance in patients under the age of 50 years.

1. **Myeloproliferative disorders**
   - Polycythaemia.
   - Abnormal plasma proteins (e.g. myeloma, Waldenström macroglobulinaemia).
2. **Acquired hypercoagulable states**
   - Hyperhomocysteinaemia.
   - Lupus anticoagulant and antiphospholipid antibodies.
   - Dysfibrinogenaemia.
3. **Inherited hypercoagulable states**
   - Activated protein C resistance (factor V Leiden mutation).
   - Protein C deficiency.
   - Protein S deficiency.
   - Antithrombin deficiency.
   - Prothrombin gene mutation.
   - Factor XII deficiency.
4. **Inflammatory disease associated with occlusive periphlebitis**
   - Behçet syndrome.
   - Sarcoidosis.
   - Wegener granulomatosis.
   - Goodpasture syndrome.
5. **Miscellaneous**
   - Oral contraceptives.
   - Chronic renal failure.
   - Causes of secondary hypertension (e.g. Cushing syndrome) or hyperlipidaemia (e.g. hypothyroidism).

NB Factors that appear to decrease the risk of venous occlusion include increased physical activity and moderate alcohol consumption.

Medical investigations

All patients

1. **Blood pressure**
2. **ECG**
3. **Blood**
   - Full-blood count and ESR.

- Fasting blood glucose and lipids.
- Plasma protein electrophoresis.

Selected patients (<50 years of age)

1. **Chest x-ray**
2. **Blood**
   - Thrombophilia screen.
   - Autoantibodies – anti-cardiolipin, lupus anticoagulant, ANA and anti-dsDNA.
   - ACE.
   - Homocysteine.

Branch retinal vein occlusion

Classification

1. **Major BRVO** may be subdivided as follows:
   - First order temporal branch at the optic disc (Fig. 16.24a).
   - First order temporal branch away from the disc but involving the branches to the macula (Fig. 16.24b).
2. **Minor macular BRVO** involving only a macular branch (Fig. 16.24c).
3. **Peripheral BRVO** not involving the macular circulation (Fig. 16.24d, e and f).

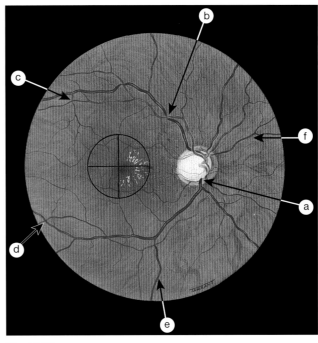

Fig. 16.24
Classification of retinal branch vein occlusion according to site of blockage. **(a)** Major at the disc; **(b)** major away from the disc; **(c)** minor macular; **(d–f)** peripheral not involving the macula

Diagnosis

1. **Presentation** depends on the amount of macular drainage compromised by the occlusion. Patients with macular involvement often present with sudden onset of blurred vision and metamorphopsia or a relative visual field defect.
2. **VA** is variable and dependent on the extent of macular involvement.
3. **Fundus** (Fig. 16.25a)
   - Dilatation and tortuosity of the venous segment distal to the site of occlusion and attenuation proximally
   - Flame-shaped and dot-blot haemorrhages, retinal oedema, and sometimes cotton-wool spots affecting the sector of the retina drained by the obstructed vein.
4. **FA** shows variable delayed venous filling, blockage by blood (Fig. 16.25b, c and d), hyperfluorescence due to leakage, hypofluorescence due to capillary non-perfusion, staining of the vessel wall and 'pruning' of vessels in the ischaemic areas.
5. **Course.** The acute features take 6–12 months to resolve and may be replaced by the following:
   - Hard exudates, venous sheathing and sclerosis peripheral to the site of obstruction with variable amount of residual haemorrhage (Fig. 16.26a).
   - Collateral venous channels, characterized by slightly tortuous vessels, develop locally or across the horizontal raphe between the inferior and superior vascular arcades (Fig. 16.26b).

Prognosis

The prognosis is reasonably good. Within 6 months about 50% of eyes develop efficient collaterals, with return of visual

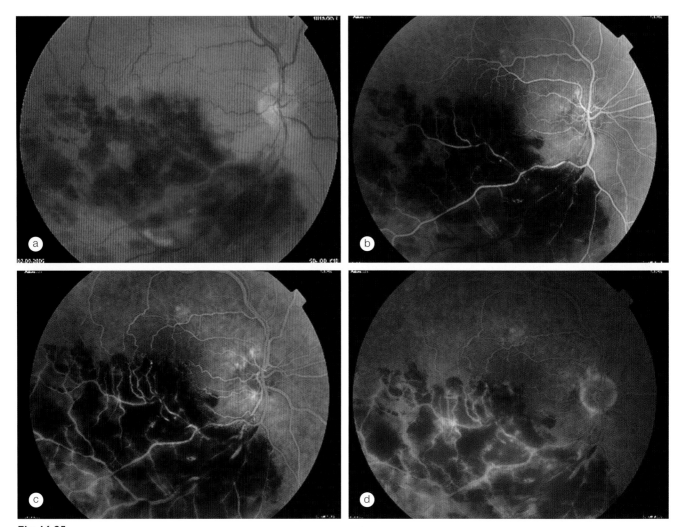

Fig. 16.25
Major inferior branch retinal vein occlusion. **(a)** Extensive intraretinal haemorrhage; **(b and c)** FA early phases shows hypofluorescence due to blockage by blood; **(d)** late phase also shows slight staining of vessel walls

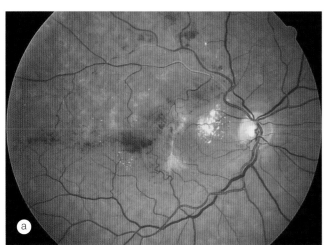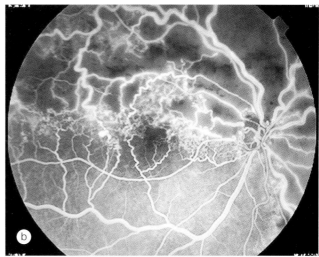

Fig. 16.26
Old branch superior branch retinal vein occlusion. **(a)** Hard exudates, venous sheathing, collaterals and residual haemorrhages; **(b)** FA shows capillary-non perfusion, and tortuous collaterals extending across the horizontal raphe between the superior and inferior arcades (Courtesy of C Barry)

acuity to at least 6/12. Eventual visual recovery depends on the amount of venous drainage involved by the occlusion (which is related to the site and size of the occluded vein) and the severity of macular ischaemia. The two main vision-threatening complications are:

1. **Chronic macular oedema** is the most common cause of persistent poor visual acuity after BRVO. Some patients with visual acuity of 6/12 or worse may benefit from laser photocoagulation, provided the macula is oedematous rather than significantly ischaemic.
2. **Neovascularization.** NVD develops in about 10% and NVE in about 25% of eyes that show at least one quadrant of capillary non-perfusion. NVE usually develops at the border of the triangular sector of ischaemic retina drained by the occluded vein. Neovascularization usually appears within 6–12 months but may develop at any time within the first 3 years. It is a serious complication because it can lead to recurrent vitreous and pre-retinal haemorrhage, and occasionally tractional retinal detachment.

Follow-up

Follow-up should be at 6–12 weeks with FA, provided the retinal haemorrhages have cleared sufficiently. Further management depends on visual acuity and angiographic findings as follows.

- Good macular perfusion and visual acuity is improving – no treatment is required.
- Macular oedema is associated with good macular perfusion and visual acuity continues to be 6/12 or worse after 3–6 months – laser photocoagulation should be considered and the FA should be studied carefully to identify the leaking areas.

- It is also very important to identify shunts, which do not leak fluorescein, because they must not be treated.
- If FA shows FAZ ring is incomplete (broken), laser is less likely to improve visual acuity.
- Macular non-perfusion and visual acuity is poor – laser treatment will not improve vision. However, if the FA shows five or more disc areas of non-perfusion the patient should be reviewed at 4-monthly intervals for 12–24 months because of the risk of neovascularization.

NB Patients with visual acuity of less than 6/60 or those with symptoms for over a year are unlikely to benefit from laser therapy.

Treatment

1. **Macular oedema**
   a. **Grid laser photocoagulation** (100–200μm size, 0.1sec duration and spaced one burn width apart) to produce a gentle reaction to the area of leakage as identified on FA. The burns should extend no closer to the fovea than the edge of the FAZ and be no more peripheral than the major vascular arcades. Care should be taken to avoid treating over intraretinal haemorrhage. Follow-up should be after 3 months. If macular oedema persists re-treatment may be considered although the results are frequently disappointing.
   b. **Intravitreal** triamcinolone acetonide may improve visual acuity. As with diabetic maculopathy the treatment effect lasts for approximately 6 months, but in some cases this may be a crucial time to protect the macula while new collateral vessels develop.

2. **Neovascularization** is not normally treated unless vitreous haemorrhage occurs because early treatment does not appear to affect the visual prognosis. If appropriate, scatter laser photocoagulation (200–500μm size, 0.05–0.1sec duration and spaced one burn width apart) is performed with sufficient energy to achieve a medium reaction covering the entire involved sector (Fig. 16.27) as defined by the colour photograph and FA. A quadrant usually requires 400–500 burns. Follow-up should be after 4–6 weeks. If neovascularization persists re-treatment is frequently effective in inducing regression.

Impending central retinal vein occlusion

Impending (partial) CRVO is an uncommon, poorly described condition which may resolve or progress to complete obstruction.

1. **Presentation** is with mild blurring of vision which is characteristically worse on waking and then improves during the day.
2. **Signs.** Mild venous dilatation and tortuosity with a few widely scattered flame-shaped haemorrhages (Fig. 16.28).
3. **FA** shows increased retinal circulation time.
4. **Treatment** is aimed at preventing complete occlusion by correcting any predisposing systemic conditions and lowering intraocular pressure to improve perfusion. A short course of systemic carbonic anhydrase inhibitors may be tried but their efficacy has not been tested in clinical trials.

Non-ischaemic central retinal vein occlusion

Non-ischaemic CRVO is the most common type, accounting for about 75% of all cases.

Diagnosis

1. **Presentation** is with sudden, unilateral blurred vision.
2. **VA** is impaired to a moderate-severe degree.
3. **Afferent pupillary defect** (APD) is absent or mild (in contrast with ischaemic CRVO).
4. **Fundus** (Fig. 16.29a)
   - Tortuosity and dilatation of all branches of the central retinal vein, dot-blot and flame-shaped haemorrhages, throughout all four quadrants and most numerous in the periphery.
   - Cotton-wool spots, optic disc and macular oedema are common.

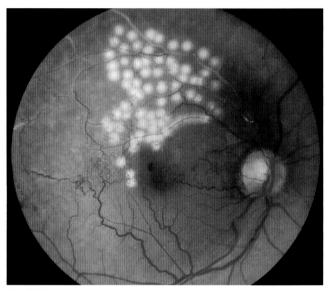

Fig. 16.27
Laser photocoagulation for neovascularization following branch retinal vein occlusion

5. **FA** shows delayed arteriovenous transit time, blockage by haemorrhages, good retinal capillary perfusion and late leakage (Fig. 16.29b and c).
6. **Course.** Most acute signs resolve over 6–12 months. Residual findings include disc collaterals (16.30a), epiretinal gliosis and pigmentary changes at the macula. Conversion to ischaemic CRVO occurs in 15% of cases within 4 months and 34% within 3 years.

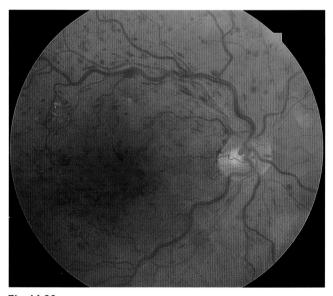

Fig. 16.28
Impending central retinal vein occlusion

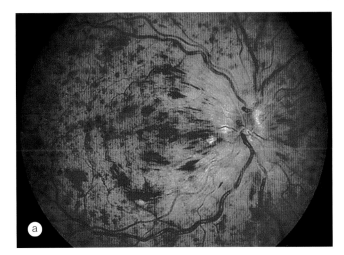

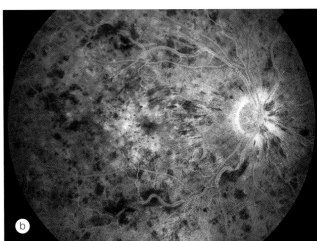

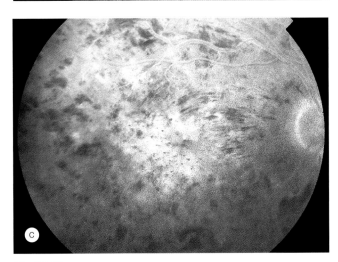

Fig. 16.29
Recent non-ischaemic central retinal vein occlusion. **(a)** Extensive flame-shaped haemorrhages, a few cotton-wool spots and disc oedema; **(b)** FA late venous phase shows scattered hypofluorescence by haemorrhages and mild hyperfluorescence at the macula due to leakage; **(c)** late phase shows more extensive hyperfluorescence due to progressive leakage but good macular perfusion (Courtesy of S Milewski)

Prognosis

In cases that do not subsequently become ischaemic, the prognosis is reasonably good with return of vision to normal or near normal in about 50%. The main cause for poor vision is chronic macular oedema (Fig. 16.30b), which may lead to secondary RPE changes. To a certain extent the prognosis is related to initial visual acuity as follows:

- 6/18 or better, it is likely to remain so.
- 6/24–6/60, the clinical course is variable, and vision may subsequently improve, remain the same, or worsen.
- Worse than 6/60, improvement is unlikely.

Treatment

Treatment is currently inadequate and laser photocoagulation for macular oedema is not beneficial. The following experimental therapies require further evaluation.

1. **Cannulation** and infusion of tissue plasminogen activator (tPA) into the vein via vitrectomy is a new modality.
2. **Intravitreal** triamcinolone acetonide for chronic macular oedema has shown good initial results and is increasingly popular but the effect is short lived.
3. **Optic nerve sheathotomy** via vitrectomy approach is advocated by some as a means of decompressing the central retinal vein. This procedure has not yet been shown to be of benefit in randomized trials and remains controversial.

Ischaemic central retinal vein occlusion

Ischaemic CRVO is characterized by rapid onset venous obstruction resulting in decreased retinal perfusion, capillary closure and retinal hypoxia. This may lead to profound vascular leakage, rubeosis iridis and neovascular glaucoma. The latter is one of the most common indications for enucleation in the Western world.

Diagnosis

1. **Presentation** is with sudden and severe visual impairment.
2. **VA** is usually CF or worse.
3. **APD** is marked.
4. **Fundus** (Fig. 16.31a)
   - Severe tortuosity and engorgement of all branches of the central retinal vein, extensive dot-blot and flame-shaped haemorrhages involving the peripheral retina and posterior pole, severe disc oedema and hyperaemia.
   - Cotton-wool spots may be present.
5. **FA** shows marked delay in arteriovenous transit time or longer than 20 seconds, central masking by retinal haemorrhages, extensive areas of capillary non-perfusion and vessel wall staining (Fig. 16.31b).
6. **ERG** is reduced.

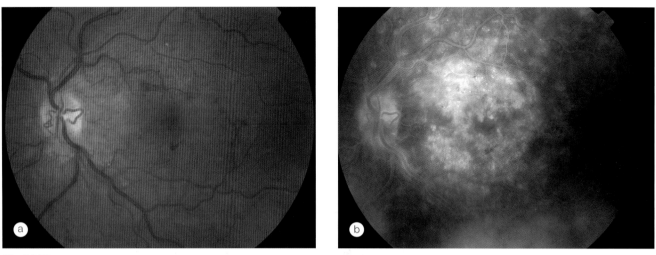

Fig. 16.30
Old non-ischaemic central retinal vein occlusion. **(a)** Disc collaterals and a few residual retinal haemorrhages; **(b)** FA late phase shows diffuse hyperfluorescence due to chronic macular oedema (Courtesy of Moorfields Eye Hospital)

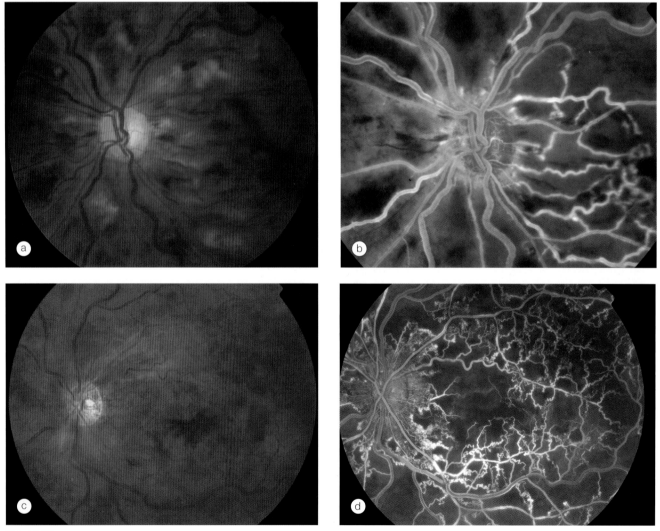

Fig. 16.31
(a) Recent ischaemic central retinal vein occlusion; **(b)** FA venous phase shows extensive hypofluorescence that also involves the fovea due to capillary-non-perfusion and staining of veins; **(c)** old ischaemic central retinal vein occlusion; **(d)** FA venous phase shows many microvascular abnormalities and extensive hypofluorescence due to capillary non-perfusion (Courtesy of A Chopdar – figs a and b; Moorfields Eye Hospital – figs c and d)

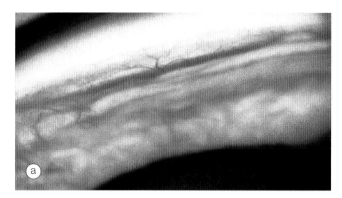

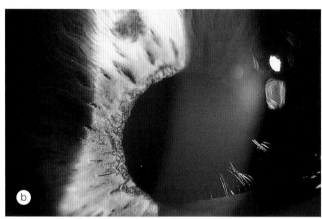

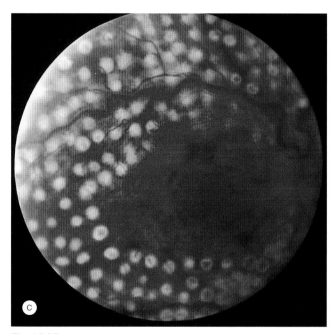

Fig. 16.32
(a) Neovascularization of an open angle; **(b)** rubeosis iridis at the pupillary border; **(c)** panretinal photocoagulation (Courtesy of E Michael Van Buskirk, from *Clinical Atlas of Glaucoma*, W B Saunders, 1986 – fig. a)

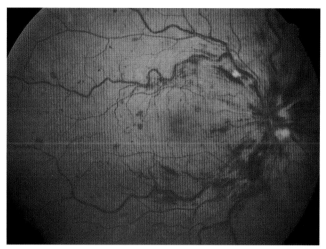

Fig. 16.33
Papillophlebitis

7. Course. Most acute signs resolve over 9–12 months. Residual findings include disc collaterals and macular epiretinal gliosis and pigmentary changes (Fig. 16.31c). Rarely subretinal fibrosis resembling that associated with exudative age-related macular degeneration may develop.

Prognosis

The prognosis is extremely poor due to macular ischaemia (Fig. 16.31d). Rubeosis iridis develops in about 50% of eyes, usually between 2 and 4 months (100-day glaucoma), and unless vigorous PRP is performed there is a high risk of neovascular glaucoma. The development of opticociliary shunts (retinochoroidal collateral veins) may protect the eye from anterior segment neovascularization. Fundus neovascularization occurs in about 5% of eyes and is therefore much less common than with BRVO.

Follow-up

The patient should be seen monthly for 6 months to detect anterior segment neovascularization. Angle neovascularization (Fig. 16.32a), while not synonymous with eventual neovascular glaucoma, is the best clinical predictor of the eventual risk of neovascular glaucoma because it may occur in the absence of rubeosis iridis (Fig. 16.32b). Routine gonioscopy of eyes at risk should therefore be performed and the pupillary margin should be examined prior to mydriasis.

Treatment

Laser PRP should be performed without delay in eyes with angle neovascularization or rubeosis iridis. This involves the application of 1500–3000 burns (0.5–0.1sec, spaced one burn width apart), with sufficient energy to produce a moderate reaction in the periphery but avoiding areas of haemorrhage (Fig. 16.32c). Some cases require further treatment if rubeosis fails to regress or continues to progress.

Prophylactic laser therapy is appropriate only if regular follow-up is not possible.

> **NB** Control of systemic cardiovascular risk factors is extremely important in order to reduce systemic morbidity and to reduce the risk of another ocular venous event.

Papillophlebitis

Papillophlebitis (optic disc vasculitis), is an uncommon condition which typically affects otherwise healthy individuals under the age of 50 years. It is thought that the underlying lesion is optic disc swelling with resultant secondary venous congestion rather than venous thrombosis occurring at the level of the lamina cribrosa as occurs in older patients.

Diagnosis

1. **Presentation** is with mild blurring of vision typically worst on waking.
2. **VA** reduction is mild to moderate.
3. **APD** is absent.
4. **Fundus** (Fig. 16.33)
   - Disc oedema, which may be associated with cotton-wool spots, is the dominant finding.
   - Also present are venous dilatation and tortuosity with variable amount of retinal haemorrhages, usually confined to the peripapillary area and posterior fundus.
5. **Blind spot is enlarged** on perimetry.
6. **FA** shows mild delay in arteriovenous transit time, hyperfluorescence due to leakage and good capillary perfusion.

Prognosis

The prognosis is excellent despite the lack of treatment and 80% of cases achieve a final visual acuity of 6/12 or better, the remainder suffer significant and permanent visual impairment as a result of macular oedema.

Hemiretinal vein occlusion

Hemiretinal vein occlusion is a variant of CRVO and may be ischaemic or non-ischaemic. It is less common than both BRVO and CRVO and involves the superior or inferior branch of the CRV. A hemispheric occlusion blocks a major branch of the CRV at or near the optic disc. A hemicentral occlusion, which is less common, involves one trunk of a dual-trunked CRV, which persists in the anterior part of the optic nerve head as a congenital variant.

1. **Presentation** is with a sudden onset altitudinal visual field defect.
2. **VA** reduction is variable.
3. **Fundus** shows the features of BRVO, involving the superior or inferior hemisphere (Fig. 16.34a).
4. **FA** shows masking by haemorrhages, hyperfluorescence due to leakage and variable capillary non-perfusion (Fig. 16.34b).
5. **Treatment** depends on the severity of retinal ischaemia. Extensive retinal ischaemia carries the risk of neovascular glaucoma and should be managed in the same way as ischaemic CRVO. Macular oedema usually responds poorly to grid laser because of extensive foveal capillary shutdown.

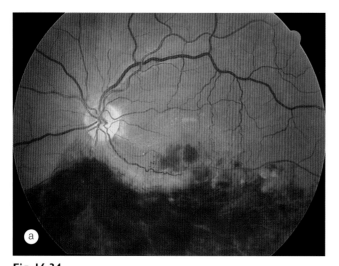
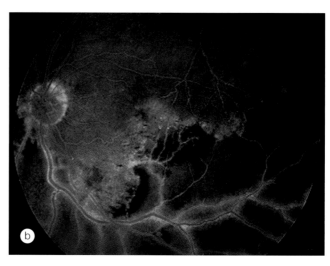

Fig. 16.34
(a) Inferior hemiretinal vein occlusion; **(b)** FA late phase shows extensive hypofluorescence due to capillary non-perfusion and mild perivascular hyperfluorescence (Courtesy of C Barry)

RETINAL ARTERIAL OCCLUSIVE DISEASE

Aetiology

Atherosclerosis-related thrombosis

Atherosclerosis-related thrombosis at the level of the lamina cribrosa is by far the most common underlying cause of central retinal artery occlusion (CRAO), accounting for about 80% of cases. Atherosclerosis is characterized by focal intimal thickening comprising cells of smooth muscle origin, connective tissue and lipid-containing foam cells (Fig. 16.35). The incidence of atherosclerosis increases with age and is accelerated by hypertension, diabetes mellitus and hyper-homocysteinaemia. Other risk factors include raised serum levels of low-density-cholesterol (LDL-cholesterol), obesity, smoking and a sedentary lifestyle.

Carotid embolism

The origin of emboli is most often an atheromatous plaque at the carotid bifurcation and less commonly from the aortic arch. The emboli may be of the following types:

1. **Cholesterol** emboli (Hollenhorst plaques) appear as intermittent showers of minute, bright, refractile, golden to yellow-orange crystals, often located at arteriolar bifurcations (Fig. 16.36a). They rarely cause significant obstruction to the retinal arterioles and are frequently asymptomatic.

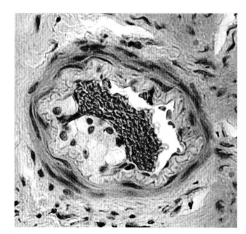

Fig. 16.35
Atherosclerosis – the arterial lumen is narrowed by lipid-containing cells within the intima (Courtesy of J Harry and G Misson, from *Clinical Ophthalmic Pathology*, Butterworth-Heinemann, 2001)

2. **Calcific** emboli may originate from atheromatous plaques in the ascending aorta or carotid arteries, as well as from calcified heart valves. They are usually single, white, non-scintillating and often on or close to the disc (Fig. 16.36b). When located on the disc itself, they may be easily overlooked because they tend to merge with the disc. Calcific emboli are much more dangerous than the other two kinds because they may cause permanent occlusion of the central retinal artery or one of its main branches.
3. **Fibrin-platelet** emboli are dull grey, elongated particles which are usually multiple (Fig. 16.36c) and occasionally fill the entire lumen (Fig. 16.36d). They may cause a retinal transient ischaemic attack (TIA), with resultant amaurosis fugax, and occasionally complete obstruction. Amaurosis fugax is characterized by painless transient unilateral loss of vision, often described as a curtain coming down over the eye, usually from top to bottom, but occasionally vice versa. Visual loss, which may be complete, usually lasts a few minutes. Recovery is in the same pattern as the initial loss, although usually more gradual. Frequency of attacks may vary from several times a day to once every few months. The attacks may be associated with ipsilateral cerebral TIA with contralateral signs.

Uncommon causes

1. **Giant cell arteritis,** whilst a common cause of anterior ischaemic optic neuropathy, it rarely causes CRAO.
2. **Cardiac embolism.** Since the ophthalmic artery is the first branch of the internal carotid artery, embolic material from the heart and carotid arteries has a fairly direct route to the eye. Emboli originating from the heart and its valves may be of the following four types:
   a. Calcific emboli from the aortic or mitral valves.
   b. Vegetations from cardiac valves in bacterial endocarditis.
   c. Thrombus from the left side of the heart, consequent to myocardial infarction (mural thrombi), and mitral stenosis associated with atrial fibrillation or mitral valve prolapse.
   d. Myxomatous material from the very rare atrial myxoma.
3. **Periarteritis** associated with dermatomyositis, systemic lupus erythematosus, polyarteritis nodosa, Wegener granulomatosis and Behçet syndrome may occasionally be responsible for branch retinal artery occlusion (BRAO), which may be multiple and bilateral.
4. **Thrombophilic disorders** that may be associated with retinal artery occlusion in young individuals include hyperhomocysteinaemia, antiphospholipid antibody syndrome and inherited defects of natural anticoagulants.
5. **Sickling haemoglobinopathies.**
6. **Retinal migraine** may very rarely be responsible for retinal artery occlusion in young individuals. However, the diagnosis should be made only after other more common causes have been excluded.

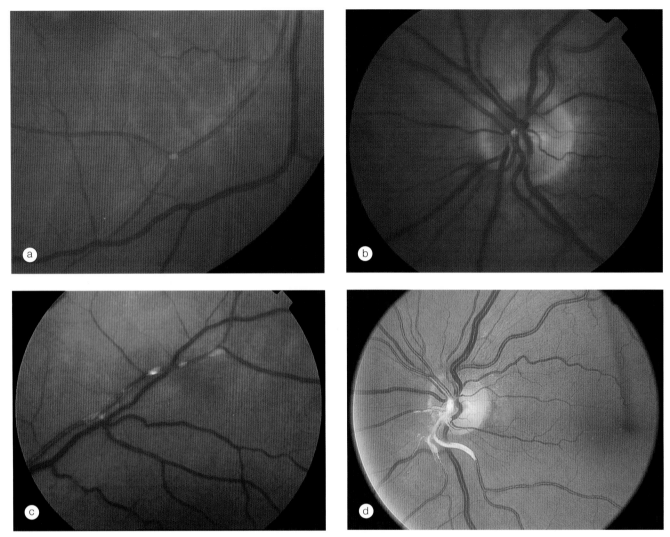

Fig. 16.36
Emboli arising from the carotid bifurcation. **(a)** Hollenhorst plaque; **(b)** calcific embolus at the disc; **(c)** fibrin-platelet emboli; **(d)** fibrin-platelet emboli extending from the disc to involve three branches (Courtesy of L Merin – fig. a; C Barry – fig. b)

7. **Susac syndrome** which is characterized by the triad of retinal artery occlusion, sensorineural deafness and encephalopathy.

Medical investigations

All patients

1. **Pulse** to detect atrial fibrillation.
2. **Blood pressure**
3. **Carotid evaluation** for stenosis by auscultation to detect a bruit, and duplex scanning.
4. **ECG**

5. **Blood**
   - Full blood count and ESR.
   - Fasting glucose and lipids.

Selected patients

1. **Echocardiogram**
2. **MR angiography**
3. **Blood**
   - Thrombophilia screen.
   - Autoantibodies – anticardiolipin, lupus anticoagulant, ANA, anti-dsDNA and ANCA.
   - Homocysteine.

Branch retinal artery occlusion

Diagnosis

1. **Presentation** is with sudden and profound altitudinal or sectoral visual field loss.
2. **VA** is variable.
3. **Fundus** (Fig. 16.37)
   - Narrowing of arteries and veins with sludging and segmentation of the blood column (cattle trucking).
   - Cloudy white retina, resulting from oedema, that corresponds to the area of ischaemia.
   - Emboli may be present.
4. **FA** shows delay in arterial filling and hypofluorescence of the involved segment due to blockage of background fluorescence by retinal swelling (Fig. 16.38).

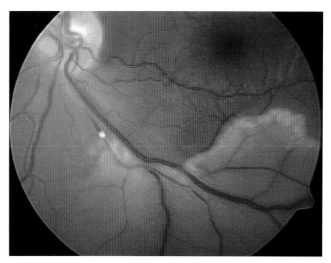

Fig. 16.37
Embolic inferotemporal branch retinal artery occlusion (Courtesy of P Gili)

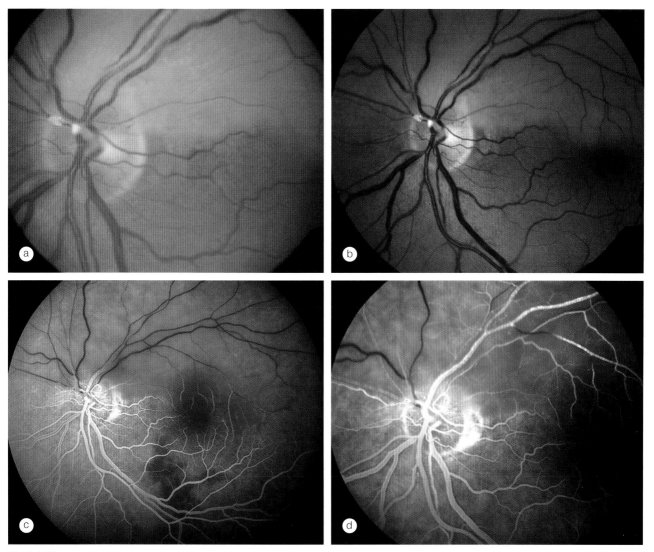

Fig. 16.38
(a) Superior branch retinal artery occlusion due an embolus at the disc; (b) red-free image shows the embolus more clearly; (c and d) FA shows delay in arterial filling and hypofluorescence of the involved segment due to blockage of background fluorescence by retinal swelling (Courtesy of P Gili)

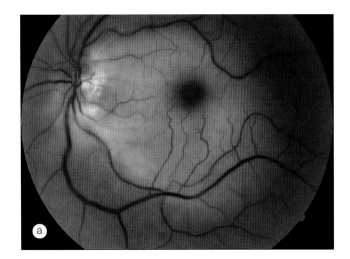

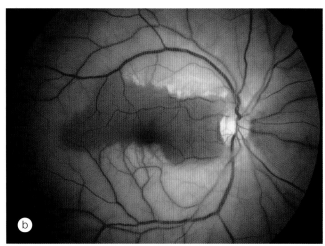

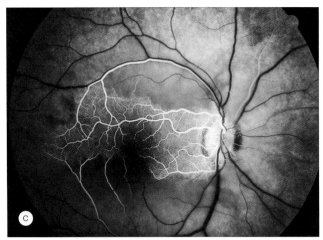

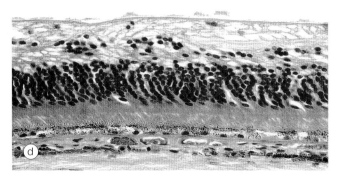

Fig. 16.39
Central retinal artery occlusion. **(a)** 'Cherry-red spot' at the macula; **(b)** patent cilioretinal artery; **(c)** FA shows blockage of background fluorescence by retinal swelling but normal perfusion at the posterior pole; **(d)** histology shows atrophy of the inner retina and ganglion cells with preservation of a few bipolar cells (Courtesy of S Milenkovic – fig. a; L Merin – figs b and c; J Harry – fig. d)

Prognosis

The prognosis is poor unless the obstruction can be relieved within a few hours (see below). The visual field defect is permanent and the affected artery remains attenuated. Occasionally, however, recanalization of the obstructed artery may leave subtle or absent ophthalmoscopic signs.

Central retinal artery occlusion

Diagnosis

1. **Presentation** is with sudden and profound loss of vision.
2. **VA** is severely reduced except if a portion of the papillomacular bundle is supplied by a cilioretinal artery, when central vision may be preserved.
3. **APD** is profound or total (amaurotic pupil).
4. **Fundus** shows similar changes to BRAO but more extensive.

- The orange reflex from the intact choroid stands out at the thin foveola, in contrast to the surrounding pale retina, giving rise to the 'cherry-red spot' appearance (Fig. 16.39a).
- In eyes with a cilioretinal artery part of the macula will remain normal in colour (Fig. 16.39b).
5. **FA** shows delay in arterial filling and masking of background choroidal fluorescence by retinal swelling. However, a patent cilioretinal artery will fill during the early phase (Fig. 16.39c).

Prognosis

The prognosis is poor due to retinal infarction. After a few weeks the retinal cloudiness and the 'cherry-red spot' gradually disappear although the arteries remain attenuated.

The inner retinal layers become atrophic (Fig. 16.39d) and consecutive optic atrophy results in permanent loss of useful vision. Some eyes develop rubeosis iridis which may require PRP, and about 2% develop NVD.

Cilioretinal artery occlusion

A cilioretinal artery, present in 20% of the population, arises from the posterior ciliary circulation but supplies the macula and papillomacular bundle.

1. **Isolated** (Fig. 16.40a) typically affects young patients with an associated systemic vasculitis.
2. **Combined with CRVO** (Fig.16.40b) has a similar prognosis to non-ischaemic CRVO.
3. **Combined with anterior ischaemic optic neuropathy** (Fig. 16.40c) typically affects patients with giant cell arteritis and carries a very poor prognosis.
4. **Presentation** is with acute, severe loss of central vision.
5. **Signs.** Cloudiness localized to that part of the retina normally perfused by the vessel.
6. **FA** shows a corresponding filling defect (Fig. 16.40d).

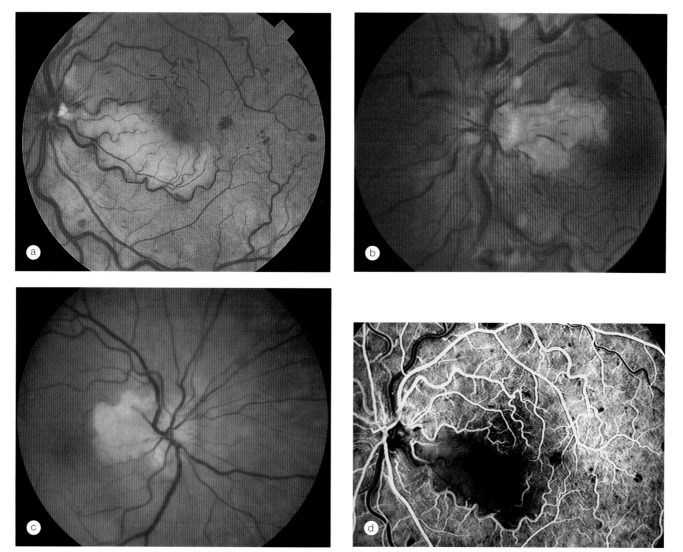

Fig. 16.40
Cilioretinal artery occlusion. **(a)** Isolated; **(b)** combined with central retinal vein occlusion; **(c)** combined with anterior ischaemic optic neuropathy; **(d)** FA shows hypofluorescence at the macula due to lack of filling and blockage by retinal swelling (Courtesy of S Milewski – figs a and d; S S Hayreh – fig. b)

Treatment of acute retinal artery occlusion

Retinal artery occlusion is an emergency because it causes irreversible visual loss unless the retinal circulation is re-established prior to the development of retinal infarction. It appears that the prognosis for occlusions caused by calcific emboli is worse than those resulting from either cholesterol or platelet emboli. Theoretically, timely dislodgement of emboli of the latter two types may prevent subsequent visual loss. The following treatment may be tried in patients with occlusions of less than 48 hours duration at presentation.

1. **Ocular massage** using a three-mirror contact lens for approximately 10 seconds, to obtain central retinal artery pulsation or cessation of flow (for BRAO), followed by 5 seconds of release. The aim is to mechanically collapse the arterial lumen and cause prompt changes in arterial flow.
2. **Anterior chamber paracentesis** should be carried out.
3. **Intravenous acetazolamide** to obtain a more prolonged lowering of intraocular pressure than with repeated paracentesis, if this was initially successful but flow has ceased.

OCULAR ISCHAEMIC SYNDROME

Pathogenesis

Ocular ischaemic syndrome is an uncommon condition which is the result of chronic ocular hypoperfusion secondary to ipsilateral atherosclerotic carotid stenosis of more than 90% resulting in 50% reduction of ipsilateral perfusion pressure. It typically affects patients during the seventh decade and may be associated with diabetes, hypertension, ischaemic heart disease and cerebrovascular disease. The 5-year mortality is in the order of 40%, most frequently from cardiac disease. Patients with ocular ischaemic syndrome may also give a history of amaurosis fugax due to retinal embolism.

Diagnosis

The ocular ischaemic syndrome is unilateral in 80% of cases and affects both anterior and posterior segments. The signs are variable and may be subtle such that the condition is missed or misdiagnosed.

1. **Presentation** is usually with gradual loss of vision over several weeks or months and occasionally with amaurosis fugax. Ocular pain may also be present.

2. **Anterior segment**
   - Diffuse episcleral injection and corneal oedema.
   - Aqueous flare with a few cells (ischaemic pseudo-iritis).
   - Iris atrophy and a mid-dilated and poorly reacting pupil.
   - Rubeosis iridis is common and often progresses to neovascular glaucoma.
   - Cataract in very advanced cases.
3. **Fundus**
   - Venous dilatation, arteriolar narrowing, haemorrhages and occasionally disc oedema (Fig. 16.41a).
   - Proliferative retinopathy with NVD and occasionally NVE.
   - Spontaneous arterial pulsation, most pronounced near the optic disc, is present in most cases or may be easily induced by exerting gentle pressure on the globe (digital ophthalmodynamometry).
4. **FA**
   - Early phase shows delayed choroidal filling and prolonged arteriovenous transit time (Fig. 16.41b and c).
   - Late phase shows disc and perivascular hyper-fluorescence, and leakage at the posterior pole (Fig.16.41d).
5. **Carotid imaging** may involve colour Doppler ultrasonography, digital subtraction angiography and MR angiography (see Chapter 2).

Management

1. **Anterior segment manifestations** are treated with topical steroids and mydriatics.
2. **Neovascular glaucoma** may be treated medically or surgically.
3. **Proliferative retinopathy** requires PRP although the results are less favourable than in diabetic retinopathy.
4. **Carotid endarterectomy** may be beneficial for proliferative retinopathy.

Differential diagnosis

1. **Non-ischaemic CRVO** is also characterized by unilateral retinal haemorrhages, venous dilatation and cotton-wool spots. However, haemorrhages are more numerous and mainly flame-shaped, and disc oedema is often present.
2. **Diabetic retinopathy** is also characterized by dot and blot retinal haemorrhages, venous tortuosity and proliferative retinopathy. However, it is usually bilateral and hard exudates are present.
3. **Hypertensive retinopathy** is also characterized by arteriolar attenuation and focal constriction, haemorrhages and cotton-wool spots. However, it is invariably bilateral and venous changes are absent.

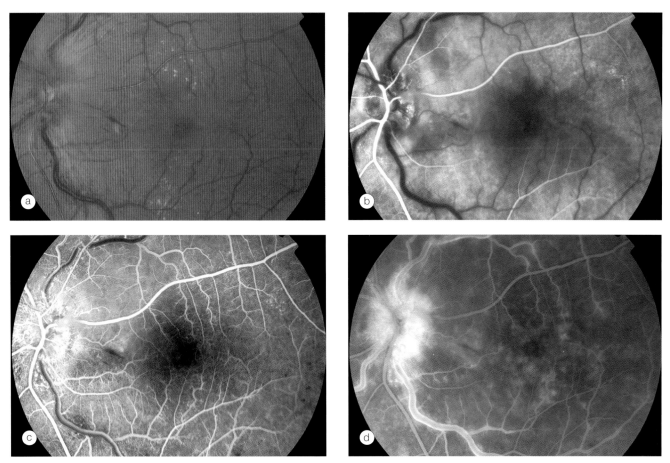

Fig. 16.41
Ocular ischaemic syndrome. **(a)** Venous dilatation, arteriolar narrowing, a few scattered flame-shaped haemorrhages and hard exudates, and disc oedema; **(b** and **c)** FA early phase shows delayed choroidal filling and prolonged arteriovenous transit; **(d)** FA late phase shows disc and perivascular hyperfluorescence, and spotty hyperfluorescence at the posterior pole due to leakage (Courtesy of Moorfields Eye Hospital)

HYPERTENSIVE DISEASE

Retinopathy

Retinopathy consists of a spectrum of retinal vascular changes that are pathologically related to microvascular damage from elevated blood pressure. The primary response of the retinal arterioles to systemic hypertension is narrowing (vasoconstriction). However, the degree of narrowing is dependent on the amount of pre-existing replacement fibrosis (involutional sclerosis). For this reason, hypertensive narrowing is seen in its pure form only in young individuals. In older patients, rigidity of retinal arterioles due to involutional sclerosis prevents the same degree of narrowing seen in young individuals. In sustained hypertension the inner blood–retinal barrier is disrupted in small areas, with increased vascular permeability. The fundus picture of hypertensive retinopathy is therefore characterized by the following.

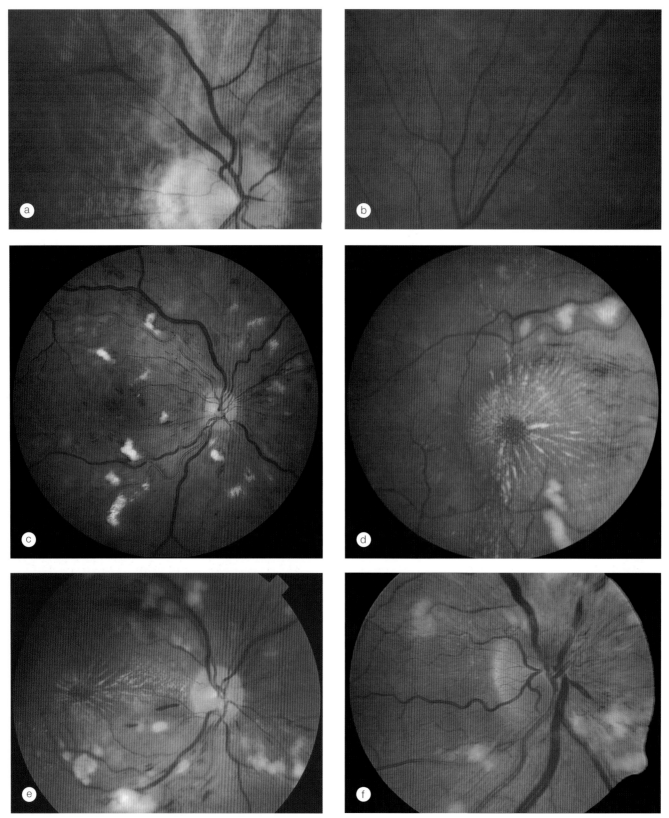

Fig. 16.42
Hypertensive retinopathy. **(a)** Focal arteriolar attenuation; **(b)** generalized arteriolar attenuation; **(c)** cotton-wool spots and flame-shaped haemorrhages; **(d)** cotton-wool spots and a macular star; **(e)** cotton-wool spots, haemorrhages and a macular star; **(f)** cotton-wool spots and disc swelling (Courtesy of P Saine – fig. c; P Gili – fig. f)

Arteriolar narrowing

Arteriolar narrowing may be focal (Fig. 16.42a) or generalized (Fig. 16.42b). Ophthalmoscopic diagnosis of generalized narrowing is difficult, although the presence of focal narrowing makes it highly probable that blood pressure is raised. Severe hypertension may lead to the development of cotton-wool spots (Fig. 16.42c).

Vascular leakage

Vascular leakage leads to flame-shaped retinal haemorrhages and retinal oedema (see Fig. 16.42c). Chronic retinal oedema may result in the deposition of hard exudates around the fovea in the Henle layer with a macular star configuration (Fig. 16.42d and e). Swelling of the optic nerve head is the hallmark of accelerated hypertension (Fig. 16.42f).

Arteriolosclerosis

Arteriolosclerosis involves thickening of the vessel wall characterized histologically by medial hypertrophy and hyalinization (Fig. 16.43a). The most important clinical sign is the presence of changes at arteriovenous crossings (AV nipping) (Fig. 16.43b). Although not necessarily indicative of the severity of hypertension, their presence makes it probable that hypertension has been present for many years. Mild changes at arteriovenous crossings are seen in patients with involutional sclerosis in the absence of hypertension. The grading of arteriolosclerosis is as follows (Fig. 16.44):

Grade 1: subtle broadening of the arteriolar light reflex, mild generalized arteriolar attenuation, particularly of small branches, and vein concealment.

Grade 2: obvious broadening of the arteriolar light reflex and deflection of veins at arteriovenous crossings (Salus sign).

Grade 3
- Copper-wiring of arterioles.
- Banking of veins distal to arteriovenous crossings (Bonnet sign).
- Tapering of veins on both sides of the crossings (Gunn sign) and right-angled deflection of veins.

Grade 4: silver-wiring of arterioles associated with grade 3 changes.

NB The presence of generalized retinal arteriolar narrowing and possibly arteriovenous nicking are related to previously elevated blood pressure, independent of concurrent blood pressure level.

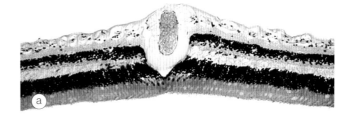
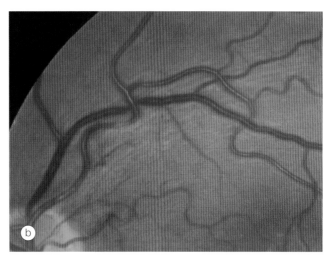

Fig. 16.43
Arteriolosclerosis. **(a)** Histology shows a thick vessel wall and narrowing of the lumen; **(b)** arteriovenous nipping (Courtesy of J Harry – fig. a)

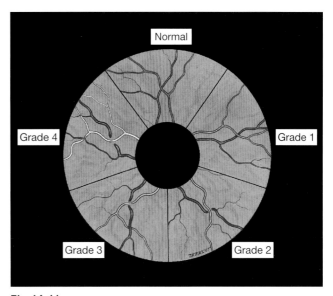

Fig. 16.44
Grading of retinal arteriolosclerosis

Choroidopathy

Choroidopathy is rare but may occur as the result of an acute hypertensive crisis (accelerated hypertension) in young adults.

1. **Elschnig spots** are small, black spots surrounded by yellow halos (Fig. 16.45a) which represent focal choroidal infarcts.
2. **Siegrist streaks** are flecks arranged linearly along choroidal vessels (Fig. 16.45b) which are indicative of fibrinoid necrosis (Fig. 16.45c).
3. **Exudative retinal detachment,** sometimes bilateral, may occur, particularly in toxaemia of pregnancy.

SICKLE-CELL RETINOPATHY

Sickling haemoglobinopathies

Sickling haemoglobinopathies are caused by one, or a combination, of abnormal haemoglobins which cause the red blood cell to adopt an anomalous shape (Fig. 16.46) under conditions of hypoxia and acidosis. Because these deformed red blood cells are more rigid than healthy cells, they may become impacted in and obstruct small blood vessels. The sickling disorders in which the mutant haemoglobins S and C are inherited as alleles of normal haemoglobin A have important ocular manifestations. These abnormal haemoglobins may occur in combination with normal haemoglobin A or in association with each other as indicated below.

1. **SS** (sickle-cell disease, sickle-cell anaemia) affects 0.4% of black Americans and is caused by a point mutation on the beta-globulin gene. The disease is characterized by severe chronic haemolytic anaemia and periodic, potentially fatal crises due to vaso-occlusive disease involving most organs, resulting in liver necrosis, painful crises (largely bone marrow infarcts), abdominal pain, acute chest syndrome and CNS symptoms. Despite the severity of systemic manifestations ocular complications are usually mild and asymptomatic.
2. **AS** (sickle-cell trait) is present in about 10% of black Americans. It is the mildest form and usually requires severe hypoxia or other abnormal conditions to produce sickling.

Fig. 16.45
Hypertensive choroidopathy. **(a)** Elschnig spots; **(b)** Siegrist streaks; **(c)** fibrinoid necrosis in a choroidal arteriole in accelerated hypertension (Courtesy of J Harry – fig. c)

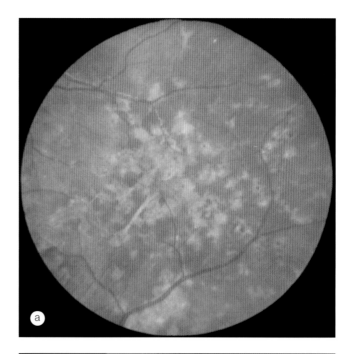

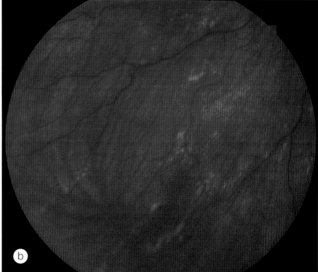

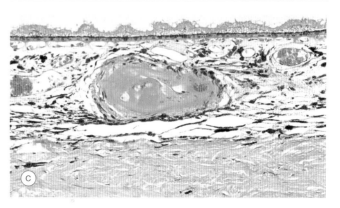

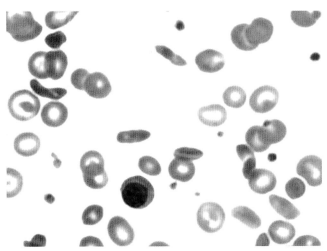

Fig. 16.46
Several sickled red cells and one nucleated red cell in a blood smear of a patient with homozygous (HbSS) sickle cell anaemia (Courtesy of N Bienz)

3. **SC** (sickle-cell C disease) is present in 0.2% of black Americans. It is characterized by haemolytic anaemia and infarctive crises that are less severe than in SS disease but may be associated with severe retinopathy.
4. **SThal** (sickle-cell thalassaemia) is characterized by mild anaemia but may be associated with severe retinopathy.

   NB Retinopathy is most severe in SC and SThal disease.

Proliferative retinopathy

Diagnosis

Figure 16.47 shows a composite of grading.
Stage 1: peripheral arterial occlusion and ischaemia.
Stage 2: peripheral arteriovenous anastomoses of dilated pre-existent capillary channels (Fig. 16.48a).
Stage 3
  • Sprouting of new vessels from the anastomoses which have a 'sea-fan' configuration and are usually fed by a single arteriole and drained by a single vein (Fig. 16.48b and 16.49a).
  • About 30–40% of 'sea-fans' involute spontaneously as a result of auto-infarction and appear as greyish fibrovascular lesions (Fig. 16.48c). Involution most frequently occurs about 2 years after the development of retinopathy.
Stage 4: in some cases the neovascular tufts continue to proliferate and bleed into the vitreous (Fig. 16.48d).
Stage 5: extensive fibrovascular proliferation (Fig. 16.48e) and retinal detachment (Fig. 16.48f).

FA in stage 3 shows filling of 'sea-fans' and peripheral capillary non-perfusion (Fig. 16.49b) followed by extensive hyperfluorescence due to leakage from new vessels (Fig. 16.49c).

   NB The development of proliferative retinopathy is usually insidious, and patients remain asymptomatic unless vitreous haemorrhage or retinal detachment occurs.

Treatment

Treatment is not required in most cases because new vessels tend to auto-infarct and involute spontaneously without treatment. Occasionally vitreoretinal surgery may be required for tractional retinal detachment and/or persistent vitreous haemorrhage.

Differential diagnosis of peripheral retinal neovascularization

1. **Vascular disease with ischaemia**
   • Proliferative diabetic retinopathy.
   • Branch retinal vein occlusion.
   • Ocular ischaemic syndrome.
   • Sickling haemoglobinopathies.
   • Retinopathy of prematurity.
   • Eales disease.
   • Familial exudative vitreoretinopathy.
   • Chronic myeloid leukaemia.
   • Encircling buckle.

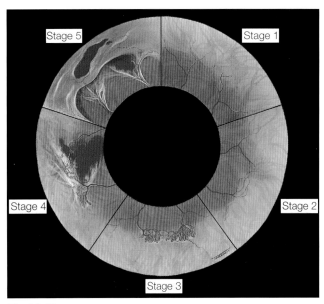

Fig. 16.47
Grading of proliferative sickle-cell retinopathy

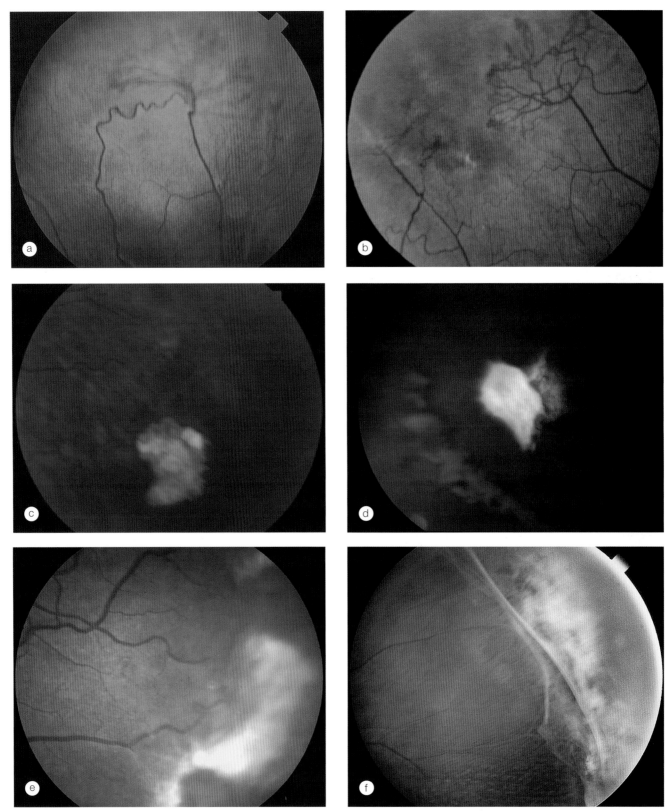

Fig. 16.48
Proliferative sickle-cell retinopathy. **(a)** Peripheral arteriovenous anastomosis; **(b)** 'sea-fan' neovascularization; **(c)** spontaneous involution of a neovascular tuft; **(d)** haemorrhage due to traction; **(e)** extensive fibrovascular proliferation; **(f)** peripheral retinal detachment (Courtesy of K Nischal – fig. a; R Marsh – figs b–f)

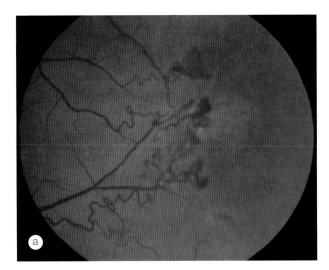

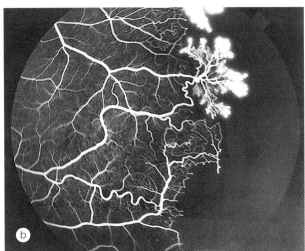

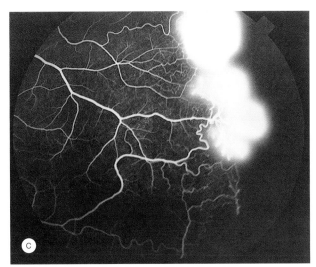

Fig. 16.49
(a) Proliferative sickle-cell retinopathy stage 3; **(b)** FA early phase shows filling of new vessels ('sea-fans') and extensive peripheral retinal capillary non-perfusion; **(c)** late phase shows leakage from new vessels

2. **Inflammatory disease with possible ischaemia**
   - Sarcoidosis.
   - Retinal vasculitis.
   - Intermediate uveitis.
   - Eales disease.
   - Acute retinal necrosis.
3. **Miscellaneous**
   - Incontinentia pigmenti.
   - Autosomal dominant vitreoretinochoroidopathy.
   - Long-standing retinal detachment.

Non-proliferative retinopathy

Asymptomatic lesions

1. **Venous tortuosity** is one of the first ophthalmic signs of sickling and is due to peripheral arteriovenous shunts.
2. **Silver-wiring of arterioles** in the peripheral retina which represent previously occluded vessels.
3. **Salmon patches** are pink, preretinal (Fig. 16.50a) or superficial intraretinal haemorrhages at the equator, which lie adjacent to arterioles and usually resolve without sequelae.
4. **Black sunbursts** are patches of peripheral RPE hyperplasia (Fig. 16.50b).
5. **Macular depression sign** is an oval depression of the bright central macular reflex due to atrophy and thinning of the sensory retina.
6. **Peripheral retinal holes** and areas of whitening similar to 'white-without-pressure' are occasionally seen (Fig. 16.50c).

Symptomatic lesions

1. **Macular arteriolar occlusion** occurs in about 30% of patients (Fig. 16.50d).
2. **Acute CRAO** is rare.
3. **Retinal vein occlusion** is uncommon.
4. **Choroidal vascular occlusion** may be seen occasionally, particularly in children.
5. **Angioid streaks** occur in a minority of patients.

Anterior segment features

1. **Conjunctival** lesions are characterized by isolated dark red vascular anomalies shaped like commas or cork-screws. They involve small calibre vessels and are most often located inferiorly.
2. **Iris** lesions consist of circumscribed areas of ischaemic atrophy, usually at the pupillary edge and extending to the collarette. Rubeosis may be seen occasionally.

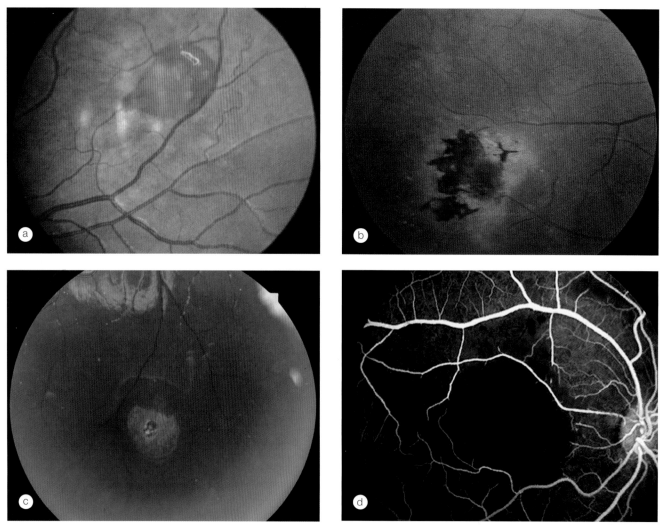

Fig. 16.50
Non-proliferative sickle-cell retinopathy. **(a)** Preretinal haemorrhage (salmon patch); **(b)** RPE hyperplasia (black sunburst); **(c)** retinal hole and an area of whitening superiorly; **(d)** FA shows macular ischaemia (Courtesy of R Marsh)

RETINOPATHY OF PREMATURITY

Pathogenesis

Retinopathy of prematurity (ROP) is a proliferative retinopathy affecting premature infants of very low birth weight, who have been exposed to high ambient oxygen concentrations (Fig. 16.51). The retina is unique among tissues in that it has no blood vessels until the fourth month of gestation, at which time vascular complexes emanating from the hyaloid vessels at the optic disc grow towards the periphery. These vessels reach the nasal periphery after 8 months of gestation, but do not reach the temporal periphery until about 1 month after delivery (Fig. 16.52). The

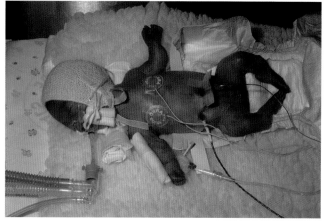

Fig. 16.51
A premature infant of low birth weight exposed to a high ambient oxygen concentration

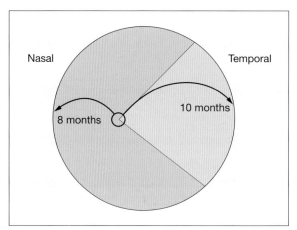

Fig. 16.52
Vascularization of the peripheral retina (see text)

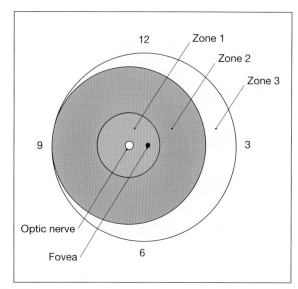

Fig. 16.53
Grading of retinopathy of prematurity according to location (see text)

incompletely vascularized retina is particularly susceptible to oxygen damage in the premature infant. A model of ROP suggests that the avascular retina produces VEGF which *in utero* is the stimulus for vessel migration in the developing retina. With premature birth the production of VEGF is down-regulated by the relative hyperoxia and vessel migration is halted. Subsequently the increased metabolic demand of the growing eye allows excessive VEGF production, which leads to ROP.

Active disease

Location of disease

For the purpose of defining the anteroposterior location of ROP, three concentric zones centred on the optic disc are described (Fig. 16.53).

Zone 1 is bounded by an imaginary circle, the radius of which is twice the distance from the disc to the macula.

Zone 2 extends concentrically from the edge of zone 1; its radius extends from the centre of the disc to the nasal ora serrata.

Zone 3 consists of a residual temporal crescent anterior to zone 2.

The approximate temporal extent of zone 1 can be determined by using a 25D condensing lens. By placing the nasal edge of the optic disc at one edge of the field of view, the limit of zone 1 is at the temporal field of view.

Extent of disease

Extent of involvement is determined by the number of clock hours of retina involved or as 30° sectors. As the observer examines each eye, the 3 o'clock position is to the right and nasal in the right eye and temporal in the left eye. The 9 o'clock position is to the left and temporal in the right eye and nasal in the left eye. The boundaries between sectors lie on the clock hour positions; the 12 o'clock sector extends from 12 o'clock to 1 o'clock.

Staging

The following five stages (Fig. 16.54) are used to describe the abnormal vascular response at the junction of immature avascular peripheral retina from vascularized posterior retina. Because more than one ROP stage may be present in the same eye, staging for the eye as a whole is determined by the most severe manifestation.

Stage 1 (demarcation line) is a thin, flat, tortuous, grey-white line running roughly parallel with the ora serrata more prominent in the temporal periphery. There is abnormal branching or arcading of vessels leading up to the line (Fig. 16.55a).

Stage 2 (ridge) arises in the region of the demarcation line, has height and width, and extends above the plane of the retina. Blood vessels enter the ridge and small isolated neovascular tufts ('popcorn') may be seen posterior to it (Fig. 16.55b).

Stage 3 (extraretinal fibrovascular proliferation) extends from the ridge into the vitreous (Fig. 16.55c). It is continuous with the posterior aspect of the ridge, causing a ragged appearance as the proliferation becomes more extensive. The severity of stage 3 can be subdivided into mild, moderate and severe depending on the extent of extra-retinal fibrous tissue infiltrating the vitreous. The highest

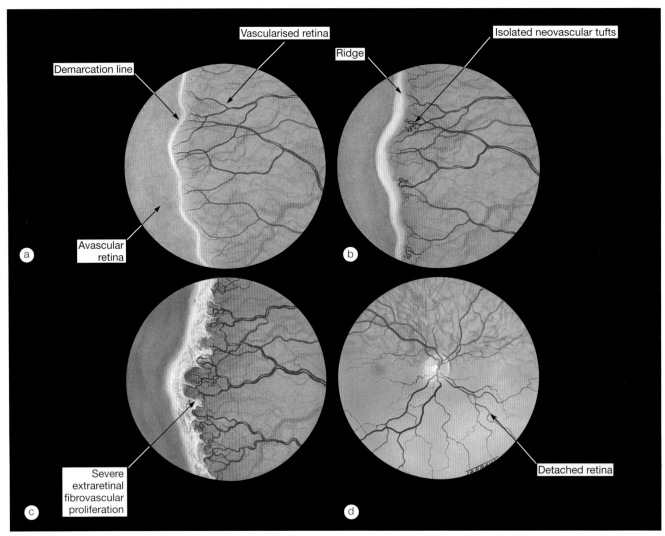

Fig. 16.54
Progression of acute retinopathy of prematurity (see text)

incidence of this stage is around the post-conceptual age of 35 weeks.

Stage 4 (partial retinal detachment) is divided into extrafoveal (stage 4a – Fig. 16.55d) and foveal (stage 4b). The detachment is generally concave and circumferentially orientated. In progressive cases the fibrous tissue continues to contract and the detachment increases in height and extends anteriorly and posteriorly.

Stage 5 is a total retinal detachment.

Other features

1. **Plus disease** signifies a tendency to progression and is characterized by the following:

- Failure of the pupil to dilate associated with gross vascular engorgement of the iris.
- Vitreous haze.
- Dilatation of veins and tortuosity of the arteries involving at least two quadrants of the posterior fundus.
- Increasing preretinal and vitreous haemorrhage.
- When these changes are present, a plus sign is added to the stage number.

2. **Pre-plus disease** is characterized by abnormal dilatation and tortuosity that is insufficient to be designated as plus disease.

3. **Threshold disease** is defined as five contiguous clock hours or eight cumulative clock hours of extraretinal neovascularization (stage 3 disease) in zone 1 or zone 2,

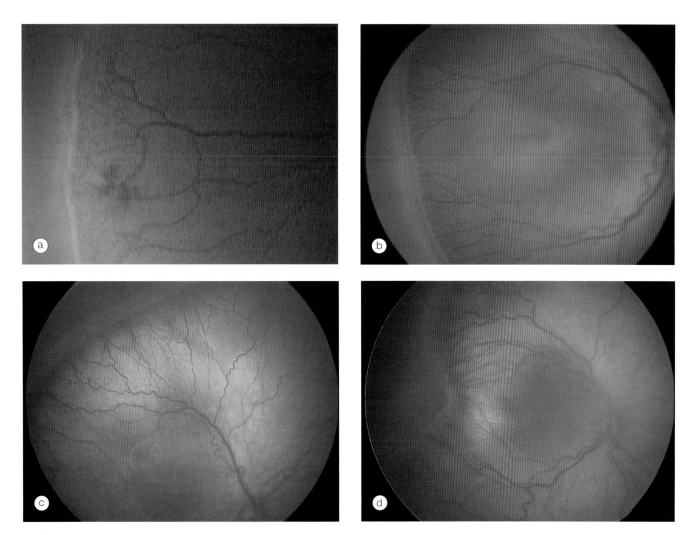

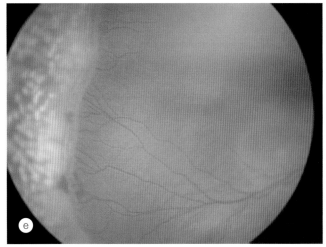

Fig. 16.55
Active retinopathy of prematurity. **(a)** Stage 1 – demarcation line; **(b)** stage 2 – ridge; **(c)** stage 3 – ridge with extraretinal vascular proliferation; **(d)** stage 4a – partial extrafoveal retinal detachment; **(e)** appearance immediately following laser photocoagulation for threshold disease (Courtesy of L MacKeen – figs a, c and d; P Watts – figs b and e)

associated with plus disease. It is an indication for treatment.

4. **Aggressive posterior (rush disease)** is uncommon but if untreated usually progresses to stage 5. It is characterized by its posterior location, prominence of plus disease and ill-defined nature of the retinopathy. It is most commonly observed in zone 1 and does not usually progress through the classical stages 1 to 3.

Regression

In about 80% of cases ROP regresses spontaneously by a process of involution or evolution from a vasoproliferative to fibrotic phase leaving few, if any, residua. Spontaneous regression may even occur in eyes with partial retinal detachments. The process of regression occurs largely at the junction of vascular and avascular retina.

Screening

Babies born at or before 31 weeks gestational age, or weighing 1500g or less, should be screened for ROP by an ophthalmologist with expertise in ROP. This may involve indirect ophthalmoscopy with a 25D lens or a wide field retinal camera (RetCam 120°). Screening should begin 4–7 weeks postnatally to detect the onset of threshold disease. Subsequent review should be at 1–2-weekly intervals, depending on severity, until retinal vascularization reaches zone 3. The pupils in a premature infant are dilated with 0.5% cyclopentolate and 2.5% phenylephrine.

> **NB** Only about 8% of babies screened actually require treatment.

Treatment

1. **Laser photocoagulation** of avascular immature retina is recommended in infants with threshold disease (Fig. 16.55e). This is successful in 85% of cases, but the remainder progress to retinal detachment in spite of treatment. Laser therapy has largely replaced cryotherapy because visual and anatomical outcomes are superior, and laser induces less myopia.

2. **Lens-sparing pars plana vitrectomy** for tractional retinal detachment not involving the macula (stage 4a) can be treated successfully with respect to anatomical and visual outcome. However, the visual outcome in stages 4b and 5, in which the macula is involved, is generally disappointing despite successful reattachment.

Cicatricial disease

About 20% of infants with active ROP develop cicatricial complications, which range from innocuous to extremely severe. In general, the more advanced or the more posterior the proliferative disease at the time of involution, the worse the cicatricial sequelae.

Stage 1: peripheral retinal pigmentary disturbance and haze at the vitreous base (Fig. 16.56a).

Stage 2: temporal vitreoretinal fibrosis and straightening of vascular arcades (Fig. 16.56b) followed by 'dragging' of the macula and disc (Fig. 16.56c). This may lead to a pseudo-exotropia due to resultant exaggeration of angle kappa.

Stage 3: more severe peripheral fibrosis with contracture and a falciform retinal fold (Fig. 16.56d).

Stage 4: partial ring of retrolental fibrovascular tissue with partial retinal detachment (Fig. 16.56e).

Stage 5: complete ring of retrolental fibrovascular tissue with total retinal detachment, a picture formerly known as 'retrolental fibroplasia' (Fig. 16.56f). Secondary angle-closure glaucoma may develop due to progressive shallowing of the anterior chamber caused by a forward movement of the iris-lens diaphragm and the development of anterior synechiae. Treatment involving lensectomy and anterior vitrectomy may be tried but the results are often poor.

> **NB** Very low birth weight infants, especially those treated for ROP, are at a higher risk of developing strabismus and myopia than term infants and require follow-up till the age of visual maturity.

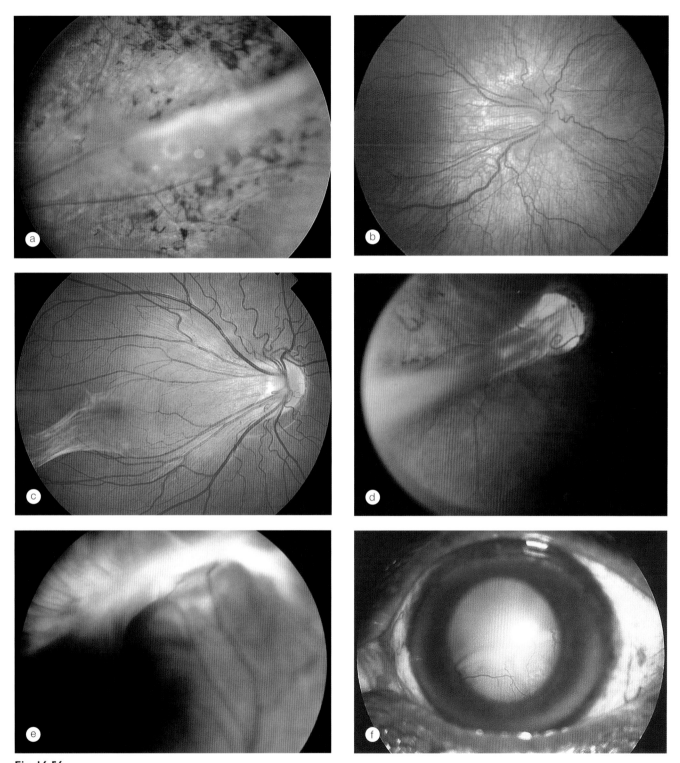

Fig. 16.56
Cicatricial retinopathy of prematurity. **(a)** Stage 1 – peripheral pigmentary disturbance; **(b)** early stage 2 – straightening of vascular arcades; **(c)** late stage 2 – 'dragging' of the disc and macula; **(d)** stage 3 – falciform fold; **(e)** stage 4 – retrolental fibrovascular tissue and partial retinal detachment; **(f)** stage 5 – total retinal detachment

RETINAL ARTERY MACROANEURYSM

A retinal artery macroaneurysm is a localized dilatation of a retinal arteriole which usually occurs in the first three orders of the arterial tree. It has a predilection for elderly hypertensive women and in 90% of cases involves one eye.

Diagnosis

1. Presentation
- Insidious impairment of central vision due to leakage involving the macula.
- Sudden visual loss resulting from haemorrhage is less common.

2. Signs
- A saccular or fusiform arteriolar dilatation, most frequently occurring at a bifurcation or an arterio-venous crossing along the temporal vascular arcades.
- The aneurysm may enlarge to several times the diameter of the artery.
- Associated retinal haemorrhage is present in 50% of cases (Fig. 16.57a).
- Multiple macroaneurysms along the same or different arterioles may occasionally be present.

3. FA findings are dependent on the patency of the lesion and any associated haemorrhage. The typical appearance is that of immediate uniform filling of the macroaneurysm (Fig. 16.57b) with late leakage (Fig. 16.57c). Incomplete filling is due to thrombosis.

4. Course
- **a. Chronic leakage** resulting in retinal oedema with accumulation of hard exudates at the fovea is common and may result in permanent loss of central vision (Fig. 16.58a).
- **b. Rupture** with haemorrhage, which may be subretinal (Fig. 16.58b), intraretinal, preretinal or vitreous (Fig. 16.58c). In these cases the underlying lesion may be overlooked and the diagnosis missed.
- **c. Spontaneous involution** following thrombosis and fibrosis is very common (Fig. 16.58d) and may precede or follow leakage or haemorrhage.

Management

1. Observation in anticipation of spontaneous involution is indicated in eyes with good visual acuity in which the macula is not threatened and those with mild retinal haemorrhage without significant oedema or exudation. In most cases following retinal or vitreous haemorrhage the macroaneurysm becomes thrombosed and laser coagulation is not required.

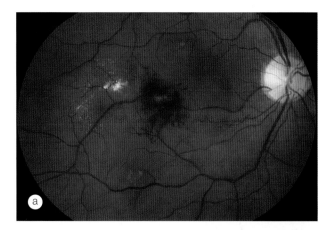

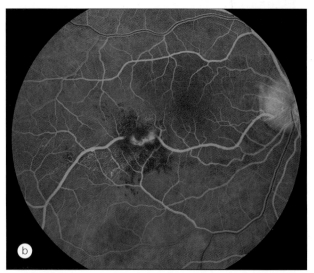

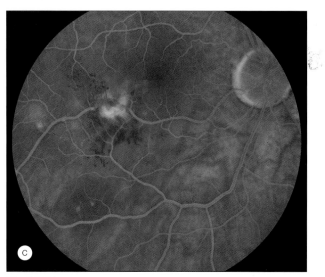

Fig. 16.57
(a) Retinal artery macroaneurysm associated with haemorrhage and hard exudates; **(b)** FA early venous phase shows partial hyperfluorescence of the microaneurysm, and surrounded blockage of fluorescence by blood; **(c)** late phase shows more hyperfluorescence due to leakage (Courtesy of P Saine)

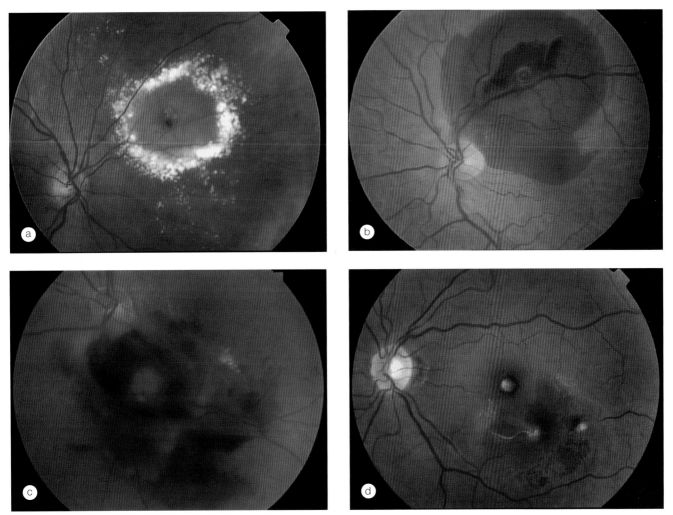

Fig. 16.58
Retinal artery macroaneurysm. **(a)** Surrounding hard exudates due to chronic leakage; **(b)** subretinal haemorrhage; **(c)** preretinal and vitreous haemorrhage; **(d)** spontaneous involution of three macroaneurysms (Courtesy of P Gili – fig. b)

2. **Laser photocoagulation** may be considered if oedema or hard exudates threaten or involve the fovea (Fig. 16.59a), particularly if there is visual deterioration. The burns may be applied to the lesion itself, the surrounding area, or both (Fig. 16.59b) although it may take several months for the oedema and hard exudates to absorb.

3. **YAG laser hyaloidotomy** may be considered in eyes with large non-absorbing preretinal haemorrhage overlying the macula (Fig. 16.59c) in order to disperse the blood into the vitreous cavity, from where it may be absorbed more quickly (Fig. 16.59d).

4. **Intravitreal injection** of expandable gas with face-down positioning to shift the submacular haemorrhage away from the macula with or without tPA.

Differential diagnosis

1. **Hard exudates at the posterior pole**

- Background diabetic retinopathy.
- Exudative age-related macular degeneration.
- Old retinal branch vein occlusion.
- Retinal telangiectasis.
- Small retinal haemangioblastoma.
- Radiation retinopathy.

2. **Deep retinal or subretinal haemorrhages at the posterior pole**
- Choroidal neovascularization.
- Valsalva retinopathy.
- Idiopathic polypoidal choroidal vasculopathy.
- Blunt trauma.
- Choroidal melanoma.
- Terson syndrome is characterized by preretinal and/or vitreous haemorrhage, typically occurring in association with a subarachnoid haemorrhage.

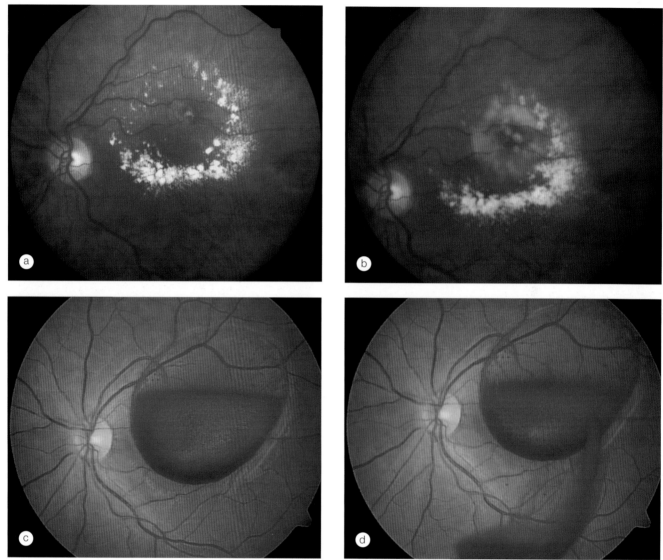

Fig. 16.59
Treatment of complications of retinal artery macroaneurysm. **(a)** Hard exudates at the macula due to chronic leakage; **(b)** following laser photocoagulation; **(c)** large preretinal haemorrhage overlying the macula; **(d)** following YAG laser hyalotomy the blood is dispersing into the vitreous (Courtesy of P Gili – figs c and d)

PRIMARY RETINAL TELANGIECTASIS

Primary retinal telangiectasis comprises a group of rare idiopathic, congenital or acquired, retinal vascular anomalies characterized by dilatation and tortuosity of retinal blood vessels, multiple aneurysms, vascular leakage and the deposition of hard exudates. Retinal telangiectasis involves the capillary bed, although the arterioles and venules may also be involved. The vascular malformations often progress and become symptomatic later in life.

Idiopathic juxtafoveolar retinal telangiectasis

Idiopathic juxtafoveolar telangiectasis is a rare congenital or acquired condition which can be divided into three groups.

1A. Unilateral congenital

1. **Presentation** is typically in a middle-aged man with mild to moderate blurring of vision.
2. **Signs.** Telangiectasis involving an area about 1.5 disc diameters temporal to the fovea (Fig. 16.60a)

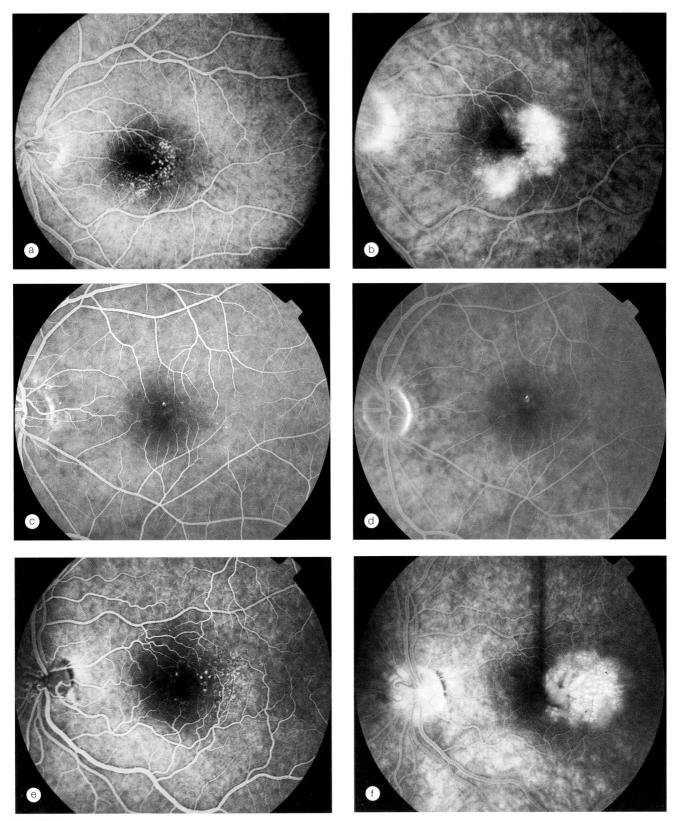

Fig. 16.60
Idiopathic juxtafoveolar retinal telangiectasis. *Group 1A* (**a**) Telangiectasis temporal to the fovea; (**b**) late leakage. *Group 1B*
(**c**) Telangiectasis confined to one clock hour of FAZ; (**d**) absence of late leakage. *Group 2A* (**e**) Telangiectasis outside and temporal to
FAZ; (**f**) late leakage

associated with leakage (Fig. 16.60b) and frequently hard exudates.
3. **Treatment** by laser photocoagulation to areas of leakage may occasionally be beneficial in preventing visual loss from CMO and exudation.

1B. Unilateral idiopathic focal

1. **Presentation** is similar to type 1A.
2. **Signs.** Telangiectasis confined to one clock hour at the edge of the foveal avascular zone (FAZ – Fig. 16.60c) without leakage (Fig. 16.60d).
3. **Treatment** is not appropriate and the prognosis good.

2A. Bilateral idiopathic acquired

1. **Presentation** is in the sixth decade with mild, slowly progressive disturbance of central vision in one or both eyes. Both sexes are affected equally.
2. **Signs**
   • Symmetrical telangiectasis, one disc area or less, involving all or a part of the parafoveal area without hard exudates.
   • Stellate pigmented plaques of RPE hyperplasia.
   • Multiple refractile white juxtafoveolar dots and solitary small yellow central deposits may be present.
   • Subretinal CNV may develop in advanced cases.
3. **FA** shows capillary dilatation outside the FAZ (Fig. 16.60e) and late leakage (Fig. 16.60f).
4. **Prognosis** is guarded although photodynamic therapy or transpupillary thermotherapy may be beneficial for subfoveal CNV.

2B. Bilateral familial occult

This is similar to 2A but presents earlier and is associated with neither superficial retinal refractile deposits nor stellate pigmented plaques.

3A. Idiopathic occlusive

This is the most severe form which is frequently associated with systemic diseases such as polycythaemia, multiple myeloma and chronic lymphatic leukaemia.

1. **Presentation** is in the sixth decade with slowly progressive loss of central vision.
2. **Signs**
   • Marked aneurysmal dilatation of terminal capillaries and progressive occlusion of parafoveal capillaries.
   • Optic atrophy may be present.

3. **FA** shows widening of the FAZ but absence of leakage.
4. **Prognosis** is usually poor as there is no effective treatment.

3B. Idiopathic occlusive

This similar to 3A but is associated with neurological disease.

Coats disease

Coats disease is an idiopathic, non-hereditary, retinal telangiectasis with intraretinal and subretinal exudation, and frequently exudative retinal detachment. About 75% of patients are males and the vast majority have involvement of only one eye. It is now considered that Coats disease and Leber miliary aneurysms represent a spectrum of the same disease, the latter being more localized and carrying a better visual prognosis.

Diagnosis

1. **Presentation** is most frequently in the first decade of life (average 5 years) with unilateral visual loss, strabismus or leukocoria. Occasionally the condition may present in later childhood and rarely in adult life.
2. **Signs**
   • Telangiectasis most often in the inferior and temporal quadrants between the equator and ora serrata (Fig. 16.61a).
   • Intraretinal (Fig. 16.61b) and subretinal exudate formation (Fig. 16.61c).
   • Sometimes the lesions are located posterior to the equator towards the vascular arcades (Fig. 16.61d).
   • Progression of intraretinal and subretinal yellowish exudation often affecting areas remote from the vascular abnormalities, particularly the macula (Fig. 16.61e).
   • Exudative retinal detachment (Fig. 16.61f).
3. **FA** in mild cases (Fig. 16.62a) shows early hyperfluorescence of the telangiectasia (Fig. 16.62b) and late staining and leakage (Fig. 16.62c).
4. **Complications** rubeosis iridis, glaucoma, uveitis, cataract and phthisis bulbi.
5. **Association.** Atypical pigmentary retinopathy is seen in a small minority of patients (see Chapter 18).

Treatment

1. **Observation** in patients with mild, non-vision threatening disease and in those with a comfortable eye with total retinal detachment in which there is no hope of restoring useful vision.
2. **Laser photocoagulation** to areas of telangiectasis should be considered if progressive exudation is documented. Frequently more than one treatment session is

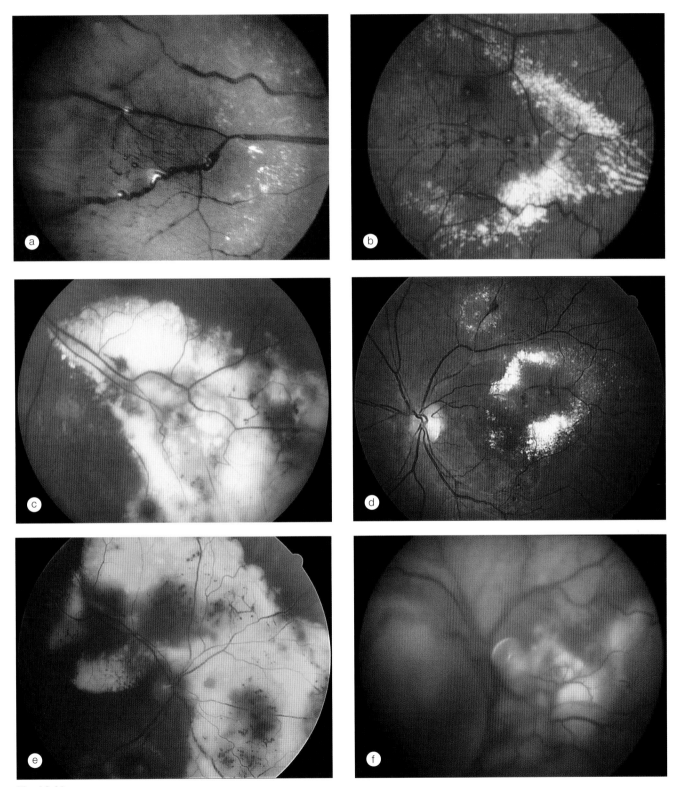

Fig. 16.61
Coats disease. **(a)** Peripheral retinal telangiectasis; **(b)** intraretinal exudates; **(c)** subretinal exudation; **(d)** central involvement; **(e)** massive subretinal exudation; **(f)** exudative retinal detachment (Courtesy of C Barry – figs d, e and f)

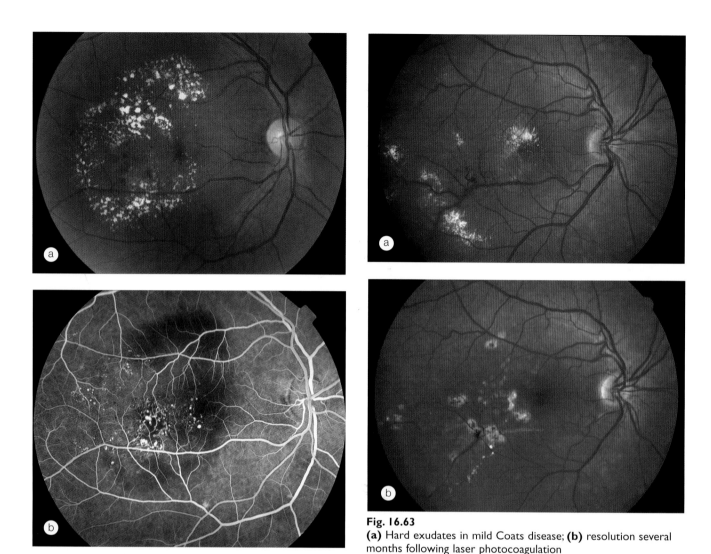

Fig. 16.63
(a) Hard exudates in mild Coats disease; **(b)** resolution several months following laser photocoagulation

Fig. 16.62
(a) Mild Coats disease; **(b)** FA venous phase shows hyperfluorescence of telangiectasis; **(c)** late phase shows staining of the lesions and mild leakage *(Courtesy of Moorfields Eye Hospital)*

required to obliterate the peripheral telangiectasis and induce resolution of remote exudation at the macula (Fig. 16.63). Photocoagulation is most effective in eyes without retinal detachment.

3. **Cryotherapy** with a double freeze-thaw method in eyes with extensive exudation or subtotal retinal detachment, although this may result in marked reaction with increased leakage. Therefore, laser photocoagulation is still the preferred option if at all possible.

4. **Vitreoretinal surgery** may be considered in eyes with total retinal detachments and a poor visual prognosis as successful retinal re-attachment often prevents the subsequent development of neovascular glaucoma.

5. **Enucleation** is frequently required in painful eyes with neovascular glaucoma.

Prognosis

The prognosis is variable and dependent on the severity of involvement at presentation. Young children, particularly those under 3 years of age, frequently have a more aggressive clinical course and often already have extensive retinal detachment at presentation. However, older children and young adults have a more benign disease with less likelihood of progressive exudation and retinal detachment and in some cases spontaneous regression may occur.

Differential diagnosis

Differential diagnosis includes other causes of unilateral leukocoria and retinal detachment in children such as late-onset retinoblastoma, toxocariasis and incontinentia pigmenti.

EALES DISEASE

The eponym 'Eales disease' is used to describe patients with bilateral, idiopathic, occlusive, peripheral periphlebitis and neovascularization. The disease is rare in Caucasians but is an important cause of visual morbidity in young Asian males and is strongly associated with tuberculoprotein hypersensitivity.

1. **Presentation** is usually in the third to fifth decades with vitreous haemorrhage.
2. **Signs**
   - Peripheral vascular sheathing associated with peripheral capillary non-perfusion, particularly superotemporally (Fig. 16.64a).
   - Peripheral neovascularization at the junction of perfused and non-perfused retina (Fig. 16.64b) and recurrent vitreous haemorrhage (16.64c).
3. **Complications** include tractional retinal detachment, rubeosis iridis, glaucoma and cataract.
4. **Treatment** involving either PRP or feeder vessel photocoagulation is useful in active disease. Persistent vitreous haemorrhage or tractional detachment may require vitreoretinal surgery. The visual prognosis is good in the majority of cases.

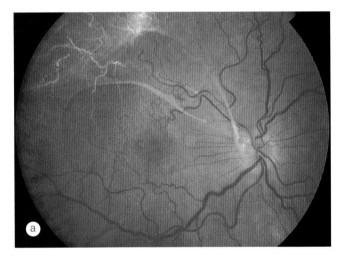

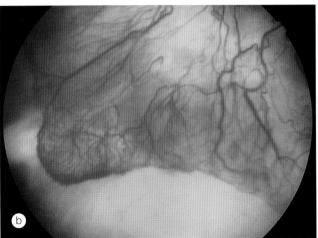

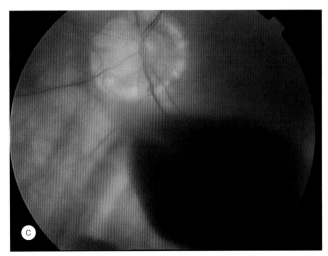

Fig. 16.64
Eales disease. **(a)** Peripheral vascular sheathing and occlusion; **(b)** peripheral neovascularization; **(c)** haemorrhage from new vessels

RADIATION RETINOPATHY

Radiation retinopathy may develop following radiotherapy of intraocular tumours or irradiation of sinus, orbital or nasopharyngeal malignancies. It is characterized by delayed retinal microvascular changes with endothelial cell loss, capillary occlusion and microaneurysm formation. As with diabetic retinopathy its progress may be accelerated by pregnancy.

1. **Presentation.** The time interval between exposure and disease is variable and unpredictable, although commonly between 6 months and 3 years.

2. **Signs**
   - Discrete capillary occlusion with the development of collateral channels and microaneurysms, best seen on FA (Fig. 16.65a and b).
   - Macular oedema, hard exudates (Fig. 16.65c and d).
   - Cotton-wool spots, papillopathy and proliferative retinopathy.
3. **Treatment** by laser photocoagulation may be beneficial for proliferative retinopathy. Papillopathy may benefit from systemic steroids and macular oedema from intravitreal injection of triamcinolone.
4. **Prognosis** depends on the severity of involvement. Poor prognostic features include papillopathy and proliferative retinopathy, which may result in vitreous haemorrhage and tractional retinal detachment.

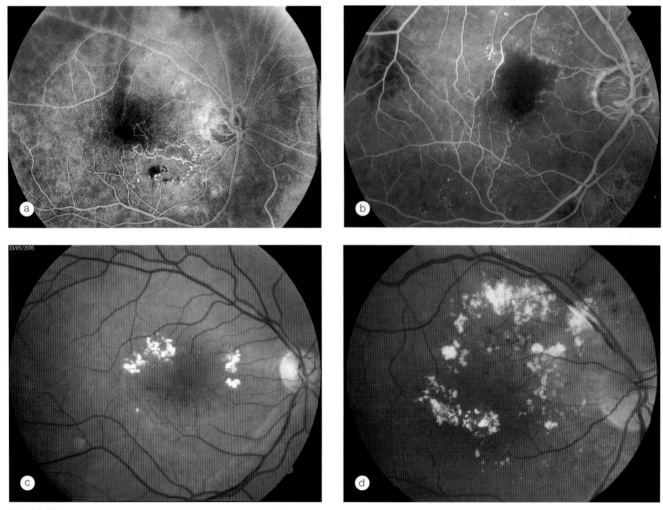

Fig. 16.65
Radiation retinopathy. **(a)** FA focal retinal capillary non-perfusion associated with microvascular abnormalities; **(b)** more severe retinal capillary non-perfusion; **(c)** microvascular abnormalities and hard exudates; **(d)** more severe involvement (Courtesy of S Milenkovic – fig. c)

PURTSCHER RETINOPATHY

Purtscher retinopathy is caused by microvascular damage with occlusion and ischaemia associated with severe trauma, especially to the head, and chest compressive injury. Other causes include embolism (fat, air or amniotic fluid) and systemic diseases (acute pancreatitis, pancreatic carcinoma, connective tissue diseases, lymphomas, thrombotic thrombocytopenic purpura and following bone marrow transplantation). Cases not associated with trauma are sometimes referred to as 'Purtscher-like retinopathy'.

1. **Presentation** is with sudden visual loss.
2. **Signs.** Multiple, unilateral or bilateral, superficial, white retinal patches, resembling large cotton-wool spots, often associated with superficial peripapillary haemorrhages (Fig. 16.66).
3. **Treatment** of the underlying cause is desirable but not always possible.
4. **Prognosis** is guarded because although the acute fundus changes usually resolve within a few weeks permanent variable visual impairment occurs in approximately 50% of cases as a result of macular or optic nerve damage.

BENIGN IDIOPATHIC HAEMORRHAGIC RETINOPATHY

Benign idiopathic haemorrhagic retinopathy is rare but important because it has a good prognosis without treatment.

1. **Presentation** is in adult life at any age with acute unilateral visual impairment.
2. **Signs.** Unilateral, multiple, large, intraretinal haemorrhages at the posterior pole and around the optic disc (Fig. 16.67).
3. **Course.** Vision recovers within 4 months.
4. **Differential diagnosis**
   - Terson syndrome, which is typically associated with subarachnoid haemorrhage.
   - Benign retinal vasculitis.
   - Valsalva retinopathy.
   - High altitude retinopathy.

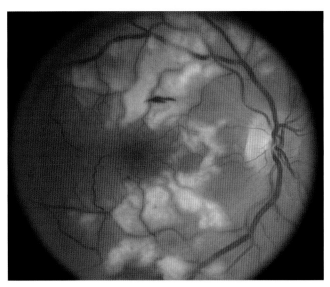

Fig. 16.66
Purtscher retinopathy (Courtesy of L Merin)

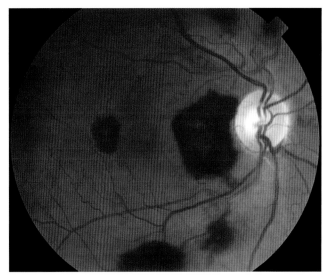

Fig. 16.67
Benign idiopathic haemorrhagic retinopathy

VALSALVA RETINOPATHY

The Valsalva manoeuvre comprises forcible exhalation against a closed glottis, thereby creating a sudden increase in intrathoracic and intra-abdominal pressure (e.g. weight lifting, blowing up balloons). The associated sudden rise in venous pressure may cause rupture of perifoveal capillaries, resulting in unilateral or bilateral premacular haemorrhage (Fig. 16.68). The blood is thought to be located under the internal limiting membrane.

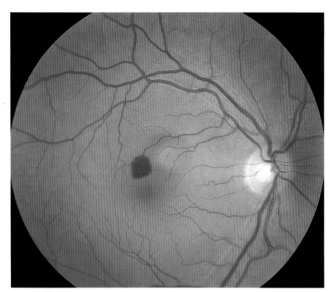

Fig. 16.68
Valsalva retinopathy

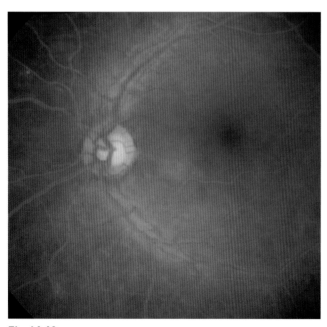

Fig. 16.69
Lipaemia retinalis

LIPAEMIA RETINALIS

Lipaemia retinalis is a rare condition characterized by creamy white coloured retinal blood vessels in patients with hypertriglyceridaemia (Fig. 16.69). The visualization of high levels of chylomicrons in blood vessels accounts for the fundus appearance. Visual acuity is usually normal but electroretinogram amplitude may be decreased.

TAKAYASU DISEASE

Takayasu disease is an extremely rare, chronic, autoimmune, inflammatory obstructive vascular disease affecting the major branches of the aorta and occurs most often in young Asian women. It carries a poor prognosis for life. The diagnosis is usually made by arteriography (Fig. 16.70).

Systemic features

1. **Early phase** is characterized by non-specific constitutional symptoms such as fever, weight loss and night sweats.

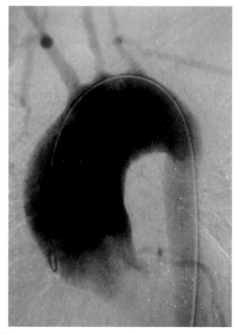

Fig. 16.70
Aortic arch angiogram shows dilatation of the ascending aorta and aortic arch, and stenosis near the origin of the left common carotid artery (Courtesy of L Goldman and D Ausiello, from *Cecil Textbook of Medicine*, Saunders, 2004)

2. **Late phase** is characterized by absence of peripheral pulse, arterial bruits, common carotid artery insufficiency, vertebrobasilar ischaemia, cardiac ischaemia, renal artery involvement with associated systemic hypertension.

Ocular features

1. **Anterior segment** manifestations include corneal oedema, anterior chamber cells and rubeosis iridis, which may result in neovascular glaucoma.
2. **Fundus** findings include arteriolar attenuation, cotton-wool spots, retinal haemorrhages, microaneurysms, arteriovenous malformations, ischaemic optic neuropathy and neovascularization, which may result in vitreous haemorrhage.
3. **Treatment** involves systemic steroids and cytotoxic agents such as methotrexate and azathioprine.

HIGH-ALTITUDE RETINOPATHY

1. **Systemic features** include progressive severe headache, followed by impaired cortical function and judgement, irrationality, projectile vomiting, diplopia, ataxia and coma. Pulmonary oedema may be rapidly life-threatening.
2. **Ocular features** in chronological order:
   - Mild venous dilation and a few small retinal haemorrhages.
   - Severe venous dilatation and multiple large retinal haemorrhages.
   - Venous engorgement, vitreous haemorrhage and disc oedema.

RETINOPATHY IN BLOOD DISORDERS

Leukaemia

The leukaemias are a group of neoplastic disorders characterized by abnormal proliferation of white blood cells (see Chapter 24). Ocular involvement is more commonly seen in the acute than the chronic forms and virtually any ocular structure may be involved. It is, however, important to distinguish the fairly rare primary leukaemic infiltration from the more common secondary changes such as those associated with anaemia, thrombocytopenia, hyperviscosity and opportunistic infections.

1. **Fundus changes**
   - Retinal haemorrhages, cotton-wool spots, which are probably caused by vascular occlusion by leukaemic cells (Fig. 16.71a), and retinal haemorrhages with white centres (Roth spots) composed either of leukaemic cells or platelet-fibrin emboli (Fig. 16.71b).
   - Peripheral retinal neovascularization is an occasional feature of chronic myeloid leukaemia (Fig. 16.71c).
   - Optic nerve infiltration may cause swelling and visual loss (Fig. 16.71d).
   - Choroidal deposits in chronic leukaemia may give rise to a 'leopard skin' appearance (Fig. 16.71e).
2. **Other ocular features**
   - Orbital involvement, particularly in children.
   - Iris thickening, iritis and pseudo-hypopyon (Fig. 16.71f).
   - Spontaneous subconjunctival haemorrhage and hyphaema.

Anaemia

The anaemias are a group of disorders characterized by a decrease in the number of circulating red blood cells, a decrease in the amount of haemoglobin in each cell, or both. Retinal changes in anaemia are usually innocuous and rarely of diagnostic importance.

1. **Retinopathy**
   - Retinal venous tortuosity is related to the severity of anaemia but may occur in isolation, particularly in patients with beta-thalassaemia major (Fig. 16.72a).
   - Dot-blot and flame-shaped haemorrhages, Roth spots and cotton-wool spots are more common with coexisting thrombocytopenia in aplastic anaemia (Fig. 16.72b). The duration and type of anaemia do not influence the occurrence of these changes.
2. **Optic neuropathy** with centrocaecal scotomas may occur in patients with pernicious anaemia. Unless treated with vitamin B_{12} supplements, permanent optic atrophy may ensue. Pernicious anaemia may also cause dementia, peripheral neuropathy and subacute combined degeneration of the spinal cord characterized by posterior and lateral column disease.

Hyperviscosity

The hyperviscosity states are a diverse group of rare disorders characterized by increased blood viscosity due to polycythaemia or abnormal plasma proteins as in Waldenström macroglobulinaemia and myeloma. Retinopathy is characterized by retinal haemorrhages, and venous dilatation, segmentation and tortuosity (Fig. 16.73a). Venous occlusion is uncommon (Fig. 16.73b).

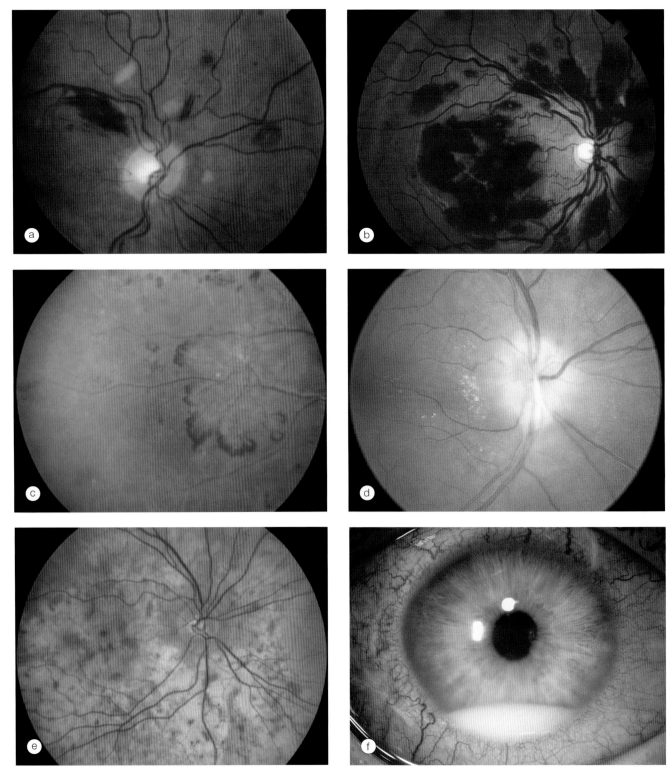

Fig. 16.71
Ocular involvement in leukaemia. **(a)** Retinal haemorrhages, cotton-wool spots and one Roth spot; **(b)** many Roth spots; **(c)** peripheral retinal neovascularization; **(d)** optic nerve infiltration; **(e)** 'leopard-skin' appearance due to choroidal infiltration; **(f)** pseudo-hypopyon
(Courtesy of C Barry – figs a and b; P Morse – fig. c)

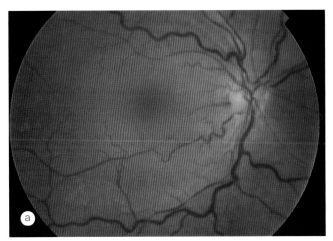
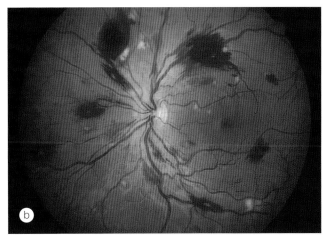

Fig. 16.72
Retinopathy in anaemia. **(a)** Venous tortuosity; **(b)** haemorrhages, cotton-wool spots and Roth spots in aplastic anaemia (Courtesy of P Saine – fig. b)

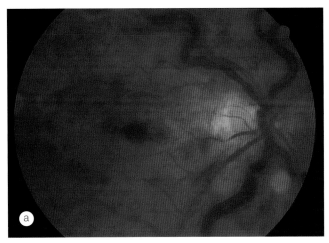
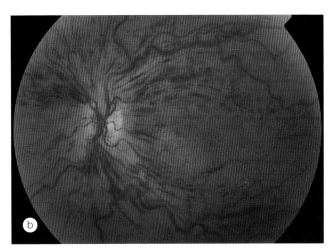

Fig. 16.73
Retinopathy in hyperviscosity. **(a)** Retinal haemorrhages and gross venous dilatation; **(b)** central retinal vein occlusion

CHAPTER 17

ACQUIRED MACULAR DISORDERS AND RELATED CONDITIONS

INTRODUCTION

Anatomy

1. **The macula** is a round area at the posterior pole measuring approximately 5.5mm in diameter (Figs 17.1 and 17.2). Histologically, it contains xanthophyll pigment and more than one layer of ganglion cells.
2. **The fovea** is a depression in the inner retinal surface at the centre of the macula with a diameter of 1.5mm (about 1 optic disc). Ophthalmoscopically it gives rise to an oval light reflex because of the increased thickness of the retina and internal limiting membrane at its border.
3. **The foveola** forms the central floor of the fovea and has a diameter of 0.35mm. It is the thinnest part of the retina,

is devoid of ganglion cells and consists only of cones and their nuclei.
4. **The foveal avascular zone** (FAZ) is located within the fovea but extends beyond the foveola. The exact diameter is variable and its limits can be determined with accuracy only by fluorescein angiography (FA).
5. **The umbo** is a tiny depression in the very centre of the foveola which corresponds to the foveolar reflex, loss of which may be an early sign of damage.

Retinal pigment epithelium

The retinal pigment epithelium (RPE) is a single layer of hexagonal cells, the apices of which manifest villous processes that envelop the outer segments of the photo-receptors. The RPE cells at the fovea are taller and contain

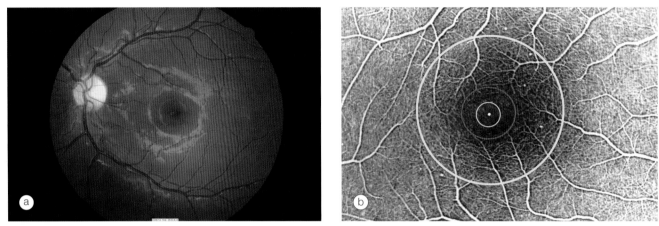

Fig. 17.1
Anatomical landmarks. **(a)** Normal foveal light reflex; **(b)** fovea (yellow circle); foveal avascular zone (red circle); foveola (lilac circle); umbo (central white spot) (Courtesy of L Merin – fig. a)

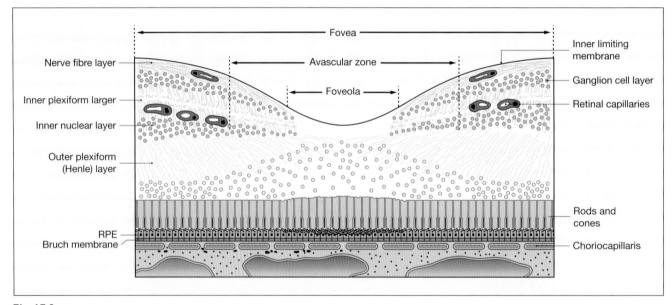

Fig. 17.2
Cross-section of the fovea

more and larger melanosomes than elsewhere in the retina. The adhesion between the RPE and sensory retina is weaker than between the RPE and Bruch membrane, which underlies the RPE. The potential space between the RPE and sensory retina is the subretinal space. The RPE prevents the accumulation of subretinal fluid in two ways:
• The RPE cells and the intervening tight junctional complexes (zonula occludens) constitute the outer blood–retinal barrier, preventing extracellular fluid, which normally leaks from the choriocapillaris, from entering the subretinal space.

• It also actively pumps ions and water out of the subretinal space.

Bruch membrane

Bruch membrane separates the RPE from the choriocapillaris. On electron microscopy it consists of five elements:
• Basal lamina of the RPE.
• Inner collagenous layer.
• Thicker band of elastic fibres.

- Outer collagenous layer.
- Basal lamina of the inner layer of the choriocapillaris.

NB Changes in Bruch membrane are relevant to the pathogenesis of many macular disorders.

Symptoms

1. **Impairment of central vision** is the main symptom. Patients with macular disease complain of 'something obstructing central vision' (positive scotoma) in contrast to those with optic neuropathy, who may notice 'something missing' or a 'hole in their central vision' (negative scotoma).
2. **Metamorphopsia** or distortion of perceived images is a common symptom of macular disease not present in optic neuropathy.
3. **Micropsia,** a decrease in image size caused by spreading apart of foveal cones, is less common.
4. **Macropsia,** an increase in image size due to crowding together of foveal cones, is uncommon.

NB Colour desaturation is not present in early macular disease, but is common in optic neuropathy, even if mild.

AGE-RELATED MACULAR DEGENERATION

Introduction

Definition

1. **Age-related maculopathy** (ARM) is an exaggeration of the 'normal' ageing process characterized by:
   - Discrete yellow spots at the macula (drusen).
   - Hyperpigmentation or depigmentation of the RPE associated with drusen.
2. **Age-related macular degeneration** (AMD) is a more advanced, sight-threatening stage of ARM characterized by one or more of the following:
   - Geographic atrophy of the RPE with visible underlying choroidal vessels.
   - Pigment epithelial detachment (PED) with or without neurosensory detachment.
   - Subretinal or sub-RPE choroidal neovascularization (CNV).
   - Fibroglial scar tissue, haemorrhage and exudates.

Prevalence

AMD is the most common cause of irreversible visual loss in the developed world in individuals over 50 years of age. The prevalence of severe visual loss increases with age. In the USA, at least 10% of individuals between the ages of 65 and 75 years have some impairment of central vision as a result of AMD. Among those over 75, 30% are affected to some degree. End stage (blinding) AMD occurs in about 1.7% of all individuals aged over 50 years and in about 18% over 85 years.

Risk factors

1. **Age** is the main risk factor.
2. **ARM,** particularly when associated with soft drusen (see below).
3. **Race** – the condition is most prevalent in Caucasians.
4. **Positive family history.**
5. **Cataract,** particularly nuclear opacity, is a risk factor for AMD. Cataract surgery may be associated with progression of macular disease in some patients with pre-existing high risk characteristics such as confluent soft drusen. It is, however, difficult to prove a link between surgery and progression of AMD since advanced disease often coexists in patients with cataracts sufficiently advanced to require surgery.
6. **Biomarkers for cardiovascular disease,** namely, smoking, obesity and hypertension. The significance of elevated C-reactive protein, homocysteine and fibrinogen levels is controversial.

Drusen

Histopathology

Loss of central vision in AMD is the result of changes that occur in response to deposition of abnormal material in Bruch membrane. This material is derived from the RPE, and its accumulation is thought to result from failure to clear the debris discharged into this region. Drusen consist of discrete deposits of the abnormal material located between the basal lamina of the RPE and the inner collagenous layer of Bruch membrane (Fig. 17.3). Thickening of Bruch membrane is compounded by excessive production of basement membrane deposit by the RPE. It has been postulated that the lipid content of drusen may be a determinant for subsequent behaviour.

Diagnosis

Drusen appear as yellow excrescences beneath the RPE, distributed symmetrically at both posterior poles. They may vary in number, size, shape, degree of elevation and extent of associated RPE changes. In some patients, drusen may be confined to the region of the fovea, whereas in others the deposits encircle but spare the fovea itself. Drusen are rarely clinically visible before the age of 45 years; they are not uncommon between the ages of 45 and 60 years and almost universal thereafter. With advancing age they increase in size and number.

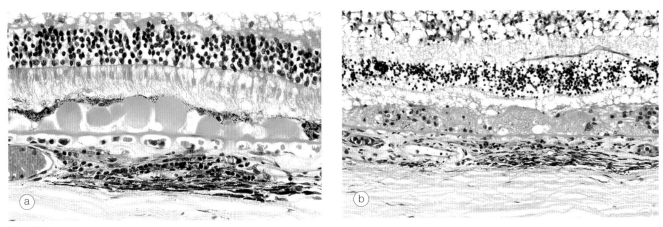

Fig. 17.3
Histology of drusen. **(a)** Hard drusen are discrete homogeneous eosinophilic nodular deposits lying between the RPE and the inner collagenous layer of Bruch membrane; **(b)** soft drusen are non-homogeneous, eosinophilic deposits with ill-defined margins
(Courtesy of J Harry)

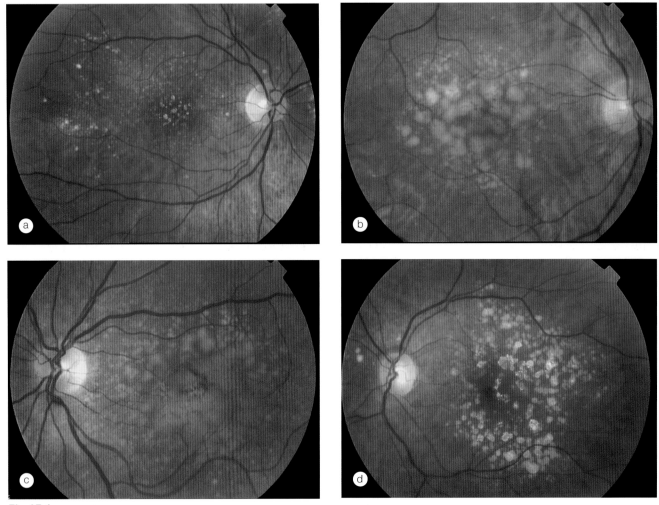

Fig. 17.4
Drusen. **(a)** Hard; **(b)** soft; **(c)** coalescence of soft drusen; **(d)** calcified

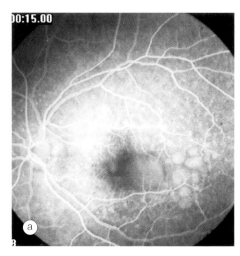
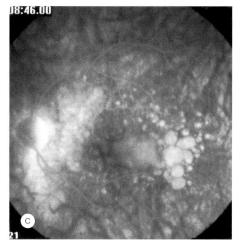

Fig. 17.5
FA of soft drusen. (**a** and **b**) Early hyperfluorescence due to a window defect; (**c** and **d**) late hyperfluorescence due to staining

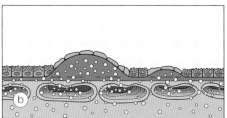
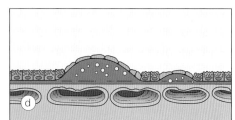

1. **Small hard drusen** are usually innocuous, round, discrete and less than half a vein width in diameter (Fig. 17.4a).
2. **Large soft drusen** have indistinct margins and are a vein width or more in diameter (Fig. 17.4b).
3. **Drusenoid RPE detachment** is caused by coalescence of large areas of soft drusen (Fig. 17.4c). It is a common precursor of AMD.
4. **Calcified drusen** have a glistening appearance and represent dystrophic calcification in hard or soft drusen (Fig. 17.4d).
5. **FA** findings depend on the state of the overlying RPE and the amount of staining.
   a. Hyperfluorescence is caused by both a window defect due to atrophy of the overlying RPE (Fig. 17.5a and b) and by late staining (Fig. 17.5c and d). The centre of the macula also shows a 'drusenoid' detachment of the RPE. It has been postulated that hyperfluorescent drusen are hydrophilic (low lipid content) and predispose to CNV.
   b. Hypofluorescent drusen are hydrophobic (high lipid content) and, if large and confluent, predispose to subsequent detachment of the RPE. A prolonged filling phase of the choroid may indicate diffuse thickening of Bruch membrane.

Differential diagnosis

1. **Familial dominant drusen** (Doyne honeycomb dystrophy) is an uncommon condition in which drusen appear during the second and third decades (see Chapter 18).

2. **Hard exudates** in diabetic retinopathy may, on cursory examination, be confused with drusen. However, unlike drusen they are arranged in rings or clumps and are associated with vascular changes such as micro-aneurysms and haemorrhages.
3. **Type 2 membranoproliferative glomerulonephritis,** also known as dense deposit disease, is a chronic disease that occurs in older children and adults. A minority of patients develop bilateral, symmetrical, diffuse yellow, drusen-like lesions scattered throughout the fundus.
4. **Other causes of retinal flecks**
   - Stargardt disease and fundus flavimaculatus.
   - Benign flecked retina.
   - North Carolina macular dystrophy.
   - Alport syndrome.

   NB In all of these, the fundus lesions develop at a much earlier age than drusen.

Drusen and age-related macular degeneration

Although many patients with drusen maintain normal vision throughout life, a significant number of elderly patients develop AMD. The exact role of drusen in the pathogenesis of AMD is still unclear, although their chemical composition may be relevant. Features associated with an increased risk of subsequent visual loss include large soft and/or confluent drusen, and focal hyperpigmentation of the RPE, particularly if the other eye has already developed AMD.

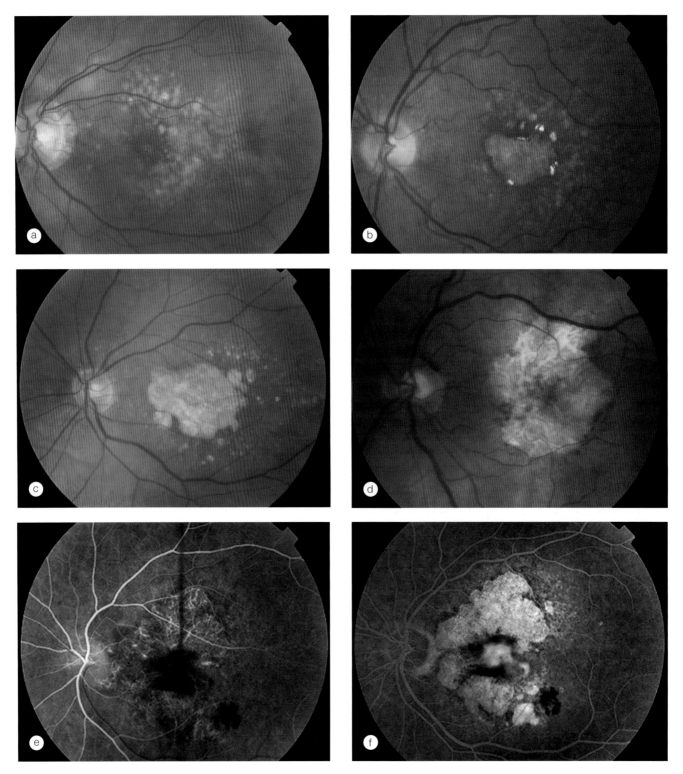

Fig. 17.6
Atrophic age-related macular degeneration. **(a)** Drusen and mild RPE changes; **(b)** drusen and atrophy; **(c)** drusen and geographic atrophy; **(d)** geographic atrophy and disappearance of drusen; **(e)** FA arteriovenous phase shows slight hyperfluorescence; **(f)** FA late phase shows intense hyperfluorescence due to a window defect

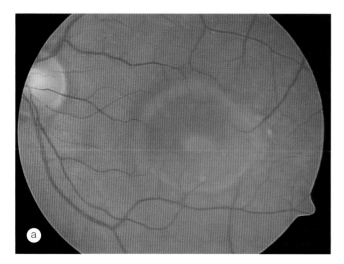

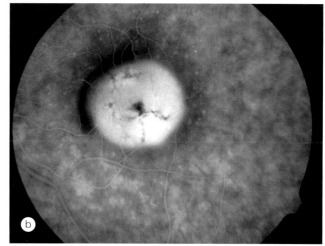

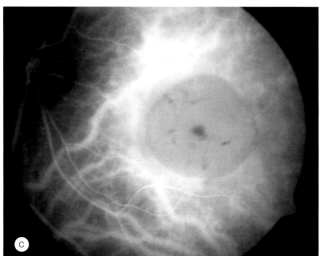

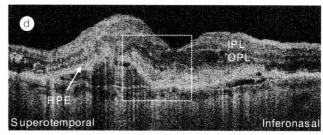

Fig. 17.7
Detachment of the RPE. **(a)** Clinical appearance; **(b)** FA shows hyperfluorescence; **(c)** ICG shows hypofluorescence with a faint ring of surrounding hyperfluorescence; **(d)** ultrahigh resolution OCT shows separation of the RPE (white arrow) from Bruch membrane (red arrow), and loss of architecture of the photoreceptors (Courtesy of P Gili – figs a, b and c; J Fujimoto – fig. d)

Prophylactic treatment

There is now substantial evidence, particularly from the AREDS study, that use of high dose multivitamins and antioxidants on a regular basis can decrease the risk of progression of ARM in those with high risk characteristics. These high risk features include visual loss in the contralateral eye from pre-existing AMD, and confluent soft drusen even in the absence of visual loss. Supplements did not provide benefit for those with early AMD. Previous studies have suggested that people who have diets rich in green, leafy vegetables have a lower risk for developing AMD. However, the high levels of dietary supplements that were evaluated in this study are difficult to achieve from diet alone. The decreased risk of progression to further visual loss at 5 years is in the order of 25% and most retinal specialists now feel these preparations have a significant benefit. The exact compounds used in the AREDS study were:

- 500mg of vitamin C
- 400IU of vitamin E
- 15mg of beta carotene
- 80mg of zinc as zinc oxide and 2mg of copper as cupric acid to prevent potential anaemia.

There is also some evidence that use of lutein may also be of benefit and many of the compounds available commercially now contain lutein. The study also found high zinc levels were associated with non-specific genitourinary tract problems. Overall the preparations seem very safe although it should be noted that taking beta-carotene is not suitable for a person who smokes due to a possible increase in the risk of lung cancer.

Atrophic age-related macular degeneration

Atrophic (dry) AMD is caused by slowly progressive atrophy of the photoreceptors, RPE and choriocapillaris, although occasionally it may follow subsidence of an RPE detachment (see later).

1. **Presentation** is with a gradual impairment of vision over months or years. Both eyes are usually affected but often asymmetrically.
2. **Signs** in chronological order:
   - Focal hyperpigmentation or atrophy of the RPE in association with macular drusen (Fig. 17.6a).
   - Sharply circumscribed, circular areas of RPE atrophy associated with variable loss of the choriocapillaris (Fig. 17.6b and c).
   - Enlargement of the atrophic areas within which the larger choroidal vessels may become visible and pre-existing drusen disappear (geographic atrophy) (Fig. 17.6d). Visual acuity is severely impaired if the fovea is involved.
3. **FA** shows a window defect characterized by hyper-fluorescence due to unmasking of background choroidal fluorescence (Fig. 17.6e and f) which may be more extensive than that apparent clinically, if the underlying choriocapillaris is still intact.
4. **Treatment** is not possible although low vision aids may be useful in many patients.

Retinal pigment epithelial detachment

PED is thought to be caused by reduction of hydraulic conductivity of the thickened Bruch membrane, thus impeding movement of fluid from the RPE towards the choroid.

Diagnosis

1. **Presentation** is with unilateral metamorphopsia and impairment of central vision.
2. **Signs**
   - Sharply circumscribed, dome-shaped elevation of varying size at the posterior pole (Fig. 17.7a).
   - The sub-RPE fluid is usually clear but may be turbid.
3. **FA** shows a well demarcated oval area of hyper-fluorescence which increases in density but not in area due to pooling of dye under the detachment (Fig. 17.7b).
4. **Indocyanine green angiography (ICG)** demonstrates an oval area of hypofluorescence with a faint ring of surrounding hyperfluorescence (Fig. 17.7c). Occult CNV is detected in 96% of cases.
5. **Optical coherence tomography (OCT)** shows separation of the RPE from Bruch membrane by fluid (Fig. 17.7d).

NB Laser photocoagulation should not be performed for PED as it may result in visual loss secondary to an RPE tear or sudden collapse of the PED with associated RPE atrophy.

Course

The course is variable and may follow one of the patterns below:

1. **Spontaneous resolution** without residua, particularly in younger patients.
2. **Geographic atrophy** may develop following spontaneous resolution in a minority of patients.
3. **Detachment of the sensory retina** may occur due to breakdown of the outer blood–retinal barrier, allowing passage of fluid into the subretinal space. Because of the relatively loose adhesion between the RPE and sensory retina, the subretinal fluid spreads more widely and is less well defined than in a pure PED.
4. **RPE tear formation** (see below).

Retinal pigment epithelial tear

A tear of the RPE may occur at the junction of attached and detached RPE if tangential stress becomes sufficient to rupture the detached tissue. Tears may occur spontaneously or, more commonly, following laser photocoagulation of CNV in eyes with PED.

1. **Presentation** is with sudden worsening of central vision.
2. **Signs.** Crescent shaped RPE dehiscence with a retracted and folded flap (Fig. 17.8a).
3. **FA** may show CNV during the early phase (Fig. 17.8b). The late phase shows relative hypofluorescence over the flap due to the folded over and thickened RPE, with adjacent hyperfluorescence due to the exposed choriocapillaris (Fig. 17.8c).
4. **ICG** shows a linear area of hypofluorescence with a hyperfluorescent outline.
5. **OCT** shows loss of the normal dome-shaped profile of the RPE in the PED, with hyper-reflectivity adjacent to the folded RPE (Fig. 17.8d).
6. **Prognosis** of subfoveal tears is poor. PEDs progressing to tears have an especially poor prog-nosis and are at particular risk of developing visual loss in the fellow eye. A minority of eyes maintain good visual acuity despite RPE tears, if the fovea is spared.

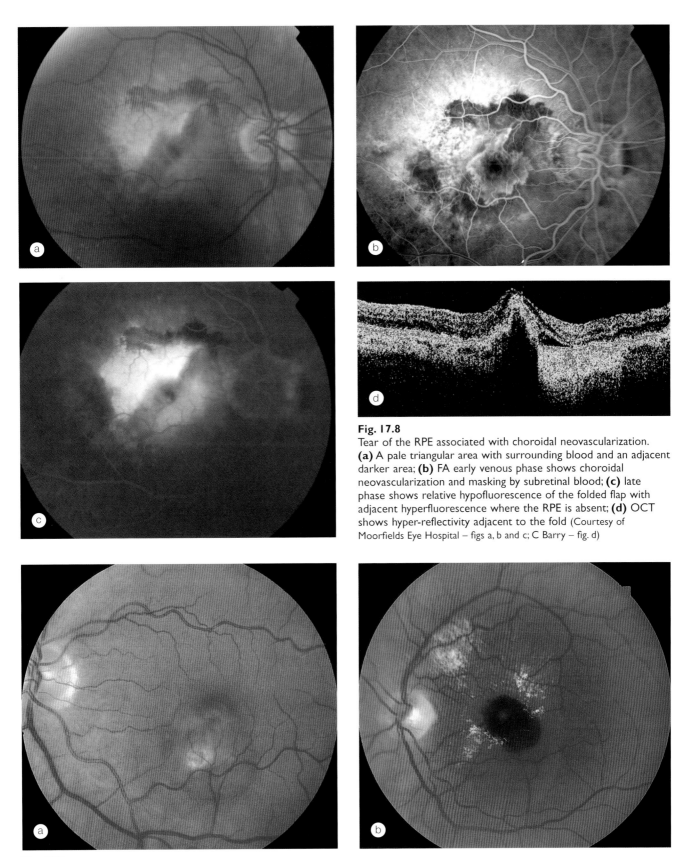

Fig. 17.8
Tear of the RPE associated with choroidal neovascularization.
(a) A pale triangular area with surrounding blood and an adjacent darker area; **(b)** FA early venous phase shows choroidal neovascularization and masking by subretinal blood; **(c)** late phase shows relative hypofluorescence of the folded flap with adjacent hyperfluorescence where the RPE is absent; **(d)** OCT shows hyper-reflectivity adjacent to the fold (Courtesy of Moorfields Eye Hospital – figs a, b and c; C Barry – fig. d)

Fig. 17.9
Choroidal neovascularization. **(a)** Below the fovea; **(b)** haemorrhage and hard exudates

Neovascular age-related macular degeneration

Pathogenesis

Neovascular (wet) AMD is caused by CNV originating from the choriocapillaris which grows through defects in Bruch membrane. This is thought to be the result of imbalance between VEGF, that stimulates vascular growth, and pigment epithelium-derived factor (PEDF), that suppresses growth. There are three basic growth patterns: sub-RPE (type 1), subretinal (type 2) and a combination of both. Type 1 is the most common in AMD, whereas type 2 is less common in AMD but tends to occur in younger individuals with myopia or chorioretinitis. Initial visual loss associated with CNV is caused by leakage of blood and serum under the retina (subretinal fluid), into the retina (macular oedema) and under the RPE (PED). This type of visual loss from fluid accumulation is potentially reversible. Eventually, persistent fluid accumulation results in loss of photo-receptors and RPE, the formation of a disciform scar and permanent visual loss.

Clinical features

1. **Presentation** is with metamorphopsia, a positive scotoma and blurring of central vision due to leakage of fluid from the CNV.
2. **Signs.** Most membranes can be identified ophthal-moscopically but occasionally they can only be seen on FA.
   - Sub-RPE (type 1) CNV appears as a grey-green or pinkish-yellow, slightly elevated lesion (Fig. 17.9a).
   - Subretinal (type 2) CNV may form a subretinal halo or pigmented plaque.
   - The most frequent signs are caused by leakage from CNV resulting in serous retinal elevation, foveal thickening, CMO, subretinal haemorrhage and hard exudates (Fig. 17.9b).

Fluorescein angiography

FA is important for the detection and precise localization of CNV in relation to the centre of the FAZ and should be performed urgently in patients with recent onset of symptoms.

1. **Classic CNV** is a well-defined membrane which fills with dye in a 'lacy' pattern during the very early phase of transit (Fig. 17.10b), fluoresces brightly during peak dye transit (Fig. 17.10c), and then leaks into the subretinal space and around the CNV within 1–2min. The fibrous tissue within the CNV then stains (Fig. 17.10d). Classic CNV is classified according to its relation to the centre of FAZ as follows:

   a. **Extrafoveal** in which the CNV is more than 200μm from the centre of the FAZ.
   b. **Juxtafoveal** in which the CNV is closer than 200μm from the centre of the FAZ but does not involve it (Fig. 17.10).
   c. **Subfoveal** in which the centre of the FAZ is involved (Fig. 17.11a–d).

   The CNV can be further subdivided into wholly classic and predominantly classic, in which 50% or more of the lesion has a classic component.

2. **Occult CNV** is poorly defined with less precise features on the early frames but gives rise to late, diffuse or multifocal leakage (Fig. 17.11e and f).
3. **Fibrovascular PED** is a combination of CNV and PED. The CNV fluoresces brighter (hot spot) than the detach-ment. In other cases, the CNV may be obscured by blood or turbid fluid.

   NB Most angiographic lesions are subfoveal and occult; about 20% of subfoveal lesions are predominantly classic; approximately half of juxtafoveal and extrafoveal lesions are predominantly classic.

Indocyanine green angiography

ICG may be superior to FA under certain circumstances. The longer, near-infrared wavelengths can penetrate the RPE and choroid, and are less absorbed by haemoglobin. These properties allow greater transmission of ICG fluorescence than that of fluorescein and are of particular value in the following circumstances:
- Occult or poorly defined CNV.
- CNV associated with overlying haemorrhage, fluid or exudate (Fig. 17.12a–c).
- Distinguishing serous from vascularized portions of a fibrovascular PED (Fig. 17.12d–f).

Course

The course of untreated CNV is often relentless and the prognosis very poor due to the following complications:

1. **Haemorrhagic PED** caused by rupture of blood vessels within the CNV. Initially, the blood is confined to the sub-RPE space and appears as a dark elevated mound. The haemorrhage may then break into the subretinal space and assumes a more diffuse outline and a lighter red colour, which may surround or be adjacent to the PED (Fig. 17.13a).
2. **Vitreous haemorrhage** may rarely occur when blood under a sensory haemorrhagic detachment breaks through into the vitreous cavity.

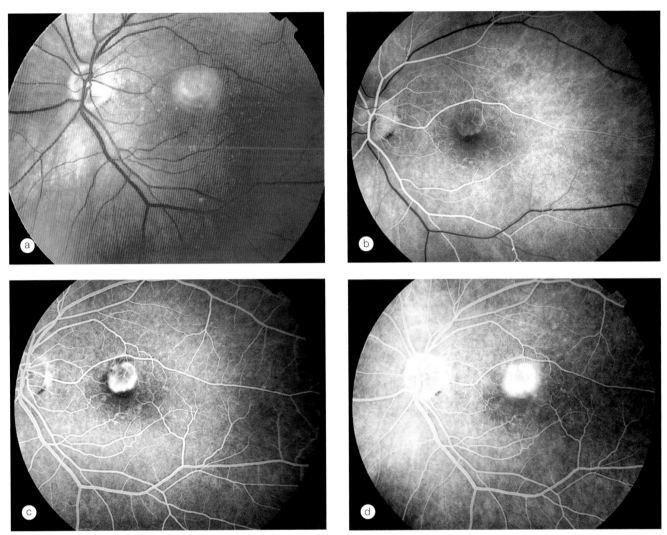

Fig. 17.10
Classic juxtafoveal choroidal neovascularization. **(a)** Small yellow elevation just above the fovea; **(b)** FA arterial phase shows 'lacy' hyperfluorescence; **(c)** venous phase shows more intense hyperfluorescence; **(d)** late phase shows persistent hyperfluorescence

3. **Subretinal (disciform) scarring** follows the haemorrhagic episode in which there is gradual organization of the blood, and further in-growth of new vessels from the choroid. Eventually, a fibrous disciform scar at the fovea causes permanent loss of central vision (Fig. 17.13b).
4. **Massive exudation** may develop in some eyes with disciform scars as a result of chronic leakage from the CNV (Fig. 17.13c). If severe, subretinal fluid may spread beyond the macula and destroy peripheral vision (Fig. 17.13d).

Photodynamic therapy

1. **Principles.** Verteporfin is a light-activated compound that is preferentially taken up by dividing cells, in this instance neovascular tissue. It is injected intravenously and is then activated locally by illumination with light from a diode laser source at a wavelength (689nm) that corresponds to an absorption peak of the compound. The main advantage of photodynamic therapy (PDT) is the ability to selectively damage tissue, attributable to both preferential localization of the photosensitizer to the CNV and irradiation confined to the target tissue. The CNV is irradiated with energy levels far lower than those required for thermal destruction by argon laser therapy, enabling treatment of subfoveal CNV with relative sparing of healthy tissue (Fig. 17.14 and 17.15).
2. **Definite indications** are subfoveal, predominantly classic CNV (area of classic CNV $\geq 50\%$ of the area of the entire lesion), not larger than 5400μm in eyes with a visual acuity of 6/60 or better. The results are encouraging in this group, with stability of visual acuity in 60% of cases over 3 years and sometimes even improvement.

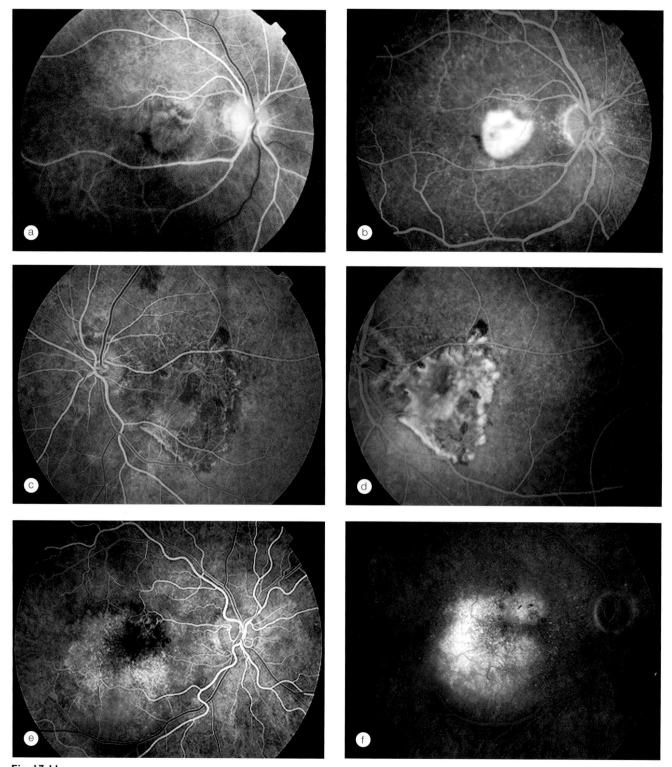

Fig. 17.11
FA of choroidal neovascularization. (**a** and **b**) Classic subfoveal; (**c** and **d**) very large subfoveal; (**e** and **f**) occult

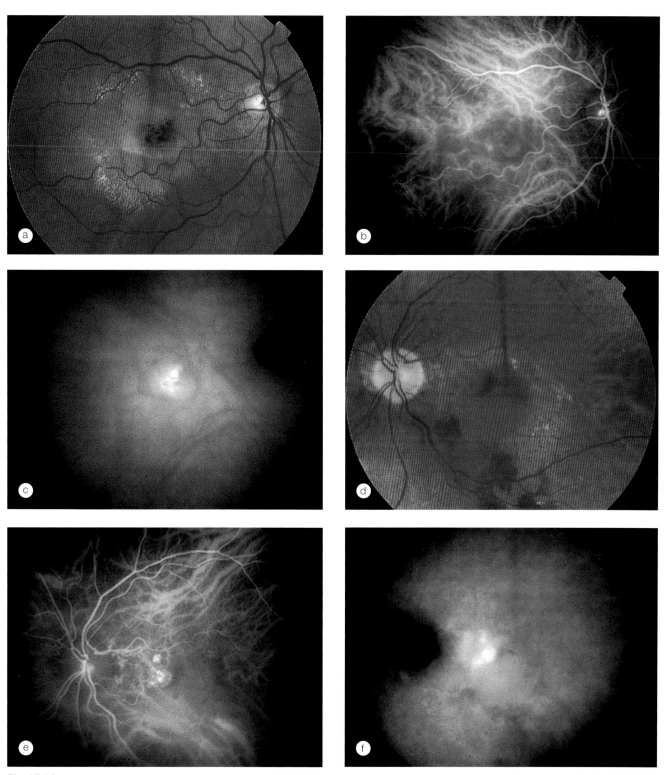

Fig. 17.12
Choroidal neovascularization. **(a)** Blood and fluid at the macula surrounded by hard exudates; **(b and c)** ICG shows a small area of increasing hyperfluorescence (hot spot) from underlying CNV; **(d)** PED with blood inferiorly; **(e and f)** ICG shows hypofluorescence of PED and two small areas of increasing hyperfluorescence (hot spots) from underlying CNV

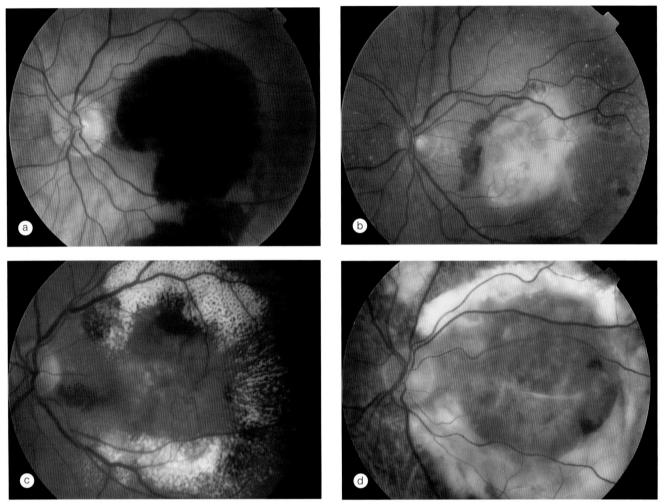

Fig. 17.13
Progression of exudative age-related macular degeneration. **(a)** Bleeding under the RPE and sensory retina; **(b)** subretinal (disciform) scarring; **(c)** subretinal exudation; **(d)** exudative retinal detachment

3. Probable indications
- Small, pure occult lesions associated with recent documented decrease in visual acuity.
- Lesions > 5400μm, juxtapapillary CNV with subfoveal extension.

4. Possible indications
- Larger occult lesions with definite decrease in visual acuity
- Mixed lesions < 50% classic if carried out with adjunctive treatment such as intravitreal triamcinolone. There is increasing evidence to suggest that all lesions may have a better outcome if PDT is preceded by intravitreal triamcinolone.

5. Contraindications are PEDs and lesions with < 50% classic CNV.

6. Technique
a. Verteporfin (6mg/kg body weight) is infused intravenously over 10 minutes.
b. Five minutes following infusion, non-thermal laser is applied to the CNV for 83 seconds. The treatment spot is 1000μm larger than the greatest linear dimension of the lesion to ensure complete closure.
c. Re-treatment is applied to areas of persistent or new leakage at 3-monthly intervals until the entire CNV is obliterated.

7. Side-effects include transient lower backache during infusion, transient decrease in vision, injection site reaction, and sensitivity to bright light for 24–48 hours.

Anti-angiogenic therapy

1. **Intravitreal steroids** (triamcinolone acetonide) may be used alone or as an adjuct to PDT. In the short term monotherapy may improve retinal thickness and decrease vascular exudation, and, in some cases, improve visual acuity, but the benefits are transient. The use of multiple steroid injections or sustained-release implants is

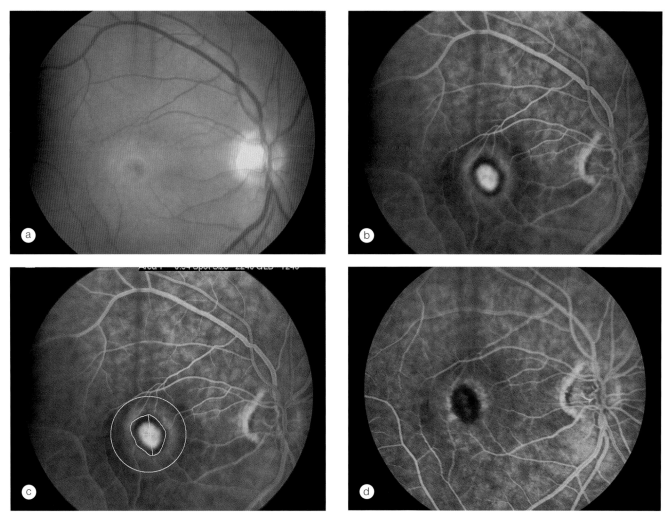

Fig. 17.14
Photodynamic therapy. **(a)** Small dirty grey lesion at the fovea surrounded by of blood; **(b)** FA venous phase shows hyperfluorescence from classic subfoveal CNV surrounded by a hypofluorescent ring; **(c)** measurement of greatest linear dimension of the lesion; **(d)** FA 3 months following successful treatment shows hypofluorescence of the lesion (Courtesy of S Milewski)

associated with a high rate of complications such as ocular hypertension and cataract but may still allow retention of better visual acuity than PDT alone.

2. **Anti-vascular endothelium growth factor (anti-VEGF) agents** such as intravitreal bevacizumab (Avastin), ranibizumab (Lucentis) and pegaptanib (Macugen) are increasingly being used to treat any type of CNV.

Surgery

1. **Submacular** surgery involves vitrectomy, posterior retinotomy and removal of the subfoveal CNV (Fig. 17.16). The procedure carries a high rate of recurrence and causes a large central scotoma because it is impossible to remove a type 1 CNV without also removing the overlying RPE. Therefore, CNV removal is not normally carried out

for patients with AMD, although results are more encouraging in younger patients with type 2 CNV in which the CNV lies anterior to the RPE.

2. **Macular translocation** is aimed at surgically moving the fovea away from the CNV. Indications and techniques are still evolving and surgery is complex requiring cataract extraction, vitrectomy, induction of retinal detachment, 360° retinotomy, removal of CNV, retinal rotation, retinopexy and silicone oil fill in conjunction with extraocular muscle surgery to correct torsion. There is a high risk of PVR and retinal detachment. With newer treatments the initial surge of enthusiasm for macular rotation surgery has declined a little, although some groups report restoration of reading acuity in a significant number of cases.

3. **Pneumatic displacement** of submacular haemorrhage involves injection of gas into the vitreous cavity followed

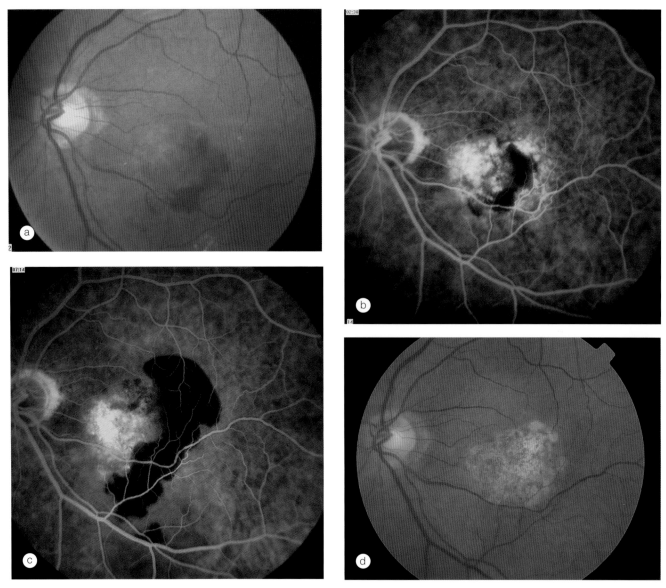

Fig. 17.15
Repeated photodynamic therapy. **(a)** Macular oedema and haemorrhage at the macula; **(b)** FA shows hyperfluorescence from mainly classic CNV and blockage by blood; **(c)** FA 4 months following treatment shows a large area of hypofluorescence due to subretinal haemorrhage with nasal hyperfluorescence from persistent CNV; **(d)** 1 year following further treatment the macula is dry and exhibits mild RPE changes (Courtesy of S Milewski)

by face-down posturing in order to displace the blood from the fovea. The procedure may also be combined with insertion of a fibrinolytic agent called tissue plasminogen activator (tPA) to aid displacement of the blood, although there is some doubt as to whether the tPA molecule is small enough to cross the blood–retinal barrier. The displacement of subretinal blood allows more accurate FA and possible PDT later.

Retinal angiomatous proliferation

Retinal angiomatous proliferation (RAP) is an uncommon cause of exudative AMD in which the neovascular process originates from the retinal vasculature as opposed to the choriocapillaris. The disease is frequently bilateral and symmetrical.

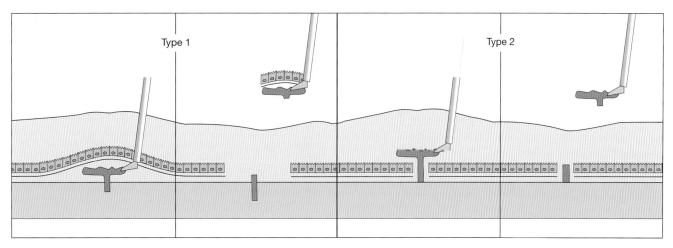

Fig. 17.16
Principles of submacular surgery (see text)

1. **Presentation** is similar to that of AMD.
2. **Signs**
   - Intraretinal neovascularization, similar to IRMA in diabetic retinopathy, that originates from the deep paramacular capillary plexus and is often accompanied by intraretinal haemorrhage and oedema (Fig. 17.17a).
   - Subretinal neovascularization beyond the photoreceptor layer into the subretinal space associated with increasing oedema, intraretinal and preretinal haemorrhage, and serous PED.
   - CNV associated with fibrovascular PED and retinochoroidal anastomoses.
3. **FA** is similar to purely occult or minimally classic CNV (Fig. 17.17b).
4. **ICG** shows a hot spot in mid or late frames (Fig. 17.17c).
5. **Treatment** with conventional laser photocoagulation is often disappointing, although PDT with adjunctive intravitreal injection of triamcinolone may be successful. Surgical section of the feeder artery and draining vein is a recently described experimental option.

POLYPOIDAL CHOROIDAL VASCULOPATHY

Polypoidal choroidal vasculopathy (PCV) is a relatively uncommon, idiopathic choroidal vascular disease in which the inner choroidal vessels consist of a dilated network and multiple terminal aneurysmal protrubences in a polypoidal configuration.

Diagnosis

1. **Presentation** is in old age with unilateral visual impairment.
2. **Signs** are often bilateral but asymmetrical in severity. Most frequently the lesions occur at the macula; 20% are peripapillary and 15% extramacular. Classically there is lack of significant drusen. Asymptomatic aneurysmal lesions or polyps appear as reddish-orange nodules beneath the RPE. Symptomatic disease has two patterns:
   a. Exudative is characterized by insidious visual impairment due to multiple, serous PED, serous retinal detachment and lipid deposits in the macula.
   b. Haemorrhagic may cause sudden visual loss due to haemorrhagic PED and subretinal haemorrhage in the macula (Fig. 17.18a).
3. **ICG** is required to make a definitive diagnosis. This shows a branching vascular network from the choroidal circulation and polypoidal and aneurysmal dilatations at the terminals of the branching vessels beneath the RPE that fill slowly and then leak intensely (Fig. 17.18b).
4. **Prognosis** is good in 50% of cases with eventual spontaneous resolution of exudation and haemorrhage. In the remainder the disorder persists for a long time with occasional repeated bleeding and leakage, resulting in macular damage and visual loss. Eyes with a cluster of grape-like vascular polypoidal dilatations have a high risk of visual loss.
5. **Differential diagnosis** of exudative pattern PCV is chronic central serous retinopathy in the elderly. Haemorrhagic pattern may mimic neovascular AMD.

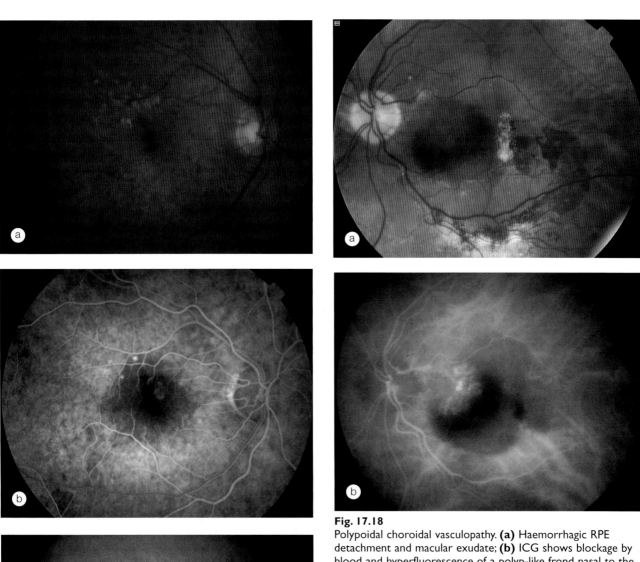

Fig. 17.17
Retinal angiomatous proliferation. **(a)** Macular drusen and a small intraretinal haemorrhage at the macula; **(b)** FA early venous phase shows faint hyperfluorescence from a small frond of intraretinal neovascularization; **(c)** ICG late phase shows hyperfluorescence of the frond (hot spot) (Courtesy of Moorfields Eye Hospital)

Fig. 17.18
Polypoidal choroidal vasculopathy. **(a)** Haemorrhagic RPE detachment and macular exudate; **(b)** ICG shows blockage by blood and hyperfluorescence of a polyp-like frond nasal to the fovea

Treatment

There is no consensus on optimal treatment although it is generally agreed that asymptomatic polyps may resolve spontaneously and can be observed. Various treatment modalities have been used to treat macular involvement although it has been suggested that PDT may be the best option.

AGE-RELATED MACULAR HOLE

Age-related (idiopathic) full-thickness macular hole (FTMH) affects approximately 3 in 1000 individuals, characteristically female, in the sixth or seventh decade. Presentation is with severe impairment of central vision or as a relatively asymptomatic deterioration, first noticed when the fellow eye is closed. The risk of involvement of the fellow eye at 5 years is about 10%.

Staging

A macular hole results from the centrifugal displacement of photoreceptors from a central dehiscence of the umbo. The primary event is probably an abnormal vitreo-foveolar attachment, with resultant anteroposterior and tangential traction initiating the following sequence.

1. **Stage 1a** (impending) macular hole is rarely seen clinically and is usually detected in a patient with a FTMH in the other eye. It is characterized by flattening of the umbo, a yellow foveolar spot 100–200μm in diameter and loss of the foveolar reflex.
2. **Stage 1b** (occult) macular hole is characterized by a yellow ring with a bridging interface of vitreous cortex that may be associated with mild decrease in visual acuity or metamorphopsia. About 50% of stage 1 holes resolve following spontaneous vitreofoveolar separation.
3. **Stage 2** (early FTMH) is characterized by a full-thickness defect, less than 300μm in diameter, with or without an overlying prefoveal opacity (pseudo-operculum) formed by the contracted prefoveal cortical vitreous. Progression from stage 1 to stage 2 takes between one week and several months.
4. **Stage 3** (established FTMH) is characterized by a full-thickness defect more than 400μm in diameter with an attached posterior vitreous face with or without an overlying pseudo-operculum.
5. **Stage 4** is characterized by a round defect more than 400μm in diameter surrounded by a cuff of subretinal fluid with tiny yellowish deposits within its crater (see Fig. 17.20a). The posterior vitreous is completely detached, often evidenced by a Weiss ring. Visual acuity is decreased primarily due to the absence of photoreceptors within the central defect, with a resultant absolute central scotoma. In addition, the surrounding cuff of subretinal fluid and secondary retinal elevation cause a surrounding relative scotoma. Vision tends to decline progressively, stabilizing at 6/60 or worse as the hole reaches its maximal diameter. Some patients may achieve better acuity by employing eccentric fixation.

NB A FTMH may rarely spontaneously resolve, with improvement of visual acuity, due to spontaneous posterior vitreous detachment and release of vitreo-macular traction.

Diagnostic tests

1. **Watzke–Allen** test is performed by projecting a narrow slit beam over the centre of the hole both vertically and horizontally. A patient with a macular hole will report that the beam is thinned or broken. Patients with a pseudo-hole or cyst usually see a beam of uniform thickness which is distorted or bent rather than thinned.
2. **Laser aiming beam** test is performed by projecting a 50μm spot of a laser aiming beam (e.g. He-Ne) at the centre of the hole. A patient with a macular hole will report that the spot has disappeared whereas those with a pseudohole or cyst will still be able to see the beam.
3. **OCT** is useful in the diagnosis and staging of macular holes (Fig. 17.19).
4. **FA** shows a corresponding area of hyperfluorescence (Fig. 17.20) resulting from unmasking of background choroidal fluorescence caused by a defect in xanthophyll due to centrifugal displacement. However, a similar appearance can also be seen with pseudoholes and cysts so FA is not usually helpful in diagnosis.

Surgical treatment

1. **Indications** are FTMH of stage 2 and above, associated with a visual acuity worse than 6/9. Best results are achieved with holes of less than one year's duration. However, it is possible to close holes of several years duration with associated improvement in visual acuity and decreased distortion.
2. **Technique** consists of removal of the cortical vitreous, relief of vitreomacular traction, peeling of the internal limiting membrane (ILM) and gas tamponade followed by strict postoperative face-down positioning. Peeling of the nearly invisible ILM may be assisted by staining it with indocyanine green or trypan blue. The potential for dramatic improvement in visual acuity, together with the (see Fig. 17.19f) restoration of normal foveal architecture on OCT scanning, suggests that closure of the hole is the result of centripetal movement of previously displaced paracentral photoreceptors and not simply re-approximation of the retinal edges to the RPE.
3. **Results.** Following successful surgery, visual improvement is achieved in 80–90% of eyes, with a final visual acuity of 6/12 or better in up to 65%.
4. **Complications** are those associated with vitrectomy, such as retinal detachment and acceleration of cataract.

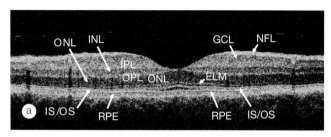
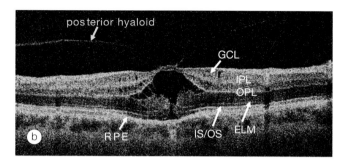
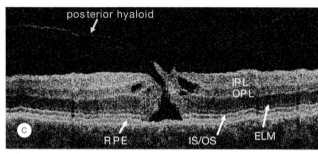
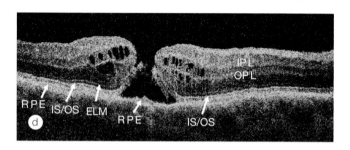
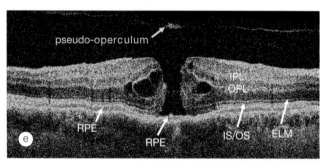
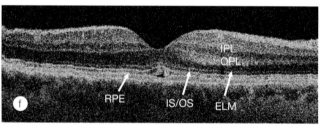

Fig. 17.19
Ultrahigh resolution OCT of macular hole. **(a)** Normal; **(b)** stage 1b shows attachment of the posterior hyaloid to the fovea, separation of a small portion of the sensory retina from the RPE in the foveolar region and intraretinal cystic changes; **(c)** eccentric stage 2 shows attachment of the vitreous to the lid of the hole and cystic changes; **(d)** stage 3 shows a full-thickness hole with cystic spaces at its border; **(e)** stage 4 shows a full-thickness macular hole with cystic spaces and an overlying pseudo-operculum; **(f)** stage 4 after surgical closure (Courtesy of J Fujimoto)

Increasingly cataract surgery is combined with vitrectomy to speed up visual rehabilitation. Occasionally, inferotemporal visual field defects may develop secondary to prolonged infusion of dry air into the ocular cavity.

Differential diagnosis

1. **Other causes of true macular hole**
   a. *High myopia*, if associated with posterior staphyloma, may be associated with macular hole formation, which can lead to retinal detachment. The subretinal fluid is confined to the posterior pole and seldom spreads to the equator.
   b. *Blunt ocular trauma* may cause a macular hole as a result of either vitreous traction or commotio retinae, in which there is disruption of photoreceptors and subsequent hole formation.

2. **Macular pseudo-hole**
   a. *Hole within a premacular membrane* that has occurred as a result of centripetal contraction.
   b. *Lamellar hole* resulting from an abortive process of macular hole formation or in long-standing severe CMO.
   c. *White dot fovea* is an uncommon asymptomatic condition in which white dots are arranged diffusely or in the form of a ring along the margin of the foveola. The latter pattern simulates the appearance of a true macular hole with a cuff of fluid.

3. **Macular microhole** (see below).

Macular microhole

Macular microholes are uncommon and may be easily overlooked without a careful history and examination. They are usually unilateral and have a favourable long-term prognosis.

1. **Presentation** is with a small central scotoma or reduced reading vision.
2. **Signs.** A very small, red, well demarcated intraretinal foveal or juxtafoveal defect that remains stationary with long-term follow-up (Fig. 17.21a).
3. **OCT** shows a well localized subtle defect that probably indicates the presence of a gap in the photoreceptors and/or the RPE (Fig. 17.21b).
4. **Differential diagnosis** includes stage 1a age-related macular hole, solar retinopathy and blunt trauma.

CENTRAL SEROUS RETINOPATHY

Central serous retinopathy (CSR), also known as central serous chorioretinopathy, is a sporadic disorder of the outer blood–retinal barrier, characterized by a localized detachment of the sensory retina at the macula secondary to focal RPE defects, usually affecting one eye. It is usually a self-limited disease typically affecting young or middle-aged men with type A personality. Factors reported to induce or aggravate CSR include emotional stress, untreated hypertension, alcohol use, systemic lupus erythematosus, organ transplantation, gastro-oesophageal reflux, Cushing disease and the administration of steroids, both by inhalation and orally. Women with CSR tend to be older than affected men, and it is also associated with pregnancy.

Typical central serous retinopathy

Diagnosis

1. **Presentation** is with unilateral blurred vision associated with a relative positive scotoma, micropsia, metamorphopsia and occasionally macropsia. There is also a delay in retinal recovery time after exposure to bright light, loss of colour saturation and diminished contrast sensitivity. Occasionally the condition is extrafoveal and asymptomatic.
2. **VA** is usually reduced to 6/9–6/12 and often correctable to 6/6 with a weak 'plus' lens. The elevation of the sensory retina gives rise to an acquired hypermetropia with disparity between the subjective and objective refraction of the eye.
3. **Signs**
   • A round or oval detachment of the sensory retina is present at the macula (Fig. 17.22a).
   • The subretinal fluid may be clear or turbid and small precipitates may be present on the posterior surface of the sensory detachment. Occasionally, an abnormal focus in the RPE can be detected, through which fluid has leaked from the choriocapillaris into the subretinal space.
   • Rare findings include yellowish subretinal deposits forming a leopard-spot pattern, as well as intraretinal or subretinal lipid.
4. **OCT** shows an elevation of full-thickness sensory retinal layer from the highly reflective RPE layer, separated by an optically empty zone (Fig. 17.22b). Sometimes a defect in the RPE may be demonstrated (Fig. 17.22c).

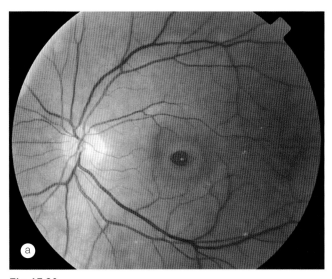
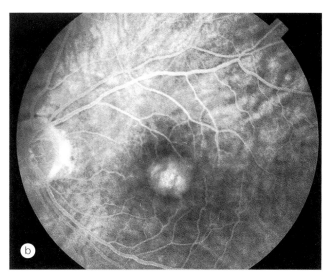

Fig. 17.20
(a) Stage 4 macular hole; **(b)** FA shows corresponding hyperfluorescence (Courtesy of S Milewski)

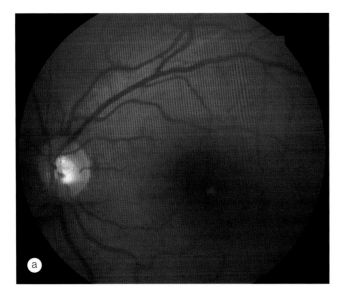

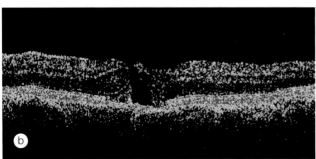

Fig. 17.21
Macular microhole. **(a)** Small red foveal lesion; **(b)** OCT shows a subtle defect in the sensory retina (Courtesy of C Barry – fig. b)

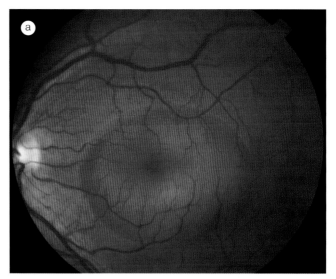

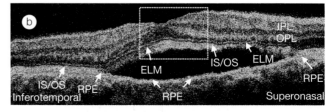

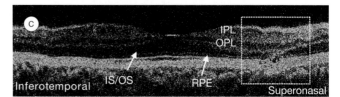

Fig. 17.22
(a) Central serous retinopathy; **(b)** ultrahigh resolution OCT shows separation of the sensory retina from the RPE; **(c)** 2 months later there is resolution of subretinal fluid and residual disruption of the RPE and overlying retina lateral to the fovea (red arrows) (Courtesy of J Fujimoto – figs b and c)

5. FA shows one of the following patterns:

   a. Smoke-stack appearance is the most common and evolves as follows:

   – The early phase shows a small hyperfluorescent spot due to leakage of dye through the RPE (Fig. 17.23a).

   – During the late venous phase, fluorescein passes into the subretinal space and ascends vertically (like a smoke-stack) (Fig. 17.23b) to the upper border of the detachment, and then spreads laterally until the entire area is filled with dye.

   b. Ink-blot appearance is less common and evolves as follows:

   – The early phase shows a small hyperfluorescent spot (Fig. 17.23c).

   – The spot gradually enlarges centrifugally (Fig. 17.23d) until the entire area is filled with dye.

6. ICG early phase shows dilated choroidal vessels at the posterior pole. The mid stages show multiple areas of hyperfluorescence due to choroidal hyperpermeability, suggesting a more generalized RPE or choroidal vascular disturbance.

Course

1. Short. Most commonly, spontaneous absorption of subretinal fluid occurs within 3–6 months with return to normal or near-normal visual acuity although mild colour and contrast sensitivity alterations may persist. Recurrences occur in about one-third to one-half of all patients.

2. Prolonged. In some patients CSR lasts longer than 6 months but spontaneously resolves within 12 months. Even if visual acuity returns to normal, some degree of subjective visual impairment such as micropsia may persist, but seldom causes any significant disability.

3. Chronic. In a minority of cases, particularly those older than 50 years, the condition lasts longer than 12 months and is characterized by progressive RPE changes, often without manifest retinal detachment, resulting in permanent impairment of visual acuity; some cases may develop CNV. FA shows granular hyperfluorescence with one or more leaks (Fig. 17.24). This may be a consequence of either multiple recurrent attacks or prolonged detachment, although a minority of patients do not have a past history of typical CSR, and in some the changes are bilateral.

Management

Most cases do not require treatment.

1. **Argon laser photocoagulation** to the RPE leak or detachment achieves speedier resolution and lowers the recurrence rate but does not influence the final visual outcome. It is advisable to wait for 4 months before considering treatment of the first attack and 1–2 months for recurrences. Treatment is contraindicated if the leak is near or within the FAZ. Two or three low- to moderate-intensity burns are applied to the leakage site (200μm, 0.2sec) to produce mild greying of the RPE. Uncommon side-effects include stimulation of CNV, localized scotoma and enlargement of the laser scar over time.

2. **PDT** may be beneficial in acute CSR with subfoveal leaks and in chronic disease.

NB Careful follow-up is required as 2–5% of treated eyes subsequently develop CNV.

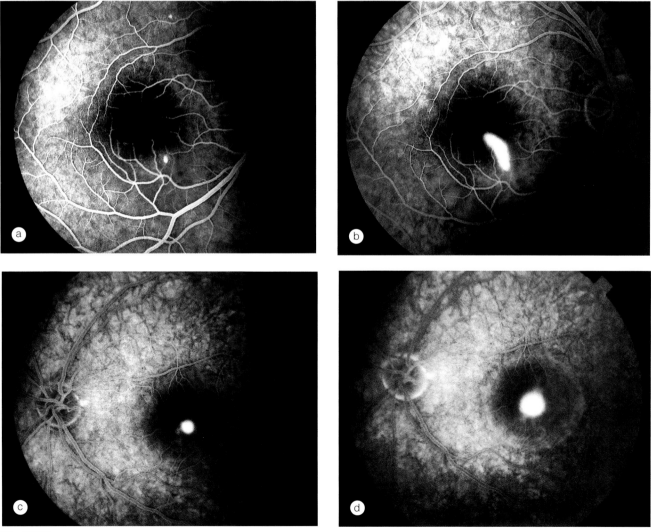

Fig. 17.23
FA in central serous retinopathy (**a** and **b**) 'Smoke-stack' appearance; (**c** and **d**) 'ink blot' appearance (Courtesy of S Milewski)

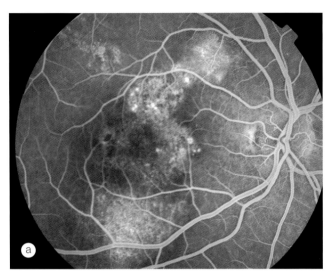 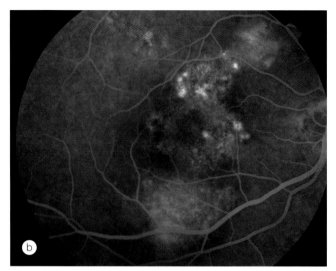

Fig. 17.24
FA in chronic central serous retinopathy. **(a)** Granular hyperfluorescence in the venous phase, **(b)** fading in the late stage (Courtesy of Moorfields Eye Hospital)

Differential diagnosis of sensory macular detachment

1. **Congenital optic disc anomalies,** most frequently optic disc pit and occasionally tilted disc, may be associated with serous macular detachment. Unless the optic disc is examined carefully the diagnosis may be missed (see Chapter 3).
2. **Choroidal tumours** with a predilection for the posterior pole such as circumscribed choroidal haemangioma and metastatic carcinoma.
3. **Unilateral acute idiopathic maculopathy** is a rare self-limiting condition that typically causes sudden unilateral visual loss in a young person (see Chapter 14).
4. **CNV,** particularly if idiopathic.
5. **Harada disease** during the stage of multifocal detachments of the sensory retina may mimic multifocal CSR (see Chapter 14).

Bullous central serous retinopathy

Bullous CSR is characterized by large, single or multiple, serous retinal and RPE detachments that are associated with an inferior bullous exudative retinal detachment. This appearance may lead to the inappropriate diagnosis of rhegmatogenous retinal detachment, or exudative detachment from some other cause.

CYSTOID MACULAR OEDEMA

CMO is the result of accumulation of fluid in the outer plexiform and inner nuclear layers of the retina with the formation of fluid-filled cyst-like changes (Fig. 17.25a). In the short term CMO is usually innocuous; however, long-standing cases usually lead to coalescence of the microcystic spaces into large cavities and subsequent lamellar hole formation at the fovea with irreversible damage to central vision. CMO is a common and non-specific condition that may occur with any type of macular oedema.

Diagnosis

1. **Presentation** varies with the cause. Visual acuity may already be impaired by pre-existing disease such as branch vein occlusion. In cases without pre-existing disease the patient complains of impairment of central vision associated with a positive central scotoma.
2. **Signs**
   - Slit-lamp biomicroscopy shows loss of the foveal depression, thickening of the retina and multiple cystoid areas in the sensory retina (Figs 17.25b).
   - In early cases cystoid changes may be difficult to discern and the main finding is a yellow spot at the foveola.

3. **OCT** shows a collection of hyporeflective spaces within the retina, with overall macular thickening and loss of the foveal depression (Fig. 17.25c). OCT is as effective at detecting CMO as FA and produces highly reproducible measurements so that serial examination may be used to assess response to treatment and lamellar hole formation (Fig. 17.25d). However, unlike FA it can also be used in eyes with opaque media and is useful in detecting vitreoretinal traction.

4. **FA**
   - The arteriovenous phase shows small hyperfluorescent spots due to early leakage (Fig. 17.26b).
   - The late phase shows a 'flower-petal' pattern of hyperfluorescence (Fig. 17.26c and d) caused by accumulation of dye within microcystic spaces in the outer plexiform layer of the retina, with its radial arrangement of fibres about the centre of the foveola (Henle layer).

Causes and treatment

Retinal vascular disease

1. **Causes** include diabetic retinopathy, retinal vein occlusion, hypertensive retinopathy, idiopathic retinal telangiectasis, retinal artery macroaneurysm and radiation retinopathy.
2. **Treatment** by laser photocoagulation may be appropriate in selected cases.

Intraocular inflammation

1. **Causes** include intermediate uveitis, birdshot retinochoroidopathy, multifocal choroiditis with panuveitis, toxoplasmosis, cytomegaloviral retinitis, Behçet syndrome and scleritis.
2. **Treatment** is aimed at controlling the inflammatory process with steroids or immunosuppressive agents. Systemic carbonic anhydrase inhibitors may be beneficial in CMO associated with intermediate uveitis. Interferon alpha 2a may be useful in CMO associated with steroid-resistant autoimmune uveitis, although discontinuation may provoke a relapse of inflammation. Side-effects include arrhythmias and disturbances in blood pressure.

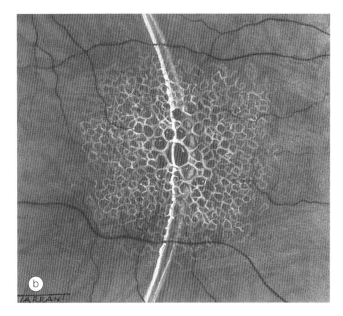

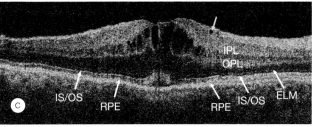

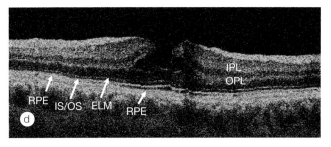

Fig 17.25
Cystoid macular oedema. **(a)** Histology shows cystic spaces in the outer plexiform and inner nuclear layer; **(b)** clinical appearance; **(c)** ultrahigh resolution OCT shows increased retinal thickness, cystoid spaces mainly in the inner nuclear layer and a small detachment of the photoreceptors from the RPE in the centre of the fovea (red arrow); **(d)** OCT shows a lamellar hole (Courtesy of J Harry and G Misson, from *Clinical Ophthalmic Pathology*, Butterworth-Heinemann, 2001 – fig. a; J Fujimoto – figs c and d)

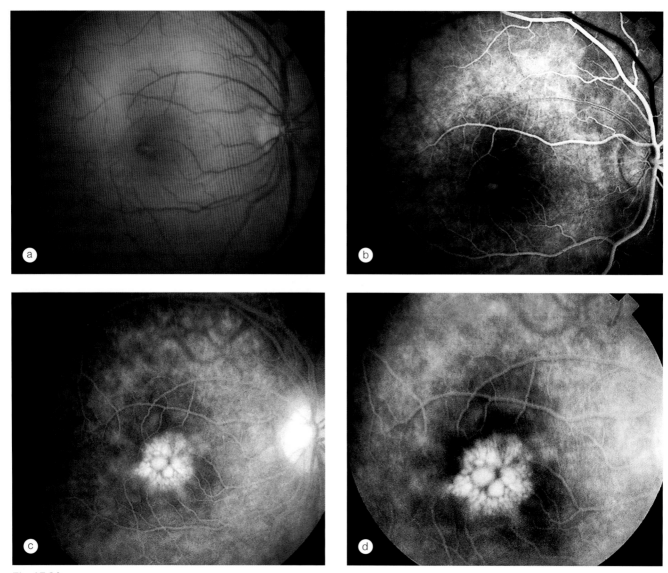

Fig. 17.26
Cystoid macular oedema. **(a)** Clinical appearance; **(b)** FA arteriovenous stage shows a hyperfluorescent spot; **(c and d)** late phase shows increasing hyperfluorescence with a 'flower-petal' pattern (Courtesy of S Milewski)

Following cataract surgery

CMO is rare following uncomplicated surgery but when it does occur spontaneous resolution is the rule.

1. **Risk factors** for visually significant CMO include operative complications such as posterior capsular rupture, vitreous loss and incarceration into the incision site, anterior chamber and secondary IOL implantation, diabetes and a history of CMO in the other eye. Peak incidence is at 6–10 weeks after surgery, although the interval may be much longer.
2. **Treatment** involves correction of the underlying cause, if possible. For example, vitreous incarceration in the anterior segment may be amenable to anterior vitrectomy or YAG laser disruption of vitreous adhesions. As a last resort it may be necessary to remove an anterior chamber IOL. If a correctable cause is not present, treatment is difficult, although many cases resolve spontaneously within 6 months. Treatment of persistent CMO involves the following measures:

   a. ***Systemic carbonic anhydrase inhibitors***.

   b. ***Steroids***, given topically or by posterior periocular injection, combined with topical non-steroidal anti-inflammatory drugs (NSAIDs) such as ketorolac 0.5% (Acular) administered q.i.d. Unfortunately, in many cases CMO recurs when treatment is discontinued so that long-term medication may be required. Intravitreal triamcinolone may reduce CMO in cases unresponsive to sub-Tenon injections.

c. Pars plana vitrectomy may be useful for CMO refractory to medical therapy, even in eyes without apparent vitreous disturbance.

Following other surgical procedures

1. **Causes** include YAG laser capsulotomy, peripheral retinal cryotherapy and laser photocoagulation. The risk of CMO may be reduced if capsulotomy is delayed for 6 months or more after cataract surgery. Rarely, CMO may develop following scleral buckling, penetrating keratoplasty and glaucoma filtration surgery.
2. **Treatment** is unsatisfactory although the CMO is often mild and self-limited.

Drug-induced

1. **Causes** include topical adrenaline 2% (especially in the aphakic eye), topical latanoprost and systemic nicotinic acid.
2. **Treatment** involves cessation of medication.

Retinal dystrophies

1. **Causes** include retinitis pigmentosa, gyrate atrophy and dominantly inherited CMO.
2. **Treatment** with systemic carbonic anhydrase inhibitors may be beneficial in retinitis pigmentosa.

Miscellaneous

1. **Vitreomacular traction syndrome** is characterized by partial peripheral vitreous separation with persistent posterior attachment to the macula. This results in anteroposterior and tangential traction vectors. Chronic CMO is common and may respond to vitrectomy.
2. **Macular epiretinal membranes** may occasionally cause CMO by disrupting the perifoveal capillaries. Surgical excision of the membrane may be beneficial in selected cases.
3. **CNV** may be associated with foveal thickening and CMO, the presence of which constitutes an adverse prognostic factor.
4. **Tumours** such as retinal haemangioblastoma and choroidal haemangioma.

MACULAR EPIRETINAL MEMBRANE

Pathogenesis

Macular epiretinal membranes that develop at the vitreoretinal interface consist of proliferation of retinal glial cells which have gained access to the retinal surface through breaks in the internal limiting membrane. It has been postulated that these breaks may be created when the posterior vitreous detaches from the macula. The causes are as follows:

1. **Idiopathic** membranes predominantly affect otherwise healthy elderly individuals and are bilateral in about 10% of cases.
2. **Secondary** membranes may be associated with the following conditions:
    a. Retinal procedures such as detachment surgery, photocoagulation and cryotherapy may either induce or worsen a pre-existing macular epiretinal membrane. Untreated, these membranes usually cause a variable but permanent reduction of vision. Very occasionally, however, the membrane may separate spontaneously from the retina.
    b. Other causes include retinal vascular disease, intra-ocular inflammation and ocular trauma.

NB The clinical appearance of epiretinal membranes depends on their density and any associated distortion of the retinal vasculature. It is convenient to divide the condition into: (a) *cellophane maculopathy* and (b) *macular pucker*.

Cellophane maculopathy

Cellophane maculopathy consists of a thin layer of epiretinal cells. It is common and usually secondary to a posterior vitreous detachment.

1. **Presentation** may be with mild metamorphopsia, although frequently the condition is asymptomatic and is discovered by chance.
2. **Signs**
    * An irregular light reflex or sheen is present at the macula.
    * The membrane itself is translucent and is best detected using 'red-free' light (Fig. 17.27a).
    * As it thickens and contracts it becomes more obvious (Fig. 17.27b) and may cause mild distortion of blood vessels (Fig. 17.27c).
3. **Treatment** is not appropriate.

Macular pucker

Macular pucker is a more serious condition caused by thickening and contraction of an epiretinal membrane and is much less common than cellophane maculopathy.

1. **Presentation** is with metamorphopsia and blurring of central vision.
2. **VA** is reduced to 6/12 or worse, depending on severity.

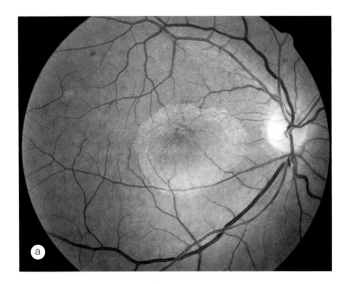

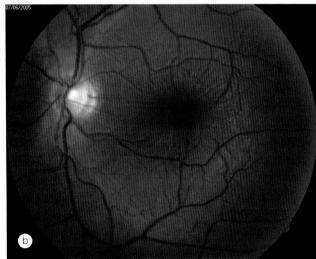

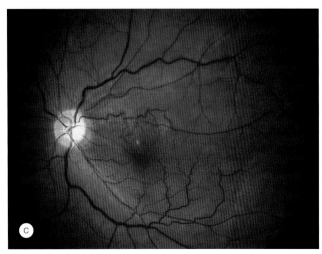

Fig. 17.27
Cellophane maculopathy. **(a)** Translucent membrane seen with red-free light; **(b)** more obvious membrane; **(c)** mild distortion of blood vessels (Courtesy of L Merin – fig. a; S Milenkovic – fig. b; C Barry – fig. c)

3. **Signs**
   - The macula shows severe distortion of the blood vessels, retinal wrinkling and white striae which may obscure underlying blood vessels (Fig. 17.28a).
   - Associated findings include macular pseudo-holes within the membrane and occasionally CMO.
4. **FA** highlights the vascular tortuosity and may show hyperfluorescence if leakage is present (Fig. 17.28b).
5. **OCT** shows a highly reflective (red) layer on the surface of the retina associated with retinal thickening (Fig. 17.28c).
6. **Treatment** by surgical removal of the membrane usually improves or eliminates distortion, and improves visual acuity in about 50% of cases.

DEGENERATIVE MYOPIA

High myopia is defined as an eye with a refractive error > −6D and an axial length of the globe > 26mm. It affects approximately 0.5% of the general population and 30% of myopic eyes. Pathological or degenerative myopia is characterized by progressive and excessive anteroposterior elongation of the globe, which is associated with secondary changes involving the sclera, retina, choroid and optic nerve head. Maculopathy is the most common cause of visual loss in highly myopic patients.

Diagnosis

1. **A pale tessellate** (tigroid) appearance due to diffuse attenuation of the RPE with visibility of large choroidal vessels (Fig. 17.29a).
2. **Focal chorioretinal atrophy** characterized by visibility of the larger choroidal vessels and eventually the sclera (Fig. 17.29b).
3. **'Lacquer cracks'** consist of ruptures in the RPE–Bruch membrane–choriocapillaris complex characterized by fine, irregular, yellow lines, often branching and criss-crossing at the posterior pole (Fig. 17.29c).
4. **CNV** which may develop in association with 'lacquer cracks' and areas of patchy atrophy (Fig. 17.29d).
5. **Subretinal 'coin' haemorrhages,** which may be intermittent, may develop from lacquer cracks in the absence of CNV (Fig. 17.29e).
6. **Fuchs spot** is a raised, circular, pigmented lesion that may develop after a macular haemorrhage has absorbed (Fig. 17.29f).

Complications

1. **Staphylomas** are due to expansion of the globe and scleral thinning (Fig. 17.30a–c). They may be peripapillary or involve the posterior pole and be associated with macular hole formation.

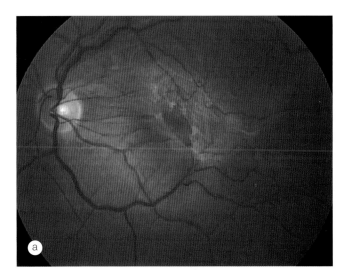

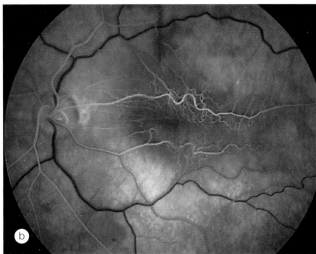

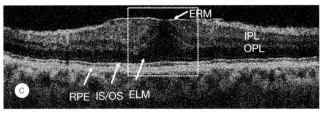

Fig. 17.28
Macular pucker. **(a)** Clinical appearance; **(b)** FA arterial phase shows highlights the vascular tortuosity; **(c)** ultrahigh resolution OCT shows a highly reflective membrane at the vitreoretinal interface associated with distortion and increased retinal thickness at the fovea (Courtesy S Milewski – figs a and b; J Fujimoto – fig. c)

2. **Rhegmatogenous retinal detachment** may occur due to vitreous liquefaction, increased frequency of posterior vitreous detachment, lattice degeneration, asymptomatic atrophic holes, macular holes (Fig. 17.30d) and occasionally giant retinal tears. The prevalence of retinal

detachment appears to be related to the severity of myopia.
3. **Foveal retinoschisis** and retinal detachment without macular hole formation may occur in highly myopic eyes with posterior staphylomas as a result of vitreous traction.
4. **Peripapillary detachment** is an asymptomatic, innocuous, yellow-orange elevation of the RPE and sensory retina at the inferior border of the myopic conus. It should be distinguished from more serious fundus pathology such as a tumour or CNV.

Associations

1. **Ocular**
   - Cataract, which may be either posterior subcapsular or early onset of nuclear sclerosis.
   - Increased prevalence of primary open-angle glaucoma, pigmentary glaucoma and steroid responsiveness.
   - Retinopathy of prematurity may be associated with the subsequent development of myopia.
   - Amblyopia is uncommon but may develop when there is a significant difference in myopia between the two eyes.
2. **Systemic**
   - Stickler syndrome.
   - Marfan syndrome.
   - Ehlers–Danlos syndrome.
   - Pierre–Robin syndrome.

Differential diagnosis

Other disorders characterized by extensive chorioretinal atrophy include the following:

1. **Choroideremia.** Differences include nyctalopia, absence of peripapillary changes and sparing of the macula until late in the disease.
2. **Gyrate atrophy.** Differences include early onset, lesions have typically scalloped edges and late macular sparing.
3. **Diffuse choroidal atrophy.** Differences include diffuse chorioretinal changes rather than punched out lesions as in myopia.
4. **Progressive bifocal chorioretinal atrophy.** Differences include early onset, specific atrophic areas confined to the macular and nasal fundus.

ANGIOID STREAKS

Angioid streaks are the result of crack-like dehiscences in thickened, calcified and abnormally brittle collagenous and elastic portions of Bruch membrane (Fig.17.31a).

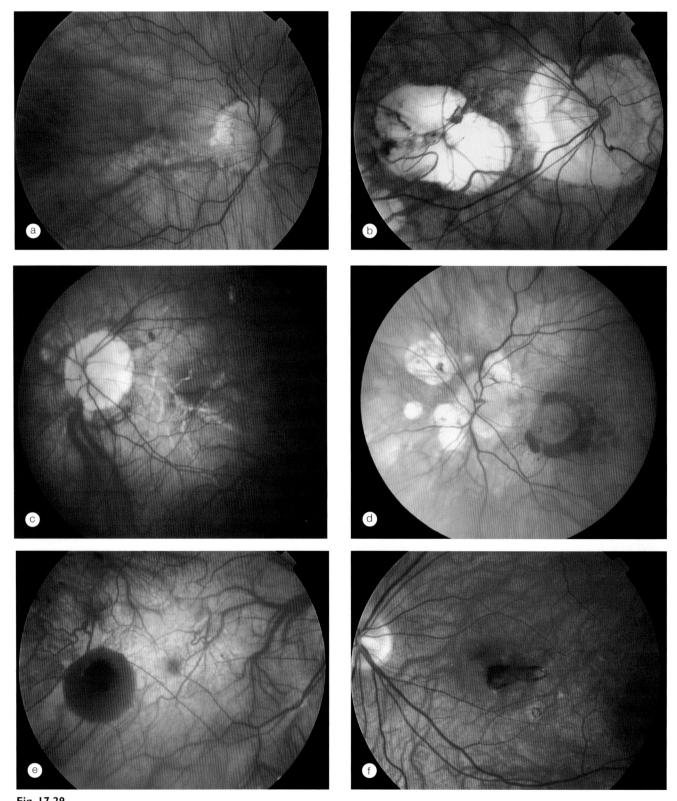

Fig. 17.29
High myopia. **(a)** Tessellated fundus; **(b)** focal chorioretinal atrophy; **(c)** lacquer cracks; **(d)** subretinal haemorrhage associated with choroidal neovascularization; **(e)** 'coin' haemorrhage; **(f)** Fuchs spot

Diagnosis

I. Signs
- 'Peau d'orange' (orange skin), consisting of mottled pigmentation is common, and subtle angioid streaks may be overlooked (Fig. 17.31b).
- Linear, grey or dark-red linear lesions with irregular serrated edges that lie beneath the normal retinal blood vessels that intercommunicate in a ring-like fashion around the optic disc and then radiate outwards from the peripapillary area (Fig. 17.31c).

2. FA shows hyperfluorescence caused by RPE window defects over the streaks associated with variable hypofluorescence corresponding to RPE hyperplasia and is primarily used to detect CNV (Fig. 17.31d).

3. Optic disc drusen are common (Fig. 17.31e).

Prognosis

The prognosis is guarded because visual impairment occurs in over 70% of patients as a result of one or more of the following:

I. CNV is by far the most common cause of visual loss. Conventional thermal laser photocoagulation may be successful in certain juxtafoveal and extrafoveal lesions although there is a high risk of aggressive recurrence. PDT for subfoveal CNV may be more effective.

2. Choroidal rupture, which may occur following relatively trivial ocular trauma and result in a subretinal haemorrhage (Fig. 17.31f). Because eyes with angioid streaks are very fragile, patients should be warned against participating in contact sports and advised to use protective spectacles for ball games.

3. Foveal involvement by a streak.

Systemic associations

Approximately 50% of patients with angioid streaks have one of the following conditions:

I. Pseudoxanthoma elasticum (PXE) is by far the most common association and approximately 85% of patients develop ocular involvement, usually after the second decade of life. The combination of the two is referred to as 'Groenblad–Strandberg syndrome' (see Chapter 24).

2. Ehlers–Danlos syndrome type 6 (ocular sclerotic) is a rare, usually AD, disorder of collagen caused by deficiency of procollagen lysyl hydroxylase. There are 11 subtypes but only type 6 is associated with ocular features (see Chapter 24).

3. Paget disease is a chronic, progressive metabolic bone disease characterized by excessive and disorganized re-

sorption and formation of bone (see Chapter 24). Angioid streaks are uncommon occurring in only about 2%.

4. Haemoglobinopathies occasionally associated with angioid streaks are: homozygous sickle-cell disease (HbSS), sickle-cell trait (HbAS), sickle-cell thalassaemia (HbS thalassaemia), sickle-cell haemoglobin C disease (HbSC), haemoglobin H disease (HbH), homozygous beta-thalassaemia major, beta-thalassaemia intermedia and beta-thalassaemia minor.

CHOROIDAL FOLDS

Causes

Choroidal (chorioretinal) folds are parallel grooves or striae involving the inner choroid, Bruch membrane, RPE and sometimes the outer sensory retina. Possible mechanisms include choroidal congestion, scleral folding and contraction of Bruch membrane. The main causes are the following:

I. Idiopathic folds may occur for no apparent reason in both eyes of healthy hypermetropic patients with normal or near-normal visual acuity.

2. Orbital diseases such as retrobulbar tumours and thyroid ophthalmopathy may cause choroidal folds that impair visual acuity.

3. Choroidal tumours such as melanomas may mechanically displace the surrounding choroid and cause folding.

4. Miscellaneous uncommon causes include chronic papilloedema, posterior scleritis and scleral buckling for retinal detachment.

Diagnosis

I. Presentation is often with metamorphopsia, although the patient may be asymptomatic. Initially visual dysfunction is caused by distortion of overlying retinal receptors, but in long-standing cases, permanent changes may develop in the RPE and sensory retina.

2. VA may be normal or variably impaired.

3. Signs
- Parallel lines, grooves or striae typically located at the posterior pole that are usually horizontally orientated (Fig. 17.32a) but may be vertical, oblique or irregular.
- The crest (elevated portion) of a fold is yellow and less pigmented as a result of stretching and thinning of the RPE and the trough is darker due to compression of the RPE.

4. FA shows alternating hyperfluorescent and hypofluorescent streaks at the level of the RPE (Fig. 17.32b). The hyperfluorescence corresponds to the crests as a result of increased background choroidal fluorescence showing through the stretched and thinned RPE. The hypofluorescence corresponds to the troughs due to blockage of choroidal fluorescence by the compressed and thickened RPE.

HYPOTONY MACULOPATHY

Hypotonous maculopathy is caused by very low intraocular pressure (usually < 6mmHg) following glaucoma filtration surgery, particularly when adjunctive antimetabolites are used. It may also occur following trauma and chronic anterior uveitis. Severe prolonged hypotony is very serious because, if sustained, it may lead to phthisis bulbi and visual loss. Chronic inflammation can lead to the development of cyclitic membranes, which both increase outflow by placing traction on the ciliary processes, and decrease secretion by directly damaging the secretory ciliary epithelium. With time the hypotonous process can itself lead to further damage, including sclerosis and atrophy of ciliary processes.

I. Signs

- Very low intraocular pressure which may be associated with shallow anterior chamber, depending on the aetiology.
- Chorioretinal folds that tend to radiate outwards in a branching fashion from the optic disc (Fig. 17.33).
- Disc oedema is a common feature.

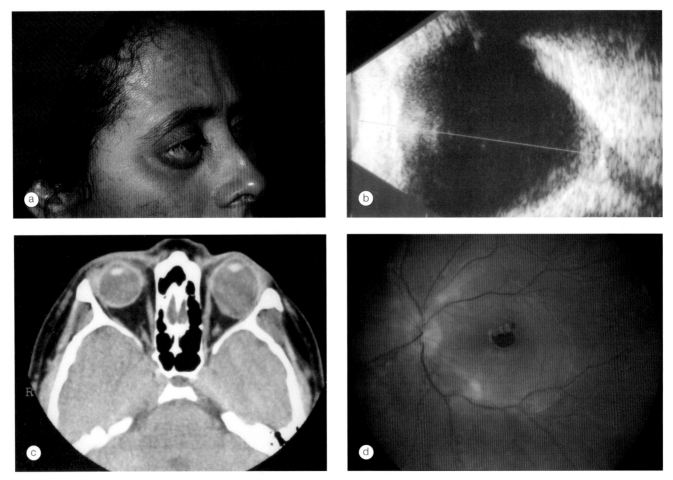

Fig. 17.30
High myopia. **(a)** Large globe; **(b)** US shows a long axial length and posterior staphyloma; **(c)** CT axial view shows a left posterior staphyloma; **(d)** shallow retinal detachment confined to the posterior pole caused by a macular hole
(Courtesy of M Khairallah–fig. d)

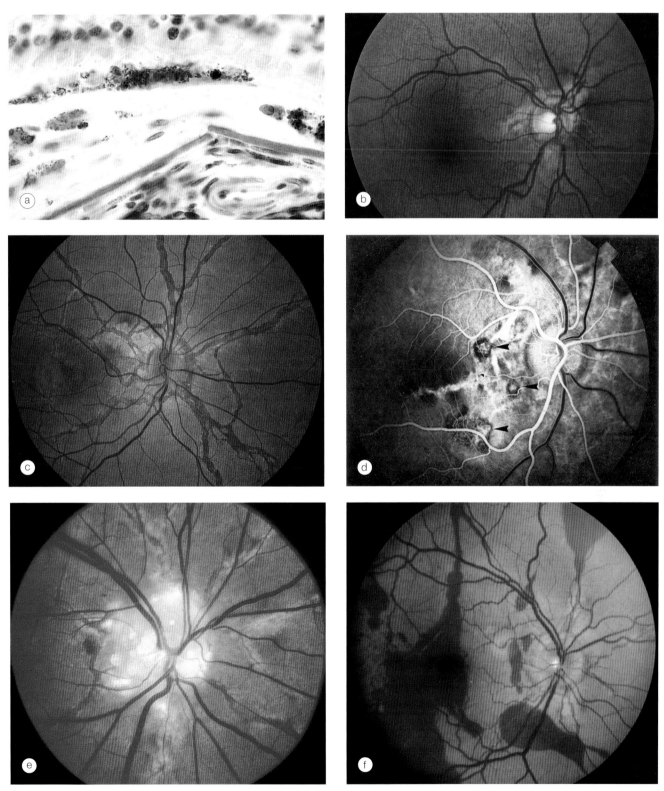

Fig. 17.31
Angioid streaks. **(a)** Histology shows a break in thickened Bruch membrane; **(b)** 'peau d'orange' and subtle angioid streaks; **(c)** advanced angioid streaks; **(d)** FA arteriovenous phase shows hypofluorescence of angioid streaks and three foci of choroidal neovascularization (arrows); **(e)** angioid streaks and optic disc drusen; **(f)** subretinal haemorrhage caused by a traumatic choroidal rupture (Courtesy of J Harry and G Misson, from *Clinical Ophthalmic Pathology*, Butterworth-Heinemann, 2001 – fig. a; P Saine – fig. c; S Milewski – fig. d)

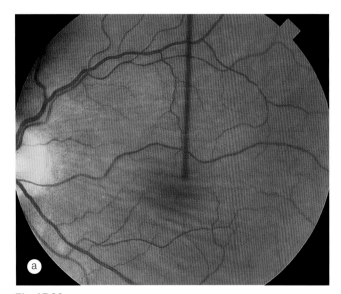

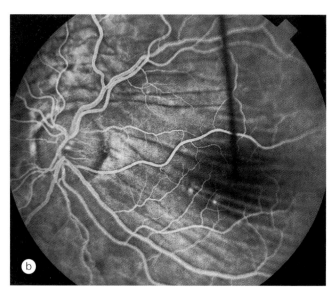

Fig. 17.32
Choroidal folds. **(a)** Clinical appearance; **(b)** FA venous phase shows alternating hypofluorescent and hyperfluorescent streaks (Courtesy of S Milewski)

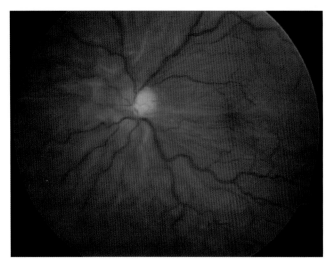

Fig. 17.33
Radial chorioretinal folds due to chronic hypotony (Courtesy of P Gili)

- Delayed normalization of intraocular pressure may result in permanent macular changes and poor vision.
2. **Treatment** depends on the cause. Hypotony following glaucoma surgery may require resuturing the scleral flap or autologous blood injection. Medical therapy may suffice in early forms of inflammatory hypotony, but persistent cases may require surgical removal of tractional membranes on the ciliary processes to prevent phthisis. Either gas or silicone oil can be used to provide post-operative tamponade. Eyes with severe atrophy of ciliary processes, as shown on US, are unlikely to benefit from surgery.

VITREOMACULAR TRACTION SYNDROME

1. **Pathogenesis.** The vitreous cortex is attached to the fovea and the optic disc but detached temporal to the fovea and the area of the papillomacular bundle. This incomplete posterior vitreous detachment exerts persistent anterior traction on the fovea, which leads to macular changes.
2. **Presentation** is usually in adult life with decreased vision, metamorphopsia, photopsia and micropsia.
3. **Signs**
   - Partial posterior vitreous detachment.
   - The macula may show retinal surface wrinkling, distortion, an epiretinal membrane or CMO.
4. **OCT** is used to confirm the diagnosis (Fig. 17.34).
5. **Treatment** involving pars plana vitrectomy to relieve macular traction is often successful.

IDIOPATHIC CHOROIDAL NEOVASCULARIZATION

Idiopathic CNV is an uncommon condition which affects patients under the age of 50 years. The diagnosis is one of exclusion of other possible associations of CNV such as AMD, angioid streaks, high myopia and presumed ocular histoplasmosis. Idiopathic CNV carries a better visual prognosis than that associated with AMD and in some cases

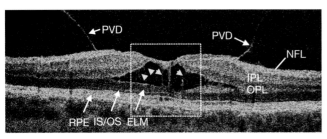

Fig. 17.34
Ultrahigh resolution OCT in vitreomacular traction syndrome shows posterior vitreous traction causing separation between the inner and outer plexiform layers with distended structures spanning the separation (yellow arrows); the red arrow points to a portion of the outer plexiform layer (Courtesy of J Fujimoto)

spontaneous resolution may occur. The CNV is of type 2 and lies predominantly above the RPE (see Fig. 17.16).

SOLAR RETINOPATHY

1. **Pathogenesis:** retinal injury caused by photochemical effects of solar radiation by directly or indirectly viewing the sun (eclipse retinopathy).
2. **Presentation** is within 1–4 hours of solar exposure with unilateral or bilateral impairment of central vision and a small central scotoma.
3. **VA** is variable according to the extent of damage.
4. **Fundus**
   - A small yellow or red foveolar spot which fades within a few weeks (Fig. 17.35).

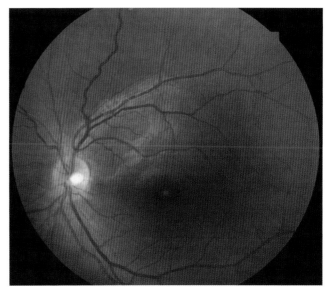

Fig. 17.35
Solar maculopathy. Yellow foveolar spot

   - The spot is replaced by a sharply defined foveolar defect with irregular borders or a lamellar hole.
5. **OCT** shows a hyporeflective space in the outer retina.
6. **Treatment** is not available; systemic steroids have no proven benefit.
7. **Prognosis** is good in most cases with improvement of visual acuity to normal or near-normal levels within 6 months, although mild symptoms may persist.

CHAPTER 18

FUNDUS DYSTROPHIES

RETINAL DYSTROPHIES

Retinitis pigmentosa

Retinitis pigmentosa (RP) defines a clinically and genetically diverse group of diffuse retinal dystrophies initially predominantly affecting the rod photoreceptor cells with subsequent degeneration of cones. Its prevalence is 1:5000.

Inheritance

The age of onset, rate of progression, eventual visual loss and associated ocular features are frequently related to the mode of inheritance. RP may occur as an isolated sporadic disorder, or be inherited as autosomal dominant (AD), autosomal recessive (AR) or X-linked (XL). Many cases are due to mutation of the rhodopsin gene. RP may also be associated with certain systemic disorders which are usually AR.

- Isolated, without any family history, is common.
- AD is also common and has the best prognosis.
- AR is less common and has an intermediate prognosis.
- XL is the least common but most severe form which may result in complete blindness by the third or fourth decades. Female carriers may have normal fundi or exhibit a golden-metallic reflex at the macula (Fig. 18.1) with atrophic and pigmentary peripheral irregularities.

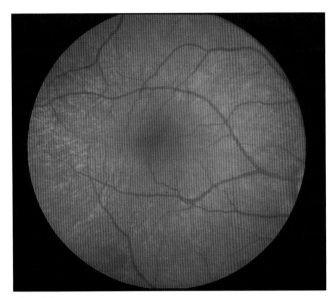

Fig. 18.1
Scintillating golden reflex at the macula in a carrier of X-linked retinitis pigmentosa

Diagnosis

The diagnostic criteria for RP comprise bilateral involvement, loss of peripheral vision and progressive deterioration of predominantly rod photoreceptor function. The classic clinical triad of RP is (a) *arteriolar attenuation*, (b) *retinal bone-spicule pigmentation* and (c) *waxy disc pallor*.

1. **Presentation** is with nyctalopia, often during the third decade, but may be sooner depending on the pedigree.
2. **Signs** in chronological order:
   - Arteriolar narrowing, mild pigmentary changes (Fig. 18.2a).
   - Mid-peripheral, coarse, perivascular 'bone-spicule' pigmentary changes (Fig. 18.2b) which gradually increase in density and spread anteriorly and posteriorly (Fig. 18.2c).
   - Tessellated fundus appearance, due to RPE atrophy and unmasking of large choroidal vessels, severe arteriolar attenuation and waxy disc pallor (Fig. 18.2d).
   - The macula may show atrophy, cellophane formation

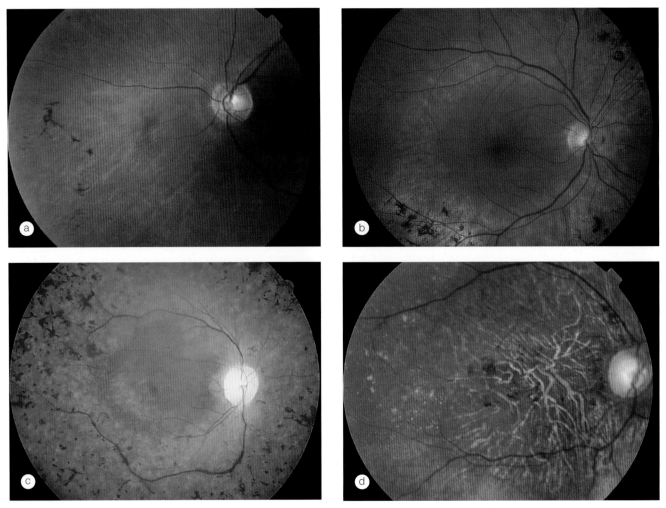

Fig. 18.2
Retinitis pigmentosa. **(a)** Vascular attenuation and mild pigmentary changes; **(b)** mid-peripheral 'bone spicule' pigmentary changes; **(c)** central spread; **(d)** advanced disease with unmasking of choroidal vessels (Courtesy P Saine – fig. b; C Barry – fig. c)

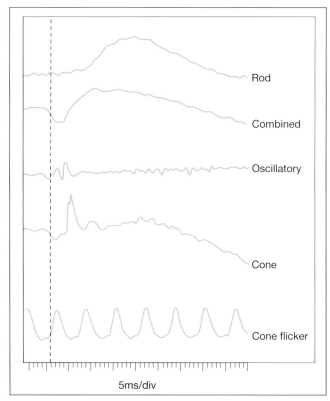

Fig. 18.3
ERG in early retinitis pigmentosa shows reduced scotopic rod and combined responses

5ms/div

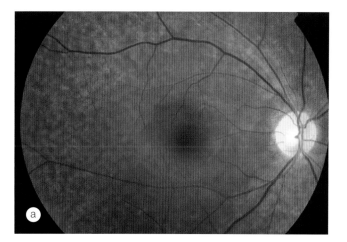

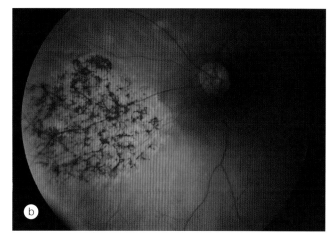

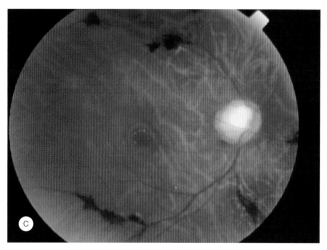

Fig. 18.4
Atypical retinitis pigmentosa. **(a)** Retinitis punctata albescens; **(b)** sector; **(c)** pericentral (Courtesy of Moorfields Eye Hospital – fig. a)

and CMO: the latter may respond to systemic acetazolamide.

3. **Electroretinography (ERG)** shows reduced scotopic rod and combined responses during the early stages of the disease in which fundus changes are minimal (Fig. 18.3); later photopic responses become reduced and eventually the ERG becomes extinguished.
4. **Electro-oculography (EOG)** is subnormal with an absence of the light rise.
5. **Dark adaptometry (DA)** (adaptation) is prolonged and may be useful in early cases where the diagnosis is uncertain.
6. **Colour vision (CV)** is normal.
7. **Visual fields (VF)** classically demonstrate an annular mid-peripheral scotoma, which expands both peripherally and centrally. It ultimately leaves a tiny island of central vision which may eventually be extinguished. Perimetry is useful in monitoring the progression of disease.

Prognosis

The long-term prognosis is poor with eventual loss of central vision due to direct involvement of the fovea by RP itself or maculopathy. Daily administration of supplemental vitamin A, if instituted early, may possibly retard progression, but because of lack of definite evidence of efficacy it is not routinely prescribed. The overall prognosis is as follows:

• About 25% of patients maintain good visual acuity and

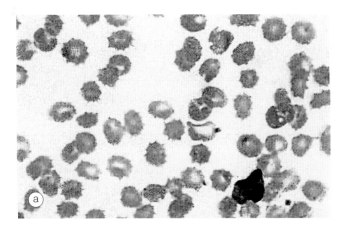

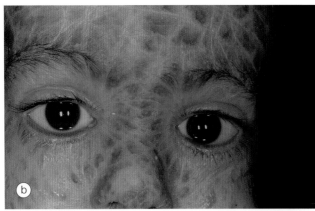

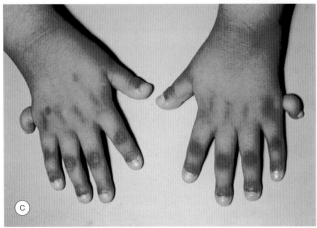

Fig. 18.5
Systemic associations or retinitis pigmentosa. **(a)** Acanthocytosis in Bassen–Kornzweig syndrome; **(b)** ichthyosis in Refsum syndrome; **(c)** polydactyly in Bardet–Biedl syndrome (Courtesy of U Raina – fig b).

are able to read throughout their working lives, despite an extinguished ERG and 2–3° central field.
- Under the age of 20 years, most patients have a visual acuity better than 6/60.
- By the age of 50 years an appreciable number have a visual acuity of worse than 6/60.

Atypical RP

1. **Retinitis punctata albescens** is characterized by scattered white dots, most numerous at the equator, usually sparing the macula, associated with vascular attenuation (Fig. 18.4a).
2. **Sector RP** is characterized by involvement of one quadrant (usually nasal – Fig. 18.4b) or one half (usually inferior). Progression is slow and many cases remain stationary.
3. **Pericentral RP** in which the pigmentary abnormalities emanate from the disc and extend along the temporal arcades and nasally (Fig. 18.4c).
4. **RP with exudative vasculopathy** is characterized by a Coats disease-like appearance with lipid deposition in the peripheral retina and exudative retinal detachment.

Ocular associations

Regular follow-up of patients with RP is essential to detect other vision-threatening complications, some of which may be amenable to treatment.

1. **Posterior subcapsular cataracts** are common in all forms of RP and surgery is often beneficial.
2. **Open-angle glaucoma** occurs in 3% of cases.
3. **Myopia** is frequent.
4. **Keratoconus** is uncommon.
5. **Vitreous changes,** which are common, consist of posterior vitreous detachment and occasionally intermediate uveitis.
6. **Optic disc drusen** occur more frequently.

Differential diagnosis

1. **End-stage chloroquine retinopathy** is also characterized by bilateral diffuse loss of RPE with unmasking of choroidal vessels and arteriolar attenuation. However, the pigmentary changes do not have a perivascular 'bone corpuscle' configuration, and the optic atrophy is not waxy.
2. **End-stage syphilitic neuroretinitis** is also characterized by gross restriction of visual fields, vascular attenuation and pigmentary changes. However, nyctalopia is mild, involvement is asymmetrical and choroidal unmasking is mild or absent.
3. **Cancer-related retinopathy** is also characterized by nyctalopia, restriction of peripheral visual field, arteriolar attenuation and extinguished ERG. However, the clinical course is more rapid and pigmentary changes are mild or absent.

Systemic associations

1. **Bassen–Kornzweig syndrome** is caused by deficiency in beta-lipoprotein resulting in intestinal malabsorption.

a. **Inheritance** is AR.

b. **Signs.** Spinocerebellar ataxia, ptosis and progressive external ophthalmoplegia.

c. **Diagnostic tests.** The blood film shows acanthocytosis (Fig. 18.5a).

d. **RP** develops towards the end of the first decade; the pigment clumps are often larger than in classic RP and are not confined to the equatorial region. Peripheral white dots are also common.

e. **Treatment** with vitamin E, if instituted early, may be beneficial for neurological disability.

2. **Refsum syndrome** (heredopathia atactica polyneuritiformis) is an inborn error of metabolism due to a deficiency in the enzyme phytanic acid 2-hydroxylase resulting in the accumulation of phytanic acid in the blood and body tissues.

a. **Inheritance** is AR.

b. **Signs** include polyneuropathy, cerebellar ataxia, deafness, anosmia, cardiomyopathy and ichthyosis (Fig. 18.5b).

c. **Diagnostic tests.** Lumbar puncture shows elevated CSF protein in the absence of pleocytosis (cytoalbuminous inversion).

d. **RP** develops in the second decade and is characterized by generalized 'salt-and-pepper' changes.

e. **Other ocular features** include cataract, miosis and prominent corneal nerves.

f. **Treatment,** initially with plasmapheresis and later with a phytanic acid-free diet, may prevent progression of both systemic and retinal involvement.

3. **Kearns–Sayre syndrome** is a mitochondrial cytopathy associated with mitochondrial DNA deletions (see Chapter 24).

a. **Presentation** is in the first to second decades with an insidious onset of bilateral and symmetrical ptosis and limitation of ocular movements in all directions of gaze (progressive external ophthalmoplegia).

b. **Signs** include ataxia, cardiac conduction defects, fatigue and proximal muscle weakness, deafness, diabetes and short stature.

c. **Diagnostic tests** Lumbar puncture shows increased CSF protein concentration (> 1g/l) and ECG demonstrates cardiac conduction defects.

d. **RP** is characterized by coarse pigment clumping which principally affects the central fundus.

4. **Bardet–Biedl syndrome**

a. **Inheritance** is AR.

b. **Signs** include obesity, brachydactyly and polydactyly (Fig. 18.5c), dental anomalies, hypogenitalism and renal disease. The syndrome is also associated with mental handicap, cardiac disease and hypertension. There is, however, considerable variation in the clinical picture. Intelligence can be nearly normal and polydactyly absent in some patients. Overlap with Laurence–Moon syndrome and Alström syndrome has also been observed.

c. **RP** is severe and almost 75% of patients are blind by the age of 20 years. Some patients develop a bull's eye maculopathy.

5. **Usher syndrome**

a. **Inheritance** is AR.

b. **Signs.** This is a distressing condition which accounts for about 5% of all cases of profound deafness in children, and is responsible for about half of all cases of combined deafness and blindness.

c. **RP** develops before puberty.

6. **Friedreich ataxia**

a. **Inheritance** is AR.

b. **Signs** include childhood spinocerebellar ataxia, dysarthria, cardiomyopathy, deafness and diabetes.

c. **RP** is common.

Progressive cone dystrophy

Progressive cone dystrophy comprises a heterogeneous group of rare disorders. Patients with pure cone dystrophy initially have only cone dysfunction. Those with cone-rod dystrophy have an associated but less severe rod dysfunction. However, in many patients with initially pure cone dysfunction the rod system subsequently becomes affected so that the term 'cone-rod dystrophy' is therefore more appropriate.

Diagnosis

1. **Inheritance.** Most cases are sporadic; of the remainder, the most frequent established inheritance pattern is AD, but it may also be AR or XL.

2. **Presentation** is in the first to second decades with gradual bilateral impairment of central and colour vision which may later be associated with photophobia and fine pendular nystagmus.

3. **Signs** in chronological order.
   - The fovea may be normal or exhibit non-specific granularity.
   - A golden sheen may be seen in XL disease (Fig. 18.6a).
   - Bull's-eye maculopathy is classically described but is not universal (Fig. 18.6b).
   - Mid-peripheral, 'bone-spicule' pigmentation, arteriolar attenuation and temporal disc pallor may develop (Fig. 18.6c).
   - Progressive RPE atrophy at the macula with eventual geographic atrophy.

4. **ERG** shows reduced photopic responses and flicker fusion frequency but rod responses are reserved until late (Fig. 18.7).

5. **EOG** is normal to subnormal.

6. **DA.** The cone segment is abnormal; the rod segment is initially normal but may become subnormal later.

7. **CV** shows a severe deuteran-tritan defect out of proportion to visual acuity.

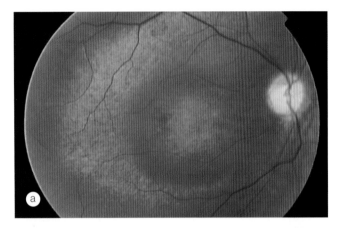

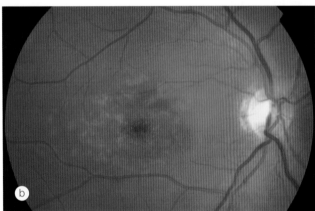

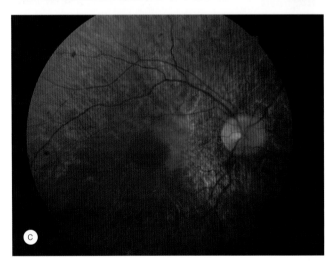

Fig. 18.6
Progressive cone dystrophy. **(a)** Golden sheen and early bull's eye maculopathy; **(b)** established bull's eye maculopathy; **(c)** mild, perivascular bone-spicule pigmentation (Courtesy of Moorfields Eye Hospital – fig. b)

Albinism

Albinism is a genetically determined, heterogeneous group of disorders of melanin synthesis in which either the eyes alone (ocular albinism) or the eyes, skin and hair (oculocutaneous

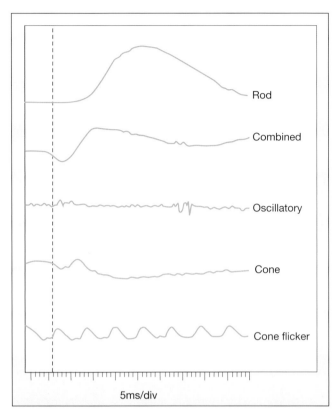

Fig. 18.7
ERG in cone dystrophy shows reduced photopic responses and flicker fusion frequency

albinism) may be affected. The latter may be either tyrosinase-positive or tyrosinase-negative. The different mutations are thought to act through a common pathway involving reduced melanin synthesis during development. Tyrosinase activity is assessed by using the hair bulb incubation test, which is reliable only after 5 years of age. Patients with albinism have an increased risk of cutaneous basal cell and squamous cell carcinoma that usually occurs before the fourth decade.

Tyrosinase-negative oculocutaneous

Tyrosinase-negative (complete) albinos are incapable of synthesizing melanin and have white hair and very pale skin throughout life with lack of melanin pigment in all ocular structures.

1. **Inheritance** is usually AR with the gene locus on 11q14-q21.
2. **Signs**
   a. **VA** is usually < 6/60 due to foveal hypoplasia.
   b. **Nystagmus** is usually pendular and horizontal. It usually increases in bright illumination and tends to lessen in severity with age.
   c. **The iris** is diaphanous and translucent (Fig. 18.8a), giving rise to a 'pink-eyed' appearance (Fig. 18.8b).

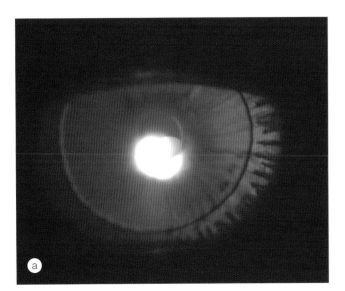

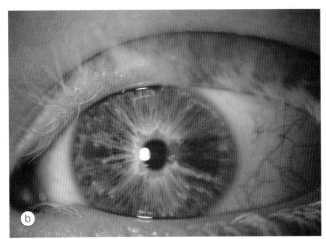

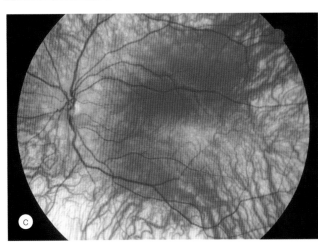

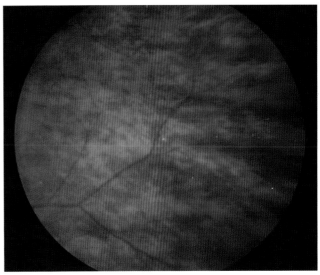

Fig. 18.9
Peripheral pigmentary changes in a carrier of ocular albinism

*d. **The fundus** lacks pigment and shows conspicuously large choroidal vessels. There is also foveal hypoplasia with absence of the foveal pit and lack of vessels forming the perimacular arcades (Fig. 18.8c). Associated optic nerve hypoplasia is uncommon.*

*e. **The optic chiasm** has fewer uncrossed nerve fibres than normal so that the majority from each eye cross to the contralateral hemisphere. This can be demonstrated by visual evoked potential.*

*f. **Other features** commonly seen include high refractive errors of various types, positive angle kappa, squint and absence of stereopsis.*

Tyrosinase-positive oculocutaneous

Tyrosinase-positive (incomplete) albinos synthesize variable amounts of melanin. The hair may be white, yellow or red and darkens with age. Skin colour is very pale at birth but usually darkens by 2 years of age.

1. **Inheritance** is usually AR with the gene locus on 15p11-q13.
2. **Signs**
   a. **VA** is usually impaired due to foveal hypoplasia.
   b. **Iris** may be blue or dark-brown with variable translucency.
   c. **Fundus** shows variable hypopigmentation.
3. **Associated syndromes**
   a. **Chediak–Higashi syndrome**
      – Inheritance is AR with the gene locus on 1q43.
      – Mild oculocutaneous albinism.
      – Leucocytic abnormalities resulting in recurrent pyogenic infections.

Fig. 18.8
Tyrosinase-negative oculocutaneous albinism. **(a)** Marked iris transillumination; **(b)** 'pink eye' appearance; **(c)** severe fundus hypopigmentation and foveal hypoplasia (Courtesy of L Merin – fig. d)

– The vast majority of patients eventually develop a lymphoproliferative syndrome (accelerated phase) characterized by fever, jaundice, hepatospleno-megaly, pancytopenia and bleeding that requires bone marrow transplantation.

– Prognosis for life is generally poor.

b. Hermansky–Pudlak syndrome is a lysosomal storage disease of the reticuloendothelial system.

– Inheritance is AR with the gene locus on 15p11-q13.

– Mild oculocutaneous albinism.

– Platelet dysfunction resulting in early bruising.

– Pulmonary fibrosis, granulomatous colitis and renal failure in some cases.

Ocular albinism

Involvement is predominantly ocular with normal skin and hair although occasionally hypopigmented skin macules may be seen.

1. **Inheritance** is usually XL and occasionally AR with the gene locus on Xp22.3.
2. **Female carriers** are asymptomatic although they may show partial iris translucency, macular stippling and mid-peripheral scattered areas of depigmentation and granularity (Fig. 18.9).
3. **Affected males** manifest hypopigmented irides and fundi.

Stargardt disease and fundus flavimaculatus

Stargardt disease (juvenile macular dystrophy) and fundus flavimaculatus are regarded as variants of the same disease, despite presenting at different times and carrying different prognoses. Inheritance is AR with the gene *ABCA4* on 1p21–22.

Fundus flavimaculatus

1. **Presentation** is in adult life, although in the absence of macular involvement the condition may be asymptomatic and discovered by chance.
2. **Signs** in chronological order:
   - Bilateral, ill-defined, yellow-white deep retinal lesions (flecks) in the posterior pole exclusively (Fig. 18.10a) or extending to the midperipheral retina (Fig. 18.10b).
   - Flecks may be round, oval, linear, semilunar or pisciform (fish-tail-like).
   - The fundus has a vermilion colour in about 50% of cases.
   - New lesions develop as older ones become ill-defined and softer.
3. **ERG.** Photopic is normal to subnormal but scotopic is normal.

Table 18.1   Other causes of bull's eye macula

1. In adults
- Chloroquine maculopathy
- Advanced Stargardt disease
- Fenestrated sheen macular dystrophy
- Benign concentric annular macular dystrophy
- Clofazimine retinopathy

2. In children
- Bardet–Biedl syndrome
- Hallervorden–Spatz syndrome
- Leber congenital amaurosis
- Lipofuscinosis
- Autosomal dominant cerebellar ataxia

4. **EOG** is subnormal.
5. **FA** shows absence of normal background choroidal fluorescence and a generalized 'dark choroid' effect due to lipofuscin deposits in the RPE. This enhances the prominence of the retinal circulation. Fresh flecks show early hypofluorescence due to blockage and late hyperfluorescence due to staining; old flecks show RPE window defects (Fig. 18.10c).
6. **Fundus autofluorescence** may be seen in some cases (Fig. 18.10d).
7. **Prognosis** is relatively good and patients may remain asymptomatic for many years unless a fleck involves the foveola or geographic atrophy (Fig. 18.10e) develops. A small minority of patients develop CNV which tends to progress rapidly and carries a very poor prognosis (Fig. 18.10f).
8. **Differential diagnosis** of retinal flecks includes dominant drusen, fundus albipunctatus, early North Carolina macular dystrophy and benign fleck retina.

Stargardt disease

Stargardt disease is the most common form of juvenile-onset macular dystrophy.

1. **Presentation** is in the first or second decades with bilateral, gradual impairment of central vision which may be out of proportion to the macular changes so that the child may be suspected of malingering.
2. **Signs**
   - The fovea may be normal or show non-specific mottling (Fig. 18.11a).
   - Oval, 'snail-slime' or 'beaten-bronze' foveal appearance, which may be surrounded by yellow-white flecks (Fig. 18.11b).
   - Geographic atrophy which may have bull's eye configuration.
3. **ERG.** Photopic is normal to subnormal but scotopic is normal.

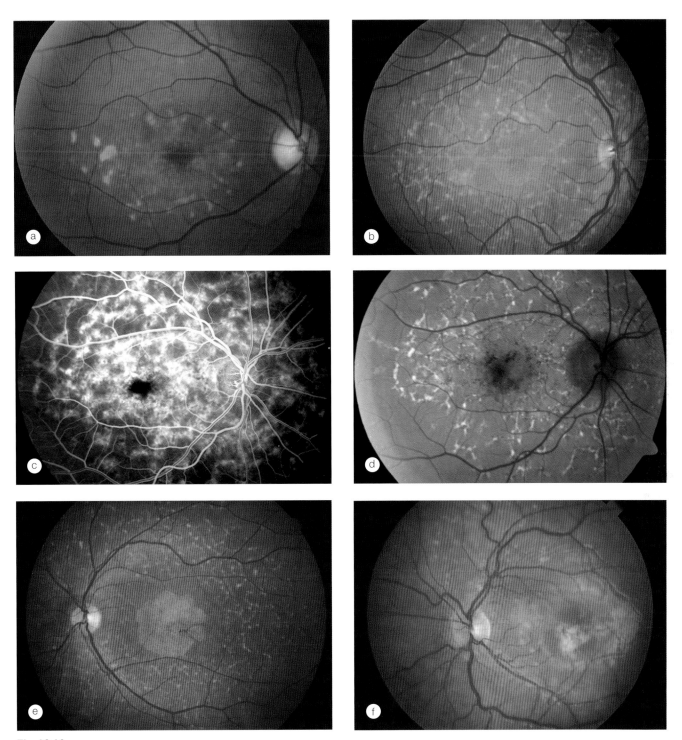

Fig. 18.10
Fundus flavimaculatus. **(a)** Macular flecks; **(b)** diffuse flecks; **(c)** FA shows dark choroid and hyperfluorescence of flecks; **(d)** autofluorescence of flecks; **(e)** geographic atrophy; **(f)** macular scar due to choroidal neovascularization (Courtesy of S Milenkovic – fig. a; P Gili – figs c and d)

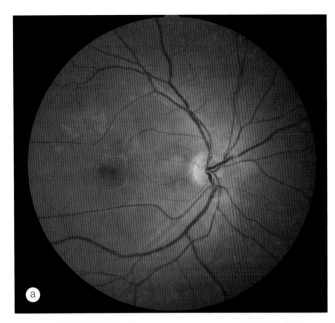

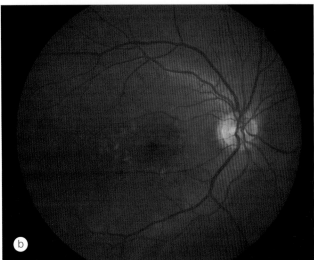

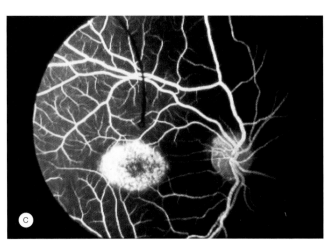

Fig. 18.11
Stargardt macular dystrophy. **(a)** Mild foveal mottling; **(b)** 'beaten-bronze' fovea surrounded by a few flecks; **(c)** FA shows disease shows a dark choroid and macular hyperfluorescence due to a window defect

4. **EOG** is subnormal in advanced cases.
5. **FA** shows a dark 'dark choroid' as in fundus flavimaculatus. Eyes with geographic atrophy show a window defect at the macula (Fig. 18.11c).
6. **Prognosis** is poor and once visual acuity drops below 6/12 it tends to decrease rapidly and stabilize at about 6/60.

Juvenile Best macular dystrophy

Juvenile Best macular (vitelliform) dystrophy is a rare condition which evolves gradually through five stages.

1. **Inheritance** is AD with variable penetrance and expressivity with the gene locus on 11q13.

2. **Signs**
   a. *Stage 0* (pre-vitelliform) is characterized by a subnormal EOG in an asymptomatic child with a normal fundus appearance.
   b. *Stage 1* is characterized by pigment mottling at the macula.
   c. *Stage 2* (vitelliform) develops in infancy or early childhood and does not usually impair visual acuity.
      – A round egg-yolk ('sunny side up') macular lesion consisting of accumulation of lipofuscin within the RPE (Fig. 18.12a and b).
      – FA shows corresponding hypofluorescence due to blockage (Fig. 18.12c). Visual acuity may be normal or slightly decreased.
      – The size of the lesions and stage of development in the two eyes may be asymmetrical and occasionally only one eye may be initially involved.
   d. *Stage 3* (pseudo-hypopyon) may occur at puberty when part of the lesion becomes absorbed (Fig. 18.12d). Occasionally, absorption continues (Fig. 18.12e) and the entire lesion becomes absorbed with little effect on vision.
   e. *Stage 4* (vitelliruptive) in which the egg yolk begins to break up ('scrambled egg') and visual acuity drops (Fig. 18.12f).
3. **EOG** is severely subnormal during all stages and in carriers with normal fundi.
4. **Prognosis** is reasonably good until the fifth decade after which visual acuity declines and some patients become legally blind due to macular scarring, CNV, geographic atrophy or, rarely, hole formation which may lead to retinal detachment.

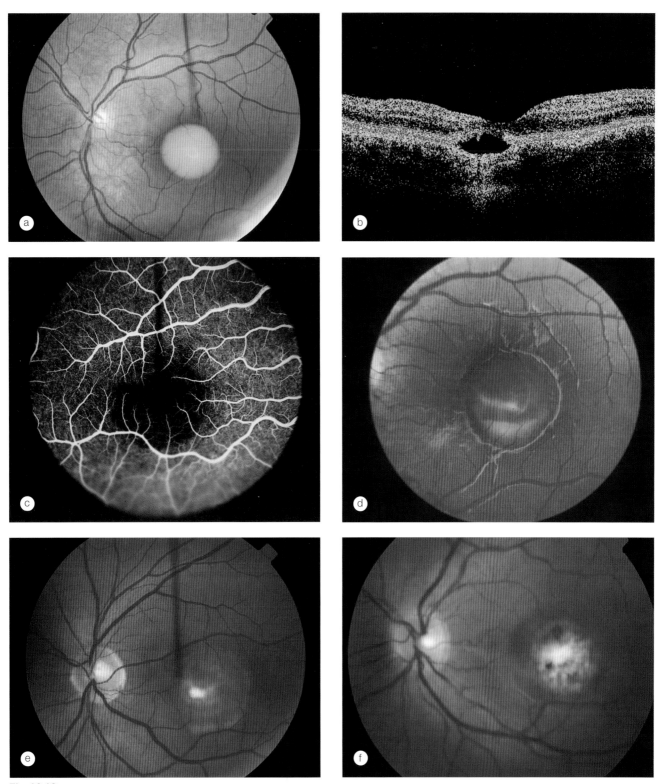

Fig. 18.12

Juvenile Best macular dystrophy. **(a)** Vitelliform stage; **(b)** OCT shows a lesion is within the RPE; **(c)** FA shows hypofluorescence due to blocked background choroidal fluorescence; **(d)** pseudo-hypopyon stage; **(e)** further absorption; **(f)** vitelliruptive stage (Courtesy of C Barry – fig. b)

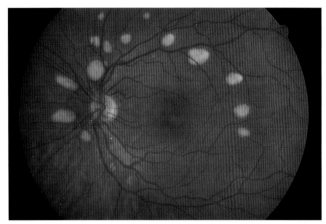

Fig. 18.13
Multifocal vitelliform disease. (Courtesy of C Barry)

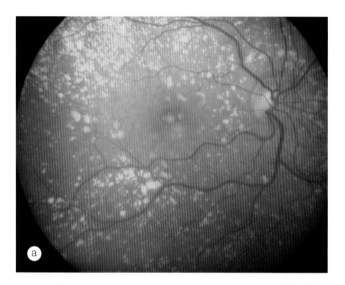

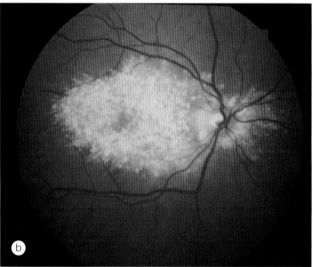

Fig. 18.14
Familial dominant drusen. **(a)** Moderately severe disease;
(b) malattia levantinese (Courtesy of Moorfields Eye Hospital –
fig. b)

NB Occasionally multifocal vitelliform lesion (Fig. 18.13), identical to those in Best disease, may become manifest in adult life and give rise to diagnostic problems. However, in these patients the EOG is normal and the family history is negative.

Familial dominant drusen

Familial drusen (Doyne honeycomb choroiditis, malattia levantinese) is thought to represent an early manifestation of age-related macular degeneration.

1. **Inheritance** is AD with full penetrance but variable expressivity and gene *EFEMP1* on 2p16-21.
2. **Signs and prognosis**
   a. *Mild disease* is characterized by a few small, discrete, innocuous, hard drusen confined to the macula that typically appear in the third decade.
   b. *Moderate disease* is characterized by large, soft drusen at the posterior pole and peripapillary region (Fig. 18.14a). The lesions appear after the third decade and are associated with normal or mild impairment of visual acuity.
   c. *Advanced disease* is uncommon and presents after the fifth decade with CNV or geographic atrophy.
   d. *Malattia leventinese* shares phenotypic overlap with familial drusen. It is characterized by numerous, small, elongated, basal laminar drusen with a spoke-like or radial distribution centered on the fovea and peripapillary area (Fig. 18.14b). Most patients are asymptomatic until the fourth or fifth decades when they may develop CNV or geographic atrophy.
3. **Investigations**
   a. *ERG* is normal.
   b. *EOG* is subnormal in patients with advanced disease.

Leber congenital amaurosis

Leber congenital amaurosis is the name ascribed to a group of inherited retinal dystrophies representing the commonest genetic cause of visual impairment in infants and children. It carries a very poor prognosis.

1. **Inheritance** is AR with the gene locus on 17p.
2. **Presentation** is with blindness at birth or shortly thereafter associated with roving eye movements.
3. **Signs** are variable and include the following:
   - The pupillary light reflexes are absent or diminished.
   - The fundi may be initially normal despite very poor vision.

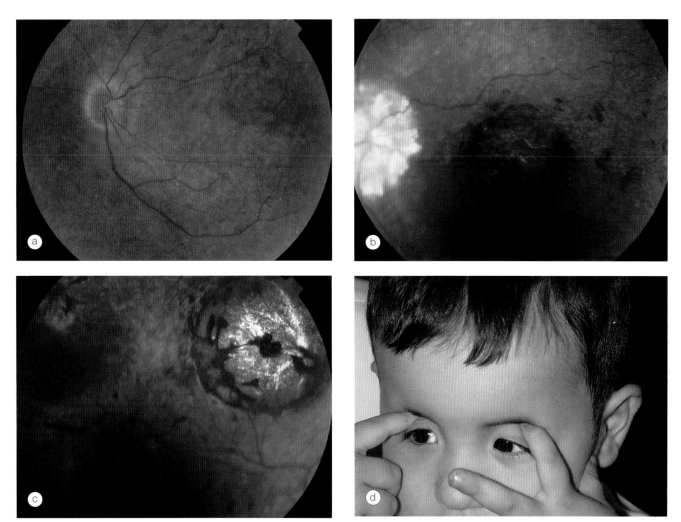

Fig. 18.15
Leber congenital amaurosis. **(a)** Mild pigmentary retinopathy; **(b)** severe macular pigmentation and optic disc drusen; **(c)** macular coloboma-like atrophy; **(d)** oculodigital syndrome (Courtesy of A Moore – figs a–c; N Rogers – fig. d)

- Patches of peripheral chorioretinal atrophy and granularity are common.
- Mild pigmentary retinopathy with arteriolar attenuation (Fig. 18.15a).
- Severe macular pigmentation (Fig. 18.15b).
- Macular coloboma-like atrophy (Fig. 18.15c).
- Other findings include disc elevation, salt-and-pepper changes, diffuse white spots and bull's eye maculopathy.
- Oculodigital syndrome in which constant rubbing of the eyes by the child causes enophthalmos as a result of resorption of orbital fat (Fig. 18.15d).
4. **Ocular associations** include strabismus, hypermetropia, keratoconus, keratoglobus and cataract.
5. **ERG** is usually non-recordable, even in early cases with normal fundi.
6. **Systemic associations** include mental handicap, deafness, epilepsy, CNS and renal anomalies, skeletal malformations and endocrine dysfunction.

Sorsby pseudo-inflammatory dystrophy

Sorsby pseudo-inflammatory macular dystrophy, also referred to as hereditary haemorrhagic macular dystrophy, is a very rare condition that results in bilateral visual loss in the fifth decade of life.

1. **Inheritance** is AD with full penetrance but variable expressivity, with the gene *TIMP3* on 22q12.13.
2. **Presentation** is in the third decade with nyctalopia or sudden visual loss due to CNV in the fifth decade.
3. **Signs** in chronological order
   - Yellow-white, confluent, drusen-like deposits along the arcades, nasal to the disc and mid-periphery (Fig. 18.16a).
   - CNV (Fig. 18.16b), and subretinal scarring (Fig. 18.16c).
   - Peripheral chorioretinal atrophy may occur by the seventh decade and result in loss of ambulatory vision.

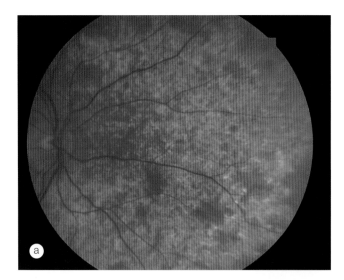

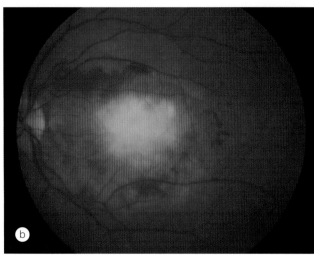

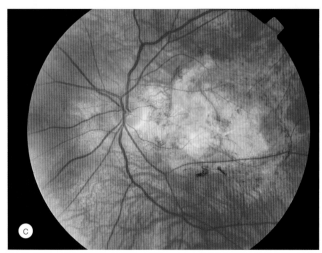

Fig. 18.16
Sorsby pseudo-inflammatory macular dystrophy. **(a)** Confluent flecks nasal to the disc; **(b)** exudative maculopathy; **(c)** subretinal scarring in end-stage disease (Courtesy of Moorfields Eye Hospital – fig. b)

4. **ERG** is initially normal but may be subnormal in late disease.
5. **Prognosis** is universally poor.

North Carolina macular dystrophy

North Carolina macular dystrophy is a very rare non-progressive condition. It was first described in families living in the mountains of North Carolina and subsequently in many unrelated families in other parts of the world.

1. **Inheritance** is AD with complete penetrance but highly variable expressivity with the gene *MCDR1* on 6q14-q16.2.
2. **Grading and prognosis**
   a. *Grade 1* is characterized by yellow-white, drusen-like peripheral (Fig. 18.17a) and macular deposits which develop during the first decade and may remain asymptomatic throughout life.
   b. *Grade 2* is characterized by deep, confluent macular deposits (Fig. 18.17b). The long-term visual prognosis is guarded because some patients develop CNV (Fig. 18.17c) and subretinal scarring.
   c. *Grade 3* is characterized by coloboma-like atrophic macular lesions (Fig.18.17d) associated with variable impairment of visual acuity.

Pattern dystrophy

Pattern dystrophy is a generic term that encompasses several retinal dystrophies exhibiting bilateral, symmetrical, yellow, orange or grey deposits at the macula that have a variety of morphologies. The lesions are associated with the accumulation of lipofuscin at the level of the RPE. Pattern dystrophy is usually present in isolation but has also been described in patients with myotonic dystrophy, Kjellin syndrome (spastic paraplegia and dementia) and pseudoxanthoma elasticum. The main phenotypes that have the following in common are: (a) *AD inheritance*, (b) *normal ERG*, (c) *bilateral symmetrical figures* and (d) *variable expressivity*.

Adult-onset foveomacular vitelliform dystrophy

In contrast to juvenile Best disease the foveal lesions are smaller, present later and do not demonstrate similar evolutionary changes.

1. **Presentation** is in the fourth to sixth decades with mild to moderate decrease of visual acuity and sometimes metamorphopsia, although often the condition is discovered by chance.
2. **Signs**
   • Bilateral, symmetrical, round or oval, slightly elevated, yellowish subfoveal deposits, about one-third of a disc

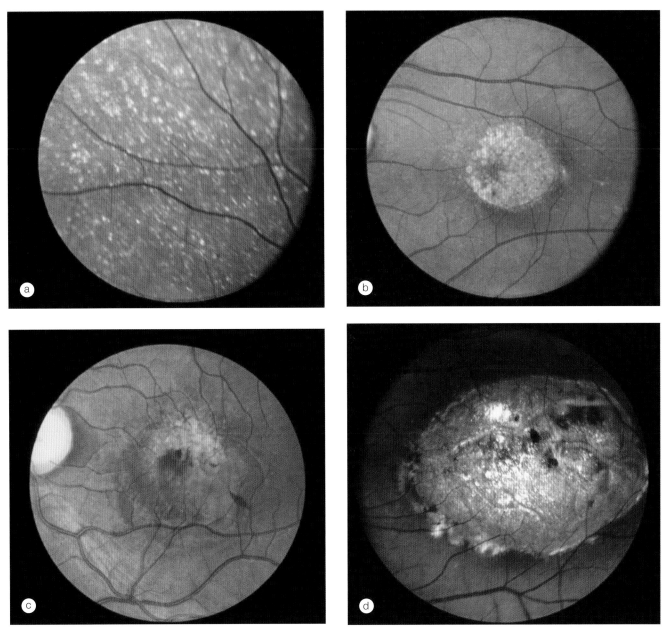

Fig. 18.17
North Carolina macular dystrophy. **(a)** Peripheral flecks; **(b)** confluent macular flecks; **(c)** early exudative maculopathy; **(d)** coloboma-like macular lesion (Courtesy of P Morse)

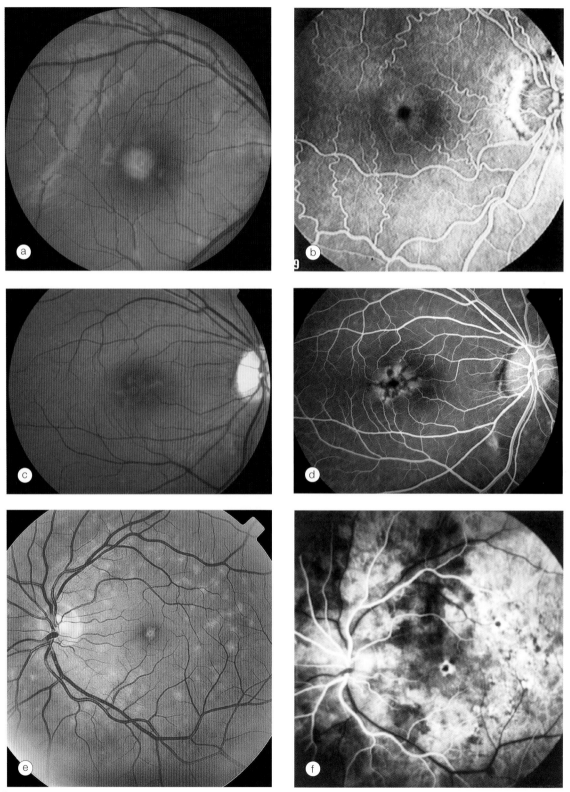

Fig. 18.18
Pattern dystrophy. **(a)** Adult-onset foveomacular vitelliform dystrophy; **(b)** FA shows central hypofluorescence with a hyperfluorescent halo; **(c)** butterfly dystrophy; **(d)** FA shows non-fluorescence of the lesions outlined by hyperfluorescence; **(e)** multifocal pattern dystrophy simulating fundus flavimaculatus; **(f)** FA shows hyperfluorescence of flecks but the choroid is not dark (Courtesy of C Barry – fig. a; Moorfields Eye Hospital – figs c and d; S Milewski – figs e and f)

diameter in size, often centered by a pigmented spot (Fig. 18.18a).

* Associated macular drusen may be seen in some cases.

3. **FA** shows central hypofluorescence surrounded by a small irregular hyperfluorescent ring (Fig. 18.18b).

4. **Prognosis** is good in the majority of cases, although some eyes may develop visual loss due to progressive foveal thinning and the possible evolution to a full-thickness macular hole.

Butterfly-shaped macular dystrophy

1. **Presentation** is in the second to third decades usually by chance and occasionally with mild impairment of central vision.

2. **Signs**
   * Yellow pigment at the fovea arranged in a triradiate manner (Fig. 18.18c).
   * Peripheral pigmentary stippling may be present.
   * Atrophic maculopathy may occasionally develop with time.

3. **FA** shows non-fluorescence of the lesions outlined by hyperfluorescence (Fig. 18.18d).

4. **Prognosis** is usually good although atrophic maculopathy may occasionally develop.

Multifocal pattern dystrophy simulating fundus flavimaculatus

1. **Presentation** is in the fourth decade with mild impairment of central vision.

2. **Signs** multiple, widely-scattered, irregular, yellow lesions

that may be similar to those seen in fundus flavimaculatus (Fig. 18.18e).

3. **FA** shows hyperfluorescence of flecks but the choroid is not dark (Fig.18.18f).

4. **Prognosis** is good.

Alport syndrome

Alport syndrome is a rare abnormality of glomerular basement membrane caused by mutations in several different genes, all of which encode particular forms of type IV collagen – a major component of basement membrane. It is characterized by chronic renal failure, often associated with sensorineural deafness.

1. **Inheritance** is XLD.

2. **Signs**
   * Scattered, yellowish, punctate flecks in the perimacular area with normal visual acuity (Fig. 18.19a).
   * Larger flecks, some of which may become confluent, in the periphery (Fig. 18.19b).

3. **ERG** is normal.

4. **Ocular associations** are anterior lenticonus and occasionally posterior polymorphous corneal dystrophy.

5. **Prognosis** for vision is excellent.

Benign familial flecked retina

Benign familial flecked retina is a very rare disorder which is asymptomatic and therefore usually discovered by chance.

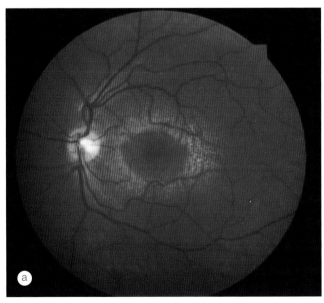
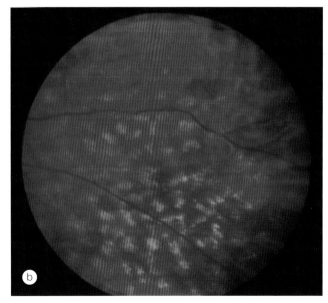

Fig. 18.19
Alport syndrome. **(a)** Perimacular flecks; **(b)** peripheral flecks (Courtesy of J Govan)

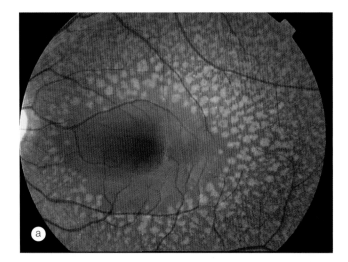

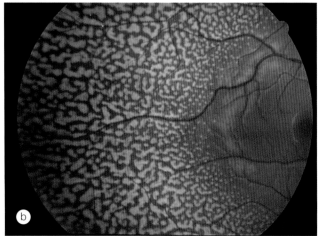

Fig. 18.20
Benign familial fleck retina. **(a)** Central flecks sparing the fovea;
(b) peripheral flecks (Courtesy of T Isaacs)

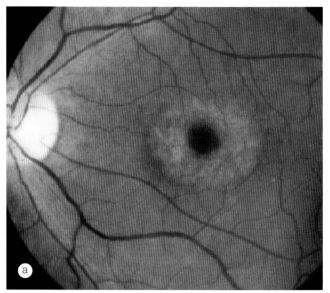

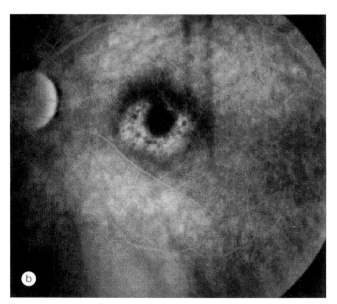

Fig. 18.21
Benign concentric annular macular dystrophy. **(a)** Bull's eye
maculopathy; **(b)** FA shows an annular RPE window defect
(Courtesy of S Milewski)

1. **Inheritance** is AR.
2. **Signs.** Widespread, discrete, yellow-white, polymorphous shapes which spare the fovea (Fig. 18.20a) and extend to the far periphery (Fig. 18.20b).
3. **ERG** is normal.
4. **Prognosis** is excellent.

Benign concentric annular macular dystrophy

1. **Inheritance** is AD.
2. **Presentation** is in adult life with very mild impairment of central vision.
3. **Signs.** Bull's-eye maculopathy associated with slight vascular attenuation but a normal disc (Fig. 18.21a).
4. **VF** shows a paracentral ring scotoma.
5. **FA** shows an annular RPE window defect (Fig. 18.21b).
6. **Prognosis** is good in the majority or cases although a minority develop progressive loss of visual acuity and nyctalopia.

Dominant macular oedema

1. **Inheritance** is AD with the gene locus on 7q.
2. **Presentation** is in the first to second decades with gradual impairment of central vision.

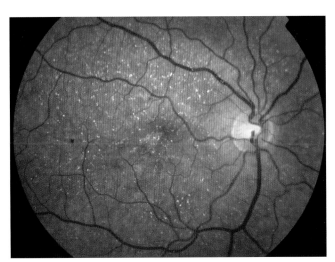

Fig. 18.22
Bietti crystalline dystrophy (Courtesy of Moorfields Eye Hospital)

3. **Signs.** Bilateral CMO.
4. **FA** shows a flower-petal pattern of leakage at the fovea.
5. **Prognosis** is poor because the oedema does not respond to treatment with systemic acetazolamide and geographic atrophy inevitably ensues.

Bietti crystalline dystrophy

Bietti crystalline dystrophy is characterized by deposition of crystals in the retina and the superficial cornea. The latter are not present in all cases of crystalline retinopathy.

1. **Inheritance** is AR with the gene locus on 4q36.
2. **Presentation** is in the third decade with slowly progressive visual loss.
3. **Signs** in chronological order:
   - Numerous fine, glistening, yellow-white crystals, located in all layers of the retina, scattered throughout the posterior fundus (Fig. 18.22).
   - Localized atrophy of the RPE and choriocapillaris at the macula.
   - Diffuse atrophy of the choriocapillaris with a decrease in size and number of the crystals.
   - Gradual confluence and expansion of the atrophic areas into the retinal periphery but normal optic discs and retinal vasculature.
4. **ERG** is subnormal.
5. **Prognosis** is variable because the rate of disease progression differs in individual cases.

Familial internal limiting membrane dystrophy

1. **Inheritance** is AD.

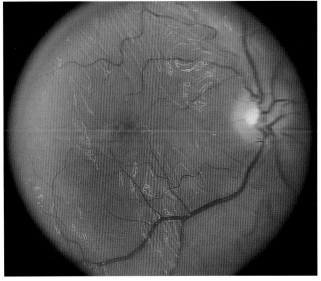

Fig. 18.23
Familial internal limiting membrane dystrophy (Courtesy of J Donald M Gass from *Stereoscopic Atlas of Macular Diseases*, Mosby 1997)

2. **Presentation** is in the third to fourth decades with visual loss.
3. **Signs.** The posterior pole manifests a glistening inner retinal surface (Fig. 18.23).
4. **ERG** shows a selective diminution of the b-wave.
5. **Prognosis** is poor with visual loss occurring by the sixth decade due to the development of retinoschisis, retinal oedema and retinal folds.

Occult macular dystrophy

Occult macular dystrophy may give rise to diagnostic problems in patients with unexplained loss of central vision, particularly in the presence of coincident ocular conditions.

1. **Presentation** is at any time between the third and seventh decades with bilateral progressive loss of visual acuity.
2. **Signs.** The fundi are normal.
3. **ERG:** full-field is normal but focal cone ERG and multifocal ERG are abnormal.
4. **FA** is normal.
5. **OCT** shows decreased foveal thickness.
6. **Prognosis** is poor.

Enhanced S-cone syndrome

The human retina has three cone photoreceptor types: short-wave sensitivity (S), middle-wave sensitivity (M) and long-wave sensitivity (L). Most inherited retinal dystrophies exhibit progressive attenuation of rods and all classes of cones. However, enhanced S-cone syndrome is unique because it is characterized by hyperfunction of S-cones and severe impairment of M and L cones, and non-recordable rod functions.

1. **Inheritance** is AR.
2. **Presentation** is with nyctalopia in childhood.
3. **Signs**
   - Pigmentary changes along the vascular arcades.
   - Cystoid maculopathy without fluorescein leakage.
4. **Prognosis** is guarded because some eyes develop CNV.

Late-onset retinal degeneration

1. **Inheritance** is AD.
2. **Presentation** is with nyctalopia in the sixth decade followed by progressive loss of central and peripheral vision over ensuing decades.
3. **Signs**
   - Normal fundus.
   - Clusters of fine yellow-white dots in the mid-periphery.
   - Pigmentary retinopathy and chorioretinal atrophy.
   - Atrophic maculopathy and optic atrophy.
4. **ERG** is initially normal; end-stage disease shows only reduced amplitude.
5. **Prognosis** is very poor.

Sjögren–Larsson syndrome

Sjögren–Larsson syndrome is a neurocutaneous disorder characterized by congenital ichthyosis, spasticity, convulsions and mental retardation with reduced life expectancy. The basic metabolic defect is deficient activity of fatty aldehyde dehydrogenase.

1. **Inheritance** is AR.
2. **Presentation** is with photophobia and poor vision.
3. **Signs**
   - Bilateral, glistening yellow-white crystalline deposits at the macula which appear during the first two years of life and become more numerous with time.
   - The presence of the macular lesions is thought to be a cardinal and perhaps pathognomonic sign of the syndrome.
4. **Visually evoked potential** is abnormal.

Cherry-red spot at macula

Pathogenesis

The cherry-red spot at the macula (Fig. 18.24) is a clinical sign seen in the context of thickening and loss of

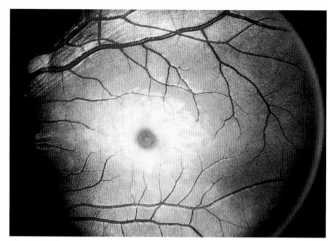

Fig. 18.24
Cherry-red spot at the macula

transparency of the retina at the posterior pole. The fovea, being the thinnest part of the retina and devoid of ganglion cells, retains relative transparency, allowing persistent transmission of the underlying highly vascular choroidal hue. This striking retinal lesion, commonly seen in occlusion of the central retinal artery, is additionally a feature of a rare group of inherited metabolic diseases, the sphingolipidoses. These are characterized by the progressive intracellular accretion of excessive quantities of certain glycolipids and phospholipids in various tissues of the body, including the retina. The lipids accumulate in the ganglion cell layer of the retina, giving the retina a white appearance. As ganglion cells are absent at the foveola, this area retains relative transparency and contrasts with the surrounding opaque retina. With the passage of time the ganglion cells die and the spot becomes less evident. The late stage of the disease is characterized by degeneration of the retinal nerve fibre layer and consecutive optic atrophy.

Systemic associations

1. **Tay–Sachs disease** (Gm2 gangliosidosis type 1), also known as infantile amaurotic familial idiocy, is an AR disease with onset during the first year of life, usually ending in death before the age of 2 years. It typically affects European Jews and is characterized by progressive neurological disease and eventual blindness. A cherry-red spot is present in about 90% of cases.
2. **Niemann–Pick disease** is divided on a clinical and chemical basis into the following four groups:
   a. *Group A* with severe early CNS deterioration.
   b. *Group B* with normal CNS function.
   c. *Group C* with moderate CNS involvement and a slow course.
   d. *Group D* with a late onset and eventual severe CNS involvement.

The incidence of a cherry-red spot is lower than in Tay–Sachs disease.

3. **Sandhoff disease** (Gm2 gangliosidosis type 2) is almost identical to Tay–Sachs disease.
4. **Generalized gangliosidosis** (Gm1 gangliosidosis type 1) is characterized by hypoactivity, oedema of the face and extremities, and skeletal anomalies from birth.
5. **Sialidosis types 1 and 2** (cherry-red spot myoclonus syndrome) are characterized by myoclonic jerks, pain in the limbs and unsteadiness. A cherry-red spot may be the initial finding.

Congenital stationary night blindness

Congenital stationary night blindness refers to a group of disorders characterized by infantile onset nyctalopia and non-progressive retinal dysfunction. The fundus appearance may be normal or abnormal.

Normal fundus

1. **AD congenital nyctalopia** (Nougaret type) is associated with a slightly impaired cone ERG and subnormal rod ERG function.
2. **AD stationary nyctalopia without myopia** (Riggs type) is associated with a normal cone ERG.
3. **AR or XL congenital nyctalopia with myopia** (Schubert–Bornschein type) is associated with a negative ERG in the maximal response, where there is selective loss of the b-wave.

Abnormal fundus

1. **Oguchi disease** is an AR condition in which the fundus has an unusual golden-yellow colour in the light-adapted state (Fig. 18.25a) which becomes normal after prolonged dark adaptation (Mizuo phenomenon) (Fig 18.25b). Rod function is absent after 30 minutes of dark adaptation but recovers to a near-normal level after a long period of dark adaptation.
2. **Fundus albipunctatus** is an AR condition characterized by a multitude of tiny yellow-white spots at the posterior pole, sparing the fovea (Fig. 18.26a), and extending to the periphery (Fig. 18.26b). The retinal blood vessels, optic disc, peripheral fields and visual acuity remain normal. The ERG and EOG may be abnormal when tested routinely but revert to normal on prolonged dark adaptation.

Congenital monochromatism

Complete rod monochromatism

1. **Inheritance** is AR.
2. **Signs**
   - VA is 6/60.
   - Macula usually appears normal but may be hypoplastic.
   - Congenital nystagmus and photophobia.
3. **Investigations**
4. **ERG.** Photopic is abnormal and flicker fusion frequency is reduced.

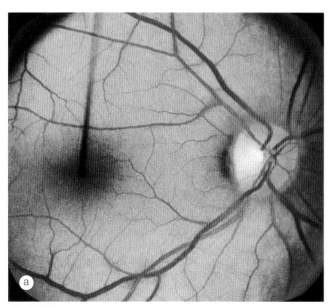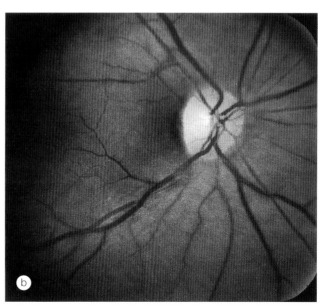

Fig. 18.25
Mizuo phenomenon in Oguchi disease. **(a)** In the light-adapted state; **(b)** in the dark-adapted state (Courtesy of J Donald M Gass, from *Stereoscopic Atlas of Macular Disease*, Mosby, 1997)

5. CV is totally absent so that all colours appear as shades of grey.

Incomplete rod monochromatism

1. Inheritance is AR or XL.
2. Signs
- VA is 6/12–6/24.
- Macula is usually normal.
- Nystagmus and photophobia may be present.

3. Investigations
4. ERG. Abnormal photopic and normal scotopic.
5. CV. Some colour vision may be present.

Cone monochromatism

1. Inheritance is uncertain.
2. Signs
- VA is 6/6–6/9.
- Normal macula.
- Nystagmus and photophobia are absent.

3. Investigations
4. ERG is normal.
5. CV is totally absent.

VITREORETINOPATHIES

Congenital retinoschisis

Congenital retinoschisis is characterized by bilateral maculopathy, with associated peripheral retinoschisis in 50% of patients. The basic defect is in the Müller cells, causing splitting of the retinal nerve fibre layer from the rest of the sensory retina. This differs from acquired (senile) retinoschisis in which splitting occurs at the outer plexiform layer.

1. **Inheritance** is XL with the implicated gene designated *RS1*.
2. **Presentation** is between the ages of 5 and 10 years with reading difficulties due to maculopathy. Less frequently the disease presents in infancy with squint or nystagmus associated with advanced peripheral retinoschisis, often with vitreous haemorrhage.
3. **Foveal schisis** is characterized by tiny cystoid spaces with a 'bicycle-wheel' pattern of radial striae (Fig. 18.27a) more apparent when examined under red-free light. Over time the radial folds become less evident, leaving a blunted foveal reflex.
4. **Peripheral schisis** predominantly involves the inferotemporal quadrant. It does not extend but may undergo the following secondary changes:
   - The inner layer, which consists only of the internal limiting membrane and the retinal nerve fibre layer, may develop oval defects (Fig. 18.27b).

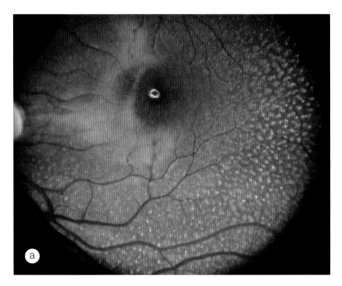

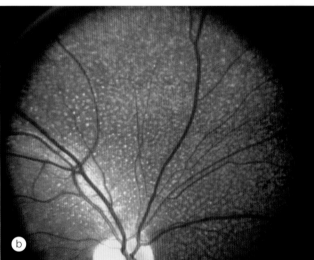

Fig. 18.26
Fundus albipunctatus. **(a)** Posterior pole flecks sparing the fovea; **(b)** peripheral flecks

- In extreme cases, the defects coalesce, leaving only retinal blood vessels floating in the vitreous ('vitreous veils') (Fig. 18.27c).
- Peripheral dendritiform lesions consisting of occluded and sheathed vessels (Fig. 18.27d).
- Other signs include nasal dragging of retinal vessels, retinal flecks, subretinal exudates and neovascularization.

5. **Complications** include vitreous and intra-schisis haemorrhage, and retinal detachment.
6. **OCT** is useful for documenting progression of maculopathy (Fig. 18.27e).
7. **ERG** is normal in eyes with isolated maculopathy. Eyes with peripheral schisis show a characteristic selective

decrease in amplitude of the b-wave as compared with the a-wave on scotopic and photopic testing (Fig. 18.28).

8. **EOG** is normal in eyes with isolated maculopathy but subnormal in eyes with advanced peripheral lesions.

9. **FA** of maculopathy may show mild window defects but no leakage.

10. **VF** in eyes with peripheral schisis shows corresponding absolute defects.

11. **Prognosis** is poor due to progressive maculopathy. Visual acuity deteriorates during the first two decades and may remain stable until the fifth or sixth decades when it further deteriorates. Patients with peripheral schisis may have sudden visual loss at any time due to haemorrhage or retinal detachment.

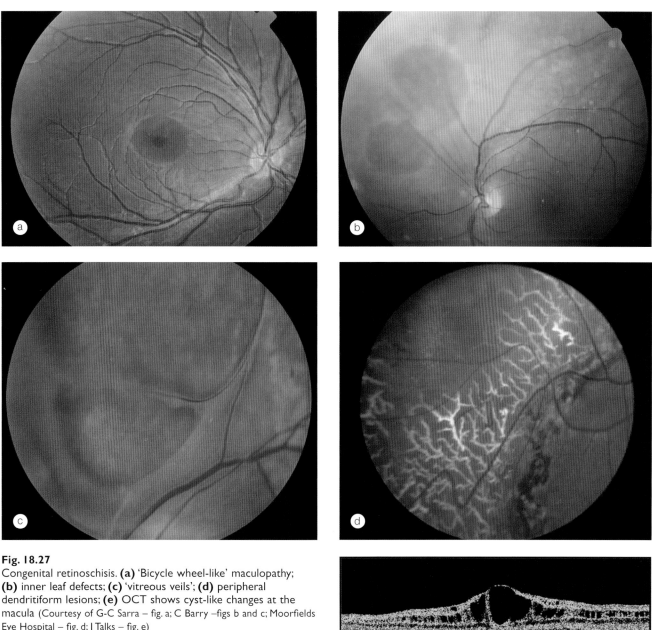

Fig. 18.27
Congenital retinoschisis. **(a)** 'Bicycle wheel-like' maculopathy; **(b)** inner leaf defects; **(c)** 'vitreous veils'; **(d)** peripheral dendritiform lesions; **(e)** OCT shows cyst-like changes at the macula (Courtesy of G-C Sarra – fig. a; C Barry –figs b and c; Moorfields Eye Hospital – fig. d; J Talks – fig. e)

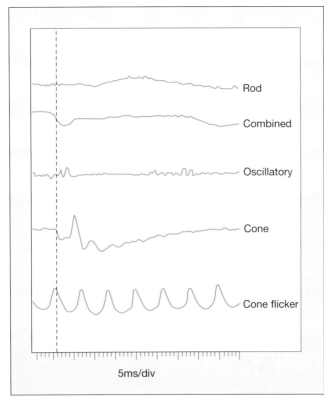

Fig. 18.28
ERG in peripheral congenital retinoschisis shows selective decrease in the b-wave amplitude

Stickler syndrome

Stickler syndrome (hereditary arthro-ophthalmopathy) is a disorder of collagen connective tissue, resulting in abnormal vitreous, myopia, and variable orofacial abnormalities, deafness and arthropathy (see Chapter 24). Inheritance is AD with complete penetrance but variable expressivity. Stickler syndrome is the commonest inherited cause of retinal detachment in children.

1. Signs
- An optically empty central vitreous cavity due to liquefaction and syneresis (contraction) associated with circumferential, equatorial, membranes extending a short way into the vitreous cavity (Fig. 18.29a).
- Radial lattice-like degeneration associated with RPE hyperplasia, vascular sheathing and sclerosis (Fig. 18.29b).

2. Complications. Retinal detachment (Fig. 18.29c) develops in approximately 30% in the first decade of life, often as a result of multiple or giant tears that may involve both eyes. Because the prognosis is poor, patients should be examined regularly and retinal breaks treated prophylactically.

3. Associations

a. Early-onset myopia, often severe but rarely progressive, is present in about 80% of cases. The remainder of patients may be either emmetropic of hypermetropic.

b. Presenile cataract characterized by frequently non-progressive peripheral cortical 'wedge' of 'fleck' opacities is very common.

c. Ectopia lentis in about 10%.

d. Glaucoma, which may be associated with a congenital angle anomaly characterized by prominent iris processes and hypoplasia of the iris root with anterior stromal iris defects, is uncommon.

Wagner syndrome

1. Inheritance is AD with the gene locus on 5q13-14.

2. Signs
- Low myopia (−3.00 or less).
- Vitreous liquefaction with complete absence of normal scaffolding (Fig. 18.30a).
- Preretinal, equatorial, avascular greyish-white membranes (Fig. 18.30b).
- Progressive chorioretinal atrophy (18.30c).

3. FA shows non-perfusion due to gross loss of the choriocapillaris (Fig. 18.30d).

4. Complications include cortical cataracts and retinal detachment in about 50% of patients by the sixth decade.

Familial exudative vitreoretinopathy

Familial exudative vitreoretinopathy (Criswick–Schepens syndrome) is a slowly progressive condition characterized by failure of vascularization of the temporal retinal periphery, similar to that seen in retinopathy of prematurity, but not associated with low birth weight and prematurity.

1. Inheritance is AD and rarely XLR, with high penetrance and variable expressivity.

2. Presentation is in late childhood.

3. Signs
- Vitreous degeneration and peripheral vitreoretinal attachments associated with areas of 'white without pressure'.
- Peripheral vascular tortuosity and telangiectasis (Fig. 18.31a).
- Fibrovascular proliferation and vitreoretinal traction resulting in ridge formation (Fig. 18.31b).
- Peripheral fibrovascular proliferation (Fig. 18.31c).
- Vascular straightening and temporal dragging of the macula and disc (Fig. 18.31d).

4. Complications include tractional retinal detachment and massive subretinal exudation (Fig. 18.31e).

5. FA shows peripheral retinal non-perfusion and highlights straightening of blood vessels (Fig. 18.31f).

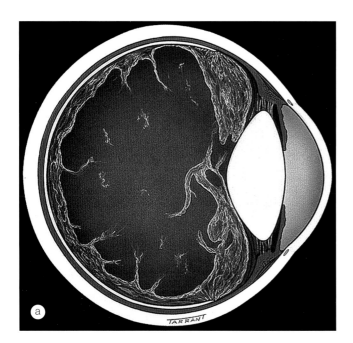

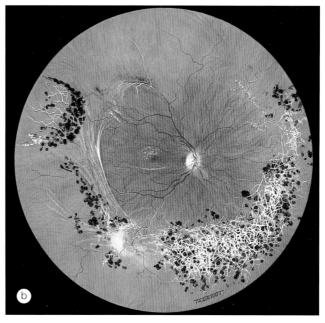

Fig. 18.29
Stickler syndrome. **(a)** Vitreous liquefaction and membranes; **(b)** radial lattice degeneration and pigmentary changes; **(c)** total retinal detachment associated with a giant retinal tear

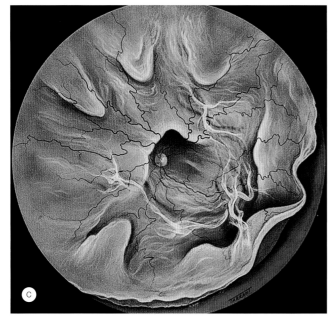

6. **Prognosis** is poor although in some cases peripheral retinal laser photocoagulation or cryotherapy may be beneficial. Vitreoretinal surgery for retinal detachment, whilst difficult, may be successful in selected cases.

Favre–Goldmann disease

Favre–Goldmann syndrome manifests features of retinoschisis and pigmentary retinopathy.

1. **Inheritance** is AR.
2. **Presentation** is in childhood with defective vision in bright light (hemeralopia).
3. **Signs**
   - Vitreous syneresis but the cavity is not optically 'empty'.
   - Peripheral and central congenital retinoschisis.
   - Atypical peripheral pigmentary dystrophy and white, arborescent retinal vessels.
   - Arteriolar attenuation and waxy disc pallor.

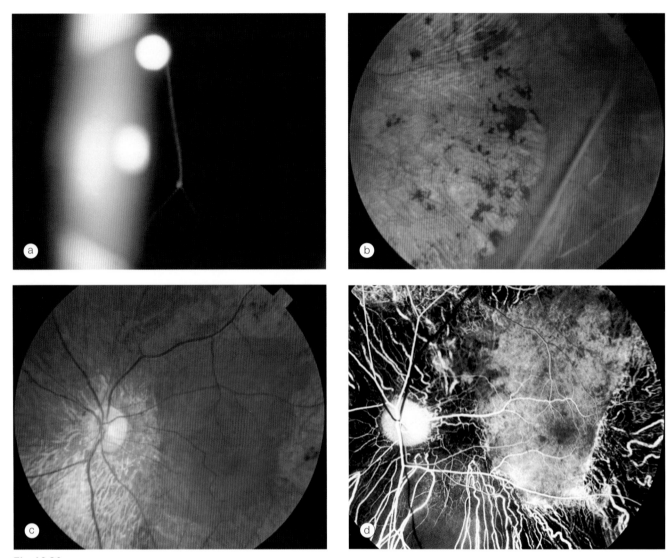

Fig. 18.30
Wagner syndrome. **(a)** Vitreous liquefaction and complete loss of normal scaffolding; **(b)** peripheral chorioretinal atrophy and pre-retinal membrane; **(c)** progressive chorioretinal atrophy; **(d)** FA shows gross loss of the choriocapillaris (Courtesy of E Messmer)

- Macular oedema and cataract are common.
4. **ERG** is markedly abnormal or extinguished. Some patients demonstrate relatively enhanced S-cone function identical to that found in the enhanced S-cone syndrome.
5. **Prognosis** is poor.

Snowflake vitreoretinal degeneration

1. **Inheritance** is AD.
2. **Signs** (Fig. 18.32)
   - Stage 1: extensive areas of 'white-without-pressure' in patients under the age of 15 years.
   - Stage 2: snowflake-like, yellow-white spots in areas of 'white-with-pressure' in patients between 15 and 25 years.
   - Stage 3: vascular sheathing and pigmentation posterior to the area of snowflake degeneration in patients between 25 and 50 years.
   - Stage 4: increased pigmentation, gross vascular attenuation, areas of chorioretinal atrophy and less apparent snowflakes in patients over the age of 60 years.
3. **Associations** include myopia, vitreous fibrillary degeneration and liquefaction.
4. **Complications** include retinal break formation, retinal detachment and presenile cataract.
5. **ERG** shows low scotopic b-wave amplitude.
6. **Prognosis** is usually good.

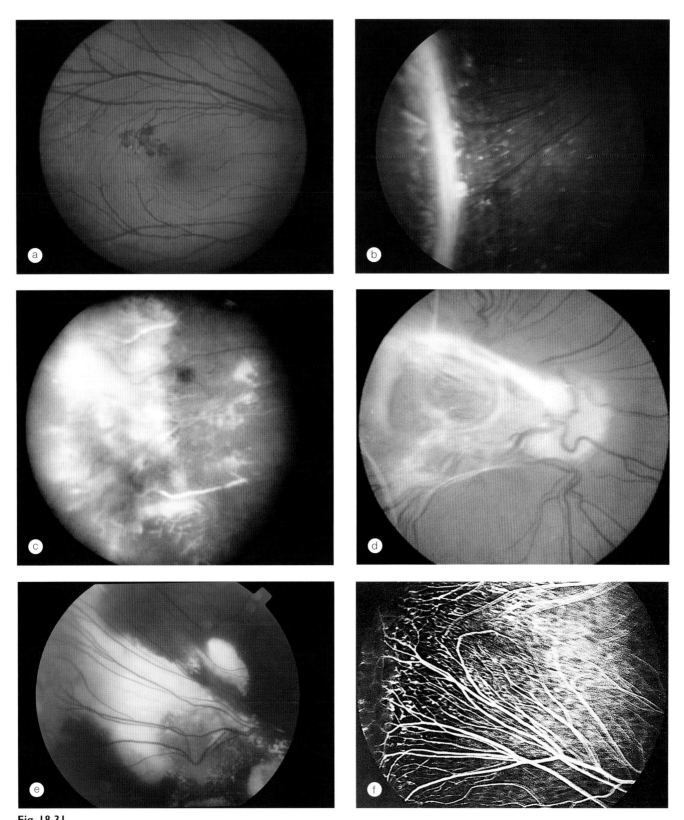

Fig. 18.31
Familial exudative vitreoretinopathy. **(a)** Peripheral retinal telangiectasis; **(b)** fibrovascular ridge; **(c)** fibrovascular proliferation; **(d)** 'dragging' of the disc and macula; **(e)** subretinal exudation; **(f)** FA shows peripheral non-perfusion with abrupt vascular termination and straightening (Courtesy of C Hoyng – fig. e)

Erosive vitreoretinopathy

1. **Inheritance** is AD with the gene locus on 5q13-14.
2. **Presentation** is in early childhood.
3. **Signs**
   - Vitreous syneresis and multiple foci of vitreoretinal traction.
   - Thinning of the RPE and progressive choroidal atrophy which may eventually involve the macula.
   - Attenuation of retinal vessels and occasionally bone spicule pigmentary changes.
4. **Complications.** Retinal detachment, which is often bilateral and due to giant tears, develops in 70% of cases.
5. **Prognosis** is guarded because retinal detachment may be difficult to treat.

Dominant neovascular inflammatory vitreoretinopathy

1. **Inheritance** is AD.
2. **Presentation** is in the second to third decade with vitreous floaters.
3. **Signs**
   - Uveitis.
   - Pigmentary retinal degeneration.
   - Peripheral vascular closure and neovascularization.
4. **Complications** include vitreous haemorrhage, tractional retinal detachment and CMO.
5. **ERG** shows selective loss of b-wave amplitude.
6. **Prognosis** is guarded. Peripheral retinal photocoagulation and vitreous surgery may be required to preserve vision.

Dominant vitreoretinochoroidopathy

1. **Inheritance** is AD.
2. **Presentation** is in adult life if symptomatic, but frequently the condition is discovered by chance.
3. **Signs**
   - An encircling band of pigmentary disturbance between the ora serrata and equator with a sharply defined posterior border.
   - Within the band there is arteriolar attenuation, neovascularization, punctate white opacities and later chorioretinal atrophy.
4. **Complications,** which are uncommon, include CMO and occasionally vitreous haemorrhage.
5. **ERG** is subnormal.
6. **Prognosis** is good.

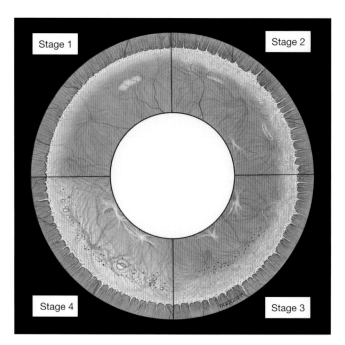

Fig. 18.32
Snowflake degeneration

CHOROIDAL DYSTROPHIES

Choroideremia

Choroideremia is a progressive, diffuse degeneration of the choroid, RPE and retinal photoreceptors.

1. **Inheritance** is XLR with the gene locus on Xq21. This has the following implications:
   - All daughters of affected fathers will be carriers.
   - Half of the sons of female carriers will develop the disease.
   - Half of the daughters of female carriers will also be carriers.
   - An affected male cannot transmit the gene to his sons.

   NB Female carriers show mild, usually innocuous, patchy peripheral atrophy and mottling of the RPE. Visual acuity, peripheral fields and ERG are usually normal although some carriers may complain of nyctalopia.

2. **Presentation** is in the first decade with nyctalopia.
3. **Signs**

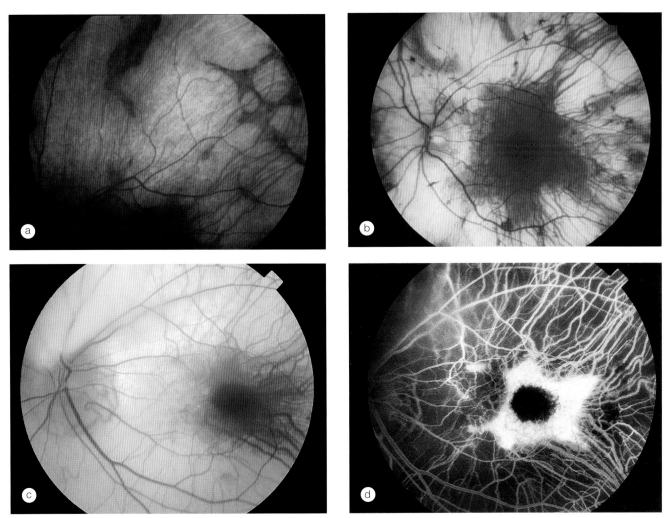

Fig. 18.33
Choroideremia. **(a)** Mid-peripheral atrophy; **(b)** advanced changes; **(c)** preservation of the fovea in end-stage disease; **(d)** FA shows filling of the retinal and large choroidal vessels but not the choriocapillaris; the intact fovea is hypofluorescent and is surrounded by hyperfluorescence due to a window defect (Courtesy of K Jordan – fig. a; K Nischal – fig. b; S Milewski – figs c and d)

- Mid-peripheral diffuse atrophy of the choriocapillaris and RPE with preservation of the intermediate and large choroidal vessels (Fig. 18.33a).
- Progressive atrophy of intermediate and large choroidal vessels rendering visible the underlying sclera (Fig. 18.33b).
- In contrast to primary retinal dystrophies, the fovea is spared until late (Fig. 18.33c) and the optic disc and retinal blood vessels remain relatively normal.

4. **ERG.** Scotopic is non-recordable but photopic is severely subnormal.
5. **FA** shows filling of the retinal and large choroidal vessels but not of the choriocapillaris. The intact fovea is hypofluorescent and is surrounded by hyperfluorescence due to a window defect (Fig. 18.33d).
6. **Prognosis** is very poor and although most patients retain useful vision until the sixth decade, very severe visual loss occurs thereafter.

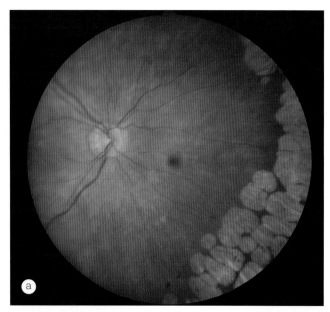

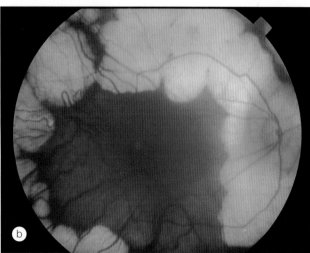

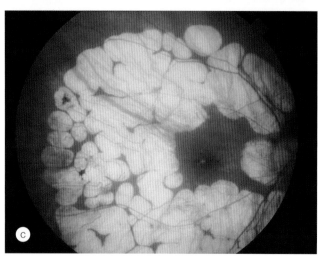

Fig. 18.34
Gyrate atrophy. **(a)** Mid-peripheral atrophic patches; **(b)** coalescence and spread; **(c)** preservation of the fovea in end-stage disease

Gyrate atrophy

1. **Inheritance** is AR.
2. **Metabolic defect** is a mutation of the gene encoding the main ornithine degradation enzyme, ornithine amino-transferase. Deficiency of the enzyme leads to elevated ornithine levels in the plasma, urine, CSF and aqueous humour.
3. **Presentation** is in the first decade with axial myopia and reduction of peripheral vision often associated with nyctalopia.
4. **Signs**
   • Peripheral patches of chorioretinal atrophy and vitreous degeneration (Fig. 18.34a).
   • Coalescence of atrophic areas.
   • Gradual peripheral and central spread (Fig. 18.34b), sparing the fovea (Fig. 18.34c) till late.
   • Areas of pigmentary change associated with numerous elongated glittering crystals.
   • Extreme attenuation of retinal blood vessels.
5. **ERG** is subnormal and later extinguished.
6. **Treatment.** There are two clinically different subtypes of gyrate atrophy based on response to pyridoxine (vitamin B6), which may normalize plasma and urinary ornithine levels. Patients responsive to vitamin B6 generally have a less severe and more slowly progressive clinical course than those who are not. Reduction in ornithine levels with an arginine-restricted diet is also beneficial.
7. **Prognosis** is generally poor with legal blindness occurring in the fourth to sixth decades from geographic atrophy, although vision may fail earlier due to cataract, CMO or epiretinal membrane formation.

Central areolar choroidal dystrophy

1. **Inheritance** is AD with the gene locus on 17p, although sporadic cases have been described.
2. **Presentation** is in the third to fourth decades with gradual impairment of central vision.
3. **Signs** in chronological order:
   • Non-specific foveal granularity.
   • Circumscribed RPE atrophy and loss of the chorio-capillaris at the macula (Fig. 18.35a).
   • Slowly expanding geographic atrophy with prominence of large choroidal vessels (Fig. 18.35b).
4. **Prognosis** is poor with severe visual loss occurring by the sixth to seventh decades.

Helicoid peripapillary chorioretinal dystrophy

1. **Inheritance** is AD with the gene locus on 11p15.
2. **Presentation** is in childhood.

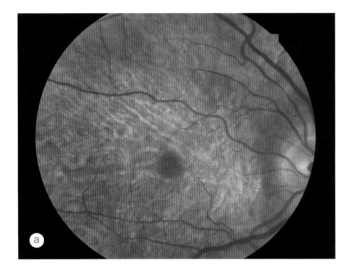

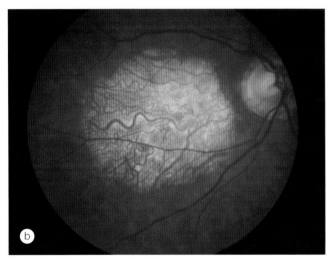

Fig. 18.35
Central areolar choroidal dystrophy. **(a)** Early; **(b)** late

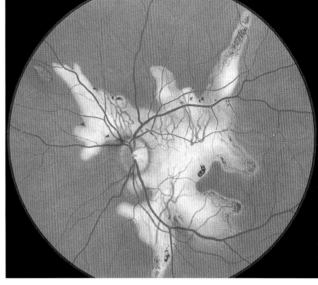

Fig. 18.36
Helicoid peripapillary chorioretinal dystrophy

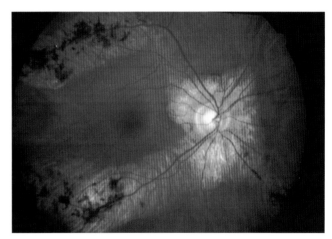

Fig. 18.37
Pigmented paravenous retinochoroidal atrophy (Courtesy of
C Barry)

3. Signs
- Slowly-enlarging, well-defined areas of chorioretinal atrophy radiating from the optic nerve head that resemble the propeller of an aeroplane (Fig. 18.36).
- Separate, peripheral, circular lesions may be present.
- Retinal vasculature is not affected.

4. ERG ranges from normal to severely abnormal.

5. Differential diagnosis includes serpiginous choroidopathy, angioid streaks, high myopia and pigmented paravenous retinochoroidal atrophy.

6. Prognosis is variable as severe disease may be seen in the young and mild disease in the elderly.

Pigmented paravenous retinochoroidal atrophy

1. Inheritance is uncertain although AD, AR and XL have been proposed.

2. Presentation is often by chance because the condition is usually asymptomatic.

3. Signs
- Bilateral, paravenous zones of chorioretinal atrophy associated with bone-spicule pigmentation (Fig. 18.37).
- CMO is rare.

4. ERG is usually normal.

5. Prognosis is excellent.

Progressive bifocal chorioretinal atrophy

1. **Inheritance** is AD with the gene locus on 6q.
2. **Presentation** is at birth.
3. **Signs** in chronological order:
   - A focus of chorioretinal atrophy temporal to the disc which extends in all directions.
   - A similar lesion develops nasally.
   - The end result manifests two separate areas of chorioretinal atrophy separated by a normal segment (Fig. 18.38).
4. **Prognosis** is poor because macular involvement is inevitable.

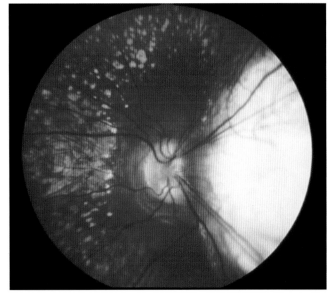

Fig. 18.38
Progressive bifocal chorioretinal atrophy (Courtesy of Moorfields Eye Hospital)

RETINAL DETACHMENT

INTRODUCTION

Anatomy

Pars plana

The pars plana starts 1mm from the limbus and extends posteriorly for about 6mm. The first 2mm consists of the pars plicata and the remaining 4mm comprises the flattened pars plana. In order not to endanger the lens or retina, the ideal location for a pars plana surgical incision is 4mm from the limbus in phakic eyes and 3.5mm from the limbus in pseudophakic eyes.

Ora serrata

The ora serrata forms the junction between the retina and ciliary body and is characterized by the following (Fig. 19.1).

1. **Dentate processes** are teeth-like extensions of retina onto the pars plana which are more marked nasally than temporally and can have extreme variations in contour.

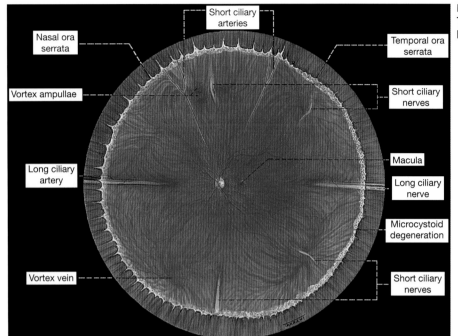

Fig. 19.1
The ora serrata and normal anatomical landmarks

2. **Oral bays** are the scalloped edges of the pars plana epithelium in between the dentate processes.
3. **A meridional fold** is a small radial fold of thickened retinal tissue in line with a dentate process, usually located in the superonasal quadrant. A fold may occasionally exhibit a small retinal hole at its apex (Fig. 19.2a). A meridional complex is a configuration in which a dentate process, usually with a meridional fold, is aligned with a ciliary process.
4. **An enclosed oral bay** is a small island of pars plana surrounded by retina as a result of meeting of two adjacent dentate processes (Fig. 19.2b). It should not be mistaken for a retinal hole because it is located anterior to the ora serrata.
5. **Granular tissue** characterized by multiple, white opacities within the vitreous base can sometimes be mistaken for small peripheral opercula (Fig. 19.2c).

> **NB** At the ora, fusion of the sensory retina with the RPE and choroid limits forward extension of subretinal fluid. However, as there is no equivalent adhesion between the choroid and sclera, choroidal detachments may progress anteriorly to involve the ciliary body (ciliochoroidal detachment).

Peripheral retina

The peripheral retina extends from the equator to the ora serrata. The anatomical equator is located approximately two disc diameters anterior to the entrance of the vortex veins.

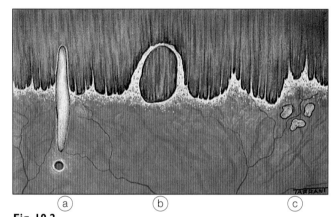

Fig. 19.2
Normal variants of the ora serrata. **(a)** Meridional fold with a small hole at its base; **(b)** enclosed oral bay; **(c)** granular tissue

The following innocuous lesions may be seen in the retinal periphery.

1. **Microcystoid degeneration** consists of tiny vesicles with indistinct boundaries on a greyish-white background which make the retina appear thickened and less transparent (Fig. 19.3a). It always starts adjacent to the ora serrata and extends circumferentially and posteriorly with a smooth undulating posterior border. Microcystoid degeneration is present in all adult eyes, increasing in severity with age, and is not in itself causally related to RD, although it may give rise to retinoschisis.

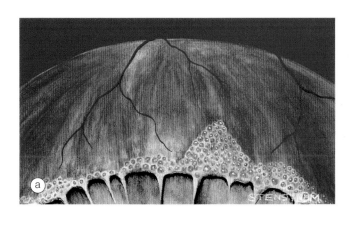
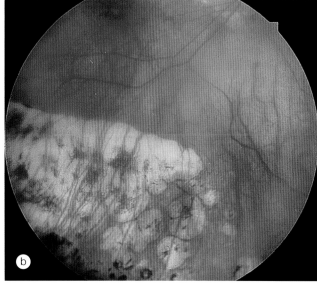
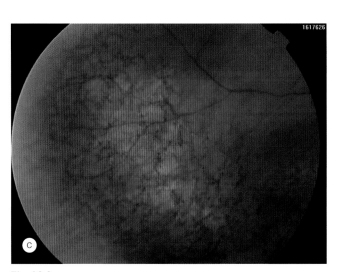
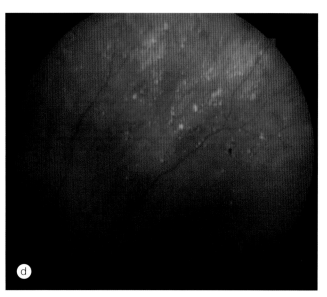

Fig. 19.3
Innocuous peripheral retinal lesions. **(a)** Microcystoid degeneration seen on scleral indentation; **(b)** pavingstone degeneration; **(c)** honeycomb (reticular) degeneration; **(d)** drusen (Courtesy of U Rutnin, CL Schepens, from *Am J Ophthalmol* 1967;64:1042 – fig. a)

2. **Pavingstone degeneration** is characterized by discrete yellow-white patches of focal chorioretinal atrophy which is present to some extent in 25% of normal eyes (Fig. 19.3b).
3. **Honeycomb (reticular) degeneration** is an age-related change characterized by a fine network of perivascular pigmentation which may extend posterior to the equator (Fig. 19.3c).
4. **Drusen** are characterized by clusters of small pale lesions which may have hyperpigmented borders (Fig. 19.3d). They are similar to drusen at the posterior pole and usually occur in the eyes of elderly individuals.

Vitreous base

The vitreous base is a 3–4mm wide zone straddling the ora serrata (Fig. 19.4). An incision through the mid-part of the pars plana will usually be located anterior to the vitreous base. The cortical vitreous is strongly attached at the vitreous base, so that following acute posterior vitreous detachment (PVD) the posterior hyaloid face remains attached to the posterior border of the vitreous base. If a blunt-ended instrument is introduced into the eye through the vitreous base it may exert traction and give rise to a peripheral retinal tear. Pre-existing retinal holes within the vitreous base do not

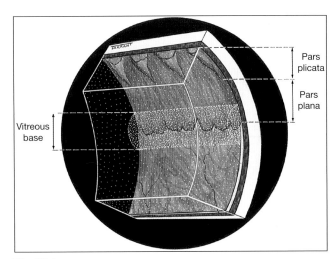

Fig. 19.4
The vitreous base

lead to RD. Severe blunt trauma may cause an avulsion of the vitreous base with tearing of the non-pigmented epithelium of the pars plana along its anterior border and of the retina along its posterior border.

Vitreous adhesions

1. **Normal.** The peripheral cortical vitreous is loosely attached to the internal limiting membrane (ILM) of the sensory retina. Stronger adhesions occur at the following sites:
   - Vitreous base, where they are very strong.
   - Around the optic nerve head, where they are fairly strong.
   - Around the fovea, where they are fairly weak, except in eyes with vitreomacular traction and macular hole formation.
   - Along peripheral blood vessels, where they are usually weak.
2. **Abnormal** adhesions at the following sites may be associated with retinal tear formation as a result of dynamic vitreoretinal traction associated with acute PVD.
   - Posterior border of islands of lattice degeneration.
   - Retinal pigment clumps.
   - Peripheral paravascular condensations.
   - Vitreous base anomalies such as tongue-like extensions and posterior islands.
   - 'White with pressure' and 'white without pressure' (see below).

Definitions

Retinal detachment

A retinal detachment (RD) describes the separation of the neurosensory retina (NSR) from the retinal pigment epithelium (RPE) caused by a breakdown of the forces that attach the NSR to the RPE. This results in the accumulation of subretinal fluid (SRF) in the potential space between the NSR and RPE. The main types of RD are:

1. **Rhegmatogenous** (*rhegma* – break), occurs secondarily to a full-thickness defect in the sensory retina, which permits fluid derived from synchytic (liquefied) vitreous to gain access to the subretinal space.
2. **Tractional** in which the NSR is pulled away from the RPE by contracting vitreoretinal membranes in the absence of a retinal break.
3. **Exudative** (serous, secondary) is caused neither by a break nor traction; the SRF is derived from fluid in the vessels of the NSR or the choroid, or both.
4. **Combined tractional-rhegmatogenous,** as the name implies, is the result of a combination of a retinal break and retinal traction. The retinal break is caused by traction from an adjacent area of fibrovascular proliferation and is most commonly seen in advanced proliferative diabetic retinopathy.

Vitreoretinal traction

Vitreoretinal traction is a force exerted on the retina by structures originating in the vitreous and may be dynamic or static.

> **NB** The difference between the two is crucial in understanding the pathogenesis of the various types of retinal detachment.

1. **Dynamic** traction is induced by eye movements and exerts a centripetal force towards the vitreous cavity. It plays an important role in the pathogenesis of retinal tears and rhegmatogenous RD.
2. **Static** traction is independent of ocular movements. It plays an important role in the pathogenesis of tractional RD and proliferative vitreoretinopathy.

Posterior vitreous detachment

A posterior vitreous detachment (PVD) is a separation of the cortical vitreous from the ILM of the sensory retina posterior to the vitreous base. PVD can be classified according to the following characteristics:

1. **Onset.** Acute PVD is by far the most common. It develops suddenly and usually becomes complete soon after onset. Chronic PVD develops gradually and may take weeks or months to become complete.
2. **Extent.** Complete PVD – in which the entire vitreous cortex detaches up to the posterior margin of the vitreous base. Incomplete PVD – in which residual vitreoretinal attachments remain posterior to the vitreous base.

NB Rhegmatogenous RD is usually associated with acute PVD; tractional RD is associated with chronic, incomplete PVD; exudative RD is unrelated to the presence of PVD.

Retinal break

A retinal break is a full-thickness defect in the sensory retina. Breaks can be classified according to (a) *pathogenesis*, (b) *morphology* and (c) *location*.

1. Pathogenesis
  a. Tears are caused by dynamic vitreoretinal traction and have a predilection for the upper fundus (temporal more than nasal).
  b. Holes are caused by chronic atrophy of the sensory retina and may be round or oval. They have a predilection for the temporal fundus (upper more than lower).
2. Morphology
  a. U-tears (horseshoe, flap or arrowhead), consist of a flap, the apex of which is pulled anteriorly by the vitreous, the base remaining attached to the retina (Fig. 19.5a). The actual tear consists of two anterior extensions (horns) running forward from the apex.
  b. Incomplete U-tears, which may be linear (Fig. 19.5b), L-shaped (Fig. 19.5c) or J-shaped, are often paravascular.

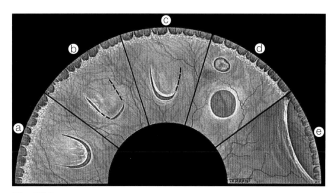

Fig. 19.5
Retinal tears. **(a)** Complete U-shaped; **(b)** linear; **(c)** L-shaped; **(d)** operculated; **(e)** dialysis

  c. Operculated tears in which the flap is completely torn away from the retina by detached vitreous gel (Fig. 19.5d).
  d. Dialyses are circumferential tears along the ora serrata with the vitreous gel attached to their posterior margins (Fig. 19.5e).
  e. Giant tears involve 90° or more of the circumference of the globe (Fig. 19.6a). They are a variant of U-shaped tears with the vitreous gel attached to the anterior margin of the break (Fig. 19.6b). Giant tears are most frequently located in the immediate post-oral retina or, less commonly, at the equator.

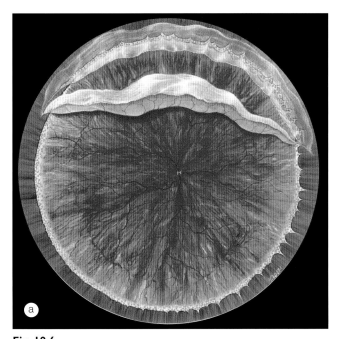
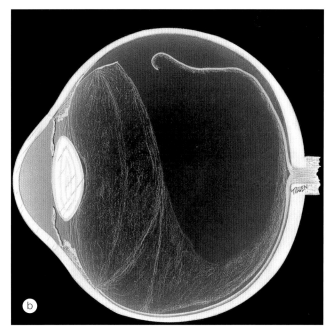

Fig. 19.6
(a) Giant retinal tear involving the immediate post-oral retina; **(b)** vitreous cortex is attached to the anterior margin of the tear
(Courtesy of C L Schepens, M E Hartnett and T Hirose, from *Schepens' Retinal Detachment and Allied Diseases*, Butterworth-Heinemann, 2000)

3. Location
   a. **Oral** breaks are located within the vitreous base.
   b. **Post-oral** breaks are located between the posterior border of the vitreous base and equator.
   c. **Equatorial** breaks are near the equator.
   d. **Post-equatorial** breaks are behind the equator.
   e. **Macular** breaks (invariably holes) are at the fovea.

How to find the primary retinal break

The primary break is the one responsible for the RD. A secondary break is not responsible for the RD because it is either present before the development of RD or forms after RD has occurred. Finding the primary break is of paramount importance and aided by the following considerations.

1. Quadrantic distribution of breaks in eyes with RD is approximately as follows: 60% in the upper temporal quadrant; 15% in the upper nasal quadrant; 15% in the lower temporal quadrant; 10% in the lower nasal quadrant.

> **NB** The upper temporal quadrant is therefore by far the most common site for retinal break formation and should be examined in great detail if a retinal break cannot be detected initially. It should also be remembered that about 50% of eyes with RD have more than one break, and in most eyes these are located within 90° of each other.

2. Configuration of SRF is of relevance because SRF spreads in a gravitational fashion, and its shape is governed by anatomical limits (ora serrata and optic nerve) and the location of the primary retinal break. If the primary break is located superiorly, the SRF first spreads inferiorly on the same side as the break and then spreads superiorly on the opposite side of the fundus. The likely location of the primary retinal break can therefore be predicted by studying the shape of the RD:

a. A shallow inferior RD in which the SRF is slightly higher on the temporal side points to a primary break located inferiorly on that side (Fig. 19.7a).
b. A primary break located at 6 o'clock will cause an inferior RD with equal fluid levels (Fig. 19.7b).
c. In a bullous inferior RD the primary break usually lies above the horizontal meridian (Fig. 19.7c).
d. If the primary break is located in the upper nasal quadrant the SRF will revolve around the optic disc and then rise on the temporal side until it is level with the primary break (Fig. 19.7d).
e. A subtotal RD with a superior wedge of attached retina points to a primary break located in the periphery nearest its highest border (Fig. 19.7e).
f. When the SRF crosses the vertical midline above, the primary break is near to 12 o'clock, the lower edge of the RD corresponding to the side of the break (Fig. 19.7f).

> **NB** The above points are important because they prevent you from treating a secondary break and overlooking the primary break. It is therefore essential to ensure that the shape of the RD corresponds to the location of the primary retinal break.

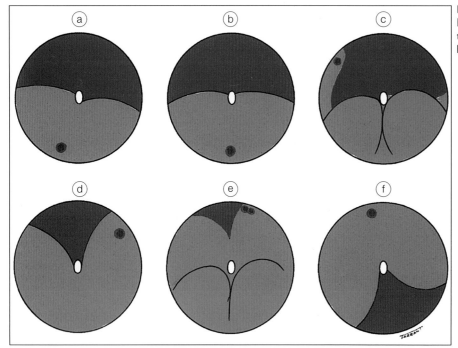

Fig. 19.7
Distribution of subretinal fluid in relation to the location of the primary retinal break (see text)

3. **History.** Although the quadrantic location of light flashes is of no value in predicting the location of the primary break, the quadrant in which the visual field defect first appears may be of considerable value. For example, if the field defect started in the upper nasal quadrant the primary break is probably located in the lower temporal quadrant.

PATHOGENESIS OF RHEGMATOGENOUS RETINAL DETACHMENT

Vitreoretinal traction

Rhegmatogenous RD affects about 1 in 10,000 of the population each year and both eyes may eventually be involved in about 10% of cases. It is characterized by the presence of a retinal break held open by vitreoretinal traction that allows accumulation of liquefied vitreous under the NSR separating it from the RPE. The retinal breaks responsible for RD are caused by interplay between dynamic vitreoretinal traction and an underlying weakness in the peripheral retina referred to as predisposing degeneration.

NB Even if a retinal break is present, a RD will not occur if the vitreous is not at least partially liquefied and if the necessary traction is not present.

Dynamic vitreoretinal traction

Synchysis is a liquefaction of the vitreous gel caused by alterations of its micromolecular structure. Some eyes with synchysis develop a hole in the posterior hyaloid membrane and fluid from within the centre of the vitreous cavity passes through this defect into the newly formed retrohyaloid space. This process forcibly detaches the posterior vitreous surface from the ILM of the sensory retina as far as the posterior border of the vitreous base. The remaining solid vitreous gel collapses inferiorly and the retrohyaloid space is occupied entirely by synchytic fluid. This process is called acute PVD with collapse and will be referred to as acute PVD henceforth. It occurs in over 60% of patients older than 70 years, and the fellow eye frequently becomes affected within 6 months to 2 years. In myopic eyes PVD tends to occur about 10 years earlier than in non-myopic eyes.

Complications of acute PVD

Following PVD, the sensory retina is no longer protected by the stable vitreous cortex, and can be directly affected by dynamic vitreoretinal tractional forces. The vision-threatening complications of acute PVD are dependent on the strength and extent of pre-existing vitreoretinal adhesions.

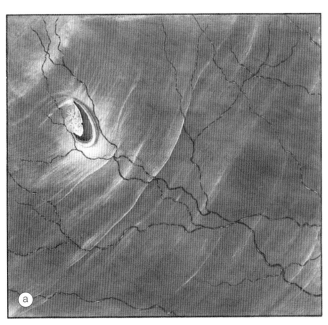
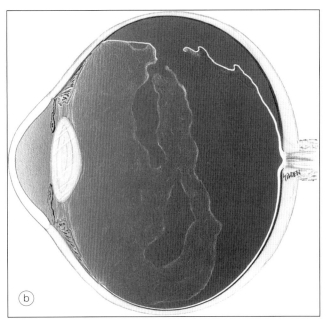

Fig. 19.8
(a) U-shaped retinal tear and localized retinal detachment associated with acute posterior vitreous detachment; **(b)** the vitreous shows syneresis, posterior detachment and partial collapse with attachment of cortical vitreous to the flap of the tear (Courtesy of C L Schepens, M E Hartnett and T Hirose, from *Schepens' Retinal Detachment and Allied Diseases*, Butterworth-Heinemann, 2000)

1. **No complications** occur in most eyes because vitreo-retinal attachments are weak so that the vitreous cortex detaches completely without sequelae.
2. **Retinal tears** may develop as a result of transmission of traction at sites of abnormally strong vitreoretinal adhesions as previously described (Fig. 19.8). Although tears usually develop at the time of PVD, very occasionally they may be delayed by several weeks. Patients with isolated PVD should therefore be re-examined 6 weeks after the onset of symptoms. Tears associated with acute PVD are usually symptomatic, U-shaped, located in the upper fundus and may be associated with vitreous haemorrhage resulting from rupture of a peripheral retinal blood vessel. After the tear has formed, the retrohyaloid fluid has direct access to the subretinal space.
3. **Avulsion of a peripheral blood vessel** resulting in vitreous haemorrhage in the absence of retinal tear formation is rare.

Predisposing peripheral retinal degenerations

About 60% of all breaks develop in areas of the peripheral retina that shows specific changes. These lesions may be associated with a spontaneous breakdown of pathologically thin retinal tissue to cause a retinal hole, or they may predispose to retinal tear formation in eyes with acute PVD. Retinal holes are round or oval, usually smaller than tears and carry a lower risk of RD. Retinal detachment without PVD is usually associated with either retinal dialysis, or round holes predominantly in young female myopes.

Lattice degeneration

1. **Prevalence.** Lattice degeneration is present in about 8% of the population. It probably develops early in life, with a peak incidence during the second and third decades. It is found more commonly in moderate myopes and is the most important degeneration directly related to RD. It is usually bilateral and most frequently located in the temporal rather than nasal fundus, and superiorly rather than inferiorly. Lattice is present in about 40% of eyes with RD and is an important cause of RD in young myopes.
2. **Pathology.** There is discontinuity of the internal limiting membrane with variable atrophy of the underlying sensory retina. The vitreous overlying an area of lattice is synchytic but the vitreous attachments around the margins are exaggerated (Fig. 19.9).
3. **Signs.**
   - Spindle-shaped areas of retinal thinning, most frequently located between the equator and the posterior border of the vitreous base.
   - A characteristic feature is an arborizing network of white lines within the islands (Fig. 19.10a)

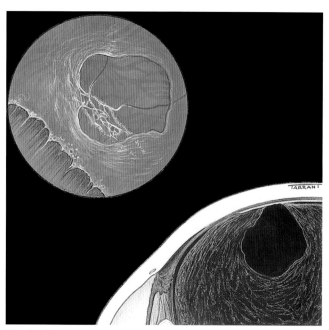

Fig. 19.9
Vitreous changes associated with lattice degeneration

   - Some lattice lesions may be associated with 'snow-flakes' (remnants of degenerate Müller cells – Fig. 19.10b).
   - Lattice associated with hyperplasia of the RPE is common (Fig. 19.10c).
   - Small holes within the lattice lesions are common and usually innocuous (Fig. 19.10d).
4. **Complications.**
   a. **No complications** are encountered in most patients (Fig. 19.11a).
   b. **Tears** may occasionally develop in eyes with acute PVD. A small area of lattice may be seen on the flap of the tear representing strong vitreoretinal attachment (Fig. 19.11b). Tears may also develop along the posterior edge of an island of lattice (Fig. 19.11c). Tears typically occur in myopes over the age of 50 years; the SRF progresses more rapidly than in RDs caused by small round holes.
   c. **Atrophic holes** (Fig. 19.11d) may rarely lead to RD, particularly in young myopes. In these patients the RD may not be preceded by symptoms of acute PVD (photopsia and floaters) and the SRF usually spreads slowly so that the diagnosis may be delayed until central vision is involved. The fellow eye often has a 'mirror-image' distribution of holes.

Snailtrack degeneration

Snailtrack degeneration is characterized by sharply demarcated bands of tightly packed 'snowflakes' which give the

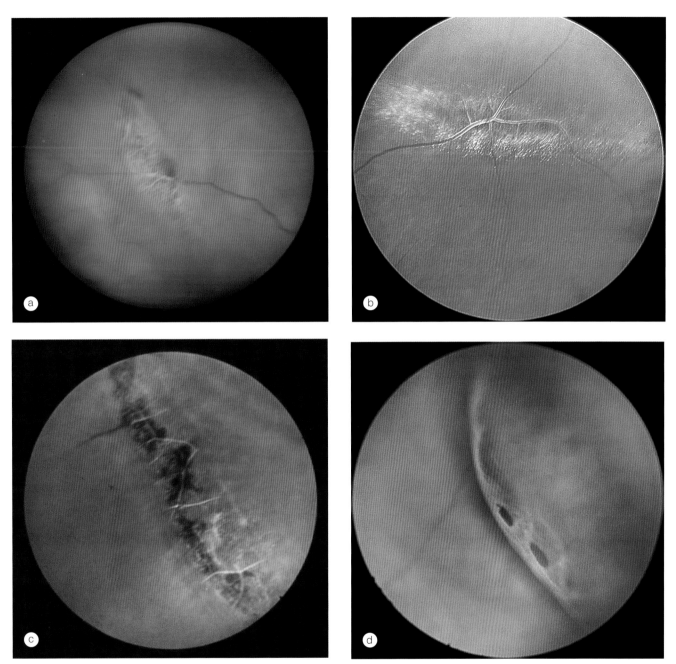

Fig. 19.10
Clinical features of lattice degeneration. **(a)** Small island of lattice with an arborizing network of white lines; **(b)** lattice associated with 'snowflakes'; **(c)** lattice associated with retinal pigment epithelial changes; **(d)** holes within lattice degeneration seen on scleral indentation (Courtesy of N E Byer, from *The Peripheral Retina in Profile, a Stereoscopic Atlas*, Criterion Press, Torrance, California, 1982 – figs b and d)

peripheral retina a white frost-like appearance (Fig. 19.12a). They are usually longer than islands of lattice and may be associated with overlying vitreous liquefaction. However, marked vitreous traction at the posterior border of the lesions is seldom present so that tractional U-tears rarely occur, although round holes within the snailtracks may be present (Fig. 19.12b).

Degenerative retinoschisis

1. **Prevalence.** Degenerative retinoschisis is present in about 5% of the population over the age of 20 years and is more prevalent in hypermetropes (70% of patients are hypermetropic). Both eyes are frequently involved.

2. **Pathology.** There is coalescence of cystic lesions as a

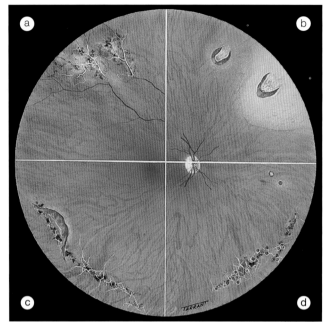

Fig. 19.11
Complications of lattice degeneration. **(a)** Atypical radial lattice not associated with breaks; **(b)** two U-shaped tears one of which exhibits a small patch of lattice on its flap and is surrounded by a small area of SRF; **(c)** linear tear along the posterior margin of lattice; **(d)** multiple small holes within islands of lattice

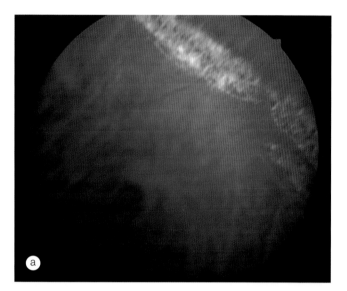

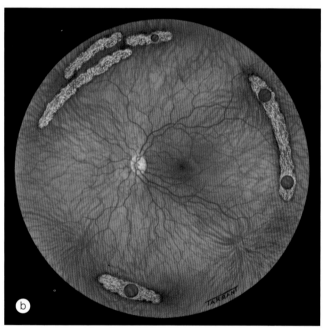

Fig. 19.12
(a) Snailtrack degeneration; **(b)** several islands of snailtrack some of which contain holes.

result of degeneration of neuroretinal and glial supporting elements within areas of peripheral cystoid degeneration (Fig. 19.13a). This eventually results in separation or splitting of the NSR into an inner (vitreous) layer and an outer (choroidal) layer with severing of neurons and complete loss of visual function in the affected area. In typical retinoschisis the split is in the outer plexiform layer, and in reticular retinoschisis, which is less common, splitting occurs at the level of the nerve fibre layer.

3. Signs

- Early retinoschisis usually involves the extreme inferotemporal periphery of both fundi, appearing as an exaggeration of microcystoid degeneration with a smooth elevation of the retina (Fig. 19.13b).
- The lesion may progress circumferentially until it has involved the entire fundus periphery. The typical form usually remains anterior to the equator, although the reticular type may spread beyond the equator.
- The surface of the inner layer may show 'snowflakes' as well as sheathing or 'silver-wiring' of blood vessels and the schisis cavity may be bridged by rows of torn grey-white tissue (Fig. 19.14).

NB Unlike RD, retinoschisis is relatively immobile.

4. Complications

  a. No complications occur in most cases and the condition is asymptomatic and innocuous.

  b. Breaks may develop in the reticular type. Inner layer breaks are small and round, whilst the less common outer layer breaks are usually larger, with rolled edges and located behind the equator (Fig. 19.15a). Eyes with only inner layer breaks do not develop RD as there is no communication with the subretinal space.

  c. RD may occasionally develop in eyes with breaks in both layers, especially in the presence of PVD. Eyes with

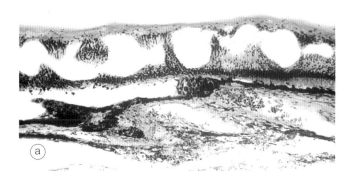

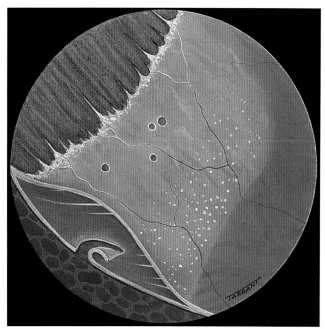

Fig. 19.14
Retinoschisis with breaks in both layers. The inner layer shows snowflakes and 'silver-wiring 'of blood vessels and the cavity is bridged by torn grey-white tissue

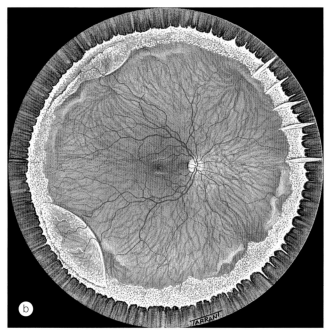

Fig. 19.13
Peripheral microcystoid degeneration. **(a)** Histology shows spaces in the neural layer delineated by delicate vertical columns of Müller cells; **(b)** circumferential microcystoid degeneration and mild retinoschisis in the inferotemporal and superotemporal quadrants (Courtesy of J Harry and G Misson, from *Clinical Ophthalmic Pathology*, Butterworth-Heinemann, 2001 – fig. a)

only outer layer breaks do not as a rule develop RD because the fluid within the schisis cavity is viscous and does not pass readily into the subretinal space. However, occasionally the schisis fluid loses its viscosity and passes through the break into the subretinal space, giving rise to a localized detachment of the outer retinal layer which is usually confined to the area of retinoschisis (Fig. 19.15b). The detachment is almost always asymptomatic, infrequently progressive and rarely requires treatment.

d. *Vitreous haemorrhage* is uncommon.

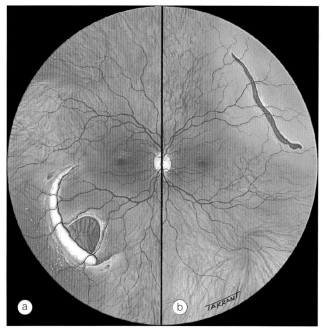

Fig. 19.15
Degenerative retinoschisis. **(a)** Large breaks in both layers; **(b)** linear break in the outer layer associated with a localized subretinal fluid

'White-with-pressure' and 'white-without-pressure'

1. **'White-with-pressure'** is a translucent grey appearance of the retina, induced by indenting the sclera (Fig. 19.16a). Each area has a fixed configuration which does

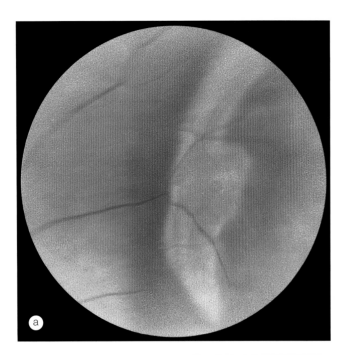

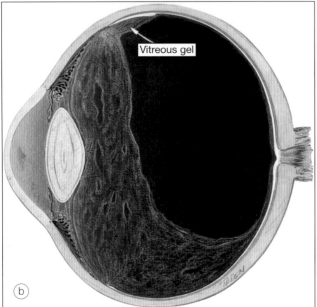

Fig. 19.16
(a) White-with-pressure; **(b)** vitreous syneresis and strong attachment of condensed vitreous gel to white-with-pressure
(Courtesy of N E Byer, from *The Peripheral Retina in Profile, a Stereoscopic Atlas*, Criterion Press, Torrance, California, 1982 – fig. a; C L Schepens, M E Hartnett and T Hirose, from *Schepens' Retinal Detachment and Allied Diseases*, Butterworth-Heinemann, 2000 – fig. b)

not change when the scleral indenter is moved to an adjacent area. It is frequently seen in normal eyes and may be associated with abnormally strong attachment of the vitreous gel (Fig. 19.16b). It is also observed along the posterior border of islands of lattice degeneration, snailtrack degeneration and outer layer of acquired retinoschisis.

2. **'White-without-pressure'** has the same appearance but is present without scleral indentation. On cursory examination a normal area of retina surrounded by white-without-pressure may be mistaken for a flat retinal hole and the appearance can be quite dramatic in heavily pigmented fundi (Fig. 19.17a). Giant tears occasionally develop along the posterior border of white-without-pressure (Fig. 19.17b). For this reason, if white-without-pressure is found in the fellow eye of a patient with a spontaneous giant retinal tear, prophylactic therapy should be performed.

> **NB** It is probably advisable to treat all fellow eyes of non-traumatic giant retinal tears prophylactically by 360° cryotherapy or indirect argon laser photocoagulation, irrespective of the presence of white-without-pressure, if they have not developed a PVD.

Diffuse chorioretinal atrophy

Diffuse chorioretinal atrophy is characterized by choroidal depigmentation and thinning of the overlying retina in the equatorial area of highly myopic eyes. Retinal holes developing in the atrophic retina may lead to RD (Fig. 19.18). Because of lack of contrast between the depigmented choroid and sensory retina, small holes may be very difficult to visualize without the help of slit-lamp biomicroscopy.

Significance of myopia

Although myopes make up 10% of the general population, over 40% of all RDs occur in myopic eyes; the higher the refractive error the greater is the risk of RD. The following interrelated factors predispose a myopic eye to RD:

1. **Lattice degeneration** is more common in moderate myopes and may give rise to either tears or atrophic holes (see Fig. 19.11d). Giant retinal tears may also develop along the posterior edge of long lattice islands (Fig. 19.19).
2. **Snailtrack degeneration** is common in myopic eyes and may be associated with atrophic holes (see Fig. 19.12b).
3. **Diffuse chorioretinal atrophy** may give rise to small round holes in highly myopic eyes (see Fig. 19.18).
4. **Macular holes** may give rise to RD in highly myopic eyes, particularly those with a posterior staphyloma.
5. **Vitreous degeneration and PVD** are more common.

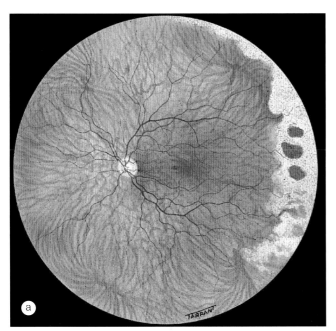

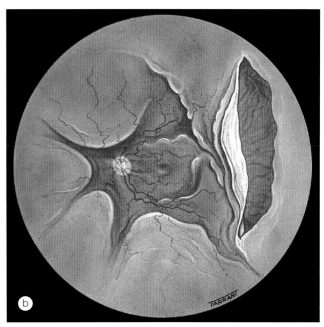

Fig. 19.17
(a) White-without-pressure with pseudoholes; **(b)** giant retinal tear causing total retinal detachment

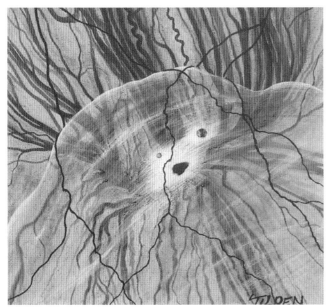

Fig. 19.18
Diffuse chorioretinal atrophy with holes and subretinal fluid
(Courtesy of C L Schepens, M E Hartnett and T Hirose, from *Schepens' Retinal Detachment and Allied Diseases*, Butterworth-Heinemann, 2000)

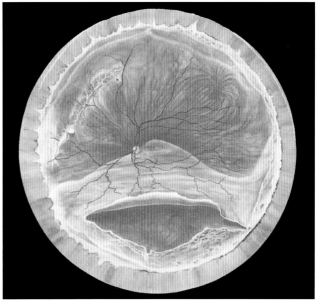

Fig. 19.19
Inferior retinal detachment in a highly myopic eye due to a giant tear along the posterior border of extensive lattice degeneration; also note extensive lattice in the superotemporal quadrant
(Courtesy of C L Schepens, M E Hartnett and T Hirose, from *Schepens' Retinal Detachment and Allied Diseases*, Butterworth-Heinemann, 2000)

6. **Vitreous loss during cataract surgery,** particularly if inappropriately managed, is associated with an increased risk of subsequent RD, particularly in highly myopic eyes.
7. **Laser posterior capsulotomy** is associated with an increased risk of RD in myopic eyes.

Trauma

Trauma is responsible for about 10% of all cases of RD and is the most common cause in children, particularly boys. A great variety of breaks may develop in traumatized eyes either at the time of impact or subsequently.

1. **Penetrating injuries** of the posterior segment carry a high risk of RD, particularly if there is vitreous incarceration at the site of penetration, which subsequently leads to vitreoretinal traction (see below).
2. **Severe blunt trauma** causes a compression of the anteroposterior diameter of the globe and a simultaneous expansion at the equatorial plane (Fig. 19.20a).

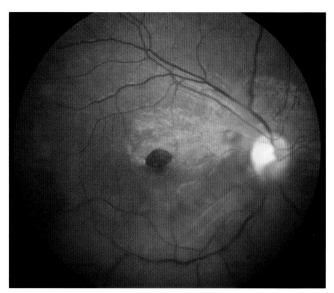

Fig. 19.21
Traumatic macular hole (Courtesy of C Barry)

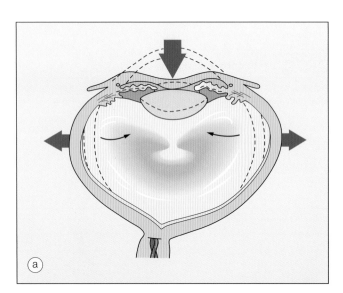

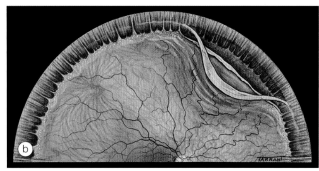

Fig. 19.20
(a) Pathogenesis of ocular damage by blunt trauma;
(b) superonasal dialysis and vitreous base avulsion associated with localized subretinal fluid

a. **Dialysis** is caused by traction of the relatively inelastic vitreous gel along the posterior aspect of the vitreous base with tearing of the retina to form a dialysis which may be associated with avulsion of the vitreous base. This gives rise to a 'bucket-handle' appearance which comprises a strip of ciliary epithelium, ora serrata and the immediate post-oral retina into which basal vitreous gel remains inserted (Fig. 19.20b). Traumatic dialyses occur most frequently in the superonasal and inferotemporal quadrants. Although they occur at the time of injury they may not result in RD because the vitreous gel is healthy in young individuals, but prophylactic treatment is recommended. In cases that do detach, the RD frequently may not develop until several months later and progression is slow.
b. **Equatorial tears** are less common and are due to direct retinal disruption at the point of scleral impact.
c. **Macular holes** may occur either at the time of injury or following resolution of commotio retinae (Fig. 19.21).

PATHOGENESIS OF TRACTIONAL RETINAL DETACHMENT

The main causes of tractional RD are (a) *proliferative retinopathy* such as diabetic and retinopathy of prematurity, and (b) *penetrating posterior segment trauma.*

Diabetic tractional retinal detachment

Pathogenesis of PVD

Tractional RD is caused by progressive contraction of fibrovascular membranes over large areas of vitreoretinal adhesion. Owing to the strong adhesions of the cortical vitreous to areas of fibrovascular proliferation, PVD is gradual and usually incomplete. In the very rare event of a complete PVD, the new blood vessels are avulsed and RD does not develop.

Vitreoretinal traction

The following three main types of static vitreoretinal traction are recognized.

1. **Tangential** traction is caused by the contraction of epiretinal fibrovascular membranes with puckering of the retina and distortion of retinal blood vessels.
2. **Anteroposterior** traction is caused by the contraction of fibrovascular membranes extending from the posterior retina, usually in association with the major arcades, to the vitreous base anteriorly (Fig. 19.22).

3. **Bridging** (trampoline) traction is the result of contraction of fibrovascular membranes which stretch from one part of the posterior retina to another or between the vascular arcades which tends to pull the two involved points together.

Traumatic tractional retinal detachment

Traumatic tractional RD may result from vitreous incarceration in the wound and bleeding within the vitreous gel which acts as a stimulus to fibroblastic proliferation along the planes of incarcerated vitreous (Fig. 19.23a). The contraction of such anterior epiretinal membranes leads to a shortening and a rolling effect on the peripheral retina in the region of the vitreous base and eventually to an anterior

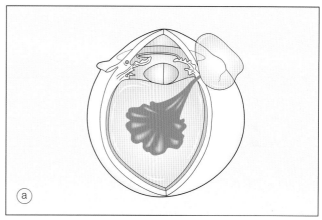

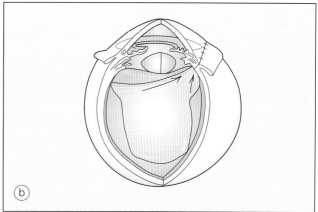

Fig. 19.22
Tractional retinal detachment associated with anteroposterior and bridging traction (Courtesy of C L Schepens, M E Hartnett and T Hirose, from *Schepens' Retinal Detachment and Allied Diseases*, Butterworth-Heinemann, 2000)

Fig. 19.23
Traumatic tractional retinal detachment. **(a)** Penetrating injury resulting in vitreous prolapse and intraocular haemorrhage; **(b)** subsequent vitreoretinal proliferation and traction resulting in retinal detachment

tractional RD (Fig. 19.23b). A retinal break may develop several weeks later leading to a sudden extension of SRF and consequent visual loss. As a rule, in penetrating trauma the traction is therefore mainly anterior whereas in diabetes it is mainly posterior.

PATHOGENESIS OF EXUDATIVE RETINAL DETACHMENT

Exudative RD is characterized by the accumulation of SRF in the absence of retinal breaks or traction. It may occur in a variety of vascular, inflammatory or neoplastic diseases involving the NSR, RPE and choroid in which fluid leaks and accumulates under the retina. As long as the RPE is able to pump the leaking fluid into the choroidal circulation, no fluid accumulates in the subretinal space and RD does not occur. However, when the normal RPE pump is overwhelmed, or if the RPE activity is decreased, then fluid starts to accumulate in the subretinal space resulting in RD.

Causes

1. **Choroidal tumours** such as melanomas, haemangiomas and metastases.

> **NB** It is important always to consider that exudative RD is caused by an intraocular tumour until proved otherwise.

2. **Inflammation** such as Harada disease and posterior scleritis.
3. **Bullous central serous retinopathy** is a rare cause.
4. **Iatrogenic** causes include retinal detachment surgery and panretinal photocoagulation.
5. **Choroidal neovascularization** which may leak and give rise to extensive subretinal accumulation of fluid at the posterior pole.
6. **Hypertensive choroidopathy,** which may occur in toxaemia of pregnancy, is now a very rare cause.
7. **Idiopathic** such as the uveal effusion syndrome (see below).

Treatment

Treatment modality depends on the cause. Some resolve spontaneously (postoperative), whilst others are treated with systemic corticosteroids (Harada disease and posterior scleritis). In some eyes with central serous choroidopathy the leak in the RPE can sometimes be sealed by argon laser photocoagulation.

DIAGNOSIS OF RHEGMATOGENOUS RETINAL DETACHMENT

Symptoms

The classic premonitory symptoms reported in about 60% of patients with spontaneous rhegmatogenous RD are flashing lights (photopsia) and vitreous floaters caused by acute PVD with collapse. After a variable period of time the patient notices a relative peripheral visual field defect which may progress to involve central vision.

Photopsia

Photopsia in eyes with acute PVD is probably caused by traction at sites of vitreoretinal adhesion. Its cessation is the result of either separation of the adhesion or complete tearing away of a piece of retina (operculum). In eyes with PVD the photopsia may be induced by eye movements and is more noticeable in dim illumination. It tends to be projected into the patient's temporal peripheral visual field and, unlike floaters, it has no lateralizing value. Photopsia caused by vitreoretinal traction should be differentiated from migraine.

Floaters

Floaters are moving vitreous opacities which are perceived when they cast shadows on the retina. Vitreous opacities in eyes with acute PVD are of the following three types:

1. **Weiss ring** is a solitary floater consisting of the detached annular attachment of vitreous to the margin of the optic disc (Fig. 19.24).

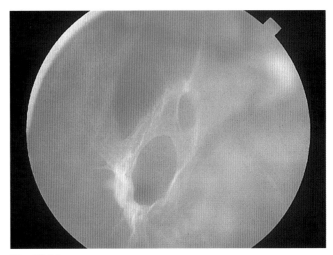

Fig. 19.24
Weiss ring

2. **Cobwebs** are caused by condensation of collagen fibres within the collapsed vitreous cortex.
3. **A sudden shower** of minute red-coloured or dark spots usually indicates vitreous haemorrhage secondary to tearing of a peripheral retinal blood vessel. Although vitreous haemorrhage associated with acute PVD is usually sparse, due to the small calibre of peripheral retinal vessels, occasionally a severe bleed may impair visualization of the fundus.

Visual field defect

A visual field defect is perceived as a 'black curtain'. In some patients it may not be present on waking in the morning, due to spontaneous absorption of SRF while lying inactive overnight, only to reappear later in the day. A lower field defect is usually appreciated more quickly by the patient than an upper field defect. The quadrant of the visual field in which the field defect first appears is useful in predicting the location of the primary retinal break (which will be in the opposite quadrant). Loss of central vision may be due either to involvement of the fovea by SRF or, less frequently, obstruction of the visual axis by a large upper bullous RD.

Signs

General signs

1. **Marcus Gunn pupil** (relative afferent pupillary defect) is present in eyes with extensive RDs irrespective of the type.
2. **The intraocular pressure** is usually lower by about 5mmHg compared with the normal eye. If extremely low, an associated choroidal detachment may be present.
3. **A mild iritis** is very common. Occasionally it may be severe enough to cause posterior synechiae. In these cases the underlying RD may be overlooked and the poor visual acuity incorrectly ascribed to some other cause.
4. **'Tobacco dust'** is seen in the anterior vitreous (Fig. 19.25).
5. **Retinal breaks** appear as discontinuities in the retinal surface. They are usually red because of the colour contrast between the NSR and underlying choroid. However, in eyes with hypopigmented choroid (as in high myopia), the colour contrast is decreased and small breaks may be overlooked unless careful slit-lamp and indirect ophthalmoscopy examination is performed.
6. **Retinal signs** depend on the duration of RD and the presence or absence of proliferative vitreoretinopathy as described next.

Fresh retinal detachment

1. **The RD** has a convex configuration and a slightly opaque and corrugated appearance as a result of intraretinal oedema. There is loss of the underlying

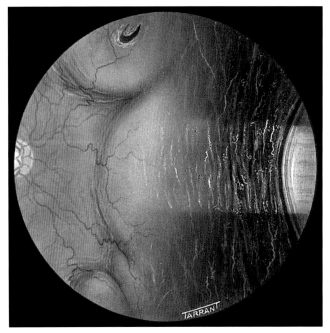

Fig. 19.25
'Tobacco dust' in the anterior vitreous associated with an extensive retinal detachment caused by a superior U-tear

choroidal pattern and retinal blood vessels appear darker than in flat retina, so the colour contrast between venules and arterioles is less apparent (Fig. 19.26).
2. **SRF** extends up to the ora serrata except in the rare cases caused by a macular hole in which the SRF is confined to the posterior pole.

NB Because of the thinness of the retina at the fovea, a pseudohole is frequently seen if the posterior pole is detached. This should not be mistaken for a true macular hole which may give rise to RD in highly myopic eyes or following blunt ocular trauma.

Long-standing retinal detachment

The following are the main features of a long-standing rhegmatogenous RD (Fig. 19.27).

1. **Retinal thinning** secondary to atrophy is a characteristic finding which must not be mistaken for retinoschisis.
2. **Secondary intraretinal cysts** may develop if the RD has been present for about one year. They tend to disappear after retinal reattachment.
3. **Subretinal demarcation lines** (high water marks) caused by proliferation of RPE cells at the junction of flat and detached retina are common and take about 3 months to develop. They are initially pigmented and then tend to lose their pigment. Demarcation lines are convex with

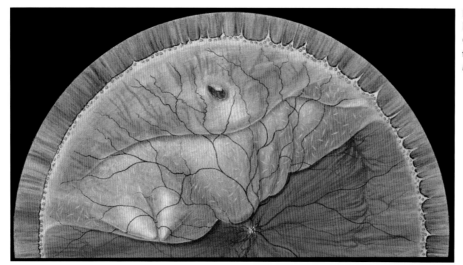

Fig. 19.26
Fresh retinal detachment (Courtesy of
C L Schepens, M E Hartnett and T Hirose,
from *Schepens' Retinal Detachment and Allied
Diseases*, Butterworth-Heinemann, 2000)

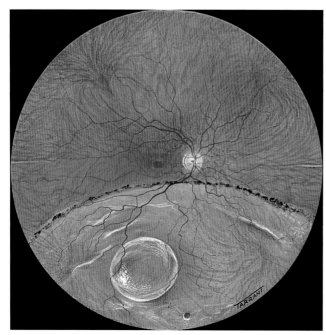

Fig. 19.27
Long-standing inferior retinal detachment associated with a
secondary intraretinal cyst and a pigmented demarcation line

respect to the ora serrata and, although they represent
sites of increased adhesion, they do not invariably limit
spread of SRF.

Proliferative vitreoretinopathy

Proliferative vitreoretinopathy (PVR) is caused by epiretinal
and subretinal membrane formation. Cell-mediated contraction of these membranes causes tangential retinal

traction and fixed retinal folds (Fig. 19.28). Usually, PVR
occurs following surgery for rhegmatogenous RD or
penetrating injury. However, it may also occur in eyes with
rhegmatogenous RD that have not had previous vitreoretinal
surgery. The main features are folds and rigidity so that
retinal mobility induced by eye movements or scleral
indentation is decreased. Classification is as follows although
it should be emphasized that progression from one stage to
the next is not inevitable.

1. **Grade A** (minimal) PVR is characterized by diffuse
   vitreous haze and 'tobacco dust'. There may also be
   pigmented clumps on the inferior surface of the retina.
   Although these findings occur in many eyes with RD, they
   are particular severe in eyes with early PVR.
2. **Grade B** (moderate) PVR is characterized by wrinkling of
   the inner retinal surface, tortuosity of blood vessels, retinal
   stiffness, decreased mobility of vitreous gel and rolled edges of
   retinal breaks (Fig. 19.29). The epiretinal membranes
   responsible for these findings cannot be identified clinically.
3. **Grade C** (marked) PVR is characterized by full-thickness
   rigid retinal folds with heavy vitreous condensation and
   strands. It can be either anterior (A) or posterior (P), the
   approximate dividing line being the equator of the globe.
   The severity of proliferation in each area is expressed by
   the number of clock hours of retina involved (1–12)
   although proliferations need not be contiguous.

DIAGNOSIS OF TRACTIONAL RETINAL DETACHMENT

1. **Symptoms.** Photopsia and floaters are usually absent
   because vitreoretinal traction develops insidiously and is
   not associated with acute PVD. The visual field defect

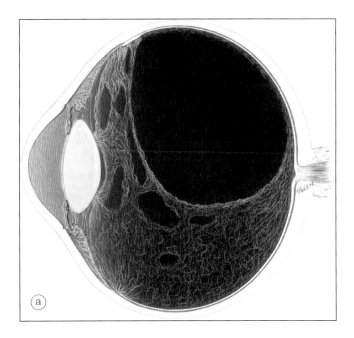
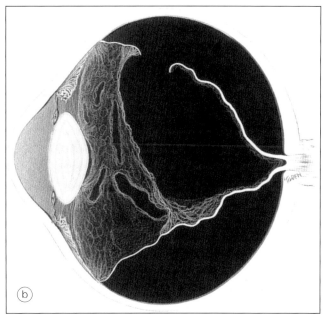
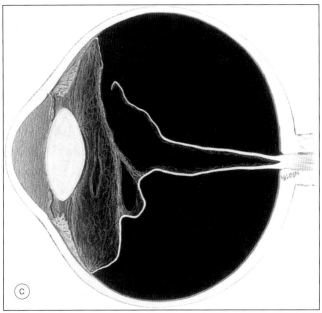
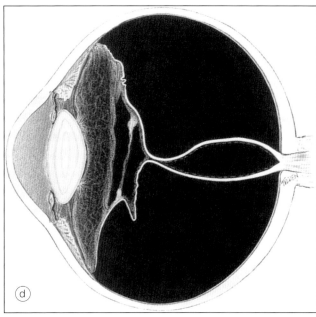

Fig. 19.28
Development of proliferative vitreoretinopathy (PVR). **(a)** Extensive vitreous syneresis; **(b)** retinal detachment but no PVR; shrunken vitreous is condensed and attached to the retinal equator; **(c)** early PVR with anteriorly retracted vitreous gel and equatorial circumferential retinal folds; **(d)** advanced PVR with funnel-like retinal detachment bridged anteriorly by dense vitreous membranes (Courtesy of C L Schepens, M E Hartnett and T Hirose, from *Schepens' Retinal Detachment and Allied Diseases*, Butterworth-Heinemann, 2000)

usually progresses slowly and may become stationary for months and even years.

2. Signs (Fig. 19.30).

- The RD has a concave configuration and breaks are absent.
- Retinal mobility is severely reduced and shifting fluid is absent.

- The SRF is less deep than in a rhegmatogenous RD and seldom extends to the ora serrata. The highest elevation of the retina occurs at sites of vitreoretinal traction.

NB If a tractional RD develops a break it assumes the characteristics of a rhegmatogenous RD and progresses more quickly (combined tractional-rhegmatogenous RD).

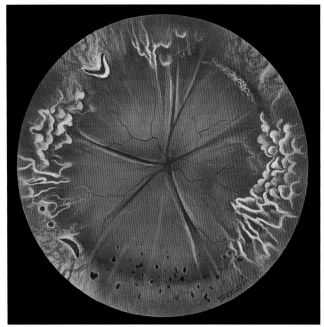

Fig. 19.29
Proliferative vitreoretinopathy grade C showing total retinal detachment with folds, large pigment clumps inferiorly, an open retinal tear at 7.30 o'clock, an open retinal tear with rolled edges at 11 o'clock and lattice degeneration between 1 and 2 o'clock

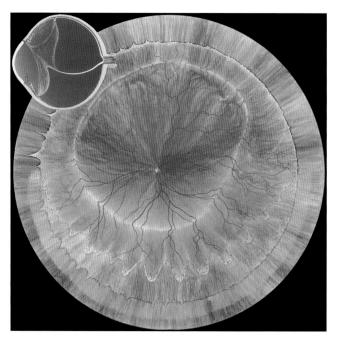

Fig. 19.30
Tractional retinal detachment following penetrating trauma and vitreous loss showing absence of retinal breaks, shallow inferior elevation that does not extend to the ora serrata and a circumferential retinal fold. The cross-section shows extensive posterior vitreous detachment and incarceration of vitreous into the wound (Courtesy of C L Schepens, M E Hartnett and T Hirose, from *Schepens' Retinal Detachment and Allied Diseases*, Butterworth-Heinemann, 2000)

DIAGNOSIS OF EXUDATIVE RETINAL DETACHMENT

1. **Symptoms.** Photopsia is absent because there is no vitreoretinal traction although floaters may be present if there is associated vitritis. The visual field defect may develop suddenly and progress rapidly. Depending on the cause both eyes may be involved simultaneously (e.g. Harada disease).
2. **Signs**
   - The RD has a convex configuration, just like a rhegmatogenous RD, but its surface is smooth and not corrugated.
   - The detached retina is very mobile and exhibits the phenomenon of 'shifting fluid' in which SRF responds to the force of gravity and detaches the area of retina under which it accumulates.
   - For example, in the upright position the SRF collects under the inferior retina (Fig. 19.31a), but on assuming the supine position for several minutes the inferior retina flattens and the SRF shifts posteriorly detaching the superior retina (Fig. 19.31b).
   - The cause of the RD, such as a choroidal tumour (Fig. 19.32), may be apparent when the fundus is examined, or the patient may have an associated systemic disease responsible for the RD (e.g. Harada disease, toxaemia of pregnancy).
   - 'Leopard spots' consisting of scattered areas of subretinal clumping may be seen after the detachment has flattened (Fig. 19.33).

DIFFERENTIAL DIAGNOSIS OF RETINAL DETACHMENT

Degenerative retinoschisis

1. **Symptoms.** Photopsia and floaters are absent because there is no vitreoretinal traction. A visual field defect is seldom observed because spread posterior to the equator is rare. If present it is absolute and not relative as in a RD. Occasionally symptoms occur as a result of either vitreous haemorrhage or development of progressive RD.

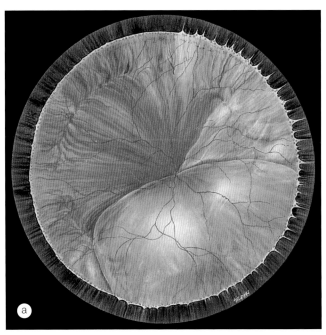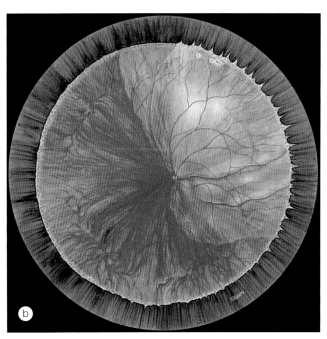

Fig. 19.31
Exudative retinal detachment with shifting fluid. **(a)** Inferior subretinal fluid with the patient sitting; **(b)** fluid shifts upwards with the patient in the supine position (Courtesy of C L Schepens, M E Hartnett and T Hirose, from *Schepens' Retinal Detachment and Allied Diseases*, Butterworth-Heinemann, 2000)

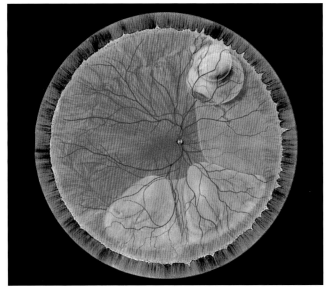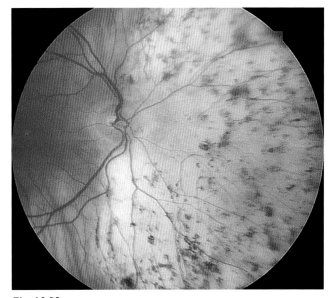

Fig. 19.32
Exudative retinal detachment. In the sitting position an inferior bullous detachment is separated by flat detachment from a smaller balloon in the upper nasal quadrant associated with a peripheral choroidal tumour (Courtesy of C L Schepens, M E Hartnett and T Hirose, from *Schepens' Retinal Detachment and Allied Diseases*, Butterworth-Heinemann, 2000)

Fig. 19.33
'Leopard spot' pigmentation following resolution of exudative retinal detachment

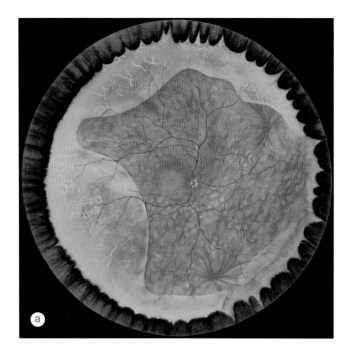

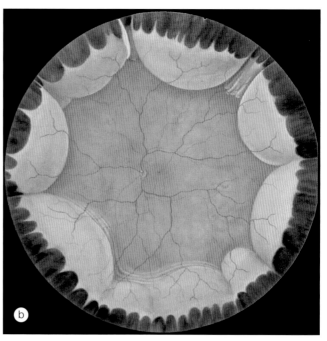

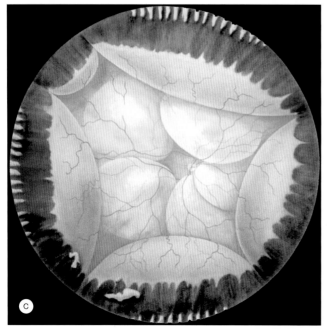

Fig. 19.34
Differential diagnosis of retinal detachment. **(a)** Degenerative retinoschisis showing peripheral vascular sheathing and 'snowflakes'; **(b)** choroidal detachment; **(c)** uveal effusion characterized by choroidal and exudative retinal detachment (Courtesy of C L Schepens, M E Hartnett and T Hirose, from *Schepens' Retinal Detachment and Allied Diseases*, Butterworth-Heinemann, 2000 – figs a and c; R J Brockhurst, C L Schepens, I D Okamura, from *Am J Ophthalmol* 1960;49:1257–1266 – fig. b)

2. Signs (Fig. 19.34a)
- Breaks may be present in one or both layers.
- The elevation is convex, smooth, thin and relatively immobile unlike the opaque and corrugated appearance of a rhegmatogenous RD. The thin inner leaf of the schisis cavity may be mistaken, on cursory examination, for an atrophic long-standing rhegmatogenous RD but demarcation lines and secondary cysts in the inner leaf are absent.

Choroidal detachment

1. Symptoms. Photopsia and floaters are absent because there is no vitreoretinal traction. A visual field defect may be noticed if the choroidal detachment is extensive.

2. Signs
- Low intraocular pressure is common as a result of concomitant detachment of the ciliary body.
- The anterior chamber may be shallow in eyes with extensive choroidal detachments.

- The elevations are brown, convex, smooth and relatively immobile (Fig. 19.34b). Temporal and nasal bullae tend to be most prominent. Large 'kissing' choroidal detachments may obscure the view of the fundus. The elevations do not extend to the posterior pole because they are limited by the firm adhesion between the suprachoroidal lamellae where the vortex veins enter their scleral canals.

Uveal effusion syndrome

The uveal effusion syndrome is a rare, idiopathic condition which most frequently affects middle-aged hypermetropic men. It is characterized by ciliochoroidal detachment followed by exudative RD (Fig. 19.34c) which may be bilateral. Following resolution, the RPE frequently shows a characteristic residual ('leopard spot') mottling. Uveal effusion may be mistaken for a RD complicated by choroidal detachment or a ring melanoma of the anterior choroid.

PROPHYLAXIS OF RHEGMATOGENOUS RETINAL DETACHMENT

Although given the right circumstances most retinal breaks can cause RD, some are more dangerous than others. Important criteria to be considered in the selection of patients for prophylactic treatment can be divided into: (a) *characteristics of the break* and (b) *other considerations*.

Characteristics of break

1. **Type:** a tear is more dangerous than a hole because it is associated with dynamic vitreoretinal traction.
2. **Size:** the larger the break the more dangerous.
3. **Symptomatic** tears associated with acute PVD are more dangerous than those detected on routine examination.
4. **Location** is important for the following reasons:
   - Superior breaks are more dangerous than inferior breaks because, as a result of gravity, SRF is likely to spread more quickly. Superotemporal tears are particularly dangerous because the macula is threatened early in the event of RD.
   - Equatorial breaks are more dangerous than oral because the latter are usually located within the vitreous base.
5. **Pigmentation** around a retinal break indicates that it has been present for a long time and the danger of progression to clinical RD is reduced, although chronicity is not a guarantee against future progression.

Other considerations

1. **Cataract surgery** is known to increase the risk of RD, particularly if associated with vitreous loss.
2. **Myopic** patients are more prone to RD. A retinal break in a myopic eye should be taken more seriously than an identical lesion in a non-myopic eye.
3. **Family history** may occasionally be relevant; any break or predisposing degeneration should be taken seriously if the patient gives a family history of RD.
4. **Systemic diseases** that are associated with an increased risk of RD include Marfan syndrome, Stickler syndrome and Ehlers–Danlos syndrome.

Clinical examples

The following clinical examples illustrate the various risk factors just discussed (Fig. 19.35):

1. **Subclinical RD** associated with a large symptomatic U-tear and located in the upper temporal quadrant (Fig. 19.35a) should be treated prophylactically without delay because the risk of progression to a clinical RD is very high. As the tear is located in the upper temporal quadrant, early macular involvement by SRF is possible. Treatment options include cryotherapy combined with an explant, and pneumatic retinopexy (see below).

   NB Argon laser photocoagulation alone is less appropriate because the break is surrounded by SRF.

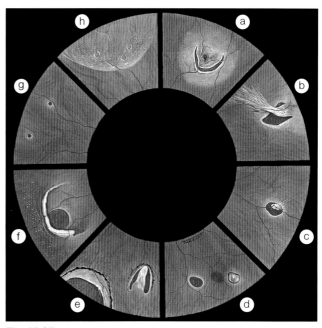

Fig. 19.35
Prophylactic treatment of retinal breaks (see text)

2. **A large U-tear** in the upper temporal quadrant in an eye with symptomatic acute PVD (Fig. 19.35b) should be treated without delay because the risk of progression to clinical RD is high. Although the tear is not associated with SRF yet, it is still dangerous because it is large. Fresh tears such as this, in patients with symptoms of acute PVD, often progress to RD within a few days or weeks unless treated prophylactically. In addition, SRF accumulates more quickly in eyes with PVD because the volume of syneretic fluid is greater than in eyes with atrophic holes or dialyses without PVD. Treatment is by cryotherapy or laser photocoagulation.

   NB 'No fluid = No explant'

3. **An operculated U-tear** bridged by a patent blood vessel (Fig. 19.35c) should be treated if persistent dynamic vitreoretinal traction on the bridging blood vessel is causing recurrent vitreous haemorrhage. Although eyes with breaks associated with avulsed or bridging blood vessels may be successfully treated by argon laser photocoagulation alone, the possibility of an explant or vitrectomy to reduce traction on the operculum and blood vessel should be considered.

4. **An operculated U-tear** in the lower temporal quadrant detected by chance (Fig. 19.35d) is much safer because there is no vitreoretinal traction. Prophylaxis is therefore not required in the absence of other risk factors.

5. **Pigment demarcation** associated with an inferior U-tear and a dialysis detected by chance are both low risk lesions (Fig. 19.35e), which have been present for a long time. However, the presence of pigmentation around a large U-tear is not always a guarantee against progression, particularly when associated with other risk factors such as aphakia, myopia or RD in the fellow eye. If necessary, treatment may involve cryotherapy or photocoagulation.

6. **Degenerative retinoschisis** with breaks in both layers (Fig. 19.35f) does not require treatment. Although this lesion represents a full-thickness defect in the sensory retina, the fluid within the schisis cavity is usually viscid and rarely passes into the subretinal space.

7. **Small asymptomatic holes** near the ora serrata (Fig. 19.35g) do not require treatment because the risk of RD is extremely small as they are probably located within the vitreous base. About 5% of the general population have such lesions.

8. **Small inner layer holes in retinoschisis** (Fig. 19.35f) also carry an extremely low risk of RD as there is no communication between the vitreous cavity and the subretinal space. Treatment is therefore inappropriate.

   NB In the absence of associated retinal breaks neither lattice nor snailtrack degenerations require prophylactic treatment. However, prophylaxis should be considered if PVD has not yet occurred and the fellow eye has suffered a RD in the past.

Choice of treatment modalities

The three modalities used for prophylaxis are: (a) *cryotherapy*, (b) *laser photocoagulation using a slit-lamp delivery system* and (c) *laser using the indirect ophthalmoscopic delivery system combined with scleral indentation*. Large areas of cryotherapy may increase the risk of pigment epithelial cell release and subsequent epiretinal membrane formation. Therefore laser is the preferred modality for extensive lesions. For small lesions there is little evidence to suggest an increased risk with cryotherapy as opposed to laser. In most cases the treatment modality is based on the surgeon's preference and experience as well as the availability of instrumentation. Other considerations are as follows:

1. **Location of lesion:** an equatorial lesion can be treated by either photocoagulation or cryotherapy. A post-equatorial lesion can be treated only by photocoagulation unless the conjunctiva is incised. Peripheral lesions near the ora serrata can be treated either by cryotherapy or laser photocoagulation using the indirect ophthalmoscope delivery system combined with indentation. Treatment of very peripheral lesions by laser photocoagulation using a slit-lamp delivery system is difficult because it may be impossible to adequately treat the base of a U-tear.

2. **Clarity of media:** eyes with hazy media are much easier to treat by cryotherapy.

3. **Pupil size:** eyes with small pupils are easier to treat by cryotherapy.

Laser photocoagulation

a. Select a spot size of 200μm and set the duration to 0.1 or 0.2 seconds.

b. Insert the triple-mirror contact lens or one of the wide field lenses.

c. Surround the lesion with two rows of confluent burns of moderate intensity (Fig. 19.36).

d. After treatment the patient should avoid strenuous physical exertion for about 7 days until an adequate adhesion has formed and the lesion is securely sealed.

Cryotherapy

a. Instil a topical anaesthetic or inject lidocaine (Xylocaine) subconjunctivally in the same quadrant as the lesion to be treated. For lesions behind the equator, a small conjunctival incision may be necessary to enable the cryoprobe to reach the required location.

b. Insert a Barraquer lid speculum.

c. Check the cryoprobe for correct freezing and defrosting and also make sure that the rubber sleeve is not covering the tip.

d. While viewing with the indirect ophthalmoscope, gently indent the sclera with the tip of the probe. In order not to

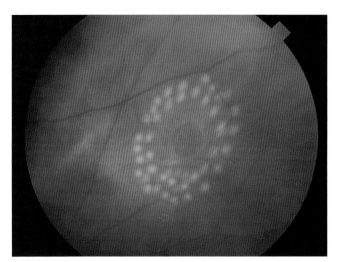

Fig. 19.36
Appearance soon after prophylactic laser photocoagulation of a retinal hole

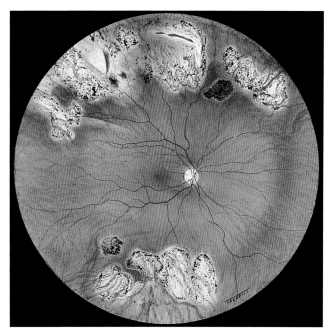

Fig. 19.37
Pigmentation and chorioretinal atrophy following prophylactic cryotherapy

mistake the shaft of the probe for the tip, start indenting near the ora serrata and then move the tip posteriorly to the lesion.

e. Surround the lesion with a single row of cryo-applications, terminating freezing as soon as the retina whitens. In most cases this can be achieved by one or two applications to the tear itself. Because recently frozen retina soon reverts to its normal colour, it is easier to inadvertently re-treat the same area with cryotherapy than with photocoagulation.

NB Do not remove the cryoprobe until it has defrosted completely because premature removal may 'crack' the choroid and give rise to choroidal haemorrhage.

f. Pad the eye for about 4 hours to help decrease chemosis and advise the patient to refrain from strenuous physical activity for 7 days. For about 2 days the treated area appears whitish due to oedema. After about 5 days pigmentation begins to appear. Initially the pigment is fine and then it becomes coarser and is associated with a variable amount of chorioretinal atrophy (Fig. 19.37).

Causes of failure

1. **Failure to surround the entire lesion,** particularly the base of a U-tear, is the most common cause of failure. If the most peripheral part of the tear cannot be reached by photocoagulation, then cryotherapy should be used.
2. **Failure to apply contiguous treatment** when treating a large break or a dialysis.
3. **Failure to use an explant** in an eye with 'subclinical RD'.
4. **New break formation** within or adjacent to treated area (Fig. 19.38) is usually caused by excessively heavy

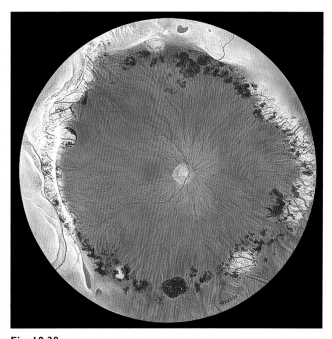

Fig. 19.38
New breaks at 7 and 12 o'clock with subretinal fluid following extensive cryotherapy of lattice degeneration

treatment, particularly of lattice degeneration. New breaks developing away from a treated area are probably not associated with the treatment itself.

SURGERY OF RHEGMATOGENOUS RETINAL DETACHMENT

Preoperative considerations

Prognosis for preservation of central vision

The main factors governing visual function following surgical reattachment of the retina are:
1. **Duration of macular involvement.**
   * If the macula is uninvolved most eyes maintain their preoperative visual acuity.
   * If the macula is detached for 10 days or less post-operative visual acuity is potentially very good, although patients may complain of distortion and altered image size.
   * If the macula is detached for over 2 months, post-operative visual acuity is usually very poor. However, it must be emphasized that, although visual acuity may be poor, the patient is frequently glad to have restoration of peripheral vision following successful retinal reattachment.
2. **Height of macular detachment,** reflected by pre-operative visual acuity, is also important. It appears that photoreceptor cell degeneration is more severe with increasing separation from the RPE.
3. **Age.** Patients 60 years of age or younger obtain better postoperative visual acuity than those older.

Indications for urgent surgery

It should be noted that the spread of SRF is governed by three factors:

1. **The position of the primary break:** SRF will spread more quickly from a superior break.
2. **The size of the break:** large breaks lead to more rapid accumulation of SRF than small ones.
3. **State of vitreous gel:** if the vitreous gel is healthy and solid, even giant retinal tears or giant dialyses may not lead to RD. However, if synchysis is advanced as in myopia, progression is usually rapid and the entire retina may become detached within 1 or 2 days.

It is therefore apparent that a patient with a fresh RD involving the superotemporal quadrant but with an intact macula should be operated on as soon as possible. In order to prevent SRF spreading to the macula, the patient should be positioned flat in bed with only one pillow and with the head turned so that the retinal break is in the most dependent position. For example, a patient with a right upper temporal RD should turn the head to the right. Preoperative bed rest is also desirable in eyes with bullous RDs because it may lessen the amount of SRF and facilitate surgery. Patients with dense fresh vitreous haemorrhage in whom visualization of the fundus is impossible should also be operated on as soon as possible if ultrasonography shows an underlying RD.

What to tell the patient

The function of the retina can be likened to the film in a camera and an RD can be explained in terms of wallpaper peeling off a wall. Simple diagrams may be helpful in explaining the principles of surgery. The patient should be informed that the other eye will also be examined and any weaknesses may be treated. It is also important to emphasize that anatomical success does not equate to visual success and occasionally a second operation is necessary. The patient should be warned that after surgery the eye will be red, tender and slightly painful. There may also be some transient double vision.

Mydriatics

The pupil is dilated with 1% cyclopentolate and 10% phenylephrine drops given at 15-minute intervals for 1 hour preoperatively; 1% atropine is also usually instilled into the operated eye at the end of the procedure to maintain good postoperative mydriasis.

> **NB** If operating under general anaesthesia it is good practice to carefully examine the fellow eye, which should therefore also be dilated preoperatively.

Choice of technique

The aim of surgery is to successfully repair the detachment with minimal trauma and attendant risks. If the retinal break has accumulated too much SRF to be suitable for pneumatic retinopexy then conventional scleral buckling techniques or vitrectomy will be necessary.

Pneumatic retinopexy

Pneumatic retinopexy is an outpatient procedure in which an intravitreal expanding gas bubble is used to seal a retinal break and reattach the retina without scleral buckling (Fig. 19.39). The most frequently used gases are sulphur hexafluoride (SF6) and perfluoropropane (C3F8). Pneumatic

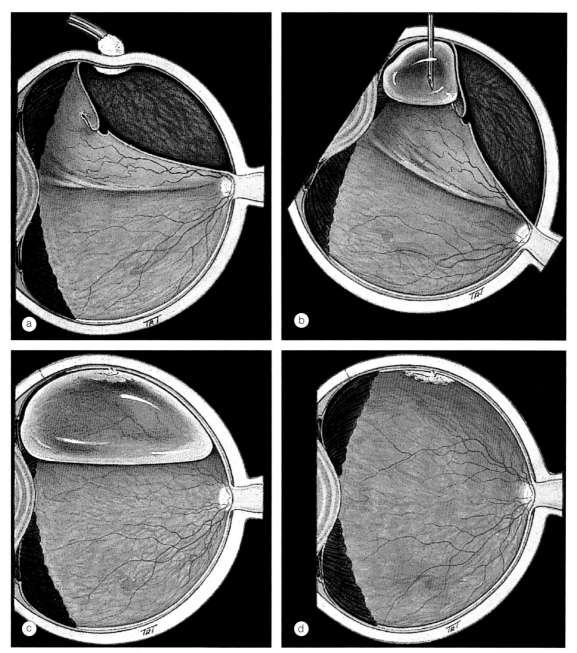

Fig. 19.39
Pneumatic retinopexy. **(a)** Cryotherapy; **(b)** gas injection; **(c)** gas has sealed the break and retina is flat; **(d)** gas has absorbed

retinopexy has the advantage of being a relatively quick, minimally invasive, 'office-based' procedure. However, success rates are usually slightly less than those achievable with conventional scleral buckling surgery. The procedure is usually reserved for treatment of uncomplicated RDs with a small retinal break or a cluster of breaks extending over an area of less than two clock hours situated in the upper two-thirds of the peripheral retina.

Principles of scleral buckling

Scleral buckling is a surgical procedure in which material sutured onto the sclera (explant) creates an inward indentation (buckle). Its purposes are to close retinal breaks by apposing the RPE to the NSR, and to reduce dynamic vitreoretinal traction at sites of local vitreoretinal adhesion.

Explants

Explants are made from soft or hard silicone. In order to adequately seal a retinal break it is essential for the buckle to have adequate length, width and height. The entire break should ideally be surrounded by about 2mm of buckle. It is also important for the buckle to involve the area of the vitreous base anterior to the tear in order to prevent the possibility of subsequent reopening of the tear and anterior leakage of SRF. The dimensions of the retinal break can be assessed by comparing it with the diameter of the optic disc (1.5mm) or the end of a scleral indenter.

Buckle configurations

1. **Radial** explants are placed at right angles to the limbus (Fig. 19.40a). They are used to seal u-tears or posterior breaks, because of inability to support them on a circumferential buckle.
2. **Segmental circumferential** explants are placed circumferentially with the limbus to create a segmental buckle (Fig. 19.40b). They may be used to seal multiple breaks located in one or two quadrants and/or at varying distances from the ora serrata, anterior breaks and dialyses.
3. **Encircling** explants are placed around the entire circumference of the globe to create a 360° buckle and,

if necessary, may be augmented by local explants (Fig. 19.40c and d). They are now seldom used unless accompanied by vitrectomy.

Technique of scleral buckling

a. A peritomy is performed appropriate to the extent of scleral exposure required and episcleral tissue is cleared (Fig. 19.41a).
b. A squint hook is inserted under a rectus muscle and a reverse mounted needle with a 4/0 black silk suture is passed under (not through) the muscle tendon (Fig. 19.41b) and the suture is secured by twisting it around mosquito forceps.
c. Breaks are localized by indenting the sclera whilst viewing the indirect ophthalmoscope and marking the site with a spot of surgical ink.
d. Cryotherapy is applied to by indenting the sclera gently with the tip of the cryoprobe and freezing is continued until the break is surrounded by a 2mm margin of ice (Fig. 19.41c).
e. With callipers, the distance separating the sutures is measured and the sclera marked and a mattress-type suture which will straddle the explant is inserted (Fig. 19.41d). As a general rule, the separation of sutures should be about 1.5× the diameter of a sponge explant.
f. The explant is fed through the sutures which are then tied (Fig. 19.41e).
g. The position of the buckle is checked in relation to the break. If the break is closed or very nearly closed, the operation can be terminated without drainage of SRF. If the buckle is incorrectly positioned it should be removed and repositioned (Fig. 19.41f).
h. 'Fishmouthing' is a tendency of certain retinal tears, typically large superior U-tears located at the equator in a bullous RD, to open widely following scleral bucking and drainage of SRF (Fig. 19.42a). Management of this problem involves insertion of an additional radial buckle and injection of air into the vitreous cavity (Fig. 19.42b).

Drainage of subretinal fluid

Indications

Although a large proportion of RDs can be treated successfully with non-drainage techniques, drainage of SRF may be required under the following circumstances:

1. **Deep SRF** beneath the retinal break. In such cases the application of cryotherapy may be difficult or impossible and the RD should be repaired using a **D-ACE** (**D**rain-**A**ir-**C**ryo-**E**xplant) although such cases are now often repaired via a vitrectomy procedure.
   • **D**rain the SRF to bring the break closer to the RPE

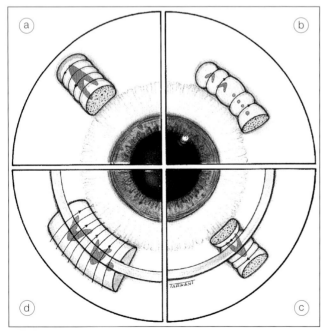

Fig. 19.40
Configuration of scleral buckles. **(a)** Radial sponge; **(b)** circumferential sponge; **(c)** encirclement augmented by a radial sponge; **(d)** encirclement augmented by a solid silicone tyre

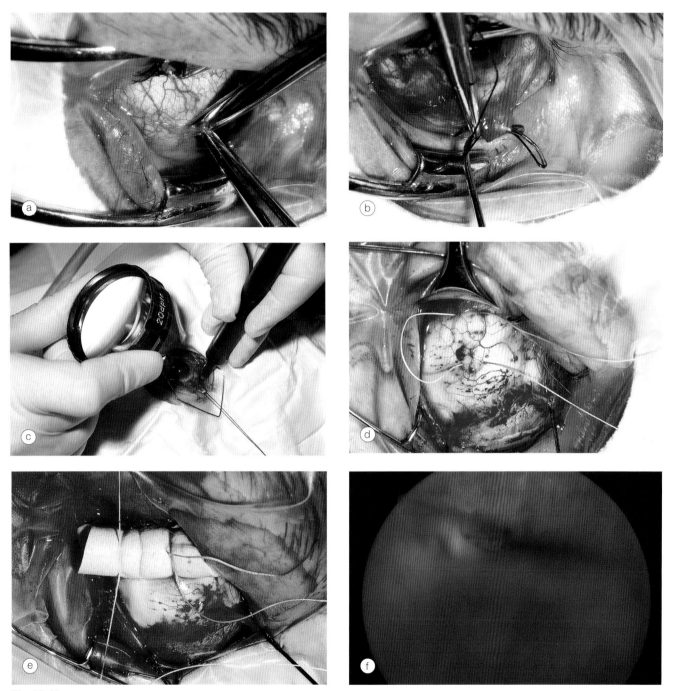

Fig. 19.41
Technique of scleral buckling. **(a)** Conjunctival incision; **(b)** insertion of bridle suture; **(c)** cryotherapy; **(d)** scleral mattress suture in place; **(e)** tying of suture over explant; **(f)** appearance of indentation – in this case the buckle is too anterior in relation to the break and must be repositioned

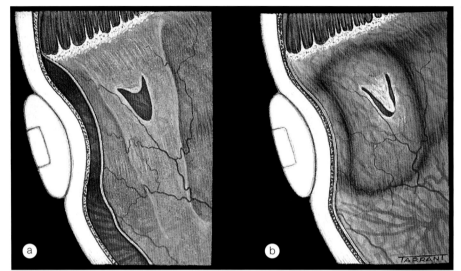

Fig. 19.42
(a) 'Fishmouthing' of a U-tear communicating with a radial fold; **(b)** insertion of radial buckle

- **A**ir injection into the vitreous cavity to counteract the hypotony induced by drainage.
- **C**ryotherapy to the localized break.
- **E**xplant insertion.

2. **Long-standing RDs** tend to be associated with viscous SRF and may take a long time (many months) to absorb. Drainage may therefore be necessary to restore macular reattachment quickly, even if the break itself can be closed without drainage.

Technique

1. 'Prang'

a. Digital pressure is applied to the globe until the central retinal artery is occluded and complete blanching of the choroidal vasculature is achieved in order to prevent haemorrhage from the drainage site.

b. A full-thickness perforation is made with the tip of a 27-gauge hypodermic needle bent 2mm at the tip in a single, swift but controlled fashion.

c. Following drainage of SRF, air is injected to restore ocular pressure.

2. 'Cut-down'

a. The sclerotomy site should be beneath the area of deepest SRF but avoiding vortex veins.

b. A radial sclerotomy is performed about 4mm long and of sufficient depth to allow herniation of a small dark knuckle of choroid.

c. A mattress suture is placed across the lips of the sclerotomy (optional).

d. The assistant holds apart the lips and the prolapsed knuckles are inspected with a +20D lens for the presence of large choroidal vessels.

e. If large choroidal vessels are absent, gentle low heat cautery is applied to the choroidal knuckle to decrease the risk of choroidal bleeding.

f. If this does not result in drainage of SRF the choroidal knuckle is perforated with a 25-gauge hypodermic needle (Fig. 19.43).

Complications

1. **Failure of drainage** of SRF ('dry tap') may be caused by one of the following:
   - Failure to perforate the full thickness of the choroid.
   - Attempted drainage in an area of flat retina – therefore always check the position of the SRF immediately prior to drainage.
   - Incarceration of the retina in the sclerotomy (see below).

2. **Haemorrhage** is usually caused by damage to a large choroidal vessel (Fig. 19.44a). Although small bleeds may be innocuous because the blood escapes with the SRF, large bleeds may give rise to postoperative maculopathy as a result of gravitation of large amounts of blood in the subretinal space to the fovea, vitreous haemorrhage and haemorrhagic choroidal detachment.

3. **Retinal incarceration** into the sclerotomy (Fig. 19.44b) is usually due to excessively elevated intraocular pressure at the time of drainage using the 'cut-down' technique. As already mentioned it is one of the causes of a dry tap although occasionally, after an initial appearance of SRF, the flow will suddenly cease despite the fact that a large amount of SRF still remains in the eye.

Clinical examples

The following clinical examples will emphasize the most important aspects of management just discussed.

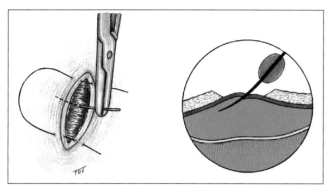

Fig. 19.43
Cut-down technique of drainage of subretinal fluid

Fresh retinal detachment

1. **Preoperative considerations.** Examination shows a localized right upper temporal RD due to a U-tear (Fig. 19.45a). The prognosis for central vision is good because the macula is uninvolved. The patient should be operated on as soon as possible because the macula is in danger as the break is located in the upper temporal quadrant and SRF will spread quickly because the break is large.
2. **Surgical technique for cryotherapy and buckle.** Peritomy should extend from 8.30 to 12.30 o'clock to expose the lateral and superior recti. The tear should close on a 5mm sponge explant. The sutures should be about 8mm apart to impart adequate height to the buckle. The sponge should be placed radially (Fig. 19.45b) to prevent 'fishmouthing'. Accurate positioning of the explant is vital in this case. Failure to close the break may be due to an undersized buckle (Fig. 19.45c) or a malposition of the buckle (Fig. 19.45d). Alternatively a solid type explant can be used, although it creates less of an indent and is associated with an increased requirement for SRF drainage to ensure closure of the break. Drainage of SRF is not otherwise required because the retina is mobile, the break can be apposed to RPE without difficulty and SRF is not viscous as the RD is fresh.

NB It is also possible to treat this case with pneumatic retinopexy.

Long-standing retinal detachment

1. **Preoperative considerations.** Examination shows an extensive right RD with macular involvement associated with a U-tear in the upper temporal quadrant and two small holes in the lower temporal quadrant (Fig. 19.46a). A partially pigmented demarcation line is present at the junction of detached and flat retina, and a secondary intraretinal cyst is present inferiorly. This is therefore a long-standing RD because demarcation marks take about 3 months to develop and secondary retinal cysts usually take about 12 months. The prognosis for restoration of good visual acuity is very poor because the fovea has probably been detached for at least 12 months. There is therefore no urgency for surgery, which can be performed at the patient's and surgeon's convenience.
2. **Surgical technique.** Peritomy should extend from 5.30 to 12.30 o'clock to expose the superior, lateral and inferior recti. The breaks can be sealed with a long 4mm wide circumferential sponge explant extending from 7 to

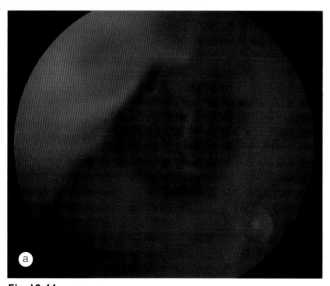
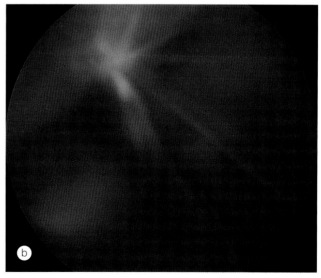

Fig. 19.44
Complications of drainage of subretinal fluid. **(a)** Haemorrhage; **(b)** retinal incarceration into the drainage site

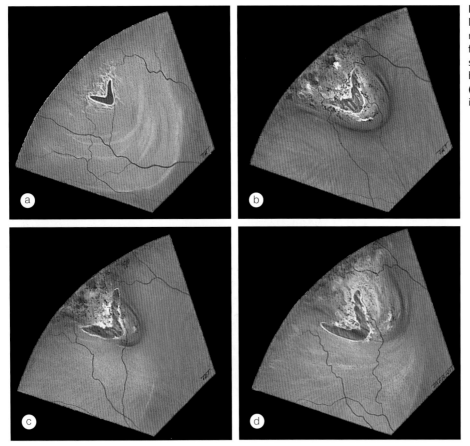

Fig. 19.45
Management of fresh upper temporal retinal detachment and causes of failure. **(a)** Prior to buckling; **(b)** tear sealed and retina is flat; **(c)** tear is open because the buckle is undersized; **(d)** tear is open because the buckle is incorrectly positioned

10.30 o'clock or a circumferential solid type explant (Fig. 19.46b). Drainage of SRF may be required because in long-standing cases SRF is viscous and may take a long time to absorb.

Causes of failure

1. **Missed breaks.** It should be emphasized that about 50% of all RDs are associated with more than one break. In most cases the breaks are located within 90° of each other. At surgery, the surgeon should therefore not be satisfied if only one break has been found until a thorough search has been made for the presence of other breaks and the configuration of the RD corresponds to the position of the primary break.
2. **Buckle failure** may be the result of the following:
   • Buckle of inadequate size – replace (see Fig. 19.45c).
   • Buckle incorrectly positioned – reposition (see Fig. 19.45d).
   • Buckle of inadequate height – drain SRF or consider intravitreal gas injection.
3. **Proliferative vitreoretinopathy** is the most common cause of late failure. The traction forces associated with

PVR can occasionally open old breaks and create new ones. Presentation is typically between the fourth and sixth postoperative weeks. After an initial period of visual improvement following successful retina reattachment the patient reports a sudden and progressive loss of vision, which may develop within a few hours.
4. **Reopening of a retinal break** in the absence of PVR as a result of inadequate cryotherapy of scleral buckling. It may occur when buckle height decreases either with time or following surgical removal.

PARS PLANA VITRECTOMY

Introduction

Instrumentation

The diameter of the shafts of most instruments is 0.9mm (20-gauge) so that they are interchangeable and can be inserted through either sclerotomy. Smaller systems are also becoming increasingly popular. The smaller sclerotomies do

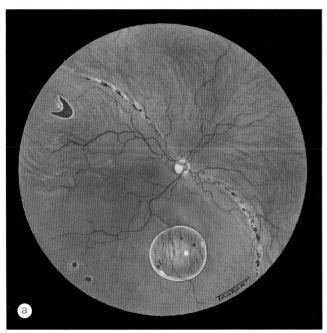
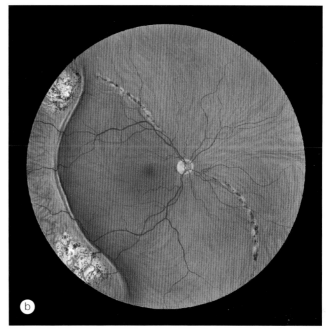

Fig. 19.46
Management of long-standing retinal detachment. **(a)** Retinal detachment with three breaks, a retinal cyst and high water marks; **(b)** successful re-attachment by circumferential buckling

not usually require suturing but there is some concern that they may seal by vitreous incarceration with an increased risk of postoperative endophthalmitis.

1. **The cutter** has an inner guillotine blade which oscillates up to 1500 times/minute (Fig. 19.47 bottom), cutting the vitreous gel into tiny pieces and simultaneously removing it by suction into a collecting cassette. Newer high speed cutters (over 2500 oscillations per minute) are increasingly being used allowing less traction on the vitreoretinal interface during surgery.
2. **The intraocular illumination source** is through a fibreoptic probe (Fig. 19.47 top) which delivers light from an 80–150 watt bulb. Brighter, high intensity halogen type light sources are also becoming available and can be inserted via a self-retaining cannula into a fourth port. These have the advantage of allowing the surgeon to carry out true bimanual surgery, which can be particularly useful in challenging cases such as advanced tractional diabetic retinal detachment.
3. **The infusion cannula** usually has an intraocular length of 4mm, although in special circumstances (such as choroidal detachment or eyes with opaque media) a 6mm cannula may be required.
4. **Accessory instruments** include scissors, forceps, flute needle, endodiathermy and endolaser delivery systems.

5. **Wide-angle viewing system** (Fig. 19.48) consists of an indirect lens beneath the operative microscope and a series of prisms to re-invert the image. The field of view is almost out to the ora serrata, and higher magnification lenses are also available for macular surgery.

Tamponading agents

1. **Purposes** are to achieve intraoperative retinal flattening by fluid-gas exchange combined with internal drainage of SRF, and to produce internal tamponade of retinal breaks during the postoperative period.

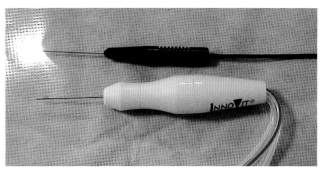

Fig. 19.47
(Top) Illumination pipe; **(bottom)** cutter (Courtesy of V Tanner)

2. **Expanding gases.** Although air can be used in certain cases one of the following expanding gases is usually preferred in order to achieve prolonged intraocular tamponade.
   - Sulphur hexafluoride (SF6), which doubles its volume if used at 100% concentration and lasts 10–14 days.
   - Perfluorethane (C2F6), which triples its volume at 100% and lasts 30–35 days.
   - Perfluoropropane (C3F8), which quadruples its volume at 100% and lasts 55–65 days.

> **NB** Because the eye is usually left almost entirely gas filled at the end of the procedure, most tamponading agents are used at an isovolumetric concentration (e.g. 20–30% for SF6 and 12–16% for C3F8).

3. **Heavy liquids** (perfluorocarbons) have a high specific gravity and thus remain in a dependent position when injected into the vitreous cavity.
4. **Silicone oils** have a low specific gravity and are thus buoyant. They allow for more controlled intraoperative retinal manipulation and may also be used for prolonged postoperative intraocular tamponade. The most commonly used liquid silicones have relatively low viscosity (1000–5000cs). The 1000-cs silicone is easy to inject and remove whilst 5000-cs silicone is less prone to the production of tiny droplets (emulsification).

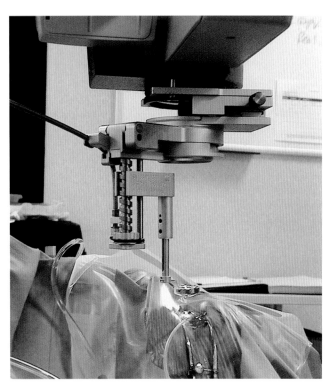

Fig. 19.48
Viewing system for pars plana vitrectomy (Courtesy of V Tanner)

5. **Long-term heavy liquid tamponade.** Although primarily developed for intraoperative use, newer perfluorocarbon compounds are now available for postoperative tamponade of the inferior retina. However, problems have been noted with potential retinal toxicity and severe postoperative inflammation.

Indications

Although the vast majority of simple rhegmatogenous RD can be treated successfully by scleral buckling, vitrectomy has greatly improved the prognosis for more complex detachments. As techniques have improved and familiarity and confidence have grown, the threshold for vitrectomy surgery has fallen. Many surgeons now feel that morbidity and success rates are better with vitrectomy for all pseudophakic, aphakic RD, and those that would otherwise require drainage of SRF. The guidelines below are therefore not absolute but intended to give some insight into the factors influencing the decision-making process.

Rhegmatogenous retinal detachment

1. **In which retinal breaks cannot be visualized** as a result of haemorrhage, vitreous debris, posterior capsular opacity, IOL edge effects. Vitrectomy is crucial to provide an adequate retinal view of all associated breaks. Scleral buckling carries a high risk of failure and PVR in such circumstances if any retinal breaks are missed.
2. **In which retinal breaks cannot be closed by scleral buckling** such as giant tears (Fig. 19.49a), posterior breaks (Fig. 19.49b) and PVR (Fig. 19.49c).

Tractional retinal detachment

1. **Indications in diabetic RD**
   a. *Tractional RD threatening or involving the macula* (Fig. 19.49d). Vitrectomy is always combined with internal panretinal photocoagulation (Fig. 19.50) to prevent postoperative neovascularization that may cause vitreous haemorrhage or rubeosis iridis. Extramacular tractional RD may be observed because, in many cases, it remains stationary for a long time, provided the proliferative retinopathy has been controlled with adequate panretinal photocoagulation.
   b. *Combined tractional-rhegmatogenous RD* should be treated urgently, even if the macula is not involved, because SRF is likely to spread quickly.
2. **Indications in penetrating trauma**
   a. *Prevention of tractional RD*. Unlike diabetic retinopathy where epiretinal membrane proliferation occurs mostly on the posterior retina, fibrocellular proliferation after penetrating trauma tends to develop

on the pre-equatorial retina and/or the ciliary body. Treatment is usually aimed at visual rehabilitation and minimizing the tractional process.

b. Late tractional RD, which may be associated with an intraocular foreign body or retinal incarceration, and occasionally develops months after otherwise successful removal of the foreign body.

Technique

Basic vitrectomy

a. Following limbal peritomy an infusion cannula is secured to the sclera 3.5mm behind the limbus in pseudophakic or aphakic eyes (4mm in phakic eyes) at the level of the inferior border of the lateral rectus muscle.

b. Two further sclerotomies are made at the 10 and 2 o'clock positions. These can be standard stab incisions made with an MVR blade or self-sealing sclerotomies.

c. The cutter and fibreoptic light pipe enter through the upper two sclerotomies (Fig. 19.51).

d. The central vitreous gel and posterior hyaloid face are excised.

The above basic steps apply to all vitrectomies although transconjunctival small gauge systems do not require a peritomy or postoperative suturing. Subsequent steps depend on the characteristics of the RD as follows.

Closure of giant tears

a. Fluid–air exchange is performed to flatten the retina (hydraulic retinal reattachment).

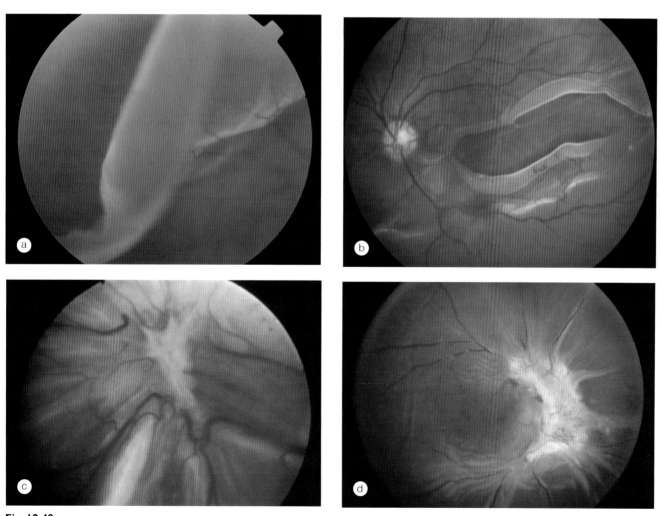

Fig. 19.49
Indications for pars plana vitrectomy. **(a)** Giant retinal tear; **(b)** large posterior tear; **(c)** severe proliferative vitreoretinopathy; **(d)** tractional retinal detachment (Courtesy of C Barry – fig. b; L Merin – fig. d)

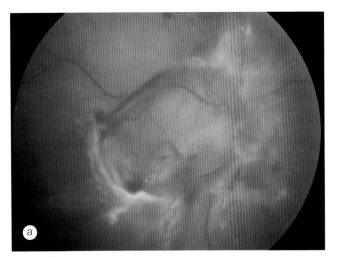
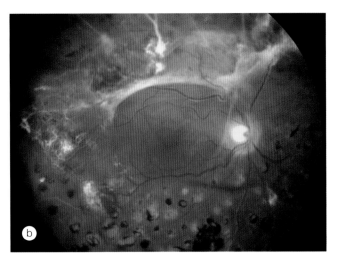

Fig. 19.50
(a) Tractional retinal detachment in severe proliferative diabetic retinopathy; **(b)** postoperative appearance following pars plana vitrectomy and endophotocoagulation (Courtesy of C Barry)

b. The flap of a giant tear is unrolled by injecting a heavy liquid over the optic disc (Fig. 19.52).

c. The now flat retinal breaks are treated with either trans-scleral cryotherapy or endolaser photocoagulation using minimal energy.

d. Prolonged internal tamponade is achieved by replacing air with a non-expansile concentration of sulphur hexafluoride (SF6) or perfluoropropane (C3F8) gases, or with silicone oil. The non-expansile mixture of gas and air is prepared in a large (50ml) syringe and the air-filled vitreous cavity is flushed with 20% or 30% SF6-air mixture or 14–16% of C3F8-air mixture.

Proliferative vitreoretinopathy

The aims of surgery in PVR are to release transvitreal traction by vitrectomy and tangential (surface) traction by membrane dissection in order to restore retinal mobility and allow closure of retinal breaks.

a. Localized fixed retinal folds ('starfolds') may be freed by the removal of the central plaque of epiretinal membrane. This can usually be achieved by engaging the tip of the vertically cutting scissors (Fig. 19.53), or other pick-type instrument, in the edge of the valley of the membrane between two adjacent retinal folds. The membrane is then either surgically dissected or simply peeled from the surface of the retina.

b. The decision to perform a relieving retinotomy (Fig. 19.54) is made after epiretinal membrane dissection has been performed as completely as possible but the retinal mobility is deemed insufficient for lasting re-attachment.

Tractional retinal detachment

The goal of vitrectomy in tractional RDs is to release anteroposterior and/or circumferential vitreoretinal traction. Because the membranes are vascularized, and the retina often friable, they cannot be simply peeled from the surface of the retina as this would result in haemorrhage and tearing of the retina. The two methods of removing fibrovascular membranes in diabetic tractional RDs are the following:

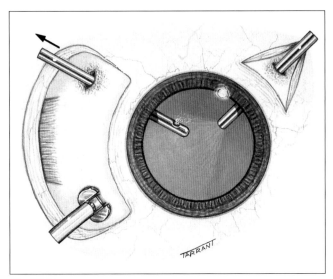

Fig. 19.51
Infusion cannula, light pipe and vitreous cutter in position

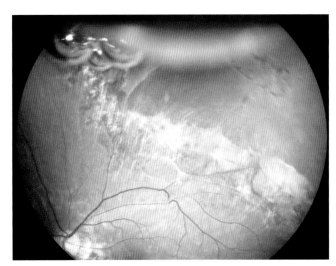

Fig. 19.52
Unrolled giant retinal tear with heavy liquid (Courtesy of C Barry)

1. **Delamination** involves the horizontal cutting of the individual vascular pegs connecting the membranes to the surface of the retina (Fig. 19.55). This is preferred to segmentation (see below) because it allows the complete removal of fibrovascular tissues from the retinal surface (en-bloc delamination).
2. **Segmentation** involves the vertical cutting of epiretinal membranes into small segments (Fig. 19.56). It is used to release circumferential vitreoretinal traction when delamination is difficult or impossible, such as in very

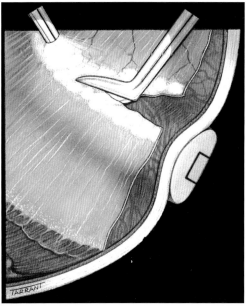

Fig. 19.54
Relieving retinotomy in proliferative vitreoretinopathy

mobile combined traction-rhegmatogenous RD associated with posterior retinal breaks.

Postoperative complications

Raised intraocular pressure

Elevation of intraocular pressure may be caused by the following mechanisms:

1. **Overexpansion of intraocular gas** may cause raised intraocular pressure as a result of complete filling of the vitreous cavity if the concentration of expansile gas used was inadvertently too high.
2. **Silicone oil-associated glaucoma**
   a. *Early glaucoma* may be caused by pupil block by anterior silicone oil face (Fig. 19.57a). This occurs particularly in the aphakic eye with an intact iris diaphragm. In aphakic eyes this can be prevented by performing an inferior ('Ando') iridotomy at the time of surgery to allow free passage of aqueous to the anterior chamber so that the silicone remains behind the iris plane and does not block the pupil.
   b. *Late glaucoma* is caused by emulsified silicone in the anterior chamber (Fig. 19.57b) which causes trabecular blockage. This complication may be reduced by an early removal of silicone oil either via the pars plana in phakic eyes or the limbus in aphakic eyes, although late glaucoma can still occur even

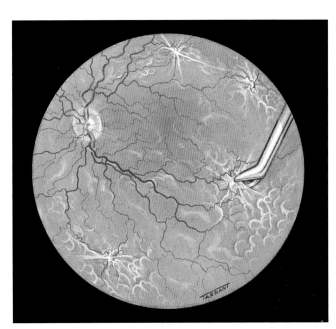

Fig. 19.53
Dissecting of star folds with vertically cutting scissors in proliferative vitreoretinopathy

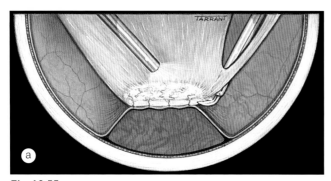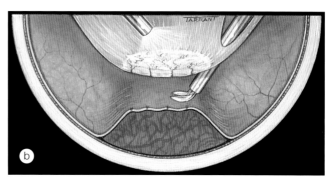

Fig. 19.55
(a) Delamination with horizontally cutting scissors; **(b)** delamination completed

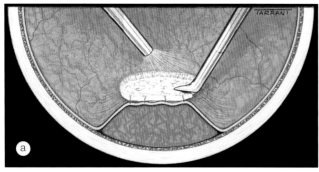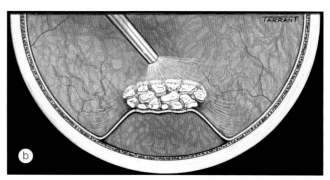

Fig. 19.56
(a) Segmentation with vertically cutting scissors; **(b)** segmentation completed

following prompt removal of apparently non-emulsified oil.
3. **Other mechanisms** are ghost cell glaucoma and steroid-induced (see Chapter 13).

Cataract

Lens opacity may be caused by the following mechanisms:

1. **Gas-induced.** The use of either a large and/or long-lasting intravitreal gas bubble almost invariably gives rise to feathering of the posterior subcapsular lens cortex. Fortunately lens opacification is usually transient in these circumstances.

2. **Silicone-induced.** Almost all phakic eyes with silicone oils eventually develop cataract (Fig. 19.57c). Treatment involves phacoemulsification, posterior capsulorhexis to allow release of oil and posterior chamber lens implantation.

3. **Delayed cataract formation.** Following successful vitrectomy a large proportion of eyes develop nuclear sclerosis within 1 year if the patient is over 50 years of age.

Band keratopathy

Band keratopathy may occur as a result of prolonged contact between silicone oil and the corneal endothelium (Fig. 19.57d).

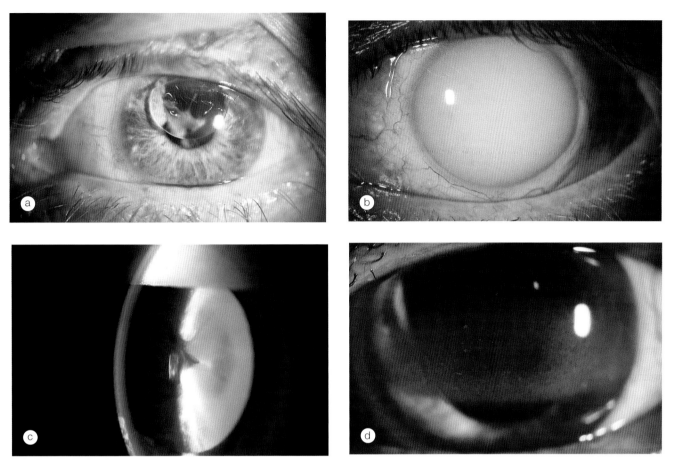

Fig. 19.57
Complications of silicone oil. **(a)** Pupil block glaucoma caused by silicone oil in the anterior chamber; **(b)** late glaucoma caused by trabecular blockage by emulsified silicone oil; **(c)** cataract with emulsified silicone oil (inverted 'pseudo-hypopyon'); **(d)** band keratopathy (Courtesy of Z Gregor – fig. d)

STRABISMUS

INTRODUCTION

Definitions

1. **Visual axis** (line of vision) passes from the fovea, through the nodal point of the eye to the point of fixation (object of regard). In normal binocular single vision (BSV) the two visual axes intersect at the point of fixation, with the images from the two eyes being aligned by the fusion reflex and combined by binocular responsive cells in the visual cortex to give BSV.

2. **Orthophoria** implies perfect ocular alignment in the absence of any stimulus for fusion which is uncommon.

3. **Heterophoria** ('phoria') implies a tendency of the eyes to deviate when fusion is blocked (latent squint). Slight phoria is present in most normal individuals and is overcome by the fusion reflex. The phoria can be either a small inward imbalance (esophoria) or an outward imbalance (exophoria). When fusion is insufficient to

control the imbalance the phoria is described as decompensating and is often associated with symptoms of binocular discomfort or double vision (diplopia).

4. **Heterotropia** ('tropia') implies a manifest deviation in which the visual axes do not intersect at the point of fixation. The images from the two eyes are misaligned so that either double vision is present or, more commonly in children, the image from the deviating eye is suppressed at cortical level. A childhood squint may occur because of failure of the normal development of binocular fusion mechanisms or as a result of oculomotor imbalance secondary to differences in refraction of the two eyes (ametropia). Failure of fusion, for example secondary to poor vision in one eye, may cause heterotropia in adulthood, or a squint may develop because of weakness or mechanical restriction of the extraocular muscles or damage to their nerve supply.
   - Horizontal deviation of the eyes (latent or manifest) is the most common form of strabismus.
   - A vertical deviation almost invariably reflects abnormal ocular motility.
   - Upward displacement of one eye relative to the other is termed a *hypertropia* and a controlled upward imbalance a *hyperphoria*.
   - Downward displacement is termed a *hypotropia* and imbalance a *hypophoria*.

5. **Anatomical axis** is a line passing from the posterior pole through the centre of the cornea. Because the fovea is usually slightly temporal to the anatomical centre of the posterior pole of the eye, the visual axis does not usually correspond to the anatomical axis of the eye.

6. **Angle kappa** is the angle subtended by the visual and anatomical axes and is usually about 5° (Fig. 20.1). The angle is positive when the fovea is temporal to the centre of the posterior pole resulting in a nasal displacement

of the corneal reflex, and negative when the converse applies. A large angle kappa may give the appearance of a squint when none is present (pseudo-squint) and is seen most commonly as a pseudo-exotropia following displacement of the macula in retinopathy of prematurity, where the angle may significantly exceed +5°.

Anatomy of extraocular muscles

Principles

The lateral and medial orbital walls are at an angle of 45° with each other (Fig. 20.2a). The orbital axis therefore forms an angle of 22.5° with both lateral and medial walls. For the sake of simplicity this angle is usually regarded as being 23°. When the eye is looking straight ahead at a fixed point on the horizon with the head erect (primary position of gaze), the visual axis forms an angle of 23° with the orbital axis (Fig. 20.2b). The actions of the extraocular muscles depend on the position of the globe at the time of muscle contraction.

1. **Primary action** of a muscle is its major effect when the eye is in the primary position.

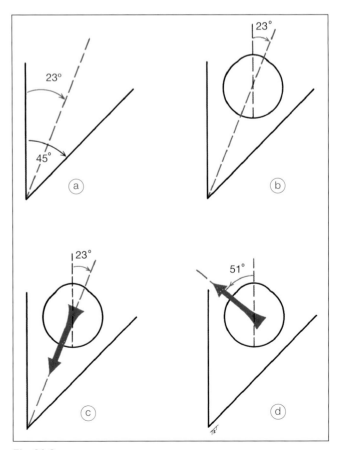

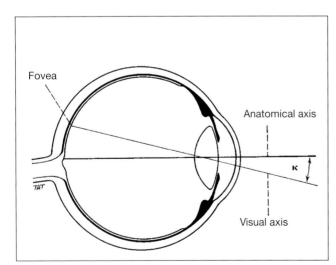

Fig. 20.1
Angle kappa

Fig. 20.2
Anatomy of extraocular muscles (see text)

2. **Subsidiary actions** are the additional effects which depend on the position of the eye.
3. **Listing plane** is an imaginary coronal plane passing through the centre of rotation of the globe. The globe rotates on the X and Z axes of Fick, which intersect in Listing plane (Fig. 20.3).
   - The globe rotates left and right on the vertical Z axis.
   - The globe moves up and down on the horizontal X axis.
   - Torsional movements (wheel rotations) occur on the Y (sagittal) axis which traverses the globe from front to back (similar to the anatomical axis of the eye).
   - Intorsion occurs when the superior limbus rotates nasally and extorsion on temporal rotation.

Horizontal rectus muscles

When the eye is in the primary position, the horizontal recti are purely horizontal movers on the vertical Z axis and have only primary actions.

1. **Medial rectus** originates at the annulus of Zinn at the orbital apex and inserts 5.5mm behind the nasal limbus. Its sole action in the primary position is adduction.
2. **Lateral rectus** originates at the annulus of Zinn and inserts 6.9mm behind the temporal limbus. Its sole action in the primary position is abduction.

Vertical rectus muscles

The vertical recti run in line with the orbital axis and are inserted in front of the equator. They therefore form an angle of 23° with the visual axis (see Fig. 20.2c).

1. **Superior rectus** originates from the upper part of the annulus of Zinn and inserts 7.7mm behind the superior limbus.
   - The primary action is elevation (Fig. 20.4a); secondary actions are adduction and intorsion.
   - When the globe is abducted 23°, the visual and orbital axes coincide (Fig. 20.4b). In this position it has no subsidiary actions and can only act as an elevator. This is therefore the optimal position of the globe for testing the function of the superior rectus muscle. If the globe were adducted 67°, the angle between the visual and orbital axes would be 90° (Fig. 20.4c). In this position the superior rectus could only act as an intortor.
2. **Inferior rectus** originates at the lower part of the annulus of Zinn and inserts 6.5mm behind the inferior limbus.
   - The primary action is depression; secondary actions are adduction and extorsion.
   - When the globe is abducted 23°, the inferior rectus acts purely as a depressor. As for superior rectus, this is the

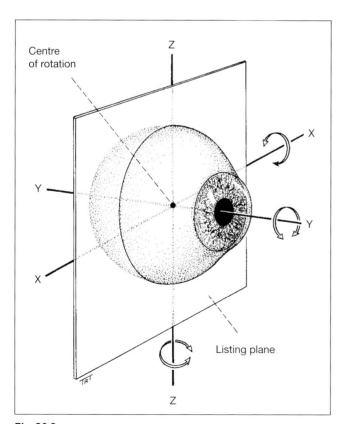

Fig. 20.3
Listing plane and axes of Fick

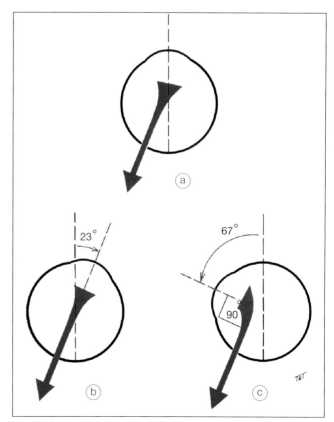

Fig. 20.4
Actions of the right superior rectus muscle (see text)

optimal position of the globe for testing the function of the inferior rectus muscle.

- If the globe were adducted 67°, the inferior rectus could only act as an extortor.

Spiral of Tillaux

The spiral is an imaginary line joining the insertions of the four recti and is an important anatomical landmark when performing surgery. The insertions get further away from the limbus and make a spiral pattern. The medial rectus insertion is closest (5.5mm) followed by the inferior rectus (6.5mm), lateral rectus (6.9mm) and superior rectus (7.7mm) (Fig. 20.5).

Oblique muscles

The obliques are inserted behind the equator and form an angle of 51° with the visual axis (see Fig. 20.2d).

1. **Superior oblique** originates superomedial to the optic foramen. It passes forwards through the trochlea at the angle between the superior and medial walls and is then reflected backwards and laterally to insert in the posterior upper temporal quadrant of the globe (Fig. 20.6).
   - The primary action is intorsion (Fig. 20.7a); secondary actions are depression and abduction.
   - The anterior fibres of the superior oblique tendon are primarily responsible for intorsion and the posterior fibres for depression, allowing separate surgical manipulation of these two actions (see below).

- When the globe is adducted 51°, the visual axis coincides with the line of pull of the muscle (Fig. 20.7b). In this position it can only act as a depressor. This is, therefore, the best position of the globe for testing the action of the superior oblique muscle. Thus, although the superior oblique has an abducting action in primary position, the main effect of superior oblique weakness is seen as failure of depression in adduction.
- When the eye is abducted 39°, the visual axis and the superior oblique make an angle of 90° with each other (Fig. 20.7c). In this position the superior oblique can only cause intorsion.

2. **Inferior oblique** originates from a small depression just behind the orbital rim lateral to the lacrimal sac. It passes

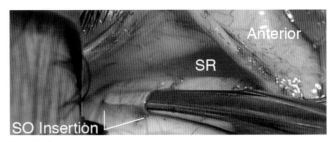

Fig. 20.6
Insertion of the superior oblique tendon

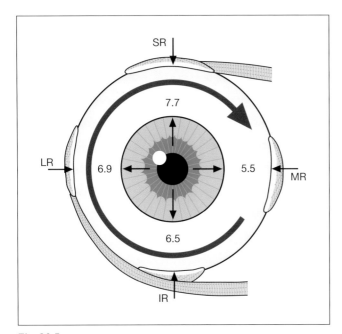

Fig. 20.5
Spiral of Tillaux

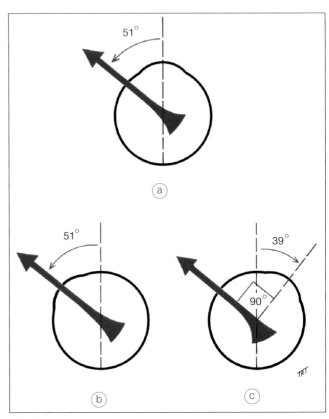

Fig. 20.7
Actions of the right superior oblique muscle (see text)

backwards and laterally, to insert in the posterior lower temporal quadrant of the globe, close to the macula.

- The primary action is extorsion; secondary actions are elevation and abduction.
- When the globe is adducted 51°, the inferior oblique acts only as an elevator.
- When the eye is abducted 39°, its main action is extorsion.

Muscle pulleys

The four rectus muscles pass through condensations of connective tissue and smooth muscle just posterior to the equator. These condensations act as pulleys and minimize upward and downward movements of the bellies of the medial and lateral rectus muscles during up-gaze and down-gaze, and horizontal movements of the superior and inferior rectus bellies in left and right gaze. Pulleys are the effective origins of the rectus muscles and play an important role in the coordination of eye movements by reducing the effect of horizontal movements on vertical muscle actions and vice versa. Displacement of the pulleys can be one cause of abnormalities of eye movements such as 'V' and 'A' patterns (see below).

Nerve supply

1. **Lateral rectus** is supplied by the 6th cranial nerve (abducent nerve – abducting muscle).
2. **Superior oblique** is supplied by the 4th cranial nerve (trochlear nerve – muscle associated with the trochlea).

3. **Other muscles** together with the levator muscle of the upper lid and the ciliary and sphincter pupillae muscles are supplied by the 3rd (oculomotor) nerve.

Ocular movements

Ductions

Ductions are monocular movements around the axes of Fick. They consist of adduction, abduction, elevation, depression, intorsion and extorsion. They are tested by occluding the fellow eye and asking the patient to follow a target in each direction of gaze. Torsional ductions are mainly observed in association with other abnormal eye movements.

Versions

Versions are binocular, simultaneous, conjugate movements (in the same direction) (Fig. 20.8, top):

- Dextroversion and laevoversion (gaze right; gaze left), elevation (up-gaze) and depression (down-gaze). These four movements bring the globe into the secondary positions of gaze by rotation around either a vertical (Z) or a horizontal (X) axis of Fick.
- Dextroelevation and dextrodepression (gaze up and right; gaze down and right) and laevoelevation and laevode-pression (gaze up and left; gaze down and left). These four oblique movements bring the eyes into the tertiary positions of gaze by rotation around oblique axes lying in the Listing plane, equivalent to simultaneous movement about both the horizontal and vertical axes.

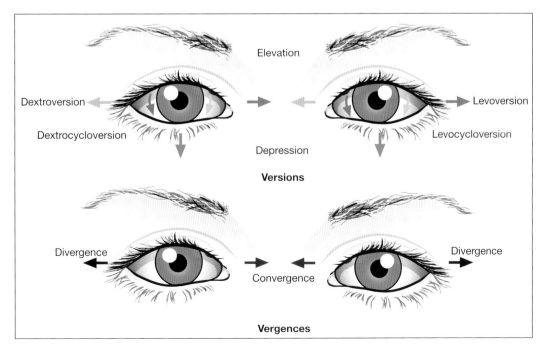

Fig. 20.8
Binocular movements

- Torsional movements to maintain upright images occur on tilting of the head. These are known as the righting reflexes. On head tilt to the right the superior limbi of the two eyes rotate to the left, causing intorsion of the right globe and extorsion of the left.

Vergences

Vergences are binocular, simultaneous, disjugate or disjunctive movements (in opposite directions) (Fig. 20.8, bottom). Convergence is simultaneous adduction (inward turning); divergence is outwards movement from a convergent position. Convergence may be voluntary or reflex. Reflex convergence has four components:

1. **Tonic** convergence, which implies inherent innervational tone to the medial recti, when the patient is awake.
2. **Proximal** convergence is induced by psychological awareness of a near object.
3. **Fusional** convergence is an optomotor reflex, which maintains BSV by ensuring that similar images are projected onto corresponding retinal areas of each eye. It is initiated by bitemporal retinal image disparity.
4. **Accommodative** convergence is induced by the act of accommodation as part of the synkinetic-near reflex. Each dioptre of accommodation is accompanied by a constant increment in accommodative convergence, giving the 'accommodative convergence by accommodation' (AC/A) ratio. This is the amount of convergence in prism dioptres (Δ) per dioptre (D) change in accommodation. The normal value is 3–5Δ. This means that 1D of accommodation is associated with 3–5Δ of accommodative convergence. It will be shown later that abnormalities of the AC/A ratio play an important role in the aetiology of strabismus.

These changes in accommodation, convergence and pupil size which occur in response to a change in the distance of viewing are known as the near triad and occur in response to both image blur and temporal retinal image disparity.

Positions of gaze

1. **Six cardinal** positions of gaze are those in which one muscle in each eye has moved the eye into that position as follows:
   - Dextroversion (right lateral rectus and left medial rectus).
   - Laevoversion (left lateral rectus and right medial rectus).
   - Dextroelevation (right superior rectus and left inferior oblique).
   - Laevoelevation (left superior rectus and right inferior oblique).
   - Dextrodepression (right inferior rectus and left superior oblique).
   - Laevodepression (left inferior rectus and right superior oblique).
2. **Nine diagnostic** positions of gaze are those in which deviations are measured. They consist of the six cardinal positions, the primary position, elevation and depression (Fig. 20.9).

Laws of ocular motility

1. **Agonist-antagonist** pairs are muscles of the same eye that move the eye in opposite directions. The agonist is the primary muscle moving the eye in a given direction. The antagonist acts in the opposite direction to the agonist. For example the right lateral rectus is the antagonist to the right medial rectus.
2. **Synergists** are muscles of the same eye that move the eye in the same direction. For example, the right superior rectus and right inferior oblique act synergistically in elevation.
3. **Yoke muscles** (contralateral synergists) are pairs of muscles, one in each eye, that produce conjugate ocular movements. For example, the yoke muscle of the left superior oblique is the right inferior rectus.
4. **Sherrington law** of reciprocal innervation (inhibition) states that increased innervation to an extraocular muscle (e.g. right medial rectus) is accompanied by a reciprocal decrease in innervation to its antagonist (e.g. right lateral rectus) (Fig. 20.10). This means that when the medial rectus contracts the lateral rectus automatically relaxes and vice versa. Sherrington law applies to both versions and vergences.
5. **Hering law** of equal innervation states that during any conjugate eye movement, equal and simultaneous innervation flows to the yoke muscles (Fig. 20.11). In the case of a paretic squint, the amount of innervation to both eyes is symmetrical, and always determined by the fixating eye, so that the angle of deviation will vary according to which eye is used for fixation. For example if, in the case of a left lateral rectus palsy, the right normal eye is used for fixation, there will be an inward deviation of the left eye due to the unopposed action of the antagonist of the paretic left lateral rectus (left medial rectus). The amount of misalignment of the two eyes in this situation is called the primary deviation (Fig. 20.12, left). If the paretic left eye is now used for fixation, additional innervation will flow to the left lateral rectus, in order to establish this. However, according to Hering law, an equal amount of innervation will also flow to the right medial rectus (yoke muscle). This will result in an overaction of the right medial rectus and an excessive amount of adduction of the right eye. The amount of misalignment between the two eyes in this situation is called the secondary deviation (Fig. 20.12, right). In a paretic squint, the secondary deviation exceeds the primary deviation.
6. **Muscle sequelae** are the effects of the interactions described by these laws. They are of prime importance

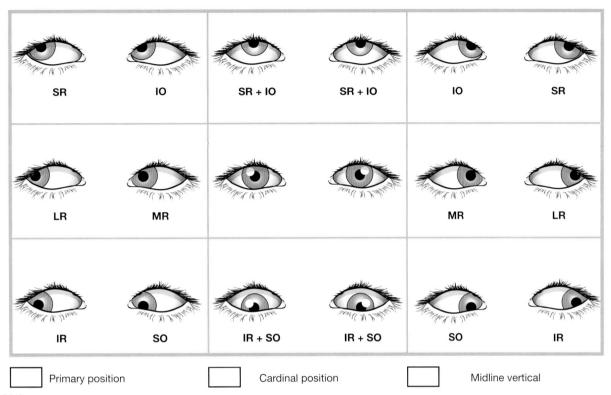

Fig. 20.9
Diagnostic positions of gaze

□ Primary position ■ Cardinal position □ Midline vertical

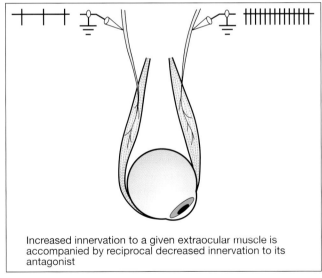

Increased innervation to a given extraocular muscle is accompanied by reciprocal decreased innervation to its antagonist

Fig. 20.10
Sherrington law of reciprocal innervation

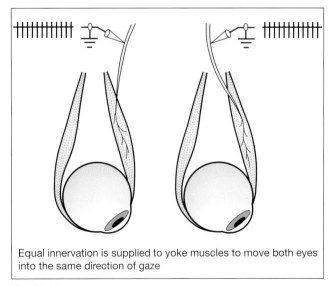

Equal innervation is supplied to yoke muscles to move both eyes into the same direction of gaze

Fig. 20.11
Hering law of equal innervation of yoke muscles

in diagnosing ocular motility disorders and in particular in distinguishing a recently acquired palsy from a long-standing one (see clinical evaluation). The full pattern of changes takes time to develop and can be summarized as follows:

- Primary underaction (e.g. left superior oblique)
- Secondary contracture of the unopposed direct antagonist (left inferior oblique).
- Secondary contracture of the contralateral synergist or yoke muscle (right inferior rectus; Hering law)

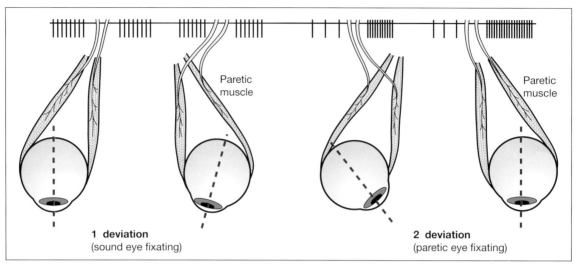

Fig. 20.12
Primary and secondary deviations in paretic strabismus

- Secondary inhibitional palsy (right superior rectus; Sherrington law)

Sensory considerations

Basic aspects

1. **Normal** BSV involves the simultaneous use of both eyes with bifoveal fixation, so that each eye contributes to a common single perception of the object of regard. This represents the highest form of binocular cooperation. Conditions necessary for normal BSV are:
   - Normal routing of visual pathways with overlapping visual fields.
   - Binocularly driven neurons in the visual cortex.
   - Normal retinal (retino-cortical) correspondence (NRC) resulting in cyclopean viewing.
   - Accurate neuromuscular development and co-ordination, so that the visual axes are directed at, and maintain fixation on, the object of regard.
   - Approximately equal image clarity and size for both eyes.

   BSV is based on NRC, which requires first an understanding of uniocular visual direction and projection.
2. **Visual direction** is the projection of a given retinal element in a specific direction in subjective space.
   a. **Principal** visual direction is the direction in external space interpreted as the line of sight. This is normally the visual direction of the fovea and is associated with a sense of direct viewing.
   b. **Secondary** visual directions are the projecting directions of extra-foveal points with respect to the principal direction of the fovea, associated with indirect (eccentric) viewing.
3. **Projection** is the subjective interpretation of the position of an object in space on the basis of stimulated retinal elements.
   - If a red object stimulates the right fovea (F), and a black object which lies in the nasal field stimulates a temporal retinal element (T), the red object will be interpreted by the brain as having originated from the straight ahead position and the black object will be interpreted as having originated in the nasal field (Fig. 20.13a). Similarly, nasal retinal elements project into the temporal field, upper retinal elements into the lower field and vice versa.
   - With both eyes open, the red fixation object is now stimulating both foveae, which are corresponding retinal points. The black object is now not only stimulating the temporal retinal elements in the right eye but also the nasal elements of the left eye. The right eye therefore projects the object into its nasal field and the left eye projects the object into its temporal field. Because both of these retinal elements are corresponding points, they will both project the object into the same position in space (the left side) and there will be no double vision.
4. **Retino-motor values.** The image of an object in the peripheral visual field falls on an extrafoveal element. To establish fixation on this object a saccadic version of accurate amplitude is required. Each extrafoveal retinal element therefore has a retino-motor value proportional to its distance from the fovea, which guides the amplitude of saccadic movements required to 'look at it'. Retino-motor value, zero at the fovea, increases progressively towards the retinal periphery.
5. **Corresponding 'points'** are areas on each retina that share the same subjective visual direction (for example, the foveae share the primary visual direction). Points on the nasal retina of one eye have corresponding points on

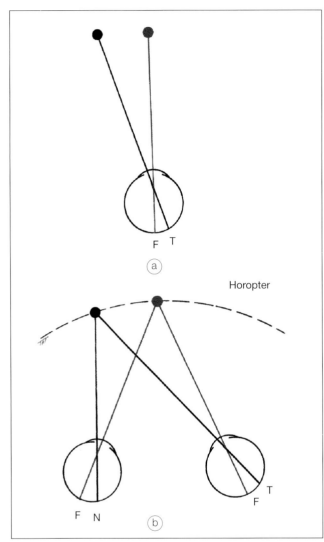

F T

(a)

Horopter

F N (b)

T

F

Fig. 20.13
Principles of projection (see text)

to produce a perception of binocular depth (stereopsis). Objects in front of and behind Panum space appear double. This is the basis of physiological diplopia. Panum space is shallow at fixation (6 seconds of arc) and deeper towards the periphery (30–40 seconds of arc at 15° from the fovea). Therefore objects on the horopter are seen singly and in one plane. Objects in Panum fusional area are seen singly and stereoscopically. Objects outside Panum fusional area appear double. Physiological diplopia is usually accompanied by physiological suppression and many subjects remain unaware of this phenomenon. The retinal areas stimulated by images falling within Panum fusional space are termed Panum fusional areas.

8. **BSV** is characterized by the ability to fuse the images from the two eyes and to perceive binocular depth:

   a. *Sensory fusion* involves the integration by the visual areas of the cerebral cortex of two similar images, one from each eye, into one image. It may be central, which integrates the image falling on the foveae, or peripheral, which integrates parts of the image falling outside the foveae. It is possible to maintain fusion with a central visual deficit in one eye, but peripheral fusion is essential to BSV and may be affected in patients with field loss as in advanced glaucoma.

   b. *Motor fusion* involves the maintenance of motor alignment of the eyes to sustain bifoveal fixation. It is driven by retinal image disparity, which stimulates fusional vergences.

9. **Fusional vergence** involves disjugate eye movements to overcome retinal image disparity. Fusional vergence amplitudes can be measured with prisms or on the synoptophore. Normal values are:
   - Convergence: about 15–20Δ for distance and 25Δ for near.
   - Divergence: about 6–10Δ for distance and 12–14Δ for near.
   - Vertical: 2–3Δ.
   - Cyclovergence: about 2–3°.

Fusional convergence helps to control an exophoria whereas fusional divergence helps to control an esophoria. The fusional vergence mechanism may be decreased by fatigue or illness, converting a phoria to a tropia. The amplitude of fusional vergence mechanisms can be improved by orthoptic exercises, particularly in the case of near fusional convergence for the relief of convergence insufficiency.

10. **Stereopsis** is the perception of depth (the third dimension, the first two being height and width). It arises when objects behind and in front of the point of fixation (but within Panum fusional space) stimulate horizontally disparate retinal elements simultaneously. The fusion of such disparate images results in a single visual impression perceived in depth. A solid object is seen stereoscopically (in 3D) because each eye sees a slightly different aspect of the object.

the temporal retina of the other eye and vice versa. For example, an object producing images on the right nasal retina and the left temporal retina will be projected into the right side of visual space. This is the basis of normal retinal correspondence. This retino-topic organization is reflected back along the visual pathways, each eye maintaining separate images until the visual pathways converge onto binocularly responsive neurons in the primary visual cortex.

6. **The horopter** is an imaginary plane in external space, all points on which stimulate corresponding retinal elements and are therefore seen singly and in the same plane (Fig. 20.13b). This plane passes through the intersection of the visual axes and therefore includes the point of fixation in BSV.

7. **Panum fusional space** is a zone in front of and behind the horopter in which objects stimulate slightly non-corresponding retinal points (retinal disparity). Objects are seen singly and the disparity information is used

11. Sensory perceptions. At the onset of a squint two sensory perceptions arise based on the normal projection of the retinal areas stimulated: confusion and pathological diplopia may result. These require simultaneous (visual) perception i.e. the ability to perceive images from both eyes simultaneously.

    a. Confusion is the simultaneous appreciation of two superimposed but dissimilar images caused by stimulation of corresponding retinal points (usually the foveae) by images of different objects (Fig. 20.14).

    b. Pathological diplopia is the simultaneous appreciation of two images of the same object in different positions and results from images of the same object falling on non-corresponding retinal points.

    • In esotropia the diplopia is homonymous (uncrossed – Fig. 20.15a).

    • In exotropia the diplopia is heteronymous (crossed – Fig. 20.15b).

Sensory adaptations to strabismus

The ocular sensory system in children has the ability to adapt to anomalous states (confusion and diplopia) by two mechanisms: (a) *suppression* and (b) *abnormal retinal correspondence*. These occur because of the plasticity of the developing visual system in children under the age of 7–8 years. Occasional adults who develop sudden-onset strabismus are able to ignore the second image after a time and therefore do not complain of diplopia.

1. Suppression involves active inhibition, in the visual cortex, of an image from one eye when both eyes are open.

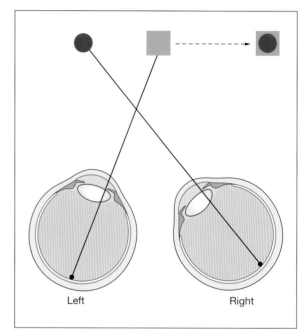

Fig. 20.14
Confusion

Stimuli for suppression include diplopia, confusion and a blurred image from one eye resulting from astigmatism/anisometropia. Clinically, suppression may be:

a. Central or *peripheral*. In central suppression the image from the fovea of the deviating eye is inhibited to avoid confusion. Diplopia, on the other hand, is eradicated by the process of peripheral suppression,

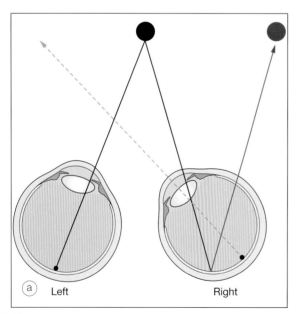
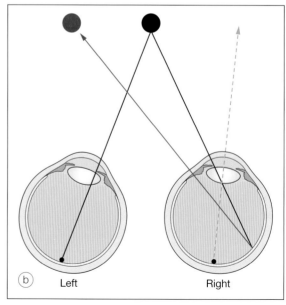

Fig. 20.15
Diplopia. **(a)** Homonymous (uncrossed) diplopia in right esotropia with normal retinal correspondence; **(b)** heteronymous (crossed) diplopia in right exotropia with normal retinal correspondence

in which the image from the peripheral retina of the deviating eye is inhibited.

b. ***Monocular*** or ***alternating***. Suppression is monocular when the image from the dominant eye always predominates over the image from the deviating (or more ametropic) eye, so that the image from the latter is constantly suppressed. This type of suppression leads to amblyopia. When suppression alternates (switches from one eye to the other) amblyopia does not develop.

c. ***Facultative*** or ***obligatory***. Facultative suppression occurs only when the eyes are misaligned. Obligatory suppression is present at all times, irrespective of whether the eyes are deviated or straight. Examples are seen in intermittent exotropia and Duane syndrome.

2. **Abnormal retinal correspondence** (ARC) is a condition in which non-corresponding retinal elements acquire a common subjective visual direction, i.e. fusion occurs in the presence of a small angle manifest squint. The fovea of the fixating eye is thus paired with a non-foveal element of the deviated eye. ARC is a positive sensory adaptation to strabismus (as opposed to suppression), which allows some anomalous binocular vision in the presence of a heterotropia. Binocular responses in ARC are never as good as in normal bifoveal BSV. ARC is most frequently present in small angle esotropia (microtropia) associated with anisometropia.

3. **Microtropia** is a small angle squint (< 10Δ) in which stereopsis is present but reduced and there is a relative amblyopia of the more ametropic eye. Microtropia has two forms.

   a. ***In microtropia with identity*** the point used for monocular fixation by the squinting eye also corresponds with the fovea of the straight eye under binocular viewing conditions. Therefore on cover test there is no movement of the squinting eye when it takes up monocular fixation.

   b. ***In microtropia without identity*** the monocular fixation point of the squinting eye does not correspond with the fovea of the straight eye in binocular viewing. There is therefore a small movement of the deviating eye when it takes up monocular fixation on cover testing. ARC is less common in accommodative esotropia because of the variability of the angle of deviation, or in large angle deviations because the separation of the images is too great.

4. **Consequences of strabismus**
   - The fovea of the squinting eye is suppressed to avoid confusion.
   - Diplopia will occur, since non-corresponding retinal elements receive the same image.
   - To avoid diplopia, the patient will develop either peripheral suppression of the squinting eye or ARC.
   - If constant unilateral suppression occurs this will subsequently lead to strabismic amblyopia.

Motor adaptation to strabismus

Motor adaptation involves the adoption of an abnormal head posture (AHP) and occurs primarily in children with congenitally abnormal eye movements who use the AHP to maintain BSV. In these children loss of an AHP may indicate loss of binocular function and the need for surgical intervention. These patients may present in adult life with symptoms of decompensation, often unaware of their AHP. Acquired paretic strabismus in adults may be consciously controlled by an AHP provided the deviation is neither too large nor too variable with gaze (incomitance). The AHP eliminates diplopia and helps to centralize the binocular visual field. The patient will turn the head into the direction of the field of action of the weak muscle, so that the eyes are then automatically turned the opposite direction and as far as possible away from its field of action (i.e. the head will turn where the eye cannot). An AHP is analysed in terms of the following three components:
- Face turn to right or left.
- Head tilt to right or left.
- Chin elevation or depression.

1. **A face turn** will be adopted to control a purely horizontal deviation. For example, if the left lateral rectus is paralyzed, diplopia will occur in left gaze; the face will be turned to the left which deviates the eyes to the right, away from the field of action of the weak muscle and area of diplopia. A face turn may also be adopted in a paresis of a vertically acting muscle to avoid the side where the vertical

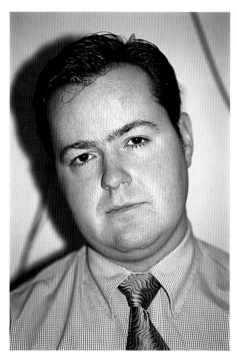

Fig. 20.16
Compensatory head tilt

deviation is greatest (e.g. in a right superior oblique weakness the face is turned to the left).

2. **A head tilt** is adopted to compensate for torsional and/or vertical diplopia. In a left superior oblique weakness the left eye is relatively elevated and the head is tilted to the right (Fig. 20.16), towards the hypotropic eye; this reduces the vertical separation of the diplopic images and permits fusion to be regained. If there is a significant torsional component preventing fusion, tilting the head in the same left direction will reduce this by invoking the righting reflexes (placing the extorted right eye in a position which requires extorsion).

3. **Chin elevation or depression** may be used to compensate for weakness of an elevator or depressor muscle or to minimize the horizontal deviation when an A or V pattern is present.

AMBLYOPIA

Classification

Amblyopia is the unilateral, or (rarely) bilateral, decrease of best-corrected visual acuity caused by form vision deprivation and/or abnormal binocular interaction, for which there is no pathology of the eye or visual pathways.

1. **Strabismic** amblyopia results from abnormal binocular interaction where there is continued monocular suppression of the deviating eye.
2. **Anisometropic** amblyopia is caused by a difference in refractive error between the eyes and may result from a difference of as little as 1D sphere. The more ametropic eye receives a blurred image which is a mild form of visual deprivation. It is frequently associated with microtropia and may coexist with strabismic amblyopia.
3. **Stimulus deprivation** amblyopia results from vision deprivation. It may be unilateral or bilateral and is caused by opacities in the media (e.g. cataract) or ptosis which covers the pupil.
4. **Bilateral ametropic** amblyopia results from high symmetrical refractive errors, usually hypermetropia.
5. **Meridional** amblyopia results from image blur in one meridian. It can be unilateral or bilateral and is caused by uncorrected astigmatism usually >1D astigmatism persisting beyond the period of emmetropization in infancy.

Diagnosis

In the absence of an organic lesion, a difference in best corrected visual acuity of two Snellen lines or more (or >1 log unit) is indicative of amblyopia. Visual acuity in amblyopia is usually better while reading single letters than letters in a row. This 'crowding' phenomenon occurs to a certain extent in normal individuals but is more marked in amblyopes and must be taken into account when testing preverbal children (see clinical evaluation).

Treatment

The sensitive period during which acuity of an amblyopic eye can be improved is usually up to 7–8 years in strabismic amblyopia and may be longer (into teens) for anisometropic amblyopia where good binocular function is present.

1. **Occlusion** of the normal eye, to encourage use of the amblyopic eye, is the most effective treatment. The regimen, full-time or part-time, depends on the age of the patient and the density of amblyopia. The younger the patient the more rapid improvement, although the greater the risk of inducing amblyopia in the normal eye. It is therefore very important to monitor visual acuity regularly in both eyes during treatment. The better the visual acuity at the start of occlusion, the shorter the duration required, although there is wide variation between patients. If there has been no improvement after 6 months of effective occlusion, further treatment is unlikely to be fruitful. Poor compliance is the single greatest barrier to improvement and must be monitored. Amblyopia treatment benefits from time spent at the outset on communication of the rationale and the difficulties involved.
2. **Penalization,** in which vision in the normal eye is blurred with atropine, is an alternative method. It is best in the treatment of relatively mild amblyopia (6/24 or better) in association with hypermetropia. Conventional occlusion is likely to produce a quicker response than atropine, which is generally used when compliance with occlusion is poor.

NB It is essential to examine the fundi to diagnose any visible organic disease prior to commencing treatment for amblyopia. Organic disease and amblyopia may coexist and a trial of patching may still be indicated in the presence of organic disease. If acuity does not respond to treatment, investigations such as electrophysiology or imaging should be reconsidered.

CLINICAL EVALUATION

History

1. **Age of onset** can give an indication as to the aetiology of a squint. The earlier the onset, the more likely the need for surgical correction. The later the onset, the greater the likelihood of an accommodative component (mostly arising between 18 and 36 months). The longer the

duration of squint in early childhood the greater the risk of amblyopia, unless fixation is freely alternating. Inspection of previous photographs may be useful for the documentation of strabismus or an AHP.

2. **Symptoms** may indicate decompensation of a pre-existent heterophoria or more significantly a recently acquired, usually paretic, condition. In the former, the patient usually complains of discomfort, blurring and possibly diplopia of indeterminate onset and duration compared to the acquired condition with sudden onset of diplopia. The type of diplopia (horizontal, cyclovertical) should be established, the direction of gaze in which it predominates and whether any BSV is retained. In adults it is very important to determine exactly what problems the squint is causing as a basis for decisions about treatment. It is not unusual for patients to present with spurious symptoms which mask embarrassment over a cosmetically noticeable squint.

3. **Variability** is significant because intermittent strabismus indicates some degree of binocularity. An alternating deviation suggests symmetrical visual acuity in both eyes.

4. **General health** or developmental problems are significant (e.g. children with cerebral palsy have an increased incidence of strabismus). In older patients poor health and stress may cause decompensation and in acquired paresis patients may report associations or causal factors (trauma, neurological disease, diabetes, etc.).

5. **Birth history,** including period of gestation, birth weight and any problems *in utero*, with delivery or in the neonatal period.

6. **Family history** is important because strabismus is frequently familial, although there is no definitive inheritance pattern. It is also important to know what therapy was necessary in other family members.

7. **Previous ocular history** including prescription and compliance with spectacles or occlusion, previous surgery or prisms is important to future treatment options and prognosis.

Visual acuity

Testing in preverbal children

The evaluation can be separated into the qualitative assessment of visual behaviour and the quantitative assessment of visual acuity using preferential looking tests. Assessment of visual behaviour is achieved as follows:

1. **Fixation and following** may be assessed using bright attention-grabbing targets (a face is often best). This method indicates whether the infant is visually alert and is of particular value in the child suspected of blindness.

2. **Comparison** between the behaviour of the two eyes may reveal a unilateral preference. Occlusion of one eye, if strongly objected to by the child, indicates poorer acuity in the other eye. However, it is possible to have good visual attention and unequal visual acuity; therefore all risk factors for amblyopia must be considered in the interpretation of these results.

3. **Fixation behaviour** can be used to establish unilateral preference if a manifest squint is present.
   a. Fixation is promoted in the squinting eye by occluding the dominant eye while the child fixates a target of interest (preferably incorporating a light).
   b. Fixation is then graded as central or non-central and steady or unsteady (the corneal reflection can be observed).
   c. The other eye is then uncovered and the ability to maintain fixation is observed.
   d. If fixation immediately returns to the uncovered eye, then visual acuity is probably impaired.
   e. If fixation is maintained through a blink, then visual acuity is probably good.
   f. If the patient alternates fixation, then the two eyes have equal vision.

4. **The 10Δ test** is similar and can be used regardless of whether a manifest squint is present. It involves the promotion of diplopia using a 10Δ vertical prism. Alternation between the diplopic targets suggests equal visual acuity.

5. **Rotation test** is a gross qualitative test of the ability of an infant to fixate with both eyes open. The test is performed as follows:
   a. The examiner holds the child facing him and rotates briskly through 360°.
   b. If vision is normal, the eyes will deviate in the direction of rotation under the influence of the vestibulo-ocular response. The eyes flick back to the primary position to produce a rotational nystagmus.
   c. When rotation stops, nystagmus is briefly observed in the opposite direction for 1–2 seconds and should then cease due to suppression of post-rotary nystagmus by fixation.
   d. If vision is severely impaired, the post-rotation nystagmus does not stop as quickly when rotation ceases because the vestibulo-ocular response is not blocked by visual feedback.

6. **Preferential looking** tests can be used from early infancy. They are based on the fact that infants prefer to look at a pattern rather than a homogenous stimulus. The infant is exposed to a stimulus and the examiner observes the eyes for fixation movements, without themselves knowing the stimulus position. Tests in common use include the Teller or Keeler acuity cards, which consist of black stripes (gratings) of varying widths, and Cardiff acuity cards, which consist of familiar pictures with variable outline width (Fig. 20.17). Low frequency (coarse) gratings or pictures with a wider outline are seen more easily than high frequency gratings or thin outline pictures, and an assessment of resolution (not recognition) visual acuity is made accordingly. Since grating acuity often exceeds

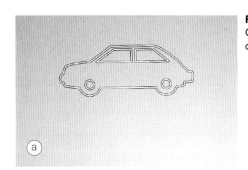

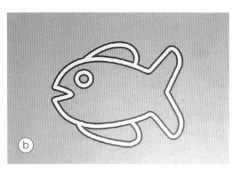

Fig. 20.17
Cardiff acuity cards

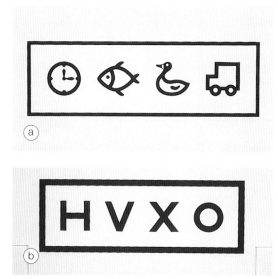

Fig. 20.18
(a) Kay pictures; **(b)** Keeler LogMAR crowded test (Courtesy of E Dawson)

Snellen acuity in amblyopia, Teller cards may overestimate visual acuity. These methods may not be reliable if a proper forced-choice staircase protocol is not followed during testing and neither method has high sensitivity to the presence of amblyopia. The results must be considered in combination with risk factors for amblyopia.

7. **Pattern visual evoked potentials** give a representation of spatial acuity but is more regularly used in the diagnosis of optic neuropathy.

Testing in verbal children

All of the tests described below are performed at 3 or 4 metres, at which it is easier to obtain compliance than at 6 metres, with little or no clinical detriment. It is important to note that amblyopia can only be accurately diagnosed using a crowded test requiring target recognition and that logMAR (logarithm of the minimal angle of resolution) tests provide the best measure against which improvement with amblyopia therapy can be assessed. These are readily available in formats suited to normal children from 2 years onwards.

1. **At age 2 years** most children will have sufficient language skills to undertake a picture naming test such as the crowded Kay pictures (Fig. 20.18a).
2. **At age 3 years** most children will be able to undertake the matching of letter optotypes as in the Keeler logMAR (Fig. 20.18b) or Sonksen crowded tests. If a crowded letter test proves too difficult it is preferable to perform the crowded Kay pictures than to use single optotype letters.
3. **Older children** may continue with the crowded letter tests, naming or matching them, or the EDTRS chart may

be used. LogMAR tests are in common usage and are preferable to Snellen for all children at risk of amblyopia.

Tests for stereopsis

Stereopsis is measured in seconds of arc ($1° = 60$ minutes of arc; 1 minute = 60 seconds of arc). It is useful to remember that normal spatial visual acuity is 1 minute and normal stereo-acuity is 60 seconds (which equals 1 minute). The lower the value the better the acuity. Various tests are employed using different test principles. Random dot tests (TNO, Frisby) provide the most definitive evidence of high grade BSV. Where this is weak and/or based on ARC, less dissociation contour based tests (e.g. Titmus) may give more reliable evidence of stereopsis.

TNO

The TNO random dot test consists of seven plates of randomly distributed paired red and green dots which are viewed with complementary red-green spectacles. Within each plate the dots of one colour forming the target shape (squares, crosses etc.) are displaced horizontally in relation to their paired dots of the other colour so that they have a different retinal disparity from those outside the target. Some control shapes are visible even without red-green spectacles (Fig. 20.19a) while the test targets are only visible to an individual with stereopsis, while wearing red-green spectacles (Fig. 20.19b). The first three plates are used to establish the presence of stereoscopic vision and subsequent plates to quantify it. Because there are no monocular clues, the TNO test provides

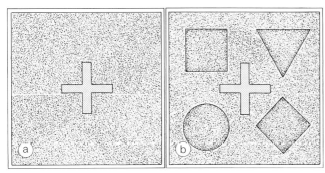

Fig. 20.19
TNO test

a truer positive measurement of stereopsis than the Titmus test, but can give false negative errors when fusion is poor. The disparities measured range from 480 to 15 seconds of arc tested at 40cm. Most children are able to do this (and the Frisby test) from the age of about 4 years.

Frisby

The Frisby stereotest consists of three transparent plastic plates of varying thickness. On the surface of each plate are printed four squares of small randomly distributed shapes (Fig. 20.20). One of the squares contains a 'hidden' circle, in which the random shapes are printed on the reverse of the plate. The patient is required to identify this hidden circle.

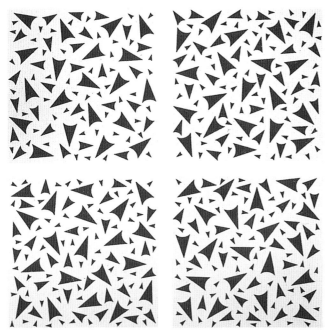

Fig. 20.20
Frisby test

The test does not require special spectacles because the disparity is created by the thickness of the plate and can be varied by increasing or decreasing the working distance, which needs to be accurately measured. The disparities measured range from 600 to 15 seconds of arc. It is important not to allow the subject to tilt the plate or move their head during testing as this gives monocular clues.

Lang

The Lang stereotest does not require special spectacles; the targets are seen alternately by each eye through the built-in cylindrical lens elements. Displacement of the dots creates disparity and the patient is asked to name or point to a simple shape, such as a star, on the card (Fig. 20.21). The Lang test can be used to assess stereopsis in very young children and babies who may reach out to touch the pictures. The examiner can also observe the child's eye movements from picture to picture on the card. However, the cards must be held exactly parallel to the plane of the face for the effect to be seen and the Frisby screening test may be superior for demonstrating stereopsis (e.g. to confirm BSV in infants with suspected squint). The degree of disparity is quite gross, ranging 1200 to 600 seconds of arc at 40cm.

Titmus

The Titmus test consists of a three-dimensional Polaroid vectograph consisting of two plates in the form of a booklet viewed through Polaroid spectacles. On the right is a large fly, and on the left is a series of circles and animals (Fig. 20.22). The test is performed at a distance of 40cm.

1. **Fly** is a test of gross stereopsis (3000 seconds of arc), and is especially useful for young children. The fly should appear to stand out from the page and the child is encouraged to pick up the tip of one of its wings between finger and thumb. In the absence of gross stereopsis the fly will appear as an ordinary flat photograph. If the book is inverted, the targets will appear to be behind the plane of the page. If the patient states that the fly's wings are still 'popping out', then they are not appreciating true stereoscopic vision.
2. **Circles** comprise a graded series which tests fine depth perception. Each of the nine squares contains four circles. One of the circles in each square has a degree of disparity and will appear forward of the plane of reference in the presence of normal stereopsis. The disparities measured range from 800 to 40 seconds of arc. If a patient perceives the circle to be shifted to the side, then they are not appreciating stereoscopic vision, but are using monocular clues instead.
3. **The animals** are similar to the circles test but consist of three rows of five animals, one of which will appear forward of the plane of reference. The degree of disparity ranges from 400 to 100 seconds of arc.

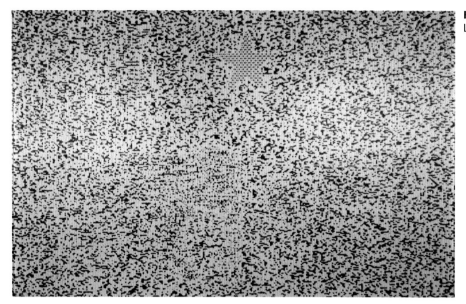

Fig. 20.21
Lang test

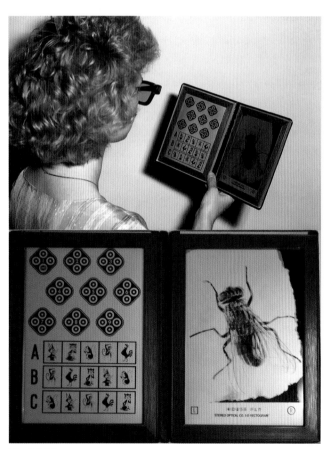

Fig. 20.22
Titmus test

Frisby–Davis distance stereotest

This consists of a large cube with an open front through which four small objects are visible. Testing is usually performed at 6 metres. The patient has to decide which of four objects within the box is closest to them.

Tests for binocular fusion in infants without manifest squint

Base-out prism

Base-out prism is a quick and easy method for detecting fusion in children. The test is performed by placing a 20Δ base-out prism in front of one eye (in this case the right). This displaces the retinal image temporally with resultant diplopia. The examiner observes corrective eye movements as follows:

    a. There will be a shift of the right eye to the left to resume fixation (right adduction) with a corresponding shift of the left eye to the left (left abduction) in accordance with Hering law (Fig. 20.23b).

    b. The left eye will then make a corrective refixational saccade to the right (left re-adduction) (Fig. 20.23c).

    c. On removal of the prism both eyes move to the right (Fig. 20.23d).

    d. The left eye then makes an outward fusional movement (Fig. 20.23e).

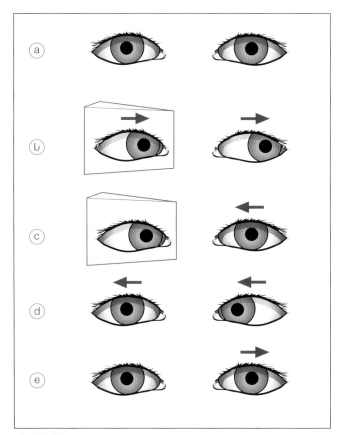

Fig. 20.23
Base-out prism test (see text)

NB Most children with good BSV should be able to overcome a 20Δ prism from the age of 6 months; if not weaker prisms (16Δ or 12Δ) may be tried but the response is harder to observe.

Binocular convergence

Simple convergence to an interesting target can be demonstrated from 3 to 4 months. Both eyes should follow the approaching target symmetrically 'to the nose'. Overconvergence in the infant may indicate an incipient esotropia. Divergence may reflect a tendency to divergence or lack of interest in the target.

Tests for sensory anomalies

Worth four-dot

This is a dissociation test which can be used with both distance and near fixation, and differentiates between BSV, or ARC and suppression. Results can only be interpreted if the presence or absence of a manifest squint is known at time of testing.

1. Procedure

   a. The patient wears a green lens in front of the right eye, which filters out all colours except green, and a red lens in front of the left eye which will filter out all colours except red (Fig. 20.24a).

   b. The patient then views a box with four lights; one red, two green and one white.

2. Results (Fig. 20.24b)

- If BSV is present all four lights are seen.
- If all four lights are seen in the presence of a manifest deviation, harmonious ARC is present.
- If two red lights are seen, right suppression is present.
- If three green lights are seen, left suppression is present.
- If two red and three green lights are seen, diplopia is present.
- If the green and red lights alternate, alternating suppression is present.

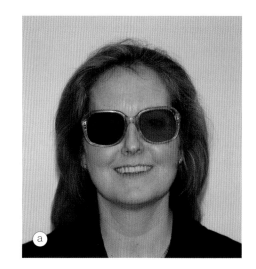

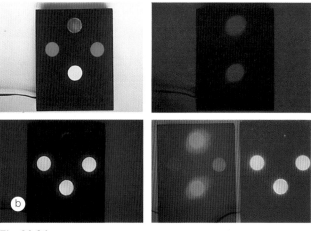

Fig. 20.24
Worth four-dot test. **(a)** Red-green glasses; **(b)** possible results

Bagolini striated glasses

This is a test for detecting BSV, ARC or suppression. Each lens has fine striations which convert a point source of light into a line, as with the Maddox rod (see below).

1. **Procedure**
   a. The two lenses are placed at 45° and 135° in front of each eye and the patient fixates a small light source (Fig. 20.25a).
   b. Each eye perceives an oblique line of light, perpendicular to that perceived by the fellow eye (Fig. 20.25b).
   c. Dissimilar images are thus presented to each eye under binocular viewing conditions.
2. **Results** (Fig. 20.25c) cannot be interpreted correctly unless it is known whether or not strabismus is present:
   - If the two streaks intersect at their centres in the form of an oblique cross (an 'X'), the patient has BSV if the eyes are straight, or harmonious ARC in the presence of manifest strabismus.

- If the two lines are seen but they do not form a cross, diplopia is present.
- If only one streak is seen, there is no simultaneous perception and suppression is present.
- In theory, if a small gap is seen in one of the streaks, a central suppression scotoma (as found in microtropia) is present. In practice this is often difficult to demonstrate and the patient describes a cross. The scotoma can be confirmed with the 4Δ test.

4Δ test

This test differentiates bifoveal fixation (normal BSV) from a central suppression scotoma (CSS) in microtropia and employs the principle described in the 20Δ test (Hering law and convergence to overcome diplopia).

1. **In bifoveal fixation** the response is as follows:
   a. The prism is placed base-out in front of the right eye with deviation of the image temporally and movement of both eyes to the left (Fig. 20.26a).
   b. The left eye converges to fuse the images (Fig. 20.26b).
2. **In left microtropia with CSS** the response is as follows:
   a. The patient fixates a distance target with both eyes open and a 4Δ prism is placed base-out in front of the left eye with suspected CSS.
   b. The image is moved temporally in the left eye but falls within the CSS and no movement of either eye is observed (Fig. 20.27a).

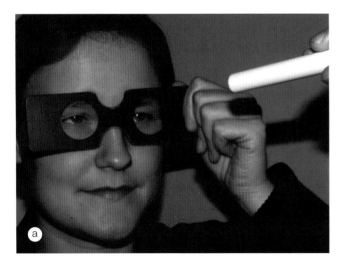

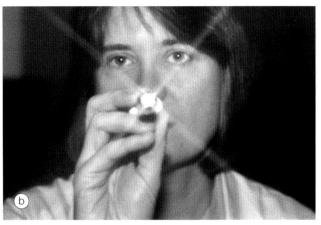

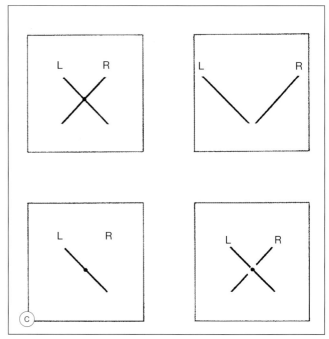

Fig. 20.25
Bagolini test. **(a)** Striated glasses; **(b)** appearance of a point of light through Bagolini lenses; **(c)** possible results (see text)

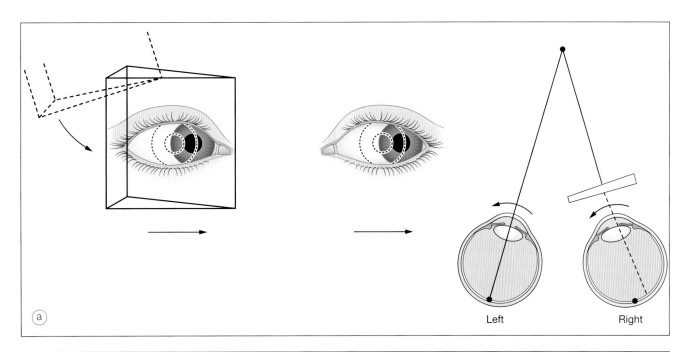

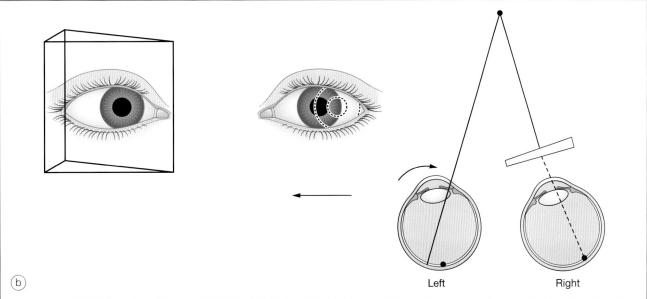

Fig. 20.26
4Δ test in bifoveal fixation. **(a)** Shift of both eyes away from the prism base; **(b)** fusional refixation movement of the left eye

c. The prism is then moved to the right eye which adducts to maintain fixation; the left eye similarly moves to the left (Hering), but the second image falls within the CSS and no refixation movement is seen (Fig. 20.27b).

Synoptophore

The synoptophore compensates for the angle of squint and allows stimuli to be presented to both eyes simultaneously (Fig. 20.28a). It can thus be used to investigate the potential for binocular function in the presence of a manifest squint and is of particular value in testing young children (from age 3 years, who find it enjoyable. It can also detect suppression and ARC. The instrument consists of two cylindrical tubes with a mirrored right-angled bend and a +6.50 D lens in each eyepiece (Fig. 20.28b, top). This optically sets the testing distance as equivalent to about 6 metres. Pictures are inserted in a slide carrier situated at the outer end of each

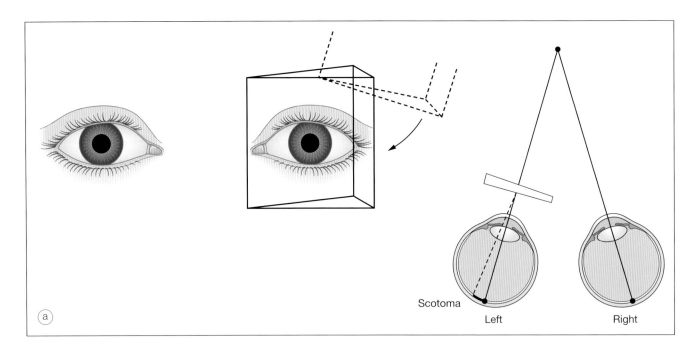

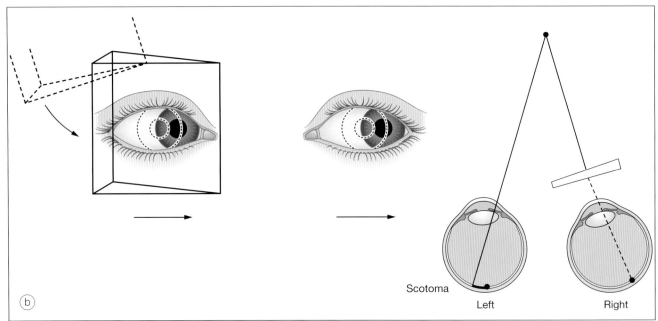

Fig. 20.27

4Δ test in left microtropia with a central suppression scotoma. **(a)** No movement of either eye; **(b)** both eyes move to the left but there is absence of re-fixation

tube. The two tubes are supported on columns which enable the pictures to be moved in relation to each other, and any adjustments are indicated on a scale. The synoptophore can measure horizontal, vertical and torsional misalignments simultaneously and is valuable in determining surgical approach by assessing the different contributions in the cardinal positions of gaze.

Grades of binocular vision

Binocular vision is graded on the synoptophore as follows (Fig. 20.28b, bottom):

1. **First grade** (simultaneous perception) is tested by introducing two dissimilar but not mutually antagonistic

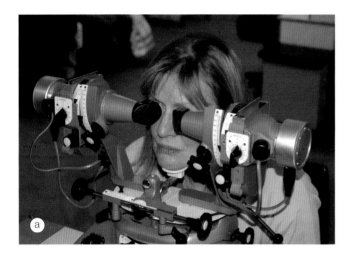

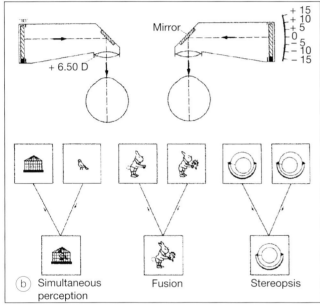

Fig. 20.28
(a) Synoptophore; **(b)** optical principles and grading of binocular vision

pictures, such as a bird and a cage. The subject is then asked to put the bird into the cage by moving the arm of the synoptophore. If the two pictures cannot be seen simultaneously, then suppression is present. Some retinal 'rivalry' will occur although one picture is smaller than the other, so that while the small one is seen foveally, the larger one is seen parafoveally (and is thus placed in front of the deviating eye). Larger macular and paramacular slides are used if foveal slides cannot be superimposed.

2. **Second grade** (fusion). If simultaneous perception slides can be superimposed then the test proceeds to the second grade which is the ability of the two eyes to produce a composite picture (sensory fusion) from two similar pictures, each of which is incomplete in one small different detail. The classic example is two rabbits, one lacking a tail

and the other lacking a bunch of flowers. If fusion is present, one rabbit complete with tail and flowers will be seen. The range of fusion (motor fusion) is then tested by moving the arms of the synoptophore so that the eyes have to converge and diverge in order to maintain fusion. The presence of simple fusion without any range is of little value in ordinary life (referred to as superimposition).

3. **Third grade** (stereopsis) is the ability to obtain an impression of depth by the superimposition of two pictures of the same object which have been taken from slightly different angles. The classic example is the bucket which is appreciated in three dimensions.

Detection of anomalous retinal correspondence

ARC can be detected on the synoptophore as follows:
a. The subjective angle of deviation is that at which the simultaneous perception slides are superimposed. The examiner determines the objective angle of the deviation by presenting each fovea alternately with a target by extinguishing one or other light and moving the slide in front of the deviating eye until no movement of the eyes is seen.
b. If the subjective and objective angles coincide then retinal correspondence is normal.
c. If the objective and subjective angles are different, ARC is present. The difference in degrees between the subjective and objective angles is the angle of anomaly. ARC is said to be harmonious when the objective angle equals the angle of anomaly and unharmonious when it exceeds the angle of anomaly. It is only in harmonious ARC that free space binocular responses can be demonstrated, the unharmonious form may be a lesser adaptation or an artefact of testing.

Measurement of deviation

Hirschberg test

The Hirschberg test gives a rough objective estimate of the angle of a manifest strabismus in young or uncooperative patients or when fixation in the deviating eye is poor. A pentorch is shone into the eyes from arm's length and the patient asked to fixate the light. The corneal reflection of the light will be (more or less) centred in the pupil of the fixating eye, but will be decentred in a squinting eye, in the direction opposite to that of the deviation. The distance of the corneal light reflection from the centre of the pupil is noted. Each mm of deviation is approximately equal to 7° (one degree ≈ 2 prism dioptres). For example, if the reflex is situated at the temporal border of the pupil (assuming a pupillary diameter of 4mm), the angle is about 15° (Fig. 20.29a); if it is at the limbus, the angle is about 45° (Fig. 20.29b and c). This test is also useful in detecting pseudo-strabismus, which may be caused by the following conditions.

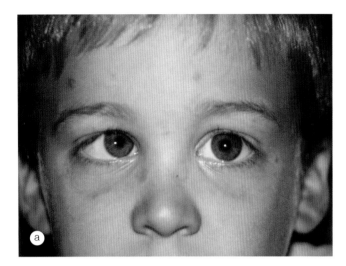

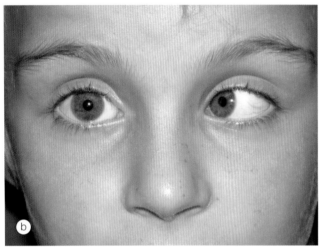

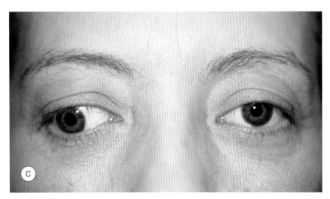

Fig. 20.29
Hirschberg test. **(a)** The right corneal reflex is near the temporal border of the pupil indicating an angle of about 15°; **(b)** the left corneal reflex at the limbus indicating an angle of about 45°; **(c)** right corneal reflex at the limbus in a divergent squint
(Courtesy of J Yanguela – fig. a)

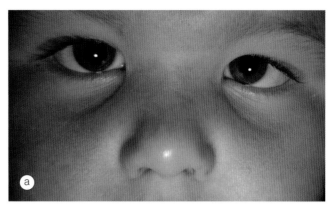

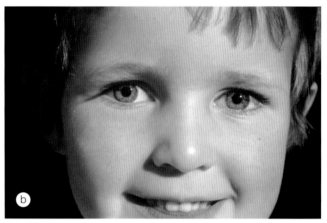

Fig. 20.30
Pseudo-strabismus. **(a)** Prominent epicanthic folds simulating esotropia; **(b)** wide interpupillary distance simulating exotropia

1. **Epicanthic folds** may simulate an esotropia (Fig. 20.30a).
2. **Abnormal inter-pupillary distance;** if short may simulate an esotropia and if wide an exotropia (Fig. 20.30b).
3. **Angle kappa** is the angle between the visual and anatomical (pupillary) axes.
   - Normally, the fovea is situated temporal to the anatomical centre of the posterior pole. The eyes are therefore slightly abducted to achieve bifoveal fixation. A light shone onto the cornea will therefore cause a reflex just nasal to the centre of the cornea in both eyes (Fig. 20.31a). This is termed a positive angle kappa.
   - A large positive angle kappa may simulate an exotropia (Fig. 20.31b).
   - A negative angle kappa occurs when the fovea is situated nasal to the posterior pole (high myopia and ectopic fovea). In this situation, the corneal reflex is situated temporal to the centre of the cornea and it may simulate an esotropia (Fig. 20.31c).

Krimsky and prism reflection tests

Corneal reflexes are used for the same indications as the Hirschberg test, but combined with prisms to give a more accurate approximation of the angle in a manifest deviation.

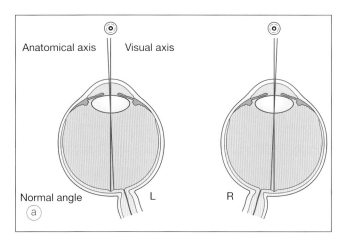

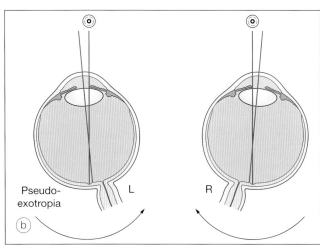

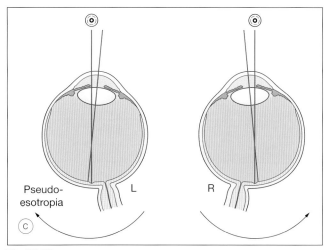

Fig. 20.31
Angle kappa. **(a)** Normal; **(b)** positive simulates an exotropia;
(c) negative simulates an esotropia

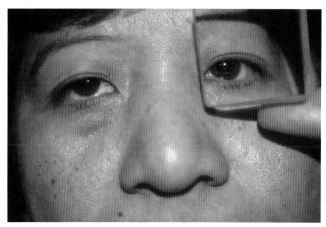

Fig. 20.32
Krimsky test (Courtesy of K Nischal)

1. **Krimsky test** involves placement of prisms in front of the fixating eye until the corneal light reflections are symmetrical (Fig. 20.32). This test reduces the problem of parallax and is more commonly used than the prism reflection test.
2. **Prism reflection test** involves the placement of prisms in front of the deviating eye until the corneal light reflections are symmetrical.

Cover tests

The cover test comprises a series of simple tests which are essential to the diagnosis of strabismus in all its forms. These tests allow the examiner to differentiate manifest from latent squint, to detect the direction and approximate size of deviation, to assess the degree of any control and to gain an indication of amblyopia. These tests are based on the patient's ability to fixate. They are performed for near and distance fixation, with and without spectacle correction or any compensatory head posture. Reasonable attention and cooperation are required but it is possible to perform the essential test in most patients regardless of age.

1. **Cover-uncover test** consists of two parts:
   a. ***Cover test*** to detect a heterotropia. It is helpful to begin the near test using a light to observe the corneal reflections and to assess the fixation in the deviating eye. It should then be repeated for near using an accommodative target and for distance as follows:
      – The patient fixates a straight-ahead target.
      – If a right deviation is suspected, the examiner covers the fixing left eye and notes any movement of the right eye to take up fixation.
      – No movement indicates orthotropia (Fig. 20.33a) or left heterotropia (Fig. 20.33b).
      – Adduction of the right eye to take up fixation indicates exotropia; abduction indicates esotropia (Fig. 20.33c).

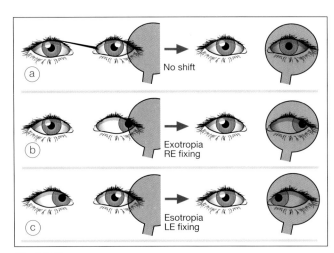

Fig. 20.33
Possible results of the cover test

- Downward movement indicates hypertropia and upward movement, hypotropia.
- The test is repeated on the opposite eye.
b. *Uncover test* to detect heterophoria should be performed both for near (using an accommodative target) and for distance as follows:
  - The patient fixates a straight-ahead distant target.
  - The examiner covers the left eye and after 2–3 seconds removes the cover.
  - No movement indicates orthophoria (Fig. 20.34a), although a keen observer will frequently detect a very slight latent deviation in most normal individuals, as very few people are truly orthophoric, particularly on near fixation.
  - If the left eye had deviated while under cover, a re-fixation movement (recovery to BSV) is observed on being uncovered.

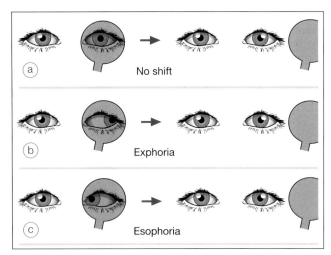

Fig. 20.34
Possible results of the uncover test

- Adduction (nasal recovery) indicates exophoria (Fig. 20.34b) and abduction esophoria (Fig. 20.34c).
- Upward or downward movement indicates a vertical phoria.
- After the cover is removed, the examiner notes the speed and smoothness of recovery as evidence of the strength of motor fusion.
- The test is repeated for the opposite eye.

NB Most examiners perform the cover test and the uncover test sequentially, hence the term cover-uncover test.

2. **Alternate cover test** is a dissociation test which reveals the total deviation when fusion is suspended. It should be performed after the cover-uncover test.
   a. The right eye is covered for several seconds.
   b. The occluder is quickly shifted to the opposite eye for 2 seconds, then back and forth several times. After the cover is removed, the examiner notes the speed and smoothness of recovery as the eyes return to their pre-dissociated state.
   d. A patient with a well compensated heterophoria will have straight eyes before and after the test has been performed whereas a patient with poor control may decompensate to a manifest deviation.
3. **Prism cover test** measures the angle of deviation on near or distance fixation and in any gaze position. It combines the alternate cover test with prisms and is performed as follows:
   a. The alternate cover test is first performed.
   b. Prisms of increasing strength are placed in front of one eye with the base opposite the direction of the deviation (i.e. point the apex of the prism in the direction of the deviation). For example, in a convergent strabismus the prism is held base-out, and in a right hypertropia, base down before the right eye.
   c. The alternate cover test is continuously performed (Fig. 20.35). As stronger prisms are brought in, the amplitude of the re-fixation movement gradually decreases.
   d. The end-point is approached when no movement is seen; to ensure the maximum angle is measured, the prism strength is increased further until a movement is observed in the opposite direction (point of reversal) and then reduced again to find the neutral value; the angle of deviation then equals the strength of the prism and is recorded as ESO or base out 16PD, or R/L (or BDRE) 16PD.

Subjective measurement tests

Subjective dissimilar image tests are of limited value in the assessment of strabismus. They require simultaneous

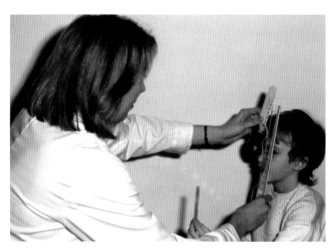

Fig. 20.35
Prism cover test

perception (cannot be used in manifest strabismus with suppression) and do not reveal the full deviation.

1. **Maddox wing** dissociates the eyes for near fixation (⅓ m) and measures heterophoria. The instrument is constructed in such a way that the right eye sees only a white vertical arrow and a red horizontal arrow, whereas the left eye sees only horizontal and vertical rows of numbers (Fig. 20.36). Measurements are made as follows:
   a. The horizontal deviation is measured by asking the patient to which number the white arrow points.

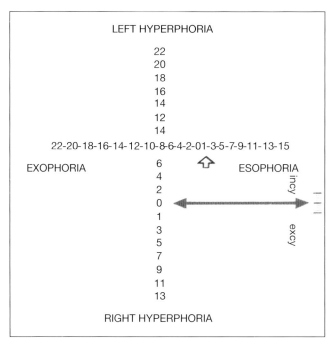

Fig. 20.36
Maddox wing

b. The vertical deviation is measured by asking the patient which number the red arrow intersects.
   c. The amount of cyclophoria is determined by asking the patient to move the red arrow so that it is parallel with the horizontal row of numbers.
2. **Maddox rod** consists of a series of fused cylindrical red glass rods which convert the appearance of a white spot of light into a red streak. The optical properties of the rods cause the streak of light to be at an angle of 90° with the long axis of the rods; when the glass rods are held horizontally, the streak will be vertical and vice versa. The test is performed as follows:
   a. The rod is placed in front of the right eye (Fig. 20.37a). This dissociates the two eyes because the red streak seen by the right eye cannot be fused with the unaltered white spot of light seen by the left eye (Fig. 20.37b).
   b. The amount of dissociation (Fig. 20.37c) is measured by the superimposition of the two images using prisms. The base of the prism is placed in the position opposite to the direction of the deviation.
   c. Both vertical and horizontal deviations can be measured in this way but the test cannot differentiate phoria from tropia.

Motility tests

Ocular movements

Examination of ocular movements involves assessment of smooth pursuit movements followed by that of saccadic movements.

1. **Versions** towards the eight eccentric positions of gaze are tested by asking the patient to follow a target, usually a pen or pen-torch (which offers the advantage of corneal light reflections to aid assessment). A quick cover test is performed in each position of gaze to confirm whether a phoria has become a tropia or the angle has increased and the patient is questioned regarding diplopia. They may also be elicited voluntarily, in response to a noise or by the doll's head manoeuvre in uncooperative patients
2. **Ductions** are assessed if reduced ocular motility is noted in either or both eyes. A pen-torch should be used with careful attention to the position of the corneal reflexes. The fellow eye is occluded and the patient asked to follow the torch into various positions of gaze. A simple numeric system may be employed using 0 to denote full movement, and −1 to −4 to denote increasing degrees of underaction (Fig. 20.38).

Near point of convergence

The near point of convergence (NPC) is the nearest point on which the eyes can maintain binocular fixation. It can be

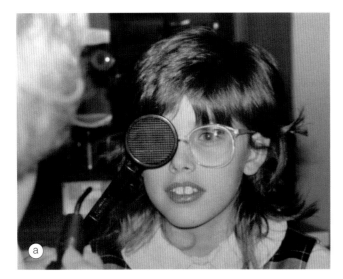

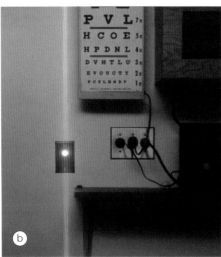

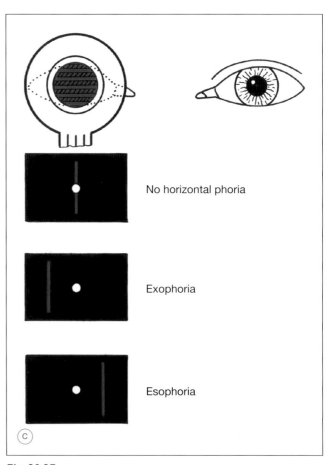

No horizontal phoria

Exophoria

Esophoria

Fig. 20.37
(a) Maddox rod test; **(b)** appearance of a point of light through Maddox rods; **(c)** possible results

measured with the RAF rule which rests on the patient's cheeks (Fig. 20.39a). A target (Fig. 20.39b) is slowly moved along the rule towards the patient's eyes until one eye loses fixation and drifts laterally (objective NPC). The subjective NPC is the point at which the patient reports diplopia. Normal NPC should be nearer than 10cm without undue effort.

Near point of accommodation

The near point of accommodation (NPA) is the nearest point on which the eyes can maintain clear focus. It can also be measured with the RAF rule. The patient fixates a line of print, which is then slowly moved towards the patient until it becomes blurred. The distance at which this is first reported is read off the rule and denotes the NPA. The NPA recedes with age; when sufficiently far away to render reading difficult without optical correction, presbyopia is present. At the age of 20 years the NPA is 8cm and by the age of 50 years

it has receded to 46cm. The amplitude of accommodation can also be assessed using concave lenses in 0.5DS steps whilst fixating the 6/6 Snellen line and reporting when the vision blurs.

Fusional amplitudes

Fusional amplitudes measure the efficacy of vergence movements. They may be tested with prisms bars or the synoptophore. Increasingly strong prisms are placed in front of one eye, which will then abduct or adduct (depending on whether the prism is base-in or base-out), in order to maintain bifoveal fixation. When a prism greater than the fusional amplitude is reached, diplopia is reported or one eye drifts the other way. This is the limit of vergence ability.

> **NB** The prism fusion range must be assessed in any binocular patient before strabismus surgery.

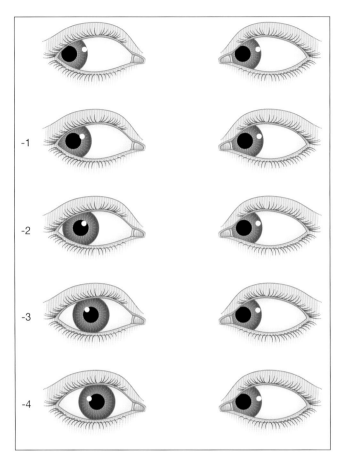

Fig. 20.38
Grading of right lateral rectus underaction

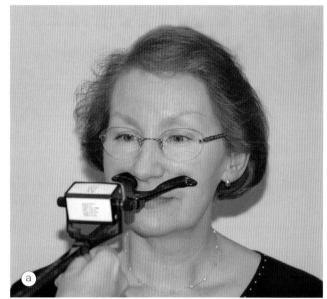

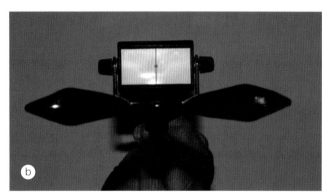

Fig. 20.39
(a) RAF rule; **(b)** convergence target

Postoperative diplopia test

This simple test is mandatory prior to strabismus surgery in all non-binocular patients over 7–8 years of age to assess the risk of diplopia after surgery. Corrective prisms are placed in front of one eye (usually the deviating eye) and the patient asked to fixate a straight ahead target with both eyes open. The prisms are slowly increased until the angle is significantly overcorrected. The patient reports if diplopia occurs. If suppression persists throughout, there is little risk of diplopia following surgery; in a consecutive exotropia of 35Δ diplopia may be reported from 30Δ and persist as the prism correction mimics an esotropia. Diplopia may be intermittent or constant but in either case this would be an indication to perform a diagnostic botulinum toxin test (see below). Diplopia is not restricted to patients with good visual acuity in the deviating eye; intractable diplopia is a difficult condition to treat and is best avoided.

Investigation of diplopia

The Hess test and the Lees screen are two similar tests that plot the dissociated ocular position as a function of the extraocular muscles. They enable differentiation of paretic strabismus caused by neurological pathology from restrictive myopathy (such as in thyroid eye disease or a blow-out fracture of the orbit), and recent-onset paresis from long-standing.

Electronic Hess test

The screen contains a tangent pattern (2D projection of a spherical surface) printed onto a dark grey background. Red lights that can be individually illuminated by a control panel indicate the cardinal positions of gaze within a central field (15° from primary position) and a peripheral field (30°); each square represents 5° of ocular rotation.

a. The patient is seated 50cm from the screen and wears red-green goggles, red lens in front of the right eye, and holds a green pointer.
b. The examiner illuminates each point in turn which is used as the point of fixation. This can now be seen only with the right eye, which therefore becomes the fixating eye.
c. The patient is asked to superimpose their green light onto the red light, so plotting the relative position of the left eye. All the points are plotted in turn.
d. In orthophoria the two lights should be more or less superimposed in all nine positions of gaze.
e. The goggles are then reversed (red filter in front of the left eye) and the procedure is repeated.
f. The relative positions are marked by the examiner on a chart and connected with straight lines.

Lees screen

The apparatus consists of two opalescent glass screens at right-angles to each other, bisected by a two-sided plane mirror which dissociates the two eyes (Fig. 20.40). Each screen has a tangent pattern marked onto the back surface which is revealed only when the screen is illuminated.

1. Procedure. The test is performed with each eye fixating in turn.
a. The patient faces the non-illuminated screen with the chin stabilized on a chin rest attached to the mirror support and fixates the dots in the mirror.
b. The examiner indicates the dot required for the patient to plot.
c. The patient positions the pointer on the non-illuminated screen perceived to be on top of the dot indicated by the examiner.
d. When all of the dots have been plotted the patient is repositioned to face the other screen and the procedure is repeated. The results are charted as before.

2. Interpretation
a. The two charts are compared (Fig. 20.41).
b. The smaller chart indicates the eye with the paretic muscle (right eye).
c. The larger chart indicates the eye with the overacting yoke muscle (left eye).
d. The smaller chart will show its greatest restriction in the main direction of action of the paretic muscle (right lateral rectus).
e. The larger chart will show its greatest expansion in the main direction of action of the yoke muscle (left medial rectus).
f. The degree of disparity between the plotted point and the template in any position of gaze gives an estimate of the angle of deviation (each square = 5°)

Changes with time

Changes with time are very useful as a prognostic guide. For example, in right superior rectus palsy, the Hess chart will show underaction of the affected muscle with an overaction of its yoke muscle (left inferior oblique) (Fig. 20.42a). Because of the great incomitance of the two charts, the diagnosis is straightforward. If the paretic muscle recovers its function, both charts will revert to normal. However, if the paresis persists, the shapes of both charts will change as follows:

- Secondary contracture of the ipsilateral antagonist (right inferior rectus) will show up on the chart as an overaction which will lead to a secondary (inhibitional) palsy of the antagonist of the yoke muscle (left superior oblique), which will show up on the chart as an underaction (Fig. 20.42b). This could lead to the incorrect impression that the left superior oblique was the primary muscle at fault.
- With further passage of time, the two charts become more and more concomitant until it may be impossible to determine which was the primary paretic muscle (Fig. 20.42c).

Clinical examples

It is worth analysing the following examples after gaining knowledge of ocular motor nerve palsies from Chapter 21.

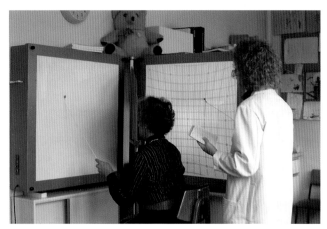

Fig. 20.40
Lees screen

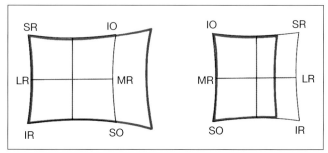

Fig. 20.41
Hess chart of a recent right lateral rectus palsy

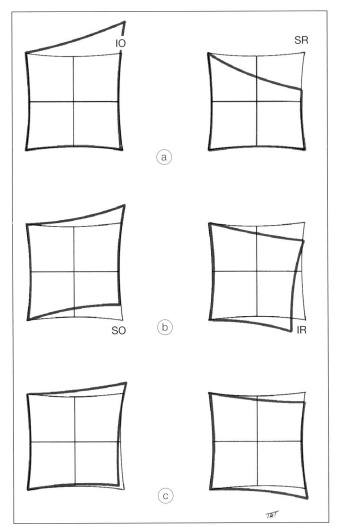

Fig. 20.42
Hess chart showing changes with time of a right superior rectus palsy (see text)

1. Left third nerve palsy (Fig. 20.43).
- The left chart is much smaller than the right.
- Left exotropia – note that the fixation spots in the inner charts of both eyes are deviated laterally. The deviation is greater on the right chart (when the left eye is fixating), indicating that secondary deviation exceeds the primary as is typical of a paretic squint.
- Left chart shows underaction of all muscles except the lateral rectus.
- Right chart shows overaction of all muscles except the medial rectus and inferior rectus, the 'yokes' of the spared muscles.
- The primary angle of deviation (fixing right eye – FR) in the primary position is −20° and R/L 10°.
- The secondary angle (fixing left eye – FL) is −28° and R/L 12°.

NB In inferior rectus palsy, the function of the superior oblique muscle can only be assessed by observing intorsion attempted depression. This is best performed by observing a conjunctival landmark on the slit-lamp.

2. Recently acquired right fourth nerve palsy (Fig. 20.44).
- Right chart is smaller than the left.
- Right chart shows underaction of the superior oblique and overaction of the inferior oblique.
- Left chart shows overaction of the inferior rectus and underaction (inhibitional palsy) of the superior rectus.
- The primary deviation (FL) is R/L 8°; the secondary deviation FR is R/L 17°.
3. Congenital right fourth nerve palsy or congenital right superior oblique weakness (Fig. 20.45).
- No differences in chart size.
- Primary and secondary deviation R/L 4°.
- Right hypertropia – note that the fixation spot of the right inner chart is deviated upwards and the left is deviated downwards.
- Hypertropia increases on laevoversion and reduces on dextroversion.
- Right chart shows underaction of the superior oblique and overaction of the inferior oblique.
- Left chart shows overaction of the inferior rectus and underaction (inhibitional palsy) of the superior rectus.
4. Right sixth nerve palsy (Fig. 20.46).
- Right chart is smaller than the left.
- Right esotropia – note that the fixation spot of the right inner chart is deviated nasally.
- Right chart shows marked underaction of the lateral rectus and slight overaction of the medial rectus.
- Left chart shows marked overaction of the medial rectus.
- The primary angle FL is +15° and the secondary angle FR +20°.

NB Inhibitional palsy of the left lateral rectus has not yet developed.

Refraction and fundoscopy

It should be emphasized that dilated fundoscopy is mandatory in the context of strabismus, to exclude any underlying ocular pathology such as macular scarring, optic disc hypoplasia or retinoblastoma. Strabismus is often secondary to refractive error. Hypermetropia, astigmatism, anisometropia and myopia may all be associated with strabismus.

Cycloplegia

The commonest refractive error causing strabismus is hypermetropia. Accurate measurements of hypermetropia

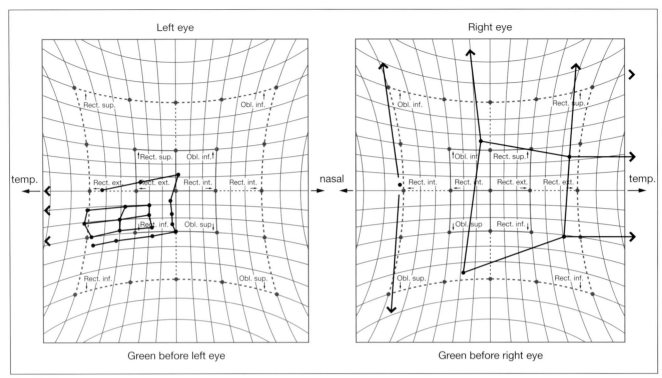

Fig. 20.43
Hess chart of a left third nerve palsy

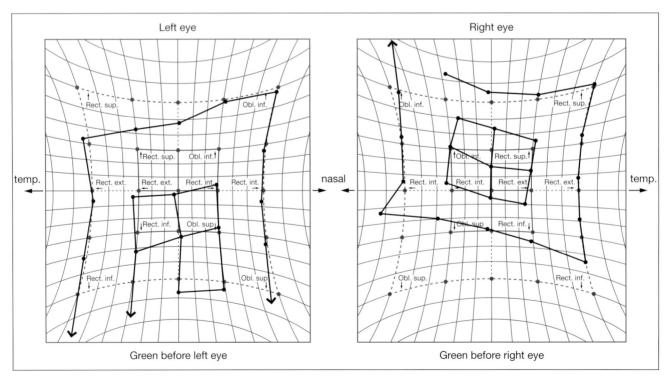

Fig. 20.44
Hess chart of a recently acquired right fourth nerve palsy

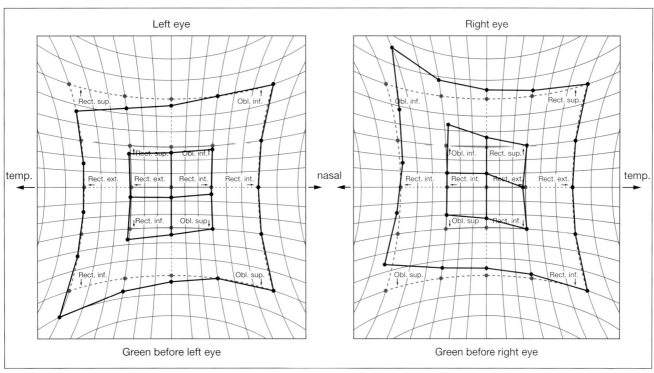

Fig. 20.45
Hess chart of a congenital right fourth nerve palsy or congenital right superior oblique weakness

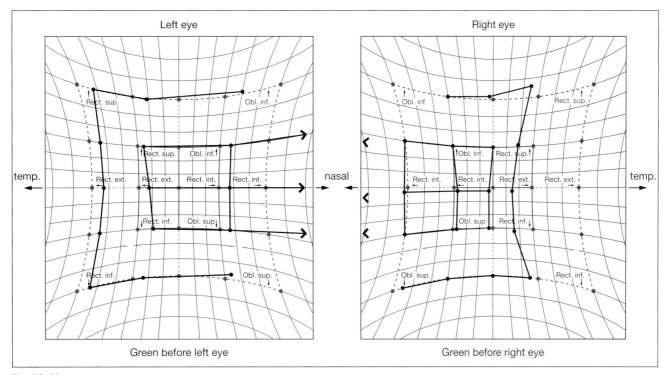

Fig. 20.46
Hess chart of a right sixth nerve palsy

necessitate effective paralysis of the ciliary muscle (cycloplegia), in order to neutralize the effect of accommodation, which masks the true degree of this refractive error.

1. **Cyclopentolate** affords adequate cycloplegia in most children. The concentration employed is 0.5% under the age of 6 months and 1% thereafter. One drop, repeated after 5 minutes, usually results in maximal cycloplegia within 30 minutes, with recovery of accommodation within 2–3 hours and of mydriasis within 24 hours. The adequacy of cycloplegia can be determined by comparing retinoscopy readings with the patient fixating for distance and then for near. If cycloplegia is adequate, there will be little or no difference. If cycloplegia is incomplete there will be a difference between the two readings and it may be necessary to wait another 15 minutes or to instil another drop.

NB Topical anaesthesia with an agent such as topical proxymetacaine, prior to instillation of cyclopentolate, is useful in preventing ocular irritation and reflex tearing, thus affording better retention of the cyclopentolate in the conjunctival sac and effective cycloplegia.

2. **Atropine** may be necessary in some children with either high hypermetropia or heavily pigmented irides, in which cyclopentolate may be inadequate. Atropine may be used as drops or ointment. Drops are easier for an untrained person to instil, but there is less risk of overdose with ointment. The concentration is 0.5% under the age of 12 months and 1% thereafter. Maximal cycloplegia occurs at 3 hours; recovery of accommodation starts after about 3 days and is usually complete by 10 days. Atropine is instilled (by the parents) b.d. for 3 days before retinoscopy, but not on the day of examination. The parents should be warned to discontinue medication if there are signs of systemic toxicity, such as flushing, fever or restlessness, and seek immediate medical attention.

Change of refraction

Because refraction changes with age, it is important to check at least every year and more frequently in smaller children and if acuity is reduced. At birth most babies are hypermetropic. After the age of 2 years there may be an increase in hypermetropia and a decrease in astigmatism. Hypermetropia may continue to increase until the age of about 6 years, and then between the ages of 6 and 8 years levels off, subsequently decreasing until the early teenage years.

When to prescribe

1. **Hypermetropia.** In general up to 4D of hypermetropia should not be corrected in a child without a squint unless they are having problems with near vision. With degrees of hypermetropia greater than this a two-thirds correction

is usually given. However, in the presence of esotropia the full cycloplegic correction should be prescribed, even under the age of 2 years.
2. **Astigmatism.** A cylinder of 1.50D or more should be prescribed, especially in cases of anisometropia after the age of 18 months.
3. **Myopia.** The necessity for correction depends on the age of the child. Under the age of 2 years, −5.00D or more of myopia should be corrected; between the ages of 2 and 4 the amount is −3.00D. Older children should have correction of even milder degrees of myopia to allow clear distance vision.
4. **Anisometropia.** After the age of 3 the full difference in refraction between the eyes should be prescribed if it is more than 1D. If there is no squint then any associated hypermetropic correction may be equally reduced for each eye.

HETEROPHORIA AND VERGENCE ABNORMALITIES

Heterophoria

Heterophoria may present clinically with associated visual symptoms, particularly at times of stress or poor health, when the fusional amplitudes are insufficient to maintain alignment. Both esophoria and exophoria can be classified by the distance at which the angle is greater (respectively: convergence excess or weakness, divergence weakness or excess, and mixed); vertical phoria are caused by abnormal ocular motility. Treatment involves the following:
* Orthoptic treatment is of most value in convergence weakness exophoria.
* Any significant refractive error should be appropriately corrected.
* Symptom relief may otherwise be obtained using temporary stick-on Fresnel prisms and may be subsequently incorporated into spectacles (maximum usually 10–12Δ split between the two eyes).
* Surgery may occasionally be required for larger deviations.

Vergence abnormalities

Convergence insufficiency

Convergence insufficiency typically affects individuals with excessive visual demand such as students.

1. **Signs.** Reduced near point of convergence independent of any heterophoria.
2. **Treatment** involves orthoptic exercises aimed at normalizing the near point and fusional amplitudes. With good

compliance, symptoms should be eliminated within a few weeks but if persistent can be treated with base-in prisms.

3. **Accommodative insufficiency** is occasionally also present. It may be idiopathic (primary) or post-viral and typically affects school age children. The minimum reading correction is prescribed to give clear vision but is often difficult to discard.

Near reflex insufficiency

1. **Paresis** of the near reflex presents as an exaggerated of convergence and accommodation insufficiency. Mydriasis may be seen on attempted near fixation. In the absence of neurological signs treatment involves reading glasses, base-in prisms and possibly Botulinum toxin (orthoptic exercises have no effect) but it is difficult to eradicate.

2. **Complete paralysis** in which no convergence or accommodation can be initiated may be of functional origin or caused by midbrain disease or follow head trauma (recovery possible).

Near reflex spasm

Spasm of the near reflex is a functional condition affecting patients of all ages (mainly females).

1. **Signs**
   - Diplopia, blurred vision and headaches are accompanied by esotropia, pseudomyopia and miosis.
   - The spasm may be triggered when testing ocular movements (Fig. 20.47a).
   - Observing miosis is the key to the diagnosis (Fig. 20.47b).
   - Refraction with and without cycloplegia confirms the pseudomyopia, which must not be corrected optically.

2. **Treatment** involves reassurance and advising the patient to look away and cease the activity that triggers the response. If persistent, atropine and a full reading correction are prescribed but it is difficult later to abandon treatment without recurrence. Patients usually seem to live a fairly normal life despite the signs and symptoms.

Divergence insufficiency

Divergence paresis or paralysis is a rare condition associated with underlying neurological disease, such as intracranial space-occupying lesions, cerebrovascular accidents and head trauma. Presentation may be at any age and may be difficult to differentiate from sixth nerve palsy, but is primarily a concomitant esodeviation with reduced or absent divergence fusional amplitudes. It is difficult to treat; prisms are the best option.

ESOTROPIA

Esotropia (manifest convergent squint) may be concomitant or incomitant. In a concomitant esotropia the variability of

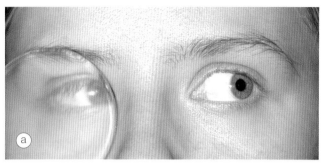
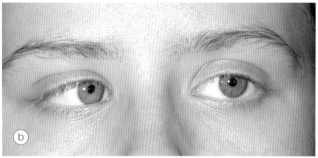

Fig. 20.47
(a) Spasm of the near reflex precipitated on testing ocular movements; **(b)** right esotropia and miosis

the angle of deviation is within 5Δ in different horizontal gaze positions. In an incomitant deviation the angle differs in various positions of gaze as a result of abnormal innervation or restriction. This section deals only with concomitant esotropia; however, all squints are different and not all fit neatly into a classification. For example a microtropia may occur with a number of the other categories. It is more important to understand the part played by binocular function, refractive error and accommodation in the pathophysiology of each individual squint and to tailor treatment accordingly.

Early onset esotropia

Up to 4 months of age infrequent episodes of convergence are normal. After 4 months ocular misalignment is abnormal. Early onset (congenital, essential, infantile) esotropia is an idiopathic condition developing within the first 6 months of life in an otherwise normal infant with no significant refractive error and no limitation of ocular movements.

Diagnosis

- The angle is usually fairly large (>30Δ) and stable.
- Fixation in most infants is alternating in the primary position (Fig. 20.48).
- There is cross-fixating in side gaze, so that the child uses the left eye in right gaze (Fig. 20.49a) and the right eye

Table 20.1   Classification of esotropia

1. Accommodative
  a. *Refractive*
    ● Fully accommodative
    ● Partially accommodative
  b. *Non-refractive*
    ● With convergence excess
    ● With accommodation weakness
  c. *Mixed*

2. Non-accommodative
  ● Essential infantile
  ● Microtropia
  ● Basic
  ● Convergence excess
  ● Convergence spasm
  ● Divergence insufficiency
  ● Divergence paralysis
  ● Sensory
  ● Consecutive
  ● Acute onset
  ● Cyclic

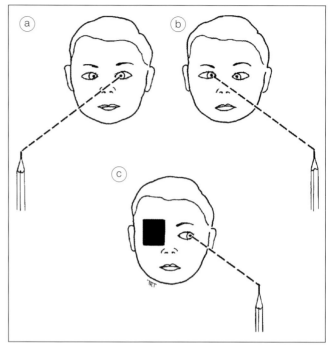

Fig. 20.49
Early onset esotropia. (**a** and **b**) Cross-fixation; (**c**) occlusion of the right eye demonstrates ability to abduct the left eye

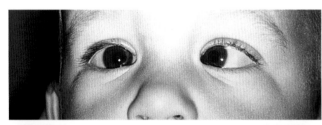
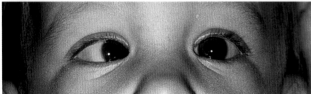

Fig. 20.48
Alternating fixation in early onset esotropia

on left gaze (Fig. 20.49b). Such cross-fixation may give a false impression of bilateral abduction deficits, as in bilateral sixth nerve palsy.
● Abduction can, however, usually be demonstrated either by the doll's head manoeuvre or by rotating the child.
● Should these fail, uniocular patching for a few hours will often unmask the ability of the other eye to abduct (Fig. 20.49c).
● Nystagmus is usually horizontal.
● Latent nystagmus is only seen when one eye is covered and the fast phase beats towards the side of the fixing eye. This means that the direction of the fast phase reverses according to which eye is covered.

● Manifest latent nystagmus is the same except that nystagmus is present with both eyes open, but the amplitude increases when one is covered.
● The refractive error is usually normal for the age of the child (about +1 to +2D).
● Asymmetry of optokinetic nystagmus.
● Inferior oblique overaction may be present initially or develop later (see Fig. 20.51).
● Dissociated vertical deviation (DVD) develops in 80% by the age of 3 years (see Fig. 20.52).

Initial treatment

Early ocular alignment gives the best chance of the child developing some form of binocular function. Ideally, the eyes should be surgically aligned by the age of 12 months, and at the very latest by the age of 2 years, but only after amblyopia or significant refractive errors have been corrected. The initial procedure can be either recession of both medial recti or unilateral medial rectus recession with lateral rectus resection. Very large angles may require recessions of 6.5mm or more. Associated inferior oblique overaction should also be addressed. An acceptable goal is alignment of the eyes to within 10Δ associated with peripheral fusion and central suppression (Fig. 20.50). This small-angle residual strabismus is often stable, even thought bifoveal fusion is not achieved.

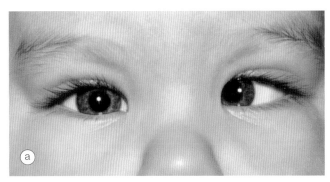

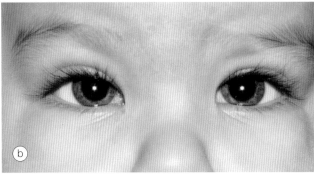

Fig. 20.50
Early onset esotropia. **(a)** Before surgery; **(b)** after surgery

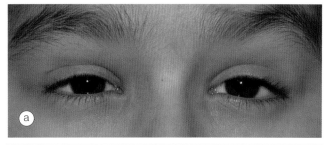

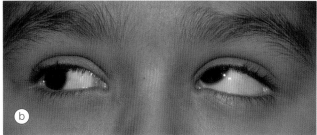

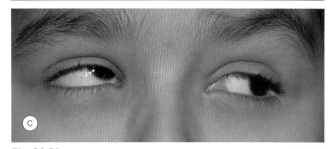

Fig. 20.51
Inferior oblique overaction. **(a)** Straight eyes in the primary position; **(b)** left inferior oblique overaction on right gaze; **(c)** right inferior oblique overaction on left gaze

Subsequent treatment

1. **Undercorrection** may require further recession of the medial recti, resection of one or both lateral recti or surgery to the other eye

2. **Inferior oblique overaction** may develop subsequently, most commonly at age 2 years (Fig. 20.51). The parents should therefore be warned that further surgery may be necessary despite an initially good result. Initially unilateral, it frequently becomes bilateral within 6 months. Inferior oblique weakening procedures include disinsertion, recession and myectomy (see later).

3. **DVD** may appear several years after the initial surgery, particularly in children with nystagmus. It is characterized by the following:
   - Up-drift with excyclorotation of the eye when under cover (Fig. 20.52b) or spontaneously during periods of visual inattention.
   - When the cover is removed the affected eye will move down without a corresponding down-drift of the other eye (Fig. 20.52c).

Thus DVD does not obey Hering law. Although it is usually bilateral, it may be asymmetrical. Surgical treatment is indicated when the condition is cosmetically unacceptable. Superior rectus recession with or without posterior fixation sutures (see below) or inferior oblique anterior transposition are useful for DVD, although full elimination is seldom possible.

4. **Amblyopia** subsequently develops in about 50% of cases as unilateral fixation preference commonly develops postoperatively.

5. **An accommodative element** should be suspected if the eyes are initially straight or almost straight after surgery and then start to reconverge. It is therefore important to perform repeated refractions on all children and to correct any new accommodative elements accordingly.

Differential diagnosis

1. **Congenital bilateral sixth nerve palsy,** which is rare and can be excluded as described above.

2. **Secondary** (sensory) esotropia due to organic eye disease.

3. **Nystagmus blockage syndrome** in which convergence dampens a horizontal nystagmus. Nystagmus can be elicited on abduction and the infant adopts a face turn to fixate in the adducted position.

4. **Duane syndrome types I and III.**

5. **Möbius syndrome.**

6. **Strabismus fixus.**

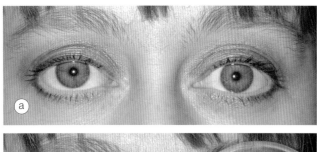
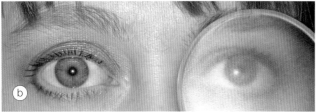
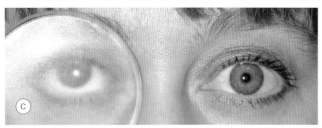

Fig. 20.52
Dissociated vertical deviation. **(a)** Straight eyes in the primary position; **(b)** up-drift of left eye under cover; **(c)** up-drift of right eye under cover and down-drift of left eye

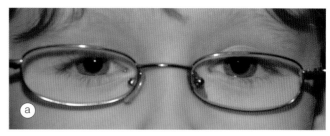
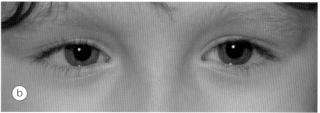

Fig. 20.53
Fully accommodative esotropia. **(a)** Eyes straight for near and distance with glasses; **(b)** right esotropia without glasses

Accommodative esotropia

Near vision involves both accommodation and convergence. Accommodation is the process by which the eye focuses on a near target, by altering the curvature of the crystalline lens. Simultaneously, the eyes converge, in order to fixate bi-foveally on the target. Both accommodation and convergence are quantitatively related to the proximity of the target, and have a fairly constant relationship to each other (AC/A ratio) as described previously. Abnormalities of the AC/A ratio are an important cause of certain types of esotropia.

Refractive accommodative esotropia

Here the AC/A ratio is normal and esotropia is a physiological response to excessive hypermetropia, usually between +2.00 and +7.00D. The considerable degree of accommodation required to focus clearly, even on a distant target, is accompanied by a proportionate amount of convergence, which is beyond the patient's fusional divergence amplitude. It cannot therefore be controlled and a manifest convergent squint results. The magnitude of the deviation varies little (usually < 10Δ) between distance and near. The deviation typically presents at the age of 18 months to 3 years (range of 6 months to 7 years).

1. **Fully accommodative** esotropia is eliminated by optical correction of hypermetropia and BSV is present at all distances with glasses (Fig. 20.53a) – but the deviation is present when glasses are not worn (Fig. 20.53b).
2. **Constant accommodative esotropia** is reduced, but not eliminated, by full correction of hypermetropia (Fig. 20.54). Amblyopia and bilateral congenital superior oblique weakness are frequent. Most cases show suppression of the squinting eye although ARC may occur, but of lower grade than in microtropia.

Non-refractive accommodative esotropia

This is associated with a high AC/A ratio in which a unit increase of accommodation is accompanied by a disproportionately large increase of convergence. This occurs independently of refractive error, although hypermetropia frequently coexists. It can be subdivided into:

1. **Convergence excess**
   - High AC/A ratio due to increased accommodative convergence (accommodation is normal, convergence is increased).
   - Normal near point of accommodation.
   - Straight eyes with BSV for distance (Fig. 20.55a).
   - Esotropia for near, usually with suppression (Fig. 20.55b).
   - Straight eyes through bifocals (Fig. 20.55c).
2. **Hypoaccommodative convergence excess**
   - High AC/A ratio due to decreased accommodation (accommodation is weak, necessitating increased effort, which produces overconvergence).
   - Remote near point of accommodation.
   - Straight eyes with BSV for distance.
   - Esotropia for near, usually with suppression.

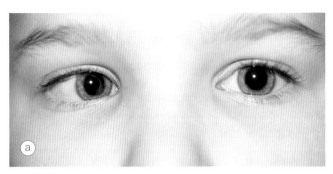

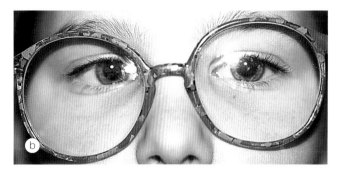

Fig. 20.54
Constant accommodative esotropia. **(a)** Right esotropia without glasses; **(b)** angle is reduced but not eliminated with glasses

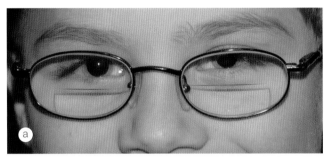

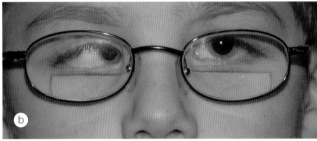

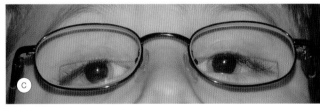

Fig. 20.55
Convergence excess esotropia. **(a)** Eyes straight for distance;
(b) right esotropia for near; **(c)** eyes straight through bifocals

Medical treatment

Refractive error should be corrected, as previously described. In children under the age of 6 years, the full cycloplegic refraction revealed on retinoscopy should be prescribed (with a deduction only for the working distance). In the fully accommodative refractive esotrope this will control the deviation for both near and distance. After the age of 8 years,

refraction should be performed without cycloplegia and the maximal amount of 'plus' that can be tolerated (manifest hypermetropia) prescribed.

For convergence excess esotropia bifocals may be prescribed to relieve accommodation (and thereby accommodative convergence), thus allowing the child to maintain bi-foveal fixation and ocular alignment at near (see Fig. 20.55c). The minimum 'add' required to achieve this is prescribed. The most satisfactory form of bifocals is the executive type in which the intersection crosses the lower border of the pupil. The strength of the lower segment should be gradually reduced and eliminated by the early teenage years. Bifocals are best suited to hypoaccommodative esotropia and where the AC/A ratio is not overly excessive, when there is a reasonable chance of discarding bifocal correction with time. At higher levels surgery is the better long-term option. The ultimate prognosis for complete withdrawal of spectacles is related to the magnitude of the AC/A ratio and also the degree of hypermetropia and associated astigmatism. Spectacles may be needed only for close work.

Surgery

The aim of surgery is to restore or enhance BSV or to improve the appearance of the squint. Surgery should only be considered if spectacles do not fully correct the deviation and after every attempt has been made to treat amblyopia.

- Bilateral medial rectus recessions are performed in patients in whom the deviation for near is greater than that for distance.
- If there is no significant difference between distance and near measurements, and equal vision in both eyes, some perform unilateral medial rectus recession combined with lateral rectus resection, whereas others prefer bilateral medial rectus recessions.
- In patients with residual amblyopia surgery is usually performed on the amblyopic eye.
- In constant accommodative esotropia surgery to improve appearance is best delayed until requested by the child to

avoid early consecutive exotropia and should only aim to correct the residual squint present with the glasses on.

NB Treatment of amblyopia is very important before contemplating surgery.

Microtropia

Microtropia (monofixation syndrome), may be primary or follow surgery for a large deviation. It may occur in apparent isolation, but it is often associated with other conditions such as anisometropic amblyopia. Microtropia is more a description of binocular status than a specific diagnosis, for example a patient with fully accommodative esotropia may control to a microtropia rather than true bifoveal BSV with glasses. It is characterized by the following:

1. **Very small angle** manifest deviation measuring 8Δ or less, which may or may not be detectable on cover testing.
2. **Central suppression scotoma,** of the deviating eye.
3. **ARC** with reduced stereopsis and variable peripheral fusional amplitudes.
4. **Anisometropia** is often present, commonly with hypermetropia or hypermetropic astigmatism.
5. **Symptoms** are rare unless there is an associated decompensating heterophoria.
6. **Treatment** involves correction of refractive errors and occlusion for amblyopia as indicated. Most patients remain stable and symptom free.

Other esotropias

Near esotropia

1. **Signs**
   - No significant refractive error.
   - Orthophoria or small esophoria with BSV for distance.
   - Esotropia for near but normal or low AC/A ratio.
   - Normal near point of accommodation.
2. **Treatment** is usually bilateral medial rectus recessions.

Distance esotropia

This typically affects healthy young adults who are often myopic.

1. **Signs**
   - Intermittent or constant esotropia for distance.
   - Minimal or no deviation for near.
   - Normal bilateral abduction.
   - Fusional divergence amplitudes may be reduced.
   - Absence of neurological disease.
2. **Treatment** is with prisms, until spontaneous resolution, or surgery in persistent cases.

NB It is important to distinguish this from sixth nerve paresis, which may be difficult on clinical grounds and investigation should be considered.

Acute (late onset) esotropia

This presents for no apparent reason around 5–6 years of age.

1. **Signs**
   - Sudden onset of diplopia and esotropia.
   - Normal ocular motility and no significant refractive error.
   - Underlying sixth nerve palsy must be excluded.
2. **Treatment** is aimed at quickly re-establishing BSV to prevent suppression with prisms, Botulinum toxin or surgery.

Secondary (sensory) esotropia

This is caused by a unilateral reduction in visual acuity which interferes with or abolishes fusion, such as cataract, optic atrophy or hypoplasia, macular scarring or retinoblastoma.

NB Fundus examination under mydriasis is therefore essential in all children with strabismus.

Consecutive esotropia

This follows surgical overcorrection of an exodeviation. If it occurs following surgery for an intermittent exotropia in a child it should not be allowed to persist for more than 6 weeks without further intervention.

Cyclic esotropia

This is a very rare condition characterized by alternating manifest esotropia with suppression and BSV, each lasting 24 hours. The condition may persist for months or years and the patient may eventually develop a constant esotropia requiring surgery. Earlier correction of the full manifest angle can be successfully performed during the intermittent phase.

EXOTROPIA

Constant (early onset) exotropia

1. **Presentation** is often at birth.
2. **Signs**
   - Normal refraction.
   - Large and constant angle.
   - DVD may be present.

3. **Neurological anomalies** are frequently present, in contrast with infantile esotropia.
4. **Treatment** is mainly surgical and consists of lateral rectus recession and medial rectus resection.

NB It is important to distinguish this from secondary exotropia which may conceal serious ocular pathology.

Intermittent exotropia

Diagnosis

1. **Presentation** is often at around 2 years with exophoria, which breaks down to exotropia under conditions of visual inattention, bright light (resulting in reflex closure of the affected eye), fatigue or ill health.
2. **Signs.** The eyes are straight with BSV at times (Fig. 20.56a) and manifest with suppression at other times (Fig. 20.56b). The control of the squint varies with the distance of fixation and other factors such as concentration.

Classification

1. **Distance** exotropia, in which the angle of deviation is greater for distance than near and increases further beyond 6 metres. There are two types:
    a. Simulated is associated with a high AC/A ratio or tenacious proximal convergence (TPC). The deviations for near and distance are similar when the near angle is remeasured with the patient looking through +3.00D lenses (high AC/A controlling exodeviation) or after a period of uniocular occlusion (TPC).
    b. True. The angle for near remains significantly less than that for distance with the above tests.
2. **Non-specific** exotropia, in which control of the squint and the angle of deviation are the same for distance and near fixation.
3. **Near** exotropia, in which the deviation is greater for near fixation. It tends to occur in older children and adults and may be associated with acquired myopia or presbyopia.

Treatment

1. **Spectacle correction** in myopic patients may, in some cases, control the deviation by stimulating accommodation, and with it, convergence. In some cases over-minus prescription may be useful.
2. **Part-time occlusion** of the deviating eye may improve control in some patients and orthoptic exercises may be helpful for near exotropia.
3. **Surgery** Patients with good and stable control of intermittent exotropia are often just observed. Surgery is indicated if control is poor or is progressively deteriorating. Unilateral lateral rectus recession and medial rectus recession are generally preferred except in true distance exotropia when bilateral lateral rectus recessions are more usual. Even after surgery the exodeviation is rarely completely eliminated.

Sensory exotropia

Secondary (sensory) exotropia is the result of monocular or binocular visual impairment by acquired lesions, such as cataract or other opacities of the media (Fig. 20.57a).

1. **Exodeviation** tends to occur in older children or adults.
2. **Esodeviation** tends to occur in infancy, but this is not invariable.
3. **Treatment** consists of correction of the visual deficit, if possible, followed by surgery, if appropriate. A minority of patients develop intractable diplopia due to loss of fusion, even when good visual acuity is restored to both eyes and the eyes are realigned.

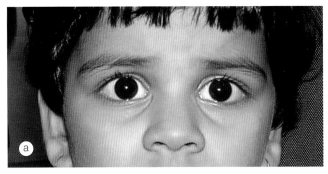
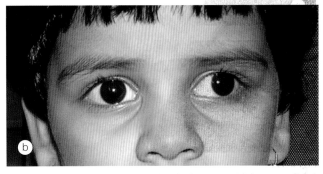

Fig. 20.56
Intermittent exotropia. **(a)** Eyes straight most of the time; **(b)** left exotropia under conditions of visual inattention or fatigue (Courtesy of M Parulekar)

Consecutive exotropia

Consecutive exotropia develops spontaneously in an amblyopic eye or, more frequently, following surgical correction of an esodeviation. In early postoperative divergence muscle slippage must be considered. Most cases present in adult life with concerns about cosmesis (Fig. 20.57b) and social function, and can be greatly helped by surgery. Careful evaluation of the risk of postoperative diplopia is required, although serious problems are uncommon. About 75% of patients are still well aligned 10 years after surgery although re-divergence may occasionally occur.

SPECIAL SYNDROMES

Recent genetic and neuropathological studies have shown that a group of *congenital neuromuscular disorders* are the result of developmental errors in innervation of ocular and facial muscles. These conditions are now referred to as congenital cranial dysinnervation disorders and include Duane syndrome, Möbius syndrome, congenital fibrosis of extraocular muscles, Marcus Gunn jaw-winking syndrome (see Chapter 4), congenital ptosis and congenital facial palsy.

Duane retraction syndrome

In Duane retraction syndrome there is failure of innervation of the lateral rectus by the sixth nerve, with anomalous innervation of the lateral rectus by fibres from the third nerve. The condition is often bilateral, although frequently

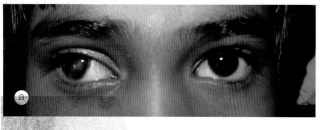

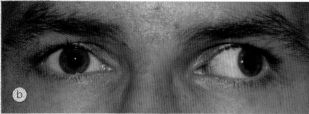

Fig. 20.57
(a) Sensory right exotropia due to traumatic corneal opacity and cataract; **(b)** large consecutive left exotropia several years following surgery for esotropia (Courtesy of M Parulekar – fig. a)

involvement in one eye may be very subtle. Some children have associated congenital defects such as perceptive deafness and speech disorder.

Diagnosis

There is usually BSV in the primary position, often with a face turn. The affected eye shows the following motility defects (Figs 20.58, 20.59 and 20.60).

1. **Restricted abduction,** which may be complete or partial.
2. **Restricted adduction** which is usually partial and rarely complete.
3. **Retraction of the globe adduction** as a result of co-contraction of the medial and lateral recti with resultant narrowing of the palpebral fissure. The degree of globe retraction may vary from gross to almost imperceptible. On attempted abduction, the palpebral fissure opens and the globe assumes its normal position.
4. **An up-shoot or down-shoot in adduction** may be present. It has been suggested that this is a 'bridle' or 'leash' phenomenon, produced by a tight lateral rectus muscle which slips over or under the globe and produces an anomalous vertical movement of the eye. However, recent studies with MR have shown that this is not always the case.
5. **Deficiency of convergence** in which the affected eye remains fixed in the primary position while the unaffected eye is converging.

Classification (Huber)

1. **Type I,** the most common, is characterized by:
   - Limited or absent abduction.
   - Normal or mildly limited adduction.
   - In the primary position, straight or slight esotropia.
2. **Type II,** the least common, is characterized by:
   - Limited adduction.
   - Normal or mildly limited abduction.
   - In primary position, straight or slight exotropia.
3. **Type III** is characterized by:
   - Limited adduction and abduction.
   - In the primary position, straight or slight esotropia.

> **NB** The underlying pathophysiology is similar in all three types, the differences being due to inequality in the degree of anomaly in the innervation to the lateral and medial recti.

Management

Most young children maintain BSV by using an abnormal head posture to compensate for their lateral rectus weakness and surgery is only needed if there is evidence of loss of binocular function, which may be indicated by failure to

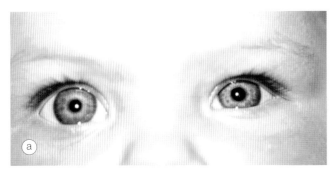
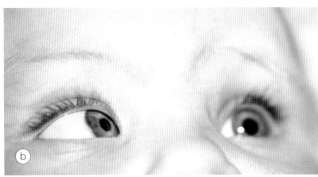
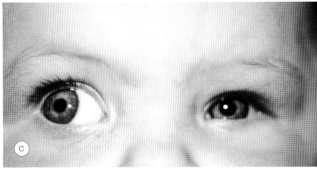

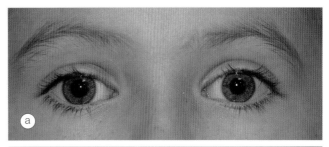
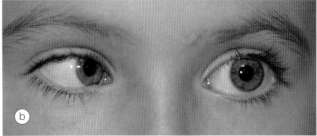
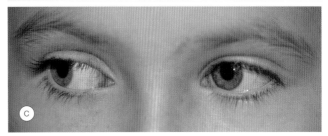

Fig. 20.59
Duane syndrome type 1 in a child. **(a)** Straight in the primary position; **(b)** grossly limited left abduction with slight widening of the left palpebral fissure; **(c)** slightly limited left adduction

Fig. 20.58
Duane syndrome type 3 in an infant. **(a)** Straight eyes in the primary position; **(b)** limited left abduction with widening of the left palpebral fissure; **(c)** grossly limited left adduction with narrowing of the left palpebral fissure (Courtesy of K Nischal)

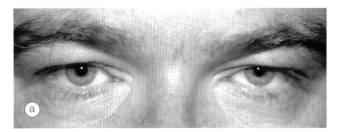
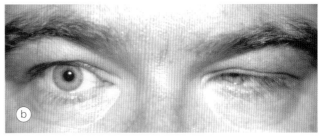

continue to use an abnormal head posture. In adults or children over the age of about 8 years surgery can reduce a cosmetically unacceptable head posture or one causing neck discomfort. Surgery may also be necessary for cosmetically unacceptable up-shoots, down-shoots or severe globe retraction. Amblyopia, when present, is usually the result of anisometropia rather than strabismus. Unilateral or bilateral muscle recession or transposition of the vertical recti are the procedures of choice.

NB The lateral rectus of the involved side should not be resected, as this increases retraction.

Fig. 20.60
Duane syndrome in an adult. **(a)** Straight in the primary position. **(b)** grossly limited right abduction with slight widening of the right palpebral fissure and marked narrowing of the left palpebral fissure

Brown syndrome

Brown syndrome is a mechanical condition which is usually congenital but occasionally may be acquired.

Classification

1. **Congenital**
   - Idiopathic.
   - Congenital click syndrome where there is impaired movement of the superior oblique tendon through the trochlea.
2. **Acquired**
   - Trauma to the trochlea or superior oblique tendon.
   - Inflammation of the tendon which may be caused by rheumatoid arthritis, pansinusitis and scleritis.

Diagnosis

A left Brown syndrome has the following characteristics:

1. **Major signs**
   - Usually straight with BSV in the primary position (Fig. 20.61a).
   - Limited left elevation in adduction (Fig. 20.61b) and occasionally also in the midline.
   - Limited left elevation on up-gaze is common (Fig. 20.61c).
   - Normal left elevation in abduction (Fig. 20.61d).
   - Absence of left superior oblique overaction (Fig. 20.61e).
   - Positive forced duction test on elevating the globe in adduction.
2. **Variable signs**
   - Down-shoot in adduction.
   - Hypotropia in primary position.
   - AHP with chin elevation and ipsilateral head tilt (Fig. 20.61f).

Treatment

1. **Congenital** cases do not usually require treatment as long as binocular function is maintained with an acceptable head posture. Spontaneous improvement is often seen towards the end of the first decade. Indications for treatment include significant primary position hypotropia, deteriorating control and/or an unacceptable head posture. The recommended procedure for congenital cases is lengthening of the superior oblique tendon.
2. **Acquired** cases may benefit from steroids, either orally or by injection near the trochlea, together with treatment of any underlying cause.

Monocular elevator deficit

Monocular elevator palsy, sometimes also referred to as double elevator palsy, is a rare sporadic condition. It is thought to be caused by either a tight or contracted inferior rectus muscle or a hypoplastic or ineffective superior rectus muscle.

1. **Signs**
   - Profound inability to elevate one eye.
   - The abnormality of up-gaze persists across the horizontal plane, from abduction to adduction (Fig. 20.62).
   - Orthophoria in the primary position in about one-third of cases.
   - Chin elevation to obtain fusion in down-gaze may be present.
2. **Treatment** involving base-up prism over the involved eye or surgery should be considered when fusion in the primary position has been compromised or a chin elevation is required to maintain fusion.

Möbius syndrome

Möbius syndrome is a very rare congenital, sporadic condition.

1. **Ocular features**
   - Horizontal gaze palsy is present in 50% of cases.
   - Bilateral sixth nerve palsy (Fig. 20.63a).
2. **Systemic features**
   - Bilateral facial palsy, usually asymmetrical and often incomplete, giving rise to a mask-like facial expression and problems with lid closure (Fig. 20.63b).
   - Paresis of the ninth and twelfth cranial nerves; the latter results in atrophy of the tongue (Fig. 20.63c).
   - Mild mental handicap.
   - Limb anomalies.

Congenital fibrosis of extraocular muscles

Congenital fibrosis of extraocular muscles syndrome is a rare non-progressive usually AD disorder characterized by bilateral ptosis and restrictive external ophthalmoplegia (Fig. 20.64).

- In the 'primary' position each eye is fixed below the horizontal by about 10°.
- The hypotropic eye may be secondarily exotropic, esotropic or neutral.
- The degree of residual horizontal movement varies from full to absent.
- Vertical movements are always severely restricted with inability to elevate the eyes above the horizontal plane.
- Absence of binocular vision and amblyopia may be present in some cases.

Strabismus fixus

Strabismus fixus is a very rare condition, in which both eyes are fixed by fibrous tightening of the medial recti (convergent

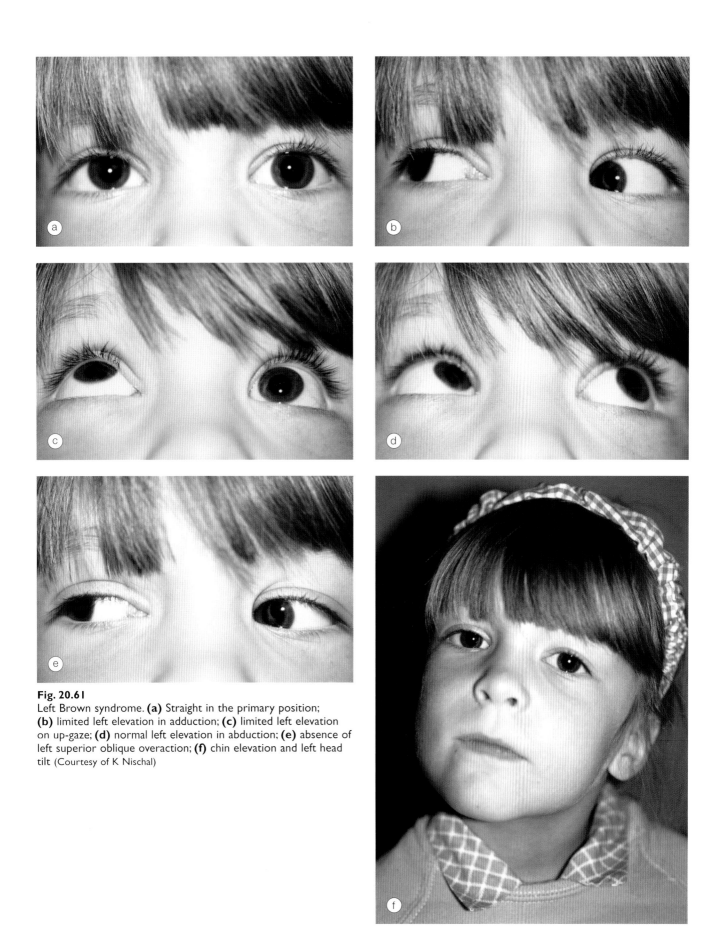

Fig. 20.61
Left Brown syndrome. **(a)** Straight in the primary position;
(b) limited left elevation in adduction; **(c)** limited left elevation
on up-gaze; **(d)** normal left elevation in abduction; **(e)** absence of
left superior oblique overaction; **(f)** chin elevation and left head
tilt (Courtesy of K Nischal)

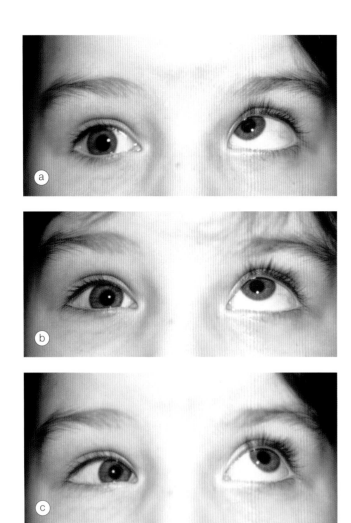

Fig. 20.62
Right monoelevation deficit. **(a)** Defective elevation in abduction;
(b) in up-gaze; **(c)** and in adduction

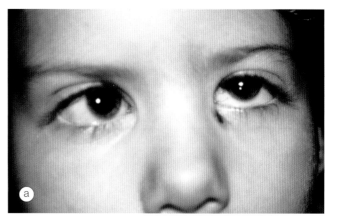

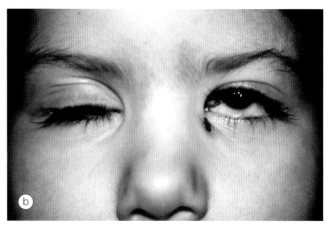

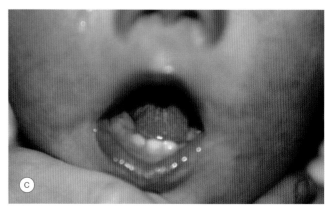

Fig. 20.63
Möbius syndrome. **(a)** Esotropia due to bilateral sixth nerve palsy;
(b) defective lid closure due to facial nerve palsy; **(c)** atrophic
tongue due to hypoglossal nerve palsy (Courtesy of K Nischal)

strabismus fixus – Fig. 20.65a) or the lateral recti (divergent
strabismus fixus – Fig. 20.65b).

ALPHABET PATTERNS

'V 'or 'A' patterns may occur when the relative contributions
of the superior rectus and inferior oblique to elevation, or of
the inferior rectus and superior oblique to depression, are
abnormal, resulting in abnormal balance of their horizontal
vectors in up- and down-gaze. They can also be caused by
anomalies in the position of the rectus muscle pulleys leading
to abnormal lines of action of the muscles. They are assessed
by measuring horizontal deviations in the primary position,
up-gaze and down-gaze and may occur regardless of whether
a deviation is concomitant or incomitant.

'V' pattern

'V' pattern is significant when difference between up-gaze
and down-gaze is ≥ 15Δ, allowing for a small physiological
variation between up- and down-gaze.

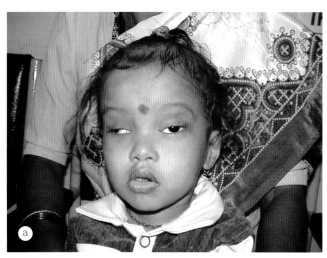
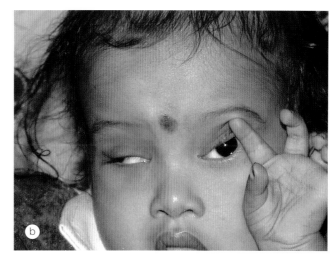

Fig. 20.64
Congenital fibrosis of extraocular muscles. **(a)** Bilateral ptosis and divergent strabismus; **(b)** compensation for severe ptosis (Courtesy of M Parulekar)

Causes

- Inferior oblique overaction associated with fourth nerve palsy.
- Superior oblique underaction with subsequent inferior oblique overaction which is seen in infantile esotropia as well as other childhood esotropias. The eyes are often straight in up-gaze with a marked esodeviation in down-gaze.
- Superior rectus underaction.
- Brown syndrome.
- Craniofacial anomalies which are associated with shallow orbits and down-slanting palpebral fissures.

Treatment

Treatment involves inferior oblique weakening or superior oblique strengthening when oblique dysfunction is present. Without oblique muscle dysfunction treatment is as follows:

1. **'V' pattern esotropia** (Fig.20.66a) can be treated by bilateral medial rectus recessions and downward transposition of the tendons.
2. **'V' pattern exotropia** (Fig. 20.66b) can be treated by bilateral lateral rectus recessions and upward transposition of the tendons.

'A' pattern

'A' pattern is significant if the difference between up-gaze and down-gaze is ≥ 10Δ. In a binocular patient it may cause problems with reading.

Causes

- Primary superior oblique overaction, which is usually associated with exodeviation in the primary position of gaze.
- Inferior oblique underaction/palsy with subsequent superior oblique overaction.
- Inferior rectus underaction.

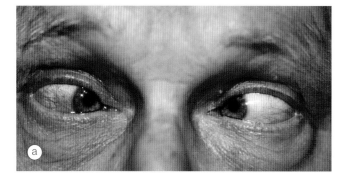
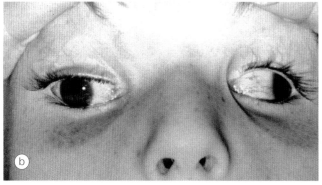

Fig. 20.65
Strabismus fixus. **(a)** Convergent; **(b)** divergent

Treatment

Patients with oblique dysfunction are treated by superior oblique posterior tenotomy. Treatment of cases without oblique muscle dysfunction is treated as follows:

1. **'A' pattern esotropia** (Fig. 20.67a) is treated by bilateral medial rectus recessions and upward transposition of the tendons.
2. **'A' pattern exotropia** (Fig. 20.67b) is treated by bilateral lateral rectus recessions and downward transposition of the tendons.

SURGERY

The most common aims of surgery on the extraocular muscles are to correct misalignment to improve appearance and, if possible, restore BSV. Surgery can also be used to reduce an AHP and to expand or centralize a field of BSV. However, the first step in the management of childhood strabismus involves correction of any significant refractive error and/or amblyopia. Once maximal visual potential is reached in both eyes, any residual deviation can be treated surgically. The three main types of procedures are: (a) weakening, which decreases the pull of a muscle, (b) strengthening, which enhances the pull of a muscle and (c) procedures that change the direction of muscle action.

Weakening procedures

The procedures for weakening the action of a muscle are: (a) *recession*, (b) *disinsertion (or myectomy)* and (c) *posterior fixation suture*.

Recession

Recession slackens a muscle by moving it away from its insertion. It and can be performed on any muscle except the superior oblique.

1. **Rectus muscle recession**
   a. The muscle is exposed and two absorbable sutures are tied through the outer quarters of the tendon.
   b. The tendon is disinserted from the sclera, and the amount of recession is measured and marked on the sclera with calipers.
   c. The detached end of the muscle is sutured to the sclera at a measured distance behind its original insertion (Fig. 20.68).
2. **Inferior oblique disinsertion or recession**
   a. The muscle belly is exposed through an inferotemporal fornix incision.
   b. A squint hook is passed behind the posterior border of the muscle, which must be clearly visualized. Care is taken to pick up the muscle without disrupting the Tenon's capsule and fat posterior to it.
   c. An absorbable suture is passed through the anterior border of the muscle at its insertion and tied.
   d. The muscle is disinserted and the cut end sutured to the sclera 3mm posterior and temporal to the temporal edge of the inferior rectus insertion (Fig. 20.69).

Disinsertion

Disinsertion involves detaching the muscle from its insertion without reattachment. It is most commonly used to weaken an overacting inferior oblique muscle, when the technique is the same as for a recession except that the muscle is not sutured. Very occasionally, the procedure is performed on a severely contracted rectus muscle.

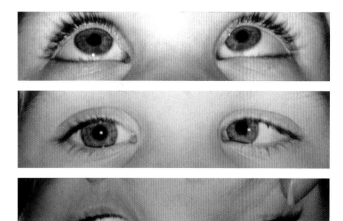
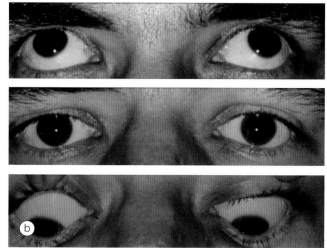

Fig. 20.66
'V' pattern. **(a)** Esotropia; **(b)** exotropia (Courtesy of Wilmer Institute)

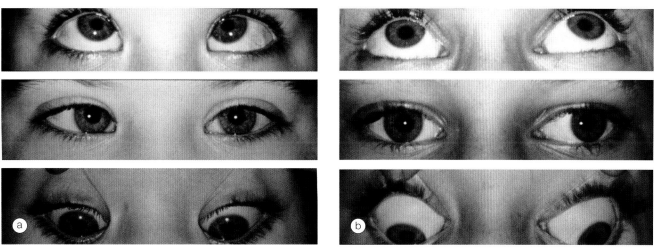

Fig. 20.67
'A' pattern. **(a)** Esotropia; **(b)** exotropia (Courtesy of Wilmer Institute)

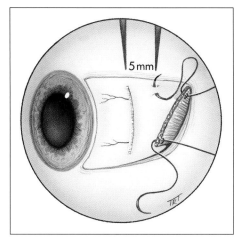

Fig. 20.68
Recession of a horizontal rectus muscle

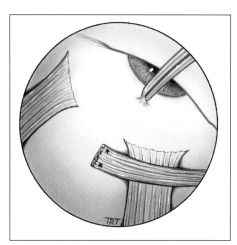

Fig. 20.69
Recession of an inferior oblique muscle

Posterior fixation suture

The principle of this (Faden) procedure is to suture the muscle belly to the sclera posteriorly so as to decrease the pull of the muscle in its field of action without affecting the eye in the primary position. The Faden procedure may be used on the medial rectus to reduced convergence in a convergence excess esotropia and on the superior rectus to treat DVD. When treating DVD, the superior rectus muscle may also be recessed. The belly of the muscle is then anchored to the sclera with a non-absorbable suture about 12mm behind its insertion.

Strengthening procedures

1. **Resection** shortens a muscle to enhance its effective pull. It is suitable only for a rectus muscle and involves the following steps:
   a. The muscle is exposed and two absorbable sutures are tied into the muscle at a measured distance behind its insertion.
   b. The muscle anterior to the sutures is excised and the cut end reattached to the original insertion (Fig. 20.70).
2. **Tucking** of a muscle or its tendon is usually reserved to enhance the action of the superior oblique muscle in congenital fourth nerve palsy.

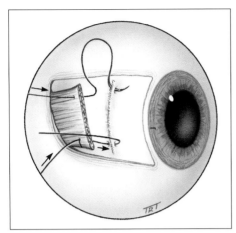

Fig. 20.70
Resection of a horizontal rectus muscle

3. Advancement of the muscle nearer to the limbus can be used to enhance the action of a previously recessed rectus muscle.

Treatment of paretic strabismus

Lateral rectus palsy

Surgical intervention for a sixth nerve palsy should be considered only when it is clear that spontaneous improvement will not occur. This is usually after at least 3 months have elapsed without improvement, usually at least 6 months in total. Treatment of partial and complete lateral rectus palsies is different

1. **Partial** palsy is treated by adjustable medial rectus recession and lateral rectus resection of the affected eye, aiming for a small exophoria in the primary position to maximize the field of BSV.
2. **Complete** palsy is treated by transposition of the superior and inferior recti to positions above and below the affected lateral rectus muscle (Fig. 20.71), coupled with an injection of Botulinum toxin to the medial rectus (toxin transposition).

NB In an adult, three rectus muscles should not be detached from the globe at the same procedure because of the risk of anterior segment ischaemia.

Superior oblique palsy

Surgical intervention should be considered to improve troublesome diplopia or an abnormal head posture. The treatment of unilateral and bilateral palsies is different. General principles are as follows:

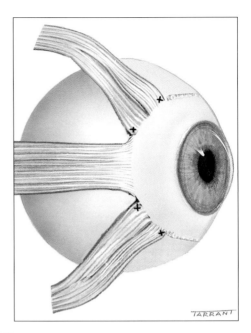

Fig. 20.71
Transposition of the superior and inferior rectus muscles in lateral rectus palsy

1. **Unilateral**
   a. **Congenital** cases can usually be treated either by inferior oblique weakening or by superior oblique tucking.
   b. **Acquired**
      – Small hypertropia is treated by ipsilateral inferior oblique weakening.
      – Moderate to large hypertropia may be treated by ipsilateral inferior oblique weakening which can be combined with, or followed by ipsilateral superior rectus weakening and/or contralateral inferior rectus weakening if required. It should be noted that weakening the inferior oblique and superior rectus of the same eye may result in defective elevation.
2. **Bilateral**
   a. Excyclotorsion should first be corrected by the Harada–Ito procedure which involves splitting and antero-lateral transposition of the lateral half of the superior oblique tendon (Fig. 20.72).
   b. Any associated vertical deviation can be either corrected at the same procedure or subsequently.

Adjustable sutures

Indications

The results of strabismus surgery can be improved by the use of adjustable suture techniques on the rectus muscles. These are particularly indicated when a precise outcome is essential and when the results with more conventional procedures are likely to be unpredictable; for example, acquired vertical

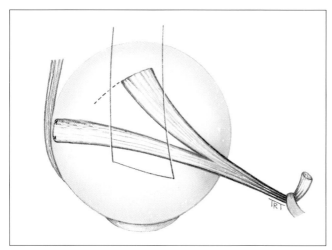

Fig. 20.72
Harada–Ito procedure for superior oblique palsy

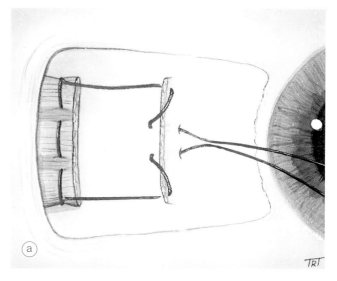

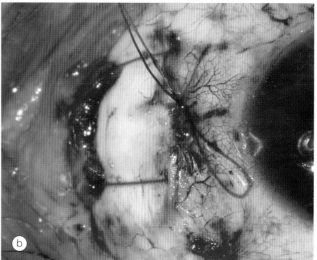

Fig. 20.73
Adjustable suture technique (see text)

deviations associated with thyroid myopathy or following a blow-out fracture of the floor of the orbit. Other indications include sixth nerve palsy, adult exotropia and re-operations in which scarring of surrounding tissues may make the final outcome unpredictable. The main contraindication is patients who are too young or unwilling to cooperate during postoperative suture adjustment.

Initial steps

a. The muscle is exposed and a double-ended absorbable suture is tied into the centre of the muscle at the insertion.
b. Each end is then passed through one muscle border and locked. The tendon is disinserted from the sclera (as for a rectus muscle recession).
c. The two ends of the suture are passed forward through the upper and lower ends of the insertion and then forward again through the centre of the insertion where they are tied in a bow (Fig. 20.73).
d. The conjunctiva is replaced in a recessed position so that it just covers the knot.

Postoperative adjustment

This is performed under topical anaesthesia, usually a few hours after surgery when the patient is fully awake.
a. The accuracy of alignment is assessed.
b. If ocular alignment is satisfactory the muscle suture is tied off and its long ends cut short.
c. If more recession is required, the bow is undone and the knot slackened so that the muscle can be further recessed.
d. If less recession is required the suture is pulled anteriorly and the bow retied.
e. Alignment is retested and adjustment repeated as required.

A similar technique can be used for rectus muscle resection.

Botulinum toxin chemodenervation

Temporary paralysis of an extraocular muscle can be created by an injection of botulinum toxin under topical anaesthesia and EMG control. The effect takes several days to develop, is usually maximal at 1–2 weeks following injection and has generally worn off by 3 months. Side-effects are uncommon, although about 5% of patients may develop some degree of temporary ptosis. The following are the main indications for chemodenervation.

1. To determine the risk of postoperative diplopia. For example, in an adult with a consecutive left divergent squint and left suppression, straightening the eyes may make suppression less effective, resulting in diplopia. If postoperative diplopia testing by correcting the angle with prisms is negative then the risk of double vision after surgery is very low. If testing is positive then the left lateral rectus muscle can be injected with toxin so that the eyes will either straighten or converge and the risk of diplopia can be assessed over several days while the eyes are straight. If diplopia does occur the patient is able to judge whether it is troublesome.

2. **To assess the potential for BSV** in a patient with a constant manifest squint by straightening the eyes temporarily. The deviation can then be corrected surgically if appropriate. A small proportion of patients maintain BSV long-term when the effects of the toxin have worn off.

3. **In lateral rectus palsy** botulinum toxin can be injected into the ipsilateral medial rectus to give symptomatic relief during recovery and to see whether there is any lateral rectus action when there is medial rectus contracture (Fig. 20.74a). The temporary paralysis of the muscle causes relaxation so that the horizontal forces on the globe are more balanced, thus allowing assessment of lateral rectus function (Fig. 20.74b).

4. **Patients with a cosmetically poor deviation** who have undergone multiple squint operations can be treated by repeated botulinum toxin injections which may reduce in frequency with time.

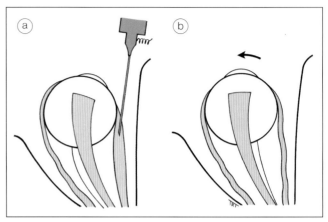

Fig. 20.74
Principles of botulinum toxin chemodenervation in left sixth nerve palsy (see text)

CHAPTER 21

NEURO-OPHTHALMOLOGY

OPTIC NERVE DISEASE

Anatomy

General structure

1. **Afferent fibres.** The optic nerve carries about 1.2 million afferent nerve fibres which originate in the retinal ganglion cells. Most of these synapse in the lateral geniculate body, although some reach other centres, notably the pre-tectal nuclei in the midbrain. Nearly one-third of the fibres subserve the central 5° of the visual field. Within the optic nerve itself the nerve fibres are divided into about 600 bundles (each containing 2000 fibres) by fibrous septae derived from the pia mater (Fig. 21.1).
2. **Oligodendrocytes** provide axonal myelination. Congenital myelination of retinal nerve fibres is the result of anomalous intraocular extension of these cells.
3. **Microglia** are immunocompetent phagocytic cells which probably modulate apoptosis (programmed death) of retinal ganglion cells.
4. **Astrocytes** line the spaces between axons and other structures. When axons are lost in optic atrophy astrocytes fill in the empty spaces.
5. **Surrounding sheaths**
   a. **The pia mater** is the delicate innermost sheath containing blood vessels.
   b. **The outer sheath** comprises the arachnoid mater and the tougher dura mater which is continuous with the sclera. Optic nerve fenestration involves incision of the outer sheath. The subarachnoid space is continuous with the cerebral subarachnoid space and contains cerebrospinal fluid (CSF).

Anatomical subdivisions

The optic nerve is approximately 50mm long from globe to chiasm and can be subdivided into four segments.

1. **Intraocular** segment (optic disc, nerve head) is the shortest being 1mm deep and 1.5mm in vertical diameter. Neurological disorders affecting this part of the optic nerve include inflammation (papillitis), oedema and abnormal deposits (drusen).
2. **Intraorbital** segment is 25–30mm long and extends from the globe to the optic foramen at the orbital apex. Its diameter is 3–4mm because of the addition of the myelin sheaths to the nerve fibres. At the orbital apex the nerve is surrounded by the tough fibrous annulus of Zinn, from which originate the four rectus muscles. Because the superior and medial rectus muscles partly originate from the nerve sheath itself, inflammatory optic neuropathy (e.g. retrobulbar neuritis) may be associated with pain on ocular movement. Within the orbit the optic nerve is slack and S-shaped, allowing for eye movements without stretching.

NB Because of this redundancy the optic nerve does not become unduly stretched until proptosis is severe.

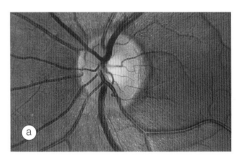
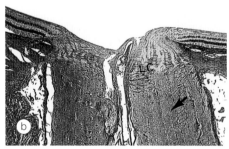
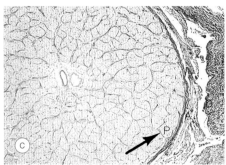
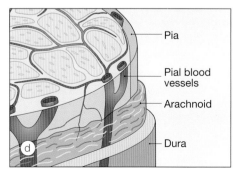

Fig. 21.1
Structure of the optic nerve.
(a) Clinical appearance; **(b)** longitudinal section, LC = lamina cribrosa, arrow points to a fibrous septum; **(c)** transverse section (P = pia, A = arachnoid, D = dura) **(d)** surrounding sheaths and pial blood vessels (Courtesy of Wilmer Institute – figs a, b and c)

Pia
Pial blood vessels
Arachnoid
Dura

3. **Intracanalicular** segment traverses the optic canal and measures about 6 mm. Unlike the intraorbital portion it is fixed to the canal, since the dura mater fuses with the periosteum.

4. **Intracranial** segment joins the chiasm and varies in length from 5 mm to 16 mm (average 10 mm). Long intracranial segments are particularly vulnerable to damage by adjacent lesions such as pituitary adenomas and aneurysms.

Axoplasmic transport

Axoplasmic transport is the movement of cytoplasmic organelles within a neuron between the cell body and the terminal synapse (Fig. 21.2a and b). Orthograde transport involves movement from the cell body to synapse and retrograde transport is characterized by the converse. Rapid axoplasmic transport is an active mechanism requiring oxygen and is energized by ATP. Axoplasmic flow may be interrupted by a variety of insults including hypoxia and toxins which interfere with ATP production. Retinal cotton-wool spots are the result of accumulation of organelles due to interruption of axoplasmic flow between the retinal ganglion cells and their terminal synapses. Papilloedema is similarly caused by hold up of axoplasmic flow at the lamina cribrosa (Fig. 21.2c).

Signs of optic nerve dysfunction

1. **Reduced visual acuity** for distance and near is common, but may also occur with a great variety of other disorders.
2. **Afferent pupillary defect** (see later).
3. **Dyschromatopsia** (impairment of colour vision), which mainly affects red and green. A simple way of detecting a uniocular colour vision defect is to ask the patient to compare the colour of a red object, such as the top of a Mydriacyl bottle (more accurate assessment is described in Chapter 1).

4. **Diminished light brightness sensitivity,** which may persist after visual acuity returns to normal, as seen after a previous attack of optic neuritis (see Chapter 1).

5. **Diminished contrast sensitivity,** which is tested by asking the patient to identify gratings of gradually decreasing contrast, over a range of spatial frequencies (the Arden plates). This is very sensitive to subtle visual loss, although it is not specific to optic nerve disease (see Chapter 1).

6. **Visual field defects,** which vary with the underlying pathology, include diffuse depression of the central visual field, central scotomas, centrocaecal scotomas, nerve fibre bundle and altitudinal (Table 21.1).

Optic atrophy

Primary optic atrophy

Primary optic atrophy occurs without antecedent swelling of the optic nerve head. It may be caused by lesions affecting the visual pathways from the retrolaminar portion of the optic nerve to the lateral geniculate body. Lesions anterior to the optic chiasm result in unilateral optic atrophy, whereas those involving the chiasm and optic tract will cause bilateral atrophy.

1. **Signs**
   - Pale, flat disc with clearly delineated margins, reduction in number of small blood vessels on the disc surface (Kestenbaum sign), attenuation of peripapillary blood vessels and thinning of the retinal nerve fibre layer (Fig. 21.3a).
   - The atrophy may be diffuse or sectoral depending on the cause and level of the lesion.
   - Temporal pallor may indicate atrophy of fibres from the papillo-macular bundle, which enters the optic nerve head on the temporal side.

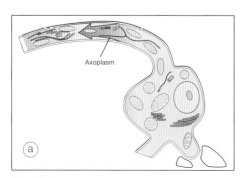
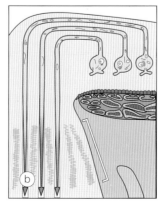
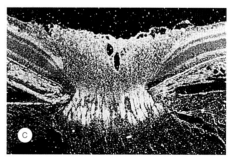

Fig. 21.2
(a and **b)** Normal axoplasmic transport; **(c)** interruption of axoplasmic transport in papilloedema (Courtesy of Wilmer Institute – fig. c)

Table 21.1 Focal visual field defects in optic neuropathies

1. *Central scotoma*
   - Demyelination
   - Toxic and nutritional
   - Leber disease
   - Compression

2. *Enlarged blind spot*
   - Papilloedema
   - Congenital anomalies

3. *Respecting horizontal meridian*
   - Anterior ischaemic optic neuropathy
   - Glaucoma
   - Disc drusen

- Band atrophy caused by involvement of the fibres entering the optic disc nasally and temporally with sparing of the superior and inferior portions occurs in lesions of the optic chiasm or tract.

2. **Causes**
   - Following retrobulbar neuritis.
   - Compression by tumours and aneurysms.
   - Hereditary optic neuropathies.
   - Toxic and nutritional optic neuropathies.

   NB Certain hereditary macular dystrophies may also present with a central scotoma, reduced colour vision and a pale disc.

Secondary optic atrophy

Secondary optic atrophy is preceded by swelling of the optic nerve head.

1. **Signs** vary according to the cause. The main features are (Fig. 21.3b):
   - White or dirty grey, slightly raised disc with poorly delineated margins due to gliosis.
   - Reduction in number of small blood vessels on the disc surface.
2. **Causes** include chronic papilloedema, anterior ischaemic optic neuropathy and papillitis.

Classification of optic neuritis

Optic neuritis is an inflammatory, infective or demyelinating process affecting the optic nerve. It can be classified both ophthalmoscopically and aetiologically as follows.

Ophthalmoscopic classification

1. **Retrobulbar neuritis,** in which the optic disc appearance is normal, at least initially, because the optic nerve head is not involved. It is the most frequent type in adults and is frequently associated with multiple sclerosis (MS).
2. **Papillitis,** in which the pathological process affects the optic nerve head primarily, or secondary to contiguous retinal inflammation. It is characterized by variable hyperaemia and oedema of the optic disc (Fig. 21.4a and b), which may be associated with peripapillary flame-shaped haemorrhages (Fig. 21.4c). Cells in the posterior vitreous may be seen. Papillitis is the most common type

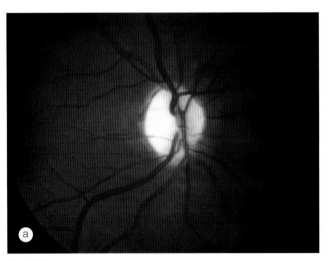
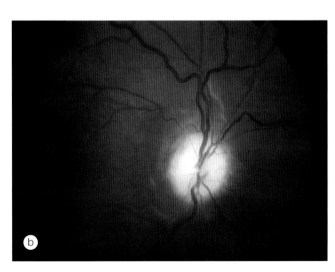

Fig. 21.3
Optic atrophy. **(a)** Primary; **(b)** secondary

of optic neuritis in children, although it can also affect adults.

3. **Neuroretinitis** is characterized by papillitis in association with inflammation of the retinal nerve fibre layer and a macular star figure (Fig. 21.4d). It is the least common type of optic neuritis and is rarely a manifestation of demyelination.

Aetiological classification

1. **Demyelinating,** which is by far the most common cause.
2. **Parainfectious,** which may follow a viral infection or immunization.
3. **Infectious,** which may be sinus-related, or associated with cat-scratch fever, syphilis, Lyme disease, cryptococcal meningitis in patients with AIDS and herpes zoster.

4. **Non-infectious** causes include sarcoidosis and systemic autoimmune diseases such as systemic lupus erythematosus, polyarteritis nodosa and other vasculitides.

Demyelinating optic neuritis

Introduction

Demyelination is a pathological process by which normally myelinated nerve fibres lose their insulating myelin layer. The myelin is phagocytosed by microglia and macrophages, subsequent to which astrocytes lay down fibrous tissue (plaque). A demyelinating disease disrupts nervous conduction within the white matter tracts within the brain, brainstem and spinal cord but peripheral nerves are not involved.

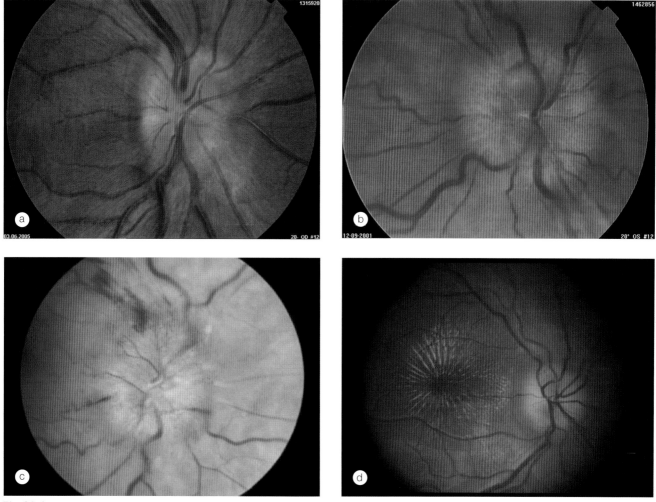

Fig. 21.4
(a) Mild papillitis; **(b)** severe papillitis; **(c)** papillitis with peripapillary haemorrhages; **(d)** neuroretinitis (Courtesy of L Merin – fig. d)

Demyelinating diseases which may cause ocular problems are the following:

1. **Isolated optic neuritis,** with no clinical evidence of generalized demyelination, although in a high proportion of cases this subsequently develops.
2. **Multiple sclerosis,** which is by far the most common.
3. **Devic disease** (neuromyelitis optica), which is a rare disease that may occur at any age. It is characterized by bilateral optic neuritis and subsequent development of transverse myelitis (demyelination of the spinal cord) within days or weeks.
4. **Schilder disease,** which is a very rare, relentlessly progressive, generalized disease with an onset prior to the age of 10 years and death within 1 to 2 years. Bilateral optic neuritis without subsequent improvement may occur.
5. **Ocular features**
   a. ***Visual pathway*** lesions most frequently involve the optic nerves and cause optic neuritis. Demyelination may occasionally involve the optic chiasm, and rarely the optic tracts or radiations.
   b. ***Brainstem*** lesions may result in gaze palsies, ocular motor cranial nerve palsies, trigeminal and facial nerve palsies and nystagmus.

Association between optic neuritis and multiple sclerosis

Although some patients with optic neuritis have no clinically demonstrable associated systemic disease, the following close association exists between optic neuritis and MS.
- Approximately 15–20% of MS patients present with optic neuritis and optic neuritis occurs at some point in 50% of patients with established MS.
- The overall 10-year risk of developing MS following an acute episode of optic neuritis is 38%.
- At the first episode of optic neuritis patients who also show T2-signal lesions on MR (Fig. 21.5), but no clinical evidence of MS, have a 56% risk of developing MS within 10 years; those with no lesions have a 22% risk.
- Even when MR lesions are present, clinical MS does not develop within 10 years in 44% of cases.
- In a patient with optic neuritis the subsequent risk of MS is increased with winter onset, HLA-DR2 positivity and Uhthoff phenomenon (worsening of symptoms on elevation of body temperature, such as with exercise or a hot bath).

Diagnosis

1. **Presentation** is usually between the ages of 20 and 50 years (mean around 30 years) with subacute monocular visual impairment. Some patients experience positive visual phenomena (phosphenes) characterized by tiny white or coloured flashes or sparkles. Discomfort or pain in or around the eye is common and frequently exacerbated by ocular movements. This may precede or accompany the

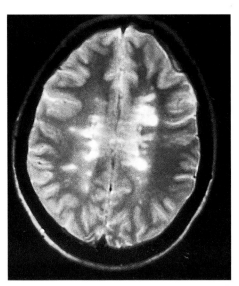

Fig. 21.5
MR axial scan shows periventricular plaques

visual loss and usually lasts a few days. Frontal headache and tenderness of the globe may also be present.
2. **Signs**
   - VA is usually between 6/18 and 6/60 although rarely it may be worse.
   - Other signs of optic nerve dysfunction (i.e. afferent pupillary defect (APD), dyschromatopsia, diminished light-brightness appreciation and impairment of contrast sensitivity).
   - The optic disc is normal in the majority of cases (retrobulbar neuritis); the remainder show papillitis.
   - Temporal disc pallor may be seen in the fellow eye, indicative of previous optic neuritis.
3. **Visual field defects**
   - The most common is diffuse depression of sensitivity in the entire central 30°.
   - This is followed by nerve fibre bundle defects and then central scotomas (Fig. 21.6).
   - Focal defects are frequently accompanied by an element of superimposed generalized depression.
4. **Course.** Vision worsens over several days to 2 weeks and then begins to recover within 2–4 weeks. Initial recovery is fairly rapid and then levels off but continues over 6–12 months.

Prognosis

Approximately 75% of patients recover visual acuity to 6/9 or better and 85% to 6/12 or better, even if vision was very bad during the attack. However, despite return of visual acuity other parameters of visual function, such as colour vision, contrast sensitivity and light brightness appreciation,

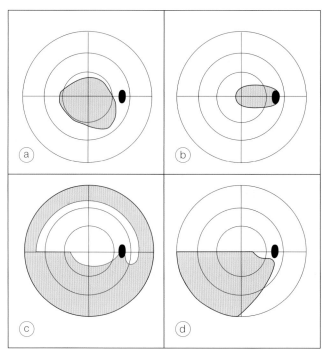

Fig. 21.6
Visual field defects in optic neuritis. **(a)** Central scotoma;
(b) centrocaecal scotoma; **(c)** nerve fibre bundle; **(d)** altitudinal

often remain abnormal. A mild APD may persist and optic atrophy may ensue, particularly following recurrent attacks. About 10% of patients develop chronic optic neuritis characterized by slowly progressive or stepwise visual loss, unassociated with periods of recovery.

Treatment

1. **Indications.** When visual acuity within the first week of onset is worse than 6/12, treatment may speed up recovery by 2–3 weeks. This may be relevant in the patients with poor vision in the fellow eye or those with occupational requirements but this small benefit must be balanced against the risks of using high-dose steroids. Treatment, however, does not influence the eventual visual outcome and the vast majority of patients do not require treatment.
2. **Regimen**
   a. *Intravenous methylprednisolone sodium succinate* 1g daily for 3 days followed by oral prednisolone (1mg/kg/day) for 11 days and then tapered for 3 days.
   b. *Intramuscular interferon beta-1a* at the first episode of optic neuritis is beneficial in reducing the development of clinical MS over the following 3 years in patients at high risk based on the presence of subclinical brain MR lesions. However, the benefit is small and most patients do not commence interferon

until they have had a second episode of clinical demyelination.

NB Oral prednisolone alone is contraindicated because it does not affect the speed of recovery and is associated with a significantly higher recurrence rate.

Parainfectious optic neuritis

Optic neuritis may be associated with various viral infections such as measles, mumps, chickenpox, rubella, whooping cough and glandular fever. It may also occur following immunization. Children are affected much more frequently than adults.

Diagnosis

1. **Presentation** is usually 1–3 weeks following a viral infection with acute severe visual loss, which may involve both eyes. This may be associated with other neurological features such as headache, seizures or ataxia (meningoencephalitis).
2. **Signs.** The optic discs most frequently manifest bilateral papillitis, although occasionally there may be a neuroretinitis or the discs may be normal.

Treatment

Treatment is not required in the vast majority of patients because the prognosis for spontaneous visual recovery is very good. However, when visual loss is severe and bilateral or involves an only seeing eye, intravenous steroids should be considered.

Infectious optic neuritis

1. **Sinus-related** optic neuritis is an infrequent condition characterized by recurrent attacks of unilateral visual loss associated with severe headache and spheno-ethmoidal sinusitis. Possible mechanisms of optic neuropathy include direct spread of infection, occlusive vasculitis and pressure by a mucocele. Treatment is with systemic antibiotics and, if appropriate, surgical drainage.
2. **Cat-scratch fever** (benign lymphoreticulosis) is caused by *Bartonella henselae* or, less commonly, *Bartonella quintana*, which is inoculated by a cat scratch or bite (see Chapter 24). Numerous ophthalmological features have been described, most notably neuroretinitis (see below).
3. **Syphilis** may cause acute papillitis or neuroretinitis during the primary or secondary stages (see Chapter 24). Involvement may be unilateral or bilateral and is frequently associated with a mild vitritis.

4. **Lyme disease** (borreliosis) is a spirochaetal infection caused by *Borrelia burgdorferi* that is transmitted by a tick bite (see Chapter 24). It may cause neuroretinitis and occasionally acute retrobulbar neuritis which may be associated with other neurological manifestations and may mimic MS. Treatment of neurological involvement is with intravenous ceftriaxone 2g daily for 14 days.

5. **Cryptococcal meningitis** in patients with AIDS may be associated with acute optic neuritis, which may be bilateral (see Chapter 24).

6. **Varicella zoster virus** most frequently causes papillitis by spread from contiguous retinitis (i.e. acute retinal necrosis, progressive outer retinal necrosis – see Chapter 14). Primary optic neuritis is uncommon but may occur in immunocompromised patients, some of who may subsequently develop viral retinitis. Treatment is with intravenous antiviral agents.

Non-infectious optic neuritis

Sarcoid

Optic neuritis affects 1–5% of patients with neurosarcoid. It may develop during the course of the disease or be its presenting manifestation. Optic nerve involvement may be indistinguishable to that in MS although the optic nerve head may exhibit a characteristic lumpy appearance suggestive of granulomatous infiltration and there may be an inflammatory reaction in the vitreous. The response to steroid therapy is often rapid although vision may decline if treatment is tapered or stopped prematurely; some patients require long-term low-dose therapy. Methotrexate may also be used as an adjunct to steroids or as monotherapy in steroid-intolerant patients.

Autoimmune

Autoimmune optic nerve involvement may be in the form of retrobulbar neuritis or anterior ischaemic optic neuropathy (see below). Some patients may also experience slowly progressive visual loss suggestive of optic nerve compression. Treatment is with systemic steroids.

Neuroretinitis

1. **Presentation** is with unilateral, painless, visual impairment which starts gradually and then becomes most marked after about a week.

2. **Signs**
   - VA is impaired to a variable degree.
   - Signs of optic nerve involvement are usually mild or absent because visual loss is largely due to macular oedema rather than optic nerve dysfunction.
   - Papillitis associated with peripapillary and macular

oedema; venous engorgement and splinter-shaped haemorrhages may be present in severe cases (Fig. 21.7a).

3. **FA** shows diffuse leakage from superficial disc vessels (Fig. 21.7b).

4. **Course**
   - A macular star then develops as the disc swelling gradually resolves (Fig. 21.7c).
   - The macular star then resolves with return to normal or near normal visual acuity in 6–12 months in the majority of cases.
   - Some patients may subsequently develop an involvement of the fellow eye.
   - Although recurrent disease is uncommon it has a different clinical profile characterized by signs of optic nerve dysfunction and carries a poor visual prognosis.

5. **Systemic associations.** About 25% of cases are idiopathic (Leber idiopathic stellate neuroretinitis). Cat-scratch fever is responsible for 60% of cases. Other notable causes include syphilis, Lyme disease, mumps and leptospirosis.

6. **Treatment** varies according to the underlying cause. Recurrent idiopathic cases may require steroids and/or azathioprine.

Non-arteritic anterior ischaemic optic neuropathy

Non-arteritic anterior ischaemic optic neuropathy (NAION) is the most common optic neuropathy in the elderly. It is the result of a partial or total infarction of the optic nerve head caused by occlusion of the short posterior ciliary arteries. It typically occurs as an isolated event in patients between the ages of 55 and 70 years with structural crowding of the optic nerve head so that the physiological cup is either very small or absent. Predisposing systemic conditions include hypertension, diabetes mellitus, hypercholesterolaemia, collagen vascular disease, antiphospholipid antibody syndrome, hyperhomocysteinaemia, sudden hypotensive events, cataract surgery, sleep apnoea syndrome and administration of sildenafil (Viagra).

Diagnosis

1. **Presentation** is with sudden, painless, monocular visual loss which is not associated with premonitory visual obscurations. Visual impairment is frequently discovered on awakening suggesting that nocturnal hypotension may play an important role.

2. **Signs**
   - VA, in about 30% of patients, is normal or only slightly reduced. The remainder has moderate-to-severe impairment.
   - Visual field defects are typically inferior altitudinal but other defects may also be seen.
   - Dyschromatopsia is proportional to the level of visual impairment in contrast with optic neuritis, in which

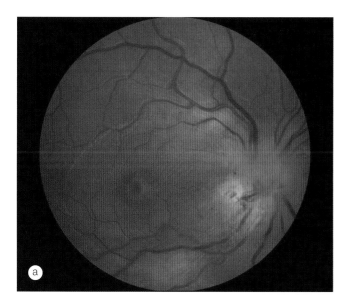

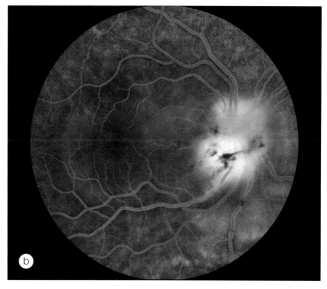

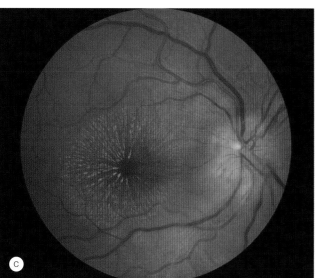

Fig. 21.7
Progression of neuroretinitis. **(a)** Severe papillitis; **(b)** FA late phase shows hyperfluorescence due to leakage; **(c)** several weeks later there is a macular star but disc swelling is less severe (Courtesy of P Saine)

colour vision may be severely impaired when visual acuity is reasonably good.

- Diffuse (Fig. 21.8a) or sectoral (Fig. 21.8b) hyperaemic disc swelling often associated with a few peripapillary splinter-shaped haemorrhages.
- The swelling gradually resolves and pallor ensues 3–6 weeks after onset.

3. FA during the acute stage shows localized disc hyperfluorescence (Fig. 21.8c) which becomes more intense and then eventually involves the entire disc (Fig. 21.8d).

4. Special investigations include serological studies, fasting lipid profile and blood glucose. It is also very important to exclude occult giant cell arteritis and other autoimmune diseases.

Treatment

There is no definitive treatment although any underlying systemic predispositions should be addressed. Although aspirin is effective in reducing systemic vascular events and is frequently prescribed in patients with NAION, it does not appear to reduce the risk of involvement of the fellow eye.

Prognosis

In most patients there is no further loss of vision although, in a small percentage, visual loss continues for 6 weeks. Recurrences in the same eye occur in about 6% of patients.

Involvement of the fellow eye occurs in about 10% of patients after 2 years and 15% after 5 years, an incidence lower than previously assumed. When the second eye becomes involved, optic atrophy in one eye and disc oedema in the other gives rise to the 'pseudo-Foster Kennedy syndrome'. Two important risk factors for fellow eye involvement are poor visual acuity in the first eye and diabetes mellitus.

Arteritic anterior ischaemic optic neuropathy

Arteritic anterior ischaemic optic neuropathy (AION) is caused by giant cell arteritis (GCA – Fig. 21.9a and b). The systemic features of GCA are described in Chapter 24.

Diagnosis

1. **Presentation** is with sudden, profound unilateral visual loss which may be accompanied by periocular pain and preceded by transient visual obscurations and flashing lights. Bilateral simultaneous involvement is rare. Most cases occur within a few weeks of the onset of GCA although at presentation about 20% of patients do not have systemic symptoms (i.e. occult GCA). Jaw claudication, headache of recent onset, scalp tenderness, weight loss and a history of polymyalgia rheumatica may be present.

2. **Signs**
   - Tenderness and loss of pulsation of one or both temporal arteries may be present.
   - A strikingly pale ('chalky white') oedematous disc is particularly suggestive of GCA (Fig. 21.9c).

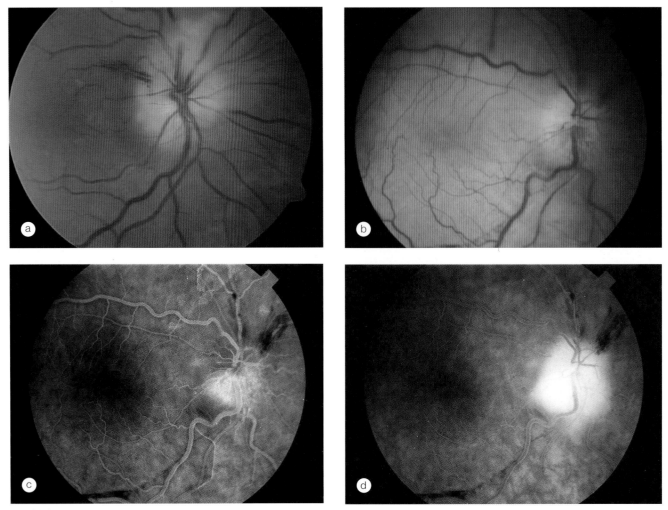

Fig. 21.8
Non-arteritic anterior ischaemic optic neuropathy. **(a)** Diffuse oedema; **(b)** inferior sectoral oedema; **(c)** FA venous phase shows localized disc hyperfluorescence and blockage by haemorrhage; **(d)** late phase shows hyperfluorescence of the entire disc (Courtesy of P Gili – fig. a; S Milewski – figs b, c and d)

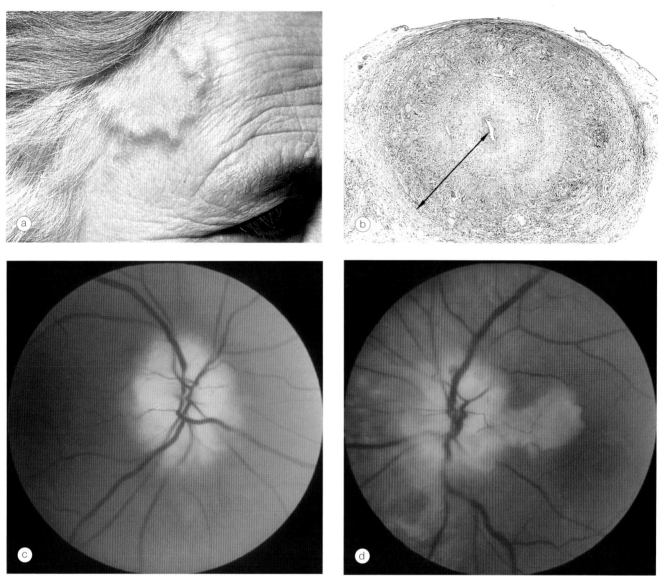

Fig. 21.9
Giant cell arteritis. **(a)** Pulseless, nodular, thickened superficial temporal artery; **(b)** histology shows granulomatous inflammation and a grossly narrowed lumen; **(c)** ischaemic optic neuropathy; **(d)** ischaemic optic neuropathy and cilioretinal artery occlusion (Courtesy of J Harry – fig. b; S S Hayreh – figs c and d)

- Occasionally AION may be combined with occlusion of the cilioretinal artery (Fig. 21.9d).
- Over 1–2 months, the swelling gradually resolves and severe optic atrophy ensues.

3. FA shows severe hypoperfusion of the choroid.

4. ESR and CRP are usually raised, as is the platelet count.

Treatment

Treatment is aimed at preventing blindness of the fellow eye, although the second eye may become involved in 25% of cases despite early and adequate steroid administration,

usually within 6 days after starting treatment. Visual loss is usually profound and is unlikely to improve even when treatment is instigated immediately.

1. The regimen is as follows:

   a. Intravenous methylprednisolone sodium succinate 1g daily for 3 days and oral prednisolone 80mg daily. After 3 days the oral dose is reduced to 60mg and then 50mg for 1 week each. The daily dose is then reduced by 5mg weekly; headache, ESR and CRP permitting, until 10mg is reached. Maintenance daily therapy is ideally 10mg, although higher doses may be required to control headache.

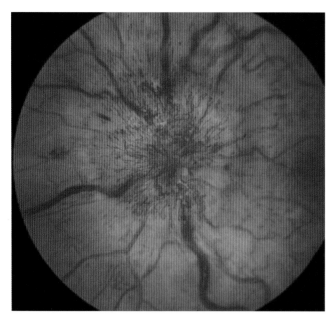

Fig. 21.10
Diabetic papillopathy (Courtesy of S S Hayreh)

b. Oral prednisolone (80–120mg daily) alone may be administered if intravenous therapy is inappropriate.

NB Temporal artery biopsy should be performed, ideally within 7 days of starting treatment. Histological confirmation of GCA will justify long-term steroid administration. Treatment should never be delayed whilst waiting for a biopsy.

2. **The duration** of treatment is governed by the patient's symptoms and the level of the ESR or CRP. Symptoms may, however, recur without a corresponding rise in ESR or CPR and vice versa. Most patients need treatment for 1–2 years, although some may require indefinite maintenance therapy. CRP may play an important role in monitoring disease activity, as the level seems to fall more rapidly in response to treatment than the ESR.

NB Injudicious use of steroids may cause greater harm than the disease itself. Steroid-induced complications may necessitate the use of steroid-sparing agents such as azathioprine although evidence that any steroid-sparing agent is effective in GCA is lacking.

Prognosis

Prognosis is very poor because visual loss is usually permanent, although very rarely, prompt administration of systemic steroids may be associated with partial visual recovery.

Posterior ischaemic optic neuropathy

Posterior ischemic optic neuropathy (PION) is much less common than the anterior variety. It is caused by ischaemia to the retrolaminar portion of the optic nerve which is supplied by the surrounding pial capillary plexus; only a small number of capillaries actually penetrate the nerve and extend to its central portion among the pial septae. The diagnosis of PION is made after other causes of retrobulbar optic neuropathy, such as compression or inflammation, have been excluded. PION occurs in the following three settings.

1. **Operative** develops following a variety of surgical procedures, most notably involving the spine. The major risk factors appear to be anaemia and hypovolaemic hypotension. Bilateral involvement is common and the visual prognosis is poor.
2. **Arteritic** is associated with giant cell arteritis and carries a poor visual prognosis.
3. **Non-arteritic** is associated with the same systemic risk factors as NAION, but is not associated with small optic discs. The visual prognosis is similar to NAION.

Diabetic papillopathy

Diabetic papillopathy is an uncommon condition characterized by transient visual dysfunction associated with optic disc swelling which may occur in both type 1 and type 2 diabetics. The underlying pathogenesis is unclear but may be the result of small-vessel disease.

1. **Presentation** is usually with milder optic nerve dysfunction and slower progression than in NAION or optic neuritis.
2. **Signs**
   - VA is usually 6/12 or better.
   - Unilateral or bilateral, mild disc swelling and hyperaemia.
   - Disc surface telangiectasis is common (Fig. 21.10), and when severe may be mistaken for neovascularization on cursory examination.
3. **Course** is usually several months with eventual spontaneous improvement but some cases develop mild to moderate visual loss.
4. **Treatment** with systemic steroids is of questionable benefit and tends to compromise diabetic control although there is anecdotal evidence that posterior sub-Tenon injections may be beneficial.

Leber hereditary optic neuropathy

Leber hereditary optic neuropathy (LHON) is a rare disease which is the result of maternally inherited mitochondrial DNA mutations, most notably 11778. The condition typically affects males between the ages of 15 and 35 years, although in atypical cases the condition may affect females and present at any age between 10 and 60 years. The diagnosis should therefore be considered in any patient with bilateral optic neuritis, irrespective of age. Unaffected carriers show thickening of temporal retinal fibres on optical coherence tomography.

Diagnosis

1. **Presentation** is typically with unilateral, acute or sub-acute, severe, painless loss of central vision. The fellow eye becomes similarly affected within weeks or months of the first.
2. **Signs** during the acute stage are often subtle and easily overlooked; in some patients the disc may be entirely normal.
   - In typical cases there is disc hyperaemia with obscuration of the disc margins.
   - Dilated capillaries on the disc surface that may extend onto adjacent retina (telangiectatic microangiopathy), swelling of the peripapillary nerve fibre layer (pseudo-oedema) and dilatation and tortuosity of posterior pole vasculature (Fig. 21.11a).
   - Subsequently, the telangiectatic vessels regress and pseudo-oedema resolves.
   - Severe optic atrophy with nerve fibre layer dropout most pronounced in the papillomacular bundle supervenes (Fig. 21.11b).
   - Telangiectatic microangiopathy may be present in asymptomatic female relatives.

   NB Surprisingly, the pupillary light reactions may remain fairly brisk.

3. **FA** shows absence of dye leakage.
4. **Visual field** defects usually consist of central or centro-caecal scotomas.

Treatment

Treatment is generally ineffective although many modalities, including steroids, hydroxocobalamin and surgical intervention, have been tried. Smoking and excessive consumption of alcohol should be discouraged, to minimize potential stress on mitochondrial energy production.

Prognosis

The prognosis is poor, although some visual recovery may occur in a minority of cases even years later. Most patients suffer severe, bilateral and permanent visual loss with a final visual acuity of 6/60 or less. The 11778 mutation carries the worst prognosis.

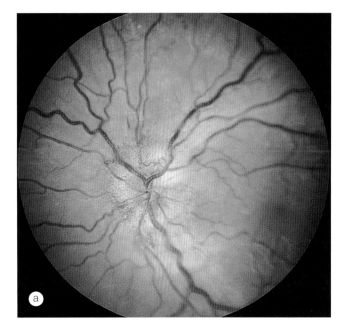

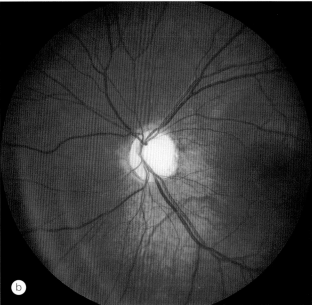

Fig. 21.11
Leber optic neuropathy. **(a)** Acute stage shows telangiectatic microangiopathy; **(b)** severe optic atrophy

Hereditary optic atrophy

The hereditary optic atrophies (neuropathies) are a very rare heterogeneous group of disorders that are primarily characterized by bilateral optic atrophy.

Kjer syndrome

1. **Inheritance** is AD.

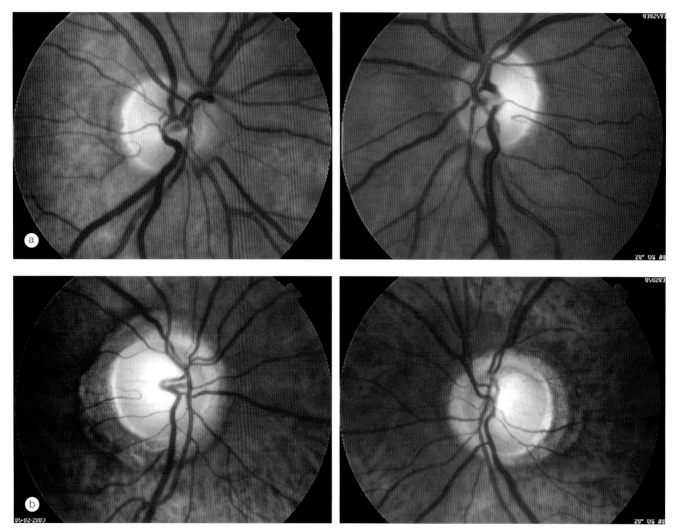

Fig. 21.12
Hereditary optic atrophy. **(a)** Bilateral temporal disc pallor; **(b)** bilateral diffuse pallor

2. **Presentation** is typically in the first or second decade with insidious visual loss, although it is occasionally in adult life.
3. **Optic atrophy** may be subtle and temporal (Fig. 21.12a) or diffuse involving the entire disc (Fig. 21.12b).
4. **Prognosis** is variable (final VA 6/12–6/60) with considerable differences within and between families. Very slow progression over decades is typical.
5. **Systemic abnormalities** are absent in the majority of cases, although some may develop sensorineural hearing loss.

Behr syndrome

1. **Inheritance** is AR.
2. **Presentation** is in the first decade with visual loss which stabilizes after a variable period of progression.
3. **Optic atrophy** is diffuse.
4. **Prognosis** is variable with moderate to severe visual loss and nystagmus.
5. **Systemic abnormalities** include spastic gait, ataxia and mental handicap.

Wolfram syndrome

Wolfram syndrome is also referred to as DIDMOAD = diabetes insipidus, diabetes mellitus, optic atrophy and deafness.

1. **Inheritance** is AR.
2. **Presentation** is between the ages of 5 and 21 years.
3. **Optic atrophy** is diffuse and severe and may be associated with disc cupping.
4. **Prognosis** is very poor (final VA is < 6/60).
5. **Systemic abnormalities** (apart from DIDMOAD) include anosmia, ataxia, seizures, mental handicap, short stature, endocrine abnormalities and elevated CSF protein.

Nutritional optic neuropathy

Nutritional optic neuropathy (tobacco-alcohol amblyopia) typically affects heavy drinkers and cigar or pipe smokers who are deficient in protein and the B vitamins. Most patients have neglected their diet, obtaining their calories from alcohol instead. Some of those affected also have defective vitamin B12 absorption and may develop pernicious anaemia.

1. **Presentation** is with insidious onset, progressive, bilateral, usually symmetrical visual impairment associated with dyschromatopsia.
2. **Signs.** The optic discs at presentation are normal in most cases. Some patients show subtle temporal pallor, splinter-shaped haemorrhages on or around the disc, or minimal disc oedema.
3. **Visual field defects** are bilateral, relatively symmetrical, centrocaecal scotomas. The margins of the defects are difficult to define with a white target but are easier to plot and larger when using a red target.
4. **Treatment** involves weekly injections of 1000 units of hydroxocobalamin for 10 weeks. Multivitamins are also administered and patients should be advised to eat a well-balanced diet and abstain from drinking and smoking.
5. **Prognosis** is good in early cases provided patients comply with treatment although visual recovery may be slow. In advanced and unresponsive cases there is permanent visual loss as a result of optic atrophy.

Papilloedema

Papilloedema is swelling of the optic nerve head, secondary to raised intracranial pressure. It is nearly always bilateral, although it may be asymmetrical. All other causes of disc oedema in the absence of raised intracranial pressure are referred to as 'disc swelling' and usually produce visual impairment. All patients with papilloedema should be suspected of having an intracranial mass unless proved otherwise. However, not all patients with raised intracranial pressure will necessarily develop papilloedema. Tumours of the cerebral hemispheres tend to produce papilloedema later than those in the posterior fossa. Patients with a history of previous papilloedema may develop a substantial increase in intracranial pressure but fail to re-develop papilloedema because of glial scarring of the optic nerve head.

Cerebrospinal fluid

1. **Circulation** (Fig. 21.13a)
   - Cerebrospinal fluid (CSF) is formed by the choroid plexus in the ventricles of the brain.
   - It leaves the lateral ventricles to enter the third ventricle through the foramina of Munro.
   - From the third ventricle, it flows through the Sylvian aqueduct to the fourth ventricle.
   - From the fourth ventricle, the CSF passes through the foramina of Luschka and Magendie to enter the subarachnoid space, some flowing around the spinal cord and the rest bathing the cerebral hemispheres.
   - Absorption is into the cerebral venous drainage system through the arachnoid villi.
2. **Normal opening pressure** of CSF on lumbar puncture is < 80mmH$_2$O in infants, < 90mm in children and < 210mm in adults.

Causes of raised intracranial pressure

Raised intracranial pressure has many mechanisms (Fig. 21.13b)
   - Obstruction of the ventricular system by congenital or acquired lesions.

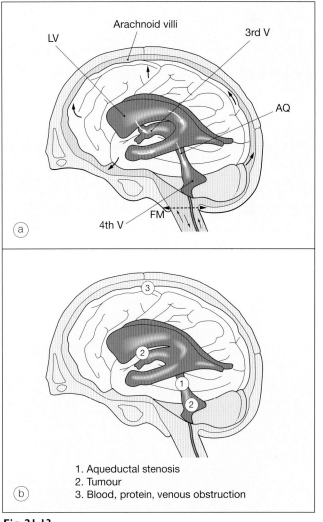

Fig. 21.13
(a) Circulation of cerebrospinal fluid; **(b)** causes of raised intracranial pressure (FM = foramen magnum; LV = lateral ventricle; AQ = aqueduct of Sylvius)

- Space-occupying intracranial lesions, including haemorrhage.
- Impairment of CSF absorption via arachnoid villi, which may be damaged by meningitis, subarachnoid haemorrhage or cerebral trauma.
- Idiopathic intracranial hypertension (pseudotumour cerebri).
- Cerebral venous sinus thrombosis.
- Diffuse cerebral oedema from blunt head trauma.
- Severe systemic hypertension.
- Hypersecretion of CSF by choroid plexus tumour, which is very rare.

Hydrocephalus

Hydrocephalus describes dilatation of the ventricles (Fig. 21.14) which may be of two types.

1. **Communicating** hydrocephalus, in which the CSF flows from the ventricular system to the subarachnoid space without impediment. The obstruction to flow lies in the basilar cisterns or in the subarachnoid space, where there is failure of absorption by the arachnoid villi.
2. **Non-communicating** hydrocephalus is caused by obstruction to CSF flow in the ventricular system or at the exit foramina of the fourth ventricle. The CSF therefore does not have access to the subarachnoid space.

Clinical features of raised intracranial pressure

1. **Headaches** characteristically occur early in the morning and may wake the patient from sleep. They tend to get progressively worse and patients usually present to hospital within 6 weeks. The headaches may be generalized or localized, and may intensify with head movement, bending or coughing. Patients with lifelong headaches often report a change in character of the headache. Very rarely, headache may be absent.
2. **Sudden nausea and vomiting,** often projectile, may partially relieve the headache. Vomiting may occur as an isolated feature or may precede the onset of headache by months, particularly in patients with fourth ventricular tumours.
3. **Deterioration of consciousness** may be slight, with drowsiness and somnolence. Dramatic deterioration is indicative of brainstem distortion and tentorial or tonsillar herniation and requires prompt attention.
4. **Visual**
   a. ***Transient obscurations*** lasting a few seconds are frequent in patients with papilloedema.
   b. ***Horizontal diplopia*** due to sixth nerve palsy caused by stretching of one or both sixth nerves over the petrous tip (Fig. 21.15). It is therefore a false localizing sign.
   c. ***Visual failure*** occurs late in patients with secondary optic atrophy due to long-standing papilloedema (see below).

Stages of papilloedema

1. **Early** (Fig. 21.16a)
   - Visual symptoms are absent and visual acuity normal.
   - Optic discs show hyperaemia and mild elevation.

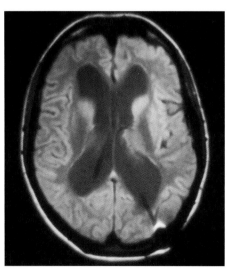

Fig. 21.14
Axial MR shows dilated ventricles due to raised intracranial pressure

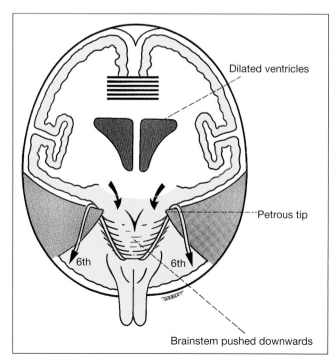

Fig. 21.15
Mechanism of sixth nerve palsy from raised intracranial pressure

- The disc margins (initially nasal, later superior, inferior and temporal) appear indistinct.
- There is loss of previous spontaneous venous pulsation.
- However, as about 20% of normal individuals do not manifest spontaneous venous pulsation, its absence does not necessarily imply raised intracranial pressure. Preserved venous pulsation renders the diagnosis of papilloedema unlikely.

2. **Established** (acute – Fig. 21.16b)
- Transient visual obscurations may occur in one or both eyes, lasting a few seconds, often on standing or bending forwards.
- VA is normal or reduced.
- Optic discs show severe hyperaemia, moderate elevation with indistinct margins and obscuration of small surface vessels.
- Venous engorgement, peripapillary flame-shaped haemorrhages and frequently cotton-wool spots.

- As the swelling increases, the optic nerve head appears enlarged and circumferential retinal folds may develop on its temporal side.
- Hard exudates may radiate from the centre of the fovea in the form of a 'macular fan' – an incomplete star with the temporal part missing.
- The blind spot is enlarged.

3. **Chronic** (Fig. 21.16c)
- VA is variable and the visual fields begin to constrict.
- Optic discs are markedly elevated (Table 21.2) with a 'champagne cork' appearance.
- Cotton-wool spots and haemorrhages are absent.
- Opto-ciliary shunts and drusen-like crystalline deposits (corpora amylacea) may be present on the disc surface.

4. **Atrophic** (secondary optic atrophy) (Fig. 21.16d)
- VA is severely impaired.
- The optic discs are a dirty grey colour, slightly elevated, with few crossing blood vessels and indistinct margins.

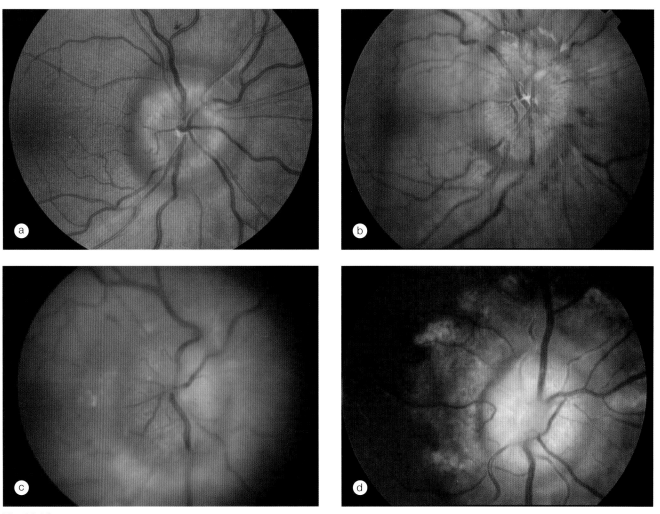

Fig. 21.16
Papilloedema. **(a)** Early; **(b)** established; **(c)** chronic; **(d)** atrophic (Courtesy of P Saine – fig. a)

Table 21.2 Causes of optic disc elevation

1. *Papilloedema*

2. *Accelerated hypertension*

3. *Anterior optic neuropathy*
   - Ischaemic
   - Inflammatory
   - Infiltrative
   - Compressive

4. *Pseudopapilloedema*
   - Optic disc drusen
   - Tilted optic disc
   - Peripapillary myelinated nerve fibres
   - Crowded disc in hypermetropia

5. *Pseudo-oedema*
   - Leber hereditary optic neuropathy
   - Methanol poisoning

6. *Intraocular disease*
   - Central retinal vein occlusion
   - Posterior uveitis
   - Posterior scleritis
   - Hypotony

Idiopathic intracranial hypertension

Idiopathic intracranial hypertension (IIH) deserves special mention, since the ophthalmologist may be involved in management. It is defined as the presence of raised intracranial pressure in the absence of an intracranial mass lesion or enlargement of the ventricles due to hydrocephalus with normal CSF constituents. Although not life-threatening, IIH may result in permanent visual damage due to papilloedema; 90% of patients are obese women of child-bearing age, who are often amenorrhoeic. Intracranial hypertension may also be caused by drugs including tetracyclines, nalidixic acid and iron therapy. It may also be associated with sleep apnoea.

Diagnosis

1. **Signs and symptoms** of raised intracranial pressure as described above.
2. **Lumbar puncture** shows an opening pressure > 250mm with no inflammatory cells and normal CSF glucose and protein. However, the pressure may be artefactually raised in obese patients with normal intracranial pressure.
3. **Neuroimaging** shows normal ventricles and often an empty sella. MR may show patulous optic nerve sheaths. Venous sinus thrombosis should be excluded.
4. **Course.** Most patients have a prolonged course with spontaneous relapses and remissions, although a few may have a short course lasting only a few months. Although mortality is low, visual loss, sometimes severe, is common.

Treatment

The two main aims are to relieve headaches and to prevent visual loss.

1. **Stop drugs** implicated in causing raised intracranial pressure.
2. **Regular perimetry** is essential to detect early or progressive visual field loss.
3. **Diuretics** such as acetazolamide or thiazides are first line treatment for headache and visual field loss. Topiramate may help if headache is particularly severe.
4. **Weight loss** in obese patients, even if relatively modest, is often associated with resolution of papilloedema. Refer to a dietician.
5. **Optic nerve fenestration,** which involves incision of the meningeal sheath around the optic nerve, is safe and effective in preserving vision provided it is performed early. However, headache is relieved only in a minority of cases.
6. **Lumboperitoneal or ventriculoperitoneal shunts** may be performed but the failure rate is high and surgical revision is frequently required.
7. **Sleep apnoea** should be treated.

PUPILLARY REACTIONS

Anatomy

Light reflex

The light reflex is mediated by the retinal photoreceptors and subserved by four neurons (Fig. 21.17).

1. **First** (sensory) connects each retina with both pretectal nuclei in the midbrain at the level of the superior colliculi. Impulses originating from the nasal retina are conducted by fibres which decussate in the chiasm and pass up the opposite optic tract to terminate in the contralateral pretectal nucleus. Impulses originating in the temporal retina are conducted by uncrossed fibres (ipsilateral optic tract) which terminate in the ipsilateral pretectal nucleus.
2. **Second** (internuncial) connects each pretectal nucleus to both Edinger–Westphal nuclei. Thus a uniocular light stimulus evokes bilateral and symmetrical pupillary constriction. Damage to internuncial neurons is responsible for light-near dissociation in neurosyphilis and pinealomas.
3. **Third** (pre-ganglionic motor) connects the Edinger–Westphal nucleus to the ciliary ganglion. The parasympathetic fibres pass through the oculomotor nerve, enter its inferior division and reach the ciliary ganglion via the nerve to the inferior oblique muscle.
4. **Fourth** (post-ganglionic motor) leaves the ciliary ganglion and passes in the short ciliary nerves to innervate the

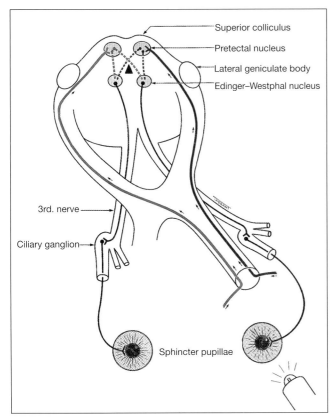

Fig. 21.17
Anatomical pathway of the pupillary light reflex

sphincter pupillae. The ciliary ganglion is located within the muscle cone, just behind the globe. It should be noted that, although the ciliary ganglion serves as a conduit for other nerve fibres, only the parasympathetic fibres synapse there.

Near reflex

The near reflex, a synkinesis rather than a true reflex, is activated when gaze is changed from a distant to a near target. It comprises accommodation, convergence and miosis. Vision is not a prerequisite, and there is no clinical condition in which the light reflex is present but the near response absent. Although the final pathways for the near and light reflexes are identical (i.e. third nerve, ciliary ganglion, short ciliary nerves), the centre for the near reflex is ill-defined. There are probably two supranuclear influences: the frontal and occipital lobes. The midbrain centre for the near reflex is probably located more ventrally than the pretectal nucleus and this may explain why compressive lesions such as pinealomas preferentially involve the dorsal internuncial neurons involved in the light reflex, sparing the ventral (near reflex) fibres until later.

Afferent pupillary defects

Absolute afferent pupillary defect

An absolute afferent pupillary defect (amaurotic pupil) is caused by a complete optic nerve lesion and is characterized by the following:
- The involved eye is completely blind (i.e. no light perception).
- Both pupils are equal in size.
- When the affected eye is stimulated by light neither pupil reacts but when the normal eye is stimulated both pupils react normally.
- The near reflex is normal in both eyes.

Relative afferent pupillary defect

A relative pupillary defect (Marcus Gunn pupil) is caused by an incomplete optic nerve lesion or severe retinal disease, but never by a dense cataract. The clinical features are those of an amaurotic pupil but more subtle. Thus the pupils respond weakly to stimulation of the diseased eye and briskly to that of the normal eye. The difference between the pupillary reactions of the two eyes is highlighted by the 'swinging flashlight test' in which a light source is alternatively switched from one eye to the other and back, thus stimulating each eye in rapid succession.
- When the normal eye is stimulated both pupils constrict (Fig. 21.18a).
- Then when the light is swung to the diseased eye, both pupils dilate instead of constricting (Fig. 21.18b).
- When the normal eye is stimulated, both pupils constrict (Fig. 21.18c).

This paradoxical dilatation of the pupils in response to light occurs because the dilatation produced by withdrawing the light from the normal eye outweighs the constriction produced by stimulating the abnormal eye.

NB In afferent (sensory) lesions, the pupils are equal in size. Anisocoria (inequality of pupillary size) implies disease of the efferent (motor) nerve, iris or muscles of the pupil.

Light-near dissociation

In this condition the light reflex is absent or sluggish but the near response is normal. The causes are shown in Table 21.3.

Argyll Robertson pupil

Argyll Robertson pupil is caused by neurosyphilis and is characterized by:
- Involvement is usually bilateral but asymmetrical.
- The pupils are small and irregular.

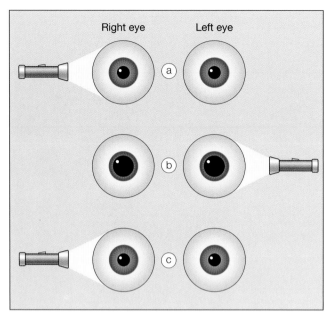

Fig. 21.18
'Swinging flashlight test' in a left afferent pupillary defect

Table 21.3 Causes of light-near dissociation

1. Unilateral
- Afferent conduction defect
- Adie pupil
- Herpes zoster ophthalmicus
- Aberrant regeneration of the third nerve

2. Bilateral
- Neurosyphilis
- Type I diabetes
- Myotonic dystrophy
- Parinaud dorsal midbrain syndrome
- Familial amyloidosis
- Encephalitis
- Chronic alcoholism

- The pupils do not dilate well in the dark but atropine or cocaine induces mydriasis unless extensive iris atrophy is present.

Adie pupil

Adie (tonic) pupil is caused by denervation of the post-ganglionic supply to the sphincter pupillae and the ciliary muscle, which may follow a viral illness. It typically affects young adults and presents as a unilateral condition in 80% of cases, although involvement of the second eye may develop within months or years.

1. Signs
- Large and regular pupil (Fig. 21.19a).
- Direct light reflex is absent or sluggish (Fig. 21.19b) and is associated with vermiform movements of the pupillary border, visible on the slit-lamp.
- Consensual light reflex is absent or sluggish (Fig. 21.19c).
- The pupil responds slowly to near, following which re-dilatation is also slow.
- Accommodation may manifest similar tonicity, in that once a near object has been fixated, the time taken to re-focus in the distance (relax the ciliary muscle) is prolonged.
- In long-standing cases the pupil may become small ('little old Adie').

2. Associations. In some cases, deep tendon reflexes are diminished (Holmes–Adie syndrome – Fig. 21.19d) and there is autonomic nerve dysfunction.

3. Pharmacological testing. If 2.5% methacholine or 0.125% pilocarpine is instilled into both eyes, the normal pupil will not constrict, but the abnormal pupil will because of denervation hypersensitivity. Some diabetic patients may also show this response.

Oculosympathetic palsy (Horner syndrome)

Anatomy

The sympathetic supply involves three neurons (Fig. 21.20).

1. First (central) starts in the posterior hypothalamus and descends, uncrossed, down the brainstem to terminate in the ciliospinal centre of Budge, in the intermedio-lateral horn of the spinal cord, located between C8 and T2.

2. Second (pre-ganglionic) passes from the ciliospinal centre to the superior cervical ganglion in the neck. During its long course, it is closely related to the apical pleura where it may be damaged by bronchogenic carcinoma (Pancoast tumour) or during surgery on the neck.

3. Third (post-ganglionic) ascends along the internal carotid artery to enter the cavernous sinus where it joins the ophthalmic division of the trigeminal nerve. The sympathetic fibres reach the ciliary body and the dilator pupillae muscle via the nasociliary nerve and the long ciliary nerves.

Causes

The causes of Horner syndrome are shown in Table 21.4.

Signs

The vast majority of cases are unilateral. Causes of bilateral involvement include cervical spine injuries and in diabetic patients as part of systemic autonomic neuropathy.

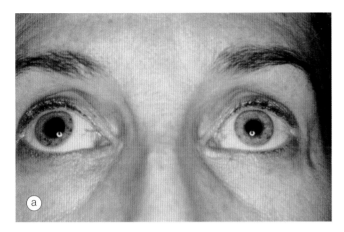
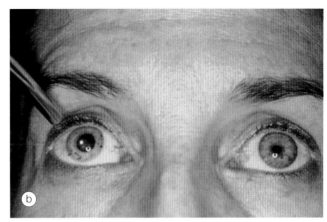
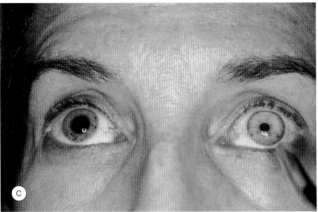
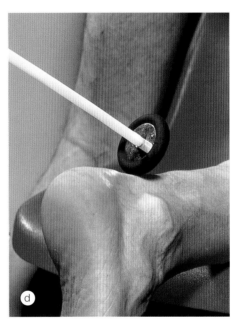

Fig. 21.19
Right Holmes–Adie pupil. **(a)** Right pupil is large and regular; **(b)** direct light reflex is absent of sluggish; **(c)** consensual light reflex is similar; **(d)** diminishes deep tendon reflex (Courtesy of D M Albert and F A Jakobiec, from *Principles and Practice of Ophthalmology*, Saunders, 1994 – figs a, b and c; M A Mir, from *Atlas of Clinical Diagnosis*, Saunders, 2003 – fig. d)

- Mild ptosis (usually 1–2mm) as a result of weakness of Müller muscle and miosis due to the unopposed action of the sphincter pupillae with resultant anisocoria (Fig. 21.21a).
- Miosis is accentuated in dim light since the Horner pupil will not dilate, unlike its fellow.
- Normal reactions to light and near.
- Hypochromic heterochromia (irides of different colour – Horner is lighter) may be seen if the lesion is congenital (Fig. 21.21b) or long-standing.
- Slight elevation of the inferior eyelid as a result of weakness of the inferior tarsal muscle.
- Reduced ipsilateral sweating, but only if the lesion is below the superior cervical ganglion, because the fibres supplying the skin of the face run along the external carotid artery.

Pharmacological tests

Cocaine confirms the diagnosis. Hydroxyamphetamine (Paredrine) may be used to differentiate a pre-ganglionic from a post-ganglionic lesion. Adrenaline may also be used to assess denervation supersensitivity.

1. **Cocaine 4%** is instilled into both eyes.
   a. ***Result***: the normal pupil will dilate but the Horner pupil will not. A post-cocaine anisocoria of > 0.8mm in a dimly lit room is significant.
   b. ***Rationale***: noradrenaline (NA) released at the post-ganglionic sympathetic nerve endings is re-uptaken by the nerve endings, thus terminating its action. Cocaine blocks this uptake. NA therefore accumulates and causes pupillary dilatation. In Horner syndrome, there is no NA being secreted in the first place – therefore

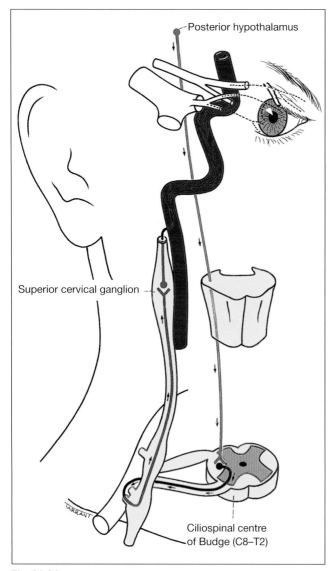

Fig. 21.20
Anatomical pathway of the sympathetic nerve supply

Table 21.4 Causes of Horner syndrome

1. *Central (first-order neuron)*
- Brainstem disease (tumour, vascular, demyelination)
- Syringomyelia
- Lateral medullary (Wallenberg) syndrome
- Spinal cord tumour
- Diabetic autonomic neuropathy

2. *Pre-ganglionic (second-order neuron)*
- Pancoast tumour
- Carotid and aortic aneurysm and dissection
- Neck lesions (glands, trauma, postsurgical)

3. *Postganglionic (third-order neuron)*
- Cluster headaches (migrainous neuralgia)
- Internal carotid artery dissection
- Nasopharyngeal tumour
- Otitis media
- Cavernous sinus mass

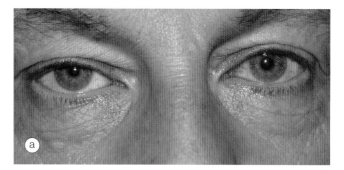

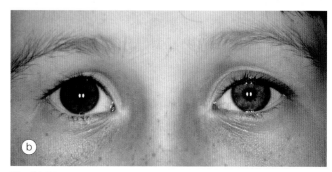

Fig. 21.21
Horner syndrome. **(a)** Right; **(b)** heterochromia iridis associated with a left congenital Horner in a child (Courtesy of A Pearson – fig. a)

cocaine has no effect. Cocaine thus confirms the diagnosis of Horner syndrome by continued constriction of the affected pupil.

2. **Hydroxyamphetamine 1%** is instilled into both eyes the next day, after the effects of cocaine have worn off.
   a. Result:
   - In a pre-ganglionic lesion both pupils will dilate (Fig. 21.22).
   - In a post-ganglionic lesion the Horner pupil will not dilate.
   b. Rationale: hydroxyamphetamine potentiates the release of NA from post-ganglionic nerve endings. If this neuron is intact (a lesion of the first or second order neuron, and also the normal eye) NA will be released and the pupil will dilate. In a lesion of the

third order neuron (post-ganglionic) there can be no dilatation since the neuron is destroyed.

3. **Adrenaline 1:1000** is instilled into both eyes.
   a. Result:
   - In a pre-ganglionic lesion neither pupil will dilate because adrenaline is rapidly destroyed by monoamine oxidase.
   - In a post-ganglionic lesion, the Horner pupil will dilate and ptosis may be temporarily relieved because

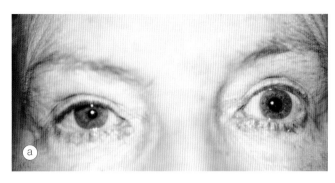

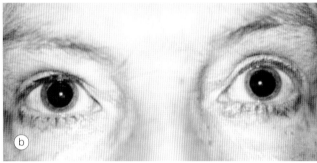

Fig. 21.22
(a) Right pre-ganglionic Horner syndrome; **(b)** bilateral mydriasis following instillation of hydroxyamphetamine into both eyes

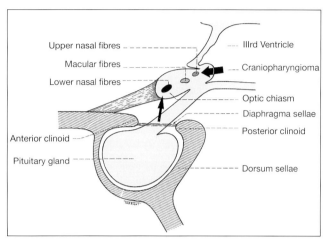

Fig. 21.23
Anatomy of the chiasm in relation to the pituitary gland

adrenaline is not broken down due to the absence of monoamine oxidase.

b. Rationale: a muscle deprived of its motor supply manifests heightened sensitivity to the excitatory neurotransmitter secreted by its motor nerve. In Horner syndrome the dilator pupillae muscle similarly manifests 'denervation hypersensitivity' to adrenergic neurotransmitters. Therefore adrenaline, even in minute concentration, produces marked dilatation of the Horner pupil.

CHIASM

Anatomy

Pituitary gland

The sella turcica (Turkish saddle) is a deep depression in the superior surface of the body of the sphenoid bone in which the pituitary gland lies (Fig. 21.23). The roof of the sella is formed by a fold of dura mater which stretches from the anterior to the posterior clinoids (diaphragma sellae). The optic nerves and chiasm lie above the diaphragma sellae; a visual field defect in a patient with a pituitary tumour therefore indicates suprasellar extension. Tumours less than 10mm in diameter (microadenomas) often remain intrasellar,

whereas those larger than 10mm (macroadenomas) tend to manifest extrasellar extension. Posteriorly the chiasm is continuous with the optic tracts and forms the anterior wall of the third ventricle.

Chiasmal nerve pathways

Optic nerve fibres passing through the chiasm are arranged as follows:

1. **Lower nasal** fibres traverse the chiasm low and anteriorly. They are therefore most vulnerable to damage from expanding pituitary lesions, so that the upper temporal quadrants of the visual fields are involved first.

   NB The inferonasal fibres loop forwards into the contralateral optic nerve, before passing posteriorly into the optic tract (anterior knee of Wilbrand) and may therefore be affected by lesions affecting the posterior part of the optic nerve.

2. **Upper nasal** fibres traverse the chiasm high and posteriorly and therefore are involved first by lesions coming from above the chiasm (e.g. craniopharyngiomas). If the lower temporal quadrants of the visual field are affected more than the upper, a pituitary adenoma is unlikely.
3. **Macular fibres** decussate throughout the chiasm.

Anatomical variants

The following anatomical variations in the location of the chiasm may have important clinical significance (Fig. 21.24):

1. **Central** chiasm, which is present in about 80% of normals, lies directly above the sella so that expanding pituitary tumours will involve the chiasm first.

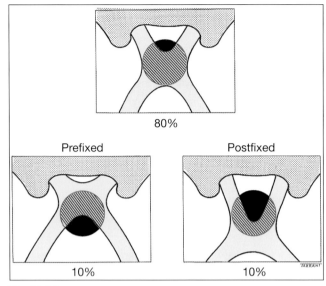

Fig. 21.24
Anatomical variations in the position of the chiasm

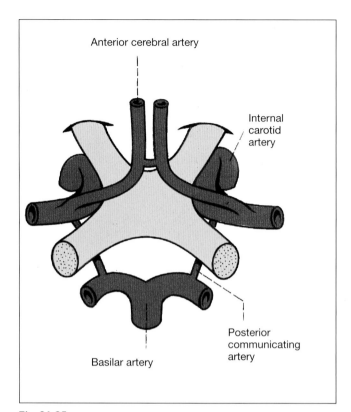

Fig. 21.25
Relationship between the chasm and adjacent structures

2. **Prefixed** chiasm, which is present in about 10% of normals, is located more anteriorly, over the tuberculum sellae, so that pituitary tumours involve the optic tracts first.
3. **Postfixed** chiasm, which is present in the remaining 10% of normals, is located more posteriorly, over the dorsum sellae, so that pituitary tumours are apt to damage the optic nerves first.

Parachiasmal vascular structures

1. **Cavernous sinuses** lie lateral to the sella so that laterally expanding pituitary tumours affect the cavernous sinus and may damage the intracavernous parts of the third, fourth and sixth cranial nerves. Conversely, aneurysms arising from the intracavernous part of the internal carotid artery may erode into the sella and mimic pituitary tumours.
2. **Internal carotid arteries** curve posteriorly and upwards from the cavernous sinus and lie immediately below the optic nerves (Fig. 21.25). They then ascend vertically alongside the lateral aspect of the chiasm. The precommunicating portion of the anterior cerebral artery is closely related to the superior surface of the chiasm and optic nerves. An aneurysm in this region can therefore compress the optic nerve or chiasm.

Physiology

Pituitary hormones

The lobules of the anterior part of the pituitary gland are composed of six cell types. Five of these secrete hormones and the sixth (follicular cell) has no secretory function. The hormones secreted by the anterior pituitary gland are follicle stimulating hormone (FSH), luteinising hormone (LH), adrenocorticotrophic hormone (ACTH), thyroid stimulating hormone (TSH), and beta-lipotrophin (C-terminal part of the ACTH precursor molecule). Although pituitary adenomas are classified as basophil, acidophil and chromophobe, tumours of mixed-cell types are common and any of the six cell types may proliferate to produce an adenoma. The anterior pituitary is itself under the control of the various inhibiting and releasing factors which are synthesized in the hypothalamus and which pass to the anterior pituitary through the hypothalamo-hypophyseal portal system. The posterior pituitary releases antidiuretic hormone (ADH) and oxytocin.

Causes of hyperpituitarism

Figure 21.26 summarizes the causes.
1. **Basophil** tumours secrete ACTH and cause Cushing disease (see Chapter 24).
2. **Acidophil** tumours secrete growth hormone, which causes gigantism in children and acromegaly in adults (see Chapter 24).
3. **Chromophobe** adenomas may secrete prolactin and are referred to as prolactinomas. Excessive levels of prolactin in women lead to the infertility-amenorrhoea-

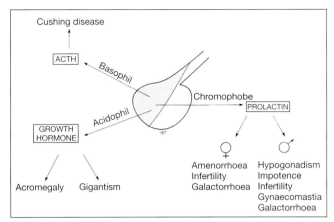

Fig. 21.26
Hormones secreted by anterior pituitary tumours

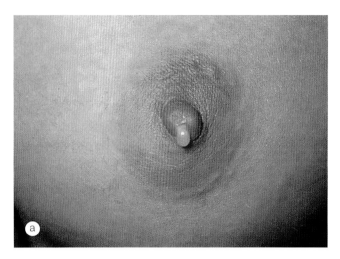

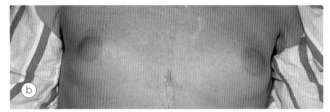

Fig. 21.27
Effects of prolactinoma. **(a)** Galactorrhoea in a female;
(b) gynaecomastia in a male (Courtesy of P-M Bouloux, from *Clinical Medicine Assessment Questions*, Wolfe, 1993 – fig. a; M A Mir, from *Atlas of Clinical Diagnosis*, Saunders, 2003 – fig. b)

galactorrhoea syndrome (Fig. 21.27a), and in men cause hypogonadism, impotence, sterility, decreased libido and occasionally gynaecomastia (Fig. 21.27b) and even galactorrhoea. Some chromophobe adenomas are non-secreting.

Causes of hypopituitarism

1. **Direct pressure** on the secreting cells in the anterior pituitary by a mass. Secondary deposits are common in the pituitary but do not normally affect hormone secretion.
2. **Vascular** damage to the pituitary (e.g. pituitary apoplexy after childbirth – Sheehan syndrome).
3. **Iatrogenic** causes such as pituitary surgery and radiotherapy.
4. **Interference** with the synthesis of inhibiting and releasing factors in the hypothalamus by gliomas or impediment of their transport in the portal system.

> **NB** The clinical features are dictated by both the pattern of hormone deficiency and the stage of growth and development of the patient at the time. Usually gonadotrophin secretion is impaired first, followed by that of growth hormone; deficiencies in other hormones occur later.

Causes of chiasmal disease

1. **Tumours** such as pituitary adenomas, craniopharyngioma, meningioma, glioma, chordoma, dysgerminoma, nasopharyngeal tumours and metastases.
2. **Non-neoplastic masses** such as aneurysms, Rathke pouch cysts, fibrous dysplasia, sphenoidal sinus mucoceles and arachnoid cysts.
3. **Miscellaneous** disorders including demyelination, inflammation, trauma, radiation-induced necrosis and vasculitis.

Pituitary adenoma

Clinical features

Chromophobe adenoma is the most common primary intracranial tumour to produce neuro-ophthalmological features. Although generally detected by endocrinologists, non-secreting tumours may first present to ophthalmologists.

1. **Presentation** is typically during early adult life or middle age with the following:
   a. **Headache** may be prominent due to involvement of pain-sensitive fibres in the diaphragma sellae. As the tumour expands upwards and breaks through the diaphragma the headaches may stop. The headache is non-specific and does not have the usual features associated with raised intracranial pressure. Diagnostic delay is therefore common in the absence of obvious endocrine disturbances.
   b. **Visual symptoms** usually have a very gradual onset and may not be noticed by the patient until well established. It is therefore essential to examine the visual function in all patients with non-specific headaches or endocrine disturbance.

2. Visual field defects depend on the anatomical relationship between the pituitary and chiasm.
- If the chiasm is central, both superotemporal fields are affected first, as the tumour grows upwards and splays the anterior chiasmal notch, compressing the crossing inferonasal fibres (Fig. 21.28).
- The defects then progress into the lower temporal fields. As tumour growth is often asymmetrical, the degree of visual field loss is usually different on the two sides.
- Patients may not present until central vision is affected from pressure on the macular fibres. The eye with the greater field loss usually also has more marked impairment of visual acuity.

NB The absence of a visual field defect does not exclude a pituitary tumour, since tumours confined to the sella are often visually asymptomatic. Acidophil adenomas do not expand beyond the sella as frequently as chromophobe adenomas, and basophil adenomas are usually small and rarely compress the chiasm.

3. Differential diagnosis of bitemporal defects includes dermatochalasis of the upper eyelids, tilted discs, optic nerve colobomas, nasal retinoschisis, nasal retinitis pigmentosa and functional visual loss.

4. Colour desaturation across the vertical midline of the uniocular visual field is an early sign of chiasmal compression which can be detected very simply with a red pin or a red Mydriacyl bottle top.
- Each eye is tested separately and the patient is asked to compare the colour and intensity of the target as it is brought from the nasal to the temporal visual field.

- Another technique is to simultaneously present red targets in precisely symmetrical parts of the temporal and nasal visual fields, and to ask if the colours appear the same.
- The patient may also miss the temporal number on Ishihara testing.

5. Optic atrophy is present in approximately 50% of cases with field defects caused by pituitary lesions. Patients are invariably more aware of difficulties with central vision (e.g. when reading) than with peripheral vision. It is therefore important to perform very careful visual field examinations on both eyes in patients with unexplained unilateral deterioration of central vision. When optic atrophy is present the prognosis for visual recovery after treatment is guarded. When nerve fibre loss is confined to fibres originating in the nasal retina (i.e. nasal to the fovea), only the nasal and temporal aspects of the disc will be involved, resulting in a band or 'bow tie' shaped atrophy.

6. Miscellaneous features include diplopia as a result of lateral expansion into the cavernous sinus and involvement of ocular motor nerves and, rarely, see-saw nystagmus of Maddox.

7. Pituitary apoplexy is a rare condition caused by a sudden increase in the size of a pituitary tumour, often secondary to haemorrhage.
- **a. Presentation** is with severe headache, diplopia, visual loss and photophobia.
- **b. Signs** include ophthalmoplegia, decreased sensation over the distribution of the first and second divisions of the trigeminal nerve, and variable visual loss.
- **c. Treatment** with systemic steroids and surgery may be necessary to prevent blindness and other neurological complications.

Special investigations

1. MR demonstrates the relationship between a mass lesion and the chiasm. The optimal study consists of coronal, axial and sagittal thin sections through the chiasm and optic nerves before and after gadolinium injection. The coronal plane is optimal for demonstrating sellar contents. Pituitary adenomas are typically hypointense on T1-weighted images, hyperintense on T2-weighted images and enhance strongly with gadolinium in a heterogeneous fashion (Fig. 21.29). Repeated MR to monitor progress is safe because there is no ionizing radiation risk.

2. CT will demonstrate enlargement or erosion of the sella.

3. Endocrinological evaluation should be tailored to the individual patient. All patients suspected of having a pituitary adenoma should have assays of serum prolactin, FSH, TSH and growth hormone. An insulin stress test may also be required in selected cases. Patients with large adenomas with visual field defects are at some risk of pituitary apoplexy if the hypoglycaemic response is profound.

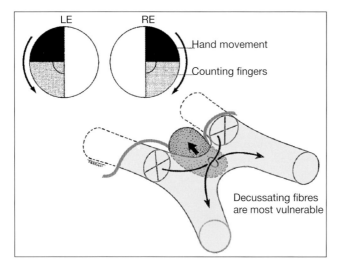

Fig. 21.28
Progression of bitemporal visual field defects caused by compression of the chiasm from below by a pituitary adenoma

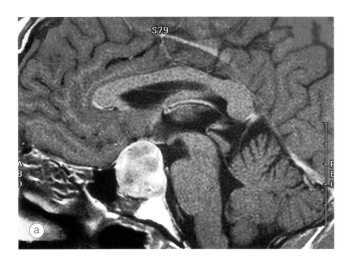

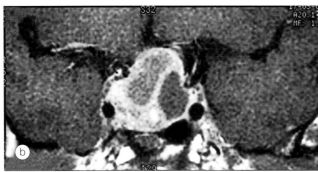

Fig. 21.29
T1-weighted gadolinium enhanced MR of a pituitary adenoma.
(a) Sagittal view; **(b)** coronal view (Courtesy of D Thomas)

Treatment

Not all tumours require treatment and observation may be appropriate for incidentally discovered and clinically silent tumours.

1. **Medical** therapy to shrink a prolactin-secreting tumour involves dopamine agonists such as cabergoline or bromocriptine. Patients with significant visual field defects should have urgent prolactin level assay and, if elevated, treatment should be started as soon as possible. Visual function may improve within hours. Endocrine function also often improves with cessation of galactorrhoea, improvement of libido and return of menstruation.
2. **Surgery**
   a. **Indications** are mass effects causing severe compressive problems or failure to respond to medical therapy or radiotherapy.
   b. **Technique.** Hypophysectomy is most frequently performed through a trans-sphenoidal approach through the upper gum under the lips. Occasionally both trans-sphenoidal hypophysectomy and a craniotomy are required to remove tissue above the diaphragma sellae.

c. **Visual recovery is tri-phasic**
   – An early fast phase in the first week may lead to normalization of visual fields in some patients.
   – A subsequent slow phase between 1 and 4 months is the period of most notable improvement.
   – A late phase (6 months to 3 years) of mild improvement follows.
3. **Radiotherapy** is often used as an adjunct following incomplete removal of tumour. It can also be used as primary treatment in selected cases. While usually effective in preventing further growth it is often less successful in controlling abnormal hormone secretion.
4. **Gamma knife stereotactic** radiotherapy is a relatively new method of delivering a concentrated dose of radiation to the tumour with little radiation to surrounding tissues. It is therefore of particular value in treating adenomas in close proximity to the optic nerve or when the cavernous sinus is invaded.

Craniopharyngioma

Craniopharyngioma is a slow-growing tumour arising from vestigial remnants of Rathke pouch along the pituitary stalk.

1. **Presentation** depends on the age of the patient:
   a. **Children** frequently present with dwarfism, delayed sexual development and obesity due to interference with hypothalamic function.
   b. **Adults** usually present with visual impairment and visual field defects.
2. **Visual field defects** are complex and may be due to involvement of the optic nerves, chiasm or tracts.
   • The initial defect frequently involves both infero-temporal fields because the tumour compresses the chiasm from above and behind, damaging the upper nasal fibres (Fig. 21.30).
   • The defects then spread to involve the upper temporal fields.
3. **MR** shows a solid tumour that appears isointense on T1-weighted images (Fig. 21.31). Cystic components appear hyperintense on T1-weighted images.
4. **Treatment** is mainly surgical, although intimacy to the chiasm may preclude complete removal. Postoperative radiotherapy may be helpful, but recurrences are common, necessitating lifelong follow-up.

Meningioma

Intracranial meningiomas typically affect middle-aged women. Visual field defects and clinical signs depend on the location of the tumour (Fig. 21.32).

1. **Tuberculum sellae** meningiomas typically compress the junction of the chiasm with the optic nerve. This

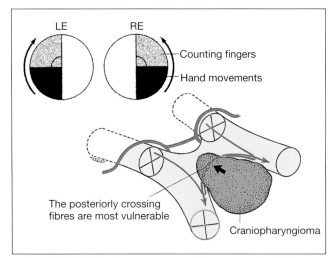

Fig. 21.30
Progression of bitemporal visual field defects caused by compression of the chiasm from above by a craniopharyngioma

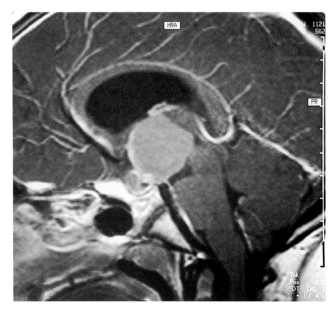

Fig. 21.31
Sagittal T1-weighted MR of a craniopharyngioma which has caused hydrocephalus (Courtesy of K Nischal)

gives rise to an ipsilateral central scotoma caused by optic nerve compression and a contralateral upper temporal defect (junctional scotoma) due to damage to the anterior knee of Wilbrand.

2. **Sphenoidal ridge** tumours compress the optic nerve early if the tumour is located medially and late if the lateral aspect of the sphenoid bone and middle cranial fossa are involved (Fig. 21.33a). A classic finding in the latter is fullness in the temporal fossa as a result of hyperostosis (Fig. 21.33b).

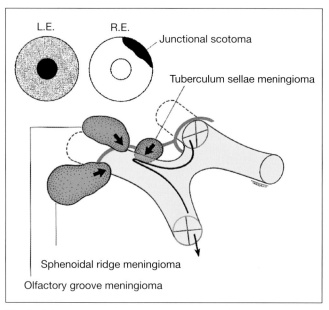

Fig. 21.32
Intracranial optic nerve compression by meningiomas and visual field defects caused by a tuberculum sellae meningioma

3. **Olfactory groove** meningioma may cause loss of the sense of smell, as well as optic nerve compression.
4. **Treatment** involves surgery but postoperative radiotherapy is used in the event of incomplete excision.

OPTIC TRACT

Introduction

Retrochiasmal pathology results in binocular visual field defects involving contralateral visual space. Both eyes therefore manifest partial or total visual hemifield loss opposite the side of a retrochiasmal lesion. Such a 'hemianopia' involving the same side of visual space in both eyes is homonymous, in contradistinction to that seen in chiasmal compression, which produces heteronymous (bitemporal) hemianopia, in which opposite sides of the visual field are affected in each eye.

Incongruity

A homonymous hemianopia may be incomplete or complete. In the context of incomplete hemianopia, congruity refers to how closely the extent and pattern of field loss in one eye matches that of the other. Almost identical field defects in either eye are therefore highly congruous, while mismatching right and left visual field defects are incongruous.

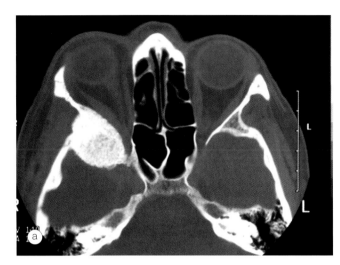

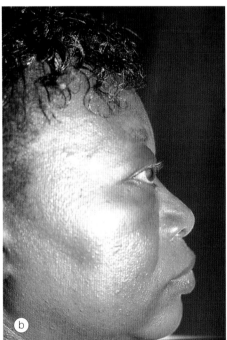

Fig. 21.33
Sphenoidal ridge meningioma. **(a)** CT axial view; **(b)** reactive hyperostosis (Courtesy of A Pearson – fig. a)

Hemianopia secondary to pathology in the anterior retrochiasmal visual pathways is characteristically incongruous, while that due to pathology further back (i.e. the posterior optic radiations) manifests a higher degree of congruity.

Clinical features

1. Homonymous hemianopia. The optic tracts arise at the posterior aspect of the chiasm, diverge and extend posteriorly around the cerebral peduncles, to terminate in the lateral geniculate bodies. Each optic tract contains crossed fibres from the contralateral nasal hemiretina, and uncrossed fibres from the ipsilateral temporal hemiretina. Nerve fibres originating from corresponding retinal elements are, however, not closely aligned. Homonymous hemianopia caused by optic tract lesions is therefore characteristically incongruous. Lesions of the lateral geniculate body also produce asymmetrical hemianopic defects. The causes of optic tract disease are similar to those affecting the chiasm but the tract is particularly vulnerable when the chiasm is pre-fixed.

2. Wernicke hemianopic pupil. The optic tracts contain both visual and pupillomotor fibres. The visual fibres terminate in the lateral geniculate body but the pupillary fibres leave the optic tract anterior to the lateral geniculate body, projecting through the brachium of the superior colliculus to terminate in the pre-tectal nuclei. An optic tract lesion may therefore give rise to an APD. Characteristically, the pupillary light reflex will be normal when the unaffected hemiretina is stimulated, and absent when the involved hemiretina is stimulated (i.e. light is shone from the hemianopic side). In practice, this Wernicke hemianopic pupillary reaction is difficult to elicit because of scatter of light within the eye – hence the need for a very fine beam of light.

3. Optic atrophy may occur when the optic tracts are damaged because the fibres in the optic tract are the axons of the retinal ganglion cells. The ipsilateral disc manifests atrophy of the superior and inferior aspects of the neuroretinal rim (fibres from the temporal retina), while the contralateral disc manifests a 'bow tie' pattern of atrophy (nasal retinal fibres).

4. Contralateral pyramidal signs may occur when an optic tract lesion also damages the ispilateral cerebral peduncle.

OPTIC RADIATIONS

Anatomy

The optic radiations extend from the lateral geniculate body to the striate cortex, which is located on the medial aspect of the occipital lobe, above and below the calcarine fissure (Fig. 21.34). The optic radiations and visual cortex have a dual blood supply from the middle and posterior cerebral arteries. As the radiations pass posteriorly, fibres from corresponding retinal elements lie progressively closer together. For this reason, incomplete hemianopia caused by lesions of the posterior radiations are more congruous than those involving the anterior radiations. Because these fibres are third-order neurons that originate in the lateral geniculate body, lesions of the optic radiations do not produce optic atrophy.

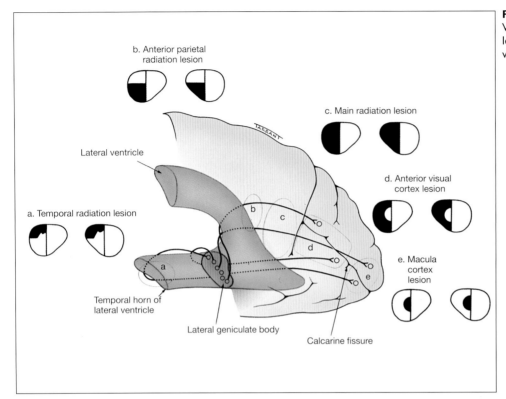

Fig. 21.34
Visual field defects caused by lesions of the optic radiations and visual cortex

b. Anterior parietal radiation lesion

c. Main radiation lesion

Lateral ventricle

d. Anterior visual cortex lesion

a. Temporal radiation lesion

e. Macula cortex lesion

Temporal horn of lateral ventricle

Lateral geniculate body

Calcarine fissure

Temporal radiations

1. **Visual field defect** consists of a contralateral, homonymous, superior quadrantanopia ('pie in the sky'), because the inferior fibres of the optic radiations, which subserve the upper visual fields, first sweep antero-inferiorly into the temporal lobe (Meyer loop) around the anterior tip of the temporal horn of the lateral ventricle (Fig. 21.34a).
2. **Associated features** include contralateral hemisensory disturbance and mild hemiparesis, because the temporal radiations pass very close to the sensory and motor fibres of the internal capsule before passing posteriorly and rejoining the superior fibres. Other features of temporal lobe disease include paroxysmal olfactory and gustatory hallucinations (uncinate fits), formed visual hallucinations, seizures and receptive dysphasia if the dominant hemisphere is involved.

Anterior parietal radiations

1. **Visual field defect** consists of a contralateral, homonymous, inferior quadrantanopia ('pie on the floor') because the superior fibres of the radiations, which subserve the inferior visual fields, proceed directly posteriorly through the parietal lobe to the occipital cortex. A lesion involving only the anterior parietal part of the radiations is, however, very rare. In general, hemianopia resulting from parietal lobe lesions tend to be relatively congruous (Fig. 21.34b).

2. **Associated features** of dominant parietal lobe disease include acalculia, agraphia, left–right disorientation and finger agnosia. Non-dominant lobe lesions may cause dressing and constitutional apraxia and spatial neglect.

Main radiations

Deep in the parietal lobe, the optic radiations lie just external to the trigone and the occipital horn of the lateral ventricle. Lesions in this area usually cause a complete homonymous hemianopia (Fig. 21.34c). Optokinetic nystagmus (OKN) may be useful in localizing a lesion causing an isolated homonymous hemianopia that does not conform to any set pattern in a patient without associated neurological deficits. Normally OKN involves smooth pursuit of a target, followed by a saccade in the opposite direction to fixate on the next target. If the optomotor pathways in the posterior hemisphere are damaged, the OKN response will be diminished when targets are rotated towards the side of the lesion (i.e. away from the hemianopia). This is explained on the basis that the occipital lobe can no longer control ipsilateral pursuit, while the contralateral hemianopia inhibits re-fixational saccades. This is called the positive OKN sign.

NB Incongruous homonymous hemianopia with asymmetrical OKN indicates a parietal lobe lesion. Congruous homonymous hemianopia with symmetrical OKN indicates an occipital lobe disease.

STRIATE CORTEX

Clinical features

1. **Visual field defects.** In the striate cortex the peripheral visual fields are represented anteriorly. This part of the occipital lobe is supplied by a branch of the posterior cerebral artery. Central macular vision is represented posteriorly just lateral to the tip of the calcarine cortex, an area supplied mainly by a branch of the middle cerebral artery. Occlusion of the posterior cerebral artery will therefore tend to produce a macular sparing congruous homonymous hemianopia (Fig. 21.34d). Damage to the tip of the occipital cortex, as might occur from a head injury, tends to give rise to congruous, homonymous, macular defects (Fig. 21.34e), although asymmetrical macular sparing may sometimes occur with vascular lesions of the occipital lobe.

   NB The anterior-most part of the calcarine cortex subserves the temporal extremity of the visual field of the contralateral eye, the area of visual space that extends beyond the field of binocular single vision and is perceived monocularly. A lesion in this area may therefore give rise to a monocular temporal field defect in the contralateral eye, known as a temporal crescent.

2. **Associated features** of visual cortex disease (cortical blindness) are:
   - Formed visual hallucinations, particularly involving the hemianopic field.
   - Denial of blindness (Anton syndrome).
   - Riddoch phenomenon, which is characterized by the ability to perceive kinetic, but not static visual targets.

Causes

1. **Vascular lesions** in the territory of the posterior cerebral artery are responsible for over 90% of isolated homonymous hemianopia with no other neurological deficits.
2. **Other causes,** which are less common, include migraine, trauma and primary or metastatic tumours.

HIGHER VISUAL FUNCTION

From the striate cortex (area 17), visual information is relayed to the visual association areas (18 and 19) of the cerebral cortex, where it is processed, analysed and interpreted. Lesions of various areas of the cerebral cortex produce characteristic clinical pictures.

Alexia and agraphia

The angulate gyrus of the dominant hemisphere (commonly the left) subserves the ability to write. Visual information from both occipital cortices is relayed to the left angulate gyrus, fibres from the right side crossing the midline in the splenium of the corpus callosum. Alexia (the inability to read), commonly accompanied by agraphia (the inability to write), may be produced by lesions of the angulate gyrus of the dominant cerebral hemisphere. Alexia may occur independently of agraphia in the context of a left occipital lesion of sufficient magnitude to involve fibres crossing the splenium, from the right occipital cortex to the left angulate gyrus. The clinical features consist of a right homonymous hemianopia with alexia, since information from the right occipital cortex (left visual field) is prevented from reaching the left angulate gyrus.

   NB It is therefore mandatory to examine reading ability in the context of a right hemianopia.

Agnosia

Lesions of the inferior occipito-temporal area may produce a wide range of clinical features. Bilateral disease may produce visual agnosia – the inability to recognize objects by sight, whilst the ability to recognize by touch is retained. Prosopagnosia implies the inability to recognize and distinguish between faces. Colour vision too has its seat in this area, each half of the visual field being represented contralaterally. Lesions here may therefore also result in contralateral (cerebral) hemi-achromatopsia with total loss or relative desaturation of colour.

Visual hallucinations

Significant visual impairment due to pathology anywhere along the visual pathway, from the eye to the primary visual cortex, may result in the emergence of complex visual hallucinations. This condition (Charles Bonnet syndrome) is thought to represent a release phenomenon, secondary to de-afferentiation of the visual association areas, which then exhibit spontaneous activity, with resultant complex (formed) visual hallucinations. Such hallucinations are often brilliantly clear and detailed, in contrast to the patient's normally indistinct vision and are recognized by the patient as unreal, often after initial deception. Hallucinatory content is usually pleasant, but may be distressing. Patients aware of the unreality of their visions often do not admit their existence for fear of being labelled insane. Sensitive history taking and reassurance are usually sufficient.

THIRD NERVE

Nuclear complex

The nuclear complex of the third (oculomotor) nerve is situated in the midbrain at the level of the superior colliculus, ventral to the Sylvian aqueduct (Fig. 21.35). It is composed of the following paired and unpaired subnuclei.

1. **Levator subnucleus** is an unpaired caudal midline structure which innervates both levator muscles. Lesions confined in this area will therefore give rise to bilateral ptosis.
2. **Superior rectus subnuclei** are paired; each innervates the respective contralateral superior rectus. A nuclear third nerve palsy will spare the ipsilateral, and affect the contralateral, superior rectus.
3. **Medial rectus, inferior rectus and inferior oblique subnuclei** are paired and innervate their corresponding ipsilateral muscles. Lesions confined to the nuclear complex are relatively uncommon. The most frequent causes are vascular disease, primary tumours and metastases. Involvement of the paired medial rectus subnuclei cause a wall-eyed bilateral internuclear ophthalmoplegia (WEBINO), characterized by exotropia, and defective convergence and adduction. Lesions involving the entire nucleus are often associated with involvement of the adjacent and caudal fourth nerve nucleus.

Fasciculus

The fasciculus consists of efferent fibres which pass from the third nerve nucleus through the red nucleus and the medial aspect of the cerebral peduncle. They then emerge from the midbrain and pass into the interpeduncular space. The causes of nuclear and fascicular lesions are similar, except that demyelination may affect the fasciculus.

1. **Benedikt** syndrome involves the fasciculus as it passes through the red nucleus and is characterized by ipsilateral third nerve palsy and contralateral extrapyramidal signs such as hemitremor.
2. **Weber** syndrome involves the fasciculus as it passes through the cerebral peduncle and is characterized by ipsilateral third nerve palsy and a contralateral hemiparesis.
3. **Nothnagel** syndrome involves the fasciculus and the superior cerebellar peduncle and is characterized by ipsilateral third nerve palsy and cerebellar ataxia. Important causes include vascular disease and tumours.
4. **Claude** syndrome is a combination of Benedikt and Nothnagel syndromes.

Basilar

The basilar part starts as a series of 'rootlets' which leave the midbrain on the medial aspect of the cerebral peduncle, before coalescing to form the main trunk. The nerve then passes between the posterior cerebral and superior cerebellar arteries, running lateral to and parallel with the posterior communicating artery (Fig. 21.36). As the nerve traverses the base of the skull along its subarachnoid course unaccompanied by any other cranial nerve, isolated third nerve palsies are commonly basilar. The following two are important causes:

1. **Aneurysm** of the posterior communicating artery at its junction with the internal carotid artery (Fig. 21.37) typically presents as acute, painful third nerve palsy with involvement of the pupil.

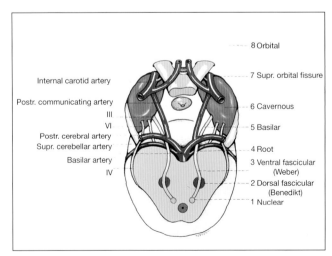

Fig. 21.35
Dorsal view of the course of the third nerve

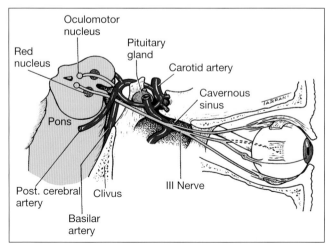

Fig. 21.36
Lateral view of the course of the third nerve

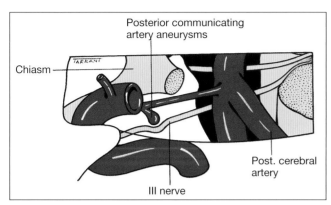

Fig. 21.37
Compression of the third nerve by a posterior communicating aneurysm

2. Head trauma, resulting in extradural or subdural haematoma, may cause a tentorial pressure cone with downward herniation of the temporal lobe. This compresses the third nerve as it passes over the tentorial edge, initially causing irritative miosis followed by mydriasis and total third nerve palsy (Fig. 21.38).

Intracavernous

The third nerve then enters the cavernous sinus by piercing the dura just lateral to the posterior clinoid process. Within the cavernous sinus, the third nerve runs in the lateral wall above the fourth nerve (Fig. 21.39). In the anterior part of the cavernous sinus, the nerve divides into superior and inferior branches which enter the orbit through the superior orbital fissure within the annulus of Zinn. The following are important causes of intracavernous third nerve palsies:

1. **Diabetes,** which may cause a vascular palsy, which usually spares the pupil.
2. **Pituitary apoplexy** (haemorrhagic infarction) may cause a third nerve palsy (e.g. after childbirth) if the gland swells laterally and impinges on the cavernous sinus.
3. **Intracavernous** pathology such as aneurysm, meningioma, carotid-cavernous fistula and granulomatous inflammation (Tolosa–Hunt syndrome) may all cause third nerve palsy. Because of its close proximity to other cranial nerves, intracavernous third nerve palsies are usually associated with involvement of the fourth and sixth nerves, and the first division of the trigeminal nerve.

Intraorbital

1. **Superior** division innervates the levator and superior rectus muscles.
2. **Inferior** division innervates the medial rectus, the inferior rectus and the inferior oblique muscles. The branch to the inferior oblique also contains preganglionic parasympathetic fibres from the Edinger–Westphal sub-

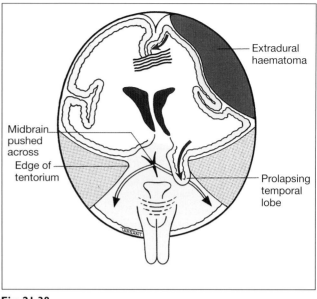

Fig. 21.38
Mechanism of third nerve palsy by extradural haematoma

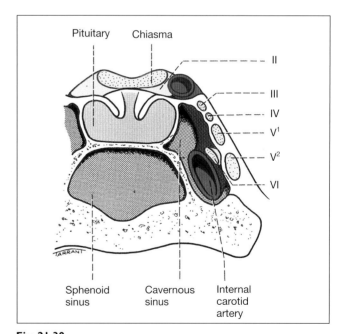

Fig. 21.39
Location of the cranial nerves in the cavernous sinus viewed from behind

nucleus, which innervate the sphincter pupillae and the ciliary muscle. Lesions of the inferior division are characterized by limited adduction and depression, and a dilated pupil. Both superior and inferior division palsies are commonly traumatic or vascular.

Pupillomotor fibres

Between the brainstem and the cavernous sinus, the pupillomotor parasympathetic fibres are located superficially in the superomedial part of the third nerve (Fig. 21.40). They derive their blood supply from the pial blood vessels, whereas the main trunk of the third nerve is supplied by the vasa nervorum. Involvement or otherwise of the pupil is of great importance because it frequently differentiates a 'surgical' from a 'medical' lesion. Pupillary involvement, like other features of third nerve palsy, may be complete or partial, and may demonstrate features of recovery. Mild mydriasis and non-reactivity may therefore be clinically significant.

1. **Surgical lesions** such as aneurysms, trauma and uncal herniation characteristically involve the pupil by compressing the pial blood vessels and the superficially located pupillary fibres.
2. **Medical lesions** such as hypertension and diabetes usually spare the pupil. This is because the microangiopathy associated with medical lesions involves the vasa nervorum, causing ischaemia of the main trunk of the nerve, sparing the superficial pupillary fibres.

NB These principles are, however, not infallible; pupil involvement may be seen in some diabetic-associated third nerve palsies, while pupillary sparing does not invariably exclude aneurysm or some other compressive lesion. Pupil involvement may develop a few days after onset of diplopia as an aneurysm expands. Sometimes pupillary involvement may be the only sign of third nerve palsy (basal meningitis, uncal herniation).

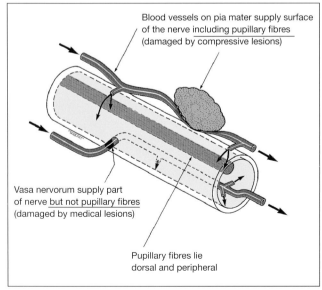

Blood vessels on pia mater supply surface of the nerve including pupillary fibres (damaged by compressive lesions)

Vasa nervorum supply part of nerve but not pupillary fibres (damaged by medical lesions)

Pupillary fibres lie dorsal and peripheral

Fig. 21.40
Location of pupillomotor fibres within the trunk of the third nerve

Diagnosis

1. **Signs** of a right third nerve palsy:
   - Weakness of the levator causing profound ptosis, due to which there is often no diplopia (Fig. 21.41a).
   - Unopposed action of lateral rectus causing the eye to be abducted in the primary position (Fig. 21.41b).
   - The intact superior oblique muscle causes intorsion of the eye at rest, which increases on attempted downgaze.
   - Normal abduction because the lateral rectus is intact (Fig. 21.41c).
   - Weakness of the medial rectus limiting adduction (Fig. 21.41d).
   - Weakness of superior rectus and inferior oblique, limiting elevation (Fig. 21.41e).
   - Weakness of inferior rectus limiting depression (Fig. 21.41f).
   - Parasympathetic palsy causing a dilated pupil associated with defective accommodation.
   - Partial involvement will produce milder degrees of ophthalmoplegia.
2. **Aberrant regeneration** may follow acute traumatic and compression, but not vascular, third nerve palsies. This is because the endoneural nerve sheaths, which may be breached in traumatic and compressive lesions, remain intact in vascular pathology. Bizarre defects in ocular motility such as elevation of the upper eyelid on attempted adduction or depression (the pseudo-Graefe phenomenon), are caused by misdirection of regenerating axons which reinnervate the wrong extraocular muscle. The pupil may also be involved.

Causes of isolated third nerve palsy

1. **Idiopathic:** about 25% have no known cause.
2. **Vascular** disease, such as due to hypertension and diabetes, is the most common cause of pupil-sparing third nerve palsy. All patients should therefore have blood pressure measurement, urinalysis and plasma glucose estimation. In most cases spontaneous recovery occurs within 3 months. Diabetic third nerve palsy is often associated with periorbital pain and may occasionally be the presenting feature of diabetes. The presence of pain is therefore not helpful in differentiating aneurysmal and diabetic third nerve palsy.
3. **Aneurysm** of the posterior communicating artery at its junction with the internal carotid (see Fig. 21.37) is a very important cause of isolated painful third nerve palsy with involvement of the pupil. Patients with a high probability of aneurysm should undergo conventional catheter angiography because other techniques (MR, MRA or CTA) may not be sufficiently sensitive. If the probability of aneurysm is low and the risk from conventional arteriography high (e.g. elderly patient, risk of stroke) then non-invasive investigations may be a reasonable approach.

758

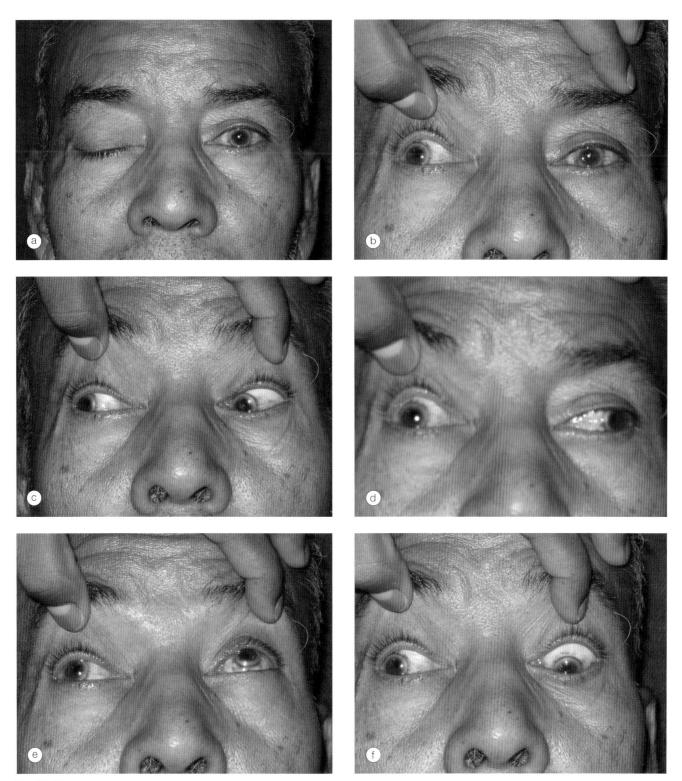

Fig. 21.41
Right third nerve palsy. **(a)** Total right ptosis; **(b)** right exotropia in the primary position; **(c)** normal abduction; **(d)** limitation of adduction; **(e)** limitation of elevation; **(f)** limitation of depression (Courtesy of S Kumar Puri)

4. **Trauma,** both direct and secondary to subdural haematoma with uncal herniation, is also a common cause (see Fig. 21.38). However, the development of third nerve palsy following relatively trivial head trauma, not associated with loss of consciousness, should alert the clinician to the possibility of an associated basal intracranial tumour which has caused the nerve trunk to be stretched and tethered.

5. **Miscellaneous** uncommon causes include tumours, syphilis, giant cell arteritis or other types of vasculitis associated with collagen vascular disorders.

> **NB** Brief episodes of third nerve dysfunction with spontaneous recovery may be idiopathic and may occur with migraine, compression, ischaemia and alterations in intracranial pressure. Myasthenia may also mimic intermittent pupil-sparing third nerve palsy.

Treatment

1. **Non-surgical** treatment options include the use of Fresnel prisms if the angle of deviation is small, uniocular occlusion to avoid diplopia (if ptosis is partial or recovering) and botulinum toxin injection into the uninvolved lateral rectus muscle to prevent its contracture before the deviation improves or stabilizes (see Chapter 20).

2. **Surgical** treatment, as with other ocular motor nerve palsies, should be contemplated only after all spontaneous improvement has ceased. This is usually not earlier than 6 months from the date of onset (see Chapter 20).

FOURTH NERVE

Anatomy

1. **Important features** of the fourth (trochlear) nerve are the following:
   - It is the only cranial nerve to emerge from the dorsal aspect of the brain.
   - It is a crossed cranial nerve; this means that the fourth nerve nucleus innervates the contralateral superior oblique muscle.
   - It is a very long and slender nerve.

2. **The nucleus** of the fourth nerve is located at the level of the inferior colliculi ventral to the sylvian aqueduct (Fig. 21.42). It is caudal to, and continuous with, the third nerve nuclear complex.

3. **The fasciculus** consists of axons which curve posteriorly around the aqueduct and decussate completely in the anterior medullary velum.

4. **The trunk** leaves the brainstem on the dorsal surface, just caudal to the inferior colliculus. It then curves laterally around the brainstem, runs forwards beneath the free

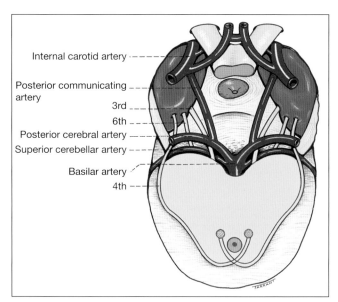

Fig. 21.42
Dorsal view of the course of the fourth nerve

edge of the tentorium, and (like the third nerve) passes between the posterior cerebral artery and the superior cerebellar artery. It then pierces the dura and enters the cavernous sinus.

5. **The intracavernous** part runs in the lateral wall of the sinus, inferiorly to the third nerve and above the first division of the fifth. In the anterior part of the cavernous sinus it rises and passes through the superior orbital fissure above and lateral to the annulus of Zinn.

6. **The intraorbital** part innervates the superior oblique muscle.

Diagnosis

Acute onset of vertical diplopia in the absence of ptosis, combined with a characteristic head posture, strongly suggests fourth nerve disease. The features of nuclear, fascicular and peripheral fourth nerve palsies are clinically identical, except that nuclear palsies produce contralateral superior oblique weakness.

1. **Signs** of a left fourth nerve palsy.
   - Left hypertropia ('left over right') in the primary position when the uninvolved right eye is fixating due to weakness of the left superior oblique (Fig. 21.43a).
   - Left limitation in depression in adduction due to superior oblique weakness (Fig. 21.43b).
   - Excyclotorsion.
   - Diplopia which is vertical, torsional and worse on looking down.
   - The left hypertropia increases on right gaze due to left inferior oblique overaction (Fig. 21.43c).

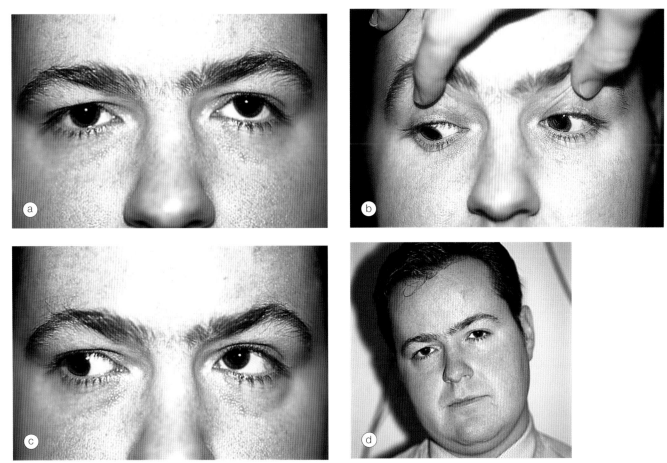

Fig. 21.43
Left fourth nerve palsy. **(a)** Left hypertropia (left-over-right) in the primary position; **(b)** left limitation of depression in adduction; **(c)** left inferior oblique overaction on right gaze; **(d)** head tilt to right, face turn to left and chin depressed

2. **Abnormal head posture** is adopted to avoid diplopia (Fig. 21.43d).
   - To intort the eye (alleviate excyclotorsion) there is contralateral head tilt.
   - To alleviate the inability to depress the eye in adduction, the face is turned to the right and the chin is depressed.

   NB The right eye cannot look down and to the left or intort – the head therefore does this and thus compensates.

3. **Bilateral involvement** should always be suspected until proved otherwise.
   - Right hypertropia in left gaze, left hypertropia in right gaze.
   - Greater than 10° of cyclodeviation on double Maddox rod test (see below).
   - 'V' pattern esotropia.
   - Bilaterally positive Bielschowsky test (see below).

Special tests

1. **Parks three-step test** is very useful in the diagnosis of fourth nerve palsy and is performed as follows:
   a. First step. Assess which eye is hypertropic in the primary position. Left hypertropia (see Fig. 21.43a) may be caused by weakness of one of the following four muscles: one of the depressors of the left eye (superior oblique or inferior rectus) or one of the elevators of the right eye (superior rectus or inferior oblique). In a fourth nerve palsy the involved eye is higher.
   b. Step two. Determine whether the left hypertropia is greater in right gaze or left gaze. Increase on right gaze (see Fig. 21.43c) implicates either the right superior rectus or left superior oblique. Increase on left gaze implicates either the right inferior oblique or left inferior rectus. (In fourth nerve palsy the deviation is Worse On Opposite Gaze – WOOG.)
   c. Step three. The Bielschowsky head tilt test is performed

with the patient fixating a straight ahead target at 3 metres. The head is tilted to the right (Fig. 21.44a) and then to the left. Increase of left hypertropia on left head tilt (Fig. 21.44b) implicates the left superior oblique and increase of right hypertropia on left head tilt implicates the right inferior rectus. (In fourth nerve palsy the deviation is Better On Opposite Tilt – BOOT.)

2. **Double Maddox rod test**
   - Red and green Maddox rods, with the cylinders vertical, are placed one in front of either eye.
   - Each eye will therefore perceive a more or less horizontal line of light.
   - In the presence of cyclodeviation, the line perceived by the paretic eye will be tilted and therefore distinct from that of the other eye.
   - One Maddox rod is then rotated till fusion (super-imposition) of the lines is achieved.
   - The amount of rotation can be measured in degrees and indicates the extent of cyclodeviation.
   - Unilateral fourth nerve palsy is characterized by less than 10° of cyclodeviation whilst bilateral fourths may have greater than 20° of cyclodeviation. This can also be measured with a synoptophore.

Causes of isolated fourth nerve palsy

1. **Congenital** lesions are frequent, although symptoms may not develop until decompensation occurs in adult life. Unlike acquired lesions patients are not usually aware of the torsional aspect. Examination of old photographs for the presence of an abnormal head posture may be helpful, as is the presence of an increased vertical prism fusional range.
2. **Trauma** frequently causes bilateral fourth nerve palsy. The long and slender nerves are vulnerable as they decussate in the anterior medullary velum through impact with the tentorial edge. Bilateral lesions are often thought to be unilateral until squint surgery is performed, following which the contralateral fourth nerve palsy may be revealed.
3. **Vascular** lesions are common but aneurysms and tumours are extremely rare.

NB Routine neuroimaging for isolated trochlear palsy is not required.

SIXTH NERVE

Nucleus

The nucleus of the sixth (abducens) nerve lies at the mid level of the pons, ventral to the floor of the fourth ventricle,

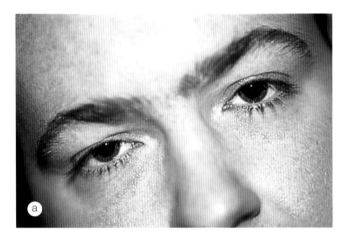
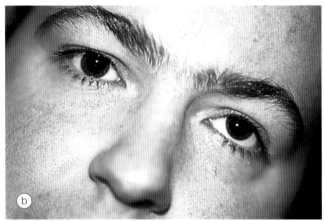

Fig. 21.44
Positive Bielschowsky test in left fourth nerve palsy. **(a)** No hypertropia on right head tilt; **(b)** marked left hypertropia on left head tilt

where it is closely related to the horizontal gaze centre. The fasciculus of the seventh nerve curves around the abducent nucleus and produces an elevation in the floor of the fourth ventricle (facial colliculus) (Fig. 21.45). Isolated sixth nerve palsy is therefore never nuclear in origin. A lesion in and around the sixth nerve nucleus causes the following signs.
- Ipsilateral weakness of abduction as a result of involvement of the sixth nerve.
- Failure of horizontal gaze towards the side of the lesion resulting from involvement of the horizontal gaze centre in the pontine paramedian reticular formation (PPRF).
- Ipsilateral lower motor neuron facial nerve palsy caused by concomitant involvement of the facial fasciculus is common.

Fasciculus

The fasciculus passes ventrally to leave the brainstem at the pontomedullary junction, just lateral to the pyramidal prominence.

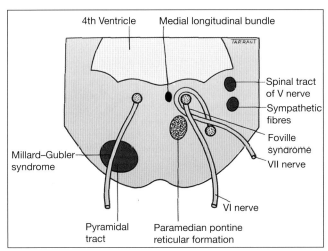

Fig. 21.45
The pons at the level of the sixth nerve nucleus

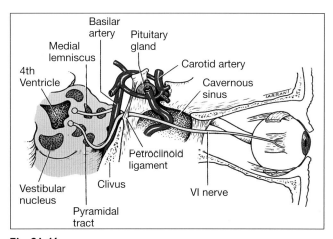

Fig. 21.46
Lateral view of the course of the sixth nerve

1. **Foville syndrome** involves the fasciculus as it passes through the PPRF and is most frequently caused by vascular disease or tumours involving the dorsal pons. It is characterized by ipsilateral involvement of the fifth to eighth cranial nerves and central sympathetic fibres.
   - Fifth nerve – facial analgesia.
   - Sixth nerve palsy combined with gaze palsy (PPRF).
   - Seventh nerve (nuclear or fascicular damage) – facial weakness.
   - Eighth nerve – deafness.
   - Central Horner syndrome.
2. **Millard–Gubler syndrome** involves the fasciculus as it passes through the pyramidal tract and is most frequently caused by vascular disease, tumours or demyelination. It is characterized by the following.
   - Ipsilateral sixth nerve palsy.
   - Contralateral hemiplegia (since the pyramidal tracts decussate further inferiorly, in the medulla, to control contralateral voluntary movement).
   - Variable number of signs of a dorsal pontine lesion.

Basilar

The basilar part leaves the brainstem at the pontomedullary junction and enters the prepontine basilar cistern. It then passes upwards close to the base of the skull and is crossed by the anterior inferior cerebellar artery (Fig. 21.46). It pierces the dura below the posterior clinoids and angles forwards over the tip of the petrous bone, passing through or around the inferior petrosal sinus, through Dorello canal (under the petroclinoid ligament), to enter the cavernous sinus. The following are important causes of damage to the basilar part of the nerve.

1. **Acoustic neuroma** may damage the sixth nerve at the pontomedullary junction (Fig. 21.47). It should be emphasized that the first symptom of an acoustic neuroma is

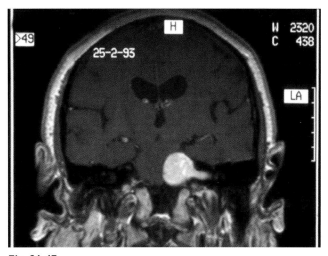

Fig. 21.47
Coronal MR with enhancement of an acoustic neuroma (Courtesy of N Rogers)

hearing loss and the first sign diminished corneal sensitivity. It is therefore very important to test hearing and corneal sensation in all patients with sixth nerve palsy.
2. **Nasopharyngeal tumours** may invade the skull and its foramina and damage the nerve during its basilar course.
3. **Raised intracranial pressure** caused by posterior fossa tumours or idiopathic intracranial hypertension may cause a downward displacement of the brainstem. This may stretch the sixth nerve over the petrous tip (see Fig. 21.15) between its point of emergence from the brainstem and its point of entry into the cavernous sinus.

NB In this situation, sixth nerve palsy, which may be bilateral, is a false localizing sign.

4. **Basal skull fracture** may cause both unilateral and bilateral palsies.

5. **Gradenigo syndrome,** most frequently caused by mastoiditis or acute petrositis, may result in damage of the sixth nerve at the petrous tip. The petrositis is frequently accompanied by facial weakness and pain, and hearing difficulties.

Intracavernous and intraorbital

1. **The intracavernous** part runs forwards below the third and fourth nerves, as well as the first division of the fifth. Although the other nerves are protected within the wall of the sinus, the sixth is most medially situated and runs through the middle of the sinus in close relation to the internal carotid artery. It is therefore more prone to damage than the other nerves. Occasionally, an intracavernous sixth nerve palsy is accompanied by a post-ganglionic Horner syndrome (Parkinson sign) because in its intracavernous course the sixth nerve is joined by sympathetic branches from the paracarotid plexus. The causes of intracavernous sixth nerve and third nerve lesions are similar.

2. **The intraorbital** part enters the orbit through the superior orbital fissure within the annulus of Zinn to innervate the lateral rectus muscle.

Diagnosis

1. **Signs** of a left sixth nerve palsy.
   - Left esotropia in the primary position due to unopposed action of the left medial rectus (Fig. 21.48a).
   - Esotropia is characteristically worse for a distant target and less or absent for near fixation.
   - Marked limitation of left abduction due to weakness of the left lateral rectus (Fig. 21.48b).
   - Normal left adduction (Fig. 21.48c).
2. **Compensatory face turn** into the field of action of the paralyzed muscle (i.e. to the right) to minimize diplopia, so that the eyes do not need to look towards the field of action of the paralyzed muscle (i.e. to the right).
3. **Causes** of isolated sixth nerve palsies have already been mentioned.

   NB In contrast with third nerve palsy, aneurysms rarely affect the sixth nerve but vascular causes are common.

Differential diagnosis

The following conditions may mimic sixth nerve palsy.

1. **Myasthenia gravis** can mimic virtually any ocular motility defect. Distinguishing features include variability

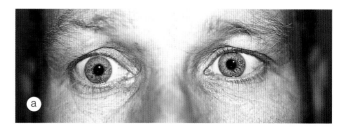
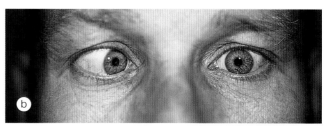
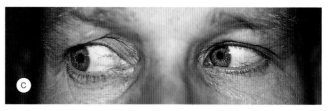

Fig. 21.48
Left sixth nerve palsy. **(a)** Slight left esotropia in the primary position; **(b)** limitation of left abduction; **(c)** normal left adduction

of diplopia and other signs such as lid fatigue and Cogan twitch sign.

2. **Restrictive thyroid myopathy** involving the medial rectus may give rise to limitation of abduction. Associated features include orbital and eyelid signs and a positive forced duction test (see Chapter 6).
3. **Medial orbital wall blowout fracture** with entrapment of the medial rectus giving rise to limitation of abduction (see Chapter 23).
4. **Orbital myositis** involving the lateral rectus is characterized by weakness of abduction and pain when this is attempted (see Chapter 6).
5. **Duane syndrome** is a congenital condition characterized by defective abduction and narrowing of the palpebral fissure on adduction (see Chapter 20).
6. **Convergence spasm** typically affects young adults and is characterized by convergence with miosis and increased accommodation.
7. **Divergence paralysis** is a rare condition which may be difficult to distinguish from unilateral or bilateral sixth nerve palsy. However, unlike sixth nerve palsy the esotropia may remain the same or diminish on lateral gaze.
8. **Infantile esotropia** (see Chapter 20).

SUPRANUCLEAR DISORDERS OF OCULAR MOTILITY

Conjugate eye movements

Conjugate eye movements or 'versions' are binocular movements in which the eyes move synchronously and symmetrically in the same direction. The three main types are: (a) *saccadic*, (b) *smooth pursuit* and (c) *non-optical reflex*. Saccadic and pursuit movements are controlled at both cerebral and brainstem levels. Supranuclear disturbances produce gaze palsies, characterized by absence of diplopia and normal vestibulo-ocular reflexes (e.g. oculocephalic movements and caloric stimulation).

Saccadic movements

1. **Function** of saccadic (fixating) movements is to place the object of interest on to the fovea rapidly or to move the eyes from one object to another. This can be done voluntarily or reflexly, triggered by the presence of an object in the peripheral visual field. Voluntary saccades are similar to the gunnery system of rapidly locating a moving target.
2. **Pathway** for horizontal saccades originates in the premotor cortex (the frontal eye fields). From there, fibres pass to the contralateral horizontal gaze centre in the PPRF. Each frontal lobe therefore initiates contralateral saccades. Irritative lesions may therefore cause ocular deviation to the opposite side.

Smooth pursuit movements

1. **Function** of pursuit movements is to maintain fixation on a target once it has been located by the saccadic system. The stimulus is movement of the image near the fovea and the movements are slow and smooth.
2. **Pathway** originates in the peristriate cortex of the occipital lobe. The fibres descend and terminate in the ipsilateral horizontal gaze centre in the PPRF. Each occipital lobe therefore controls pursuit to the ipsilateral side.

Non-optical reflexes

1. **Function** of non-optical (vestibular) reflexes is to maintain eye position with respect to any changes of head and body position.
2. **Pathway** originates in the labyrinths and proprioceptors in the neck muscles which mediate information concerning head and neck movements. Afferent fibres synapse in the vestibular nuclei and pass to the horizontal gaze centre in the PPRF.

Horizontal gaze palsy

Anatomy

- Horizontal eye movements are generated from the horizontal gaze centre in the PPRF (Fig. 21.49). From here motor neurons connect to the ipsilateral sixth nerve nucleus which innervates the lateral rectus.
- From the sixth nerve nucleus internuclear neurons cross the midline at the level of the pons and pass up the contralateral medial longitudinal fasciculus (MLF) to synapse with motor neurons in the medial rectus subnucleus in the third nerve complex which innervates the medial rectus.
- Stimulation of the PPRF on one side therefore causes a conjugate movement of the eyes to the same side.
- Loss of normal horizontal eye movements occurs when these pathways are disrupted. The causes are shown in Table 21.5.

Diagnosis

1. **PPRF** lesion gives rise to ipsilateral horizontal gaze palsy with inability to look in the direction of the lesion.
2. **MLF** lesion is responsible for the clinical syndrome of internuclear ophthalmoplegia (INO). A left internuclear ophthalmoplegia is characterized by:
   - Straight eyes in the primary position (Fig. 21.50a).

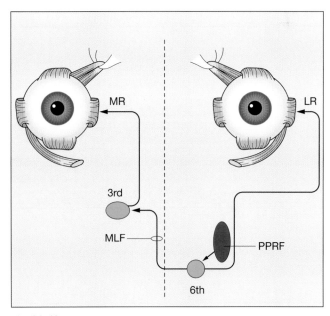

Fig. 21.49
Anatomical pathways for horizontal eye movements (PPRF = pontine paramedian reticular formation; MLF = medial longitudinal fasciculus; MR = medial rectus; LR = lateral rectus)

Table 21.5 Causes of internuclear ophthalmoplegia

- Demyelination
- Vascular disease
- Tumours of the brainstem and fourth ventricle
- Trauma
- Encephalitis
- Hydrocephalus
- Progressive supranuclear palsy
- Drug-induced
- Remote effects of carcinoma

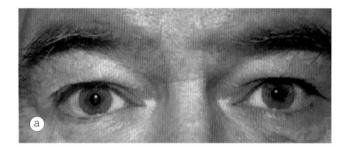

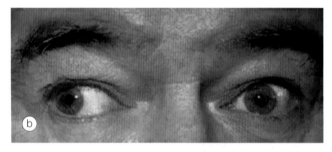

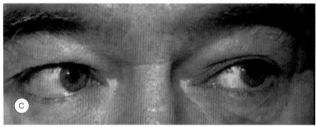

Fig. 21.50
Left internuclear ophthalmoplegia. **(a)** Straight in the primary position; **(b)** limitation of left adduction on right gaze; **(c)** normal left abduction on left gaze

- Defective left adduction and ataxic nystagmus of the right eye on right gaze (Fig. 21.50b).
- Left gaze is normal (Fig. 21.50c).
- Convergence is intact if the lesion is discrete; this may help to differentiate INO from myasthenia.
- Vertical nystagmus on attempted upgaze.

3. **Bilateral INO** is characterized by:
   - Limitation of right adduction and ataxic nystagmus of the left eye on left gaze (Fig. 21.51a).

- Limitation of left adduction and ataxic nystagmus of the right eye on right gaze (Fig. 21.51b).
- Convergence is usually intact if the lesion is discrete but may be absent if the lesion is extensive (Fig. 21.51c).

4. **PPRF and MLF** combined lesions on the same side give rise to the 'one-and-a-half syndrome' which is characterized by a combination of ipsilateral gaze palsy and INO so that the only residual movement is abduction of the contralateral eye which also exhibits ataxic nystagmus.

Vertical gaze palsy

Anatomy

Vertical eye movements are generated from the vertical gaze centre (rostral interstitial nucleus of the MLF) which lies in the midbrain just dorsal to the red nucleus. From the vertical gaze centre, impulses pass to the subnuclei of the eye muscles controlling vertical gaze in both eyes. Cells mediating upward and downward eye movements are intermingled in the vertical gaze centre, although selective paralysis of up-gaze and down-gaze may occur in spite of this.

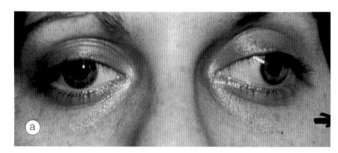

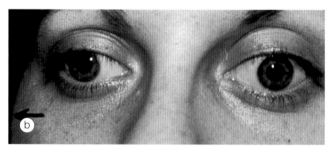

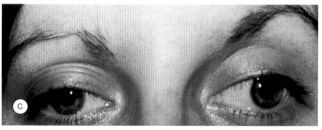

Fig. 21.51
Bilateral internuclear ophthalmoplegia. **(a)** Limitation of right adduction on left gaze; **(b)** limitation of left adduction on right gaze; **(c)** absence of convergence because the lesion is extensive

Parinaud dorsal midbrain syndrome

1. Signs
- Straight eyes in the primary position (Fig. 21.52a).
- Supranuclear up-gaze palsy (Fig. 21.52b).
- Defective convergence (Fig. 21.52c).
- Large pupils with light-near dissociation.
- Lid retraction (Collier sign).
- Convergence-retraction nystagmus.

2. Causes
- **a. *In children:*** aqueduct stenosis, meningitis and pinealoma (Fig. 21.52d).
- **b. *In young adults:*** demyelination, trauma and arteriovenous malformations.
- **c. *In the elderly:*** midbrain vascular accidents, mass lesions involving the periaqueductal grey matter and posterior fossa aneurysms.

Progressive supranuclear palsy

Progressive supranuclear palsy (Steele–Richardson–Olszewski syndrome) is a severe degenerative disease which presents in old age and is characterized by:

- Supranuclear gaze palsy, which initially primarily affects down-gaze.
- As the disease progresses up-gaze is also affected.
- Horizontal movements subsequently become impaired and eventually global gaze palsy develops.
- Pseudobulbar palsy.
- Extrapyramidal rigidity, gait ataxia and dementia.
- Paralysis of convergence.

CHRONIC PROGRESSIVE EXTERNAL OPHTHALMOPLEGIA

Chronic progressive external ophthalmoplegia (CPEO) refers to a group of disorders characterized by ptosis and slowly progressive bilateral ocular immobility.

Classification

1. Isolated presents in adult life and is the mildest.

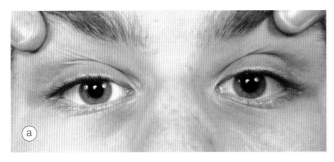
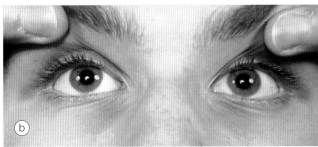
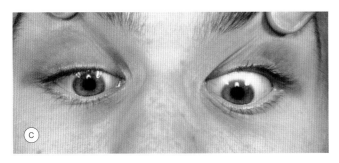
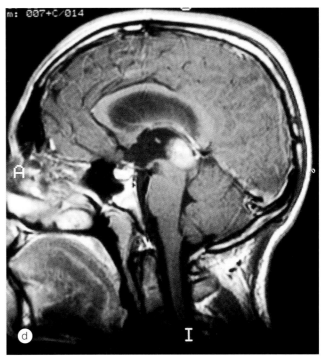

Fig. 21.52
Parinaud syndrome. **(a)** Eye straight in the primary position; **(b)** defective up-gaze; **(c)** defective convergence; **(d)** MR sagittal view shows a pinealoma and a dilated third ventricle (Courtesy of D Thomas)

2. **Oculopharyngeal dystrophy** is of intermediate severity and presents in adolescence or early childhood. It is characterized by weakness of the pharyngeal muscles and wasting of the temporalis.
3. **Kearns–Sayre syndrome,** the most severe, presents in childhood and is associated with pigmentary retinopathy, heart block and ragged-red fibre myopathy (see Chapter 24).

Diagnosis

1. **Ptosis,** usually the first sign, is bilateral and may be asymmetrical (Fig. 21.53a). Surgical correction may improve compensatory head posture but does not restore normal movements and is associated with a risk of corneal exposure. Pupils are usually not involved.
2. **External ophthalmoplegia** begins in young adulthood and typically is symmetrical. It is characterized by progressive course without remission or exacerbation. Initially up-gaze is involved (Fig. 21.53b); subsequently lateral gaze is affected (Fig. 21.53c and d) so that the eyes may become virtually fixed. Because of this

symmetrical loss of eye movements diplopia is rare, although reading may be a problem due to inadequate convergence. A minority of patients with diplopia may benefit from surgery.

NB Saccades are slow in CPEO unlike ocular myasthenia, in which saccades over a short distance are quick.

INTRACRANIAL ANEURYSM

Anatomy

The arterial supply to the brain comes from the internal carotid and vertebral arteries.

1. **Vertebral arteries** enter the cranial cavity through the foramen magnum and unite into the basilar artery, which ascends on the ventral surface of the brainstem. After

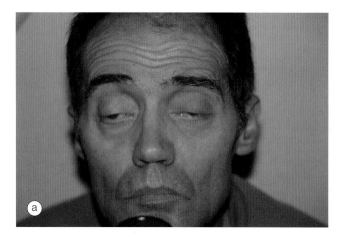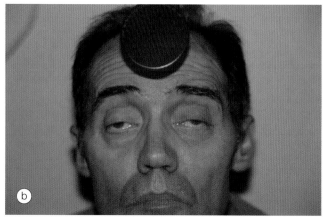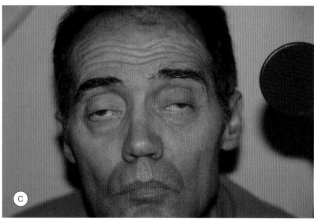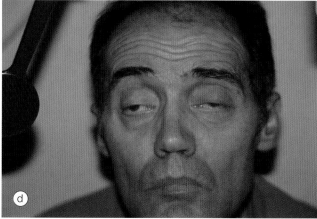

Fig. 21.53
Progressive external ophthalmoplegia. **(a)** Severe bilateral ptosis; **(b)** defective up-gaze; **(c)** defective left gaze; **(d)** defective right gaze
(Courtesy of J Yanguela)

giving rise to branches to the brainstem, the basilar artery divides into its terminal branches: the posterior cerebral arteries.

2. **Internal carotid arteries** enter the base of the skull through the carotid canal and the cranial cavity through the foramen lacerum, at the apex of the petrous part of the temporal bone. They then run forwards in the cavernous sinus, lateral to the pituitary gland before ascending, lateral to the optic chiasm and dividing into the anterior and middle cerebral arteries.

3. **Circle of Willis.** The anterior cerebral arteries are connected by the anterior communicating artery. The middle and posterior cerebral arteries are connected by the posterior communicating artery. This anastomosis forms the circle of Willis, which lies in the subarachnoid space on the ventral surface of the brain (Fig. 21.54).

Neurological considerations

Intracranial aneurysms are saccular arterial out-pouchings that most commonly develop at the branching points of the major arteries coursing through the subarachnoid space at the base of the brain; 85% arise from the anterior half of the circle of Willis. Their prevalence ranges from 1% to 6% among adults in large autopsy series. Aneurysms are multiple (usually two or three) in about 25% of cases.

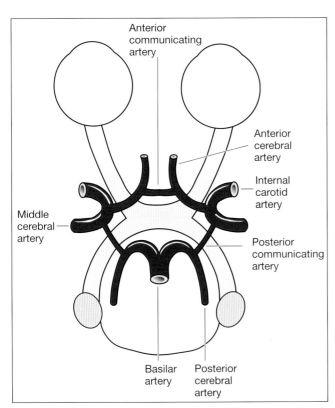

Fig. 21.54
Dorsal view of the circle of Willis (Courtesy of G Robertson)

The majority remain asymptomatic during life although occasionally they may cause the following life-threatening complications.

1. **Subarachnoid haemorrhage** due to rupture is by far the most frequent complication which presents with sudden onset of severe headache, photophobia, clouding consciousness, vomiting and signs of meningeal irritation, including neck stiffness and positive Kernig sign. Blood-stained CSF is revealed on lumbar puncture. Approximately 12% of patients die before receiving medical attention, 40% of hospitalized patients die within one month and more than one-third of those that survive suffer major neurological deficits.

2. **Pressure effects** are less frequent and associated with 'giant' aneurysms (>25mm). The most common symptom is headache and associated signs depend on the location of the lesion and are frequently neuro-ophthalmological. Such aneurysms also have a high subsequent rupture rate with an estimated frequency of 6% per year. The interval between warning mass signs and rupture varies from 1 day to 4 months so that early diagnosis is paramount.

Neuroimaging

MR, MRA or conventional (intra-arterial) angiography are useful in diagnosis. Whilst the first two are capable of demonstrating large to medium-sized aneurysms, they often fail to detect those smaller than 5mm. Despite infrequent but potentially serious risks including vascular damage and permanent neurological deficits, conventional angiography is still the 'gold standard', particularly prior to surgical intervention.

Treatment

Definitive treatment is surgical, aimed at excluding the aneurysmal sac from the intracranial circulation while preserving the parent artery. This involves placing a clip around the neck of the aneurysm or, less frequently, the insertion of soft metallic coils within the lumen of the aneurysm (Fig. 21.55).

Ocular motor nerve palsies

1. **Isolated third nerve palsy** may be caused by compression by an aneurysm of the posterior communicating artery at its junction with the internal carotid artery in the subarachnoid space. Presentation is typically with ipsilateral frontal headache and total third nerve palsy (with internal ophthalmoplegia).

2. **Isolated sixth nerve palsy** can occur with aneurysms of the intracavernous part of the internal carotid artery, but very rarely from involvement within the subarachnoid space.

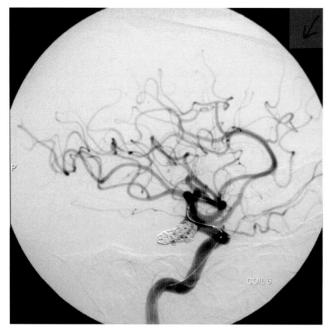

Fig. 21.55
Coil occlusion of an aneurysm (Courtesy of E Pringle)

3. **Combined palsies** of the third and sixth nerves occur with intracavernous carotid aneurysms, although this may also occur in other cavernous sinus lesions. The fourth nerve may also be involved but this is frequently obscured by the other lesions. Although parasympathetic innervation is commonly damaged, mydriasis may not occur and the pupil may even be miosed because of coexistent damage to the sympathetic fibres.

NB An important sign of cavernous sinus lesions is sensory loss over the distribution of the first division of the trigeminal nerve.

Visual loss

1. **Monocular** visual loss is most frequently caused by compression of the intracranial part of the optic nerve by aneurysms arising from the internal carotid artery near the origin of the ophthalmic artery, at its terminal bifurcation. The clinical picture is that of unilateral acute or progressive visual loss occasionally associated with orbital pain, which may initially be misdiagnosed as retrobulbar neuritis.
2. **Visual field defects** involving the nasal field may be caused by a giant aneurysm at or near the origin of the ophthalmic artery. Rarely, a giant aneurysm may compress the lateral aspect of the chiasm and cause a nasal field defect which is initially unilateral but may become bilateral if the chiasm is pushed across against the opposite carotid artery. Homonymous defects and cortical blindness may be caused by transient or permanent ischaemia of the retrochiasmal visual pathways.

NB Carotid aneurysms may also invade the sella and mimic pituitary adenomas.

Terson syndrome

Terson syndrome refers to the combination of intraocular haemorrhage and subarachnoid haemorrhage secondary to aneurysmal rupture, most commonly arising from the anterior communicating artery. However, intraocular haemorrhage may also occur with subdural haematoma and acute elevation of intracranial pressure from other causes. The haemorrhage is frequently bilateral and is typically intraretinal and/or preretinal (subhyaloid – Fig. 21.56), although occasionally subhyaloid blood may break into the vitreous. It is probable that intraocular bleeding is due to retinal venous stasis secondary to increase in cavernous sinus pressure. Vitreous haemorrhage usually resolves spontaneously with a few months and the long-term visual prognosis is good in the majority of cases. Early vitrectomy may be considered for dense bilateral vitreous involvement.

NB Papilloedema may be a feature of subarachnoid haemorrhage. Elevation of intracranial pressure may be caused by blockage of CSF flow within the ventricular system (obstructive hydrocephalus) or defective CSF absorption by the arachnoid villi.

NYSTAGMUS

Introduction

Physiological principles

Nystagmus is a repetitive, involuntary, to-and-fro eye oscillation of the eyes, which may be physiological or pathological. Thus, nystagmus that occurs in response to rotation of an optokinetic drum or of the body in space is normal and acts to preserve clear vision. Ocular movements that bring about fixation on an object of interest are called foveating and those that move the fovea away from the object are defoveating. In pathological nystagmus, each cycle of movement is usually initiated by an involuntary, defoveating drift of the eye away from the object of interest, followed by a returning refixation saccadic movement. The plane of nystagmus may be horizontal, vertical, torsional or non-specific. The amplitude of nystagmus refers to how far the eyes move, while the frequency refers to how often the eyes oscillate. On the basis of amplitude, nystagmus

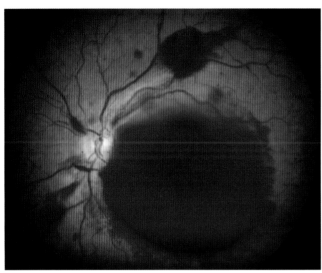

Fig. 21.56
Intraretinal and subhyaloid haemorrhages in Terson syndrome

nystagmus can be divided into gaze-evoked (i.e. vestibular) and gaze-paretic, which is slow and usually indicates brainstem damage.

2. **Pendular** nystagmus is non-saccadic in that both the foveating and defoveating movements are slow (i.e. the velocity of nystagmus is equal in both directions).
   * Congenital pendular nystagmus is horizontal, conjugate and tends to convert to jerk on lateral gaze.
   * Acquired pendular nystagmus has horizontal, vertical and torsional components.
   * If the horizontal and vertical components of pendular nystagmus are in phase (i.e. occur simultaneously) the perceived direction becomes oblique.
   * If the horizontal and vertical components are out of phase the direction becomes elliptic or rotary.
3. **Mixed** nystagmus involves pendular nystagmus in the primary position and jerk nystagmus on lateral gaze.

The characteristics of any form of nystagmus can be documented using the schematic shown in Figure 21.57.

Physiological nystagmus

1. **End-point** nystagmus is a fine jerk nystagmus of moderate frequency found when the eyes are in extreme positions of gaze. The fast phase is in the direction of gaze.
2. **Optokinetic** nystagmus is a jerk nystagmus induced by moving repetitive targets across the visual field. The slow phase is a pursuit movement in which the eyes follow the target; the fast phase is a saccadic movement in the opposite direction as the eyes fixate on the next target.

may be fine or coarse; while the frequency may be high, moderate or low.

Classification

1. **Jerk** nystagmus is saccadic with a slow defoveating 'drift' movement and a fast corrective refoveating saccadic movement. The direction of nystagmus is described in terms of the direction of the fast component, so that jerk nystagmus may be right, left, up, down or rotatory. Jerk

Fig. 21.57
Schematic for documenting nystagmus

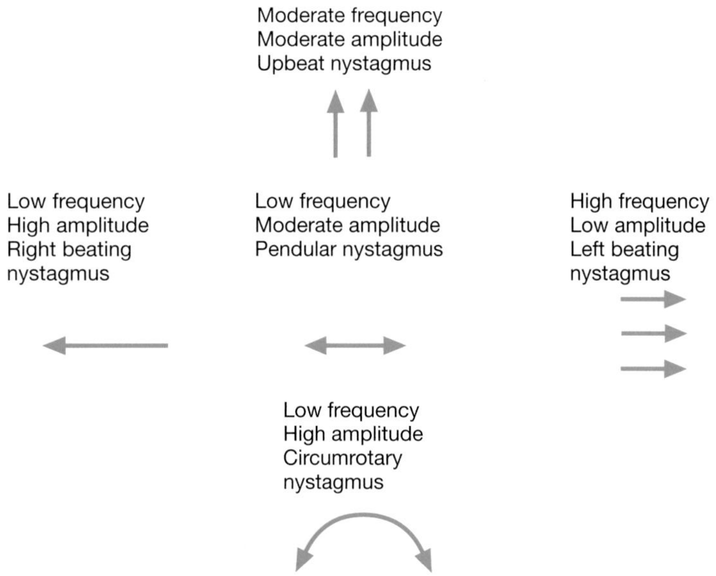

Moderate frequency
Moderate amplitude
Upbeat nystagmus

Low frequency
High amplitude
Right beating
nystagmus

Low frequency
Moderate amplitude
Pendular nystagmus

High frequency
Low amplitude
Left beating
nystagmus

Low frequency
High amplitude
Circumrotary
nystagmus

If the optokinetic tape or drum is moved from right to left, the left parieto-occipital region controls the slow (pursuit) phase to the left, and the left frontal lobe controls the rapid (saccadic) phase to the right. Optokinetic nystagmus is useful for detecting malingerers who feign blindness and for testing visual acuity in the very young. It may also be helpful in determining the cause of an isolated homonymous hemianopia.

3. **Vestibular** nystagmus is a jerk nystagmus caused by altered input from the vestibular nuclei to the horizontal gaze centres. The slow phase is initiated by the vestibular nuclei and the fast phase by the brainstem and frontomesencephalic pathway. Rotatory nystagmus is usually caused by pathological conditions affecting the vestibular system. Vestibular nystagmus may be elicited by caloric stimulation as follows:
   - When cold water is poured into the right ear the patient will develop left jerk nystagmus (i.e. fast phase to the left).
   - When warm water is poured into the right ear the patient will develop right jerk nystagmus (i.e. fast phase to the right). A useful mnemonic is 'COWS' (cold-opposite, warm-same) indicating the direction of the nystagmus.
   - When cold water is poured into both ears simultaneously, a jerk nystagmus with the fast phase upwards develops; warm water in both ears elicits nystagmus with the fast phase downwards (cold 'slows things down').

Motor imbalance nystagmus

Motor imbalance nystagmus is the result of primary defects in the efferent mechanisms.

Primary congenital nystagmus

1. **Inheritance** is XLR or AD.
2. **Presentation** is about 2–3 months after birth and persists throughout life.
3. **Signs** Uniplanar horizontal nystagmus, usually of the jerk type. The plane remains horizontal on up-gaze and down-gaze.
   - It may be dampened by convergence and is not present during sleep.
   - There is usually a null point – a position of gaze in which nystagmus is minimal.
   - In order to move the eyes into the null point, an AHP may be adopted.

NB Adults with congenital forms of nystagmus do not notice oscillopsia but it is noticed by adults with acquired nystagmus.

Spasmas nutans

1. **Presentation** of this rare condition is between 3 and 18 months.
2. **Signs**
   - Unilateral or bilateral, small-amplitude, high-frequency horizontal nystagmus associated with head nodding.
   - It is frequently asymmetrical with increased amplitude in abduction.
   - Vertical and torsional components may be present.
3. **Causes**
   - Idiopathic which spontaneously resolves by age 3 years.
   - Glioma of anterior visual pathway, empty sella syndrome and porencephalic cyst.

Latent nystagmus

Latent nystagmus is associated with infantile esotropia and dissociated vertical deviation (see Chapter 20). It is characterized by the following:
- With both eyes open there is no nystagmus.
- Horizontal nystagmus becomes apparent on covering one eye or reducing the amount of light reaching the eye.
- Fast phase is in the direction of the uncovered fixating eye.
- Occasionally, an element of latency may be superimposed on a manifest nystagmus so that when one eye is covered the amplitude of nystagmus increases (latent-manifest nystagmus).

Periodic alternating nystagmus

1. **Signs**
   - Conjugate horizontal jerk nystagmus that periodically reverses its direction.
   - Each cycle may be divided into active and quiescent phases as follows:
   - During the active phase, the amplitude, frequency and slow-phase velocity of nystagmus first progressively increase then decrease.
   - This is followed by a short, quiet interlude, lasting 4–20 seconds, during which time the eyes are steady and show low-intensity, often pendular movements.
   - A similar sequence in the opposite direction occurs thereafter, the whole cycle lasting 1–3 minutes.
2. **Causes** include congenital, cerebellar disease, ataxia telangiectasia (Louis-Bar syndrome) and drugs such as phenytoin.

Convergence-retraction nystagmus

Convergence-retraction nystagmus is caused by co-contraction of the extraocular muscles, particularly the medial recti.

I. Signs
- Jerk nystagmus is induced by passing an optokinetic tape or drum downwards.
- The upward refixation saccade brings the two eyes towards each other in a convergence movement.
- Associated retraction of the globe into the orbit.

2. Causes include lesions of the pre-tectal area such as pinealoma and vascular accidents (dorsal midbrain syndrome).

Downbeat nystagmus

I. Signs. Vertical nystagmus with the fast phase beating downwards, which is more easily elicited in lateral gaze and down-gaze.

2. Causes
- Lesions of the craniocervical junction at the foramen magnum such as Arnold–Chiari malformation and syringobulbia.
- Drugs such as lithium, phenytoin, carbamazepine and barbiturates.
- Wernicke encephalopathy, demyelination and hydrocephalus.

Upbeat nystagmus

I. Signs. Vertical nystagmus with the fast phase beating upwards.

2. Causes include posterior fossa lesions, drugs and Wernicke encephalopathy.

See-saw nystagmus of Maddox

I. Signs. Pendular nystagmus, in which one eye elevates and intorts while the other depresses and extorts; the eyes then reverse direction.

2. Causes include parasellar tumours often producing bitemporal hemianopia, syringobulbia and brainstem stroke.

Ataxic nystagmus

Ataxic nystagmus is a horizontal jerk nystagmus which occurs in the abducting eye of a patient with an INO.

Sensory deprivation nystagmus

Sensory deprivation (ocular) nystagmus is caused by defective vision. Horizontal and pendular, it can often be dampened by convergence. The severity depends on the degree of visual loss. An AHP may be adopted to decrease the amplitude of the nystagmus. It is caused by severe impairment of central vision in early life (e.g. congenital cataract, macular hypoplasia). In general, children who sustain bilateral loss of central vision before the age of 2 years develop nystagmus.

Nystagmoid movements

Nystagmoid movements resemble nystagmus but differ in that the initial, pathological defoveating movement is a saccadic intrusion.

Ocular flutter and opsoclonus

I. Signs
- Saccadic oscillations with no intersaccadic interval.
- In ocular flutter they are purely horizontal and in opsoclonus they are multiplanar.

2. Causes include viral encephalitis, myoclonic encephalopathy in infants ('dancing eyes and dancing feet'), transient (idiopathic) in healthy neonates and drug-induced (lithium, amitriptyline, and phenytoin).

Ocular bobbing

I. Signs. Rapid, conjugate, downward eye movements with a slow drift up to the primary position.

2. Causes include pontine lesions (usually haemorrhage), cerebellar lesions compressing the pons and metabolic encephalopathy.

MIGRAINE

Clinical features

Migraine is an often familial disorder, more common in females, characterized by recurrent attacks of headache widely variable in intensity, duration and frequency. The headache is commonly unilateral, associated with nausea and vomiting and may be preceded by, or associated with, neurological and mood disturbances. However, all these characteristics are not necessarily present during each attack or in every patient. The main types of migraine are as follows.

Common migraine

Common migraine (migraine without aura) is characterized by headache with autonomic nervous system dysfunction (e.g. pallor and nausea), but without the stereotypical neurological or ophthalmic features seen in classical migraine (see below).
- Premonitory features include changes in mood, frequent yawning or other non-specific prodromal symptoms such as poor concentration.
- The headache starts anywhere on the cranium and is pounding or throbbing. It usually spreads to involve one half or even the whole head. If retro-orbital, the pain may be mistaken for ocular or sinus disease.
- During the attack, which lasts from hours to a day or more, the patient is frequently photophobic and

phonophobic and seeks relief in a quiet dark environment or through sleep.

- Because of the absence of the well-known migrainous visual distortions, severe nausea and vomiting, common migraine often goes unrecognized.

Classical migraine

Classical migraine (migraine with aura) is less common but better recognized.

- The attack is heralded by a visual aura which lasts about 20 minutes. This may consist of bright or dark spots, zig-zags (fortification spectra), heat haze distortions, jig-saw puzzle effects, scintillating scotomas or tunnel vision, which may progress to homonymous hemianopia.
- A small bright positive paracentral scotoma develops, lined on one side with luminous zig-zag lines (Fig. 21.58a).
- After several minutes the fortification spectrum gradually enlarges with the open end pointing centrally (Fig. 21.58b). It is often lined on the inner edge by an absent area of vision (negative scotoma–Fig. 21.58c).
- As the scotoma expands it may drift towards the temporal periphery before breaking up (Fig. 21.58d).
- Full visual recovery within 30 minutes is the rule and symptoms persisting longer than an hour should make you consider an alternative diagnosis.

> **NB** These visual features, supposedly pathognomonic of migraine, may rarely be caused by degenerative arterial disease or arteriovenous malformation in the occipital poles.

- The headache follows the aura by about 30 minutes and is usually hemicranial, opposite the hemianopia and is accompanied by nausea and photophobia. It may, however, be absent, trivial or very severe, with considerable variation between attacks even in the same individual.
- Visual aura without headache is not uncommon in the over 40s but there should always be a history of common or classical migraine in the patient's early 20s.

Cluster headache

Cluster headache (migrainous neuralgia) is a migraine variant which typically affects men during the fourth and fifth decades of life. It is of particular interest to ophthalmologists because it is associated with ocular features and may initially be misdiagnosed as an ocular problem. The condition is characterized by a stereotyped headache accompanied by various autonomic phenomena occurring almost every day for a period of some weeks. The headache is unilateral, oculotemporal, excruciating, sharp and deep. It begins relatively abruptly, lasts between 10 minutes and 2 hours, and then clears quickly.

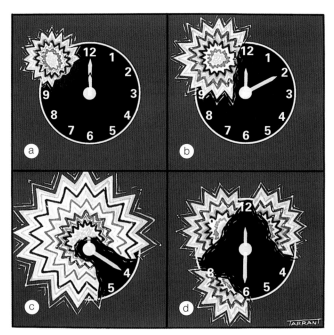

Fig. 21.58
Progression of classic migrainous fortification spectrum and scintillating scotoma (see text)

> **NB** The patient cannot keep still and is very agitated, unlike a patient with migraine who would rather lie quietly in a dark room.

- It may occur several times in a 24-hour period, often at particular times and not infrequently at around 2am.
- Once the 'cluster' is over, there may be a long headache-free interval of several years.
- Associated autonomic phenomena include lacrimation, conjunctival injection and rhinorrhoea.

> **NB** Cluster headaches are also a common cause of a transient or permanent post-ganglionic Horner syndrome.

Other types of migraine

1. **Focal migraine** is characterized by transient dysphasia, hemisensory symptoms or even focal weakness in addition to other symptoms of migraine.
2. **Migraine sine migraine** is characterized by episodic visual disturbances without headache. Elderly patients with a past history of classical migraine are typically affected.
3. **Retinal migraine** is characterized by acute, transient unilateral visual loss. Since this may occur in middle-aged patients without past history of migraine, it is prudent to investigate such individuals as undergoing attacks of retinal embolization until proved otherwise.

4. **Ophthalmoplegic migraine** is rare and typically starts before the age of 10 years. It is characterized by a recurrent transient third nerve palsy which begins after the headache.
5. **Familial hemiplegic migraine** is characterized by a failure of full recovery of focal neurological features after an attack of migraine subsides.
6. **Basilar migraine** occurs in children. It is characterized by a typical migrainous aura associated with numbness and tingling of the lips and extremities which is often bilateral. Ataxia of gait and speech also occur, with occasional impairment of consciousness.

Treatment

1. **General measures** include the elimination of conditions and agents that may precipitate an attack of migraine, such as coffee, chocolate, alcohol, cheese, oral contraceptives, stress, lack of sleep and long intervals without food.
2. **Prophylaxis** is indicated if the frequency and/or severity of the attacks are beyond the patient's tolerance. This may involve beta-adrenergic blockers, calcium channel blockers, amitriptyline, clonidine, pizotifen and low-dose aspirin.
3. **Treatment of an acute attack** may be with simple analgesics (aspirin, codeine analogues, paracetamol or NSAID) and, if appropriate, an anti-emetic such as metoclopramide. Other drugs, usually reserved for patients refractory to analgesics, include sumatriptan and ergotamine tartrate.

Differential diagnosis

Visual phenomena

The visual phenomena of migraine are typically binocular, zig-zag, scintillating and migrate within the visual field. This is often followed by a scotoma and/or homonymous visual loss. The patient may report loss of vision in the eye ipsilateral to the hemianopia. The following conditions should be considered in the differential diagnosis.

1. **Acute posterior vitreous detachment** is characterized by photopsia, usually associated with the sudden onset of floaters. The flashing lights are usually projected into the temporal visual field and may be precipitated by movements of the head or eyes.
2. **Transient ischaemic attacks** due to retinal microembolization are unilateral and not scintillating. The patient often describes a 'shade' or 'cloud' which typically starts in the upper or lower parts of the visual field and spreads centrally. It lasts several minutes and clears from the centre to the periphery.

3. **Transient visual obscurations** last only a few seconds and are characterized by a 'greying out' or 'darkening' of vision in one or both eyes. They classically occur in patients with papilloedema and are often precipitated by changes in posture. They may also precede anterior ischaemic optic neuropathy in patients with giant cell arteritis.
4. **Occipital epilepsy** is very rare; the patient typically sees coloured circles during an attack.

Neuralgias

The following conditions should be considered in the differential diagnosis of ocular or periocular pain in the absence of apparent physical disease.

1. **Herpes zoster ophthalmicus** frequently presents with pain 2–3 days before the onset of the characteristic vesicular rash.
2. **Trigeminal neuralgia** is characterized by brief attacks of severe pain that start in the distribution of one of the divisions of the trigeminal nerve. The pain is paroxysmal and sharp, like an electric shock, usually occurring in multiple bursts lasting a few seconds, in rapid succession. Attacks can be triggered either by cutaneous stimulation such as touching the face whilst shaving or by motor activity such as chewing, but sleep is usually undisturbed by pain. Facial sensation is normal. Treatment involves anti-epileptic drugs such as carbamazepine, phenytoin and sodium valproate. Trigeminal neuralgia of compressive aetiology may necessitate intra-cranial surgical decompression of the trigeminal nerve.
3. **Raeder paratrigeminal neuralgia** occurs in middle-aged men. It is characterized by severe unilateral headache with periocular pain in the distribution of the first division of the trigeminal nerve associated with an ipsilateral Horner syndrome. The pain may last from hours to weeks before it resolves spontaneously.

   NB Carotid dissection needs to be excluded before making the diagnosis.

4. **Greater occipital neuralgia** is characterized by attacks of pain that begin in the occipital region and then spread to the eye, temple and face. The attacks frequently occur at night and are associated with flushing of the face, dizziness and sometimes ipsilateral nasal obstruction. Examination during an attack may reveal extreme tenderness between the mastoid process and occipital protuberance.
5. **Ophthalmodynia periodica** is characterized by short, sharp stabbing ocular pain which often causes the patient to place the hand over the involved eye. A second series of episodes may immediately follow the initial attack.
6. **Ice-pick syndrome** is characterized by attacks of momentary, multifocal, sharp, pain around the skull, face

and eyes. Unlike trigeminal neuralgia there are no specific trigger points; the pain also does not conform to the anatomical distribution of the trigeminal nerve.

FACIAL SPASM

Essential blepharospasm

Diagnosis

Essential blepharospasm is an uncommon but distressing, idiopathic disorder which presents in the sixth decade and affects women more commonly than men by a 3:1 ratio. It is characterized by progressive bilateral involuntary spasm of the orbicularis oculi and upper facial muscles. In severe cases blepharospasm is disabling because it may temporarily render the patient functionally blind (Fig. 21.59a). Spasms may be precipitated by reading, driving, stress or bright light, and alleviated by talking, walking and relaxation, but it does not occur during sleep.

1. **Meige syndrome** is a combination of blepharospasm and involvement of the lower facial and neck muscles.
2. **Brueghel syndrome** is associated with severe mandibular and cervical muscle involvement.

Treatment

Prior to commencing treatment it is important to exclude reflex blepharospasm, most commonly due to ocular surface disease such as filamentary keratitis, as well as extrapyramidal disease such as Parkinsonism.

1. **Medical** treatment with a great variety of drugs has been reported to ameliorate specific types of blepharospasm, but their efficacy is disappointing.
2. **Botulinum toxin injected** along the upper and lower eyelid and eyebrow affords temporary relief in most patients (Fig. 21.59b). By interference with acetylcholine release from nerve terminals it results in temporary paralysis of the injected muscles. Most patients require

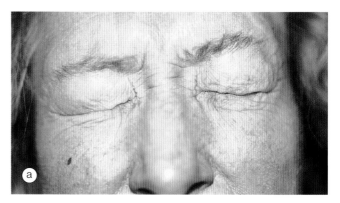
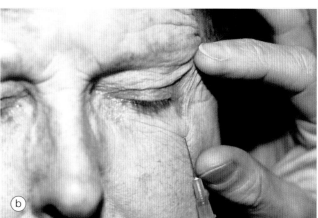

Fig. 21.59
(a) Essential blepharospasm; **(b)** botulinum injection

repeat injections every 3–4 months; progressively larger doses may be needed. Side effects include lagophthalmos and ectropion or entropion, depending on the tone of the eyelids before the injection. Accidental migration of the toxin into the orbit may result in ptosis and diplopia due to paralysis of the levator or extraocular muscles.
3. **Surgical** treatment involves removal of the entire orbicularis, corrugator and procerus muscles. Such radical surgery is reserved for patients who cannot tolerate or are unresponsive to botulinum toxin.

Facial hemispasm

Facial hemispasm is a unilateral condition that presents in the fifth to sixth decades of life. It is characterized by brief spasm of the orbicularis oculi which later spreads along the distribution of the facial nerve (Fig. 21.60). The condition may be idiopathic or the result of irritation at any region from the facial nucleus to the peripheral nerve. Neuroimaging should be performed to exclude a compressive aetiology. Facial hyperkinesia may occur several months or years after a Bell palsy. Treatment is similar to essential blepharospasm.

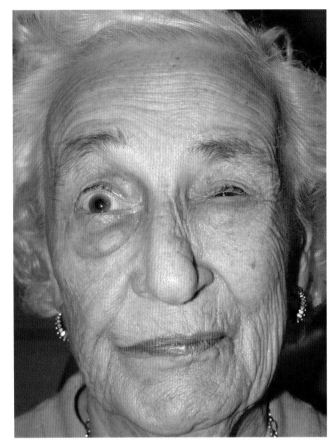

Fig. 21.60
Hemifacial spasm

DRUG-INDUCED DISORDERS

KERATOPATHY

Vortex keratopathy

Vortex keratopathy (cornea verticillata) is characterized by whorl-like corneal epithelial deposits.

1. **Signs** in chronological order:
   - Bilateral, fine greyish or golden-brown opacities in the inferior corneal epithelium.
   - Arborizing horizontal lines in a pattern resembling cat's whiskers, similar to the more common Hudson–Stahli line.
   - A whorl-like pattern which originates from a point below the pupil and swirls outwards, sparing the limbus (Fig. 22.1a).

   NB Although deposits may involve the visual axis, vision is not impaired but some patients may experience haloes around lights.

2. **Causes**
   a. **Antimalarials** (chloroquine and hydroxychloroquine) are common causes. Unlike retinopathy (see below),

keratopathy bears no relationship to dosage or duration of treatment. The changes are usually reversible on cessation of therapy, although they may clear despite continued administration.
   b. **Amiodarone**. Virtually all patients develop keratopathy which is reversible on discontinuation of medication. In general the higher the dose and the longer the duration of administration the more advanced the corneal deposits. Other toxic effects are anterior subcapsular lens deposits and optic neuropathy (see below).

Chlorpromazine

Chlorpromazine (Largactil) is used as a sedative and to treat psychotic illnesses. Some patients on long-term therapy may develop innocuous, subtle, diffuse, yellowish-brown granular deposits in the endothelium and deep stroma (Fig. 22.1b). Other toxic effects are anterior lens capsule deposits and retinopathy (see below).

Argyrosis

Argyrosis is a discolouration of ocular tissues secondary to silver deposits which may be iatrogenic or from occupational

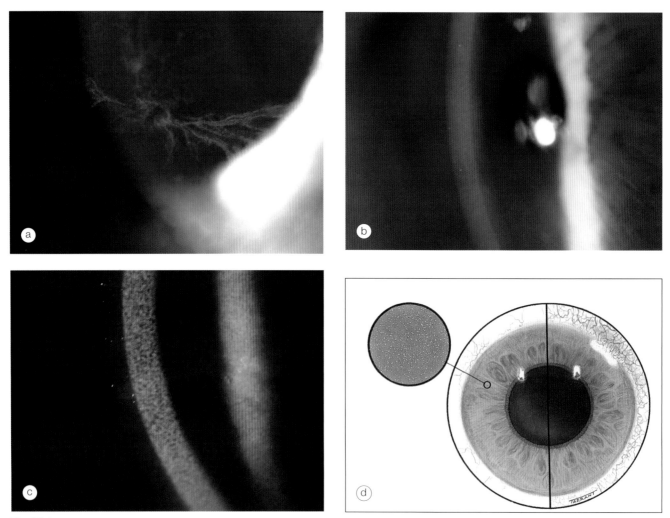

Fig. 22.1
Drug-induced keratopathies. **(a)** Vortex keratopathy; **(b)** chlorpromazine; **(c)** argyrosis; **(d)** chrysiasis (left), marginial keratitis (right)
(Courtesy of L Zografos – fig. c)

exposure. Keratopathy is characterized by greyish-brown, granular deposits in Descemet membrane (Fig. 22.1c). The conjunctiva may also be affected.

Chrysiasis

Chrysiasis is the deposition of gold in living tissue, occurring after prolonged administration of gold, usually in the treatment of rheumatoid arthritis. Virtually all patients on continuous chrysotherapy who have received a total dose of gold compound exceeding 1000mg develop corneal deposits. Corneal chrysiasis is characterized by dust-like or glittering purple granules throughout the corneal stroma, more concentrated in the deep layers and the periphery (Fig. 22.1d left). These findings are innocuous and therefore not an indication for cessation of therapy. Other toxic effects are innocuous lens deposits and occasionally marginal keratitis (Fig. 22.1d right).

CATARACT

Steroids

Steroids, both systemic and topical, are cataractogenic. The lens opacities are initially posterior subcapsular (Fig. 22.2a) and later the anterior subcapsular region becomes affected. The relationship between weekly systemic dose, duration of administration, total dose and cataract formation is unclear. It is thought that patients on less than 10mg prednisolone (or equivalent), or treated for less than 4 years may be immune. Although it is believed that children may be more susceptible to the cataractogenic effects of systemic steroids, individual (genetic) susceptibility may also be of relevance. It has therefore been suggested that the concept of a safe dose be abandoned. Patients who develop lens changes should have their dosage reduced to a minimum consistent with

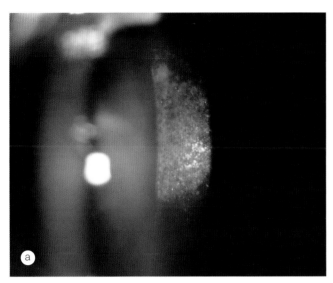

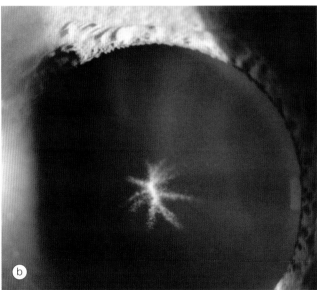

Fig. 22.2
(a) Steroid-induced posterior subcapsular cataract; **(b)** anterior capsular deposits due to chlorpromazine

control of the underlying disease, and if possible be considered for alternate day therapy. Early opacities may regress if therapy is discontinued; alternatively progression may occur despite withdrawal and warrant surgical intervention.

Other drugs

1. **Chlorpromazine** may cause the deposition of innocuous, fine, stellate, yellowish-brown granules on the anterior lens capsule within the pupillary area (Fig. 22.2b).
2. **Busulphan** (Myleran), used in the treatment of chronic myeloid leukaemia, may occasionally cause lens opacities.
3. **Gold,** used in the treatment of rheumatoid arthritis, causes innocuous anterior capsular deposits in

about 50% of patients on treatment for longer than 3 years.
4. **Allopurinol,** used in the treatment of hyperuricaemia and chronic gout, increases the risk of cataract formation in elderly patients, if the cumulative dose exceeds 400g or duration of administration exceeds 3 years.

UVEITIS

Rifabutin

Rifabutin is used mainly in the management and prophylaxis of *Mycobacterium avium* complex infections in AIDS patients with low CD4 counts. It is also used to treat tuberculosis with other drugs in immunocompetent patients.

1. **Acute anterior uveitis** is typically unilateral and frequently associated with hypopyon; associated vitritis may be mistaken for endophthalmitis.
2. **Treatment** involves withdrawal of the drug or reduction of dose.

> **NB** Drugs that inhibit metabolism of rifabutin through cytochrome p-450 pathway, such as clarithromycin and fluconazole, will increase the risk of uveitis.

Cidofovir

Cidofovir is used in the management of cytomegalovirus retinitis in AIDS patients.

1. **Acute anterior uveitis** with few cells but a marked fibrinous exudate may develop following several intravenous infusions. Vitritis is common and hypopyon may occur with long-term administration.
2. **Treatment** with topical steroids and mydriatics is usually successful, avoiding the need to discontinue therapy.

> **NB** Intravitreal injection of cidofovir should be used with caution because it carries a high risk of hypotony.

RETINOPATHY

Antimalarials

Drugs

Chloroqine (Nivaquine, Avlocor) and hydroxychloroquine (Plaquenil) are quinolone antimalarial drugs used in the prophylaxis and treatment of malaria as well as in the treatment of certain rheumatological disorders (e.g. rheumatoid arthritis, juvenile idiopathic arthritis, systemic lupus erythematosus). The use of chloroquine has also been advocated in the treatment of calcium abnormalities associated with sarcoidosis. Antimalarials are excreted from the body very slowly and are melanotropic drugs that become concentrated in melanin-containing structures of the eye such as the retinal pigment epithelium (RPE) and choroid.

1. **Chloroquine** retinotoxicity is related to the total cumulative dose. The normal daily dose is 250mg; a cumulative dose of less than 100g or treatment duration under 1 year is rarely associated with retinal damage. The risk of toxicity increases significantly when the cumulative dose exceeds 300g (i.e. 250mg daily for 3 years). However, there have been reports of patients receiving cumulative doses exceeding 1000g who did not develop retinotoxicity.

If possible, chloroquine should be used only if other agents are ineffective.

2. **Hydroxychloroquine** is much safer than chloroquine and if the daily dose does not exceed 400mg the risk of retinotoxicity is negligible. Physicians should therefore be encouraged to use hydroxychloroquine instead of chloroquine whenever possible. The risk of toxicity is increased if a daily dose is over 6.5mg/kg is administered for longer than 5 years, although even then the risk is still very small.

Retinopathy

Chloroquine retinopathy can be divided into the following stages:

1. **Premaculopathy** is characterized by normal visual acuity and a scotoma to a red target located between 4° and 9° from fixation. Amsler grid testing may also show a defect.

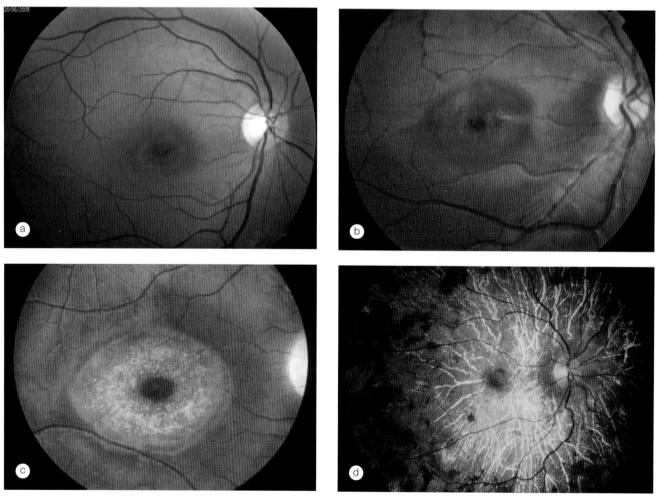

Fig. 22.3
Progression of chloroquine retinopathy (Courtesy of S Milenkovic – fig. a; Moorfields Eye Hospital – fig. b)

If the drug is discontinued, visual function usually returns to normal.

2. **Early maculopathy** is the next stage, if treatment is not discontinued. It is characterized by a modest reduction of visual acuity (6/9–6/12). Fundus examination shows a subtle 'bull's eye' macular lesion characterized by central foveolar island of pigment surrounded by a depigmented zone of RPE atrophy which is itself encircled by a hyperpigmented ring (Fig. 22.3a). The lesion may be more obvious on FA than ophthalmoscopy because the RPE atrophy gives rise to a RPE 'window' defect. This stage may progress even if the drug is stopped.

3. **Moderate maculopathy** is characterized by moderate reduction of visual acuity (6/18–6/24) and an obvious 'bull's eye' macular lesion (Fig. 22.3b).

4. **Severe maculopathy** is characterized by marked reduction of visual acuity (6/36–6/60) with widespread RPE atrophy surrounding the fovea (Fig. 22.3c).

5. **End-stage maculopathy** is characterized by severe reduction of visual acuity and marked atrophy of the RPE with unmasking of the larger choroidal blood vessels. The retinal arterioles may also become attenuated and pigment clumps develop in the peripheral retina (Fig.22.3d).

Screening

Screening of patients on hydroxychloroquine is unnecessary although some have recommended annual screening if the patient has been on medication for over 6 years. In clinical practice chloroquine can also be given safely to patients without the need for repetitive routine examinations by ophthalmologists or the use of complicated tests. Recording of visual acuity and ophthalmoscopy by the prescribing doctor is all that is required. The patient can be given an Amsler grid to use once a week. If symptoms occur or an abnormality is found, then the opinion of an ophthalmologist should be sought. The ophthalmologist can, if necessary, perform more sophisticated tests such as visual fields, macular threshold, colour vision testing, contrast sensitivity, FA and electro-oculography. Recent reports suggest that multifocal electroretinography (see Chapter 1) may be useful in detecting early toxicity.

Phenothiazines

Thioridazine

Thioridazine (Melleril) is used to treat schizophrenia and related psychoses. The normal daily dose is 150–600mg. Doses which exceed 800mg/day for just a few weeks may be sufficient to cause reduced visual acuity and impairment of dark adaptation. The clinical signs of progressive retinotoxicity are as follows:

- Salt-and-pepper pigmentary disturbance involving the mid-periphery and posterior pole.

- Plaque-like pigmentation and focal loss of the RPE and choriocapillaris (Fig. 22.4a).
- Diffuse loss of the RPE and choriocapillaris (Fig. 22.4b).

Chlorpromazine

The normal daily dose is 75–300mg. Retinotoxicity may occur if very much larger doses are used over a prolonged period. It is characterized by non-specific pigmentary granularity and clumping.

Crystalline maculopathies

Tamoxifen

Tamoxifen (Nolvadex, Emblon, Noltan and Tamofen) is a specific anti-oestrogen used in the treatment of selected

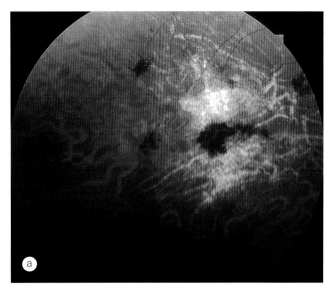
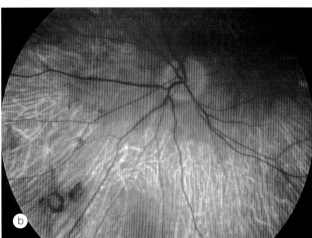

Fig. 22.4
Thioridazine retinopathy. **(a)** Pigmented plaques and focal loss of retinal pigment epithelium (the choriocapillaris); **(b)** diffuse atrophy of the retinal pigment epithelium and choriocapillaris (Courtesy of K Jordan)

patients with breast carcinoma. It has few systemic side-effects and ocular complications are uncommon. The normal daily dose is 20–40mg. Retinotoxicity and visual impairment may develop in some patients on higher doses and rarely in patients on normal doses. Retinopathy is characterized by bilateral, fine, superficial, yellow, crystalline deposits in theinner layers of the retina and punctate grey lesions in the outer retina and RPE (Fig. 22.5a). Visual impairment is thought to be caused by maculopathy associated with foveolar cyst formation. Other rare side-effects are optic neuritis, which is reversible on cessation of therapy.

Canthaxanthin

Canthaxanthin is a carotenoid used to enhance sun tanning. If used over prolonged periods of time it may cause the deposition of innocuous, inner retinal, tiny, glistening, yellow deposits, arranged symmetrically in a doughnut shape at the posterior poles (Fig. 22.5b). The deposits are slowly reversible.

Methoxyflurane

Methoxyflurane (Penthrane) is an inhalant general anaesthetic. It is metabolized to oxalic acid which combines with calcium to form an insoluble salt which is deposited in tissues including the RPE. Prolonged administration may lead to renal failure and secondary hyperoxalosis. It may also result in mild visual impairment associated with calcium oxalate crystals at the level of the RPE, sensory retina and along retinal arteries (Fig. 22.5c).

Nitrofurantoin

Nitrofurantoin is an antibiotic used in the treatment of urinary tract infections. Long-term use may result in slight visual impairment associated with superficial and deep intraretinal glistening deposits distributed in a circinate pattern throughout the posterior pole.

> **NB** Other causes of macular crystals include: primary hyperoxaluria, Bietti crystalline dystrophy, cystinosis, Sjögren–Larsson syndrome, gyrate atrophy, acquired parafoveal telangiectasis, talc-cornstarch emboli and West African crystalline maculopathy.

Miscellaneous agents

Interferon alpha

Interferon alpha is used in a variety of systemic conditions including Kaposi sarcoma, haemangioma in infancy, cutaneous

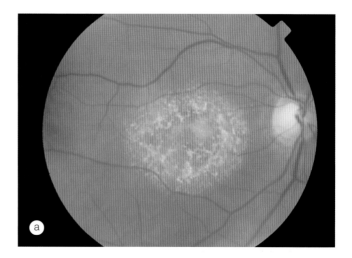

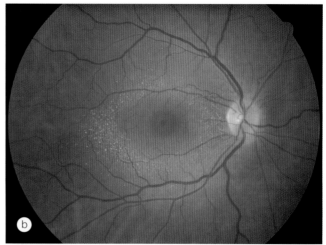

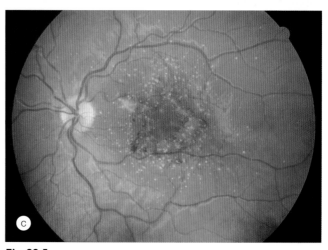

Fig. 22.5
Toxic crystalline retinopathies. (**a**) Tamoxifen; (**b**) canthaxanthin; (**c**) oxalosis (Courtesy of L Merin – figs b and c)

melanomas, metastatic renal cell carcinoma, leukaemia, lymphoma and chronic hepatitis C. Systemic adverse effects include constitutional symptoms, neutropenia and thrombocytopenia. Retinopathy characterized by cotton-wool spots and intraretinal haemorrhages may develop in some patients, particularly those on high-dose therapy (Fig. 22.6). The condition usually resolves spontaneously with cessation of therapy and in the majority of patients the visual prognosis is good. Less common ocular side-effects include cystoid macular oedema (CMO), oculomotor nerve palsy, optic disc oedema and retinal vein occlusion.

Desferrioxamine mesylate

Desferrioxamine mesylate is an iron chelator used in the treatment of chronic iron overload, to prevent haemosiderosis, in patients with haematological conditions requiring regular transfusion. It is most commonly administered as a slow subcutaneous infusion. Retinopathy is characterized by macular and/or equatorial pigmentary degeneration associated with low electroretinogram amplitudes and reduced electro-oculogram light-peak to dark-trough ratios.

Nicotinic acid

Nicotinic acid, a cholesterol-lowering agent, has a number of side-effects, including cutaneous flushing, pruritus, nausea and abdominal pain. A small minority of patients develop cystoid maculopathy suggestive of CMO but without leakage on fluorescein angiography. The macular changes cause a mild reduction of visual acuity and occur when doses greater than 1.5g daily are used but resolve with discontinuation of the drug.

Gentamicin

Gentamicin may cause severe retinal ischaemia when injected intravitreally for the treatment of bacterial endophthalmitis (Fig. 22.7). Rarely, retinal toxicity may result from periocular injection.

OPTIC NEUROPATHY

Ethambutol

Ethambutol (Myambutol, Mynah) is used in combination with isoniazid and rifampicin in the treatment of tuber-

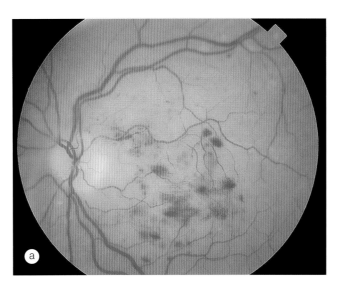

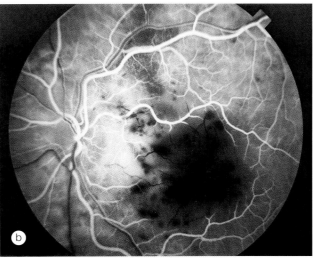

Fig. 22.7
Gentamicin retinopathy. **(a)** Retinal pallor and haemorrhages; **(b)** FA shows corresponding hypofluorescence due to ischaemia (Courtesy of S Milweski)

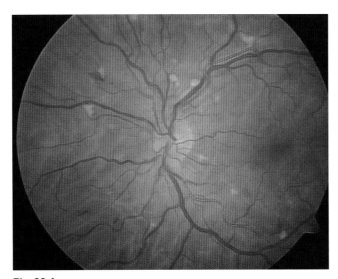

Fig. 22.6
Interferon retinopathy (Courtesy of P Gilli)

culosis. Ocular toxic effects include optic neuritis, colour vision abnormalities and visual field defects. Toxicity is dose and duration dependent, the incidence is up to 6% at a daily dose of 25mg/kg and rare with a daily dose not exceeding 15mg/kg. Toxicity typically occurs between 3 and 6 months of starting treatment.

> **NB** Isoniazid may also rarely cause toxic optic neuropathy, particularly in combination with ethambutol.

1. **Presentation** of optic neuritis is with abrupt visual impairment.
2. **Signs** include normal or slightly swollen optic discs with splinter-shaped haemorrhages.
3. **Visual field defects** usually consist of central or centrocaecal scotomas although bitemporal or peripheral constriction may occur.
4. **Prognosis** is good following cessation of treatment although recovery may take up to 12 months. A minority of patients develop permanent visual impairment as a result of optic atrophy.
5. **Screening** should be every 4 weeks when the dose is more than 15mg/kg and every 3–6 months for lower doses. The drug should be stopped immediately if symptoms develop.

Amiodarone

Amiodarone is an anti-arrhythmia drug used in the treatment of ventricular tachycardia and fibrillation, and in restoration of sinus rhythm in atrial fibrillation. Common systemic side-effects include thyroid dysfunction, pulmonary toxicity, peripheral neuropathy and gastrointestinal problems. Vortex keratopathy (see Fig. 22.1a), which is innocuous, is virtually universal. Other uncommon ocular side-effects include anterior subcapsular lens deposits and optic neuropathy. The latter affects only 1–2% of patients and is not dose-related.

1. **Presentation** is with insidious unilateral or bilateral visual impairment.
2. **Signs** are bilateral optic disc swelling that may persist for a few months after medication is stopped.
3. **Visual field defects** may be mild and reversible or severe and permanent.
4. **Prognosis** is variable because cessation of the drug may not inevitably bring about improvement.
5. **Screening** is not appropriate because there is no way to identify those at risk. Patients should, however, be warned of the small risk of toxicity and to report any suggestive symptoms.
6. **Differential diagnosis** includes non-arteritic anterior ischaemic optic neuropathy (NAION) which also affects patients with systemic vascular disease. However, amiodarone optic neuropathy typically has a more insidious onset, milder visual loss, a longer duration of disc oedema and is more commonly bilateral than NAION.

Vigabatrin

Vigabatrin is used as a second-line antiepileptic drug for the treatment of uncontrolled complex partial seizures and as first-line monotherapy for infantile spasms (West syndrome). Some patients develop bilateral concentric or binasal visual field defects, often asymptomatic, months or years after starting treatment. The defects persist if treatment is stopped but do not progress if medication is continued. This suggests that toxicity is idiosyncratic rather than a dose-related effect. Ophthalmoscopy is usually normal although a small percentage of patients may show a variety of changes including nasal (inverse) optic disc atrophy, arteriolar narrowing, abnormal macular reflexes and surface wrinkling. Baseline visual field examination is recommended prior to starting treatment. Reassessment is made thereafter every 6 months for 3 years and then annually if no abnormality is detected.

TRAUMA

EYELID TRAUMA

Haematoma

A haematoma (black eye) is the most common result of blunt injury to the eyelid or forehead and is generally innocuous. It is, however, very important to exclude the following more serious conditions:

1. **Trauma to the globe or orbit.** It is easier to examine the integrity of the globe before the lids become oedematous (Fig. 23.1a).
2. **Orbital roof fracture,** if the black eye is associated with a subconjunctival haemorrhage without a visible posterior limit (Fig. 23.1b).
3. **Basal skull fracture,** which may give rise to characteristic bilateral ring haematomas ('panda eyes' – Fig. 23.1c).

Laceration

The presence of a lid laceration, however insignificant, mandates careful exploration of the wound and examination of the globe. Any lid defect should be repaired by direct closure whenever possible, even under tension, since this affords the best functional and cosmetic results.

1. **Superficial** lacerations parallel to the lid margin without gaping can be sutured with 6-0 black silk. The sutures are removed after 5 days.
2. **Lid margin** lacerations invariably gape (Fig. 23.2a) and must therefore be very carefully sutured with perfect alignment to prevent notching (Fig. 23.2b).
3. **With mild tissue loss** just sufficient to prevent direct primary closure can usually be managed by performing a lateral cantholysis in order to increase lateral eyelid mobility.
4. **With extensive tissue** loss (Fig. 23.2c) may require major reconstructive procedures (Fig. 23.2d) such as used following lid resection for malignant tumours (see Chapter 4).
5. **Canalicular** lacerations should be repaired within 24 hours. The laceration is bridged by silicone tubing, which is threaded down the lacrimal system and tied in the nose, and the laceration is sutured. The tubing is left *in situ* for 3–6 months.

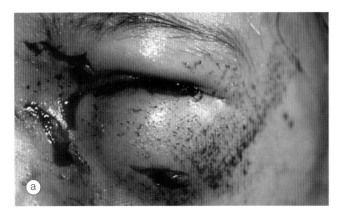

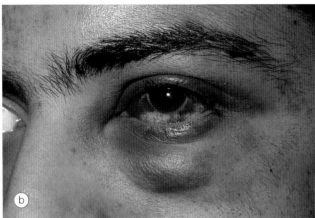

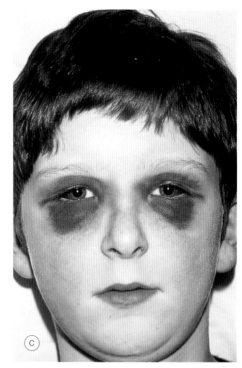

Fig. 23.1
Periocular haematoma. **(a)** Severe periocular haematoma and oedema; **(b)** periocular haematoma and subconjunctival haemorrhage; **(c)** 'panda eyes'

ORBITAL FRACTURES

Blow-out orbital floor fracture

A 'pure' blow-out fracture of the orbit does not involve the orbital rim, whereas an 'impure' fracture involves the orbital rim and adjacent facial bones. A blow-out fracture of the orbital floor is typically caused by a sudden increase in the orbital pressure by a striking object which is greater than 5cm in diameter, such as a fist or tennis ball (Fig. 23.3). Since the bones of the lateral wall and the roof are usually able to withstand such trauma, the fracture most frequently involves the floor of the orbit along the thin bone covering the infraorbital canal. Occasionally, the medial orbital wall may also be fractured. Clinical features vary with the severity of trauma and the time interval between injury and examination.

Diagnosis

1. **Periocular signs** include variable ecchymosis (Fig. 23.4a), oedema and occasionally subcutaneous emphysema.
2. **Infraorbital nerve anaesthesia** involving the lower lid, cheek, side of nose, upper lip, upper teeth and gums is very common because the fracture frequently involves the infraorbital canal.
3. **Diplopia** may be caused by one of the following mechanisms:
   - Haemorrhage and oedema in the orbit may cause the septa, which connect the inferior rectus and inferior oblique muscles to the periorbita, to become taut and thus restrict movements of the globe. Ocular motility usually improves as the haemorrhage and oedema resolve.
   - Mechanical entrapment within the fracture of the inferior rectus or inferior oblique muscle, or adjacent connective tissue and fat. Diplopia typically occurs in both up-gaze (Fig. 23.4b) and down-gaze (double diplopia). In these cases forced duction and the differential intraocular pressure tests are positive. Diplopia may subsequently improve if mainly due to entrapment of connective tissue and fat, but usually persists if there is significant involvement of the muscles themselves.
   - Direct injury to an extraocular muscle is associated with a negative forced duction test. The muscle fibres usually regenerate and normal function returns within about 2 months.
4. **Enophthalmos** (Fig. 23.4c) may be present if the fracture is severe, although it tends to manifest after a few days, as the initial oedema resolves. In the absence of surgical intervention, enophthalmos may continue to

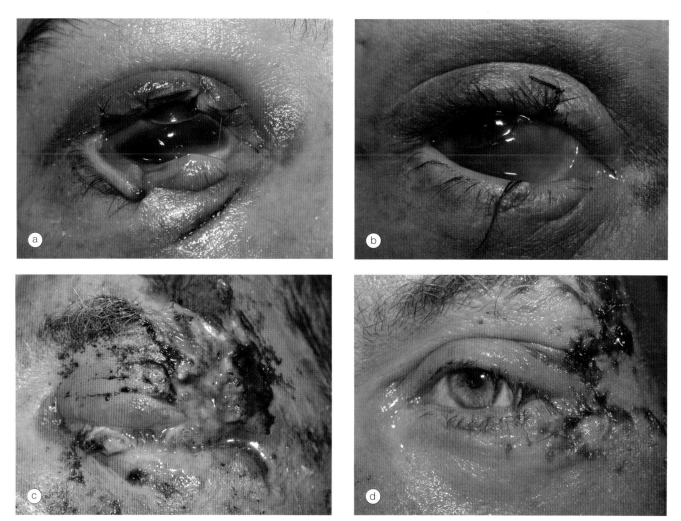

Fig. 23.2
Lid lacerations. **(a)** Two lid margin lacerations without tissue loss; **(b)** following repair; **(c)** lid laceration with extensive tissue loss; **(d)** following repair (Courtesy of A Pearson)

increase for about 6 months as post-traumatic orbital degeneration and fibrosis develop.

5. **Ocular damage** (e.g. hyphaema, angle recession, retinal dialysis), although uncommon, should be excluded.

6. **CT** with coronal sections (Fig. 23.4d) is particularly useful in evaluating the extent of the fracture, as well as determining the nature of maxillary antral soft-tissue densities which may represent prolapsed orbital fat, extraocular muscles, haematoma or unrelated antral polyps.

7. **Hess test** (Fig. 23.5) is useful in assessing and monitoring the progression of diplopia.

Treatment

1. **Initial** treatment is conservative with antibiotics if the fracture involves the maxillary sinus. The patient should also be instructed not to blow the nose.

2. **Subsequent** treatment is aimed at prevention of perma-

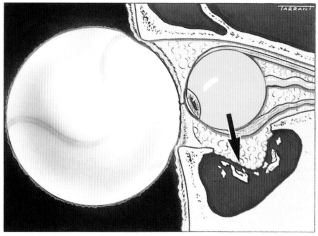

Fig. 23.3
Mechanism of an orbital floor blow-out fracture

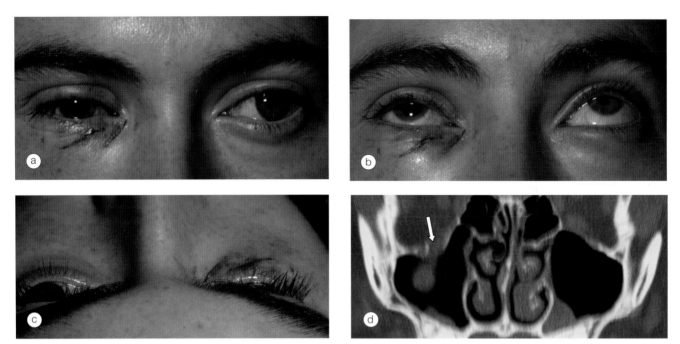

Fig. 23.4
Right orbital floor blow-out fracture. **(a)** Mild bruising and superficial laceration; **(b)** restricted elevation; **(c)** mild enophthalmos; **(d)** CT coronal view shows a defect in the orbital floor (arrow) and the 'tear drop' sign in the antrum (Courtesy of A Pearson – fig. d)

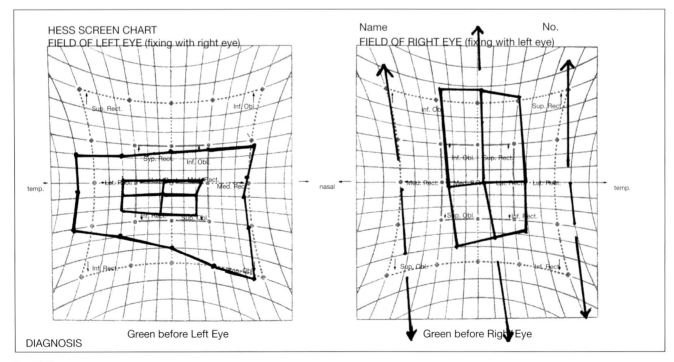

Fig. 23.5
Hess chart of a left orbital floor blow-out fracture shows restriction of left up-gaze (superior rectus and inferior oblique) and restriction on down-gaze (inferior rectus); there is also secondary overaction of the right eye

nent vertical diplopia and cosmetically unacceptable enophthalmos. The three factors that determine the risk of these late complications are fracture size, herniation of orbital contents into the maxillary sinus and muscle entrapment. Although there may be some overlap, most fractures fall into one of the following categories:

- Small cracks unassociated with herniation do not require treatment as the risk of permanent complications is small.
- Fractures involving less than half the orbital floor, with little or no herniation, and improving diplopia also do not require treatment, unless there is more than 2mm of enophthalmos.
- Fractures involving half or more of the orbital floor with entrapment of orbital contents, and persistent diplopia in the primary position should be repaired within 2 weeks. If surgery is delayed, the results are less satisfactory because of secondary fibrotic changes in the orbit.

3. Technique of surgical repair (Fig. 23.6)
   a. A transconjunctival or subciliary incision is made (Fig. 23.6a).
   b. The periosteum is elevated from the floor of the orbit and orbital contents are removed from the antrum (Fig. 23.6b).
   c. The defect in the floor is repaired using synthetic material such as Supramid, silicone or Teflon (Fig. 23.6c).
   d. The periosteum is sutured (Fig. 23.6d).

Blow-out medial wall fracture

Most medial wall orbital fractures are associated with floor fractures.

1. Signs
   - Periorbital haematoma (Fig. 23.7a) and frequently subcutaneous emphysema, which typically develops on blowing the nose.
   - Defective ocular motility involving abduction (Fig. 23.7b) and adduction (Fig. 23.7c), if the medial rectus muscle is caught in the fracture.
2. CT will show the extent of damage (Fig. 23.7d).
3. Treatment involves release of the entrapped tissue and repair of the bony defect.

   NB Because of the possibility of forcing infected sinus contents into the orbit, blowing of the nose should be discouraged.

Roof fracture

Roof fractures are rarely encountered by ophthalmologists. Isolated fractures, caused by minor trauma such as falling on a sharp object or a blow to the brow or forehead, are most common in young children. Complicated fractures, caused by major trauma with associated displacement of the

Fig. 23.6
Technique of repair of an orbital floor blow-out fracture (see text)

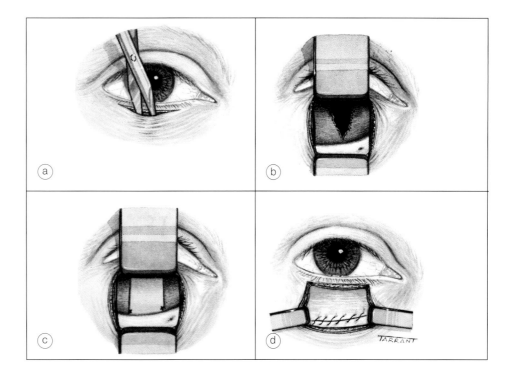

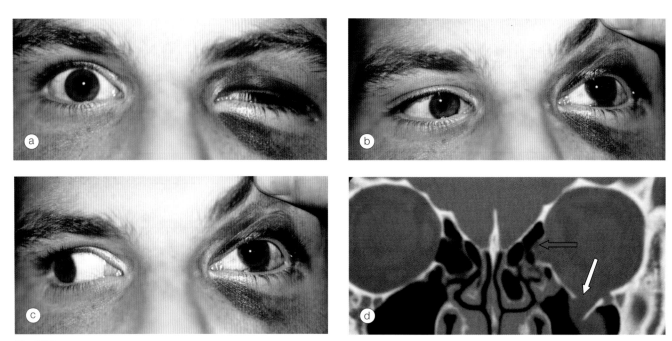

Fig. 23.7
Blowout fracture of the left medial wall and floor. **(a)** Periorbital haematoma and ptosis; **(b)** defective left abduction; **(c)** defective left adduction; **(d)** CT coronal view shows fractures of the medial wall (red arrow) and floor (white arrow) (Courtesy of A Pearson)

orbital rim or significant disturbance of other craniofacial bones, most commonly affect adults.

1. **Presentation** is with a haematoma of the upper eyelid and periocular ecchymosis which develop after a few hours and may later spread to the opposite side (see Fig. 23.1c).
2. **Signs**
   - Inferior or axial displacement of the globe.
   - Large fractures may be associated with pulsation of the globe unassociated with a bruit, due to transmission of CSF pulsation, best detected on applanation tonometry.
3. **Treatment**
   - Small fractures may not require treatment but it is important to observe the patient for the possibility of a CSF leak which may lead to meningitis.
   - Sizeable bony defects with downwardly displaced fragments usually require reconstructive surgery.

Lateral wall fracture

Acute lateral wall fractures are also rarely encountered by ophthalmologists. Because the lateral wall of the orbit is more solid than the other walls, a fracture is usually associated with extensive facial damage (Fig. 23.8).

TRAUMA TO THE GLOBE

Introduction

Definitions

1. **Closed injury** is commonly due to blunt trauma. The corneo-scleral wall of the globe is intact but intraocular damage may be present.
2. **Open injury** involves a full-thickness wound of the corneo-scleral wall.
3. **Contusion** is a closed injury resulting from blunt trauma. Damage may occur at the site of impact or at a distant site.
4. **Rupture** is a full-thickness wound caused by blunt trauma. The globe gives way at its weakest point, which may not be at the site of impact.
5. **Laceration** is a full-thickness wound caused by a sharp object at the site of impact.
6. **Lamellar** laceration is a partial-thickness wound caused by a sharp object.
7. **Penetration** is a single full-thickness wound, usually caused by a sharp object, without an exit wound. Such a wound may be associated with intraocular retention of a foreign body.
8. **Perforation** consists of two full-thickness wounds, one entry and one exit, usually caused by a missile.

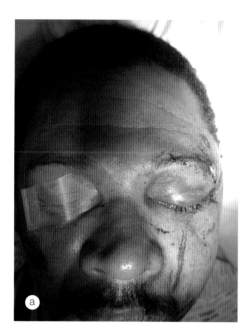

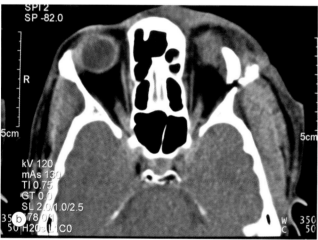

Fig. 23.8
Lateral wall fracture. **(a)** Severe facial trauma; **(b)** CT axial view
shows a left lateral wall fracture (Courtesy of A Pearson)

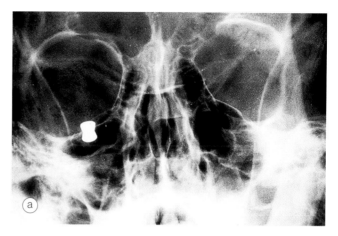

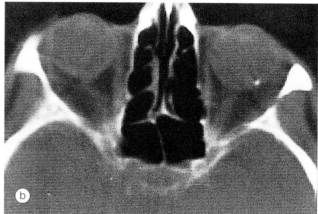

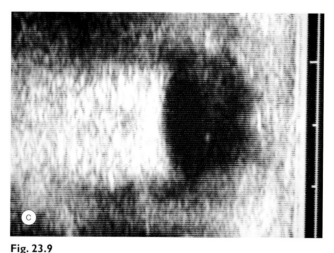

Fig. 23.9
Imaging of foreign bodies. **(a)** Plain radiograph shows an air gun
pellet; **(b)** CT axial view shows an intraocular foreign body; **(c)**
US shows an intraocular foreign body

Principles of management

1. Initial assessment should be performed in the following
order:
- Determination of the nature and extent of any life-
  threatening problems.
- History of the injury, including the circumstances,
  timing and likely object.
- Thorough examination of both eyes and orbits.

2. Special investigations

a. Plain radiographs may be taken when a foreign body
is suspected (Fig. 23.9a).

b. CT is superior to plain radiography in the detection and
localization of intraocular foreign bodies (Fig. 23.9b).
It is also of value in determining the integrity of
intracranial, facial and intraocular structures.

NB MR should never be performed if a metallic foreign body is suspected.

   c. ***US*** may be useful in the detection of intraocular foreign bodies (Fig. 23.9c), globe rupture, suprachoroidal haemorrhage and retinal detachment. It is also helpful in planning surgical repair, for example regarding placement of infusion ports during vitrectomy and whether drainage of suprachoroidal haemorrhage is required.

   d. ***Electrophysiological tests*** may be useful in assessing the integrity of the optic nerve and retina, particularly if some time has passed since the original injury and there is suspicion of a retained intraocular foreign body.

Blunt trauma

The most common causes of blunt trauma are squash balls, elastic luggage straps and champagne corks. Severe blunt trauma results in anteroposterior compression with simultaneous expansion in the equatorial plane associated with a transient but severe increase in intraocular pressure. Although the impact is primarily absorbed by the lens-iris diaphragm and the vitreous base, damage can also occur at a distant site such as the posterior pole. The extent of ocular damage depends on the severity of trauma and for unknown reasons is largely concentrated to either anterior or posterior segment. Apart from obvious ocular damage, blunt trauma may result in long-term effects so that the prognosis is necessarily guarded.

Cornea

1. **Corneal abrasion** involves a breach of the epithelium, which stains with fluorescein (Fig. 23.10a). If over the pupillary area, vision may be grossly impaired. This exquisitely painful condition is treated with topical cycloplegia (to promote comfort) and antibiotic ointment. Although patching has been standard treatment in the past it has become apparent that the cornea heals faster with less pain when not patched.
2. **Acute corneal oedema** may develop, secondary to focal or diffuse dysfunction of the corneal endothelium. It is commonly associated with folds in Descemet membrane and stromal thickening (Fig. 23.10b), which clear spontaneously.
3. **Tears in Descemet membrane** are usually vertical and associated with birth trauma (Fig. 23.10c).

Hyphaema

Hyphaema (haemorrhage into the anterior chamber) is a common complication. The source of the bleeding is the iris or ciliary body (Fig. 23.11a).

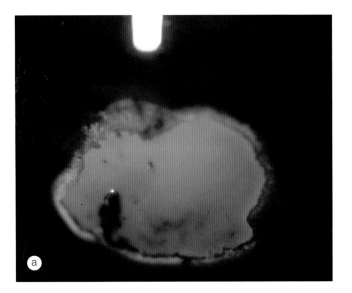

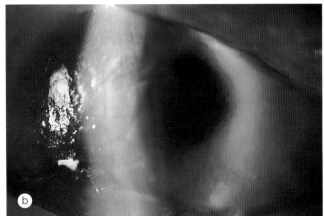

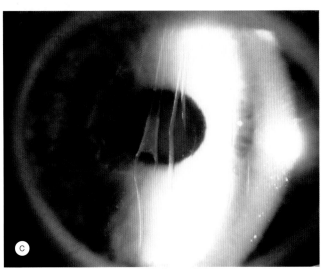

Fig. 23.10
Corneal complications of blunt trauma. **(a)** Abrasion stained with fluorescein; **(b)** stromal oedema and folds in Descemet membrane; **(c)** tears in Descemet membrane
(Courtesy of R Curtis – fig. c)

1. **Signs.** Characteristically, the red blood cells sediment inferiorly with a resultant 'fluid level', the height of which should be measured and documented (Fig. 23.11b).
2. **Observation** is all that is required in most cases because most hyphaemas are small, innocuous and transient. The immediate risk is that of secondary haemorrhage, often larger than the original hyphaema (Fig. 23.11c), which may occur at any time up to a week after the original injury (most commonly within the first 24 hours).
3. **Treatment** of significant hyphaemas with oral tranexamic acid 25mg/kg t.i.d., an anti-fibrolytic agent, is useful for the prevention of secondary haemorrhage. Opinions vary, but it would appear sensible to immobilize the pupil in the dilated state, with atropine to both prevent further haemorrhage and treat associated uveitis. Hospital admission for a few days may be advisable so that intraocular pressure may be monitored, and if elevated, treated appropriately (see Chapter 13) so as to prevent secondary corneal blood-staining (Fig. 23.11d).

Anterior uvea

1. **Pupil.** Severe contusion may cause miosis and pigment imprinting on the anterior lens capsule (Vossius ring), which corresponds to the size of the miosed pupil (Fig. 23.12a). Alternatively, damage to the iris sphincter may result in traumatic mydriasis, which is often permanent – the pupil reacts sluggishly or not at all to both light and accommodation. Radial tears in the pupillary margin are common (Fig. 23.12b).
2. **Iridodialysis** is a dehiscence of the iris from the ciliary body at its root. The pupil is typically 'D' shaped and the dialysis is seen as a dark biconvex area near the limbus (Fig. 23.12c). An iridodialysis may be asymptomatic if covered by the upper lid, but if exposed in the palpebral aperture, uniocular diplopia and glare may ensue, sometimes necessitating surgical repair. Traumatic aniridia (360° iridodialysis) is rare.
3. **The ciliary body** may react to severe blunt trauma by temporary cessation of aqueous secretion (ciliary shock)

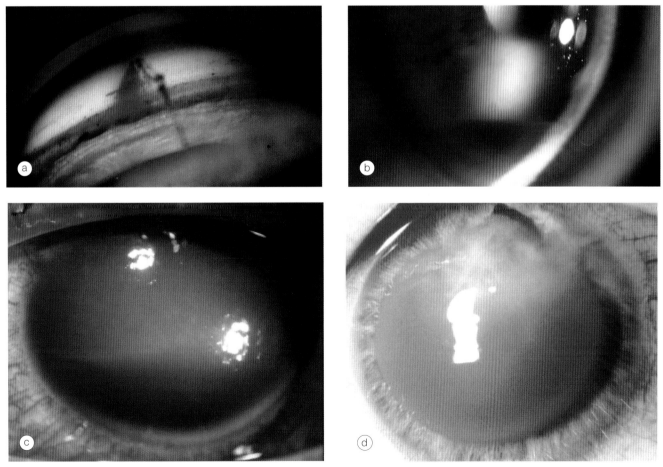

Fig. 23.11
Traumatic hyphaema. **(a)** Bleeding from the ciliary body; **(b)** small hyphaema; **(c)** secondary total hyphaema; **(d)** corneal blood staining
(Courtesy of R Curtis – fig. a; Krachmer, Mannis and Holland, from *Cornea*, Mosby, 2005 – fig. d)

resulting in ocular hypotony. Tears extending into the face of the ciliary body (angle recession) are associated with a risk of late glaucoma (see Chapter 13).

Lens

1. **Cataract** formation is a common sequel to severe blunt trauma. Postulated mechanisms include traumatic damage to the lens fibres themselves and minute ruptures in the lens capsule with influx of aqueous humour, hydration of lens fibres and consequent opacification. A ring-shaped faint anterior subcapsular opacity may underlie Vossius ring. Commonly, opacification occurs in the posterior subcapsular cortex along the posterior sutures resulting in a flower-shaped ('rosette') opacity (Fig. 23.13a), which may subsequently disappear, remain stationary or progress to maturity. Cataract surgery may be necessary for visually significant opacity.

2. **Subluxation** may occur, secondary to tearing of the suspensory ligament. A subluxated lens tends to deviate towards the meridian of intact zonule and the anterior chamber may deepen over the area of zonular dehiscence, if the lens rotates posteriorly. The edge of a subluxated lens may be visible under mydriasis and the iris may tremble on ocular movement (iridodonesis). Subluxation of magnitude sufficient to render the pupil partly aphakic (Fig. 23.13b) may result in uniocular diplopia. Lenticular astigmatism due to lens tilt may also occur.

3. **Dislocation** due to 360° rupture of the zonule is rare and may be into the vitreous or, less commonly, into the anterior chamber (Fig. 23.13c).

Globe rupture

Rupture of the globe (Fig. 23.14a) may result from very severe blunt trauma. The rupture is usually anterior, in the vicinity of Schlemm canal, with prolapse of intraocular structures such as lens, iris, ciliary body and vitreous (Fig. 23.14b). Occasionally, the rupture is posterior (occult) with little visible damage to the anterior segment. Clinically, occult rupture should be suspected if there is asymmetry of anterior chamber depth and intraocular pressure in the affected eye is low. The principles of repairing scleral ruptures are described later.

Vitreous

Posterior vitreous detachment, which may be associated with vitreous haemorrhage, may occur. Pigment cells similar to tobacco dust may be seen floating in the anterior vitreous.

Retina and choroid

1. **Commotio retinae** is caused by concussion of the sensory retina resulting in cloudy swelling which gives

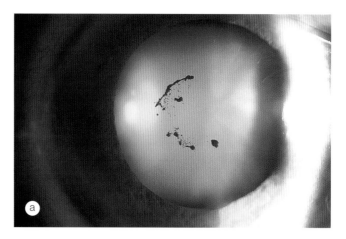
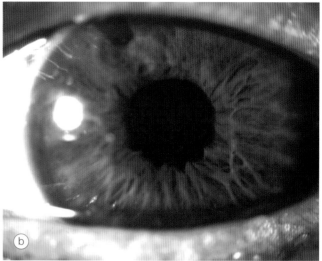
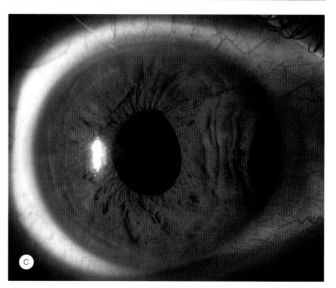

Fig. 23.12
Iris complications of blunt trauma. **(a)** Vossius ring; **(b)** radial sphincter tears; **(c)** iridodialysis (Courtesy of P Gili – fig. c)

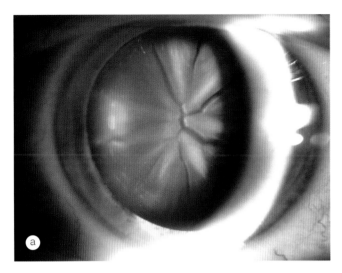

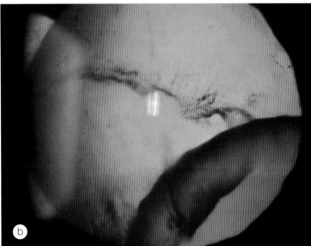

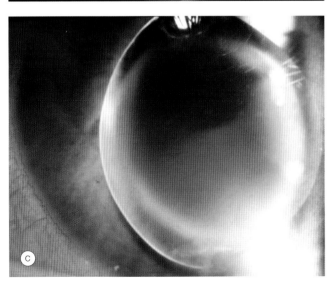

Fig. 23.13
Lens complications of blunt trauma. **(a)** Flower-shaped cataract; **(b)** inferior subluxation; **(c)** dislocation into the anterior chamber (Courtesy of C Barry – fig. b)

the involved area a grey appearance. Commotio most frequently involves the temporal fundus (Fig. 23.15a) and occasionally the macula, when a 'cherry red spot' may be seen at the fovea (Fig. 23.15b). The prognosis in mild cases is good with spontaneous resolution without sequelae within 6 weeks. Severe involvement of the macula may be associated with intraretinal haemorrhage. Subsequent post-traumatic macular changes include progressive RPE degeneration and macular hole formation (Fig. 23.15c).

2. **Choroidal rupture** involves the choroid, Bruch membrane and RPE and may be direct or indirect. Direct ruptures are located anteriorly at the site of impact and run parallel with the ora serrata. Indirect ruptures occur opposite the site of impact. A fresh rupture may be partially obscured by subretinal haemorrhage (Fig. 23.15d), which may break through the internal limiting membrane with a resultant subhyaloid or vitreous bleed. Weeks to months later, a white, crescent-shaped, vertical streak of exposed underlying sclera concentric with the optic disc becomes visible (Fig. 23.15e). The visual prognosis is poor if the fovea is involved. An uncommon late complication is secondary choroidal neovascularization which may result in haemorrhage, scarring and further visual deterioration.

3. **Retinal breaks and retinal detachment** (see Chapter 19).

Optic nerve

1. **Optic neuropathy** presents as sudden visual loss secondary to either blunt or penetrating trauma to the orbit that cannot be explained by other ocular pathology. The damage to the optic nerve is either direct (haemorrhage or compression), shearing (acceleration of the nerve at the optic canal where it is tethered to the dural sheath) or transmission of a shock wave through the orbit. Typically the optic nerve head and fundus are initially normal, the only objective finding being a relative afferent pupillary defect. Many treatments have been advocated (high-dose intravenous steroids, optic canal decompression and optic nerve sheath fenestration) but none appear to be effective and most patients develop permanent visual impairment due to optic atrophy.

2. **Optic nerve avulsion** is rare and typically occurs when an object intrudes between the globe and the orbital wall, displacing the eye. Postulated mechanisms include sudden extreme rotation or anterior displacement of the globe. Avulsion may be isolated or occur in association with other injuries to the globe or orbit. Fundus examination shows a striking cavity where the optic nerve head has retracted from its dural sheath (Fig. 23.15f). There is no treatment; the visual prognosis depends on whether avulsion is partial or complete.

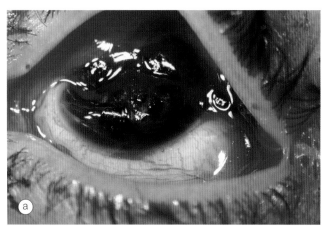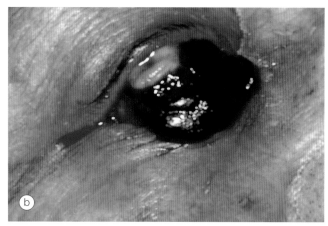

Fig. 23.14
(a) Ruptured globe; **(b)** extremely severe rupture with extrusion of all intraocular contents

Non-accidental injury

Non-accidental injury (shaken baby syndrome) indicates physical abuse in children usually under the age of 2 years, and should be suspected whenever characteristic ophthalmic features are identified in the absence of a convincing alternative explanation. The diagnosis should be considered with the help of a specialist paediatrician; most hospitals dealing with children will have a child abuse team. The injury may be caused by violent shaking alone. However, careful examination also frequently reveals signs of impact injuries. Brain damage is thought to be the result of hypoxia and ischaemia resulting from apnoea, rather than shearing or impact.

1. **Presentation** is frequently with irritability, lethargy and vomiting which may be initially misdiagnosed as gastroenteritis or other infection because the history of injury is withheld.
2. **Systemic features** include subdural haematoma and impact injuries to the head, ranging from skull fractures to soft tissue bruises. Many survivors suffer significant permanent neurological handicap.
3. **Ocular features** are many and varied. The most important are:
   • Retinal haemorrhages, unilateral or bilateral, are the most common feature. They typically involve different layers of the retina and are most obvious in the posterior pole, although they often extend to the periphery.
   • Periocular bruising and subconjunctival haemorrhages.
   • Poor visual responses and afferent pupillary defect.
   • Visual loss occurs in about 20% of cases, largely as a result of cerebral damage.

Penetrating trauma

Causes

Penetrating injuries are three times more common in males than females, and in the younger age group. The most frequent causes are assault, domestic accidents and sport. The extent of the injury is determined by the size of the object, its speed at the time of impact and its composition. Sharp objects such as knives cause well-defined lacerations of the globe. However, the extent of damage caused by flying foreign bodies is determined by their kinetic energy. For example, an air gun pellet is large and, although relatively slow moving, has a high kinetic energy, and can thus cause considerable ocular damage. In contrast, a fast moving fragment of shrapnel has a low mass and therefore will cause a well-defined laceration with relatively less intraocular damage than an air gun pellet.

NB Of paramount immediate importance is the introduction of infection with any penetrating injury. Endophthalmitis or panophthalmitis, often more severe than the initial injury, may ensue with loss of the eye. Risk factors include delay in primary repair, ruptured lens capsule and a contaminated wound.

Corneal

The technique of primary repair depends on the extent of the wound and associated complications such as iris incarceration, flat anterior chamber and damage to intraocular contents.

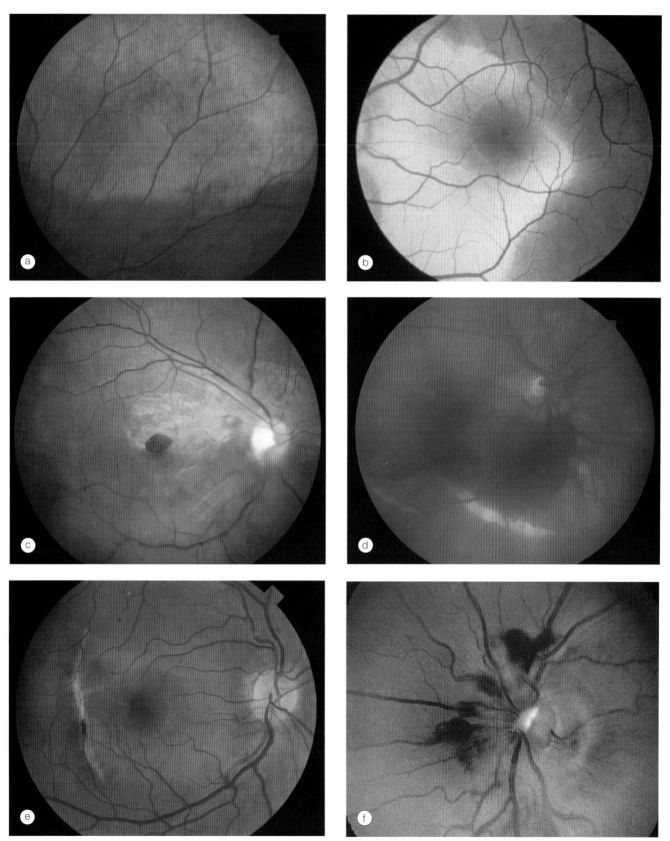

Fig. 23.15
Fundus complications of blunt trauma. **(a)** Peripheral commotio retinae; **(b)** commotio involving the macula; **(c)** macular hole following resolution of commotio retinae; **(d)** acute choroidal rupture with subretinal haemorrhage; **(e)** old choroidal rupture; **(f)** optic nerve avulsion (Courtesy of C Barry – fig. c; E M Eagling and M J Roper-Hall, from *Eye Injuries*, Butterworths, 1986 – fig. f)

1. **Small shelving** wounds (Fig. 23.16a) with formed anterior chamber may not require suturing as they often heal spontaneously or with the aid of a soft bandage contact lens.
2. **Medium-sized** wounds usually require suturing, especially if the anterior chamber is shallow or flat (Fig. 23.16b). A postoperative bandage contact lens may also be useful for a few days to ensure that the anterior chamber remains deep.
3. **With iris involvement** (Fig. 23.16c) usually require iris abscission.
4. **With lens damage** (Fig. 23.16d) is treated by suturing the laceration and removing the lens by phacoemulsification or with a vitreous cutter. Primary implantation of an intraocular lens is frequently associated with a favourable visual outcome.

Scleral

1. **Anterior** scleral lacerations have a better prognosis than those posterior to the ora serrata. An anterior scleral wound may, nevertheless, be associated with serious complications such as iridociliary prolapse (Fig. 23.17a) and vitreous incarceration (Fig. 23.17b). The latter, unless appropriately managed, may result in subsequent fibrous proliferation along the plane of incarcerated vitreous (Fig. 23.17c) and tractional retinal detachment. Every attempt should be made to reposit viable uveal tissue and cut prolapsed vitreous flush with the wound.
2. **Posterior** scleral lacerations are frequently associated with retinal breaks that require prophylactic treatment after the wound has been sutured.

Superficial foreign bodies

Subtarsal

Small foreign bodies such as particles of steel, coal or sand often impact on the corneal or conjunctival surface. They may be washed along the tear film into the lacrimal drainage system or adhere to the superior tarsal conjunctiva (Fig. 23.18a) and abrade the cornea with every blink. A pathognomonic pattern of linear corneal abrasions may be seen (Fig. 23.18b).

Corneal

1. **Clinical features.** Corneal foreign bodies are extremely common and cause considerable irritation. Leukocytic infiltration may also develop around any foreign body of some duration (Fig. 23.18c). If a foreign body is allowed to remain, there is a significant risk of secondary infection and corneal ulceration. Mild secondary uveitis is common with irritative miosis and photophobia. Ferrous foreign bodies of even a few days duration often result in rust staining of the bed of the abrasion.

2. **Management**
   a. The foreign body is removed under slit-lamp visualization using a sterile 26-gauge needle.
   b. Magnetic removal may be useful for a deeply embedded metallic foreign body.
   c. A residual 'rust ring' is easiest to remove with a sterile 'burr', if available.
   d. Antibiotic ointment is instilled together with a cycloplegic and/or ketorolac to promote comfort.

> **NB** Any discharge, infiltrate or significant uveitis, should raise suspicion of secondary bacterial infection and be managed as for a corneal ulcer. Metallic foreign bodies are often sterile due to acute rise in temperature during transit through the air but organic and stone foreign bodies, however, carry a higher risk of infection.

Intraocular foreign bodies

An intraocular foreign body may traumatize the eye mechanically, introduce infection or exert other toxic effects on the intraocular structures. Once in the eye, the foreign body may lodge in any of the structures it encounters (Fig. 23.19). Notable mechanical effects include cataract formation secondary to capsular injury, vitreous liquefaction, and retinal haemorrhages and tears. Stone and organic foreign bodies are particularly prone to result in infection. Many substances including glass, many plastics, gold and silver are inert. However, iron and copper may undergo dissociation and result in siderosis and chalcosis respectively.

Initial management

1. **Accurate history** is vital to determine the origin of the foreign body and it may be helpful for the patient to bring any causative objects such as a chisel.
2. **Eye examination** is performed, paying special attention to possible sites of entry or exit. Topical fluorescein may be helpful to identify an entry wound. Alignment and projection of identified wounds may allow logical deduction of the probable location of a foreign body. Gonioscopy and fundoscopy must be performed, and associated signs such as lid laceration and damage to anterior segment structures noted.
3. **CT** with axial and coronal cuts is used to detect and localize metallic intraocular foreign bodies (see Fig. 23.9b), providing cross-sectional images with a sensitivity and specificity that is superior to plain radiography and ultrasonography.

> **NB** MR is contraindicated in the context of metallic intraocular foreign body.

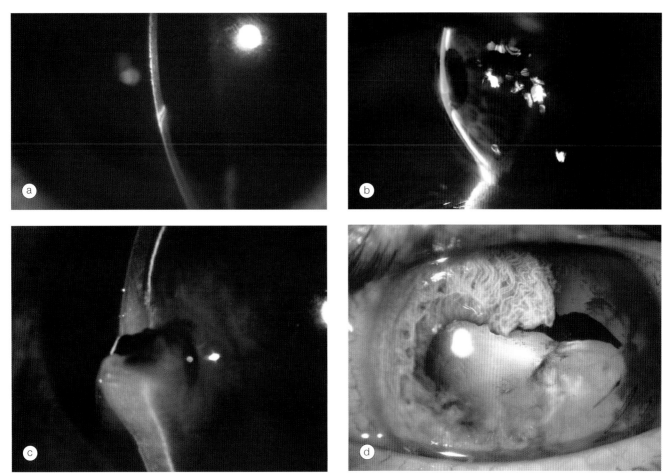

Fig. 23.16
Corneal wounds. **(a)** Small shelving with formed anterior chamber; **(b)** with flat anterior chamber; **(c)** with iris involvement; **(d)** with lens damage

Technique of removal

1. **Magnet** removal of ferrous foreign bodies involves a sclerotomy adjacent to the foreign body, application of a magnet, followed by cryotherapy to the retinal break. Scleral buckling may be performed to reduce the risk of retinal detachment, but this is optional.
2. **Forceps** removal may be used for non-magnetic foreign bodies and magnetic foreign bodies that cannot be safely be removed with a magnet. It involves pars plana vitrectomy and removal of the foreign body with forceps either through the pars plana or limbus, dependent on its size.

   NB Prophylaxis of endophthalmitis with intravitreal antibiotics is required in high-risk cases such as soil-contaminated or vegetable matter.

Siderosis

Perhaps the commonest foreign body is a piece of steel. An intraocular ferrous foreign body undergoes dissociation resulting in the deposition of iron in the intraocular epithelial structures – notably the lens epithelium, iris and ciliary body epithelium, and sensory retina (Fig. 23.20a), where it exerts a toxic effect on cellular enzyme systems, with resultant cell death.

1. **Signs** include anterior capsular cataract, consisting of radial iron deposits on the anterior lens capsule (Fig. 23.20b) and reddish brown staining of the iris (Fig. 23.20c) that may give rise to heterochromia iridis (Fig. 23.20d).
2. **Complications** include secondary glaucoma due to trabecular damage and pigmentary retinopathy. The latter has a profound effect on vision and electroretinography manifests progressive attenuation of the b-wave over time.

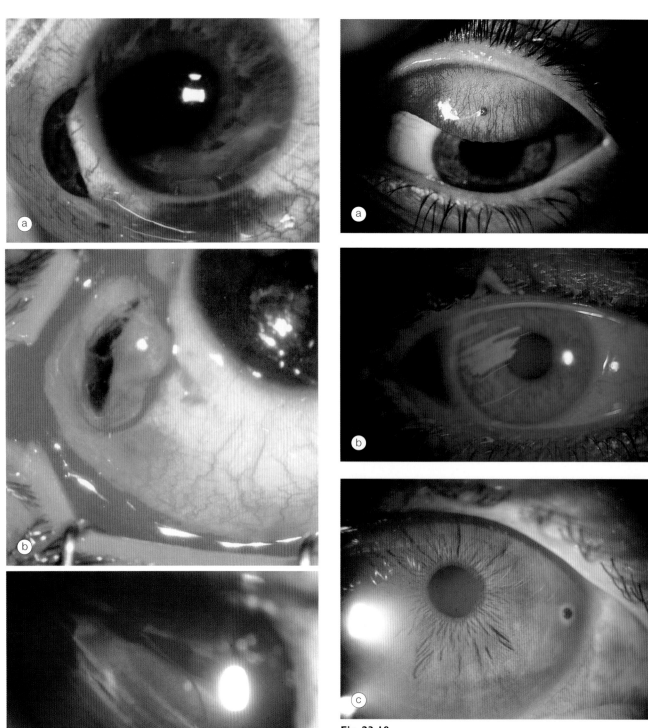

Fig. 23.17
Scleral wounds. **(a)** Anterior circumferential scleral laceration
with iridociliary prolapse; **(b)** radial anterior scleral laceration
with ciliary and vitreous prolapse; **(c)** fibrous proliferation
(Courtesy of Wilmer Institute – fig. a; E M Eagling and M J Roper-Hall,
from *Eye Injuries*, Butterworths, 1986 – fig. b)

Fig. 23.18
(a) Subtarsal foreign body; **(b)** linear abrasions stained with
fluorescein; **(c)** corneal foreign body (Courtesy of R Fogla –
fig. c)

Chalcosis

The ocular reaction to an intraocular foreign body with a high copper content involves a violent endophthalmitis-like picture, often with progression to phthisis bulbi. On the other hand, an alloy such as brass or bronze, with a relatively low copper content, results in chalcosis. Electrolytically dissociated copper becomes deposited intraocularly, resulting in a picture similar to that seen in Wilson disease. Thus a Kayser–Fleischer ring develops, as does an anterior 'sunflower' cataract. Retinal deposition results in golden plaques but, since copper is less retinotoxic than iron, degenerative retinopathy does not develop and visual function may be preserved.

Enucleation

Primary enucleation should be performed only for very severe injuries, with no prospect of retention of vision when it is impossible to repair the sclera (see Fig. 23.14b). Secondary enucleation may be considered following primary repair if the eye is severely and irreversibly damaged, particularly if it is also unsightly and uncomfortable. The time delay also allows the patient valuable time to mentally and emotionally adapt to the prospect of losing an eye. Based on anecdotal evidence, it has been recommended that enucleation should be performed within 10 days of the original injury in order to prevent the very remote possibility of sympathetic ophthalmitis. However, objective evidence for this is lacking.

Sympathetic ophthalmitis

Sympathetic ophthalmitis is a bilateral granulomatous panuveitis occurring after penetrating trauma, often associated with uveal prolapse (Fig. 23.21a) or, less frequently, following intraocular surgery, usually multiple vitreoretinal procedures. The traumatized eye is referred to as the *exciting* eye and the fellow eye, which also develops uveitis, is the *sympathizing* eye. Since histological proof is frequently lacking the diagnosis is mostly presumptive.

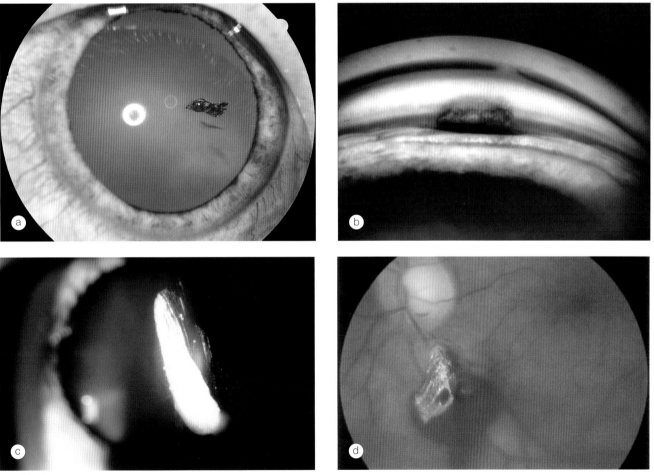

Fig. 23.19
Intraocular foreign bodies. **(a)** In the lens; **(b)** in the angle; **(c)** in the anterior vitreous; **(d)** on the retina with associated preretinal haemorrhage (Courtesy of R Curtis – fig. b; E M Eagling and M J Roper-Hall, from *Eye Injuries*, Butterworths, 1986 – fig. d)

Histology

The characteristic feature is a diffuse and massive lymphocytic infiltration of the choroid, and scattered aggregates of epithelioid cells, many of which contain fine granules of phagocytosed melanin (Fig. 23.21b). Dalen–Fuchs nodules are granulomas located between Bruch membrane and the RPE (Fig. 23.21c).

Diagnosis

1. **Presentation** in 65% of cases is between 2 weeks and 3 months after initial injury and 90% of all cases occur within the first year.
2. **Signs** in chronological order:
   • The exciting eye shows evidence of the initial trauma and is frequently very red and irritable.
   • The sympathizing eye then becomes photophobic and irritable.
   • Both eyes develop anterior uveitis which may be mild or severe and granulomatous (Fig. 23.21d). Because the severity of may be asymmetrical, mild involvement in one eye may be missed.
   • Multifocal choroidal infiltrates in the midperiphery and sub-RPE infiltrates (Fig. 23.21e), corresponding to Dalen–Fuchs nodules seen on histology.
   • Exudative retinal detachment may occur in severe cases.
   • Residual chorioretinal scarring may cause for visual loss when involving the macula.
   • 'Sunset-glow' appearance, similar to Vogt–Koyanagi–Harada syndrome (V-K-H).
3. **FA** shows multiple foci of leakage at the level of RPE, with subretinal pooling in the presence of exudative retinal detachment.
4. **ICG** shows dark spots in the choroid that indicate the presence of active disease. They tend to disappear if treated aggressively in the early stages.
5. **US** may show choroidal thickening and retinal detachment.
6. **Systemic manifestations** are the same as in V-K-H (headache, pleocytosis in the CSF, dysacousis, tinnitus, alopecia, poliosis and vitiligo) but are less common.

Treatment

1. **Enucleation** within first 10 days following trauma should be considered only in eyes with a hopeless visual prognosis because the exciting eye may eventually have better vision than the sympathizing eye.

   NB Evisceration does not seem to protect against sympathetic ophthalmitis.

2. **Topical** treatment of anterior uveitis is with steroids and cycloplegics.

3. **Systemic** treatment with steroids (1–1.5mg/kg) is usually effective although occasionally ciclosporin or azathioprine may be required. Treatment is often required for at least a year with gradual tapering of the dose to reduce the risk of relapse. With aggressive therapy the prognosis is good with 75% of eyes having a visual acuity of better that 6/12.

   NB Long-term follow-up is mandatory because relapses occur in 50% of cases which may be delayed for several years.

Bacterial endophthalmitis

Pathogenesis

Endophthalmitis develops in about 8% of cases of penetrating trauma with retained foreign body.

1. **Risk factors** include delay in primary repair, retained intraocular foreign body, and the position and extent of the laceration. Clinical signs are the same as acute postoperative endophthalmitis.
2. **Pathogens.** *Staphylococcus* spp. and *Bacillus* spp. are isolated from about 90% of culture positive cases.

Management

1. **Prophylaxis**
   • Ciprofloxacin 750mg b.d. is given for open globe injuries.
   • Prompt removal of retained intraocular foreign bodies.
   • Intravitreal antibiotics for high-risk cases requiring vitrectomy (e.g. agricultural injuries).
2. **Culture** of removed intraocular foreign bodies (do not stick them in the clinical notes!).
3. **Treatment** for established cases is the same as for acute bacterial endophthalmitis (see Chapter 12).

CHEMICAL INJURIES

Causes

Chemical injuries range in severity from trivial to potentially blinding. The majority are accidental and a few the result of assault. Two-thirds of accidental burns occur at work and the remainder at home. Alkali burns are twice as common as acid burns since alkalis are more widely used at home and in industry. The most common involved alkalis are ammonia, sodium hydroxide and lime. The commonest acids implicated are sulphuric, sulphurous, hydrofluoric,

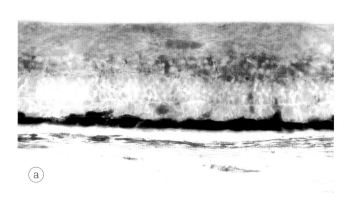

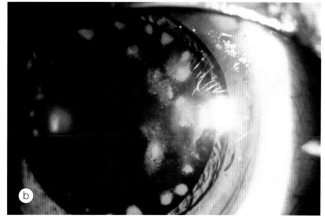

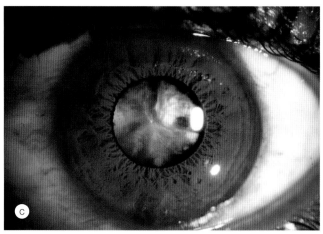

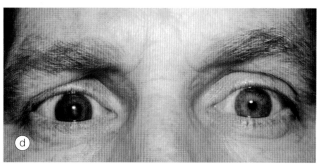

Fig. 23.20
Siderosis oculi. **(a)** Iron deposition in the retina; **(b)** lenticular deposits; **(c)** severe iris involvement and advanced cataract; **(d)** heterochromia iridis (Courtesy of J Harry and G Misson, from *Clinical Ophthalmic Pathology*, Butterworth-Heinemann, 2001–fig. a)

acetic, chromic and hydrochloric. The severity of a chemical injury is related to the properties of the chemical, the area of affected ocular surface, duration of exposure (retention of particulate chemical on the surface of the globe) and related effects such as thermal damage. Alkalis tend to penetrate deeper than do acids, which coagulate surface proteins, resulting in a protective barrier. Ammonia and sodium hydroxide may produce severe damage because of rapid penetration. Hydrofluoric acid used in glass etching and cleaning also tends to rapidly penetrate the eye whilst sulphuric acid may be complicated by thermal effects and high velocity impact after car battery explosions.

Pathophysiology

1. **Damage** by severe chemical injuries occurs in the following order:
   - Necrosis of the conjunctival and corneal epithelium with disruption and occlusion of the limbal vasculature.

- Loss of limbal stem cells may subsequently result in conjunctivalization and vascularization of the corneal surface or persistent corneal epithelial defects with sterile corneal ulceration and perforation. Other long-term effects include ocular surface wetting disorders, symblepharon formation and cicatricial entropion.
- Deeper penetration causes breakdown and precipitation of glycosaminoglycans and stromal corneal opacification.
- Anterior chamber penetration results in iris and lens damage.
- Ciliary epithelial damage impairs secretion of ascorbate which is required for collagen production and corneal repair.
- Hypotony and phthisis bulbi may ensue.
2. **Healing** of the corneal epithelium and stroma as follows:
   - The epithelium heals by migration of epithelial cells which originate from limbal stem cells.
   - Damaged stromal collagen is phagocytosed by keratocytes and new collagen is synthesized.

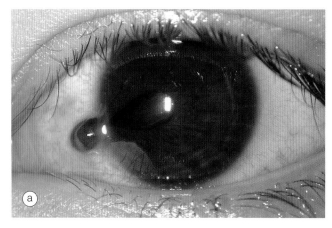

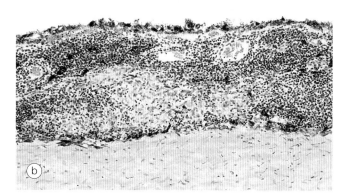

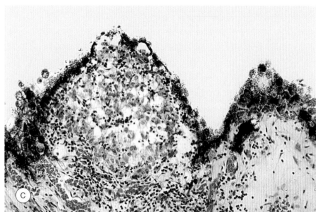

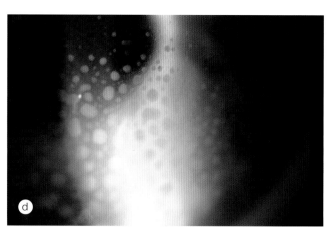

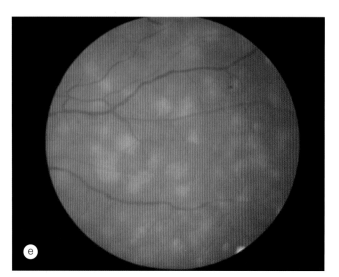

Fig. 23.21
Sympathetic ophthalmitis. **(a)** Penetrating injury with iris prolapse; **(b)** lymphocytic infiltration and granuloma formation in the choroid; **(c)** Dalen–Fuchs nodule – a granuloma situated between Bruch membrane and the retinal pigment epithelium; **(d)** mutton fat keratic precipitates in granulomatous anterior uveitis; **(e)** multifocal choroiditis (Courtesy of N Rogers fig. a; J Harry – figs b and c; C Pavesio – fig. e)

Management

Emergency treatment

A chemical burn is the only eye injury that requires immediate treatment without first taking a history and performing a careful examination. Immediate treatment is as follows:

1. **Copious irrigation** is crucial to minimize duration of contact with the chemical and normalize the pH in the conjunctival sac as soon as possible. Normal saline (or equivalent) should be used to irrigate the eye for 15–30 minutes or until pH is normalized.
2. **Double-eversion of the eyelids** should be performed so that any retained particulate matter trapped in the fornices, such as lime or cement, may be removed.
3. **Debridement** of necrotic areas of corneal epithelium should be performed to allow for proper re-epithelialisation.

Grading of severity

Acute chemical injuries are then graded to plan appropriate subsequent treatment and afford an indication of likely ultimate prognosis. Grading is performed on the basis of corneal clarity and severity of limbal ischaemia. The latter is assessed by observing the patency of the deep and superficial vessels at the limbus (Fig. 23.22a).

1. **Grade 1:** clear cornea and no limbal ischaemia (excellent prognosis).
2. **Grade 2:** hazy cornea but with visible iris details (Fig. 23.22b) and less than one-third of limbal ischaemia (good prognosis).
3. **Grade 3:** total loss of corneal epithelium, stromal haze obscuring iris details (Fig. 23.22c) and between one-third and half of limbal ischaemia (guarded prognosis).
4. **Grade 4:** opaque cornea (Fig. 23.22d) and more than half of limbal ischaemia (very poor prognosis).

Other features to note at initial assessment are the extent of corneal and conjunctival epithelial loss, iris changes, status of the lens and intraocular pressure.

Medical treatment

Mild (grade 1 and 2) injuries are treated with a short course of topical steroids, cycloplegics and prophylactic antibiotics for about 7 days. The main aims of treatment for more severe burns are to reduce inflammation, promote epithelial regeneration and prevent corneal ulceration.

1. **Steroids** reduce inflammation and neutrophil infiltration. However, they also impair stromal healing by reducing collagen synthesis and inhibiting fibroblast migration. For this reason topical steroids may be used initially but must be tailed off after 7–10 days when sterile corneal ulceration is most likely to occur. They may be replaced by topical NSAIDs, which do not affect keratocyte function.
2. **Ascorbic acid** reverses a localized tissue scorbutic state and improves wound healing by promoting the synthesis of mature collagen by corneal fibroblasts. Topical sodium ascorbate 10% is given 2-hourly in addition to a systemic dose of 2g q.i.d.
3. **Citric acid** is a powerful inhibitor of neutrophil activity and reduces the intensity of the inflammatory response. Chelation of extracellular calcium by citrate also appears to inhibit collagenase. Topical sodium citrate 10% is given 2-hourly for about 10 days. The aim is to eliminate the second wave of phagocytes, which normally occurs 7 days after the injury.
4. **Tetracyclines** are effective collagenase inhibitors and also inhibit neutrophil activity and reduce ulceration. They are administered both topically and systemically (doxycycline 100mg b.d.).

Surgery

1. **Early** surgery may be necessary to revascularize the limbus, restore the limbal cell population and re-establish the fornices. One or more of the following procedures may be used:
   - Advancement of Tenon capsule and suturing to the limbus is aimed at re-establishing limbal vascularity thus preventing the development of corneal ulceration.
   - Limbal stem cell transplantation from the patient's other eye (autograft) or from a donor (allograft) is aimed at restoring normal corneal epithelium.
   - Amniotic membrane grafting to promote epithelialisation and suppression of fibrosis.
2. **Late** surgery may involve the following procedures:
   - Division of conjunctival bands (Fig. 22.23e) and symblepharon (Fig. 22.23f).
   - Conjunctival or mucous membrane grafts.
   - Correction of eyelid deformities.
   - Keratoplasty should be delayed for at least 6 months, and preferably longer, to allow maximal resolution of inflammation.
   - Keratoprosthesis (see Fig. 10.5a) may be required in very severely damaged eyes because the results of conventional grafting are poor.

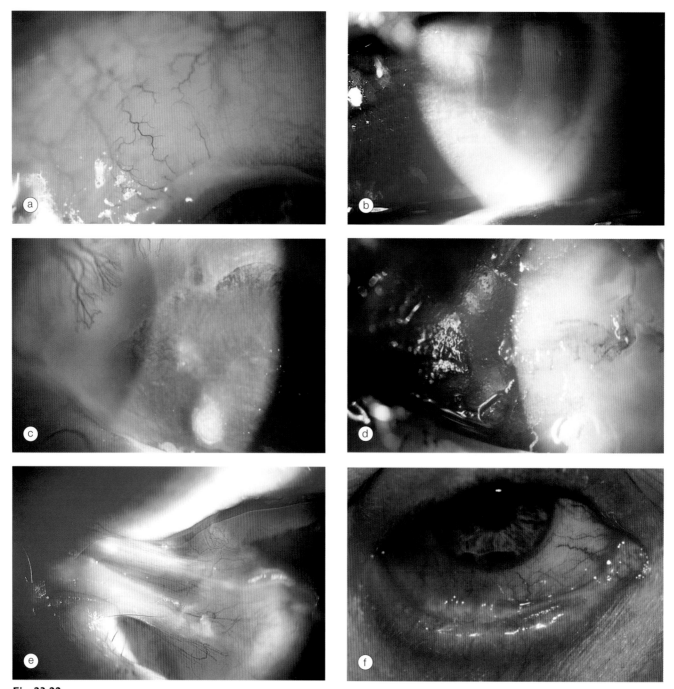

Fig. 23.22
Chemical burns. **(a)** Limbal ischaemia; **(b)** grade 2 − corneal haze but visible iris details; **(c)** grade 3 − corneal haze obscuring iris details; **(d)** grade 4 − total corneal opacification; **(e)** conjunctival bands; **(f)** symblepharon

CHAPTER 24

SYSTEMIC DISEASES

CONNECTIVE TISSUE DISEASES

Rheumatoid arthritis

Rheumatoid arthritis (RA) is an autoimmune systemic disease characterized by a symmetrical, destructive, deforming, inflammatory polyarthropathy, in association with a spectrum of extra-articular manifestations and circulating antiglobulin antibodies, termed rheumatoid factors. It is much more common in females than males.

1. **Presentation** is often in the fourth decade with joint swelling, usually of the hands (Fig. 24.1a).
2. **Signs**
   - Symmetrical arthritis of the small joints of the hands typically involving the proximal interphalangeal and sparing the distal interphalangeal joints. The metacarpophalangeal and wrist joints are also commonly involved.
   - Joint instability secondary to chronic inflammation may result in subluxation and deformities, such as ulnar deviation of the metacarpophalangeal joints (Fig. 24.1b).
   - Less frequent involvement of the feet, shoulders, elbows, hips and cervical spine.
   - Skin manifestations include 'rheumatoid' nodules over bony prominences (Fig. 24.1c), vasculitis which may cause ulceration (Fig. 24.1d), and occasionally pyoderma gangrenosum.
3. **Complications**
   - Pulmonary nodules and fibrosis.
   - Multifocal neuropathy.
   - Septic arthritis.
   - Secondary amyloidosis.
   - Carpal tunnel syndrome.
4. **Treatment** options include NSAIDs, gold salts, D-penicillamine, hydroxychloroquine, sulfasalazine, steroids and cytotoxic agents.
5. **Ocular features:** keratoconjunctivitis sicca (secondary Sjögren syndrome), scleritis, ulcerative keratitis, and rarely, acquired superior oblique tendon sheath syndrome.

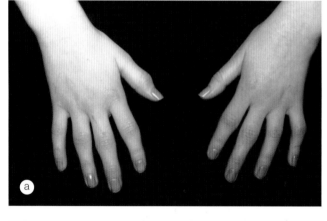

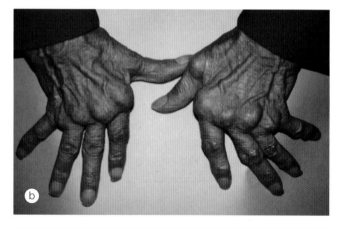

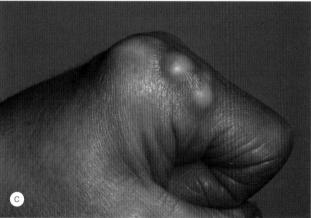

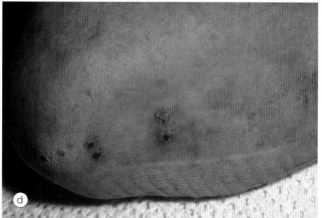

Fig. 24.1
Rheumatoid arthritis. **(a)** Swelling of the fingers in early active disease; **(b)** ulnar deviation of the fingers in longstanding disease; **(c)** 'rheumatoid' nodules; **(d)** cutaneous vasculitis

Juvenile idiopathic arthritis

Juvenile idiopathic arthritis (JIA) is an inflammatory arthritis of at least 6 weeks duration occurring before the age of 16 years. Girls are affected more commonly than boys by a 3:2 ratio. JIA is by far the most common disease associated with childhood anterior uveitis.

NB JIA is not the same as juvenile rheumatoid arthritis (JRA); the former is negative for rheumatoid factor whereas the latter is positive. JRA is the same disease as rheumatoid arthritis except that it occurs before the age of 16 years.

1. **Presentation** is based on the onset and the extent of joint involvement during the first 6 months as follows:
   a. **Pauciarticular onset** JIA involves four or fewer joints and accounts for about 60% of cases.

- Girls are affected five times as often as boys, with a peak age of onset around 2 years.
- The arthritis involves most commonly the knees (Fig. 24.2a), although the ankles and wrists may also be affected.
- Some patients in this subgroup remain pauci-articular others subsequently develop a polyarthritis.
- About 75% of children are antinuclear antibody (ANA) positive.
- Uveitis is common in this group and affects about 20% of children.
- Risk factors for uveitis are early-onset of JIA, and positive findings for ANA and HLA-DR5.

   b. **Polyarticular onset** JIA affects five or more joints and accounts for a further 20% of cases.
- Girls are affected about three times as often as boys and the disease may commence at any age throughout childhood.
- The arthritis involves both small and large joints symmetrically (Fig. 24.2b).

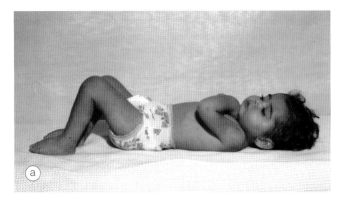
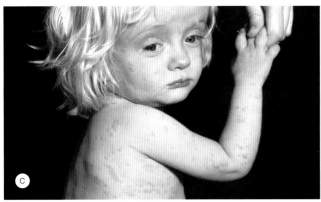
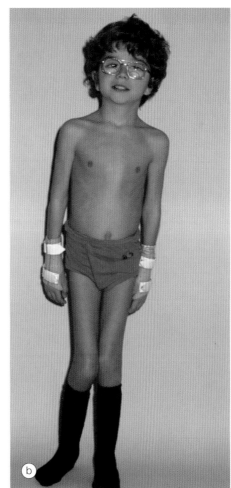

Fig. 24.2
Juvenile idiopathic arthritis. **(a)** Early-onset pauciarticular disease affecting the knees; **(b)** severe polyarticular disease; **(c)** maculopapular rash in systemic onset disease

– Systemic features such as fever and rash are mild or absent.
– About 40% of children are ANA positive.
– Uveitis occurs in about 5% of cases.

c. _Systemic onset_ JIA accounts for about 20% of cases.
– The disease occurs with equal frequency in boys and girls and may occur at any age throughout childhood.
– Systemic features include a high remittent fever, transient maculopapular rash (Fig. 24.2c), generalized lymphadenopathy, hepatosplenomegaly and serositis.
– Initially, arthralgia or arthritis may be absent or minimal and a minority of patients subsequently develops progressive polyarthritis.
– The vast majority are negative for ANA.
– Uveitis does not occur.

NB The term 'Still disease' is reserved for patients in this subgroup.

2. **Treatment** options include physiotherapy, NSAIDs, intra-articular triamcinolone hexacetonide injection and low dose methotrexate.
3. **Ocular feature:** chronic anterior uveitis.

Systemic lupus erythematosus

Systemic lupus erythematosus (SLE) is an autoimmune, non-organ specific connective tissue disease characterized by numerous autoantibodies and circulating immune complexes which mediate widespread vasculitis and tissue damage. It predominantly affects young females.

1. **Presentation** is in the third to fifth decades with fatigue without specific organ involvement. Alternatively, the disease may present with symmetrical arthralgia.
2. **Signs**
   • Mucocutaneous features include a 'butterfly' facial rash (Fig. 24.3a), discoid rash, vasculitis, telangiectasis, photosensitivity, alopecia, oral ulceration and Raynaud phenomenon (Fig. 24.3b).
   • Arthritis, myositis and tendonitis.
   • Glomerulonephritis.
   • Pericarditis, endocarditis, myocarditis, and arterial and venous occlusion.
   • Pleurisy, atelectasis and 'shrinking lungs'.
   • Anaemia, thrombocytopenia, lymphopenia and leucopenia.
   • Splenomegaly and lymphadenopathy.
   • Polyneuritis, cranial nerve palsies, spinal cord lesions, epilepsy, stroke and psychosis.
3. **Diagnostic tests**
   • The ESR is raised, but C-reactive protein is usually not.

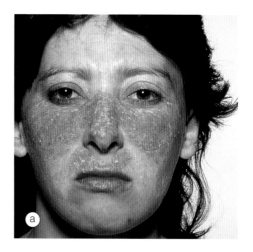

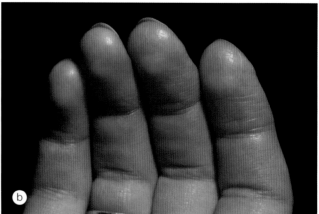

Fig. 24.3
Systemic lupus erythematosus. **(a)** Butterfly facial skin rash; **(b)** Raynaud phenomenon involving the finger tips

   • A variety of autoantibodies including lupus anti-coagulant, antiphospholipid and antinuclear may be present.
4. **Treatment** options include antimalarials, NSAIDs, steroids and cytotoxic agents.
5. **Ocular features:** madarosis, keratoconjunctivitis sicca, scleritis, peripheral ulcerative keratitis, retinal vasculitis and optic neuropathy.

Wegener granulomatosis

Wegener granulomatosis is an idiopathic, multisystem disorder characterized by small vessel vasculitis affecting predominantly the respiratory tract and kidneys. It affects males more commonly than females. Because it can be localized to the eye and the orbit, without any systemic involvement, orbital biopsy may be required for diagnosis.

1. **Presentation** is in the fifth decade, often with pulmonary symptoms.
2. **Signs**
   - Upper respiratory tract involvement by necrotizing granulomatous inflammation may result in perforation of the nasal septum, saddle-shaped nasal deformity and nasal-paranasal fistulae.
   - Lower respiratory tract involvement may result in nodular lesions, infiltrates and cavitation with fluid levels (Fig. 24.4a).
   - Necrotizing glomerulonephritis, with renal failure.
   - Cutaneous vasculitis and bullae (Fig. 24.4b).
   - Focal vasculitis involving the spleen, heart and adrenals.
   - Polyneuritis and meningoencephalitis.
3. **Diagnostic tests.** Anti-neutrophil cytoplasmic antibodies (c-ANCA) are found in over 90% of patients with active disease.

4. **Treatment** is with systemic steroids and cyclophosphamide.
5. **Ocular features:** necrotizing scleritis, peripheral ulcerative keratitis, occlusive retinal periarteritis, orbital inflammatory disease, nasolacrimal obstruction, dacryocystitis and rarely tarsal-conjunctival disease.

Polyarteritis nodosa

Polyarteritis nodosa (PAN) is an idiopathic, potentially lethal, collagen vascular disease affecting medium-sized or small arteries. It is three times more common in males than in females. Ocular involvement may precede the systemic manifestations by several years.

1. **Presentation** is in the third to sixth decades with tachycardia, myalgia, arthralgia, fever and weight loss.
2. **Signs**
   - Cutaneous signs include purpura, dermal infarcts (Fig. 24.5a) and livedo reticularis (Fig. 24.5b).
   - Muscular weakness and tenderness.

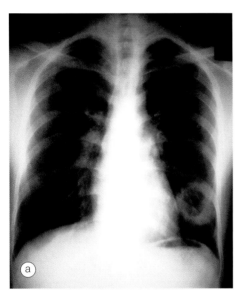

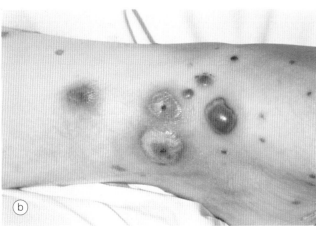

Fig. 24.4
Wegener granulomatosis. **(a)** Pulmonary cavitation; **(b)** vasculitis and bullae (Courtesy of M A Mir, from *Atlas of Clinical Diagnosis*, Saunders, 2003 – fig. b)

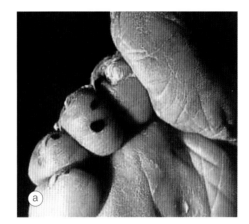

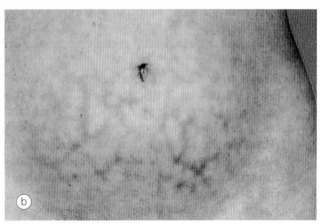

Fig. 24.5
Polyarteritis nodosa. **(a)** Dermal infarcts; **(b)** livedo reticularis

- Renal involvement and hypertension.
- Coronary arteritis which may lead to heart failure and myocardial infarction.
- Gastrointestinal bleeding or an acute abdominal crisis.
- Stroke or multifocal neuropathy.

3. **Diagnostic tests** show eosinophilia, hypergammaglobulinaemia and necrotizing lesions on skin biopsy.
4. **Treatment** is with systemic steroids and cytotoxic agents.
5. **Ocular features:** necrotizing scleritis, peripheral ulcerative keratitis, orbital inflammatory disease and occlusive retinal periarteritis.

Relapsing polychondritis

Relapsing polychondritis is a rare idiopathic condition characterized by small vessel vasculitis involving cartilage resulting in recurrent, often progressive, inflammatory episodes involving multiple organ systems.

1. **Presentation** is in the fifth and sixth decades.
2. **Signs**
   - Recurrent swelling of the pinnae (Fig. 24.6a).
   - Involvement of the tracheobronchial cartilage may give rise to hoarse voice, cough and stridor.
   - Collapse of the nasal bridge resulting in a 'saddle-shaped' deformity (Fig. 24.6b).
   - Cardiac valve dysfunction.
   - Non-erosive inflammatory polyarthritis.
   - Cochlear or vestibular damage resulting in neurosensory hearing loss, tinnitus, or vertigo.

3. **Treatment.** Mild ear disease usually responds to systemic NSAIDs but major organ involvement requires high-dose systemic steroids in combination with cytotoxic agents.
4. **Ocular features:** scleritis and acute anterior uveitis.

Sjögren syndrome

Sjögren syndrome is characterized by autoimmune inflammation and destruction of lacrimal and salivary glands (Fig. 24.7a). The condition is classified as primary when it exists in isolation, and secondary when associated with other diseases such as RA, SLE, systemic sclerosis, primary biliary cirrhosis, chronic active hepatitis and myasthenia gravis. Primary Sjögren syndrome affects females more commonly than males.

1. **Presentation** is in adult life with grittiness of the eyes and dryness of the mouth.
2. **Signs**
   - Enlargement of salivary glands (Fig. 24.7b), and occasionally lacrimal glands, with secondary diminished salivary flow rate and a dry fissured tongue (Fig. 24.7c).
   - Dry nasal passages, diminished vaginal secretions and dyspareunia.
   - Raynaud phenomenon and cutaneous vasculitis.
3. **Complications**
   - Dental caries (Fig. 24.7d).
   - Reflux oesophagitis and gastritis.
   - Malabsorption due to pancreatic failure.
   - Pulmonary and renal disease, and polyneuropathy.
   - Lymphoma.

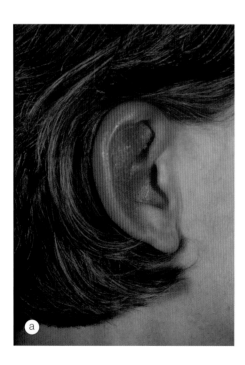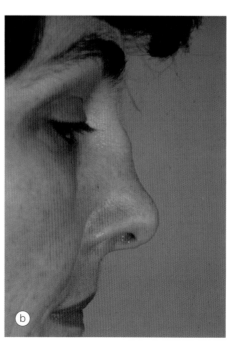

Fig. 24.6
Relapsing polychondritis. **(a)** Swelling of the pinna; **(b)** 'saddle-shaped' nasal deformity (Courtesy of C Pavesio)

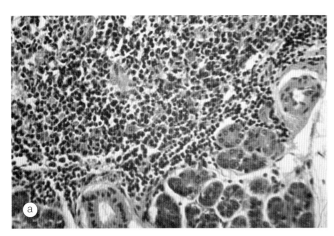

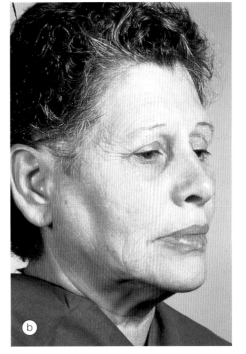

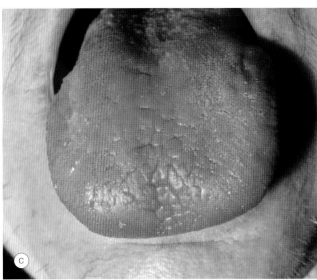

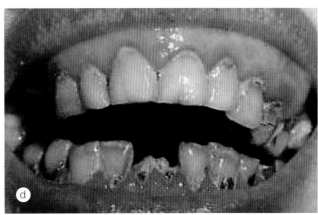

Fig. 24.7
Sjögren syndrome. **(a)** Histology of a lacrimal gland shows lymphocytic infiltration; **(b)** parotid gland enlargement; **(c)** dry fissured tongue; **(d)** severe dental caries (Courtesy of M A Mir, from *Atlas of Clinical Diagnosis*, Saunders, 2003 – figs b and d).

4. Diagnostic tests: serum autoantibodies, Schirmer test and biopsy of minor salivary glands.

5. Treatment options include systemic steroids and cytotoxic agents.

6. Ocular features: keratoconjunctivitis sicca and Adie pupil (rare).

Systemic sclerosis

Systemic sclerosis is an idiopathic, chronic connective tissue disease affecting the skin (scleroderma) and internal organs,

occurring most commonly in females. The risk of internal organ disease is proportional to the extent of skin involvement. Systemic sclerosis may be (a) *limited*, (b) *diffuse*, (c) *sine scleroderma* and (d) *overlap with other autoimmune diseases.*

1. Presentation is in the fourth to sixth decades with Raynaud phenomenon.

2. Signs

  a. Skin

  – A typical facial appearance characterized by a fixed expression, restrictive movements of the lips and 'beaking' of the nose (Fig. 24.8a).

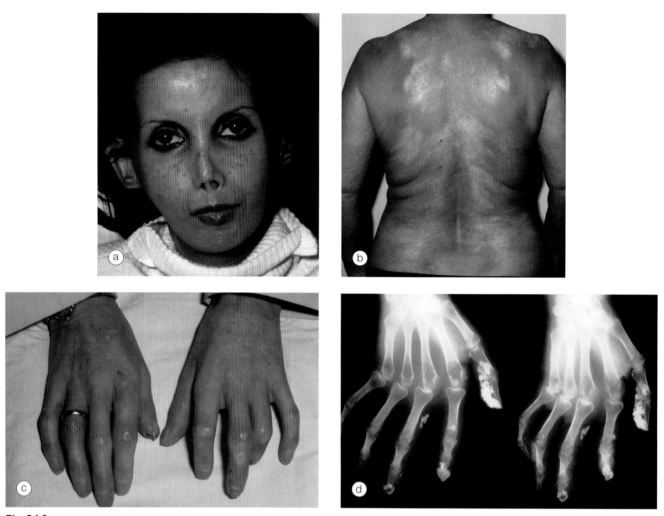

Fig. 24.8
Systemic sclerosis. **(a)** Fixed facial expression and a 'beaked' nose; **(b)** morphea; **(c)** sclerodactyly; **(d)** calcinosis cutis

- Tightening and thickening of the skin gives rise to a waxy appearance (Fig. 24.8b).
- Subcutaneous fibrosis causes binding-down of skin, tapering of the fingers with loss of pulps (sclerodactyly – Fig. 24.8c) and subcutaneous deposition of calcium (calcinosis cutis – Fig. 24.8d).

   b. Organs
- Oesophageal dysmobility.
- Cardiac, pulmonary and renal disease.
- Mild arthritis and myositis.

3. Diagnostic tests. Positive serum ANA and other autoantibodies; skin biopsy.

4. Treatment is unsatisfactory.

5. Ophthalmic features
   a. Common. Eyelid tightening and telangiectasis.
   b. Uncommon. Keratoconjunctivitis sicca.

c. Rare. Conjunctival forniceal shortening and vascular changes, nodular episcleritis, scleral pits, retinal cotton-wool spots, and patches of choroidal non-perfusion seen only on fluorescein angiography

Giant cell arteritis

Giant cell arteritis (GCA) is a granulomatous necrotizing arteritis (Fig. 24.9a and b) with a predilection for large and medium-size arteries, particularly the superficial temporal, ophthalmic, posterior ciliary and proximal vertebral. The severity and extent of involvement are associated with the quantity of elastic tissue in the media and adventitia. Intra-cranial arteries, which possess little elastic tissue, are usually spared.

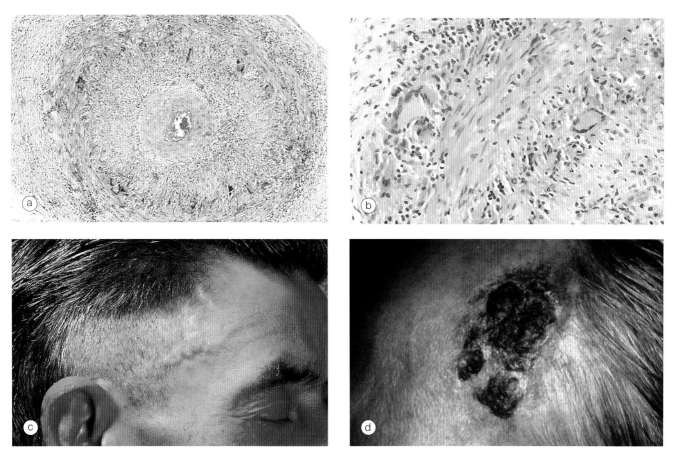

Fig. 24.9
Giant cell arteritis. **(a)** Histology shows transmural granulomatous inflammation, disruption of the internal elastic lamina, proliferation of the intima and gross narrowing of the lumen; **(b)** high power view shows giant cells and infiltration with small round cells; **(c)** superficial temporal arteritis and shaved hair prior to biopsy; **(d)** scalp gangrene (Courtesy of J Harry – fig. a; J Harry and G Misson, from Clinical Ophthalmic Pathology, Butterworth-Heinemann, 2001 – figs a and b)

Clinical features

1. Presentation is usually in the seventh to eighth decades with the following:

- Scalp tenderness, first noticed when combing the hair, is a frequent presenting complaint.
- Headache, sometimes severe, may be localized to the frontal, occipital or temporal areas, or more generalized.
- Jaw claudication is virtually pathognomonic. It is caused by ischaemia of the masseter and causes pain on speaking and chewing.
- Polymyalgia rheumatica is characterized by pain and stiffness in proximal muscle groups (typically the shoulders). It is typically worse in the morning and after exertion, and may precede other symptoms by many months.
- Non-specific manifestations such as neck pain, weight loss, fever, night sweats, malaise and depression are common.

- Blindness of sudden onset with minimal systemic upset (occult arteritis) is uncommon.

2. Other features

- Superficial temporal arteritis is characterized by thickened, tender inflamed and nodular arteries (Fig. 24.9c), which cannot be flattened against the skull. Pulsation is initially present, but later ceases, a sign strongly suggestive of GCA, since a non-pulsatile superficial temporal artery is highly unusual in a normal individual. In very severe cases, scalp gangrene may ensue (Fig. 24.9d).

NB The best location to examine pulsation is directly in front of the pinna.

- Complications include dissecting aneurysms, aortic incompetence, myocardial infarction, renal failure and brainstem stroke.

Investigations

1. **Erythrocyte sedimentation rate** (ESR) is often very high, with levels of > 60mm/h. In interpreting the ESR the following should be borne in mind.
   - The normal ESR equals roughly half the age in men and is 5 mm higher in women.
   - ESR levels of 40mm/h may be 'normal' in diabetics and in the elderly.
   - Approximately 20% of patients with CGA have a normal ESR.
2. **C-reactive protein** (CRP) is invariably raised and may be helpful when ESR is equivocal.
3. **Platelet counts** tend to be elevated and the presence of thrombocytosis makes the diagnosis of GCA more likely, particularly if the ESR is also elevated.
4. **Temporal artery biopsy** (TAB) should be performed if GCA is suspected.
   - Steroids should never be withheld pending biopsy, which should ideally be performed within 3 days of commencing steroids.
   - Systemic steroids for more than 7 days may suppress histological evidence of active arteritis; however, this is not invariable and biopsy should still be performed even if steroid therapy has been commenced considerably earlier. This is for two reasons; (a) if positive, it justifies long-term administration of steroids in a population highly prone to their adverse effects, and (b) if negative, it provides justification for tailing off and stopping steroid therapy.
   - In patients with ocular involvement it is advisable to take the biopsy from the ipsilateral side. The ideal location is the temple because it avoids damage to a major branch of the auriculotemporal nerve.
   - At least 2.5cm of the artery should be taken and serial sections examined because of the phenomenon of 'skip lesions' in which segments of histologically normal arterial wall may alternate with segments of granulomatous inflammation.
   - Lack of pulsation may render TAB difficult, especially in inexperienced hands; not uncommonly, a segment of nerve is excised and sent for histological examination.

Treatment

Treatment involves systemic steroids. The duration of treatment is governed by the patient's symptoms and the level of the ESR or CRP. Symptoms may, however, recur without a corresponding rise in ESR or CRP and vice versa. Most patients need treatment for 1–2 years, although some may require indefinite maintenance therapy. CRP may play an important role in monitoring disease activity, as the level seems to fall more rapidly than the ESR in response to treatment.

Ophthalmic features

1. **Arteritic anterior ischaemic optic neuropathy** (AION) is the most common. In untreated patients the incidence is 30–50%, of which one-third develop involvement of the fellow eye usually within one week of the first. Posterior ischaemic optic neuropathy is much less common.
2. **Transient ischaemic attacks** (amaurosis fugax) may precede AION.
3. **Cotton-wool spots** are uncommon. They are probably caused by platelet microembolization from the partially thrombosed ophthalmic or central retinal artery. Because GCA is a disease of medium-sized or large arteries, it cannot involve terminal arterioles to produce cotton-wool spots.
4. **Cilioretinal artery occlusion** may be combined with AION.
5. **Central retinal artery occlusion** is usually combined with occlusion of a posterior ciliary artery. This is because the central retinal artery often arises from the ophthalmic artery by a common trunk with one or more of the posterior ciliary arteries. However, ophthalmoscopy shows occlusion of only the central retinal artery and the associated ciliary occlusion can be detected only on fluorescein angiography.
6. **Ocular ischaemic syndrome** due to involvement of the ophthalmic artery is rare.
7. **Diplopia,** transient or constant, may be caused by ischaemia of the ocular motor nerves or extraocular muscles.

Ehlers–Danlos syndrome type 6

Ehlers–Danlos syndrome type 6 (ocular sclerotic) is a rare, usually AR disorder of collagen caused by deficiency of procollagen lysyl hydroxylase. There are nine distinct subtypes but only type 6, and rarely type 4, are associated with ocular features.

1. **Skin** is thin and hyperelastic (Fig. 24.10a). It bruises easily, heals slowly and with a tendency to (papyraceous) scarring (Fig. 24.10b).
2. **Joints** are hypermobile with lax ligaments (Fig. 24.10c). This may lead to recurrent dislocation, repeated falls, hydroarthrosis and pseudotumour formation over the knees and elbows.
3. **Cardiovascular disease** consists of a bleeding diathesis, dissecting aneurysms, spontaneous rupture of large blood vessels and mitral valve prolapse.
4. **Other systemic manifestations** include scoliosis, diaphragmatic hernias, and diverticula of the gastro-intestinal and respiratory tracts.
5. **Ocular features**
   a. Common. Ocular fragility with increased vulnerability to mild trauma, high myopia, retinal detachment and keratoconus.

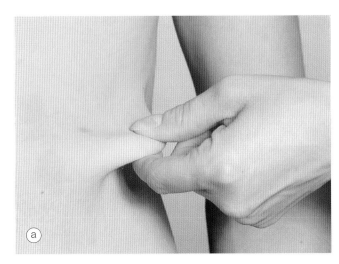

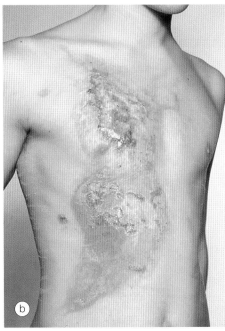

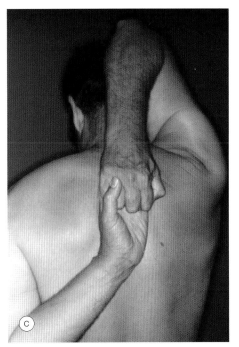

Fig. 24.10
Ehlers–Danlos syndrome type 6. **(a)** Cutaneous hyperelasticity; **(b)** papyraceous scarring; **(c)** joint hypermobility (Courtesy of M A Mir, from *Atlas of Clinical Diagnosis*, Saunders, 2003 – figs a and b)

- Disproportionately long limbs compared with the trunk (arm span > height – Fig. 24.11a).
- Long spider-like fingers and toes (arachnodactyly – Fig. 24.11b) and mild joint hypermobility.
- A narrow high-arched (gothic) palate (Fig. 24.11c).
- Muscular underdevelopment and predisposition to hernias.

2. Cardiovascular
- Dilatation of the ascending aorta leading to aortic incompetence and heart failure.
- Mitral valve disease and aortic dissection.

3. Skin may show striae, fragility and easy bruising.

4. Ophthalmic features
   a. Common. Ectopia lentis, hypoplasia of dilator pupillae, angle anomaly, myopia and retinal detachment.
   b. Uncommon. Microspherophakia, keratoconus and cornea plana.
   c. Rare. Megalocornea.

b. Uncommon. Epicanthic folds, microcornea, blue sclera, ectopia lentis and angioid streaks.

Marfan syndrome

Marfan syndrome is a widespread disorder of connective tissue associated with mutation of the fibrillin gene on chromosome 15q. Inheritance is AD with variable expressivity.

1. Musculoskeletal features
- Tall, thin stature, scoliosis, sternal deformity (prominence or depression).

Stickler syndrome

Stickler syndrome (hereditary arthro-ophthalmopathy) is a disorder of collagen connective tissue, resulting in abnormal vitreous, myopia (Fig. 24.12a), and a variable degree of orofacial abnormality, deafness and arthropathy. Inheritance

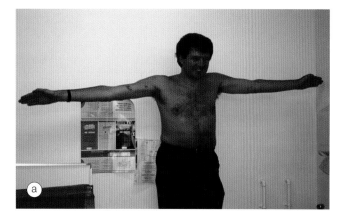

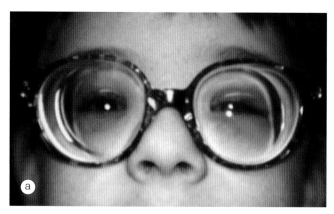

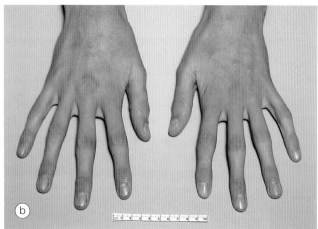

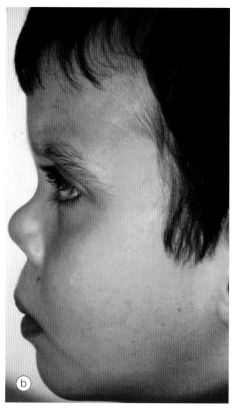

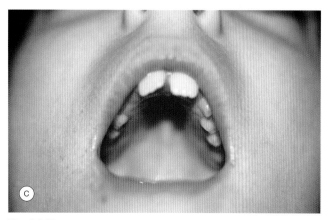

Fig. 24.11
Marfan syndrome. **(a)** Arm span greater than height;
(b) arachnodactyly; **(c)** high-arched palate

Fig. 24.12
Stickler syndrome. **(a)** High myopia; **(b)** flat nasal bridge and
maxillary hypoplasia (Courtesy of K Nischal – fig. a)

is AD with complete penetrance but variable expressivity.
Stickler syndrome is the commonest inherited cause of
retinal detachment in children.

Classification

1. Type 1 is the result of mutations in the *COL2A1* gene

and accounts for approximately 60% of cases. These
subjects have the classic ocular and systemic features as
originally described by Stickler.

2. Type 2 is caused by mutations in the *COL11A1* gene.
These subjects have congenital non-progressive high
myopia, sensorineural deafness, and other features of
Stickler syndrome type 1.

3. Type 3 is caused by mutations in the *COL11A2* gene. These subjects have the typical systemic features, but no ocular manifestations.

Systemic features

1. **Facial** anomalies include a flat nasal bridge and maxillary hypoplasia (Fig. 24.12b).
2. **Skeletal** involvement includes a Marfanoid habitus, arachnodactyly, arthropathy and joint hyperextensibility.
3. **Robin sequence** is characterized by micrognathia, small tongue, cleft soft palate and high-arched palate.
4. **Deafness.**
5. **Mitral valve prolapse.**

Pseudoxanthoma elasticum

Pseudoxanthoma elasticum is a hereditary disorder of connective tissue in which there is progressive calcification, fragmentation and degeneration of elastic fibres in the skin (Fig. 24.13a), eye and cardiovascular system. There are four distinctive types in which ocular manifestations are common but of variable severity.

1. Dominant type 1
- 'Plucked chicken' appearance of the skin resulting from small, yellowish macules, papules or plaques most commonly on the neck (Fig. 24.13b), axillae, antecubital fossae, groins and paraumbilical area.
- Involved skin becomes progressively loose (Fig. 24.13c), thin and delicate.
- Calcification of elastic media and intima of arteries and heart valves causes renal artery stenosis, intermittent claudication and mitral valve prolapse.
- Gastric haemorrhage is due to bleeding from fragile calcified submucosal vessels.
- Occasional bleeding in the urinary tract or cerebrovascular system.
- Severe angioid streaks (Groenblad–Strandberg syndrome).

2. Dominant type 2
- Fewer and flatter skin papules than in dominant type 1.
- Skin hyperelasticity and high-arched palate.
- Mild angioid streaks and blue sclera.

3. Recessive type 1
- Skin changes are similar to dominant type 1.
- Mild vascular disease but frequent gastric bleeding.

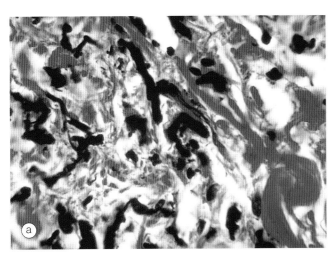

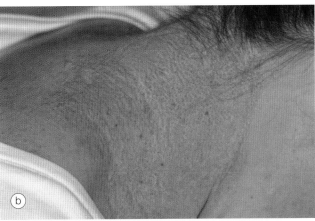

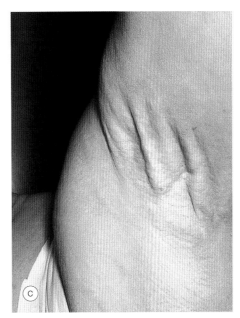

Fig. 24.13
Pseudoxanthoma elasticum. **(a)** Histology shows thickened fragmented fibres in the dermis; **(b)** 'chicken-skin' papules; **(c)** loose skin (Courtesy of J Harry and G Misson, from *Clinical Ophthalmic Pathology*, Butterworth-Heinemann, 2001 – fig. a; P Saine – fig. b)

- Mild angioid streaks.
4. **Recessive type 2**
   - Severe generalized skin changes.
   - No systemic complications.
   - Angioid streaks.

SPONDYLOARTHROPATHIES

Ankylosing spondylitis

Ankylosing spondylitis (AS) is characterized by inflammation, calcification and finally ossification of ligaments and capsules of joints with resultant bony ankylosis of the axial skeleton. It typically affects males, about 95% of whom are HLA-B27 positive; some patients also have inflammatory bowel disease (enteropathic arthritis).

1. **Presentation** is in early adulthood with insidious onset of pain and stiffness in the lower back or buttocks. This is initially worse after inactivity, but may be aggravated by weight bearing.
2. **Signs**
   a. Arthritis. In order of frequency, the joints most affected are the sacroiliac, spine, hips, ribs and shoulders. Progressive limitation of spinal movements occurs and then the spine becomes fixed in flexion (Fig. 24.14a). Reduced mobility of the thoracic cage may predispose to pulmonary infection.
   b. Enthesopathy characterized by inflammation and pain at ligamentous attachments to bone.
3. **Complications** include apical pulmonary fibrosis, aortic incompetence and cardiac conduction defects.
4. **Investigations.** The ESR is raised. Radiology of the sacroiliac joints reveals juxta-articular osteoporosis in the early stages, later followed by sclerosis and bony obliteration of the joint. The spinal ligaments may also manifest calcification ('bamboo spine' – Fig. 24.14b), as may other joints.

   NB Radiological changes often pre-date clinical symptoms.

5. **Treatment** options include physiotherapy, NSAIDs, sulfasalazine and intra-articular steroid injections. Surgical correction of bony deformities may be necessary.
6. **Ocular features:** acute anterior uveitis is very common, scleritis is rare.

Reiter syndrome

Reiter syndrome (RS), also referred to as reactive arthritis, is characterized by the triad of non-specific (non-gonococcal) urethritis, conjunctivitis and arthritis. Although relatively rare, RS develops in 1–3% of men following an attack of non-

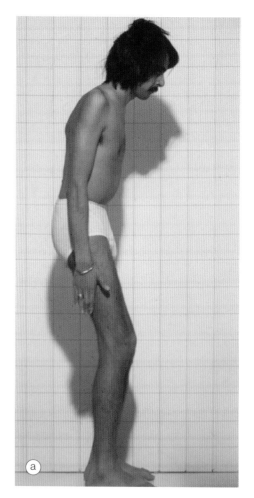
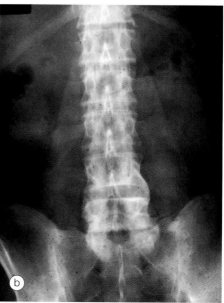

Fig. 24.14
Ankylosing spondylitis. **(a)** Flexion spine deformity in moderately severe disease; **(b)** radiological changes in advanced disease show bilateral sclerosis and erosion of the sacroiliac joints and bony fusion of the spine (Courtesy of B Ansell – fig. a; A Hall – fig. b)

specific urethritis, up to 4% of persons after enteric infections caused by *Shigella*, *Salmonella* and *Campylobacter*, and in a higher proportion of patients with *Yersinia* enteric infections. Post-dysenteric RS affects males and females equally, whereas post-venereal RS is more common in men. About 85% of patients with RS are positive for HLA-B27 but the diagnosis is clinical and is based on the presence of arthritis and other characteristic manifestation.

1. **Presentation** is between the second and fourth decades with non-specific urethritis, conjunctivitis and arthritis, occurring within a short period of each other, classically a month after dysentery or sexual intercourse.
2. **Signs**
   a. ***Peripheral arthritis*** is typically acute in onset, asymmetrical and migratory. Two to four joints tend to be involved, most commonly the knees, ankles and toes. In some patients peripheral arthritis may be recurrent or become chronic.
   b. ***Spondyloarthritis*** (spondylitis and sacroiliitis) affects about 30% of patients with severe chronic RS and is related to the presence of HLA-B27.
   c. ***Enthesopathy*** may manifest as plantar fasciitis, Achilles tenosynovitis, bursitis and calcaneal periostitis; reactive bone formation in the latter may result in a calcaneal spur.
   d. ***Mucocutaneous*** features include painless mouth ulceration, circinate balanitis (Fig. 24.15a), keratoderma blenorrhagica involving the palms and soles (Fig. 24.15b) and nail dystrophy.
   e. ***Genitourinary:*** cystitis, cervicitis, prostatitis, epididymitis and orchitis.
   f. ***Other manifestations*** include cardiac disease, amyloidosis, thrombophlebitis, pleurisy, diarrhoea, neuropathy and meningoencephalitis.
3. **Treatment** is with NSAIDs.
4. **Ocular features:** conjunctivitis, acute anterior uveitis, nummular keratitis, episcleritis, scleritis, papillitis and retinal vasculitis.

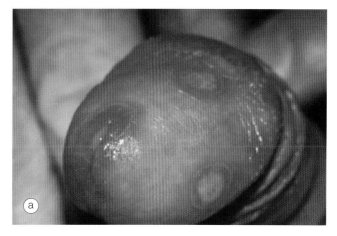
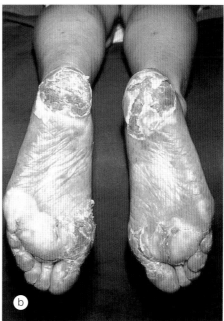

Fig. 24.15
Reiter syndrome. **(a)** Urethral discharge and circinate balanitis; **(b)** keratoderma blenorrhagica (Courtesy of M A Mir, from *Atlas of Clinical Diagnosis*, Saunders, 2003 – fig. b)

Psoriatic arthritis

About 7% of patients with psoriasis develop arthritis. Psoriatic arthritis affects both sexes equally and is associated with an increased prevalence of HLA-B27 and HLA-B17.

1. **Presentation** is in the third to fourth decades.
2. **Signs**
   a. ***Skin***
      - Plaque psoriasis (most common) is characterized by well-demarcated, salmon-pink areas covered with thick, silvery plaques (Fig. 24.16a).
      - Flexural psoriasis manifests non-scaly pink lesions usually affecting the groin and perineum.
   b. ***Arthritis*** may take one of the following patterns
      - Asymmetrical involvement of the distal interphalangeal joints (Fig. 24.16b).
      - Pauciarticular peripheral involvement.
      - Symmetrical peripheral involvement similar to RA.
      - Arthritis mutilans affecting a few digits is rare.
      - Associated AS.
   c. ***Nail dystrophy*** consists of pitting, transverse depression and onycholysis (Fig. 24.16b).
3. **Treatment** involves NSAIDs, intra-articular steroids and cytotoxic drugs for severe disease.
4. **Ocular features:** anterior uveitis, conjunctivitis, marginal corneal infiltrates and secondary Sjögren syndrome.

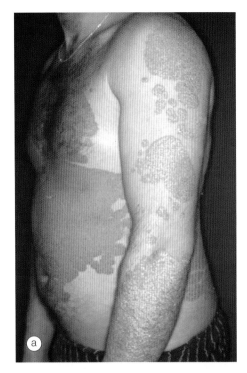

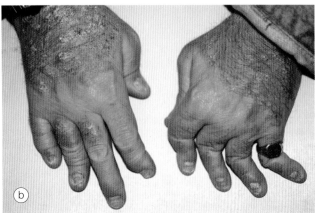

Fig. 24.16
Psoriatic arthritis. **(a)** Plaque psoriasis; **(b)** psoriasis of the hands, nail dystrophy and asymmetrical arthritis with ulnar deviation of fingers

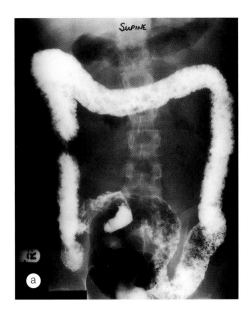

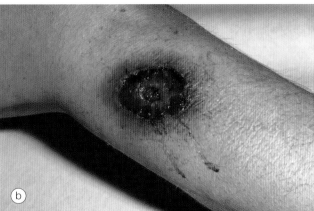

Fig. 24.17
Ulcerative colitis. **(a)** Barium enema shows pseudopolyposis, lack of haustral markings and straightening of the ascending colon; **(b)** pyoderma gangrenosum

INFLAMMATORY BOWEL DISEASE

Ulcerative colitis

Ulcerative colitis is an idiopathic, chronic, relapsing disease, involving the rectum and extending proximally to involve part or all of the large intestine. The disease is characterized by diffuse surface ulceration of the mucosa with the development of crypt abscesses and pseudopolyps (Fig. 24.17a). Patients with long-standing disease carry an increased risk of developing carcinoma of the colon.

1. **Presentation** is in the second to third decades with bloody diarrhoea, lower abdominal cramps, urgency and tenesmus. Constitutional symptoms include tiredness, weight loss, malaise and fever.
2. **Extra-intestinal manifestations**
   a. ***Mucocutaneous*** features include oral aphthous ulceration, erythema nodosum and pyoderma gangrenosum (Fig. 24.17b).
   b. ***Skeletal*** manifestations include asymmetrical lower limb arthritis of large joints; sacroiliitis and AS spondylitis may develop in HLA-B27 positive patients.

c. **Hepatic disease** may be in the form of autoimmune hepatitis, sclerosing cholangitis and cholangiocarcinoma.

d. **Thromboses** which may involve both arteries and veins.

e. **Secondary amyloidosis.**

3. **Investigations** involve endoscopy and biopsy.

4. **Treatment** options include systemic steroids, sulfasalazine, cytotoxic agents and colectomy.

5. **Ocular features:** acute anterior uveitis, peripheral corneal infiltrates, conjunctivitis, episcleritis, scleritis, papillitis and retinal vasculitis.

Crohn disease

Crohn disease (regional ileitis) is an idiopathic, chronic, relapsing disease characterized by multifocal, full-thickness, non-caseating granulomatous inflammation of the intestinal wall most frequently involving the ileocaecal region.

1. **Presentation** is in the second to third decades with fever, weight loss, diarrhoea and abdominal pain.

2. **Extra-intestinal manifestations**

a. **Oral** lesions include glossitis and aphthous ulceration.

b. **Cutaneous** lesions consist of erythema nodosum, pyoderma gangrenosum and psoriasis.

c. **Skeletal** findings include finger clubbing, acute peripheral arthritis, sacroiliitis and AS.

3. **Complications** include intestinal obstruction due to stricture formation (Fig. 24.18a), perirectal abscesses and fistulae (Fig. 24.18b), and liver disease.

4. **Investigations** involve endoscopy and biopsy.

5. **Treatment** options include nutritional support, steroids, antibiotics, cytotoxic agents and surgery.

6. **Ocular features:** acute anterior uveitis, conjunctivitis, episcleritis, peripheral corneal infiltrates and retinal periphlebitis.

NON-INFECTIOUS MULTISYSTEM DISEASES

Sarcoidosis

Sarcoidosis is an idiopathic T-lymphocyte-mediated non-caseating granulomatous inflammatory disease. The clinical spectrum varies from mild single organ involvement to potentially fatal multisystem disease. The tissues most commonly involved are the mediastinal and superficial lymph nodes, lungs, liver, spleen, skin, parotid glands, phalangeal bones and the eye.

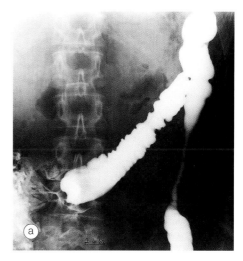

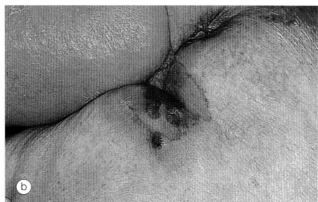

Fig. 24.18
Crohn disease. **(a)** Barium enema shows a stricture in the descending colon; **(b)** perianal abscess and fistula (Courtesy of P C Hayes and N D C Finlayson, from *Colour Guide Medicine*, Churchill Livingstone, 1994 – fig. b)

Presentation

1. **Acute-onset** sarcoidosis presents in one of the following ways:

a. **Löfgren syndrome** is characterized by erythema nodosum and bilateral hilar lymphadenopathy, often accompanied by fever and/or arthralgia.

b. **Heerfordt syndrome** (uveoparotid fever) manifests uveitis, parotid gland enlargement, fever and cranial nerve palsy, often facial.

2. **Insidious-onset** sarcoidosis typically presents during the fifth decade with pulmonary involvement resulting in cough and dyspnoea, or extrapulmonary signs.

Pulmonary disease

Stage 1: Bilateral asymptomatic hilar lymphadenopathy (Fig. 24.19a); spontaneous resolution occurs within 1 year in most cases.

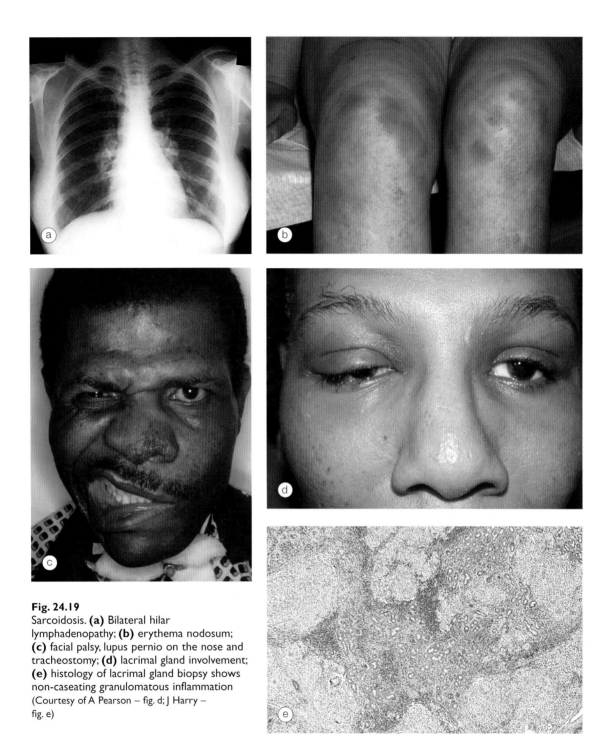

Fig. 24.19
Sarcoidosis. **(a)** Bilateral hilar
lymphadenopathy; **(b)** erythema nodosum;
(c) facial palsy, lupus pernio on the nose and
tracheostomy; **(d)** lacrimal gland involvement;
(e) histology of lacrimal gland biopsy shows
non-caseating granulomatous inflammation
(Courtesy of A Pearson – fig. d; J Harry –
fig. e)

Stage 2: Bilateral hilar lymphadenopathy and diffuse parenchymal reticulonodular infiltrates; spontaneous resolution occurs in the majority.

Stage 3: Reticulonodular infiltrates alone; spontaneous resolution is less common.

Stage 4: Pulmonary fibrosis which may result in progressive ventilatory failure, pulmonary hypertension and cor pulmonale.

Skin lesions

The skin is involved in about 25% of patients by one of the following:

1. **Erythema nodosum** is characterized by erythematous plaques typically involving the knees and shins (Fig. 24.19b) and occasionally the thighs and forearms.

2. **Granulomas** are scattered papules, plaques or nodules.
3. **Lupus pernio** is characterized by indurated, violaceous lesions involving exposed parts of the body such as the nose, cheeks, fingers or ears (Fig. 24.19c).
4. **Granulomatous deposits** in long-standing scars or tattoos.

Other manifestations

1. **Neurological** disease affects about 5–10% of patients. The most common lesion is unilateral facial nerve palsy (Fig. 24.19c); less common manifestations include seizures, meningitis, peripheral neuropathy and psychiatric symptoms.
2. **Arthritis** in chronic sarcoidosis is symmetrical and may involve both small and large joints.

NB In children the presentation can be very similar to juvenile idiopathic arthritis because arthropathy tends to be more prominent than pulmonary disease.

3. **Renal disease** in the form of nephrocalcinosis, hypercalciuria and renal stones.
4. **Miscellaneous** involvement includes lymphadenopathy, granulomatous liver disease, splenomegaly and cardiac arrhythmias.

Investigations

1. **Chest radiographs** are abnormal in 90%.
2. **Biopsy**
   - Lungs give the greatest yield (90%) even in asymptomatic patients with normal chest radiograms.
   - Conjunctiva is positive in about 70% of patients with conjunctival nodules, which resemble follicular conjunctivitis.
   - Lacrimal glands are positive in 25% of un-enlarged and 75% of enlarged glands (Fig. 24.19d and e).
   - Superficial lymph node or skin lesion.
3. **Serum angiotensin-converting enzyme (ACE)** is raised in up to 80% of patients with acute sarcoidosis but may be normal during remissions. The normal serum level in adults is 32.1 ± 8.5 IU. In children the levels tend to be higher and diagnostically less useful. In patients with suspected neurosarcoid ACE can be measured in the cerebrospinal fluid.

NB ACE may also be elevated in other conditions such as tuberculosis, lymphoma and leprosy.

4. **Lysozyme assay** has good sensitivity but less specificity than ACE but both tests seem to increase sensitivity and specificity.
5. **Bronchoalveolar lavage** shows a raised proportion of activated T-helper lymphocytes. Sputum examination may also show increased CD4/CD8 ratios.

6. **Pulmonary function tests** reveal a restrictive lung defect with reduced total lung capacity and are very useful for monitoring disease activity and the need for systemic therapy.
7. **Mantoux test** is negative in most patients; a strongly positive reaction to one tuberculin unit makes the diagnosis of sarcoidosis highly unlikely.

Treatment

Patients with stage 1 and 2 pulmonary disease seldom require treatment because spontaneous resolution is the rule. Troublesome erythema nodosum, pyrexia and arthralgia may benefit from NSAIDs. Systemic corticosteroids are usually effective in patients with symptomatic stage 3 pulmonary disease or involvement of vital organs. Methotrexate may be used as a steroid-sparing agent.

Ocular features

Uveitis is the most common and may be in the form of anterior, posterior or intermediate. Other manifestations include keratoconjunctivitis sicca and conjunctival nodules.

Behçet syndrome

Behçet syndrome (BS) is an idiopathic disease characterized by recurrent episodes of orogenital ulceration and vasculitis which may involve small, medium and large veins and arteries. The disease typically affects patients from the eastern Mediterranean region and Japan and is strongly associated with HLA-B51. The peak age of onset of BS is in the third decade, although rarely it presents in childhood or old age; males are affected more frequently than females.

Diagnostic criteria

1. **Painful oral aphthous ulceration** (Fig. 24.20a) that has recurred at least three times in a 12-month period.
2. **Plus at least two of the following:**
   - Recurrent genital ulceration (Fig. 24.20b).
   - Uveitis.
   - Skin lesions include erythema nodosum, folliculitis, acneiform nodules or papulopustular lesions (Fig. 24.20c).
   - Positive pathergy test which is characterized by the formation of a pustule after 24–48 hours at the site of a sterile needle prick.

Non-diagnostic manifestations

1. **Major vascular complications**
   - Aneurysms of the pulmonary and or systemic arterial system.
   - Coronary artery disease, cardiomyopathy and valvular disease.

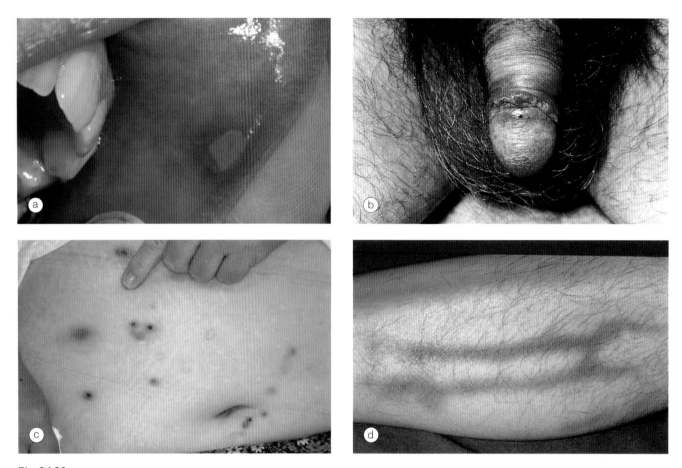

Fig. 24.20
Behçet disease. **(a)** Aphthous ulceration; **(b)** genital ulceration; **(c)** papulopustular skin lesions; **(d)** thrombophlebitis (Courtesy of
P Saine – fig. c; M A Mir, from *Atlas of Clinical Diagnosis*, Mosby, 2003 – fig. d)

- Venous thrombosis which may involve superficial vein (Fig. 24.20d), deep veins, vena cava, portohepatic vein and cerebral sinuses.
2. **Arthritis** occurs in 50% of patients. It is typically mild and involves a few large joints, particularly the knees.
3. **Skin**
   - Hypersensitivity demonstrated by the formation of erythematous lines following stroking of the skin (dermatographia).
   - Vasculitis.
4. **Gastrointestinal ulceration** is less uncommon and may involve the oesophagus, stomach or intestines.
5. **Neurological manifestations** occur in 5% of patients and mainly involve the brainstem, although meningo-encephalitis and spinal cord disease may also occur.
6. **Other** uncommon manifestations include glomerulo-nephritis and epididymitis.

Treatment

Annoying oral ulceration is treated with steroid mouth-washes or pastes. Systemic disease requires systemic steroids in combination with other immunosuppressive agents.

Ocular features

Panuveitis is common. Other less common manifestations include conjunctivitis, conjunctival ulceration, episcleritis, scleritis, and ophthalmoplegia from neurological involvement.

Vogt–Koyanagi–Harada syndrome

Vogt–Koyanagi–Harada (V-K-H) syndrome is an idiopathic autoimmune disease against melanocytes causing inflammation of melanocyte-containing tissues such as the uvea, ear and meninges. V-K-H predominantly affects Hispanics, Japanese and pigmented individuals. In different racial groups the disease is associated with HLA-DR1 and HLA-DR4, suggesting a common immunogenic predisposition. In practice, V-K-H can be subdivided into Vogt–Koyanagi disease, characterized mainly by skin changes and anterior uveitis, and Harada disease, in which neurological features and

Table 24.1 Modified diagnostic criteria for V-K-H syndrome

1. Absence of a history of penetrating ocular trauma.

2. Absence of other ocular disease entities.

3. Bilateral uveitis.

4. Neurological and auditory manifestations.

5. Integumentary findings not preceding onset of central nervous system or ocular disease such as alopecia, poliosis and vitiligo.
   - In complete V-K-H, criteria 1 to 5 must be present.
   - In incomplete V-K-H, criteria 1 to 3 and either 4 or 5 must be present.
   - In probable V-K-H (isolated ocular disease), criteria 1 to 3 must be present.

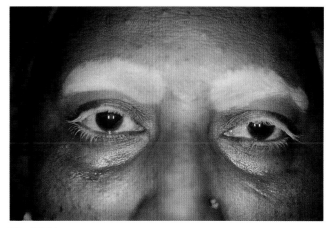

Fig. 24.21
Localised vitiligo and poliosis in Vogt–Koyanagi–Harada syndrome (Courtesy of U Raina)

exudative retinal detachments predominate. Possible trigger factors include cutaneous injury or a viral infection which may lead to sensitization of melanocytes.

Phases

1. **Prodromal** phase lasting a few days is characterized by neurological and auditory manifestations.
   - Meningitis causing headache and neck stiffness.
   - Encephalopathy is less frequent and may manifest as convulsions, paresis and cranial nerve palsies.
   - Auditory features include tinnitus, vertigo and deafness.
2. **Acute uveitic** phase follows soon thereafter and is characterized by bilateral granulomatous anterior or multifocal posterior uveitis and exudative retinal detachments.
3. **Convalescent** phase follows several weeks later and is characterized by:
   - Localized alopecia, poliosis and vitiligo (Fig. 24.21).
   - Focal depigmented fundus lesions (sunset glow fundus) and depigmented limbal lesions (Sugiura sign).
4. **Chronic-recurrent** phase is characterized by smoldering anterior uveitis with exacerbations.

SYSTEMIC INFECTIONS AND INFESTATIONS

Acquired immunodeficiency syndrome

Pathogenesis

Acquired immunodeficiency syndrome (AIDS) is caused by the human immunodeficiency virus (HIV). On a worldwide basis, heterosexual intercourse is the predominant mode of transmission; in the western world, however, AIDS is commonly transmitted by homosexual contact. Transmission may also occur by contaminated blood or needles, transplacentally or via breast milk. HIV targets CD4+T (helper) lymphocytes, which are vital to the initiation of the immune response to pathogens. A steady decline in the absolute number of CD4+T-lymphocytes therefore occurs, resulting in progressive immune deficiency, particularly of cell mediated immunity. Regular estimation of the CD4+T count is therefore a useful measure of disease progression.

Systemic features

1. **Progression of HIV infection**
   a. **Acute seroconversion illness**. HIV infection is sometimes followed a few weeks later by constitutional symptoms such as fever, headache, malaise, maculopapular rash associated with generalized lymphadenopathy, soon after which anti-HIV antibodies appear.
   b. **An asymptomatic phase**, often lasting many years, then follows, during which steady depletion of CD4+T-lymphocytes occurs.
   c. **Symptomatic HIV infection** (AIDS) then ensues, characterized by opportunistic infections, neoplasms and tissue damage directly due to HIV infection.
2. **Opportunistic infections** with protozoa (e.g. *Pneumocystis carinii* and *Cryptosporidium* spp.), viruses (e.g. CMV, HSV) fungi (e.g. *Cryptococcus neoformans* and *Candida albicans* – Fig. 24.22a) and bacteria (e.g. *M. avium-intracellulare* and *Bartonella henselae*).
3. **Tumours** include Kaposi sarcoma (Fig. 24.22b), non Hodgkin B-cell lymphoma and squamous cell carcinoma of the conjunctiva (in Africa), cervix and anus.

4. Other manifestations include HIV wasting syndrome (Fig. 24.22c), HIV encephalopathy (Fig. 24.22d) and progressive multifocal leucoencephalopathy

Serology

- Serological testing for HIV infection should be performed only with informed consent after proper counselling, due to the profound implications of a positive result. HIV is confirmed most commonly by the demonstration of anti-HIV antibodies in the serum by the ELISA and Western Blot tests.
- 'Seroconversion' may take 3 months or longer to occur following exposure to the virus, sometimes necessitating serial testing in individuals at high risk.
- Subsequent to the establishment of HIV positivity,

CD4+T-lymphocyte counts are measured every 3 months. A CD4+T-lymphocyte count < 200/mm^3 implies a high risk of HIV related disease. AIDS is diagnosed when a HIV positive subject develops one or more of a defined list of indicator diseases.

Treatment

Although there is no cure for AIDS, the progression of disease can be slowed by a number of drugs. The aim of treatment is to reduce the plasma viral load. Ideally therapy should be commenced before the development of irreversible damage to the immune system.

I. Indications for commencement of anti-HIV therapy include:

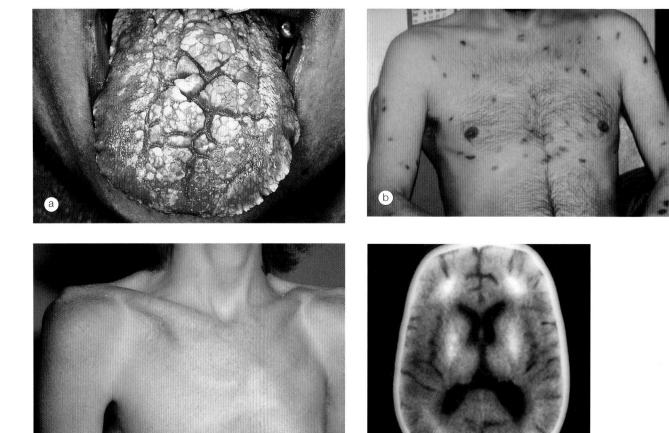

Fig. 24.22
Acquired immunodeficiency syndrome. **(a)** Candidiasis; **(b)** Kaposi sarcoma; **(c)** HIV wasting syndrome; **(d)** axial CT in advanced HIV encephalopathy shows increase in ventricular size secondary to brain atrophy, and calcification in the basal ganglia and frontal lobes
(Courtesy of Emond, Welsby and Rowland from, *Colour Atlas of Infectious Diseases*, Mosby, 2003 – fig. a; B J Zitelli and H W Davis, from *Atlas of Pediatric Physical Diagnosis*, Mosby, 2002 – fig. d)

- Symptomatic HIV disease.
- Rapidly falling CD4+T-lymphocyte count.
- Viral load > 10,000/ml of plasma.

2. **Drug treatment** is with 'highly active antiretroviral therapy' (HAART), which involves two nucleoside reverse transcriptase inhibitors with either a non-nucleoside reverse transcriptase inhibitor or one or two protease inhibitors.

   a. *Nucleoside reverse transcriptase inhibitors* include zidovudine, lamivudine and zalcitabine.

   b. *Protease inhibitors* include amprenavir, indinavir and nelfinadir.

   c. *Non-nucleoside reverse transcriptase inhibitors* include efavirenz and nevirapine.

NB Antiretroviral therapy is continuously evolving and should therefore be left to a trained physician.

Ocular features

1. **Eyelid:** blepharitis, Kaposi sarcoma, multiple molluscum lesions and severe herpes zoster ophthalmicus.
2. **Orbital:** cellulitis, usually from contiguous sinus infection, and B-cell lymphoma.
3. **Anterior segment**
   - Conjunctival Kaposi sarcoma, squamous cell carcinoma and microangiopathy.
   - Keratitis due to microsporidium, herpes simplex and herpes zoster.
   - Keratoconjunctivitis sicca.
   - Anterior uveitis (usually secondary to systemic drug toxicity: rifabutin, cidofovir).
4. **Posterior segment**
   - HIV retinopathy.
   - Cytomegalovirus retinitis.
   - Progressive outer retinal necrosis.
   - Toxoplasmosis, frequently atypical.
   - Choroidal cryptococcosis.
   - Choroidal pneumocystosis.
   - B-cell intraocular lymphoma.

Tuberculosis

Tuberculosis (TB) is a chronic granulomatous infection caused by the tubercle bacillus which is of the genus *Mycobacterium*, which are non-motile, non-sporing, strictly aerobic rods. The two species responsible for TB in humans are the human strain *M. tuberculosis*, which is acquired by inhaling infected airborne droplets, and the bovine strain *M. bovis*, which is acquired by drinking unpasteurised milk from infected cattle. TB is primarily a pulmonary disease but it may spread by the blood stream to other sites of form a generalized (miliary) infection. Human immunodeficiency virus increases the risk of developing TB. In addition,

infection with atypical mycobacteria *M. avium complex* may cause disease in immunocompromised individuals.

Stages

1. **Primary TB** usually occurs in children not previously exposed to *M. tuberculosis*. It is characterized by a small subpleural lesion (Ghon focus) and regional lymphadenopathy (primary complex) which causes few, if any, symptoms. This usually heals spontaneously, often with calcification, within 1–2 months.
2. **Latent TB** is characterized by lack of clinical manifestations, but a positive tuberculin skin test or radiological evidence of self-healed TB.
3. **Post-primary (secondary) TB** is the result of re-infection or recrudescence of a primary lesion. Clinical features include erythema nodosum, fibrocaseous pulmonary lesions and lymph node involvement – scrofula describes massive lymph node enlargement with discharging sinuses (Fig. 24.23). Miliary (like millet seeds on chest x-ray) TB may involve internal organs, central nervous system and bone.

Investigations

1. **Sputum examination** for acid-fast bacilli using Ziehl–Neelsen stain.
2. **Cultures.** Mycobacteria require special media, such as Lowenstein–Jensen, and grow slowly (2–6 weeks) to produce a friable tenacious mass of adherent organisms.
3. **Tuberculin skin tests (Mantoux and Heaf)** involve the intradermal injection of purified protein derivative of *M. tuberculosis*.

   a. *Positive* result is characterized by the development of an induration of 5–14mm within 48 hours.

   b. *Negative* result usually excludes TB, but may also occur in patients with advanced disease.

   c. *Weakly positive* result does not necessarily distinguish between previous exposure and active disease. This is because most individuals have already received BCG (Bacille Calmette-Guérin) vaccination and will therefore exhibit a hypersensitivity response.

   d. *Strongly positive* result (induration > 15mm) is usually indicative of active disease since this level of response is not expected after long exposure to the vaccine (see Fig. 14.2b).

Treatment

Treatment is initially with at least three drugs (isoniazid, rifampicin, pyrazinamide or ethambutol) and then with isoniazid and rifampicin. Quadruple therapy is sometimes necessary in resistant cases, more frequently seen in highly endemic areas such as India.

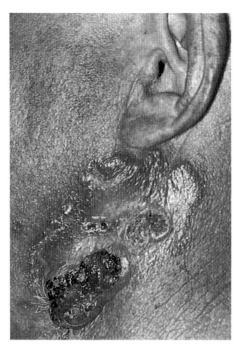

Fig. 24.23
Scrofula (Courtesy of Emond, Welsby and Rowland from *Colour Atlas of Infectious Diseases*, Mosby, 2003)

Ocular features

- Eyelid lesions may be reddish-brown nodules (lupus vulgaris) or a 'cold abscess'.
- Tuberculous conjunctivitis is uncommon and may be associated with lymphadenopathy, as in Parinaud syndrome.
- Keratitis may be phlyctenular or interstitial.
- Scleritis is rare.
- Anterior uveitis is often granulomatous.
- The posterior segment may manifest focal or multifocal choroiditis, serpiginous-like choroiditis, diffuse choroiditis in patients with AIDS, occlusive retinal periphlebitis and Eales disease.
- Neuro-ophthalmic disease may result in pupillary abnormalities, optic neuropathy and ocular motor palsies.

Acquired syphilis

Syphilis is caused by the spirochaete *Treponema pallidum* which is thin and has a spiral shape resulting in corkscrew movements. It is very fragile, does not live in culture and dies quickly on drying or warm temperature. In adults the disease is usually sexually acquired when the treponemes enter through an abrasion of the skin or a mucous membrane. Transmission by kissing, blood transfusion or percutaneous injury is rare. Transplacental infection of the fetus can occur from a mother who has become infected during or shortly before pregnancy. Although the infection is systemic from onset, in some cases clinical manifestations may be minimal or absent. The natural history of untreated syphilis is variable and may remain latent throughout, although overt disease may develop at any time.

Stages

1. **Primary** syphilis occurs after an incubation period, usually lasting 2–4 weeks, and is characterized by a painless ulcer (chancre) at the site of infection. The most common site in males is the penis (Fig. 22.24a) and in females the vulva. In homosexual men the anus is a major site. The chancre is associated with discrete, mobile, rubbery, enlargement of inguinal lymph nodes. Without treatment the chancre resolves within 2–6 weeks leaving an atrophic scar.
2. **Secondary** syphilis usually develops 6–8 weeks after the chancre and is characterized by:
   - Generalized lymphadenopathy with mild or absent constitutional symptoms.
   - Symmetrical maculopapular rash on the trunk (Fig. 24.24b), palms and soles.
   - Condylomata lata in the anal region.
   - Mucous patches in the mouth, pharynx and genitalia consisting of painless greyish-white circular erosions ('snail-track ulcers').
   - Meningitis, nephritis and hepatitis may occur.
3. **Latent** syphilis follows resolution of secondary syphilis, may last for years and can be detected only by serological tests
4. **Tertiary** syphilis occurs in about 40% of untreated cases and is characterized by:
   - Cardiovascular manifestations: aortitis with aneurysm formation and aortic regurgitation.
   - Neurosyphilis: tabes dorsalis, Charcot joints and general paralysis of the insane.
   - Gummatous infiltration of bone and viscera. Gummatous infiltration of the tongue may lead to leukoplakia and an increased risk of carcinoma (Fig. 24.24c).

Investigations

1. **Serological tests** rely on detection of non-specific antibodies (cardiolipin) or specific treponemal antibodies.
2. **Dark-ground microscopy** of exudate from a mucocutaneous lesion is reliable if positive.

Treatment

Treatment is with procaine penicillin (10 days in primary and secondary syphilis; 4 weeks in tertiary syphilis); alternatives in penicillin-allergic patients include doxycycline, tetracycline and erythromycin.

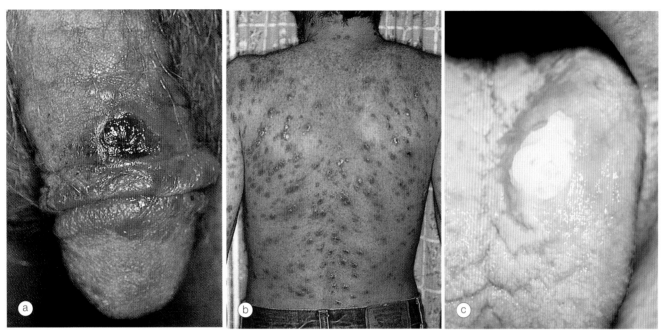

Fig. 24.24
Acquired syphilis. **(a)** Chancre in primary syphilis; **(b)** symmetrical maculopapular rash in secondary syphilis; **(c)** gummatous infiltration of the tongue in tertiary syphilis (Courtesy of Emond, Welsby and Rowland, from *Colour Atlas of Infectious Diseases*, Mosby, 2003)

Ocular features

Uveitis, interstitial keratitis, madarosis, optic neuritis, Argyll Robertson pupils and ocular motor nerve palsies.

Congenital syphilis

Transplacentally acquired infection may result in stillbirth, stigmata of congenital syphilis or be sub-clinical.

1. **Early features**
   - Rhinitis and failure to thrive.
   - Maculopapular rash, especially on the buttocks and thighs, and mucosal ulcers.
   - Fissures around the lips, nares and anus.
   - Pneumonia, hepatosplenomegaly, lymphadenopathy and jaundice.
2. **Late features**
   - Sensorineural deafness.
   - Stigmata include saddle-shaped nose (Fig. 24.25a), sabre tibia (Fig. 24.25b), malformed incisors (Hutchinson teeth – Fig. 24.25c) and mulberry molars.
3. **Ophthalmic features**
   - *a. Common.* Anterior uveitis and interstitial keratitis in early cases.
   - *b. Uncommon.* Pigmentary retinopathy in late cases.

Lyme disease

Lyme disease (borreliosis) is an infection caused by a flagellated spirochaete, *Borrelia burgdorferi*, transmitted through the bite of a hard-shelled tick (Fig. 24.26a) of the genus *Ixodes* (Fig. 24.26b) which feeds on a variety of large mammals, particularly deer. The disease is endemic in temperate regions of North America, Europe and Asia. It is the commonest vector-borne disease in many areas. Systemic manifestations are complex and are best conceptualized as early and late.

1. **Early stage** presents several days after the bite with a pathognomonic annular expanding skin lesion – erythema chronicum migrans (Fig. 24.26c), which may be accompanied by constitutional symptoms and lymphadenopathy. This may last for several weeks and resolve even without treatment. Complications, both neurological (cranial nerve palsies, meningitis) and cardiac (conduction defects, myocarditis), may follow within 3–4 weeks of the initial manifestations.
2. **Late complications** include chronic arthritis of large joints, polyneuropathy and encephalopathy. Some patients develop a doughy, patchy, skin discoloration which eventually results in shiny atrophy (acrodermatitis chronica atrophicans).
3. **Investigations** include PCR and ELISA.
4. **Treatment** of acute disease involves oral doxycycline or

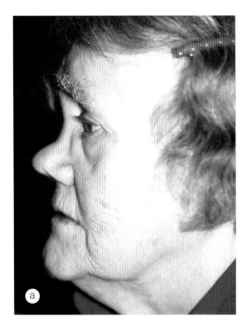

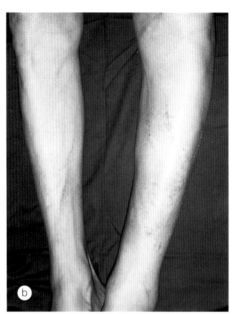

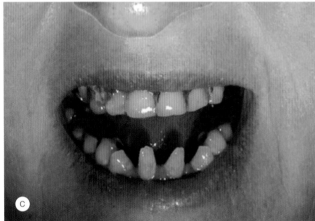

Fig. 24.25
Stigmata of congenital syphilis. **(a)** Saddle-shaped nasal deformity; **(b)** 'sabre' tibia; **(c)** Hutchinson teeth (Courtesy of R Marsh and S Ford – fig. c)

amoxicillin. Patients with ocular, cardiac, joint or neurological disease require intravenous ceftriaxone 2g daily for 14–28 days. Prophylaxis with doxycycline should be given within 72 hours of the tick bite.

NB Protective clothing and insect repellents should be used in tick-infested areas.

5. Ocular features: transient follicular conjunctivitis, keratitis, episcleritis, scleritis, uveitis, orbital myositis, optic neuritis, neuroretinitis, ocular motor nerve palsies and reversible Horner syndrome.

Leprosy

Leprosy (Hansen disease) is a chronic granulomatous infection caused by an intracellular acid-fast bacillus *Mycobacterium leprae* which has an affinity for skin, peripheral nerves and the anterior segment of the eye. The exact mode of infection is unknown although the upper respiratory tract appears the most likely portal of entry.

1. **Lepromatous** leprosy is a generalized infection with widespread lesions of skin, peripheral nerves, upper respiratory tract, reticuloendothelial system, eyes, bones and testes. Important signs include:
   - Erythema nodosum leprum consisting of multiple painful red nodules.
   - Leonine facies characterized by cutaneous thickening and ridging, nasal widening and thickening of ear lobes (Fig. 24.27a).
   - Peripheral cutaneous plaques and nodules.
   - Mucosal thickening and saddle-shaped nasal deformity.
   - Motor neuropathy as exemplified by the 'claw hand' deformity due to ulnar nerve palsy (Fig. 24.27b).
   - Sensory peripheral neuropathy facilitates trauma which may result in shortening and loss of digits (Fig. 24.27c).
   - Autonomic neuropathy leads to dry, cracked, infection prone skin; often superimposed on this is secondary bacterial infection, with gross tissue destruction.
2. **Tuberculoid** leprosy is restricted to the skin and peripheral nerves.
   - Annular, anaesthetic, hypopigmented lesions with raised edges.
   - Thickening of cutaneous sensory nerves.

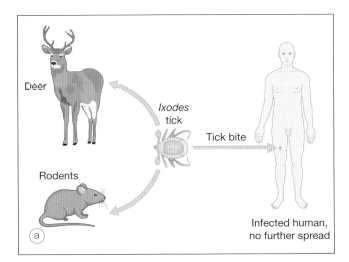

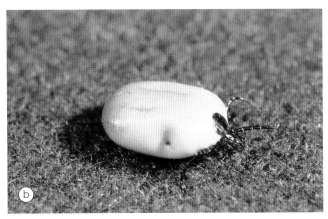

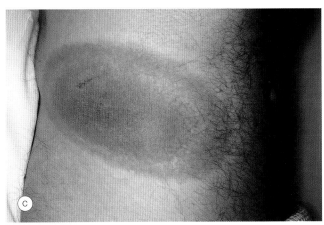

Fig. 24.26
Lyme disease. **(a)** Transmission; **(b)** engorged tick; **(c)** erythema chronicum migrans (Courtesy of Emond, Welsby and Rowland, from *Colour Atlas of Infectious Diseases*, Mosby, 2003 – figs b and c)

3. **Leprin test** involves intradermal injection of an extract of leprosy bacilli. It is strongly positive in tuberculoid leprosy and negative in lepromatous disease.
4. **Treatment** is with dapsone, rifampicin and clofazimine.

5. **Ocular features:** anterior uveitis, keratitis, madarosis, trichiasis, conjunctivitis, episcleritis, keratitis and scleritis.

Cat-scratch disease

Cat-scratch disease (benign lymphoreticulosis) is a subacute infection caused by *Bartonella henselae*, a Gram-negative rod. The infection is transmitted by the scratch or bite of an apparently healthy cat. Ocular involvement occurs in about 6% of cases.

1. **Presentation** is with a red papule or pustule at the site of inoculation followed by fever, malaise and regional lymphadenopathy (Fig. 24.28). However, general symptoms are frequently absent or unremarkable and a history of contact with a cat not always present.
2. **Disseminated** disease is rare but may affect immunocompromised individuals in the form of endocarditis, encephalopathy, meningitis, splenomegaly, splenic abscess formation and osteomyelitis.
3. **Investigations** include serology for *B. henselae* and PCR.
4. **Treatment** is with oral doxycycline or erythromycin, with or without rifampicin; the organism is also sensitive to ciprofloxacin and cotrimoxazole.
5. **Ocular features:** neuroretinitis, Parinaud oculoglandular syndrome, focal choroiditis, intermediate uveitis, exudative maculopathy, retinal vascular occlusion and panuveitis.

Toxoplasmosis

Toxoplasmosis is causes by *Toxoplasma gondii*, an obligate intracellular protozoan. It is estimated to infest at least 10% of adults in northern temperate countries and more than half of adults in Mediterranean and tropical countries.

Pathogenesis

The cat is the definitive host of the parasite and other beings, such as mice, livestock and humans, are intermediate hosts (Fig. 24.29).

1. **Organisms** exist in the following three forms:
   a. **Sporozoites** are contained within an oocyst (sporocyst) and are the result of sexual reproduction of the organisms with the intestinal mucosa of the cat. They are excreted in the faeces and spread to intermediate hosts.
   b. **Bradyzoites** are relatively inactive and are contained within tissue cysts (Fig. 24.30a) that most commonly develop in the brain, eye, heart, skeletal muscles and lymph nodes. They may lie dormant for many years without provoking an inflammatory reaction.
   c. **Tachyzoites** (trophozoites) are the proliferating active form responsible for tissue destruction and inflam-

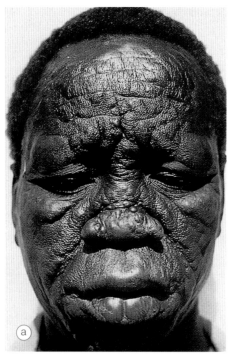

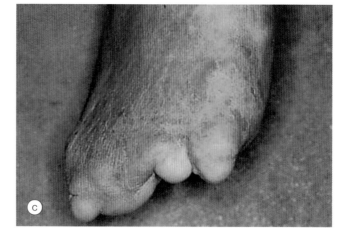

Fig. 24.27
Lepromatous leprosy. **(a)** Leonine facies; **(b)** 'claw hand' due to
motor neuropathy; **(c)** loss of digits due to sensory neuropathy
(Courtesy of Emond, Welsby and Rowland, from *Colour Atlas of Infectious
Diseases*, Mosby, 2003 – figs a and b; C D Forbes and W F Jackson, from
Color Atlas and Text of Clinical Medicine, Mosby, 2003 – fig. c)

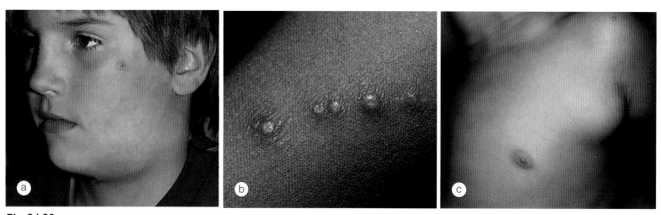

Fig. 24.28
Cat-scratch disease. **(a)** Ulcerated papule on the cheek, caused by the scratch of a cat two weeks previously, and enlargement of
submandibular lymph nodes; **(b)** a line of papules on the forearm of another patient at the site of a cat scratch three weeks previously;
(c) marked enlargement of ipsilateral axillary lymph nodes (Courtesy of Zitelli and Davis, from *Atlas of Pediatric Physical Diagnosis*,
Mosby, 2002)

mation following rupture of cell wall containing bradyzoites (Fig. 24.30b).

2. Mode of human infection

a. ***Ingestion of undercooked*** meat (lamb, pork, beef) containing bradyzoites of an intermediate host.

b. ***Ingestion of sporocysts*** following accidental contamination of hands when disposing of cat litter trays and then subsequent transfer on to food. Infants may also become infested by eating dirt (pica) containing sporocysts. It is likely that water contamination plays an important role in the transmission of the disease in rural areas.

c. ***Transplacental spread*** of the parasite (tachyzoite) can occur if a pregnant woman becomes infected.

Congenital toxoplasmosis

Toxoplasmosis is transmitted to the fetus through the placenta when a pregnant woman becomes infested. If the mother is infected before pregnancy, the fetus will be unscathed.

1. Severity of involvement of the fetus is dependent on the duration of gestation at the time of maternal infestation. For example, involvement during early pregnancy may result in stillbirth, whereas if it occurs during late pregnancy it may result in convulsions, paralysis, hydrocephalus (Fig. 24.31a) and visceral disease.

2. Manifestations

- Intracranial calcification may be seen on CT (Fig. 24.31b).
- However, just as in the acquired form, most cases of congenital systemic toxoplasmosis are subclinical. In these children, bilateral healed chorioretinal scars may be discovered later in life, either by chance or when the child is found to have defective vision.
- Infestation occurring towards the end of the second trimester usually results in disease that can be detected at birth such as macular scars. That occurring later in the third trimester may result in normal examinations at birth, but the development of uveitis or neurological disease in the future.
- The risk of disease later in life can be modified by early recognition of the transmission and long-term therapy.

3. Serological tests (see Chapter 14).

Acquired toxoplasmosis

1. In immunocompetent patients may have the following manifestations.

a. ***Subclinical*** is the most frequent.

b. ***Lymphadenopathic syndrome***, which is uncommon and self-limiting, is characterized by cervical lymphadenopathy, fever, malaise and pharyngitis.

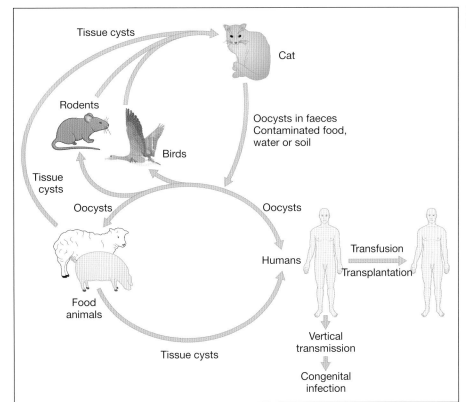

Fig. 24.29
Life cycle of *Toxoplasma gondii*

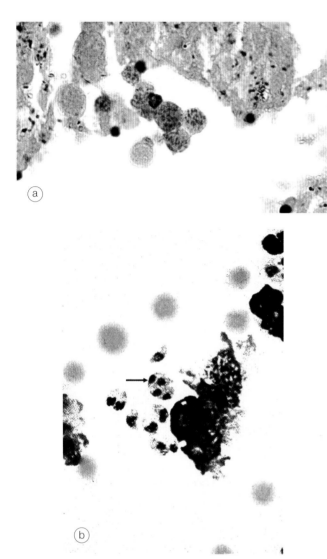

Fig. 24.30
Toxoplasma gondii. **(a)** Tissue cysts containing bradyzoites;
(b) release of tachyzoites (arrow) following rupture of the cell
wall (Courtesy of J Harry – fig. a; Emond, Welsby and Rowland, from
Colour Atlas of Infectious Diseases, Mosby, 2003 – fig. b)

  c. Meningoencephalitis, which is characterized by
  convulsions and altered consciousness, occurs in a
  minority of patients.
  d. The exanthematous form, resembling a rickettsial
  infection, is the rarest.
2. **In immunocompromised** patients toxoplasmosis may
  be life-threatening. The most common manifestation in
  AIDS patients is an intracerebral space occupying lesion
  which resembles a cerebral abscess on MR (Fig. 24.31c).

Ocular features

Toxoplasmosis is the most frequent cause of infectious
retinitis in immunocompetent individuals. Although some

cases may occur as a result of reactivation of prenatal
infestation the vast majority are acquired postnatally.

Toxocariasis

Toxocariasis is caused by infestation with a common
intestinal ascarid (roundworm) of dogs called *Toxocara canis*
(Fig. 24.32a). About 80% of puppies between the ages of 2
and 6 months are infested with this worm. Human infestation
is by accidental ingestion of soil or food contaminated with
ova shed in dog faeces. Very young children who eat dirt
(pica) or are in close contact with puppies are at particular
risk of acquiring the disease. In the human intestine, the ova
develop into larvae which penetrate the intestinal wall and
travel to various organs, such as the liver, lungs, skin, brain
and eyes (Fig. 24.32b). When the larvae die, they disintegrate
and cause an inflammatory reaction followed by granulation.
Clinically, human infestation can take one of the following
forms:

1. **Visceral larva migrans** (VLM) is caused by severe
  systemic infection which usually occurs at about the age
  of 2 years. The clinical features, which vary in severity,
  include a low-grade fever, hepatosplenomegaly, pneumonitis, convulsions and, rarely, death. The blood shows a
  leucocytosis and marked eosinophilia.
2. **Ocular toxocariasis** differs markedly from VLM because
  it involves otherwise healthy individuals who have a
  normal white cell count with absence of eosinophilia. A
  history of pica is less common, and the average age at
  presentation is considerably older (7.5 years) compared
  with VLM (2 years).

Onchocerciasis

Onchocerciasis, or river blindness, is caused by infestation
with the parasitic helminth *Onchocerca volvulus.* The normal
vector is the black fly *Simulium spp,* an obligate intermediate
host, which breeds in fast flowing water. Larvae are transmitted when the fly bites to obtain blood, and then mature
into adult worms that produce millions of microfilariae over
years (Figs 24.33 and 24.34a). *Wolbachia* (a rickettsia) lives
symbiotically in the coat of the microfilaria and is important
for fertility of the female filarial worm. Lipopolysaccharide
endotoxins released by the bacteria may be important in the
pathogenesis of the disease and the adverse response to
treatment in some individuals. Onchocerciasis is endemic in
West, Central and East Africa, with small foci in central and
South America, Sudan and Yemen, infecting over 17.7
million people, most of whom are asymptomatic but with an
estimated 270,000 blind and half a million visually
impaired.

1. **Signs**
  • The most common early manifestation is pruritus

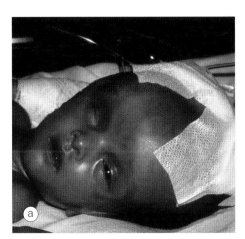

Fig. 24.31
Cerebral toxoplasmosis. **(a)** Hydrocephalus in congenital toxoplasmosis – note right anophthalmos; **(b)** axial CT shows cerebral calcification in congenital disease; **(c)** axial MR in acquired cerebral toxoplasmosis in AIDS shows several round lesions resembling abscesses (Courtesy of M Szreter – fig. a, Emond, Welsby and Rowland, from *Colour Atlas of Infectious Diseases*, Mosby, 2003 – fig. c).

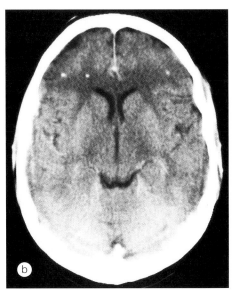

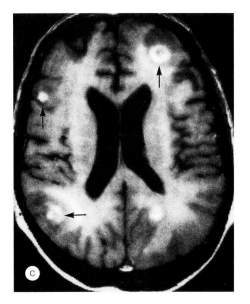

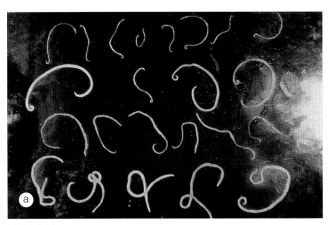

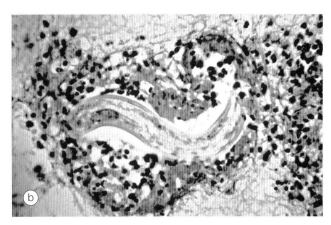

Fig. 24.32
Toxocara canis. **(a)** Adult worms from dog faeces; **(b)** larva in tissue surrounded by an inflammatory reaction (Courtesy of Hart and Shears, from *Color Atlas of Medical Microbiology*, Mosby, 2004 – fig. a).

which is followed by a maculopapular rash often involving the buttocks and extremities (Fig. 24.34b).

- Chronic lesions are characterized by focal areas of hypo- and hyperpigmentation on the shins ('leopard' skin – Fig. 24.34c).
- With time the skin may become thickened and wrinkled as a result of constant scratching ('lizard' skin – Fig. 24.34d).
- Subcutaneous nodules (onchocercomas) consisting of encapsulated worms develop over bony prominences (Fig. 24.34e) and the head.
- Occasionally the lymph nodes become grossly enlarged resulting in chronic lymphatic obstruction and lymphoedema.

2. **Treatment** is with ivermectin 12mg given as an annual single dose. Although it acts rapidly to reduce the number of skin microfilariae it depletes them for only a few months after which they reappear at 20% or more of pre-treatment numbers within 1 year, which is sufficient for transmission to continue. New therapies are being developed targeting *Wolbachia*.

3. **Ocular features:** microfilariae in the aqueous, anterior uveitis, keratitis and chorioretinitis.

Cysticercosis

Cysticercosis refers to a parasitic infestation by *Cysticercus cellulosae*, the larval form of the pork tapeworm *Taenia solium*. Pigs are the intermediate hosts and humans are the definitive hosts acquiring the disease by ingesting cysts of *T. solium* from contaminated pork, vegetables or water.

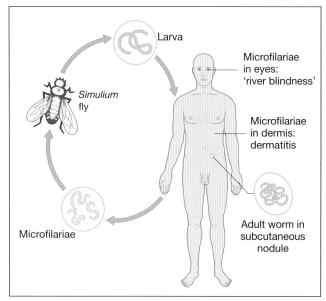

Fig. 24.33
Life cycle of *Onchocerca volvulus*

1. **Systemic disease** often involves the lungs, muscles and brain.
2. **Investigations** involve radiology of the chest (Fig. 24.35) and muscles to detect calcified cysts.
3. **Ocular disease** primarily involves the vitreous and retina.

Cryptococcosis

Cryptococcus neoformans is a diamorphic yeast that enters the body through inhalation. Infection primarily affects patients with cell-mediated immune deficiency and affects 5–10% of patients with AIDS. Other predisposing factors include lymphoma, active hepatitis with use of prednisone and azathioprine, alcoholism, uremia, systemic lupus erythematosus, organ transplantation with immuno-suppression and exposure to pigeons.

1. **Systemic disease** primarily involves the CNS (meningitis, meningoencephalitis and cryptococcoma) but may also cause pneumonia, mucocutaneous lesions, pyelonephritis, endocarditis and hepatitis.
2. **Investigations** involve culture or recognition of spores in cerebrospinal fluid, and serological detection of antigen.
3. **Treatment** is with intravenous amphotericin B and oral flucytosine.
4. **Ocular disease,** most notably choroiditis, is present in approximately 6% of patients with cryptococcal meningitis.

Congenital rubella

Rubella (German measles) is usually a benign febrile exanthema. Congenital rubella results from transplacental transmission of virus to the fetus from an infected mother, usually during the first trimester of pregnancy. This may lead to serious chronic fetal infection and malformations. It appears that the risk to the fetus is closely related to the stage of gestation at the time of maternal infection.

1. **Fetal infection** occurs in about 50% of cases during the first 8 weeks, 33% between weeks 9 and 12, and about 10% between weeks 13 and 24. Each of the various organs affected has its own period of susceptibility, after which no gross malformations are produced.
2. **Systemic complications** include: spontaneous abortion, stillbirth, congenital heart malformations, deafness, micro-cephaly, mental handicap, hypotonia, hepatosplenomegaly, thrombocytopenic purpura, pneumonitis, myocarditis and metaphyseal bone lesions.
3. **Ocular features:** cataract, microphthalmos, glaucoma, retinopathy, keratitis, anterior uveitis and iris atrophy, severe refractive errors, pendular nystagmus and strabismus secondary to poor vision.

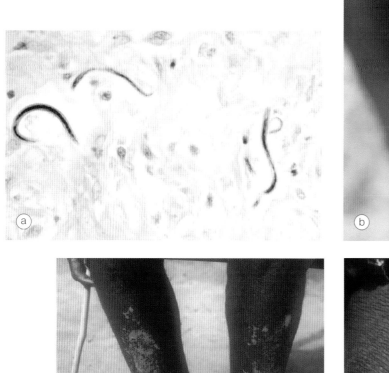

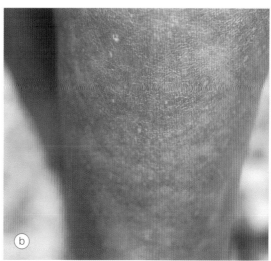

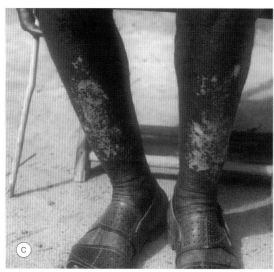

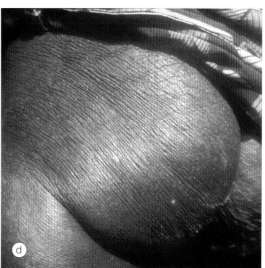

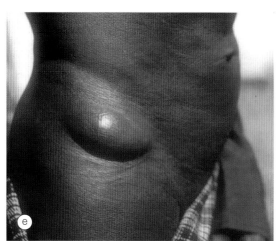

Fig. 24.34
Onchocerciasis. **(a)** Giemsa stain of microfilariae; **(b)** maculopapular rash; **(c)** 'leopard' skin; **(d)** 'lizard' skin; **(e)** subcutaneous nodule (onchocercoma) (Courtesy of J Harry and G Misson, from *Clinical Ophthalmic Pathology*, Butterworth-Heinemann, 2001 – fig. a; C Gilbert – figs b, c, d and e)

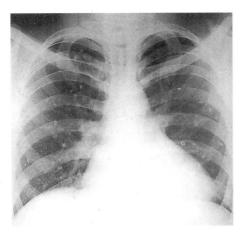

Fig. 24.35
Chest radiograph showing calcified cysticercus cysts (Courtesy of Hart and Shears from *Color Atlas of Medical Microbiology*, Mosby, 2004).

Whipple disease

Whipple disease (intestinal lipodystrophy) is a rare, chronic, bacterial infection with *Tropheryma whippelii* that primarily involves the gastrointestinal tract and its lymphatic drainage. It occurs mostly in white middle-aged men and is fatal if untreated.

1. **Presentation** is with weight loss, arthralgia, diarrhoea and abdominal pain.
2. **Extraintestinal manifestations** primarily involve the CNS, lungs, heart, joints and eyes.
3. **Diagnostic tests:** jejunal biopsy shows infiltration of small intestinal mucosa by 'foamy' macrophages which stain positive with periodic acid-Schiff. Electron microscopy shows small rod-shaped bacilli within the macrophages.
4. **Treatment** is with trimethoprim-sulfamethoxazole; the organism is also usually sensitive to tetracycline, erythromycin, penicillin, streptomycin and chloramphenicol.
5. **Ocular features** may be secondary to CNS involvement or caused by various types of intraocular inflammation.

Chlamydial genital infection

Chlamydial genital infection is sexually transmitted and caused by serotypes D-K of *Chlamydia trachomatis*.

1. **In males** chlamydial infection is the most common cause of 'non-specific urethritis' (NSU) and 'non-gonococcal urethritis' (NGU). It may also cause epididymitis and act as a trigger for Reiter disease.
2. **In females** chlamydia may cause abacterial pyuria, cervicitis, salpingitis, peritonitis and perihepatitis (Fitz-

Hugh-Curtis syndrome). Chronic salpingitis may result in infertility.
3. **Treatment** is with doxycycline 100mg b.d. for 7 days or a single dose of azithromycin 1g.
4. **Ophthalmic features**
   a. Uncommon. Adult conjunctivitis.
   b. Rare. Neonatal conjunctivitis.

Nocardia

Nocardia asteroides (a Gram-positive, aerobic, filamentous bacterium) is a cause of opportunistic infections in immuno-compromised patients, particularly with lymphomas, long-term pulmonary disease and long-term systemic steroid therapy. The organism is usually acquired by inhalation.

1. **Systemic disease** has a predilection for the lungs, brain and skin with suppurative necrosis and abscess formation.
2. **Ocular disease** is characterized by intraocular inflammation.

MUCUTANEOUS DISEASES

Mucous membrane pemphigoid

Mucous membrane pemphigoid is an autoimmune muco-cutaneous blistering disease that may affect the mouth, nose, pharynx, trachea, genitalia and anus. The condition affects women more commonly than men (2:1) with a peak age of onset after 70 years of age. Conjunctival disease (ocular cicatricial pemphigoid – OCP) is seen in 75% of cases with oral involvement but only 25% of those with skin lesions and occasionally it occurs in isolation. OCP is always bilateral, but frequently asymmetrical with regard to time of onset, severity and rate of progression. Patients who develop OCP before the age of 60 years tend to have more severe ocular and systemic involvement and, despite immunosuppressive therapy, progress more rapidly.

Pathogenesis

An unknown trigger in genetically susceptible individuals causes auto-antibody production against components of the basement membrane and hemidesmosomes. The result is a type II hypersensitivity response with IgG or IgA antibodies binding to the basement membrane zone and causing complement activation. Inflammatory cells are recruited by this reaction, causing separation of the epithelium from the underlying tissue. The release of cytokines causes fibroblast activation and scarring, resulting in conjunctival shrinkage and loss of components of the ocular surface. The resultant damage to the ocular environment causes keratinization, corneal drying resulting in epithelial defects, vascularization and scarring. Dry eye is caused by a combination of destruction of goblet cells and accessory lacrimal glands as well as occlusion of the main lacrimal ductules.

Clinical features

1. **Mucosal** subepidermal blisters, most frequently oral (Fig. 24.36a), rupture within a day or two leaving erosions and ulcers that heal without significant scarring. Ulcers in other sites typically heal with scarring that may result in stricture formation. Stricture of the oesophagus can result in potentially lethal inhalation of food. Laryngeal or tracheal stenosis is a medical emergency.
2. **Skin** lesions are less common and present as tense blisters and erosions. They typically involve the head and neck (Fig. 24.36b), the groins and extremities (Fig. 24.36c) but generalized involvement is uncommon (Fig. 24.36d).

Stevens–Johnson syndrome and toxic epidermal necrolysis

Stevens–Johnson syndrome and toxic epidermal necrolysis (Lyell disease) reflect different severity of the same muco-cutaneous blistering disease process. Both are uncommon but potentially lethal conditions that may be associated with severe ocular complications. They have the same clinical signs, treatment and prognosis, although ocular changes are much less common in toxic epidermal necrolysis. Males are affected more often than females with a mean age of onset of 25 years.

Pathogenesis

The disease is thought to be either a delayed hypersensitivity response to drugs or a response to epithelial cell antigens

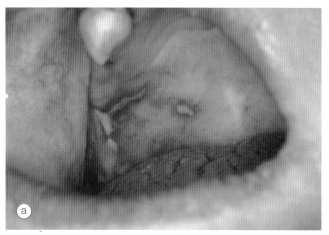

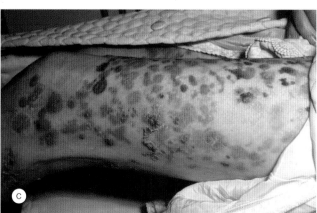

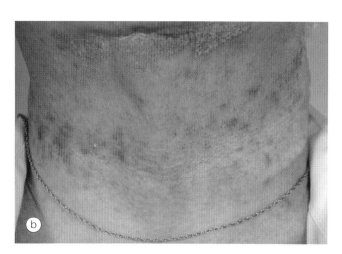

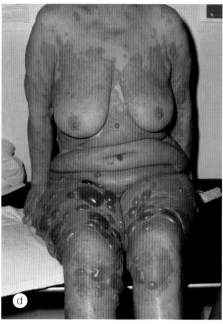

Fig. 24.36
Mucous membrane pemphigoid. **(a)** Oral blisters; **(b)** mild involvement of the neck; **(c)** severe involvement of the leg; **(d)** generalized involvement (Courtesy of S Tuft – figs a and b)

modified by drug exposure. Specific drug metabolites may also play a role, suggesting a genetically determined enzyme deficiency. A wide range of drugs have been incriminated including antibiotics (especially trimethoprim), analgesics, cold remedies, NSAIDs, phenytoin, allopurinol and acetazolamide. Infection with *Mycoplasma pneumoniae* also appears to be a risk factor. However, because symptoms often take 3 weeks to develop after exposure, the precipitating cause cannot be identified with certainty in over 50% of cases.

Clinical features

1. **Presentation** is fever, malaise, sore throat, and possibly cough and arthralgia, which may last up to 14 days before the appearance of mucocutaneous lesions. In many case the patient is very ill and hospitalization required.
2. **Signs**
   - Mucosal blisters of the mouth and nose, which rupture, forming erosions.

- Haemorrhagic crusting of the lips is characteristic (Fig. 24.37a); genital involvement is less common (Fig. 24.37b).
- A generalized erythematous papular skin rash which evolves into 'target' lesions, consisting of erythematous centres surrounded by pale areas, in turn encircled by erythematous rings (Fig. 24.37c).
- Blisters are usually transient but may be widespread and associated with haemorrhage and necrosis (Fig. 24.37d). Healing occurs within 1–4 weeks, usually leaving a pigmented scar.
- In toxic epidermal necrolysis there may be widespread sloughing of the epidermis.

Atopic eczema

Atopic eczema (dermatitis) is an idiopathic, often familial, skin condition, which may be associated with asthma and hay fever.

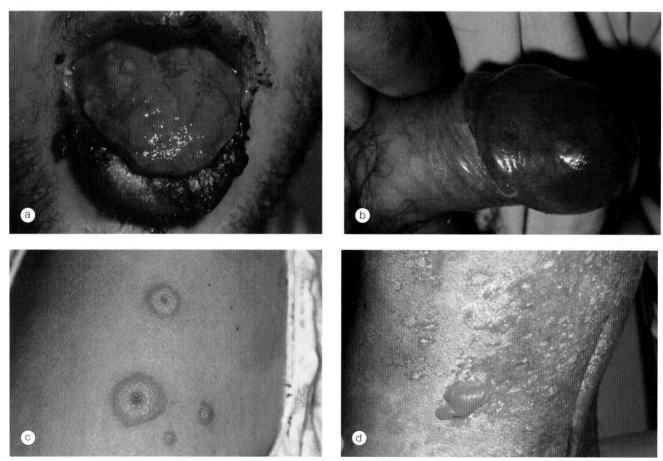

Fig. 24.37
Stevens–Johnson syndrome. **(a)** Involvement of the mouth and haemorrhagic crusting of the lips; **(b)** involvement of the glans penis; **(c)** 'target' lesions; **(d)** widespread haemorrhagic blisters (Courtesy of Emond, Welsby and Rowland, from *Colour Atlas of Infectious Diseases*, Mosby, 2003 – fig. c)

I. Presentation is with intense pruritus, usually in infancy but may be at any age.
2. Signs
- Facial eczema is usually seen in infants and consists of itchy, dry, erythematous papules (Fig. 24.38a).
- Flexural eczema usually develops later with symmetrical involvement of the elbow and knee flexures, wrists (Fig. 24.38b) and ankles by dry, lichenified or excoriated skin.

3. Treatment options include emollients, coal tar preparations and topical steroids.
4. Ophthalmic features
   a. Common. Madarosis and staphylococcal blepharitis.
   b. Uncommon. Chronic keratoconjunctivitis, keratoconus and early-onset cataract.
   c. Rare. Retinal detachment.

Acne rosacea

Acne rosacea is a common, idiopathic, chronic dermatosis involving the sun-exposed skin of the face and upper neck.

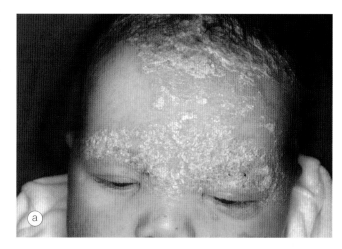
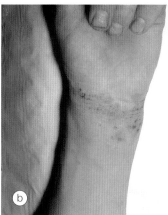
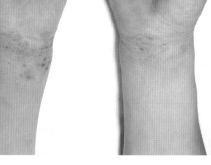

Fig. 24.38
Atopic eczema. **(a)** Facial; **(b)** flexural

Pathogenesis

The papules and pustules may be precipitated by lipases secreted by *S. epidermidis*. Lipases may break down the wax and sterol esters of the meibomian glands to release inflammatory free fatty acids. Co-infection with *Helicobacter pylori* has been implicated as an aggravating factor. Tetracyclines reduce the bacterial flora on the lids and thereby decrease lipase production.

Diagnosis

I. Presentation is in adult life with itching and flushing of the forehead, cheeks, nose and chin. Symptoms are often precipitated by ingestion of alcohol, hot drinks or spicy food.
2. Signs
- Erythema progressing to telangiectasia (Fig. 24.39a).
- Papules and pustules (Fig. 24.39b).
- Sebaceous gland hypertrophy (Fig. 24.39c).
- Rhinophyma (Fig. 24.39d).

   NB In contrast to acne vulgaris, comedones (blackheads and whiteheads) are absent.

Treatment

Treatment involves topical metronidazole gel and azelaic acid cream, and oral tetracycline. Other measures include oral isotretinoin and laser therapy.

CARDIOVASCULAR DISEASE

Systemic hypertension

Hypertension is most commonly idiopathic (essential) and occasionally secondary to a renal or metabolic disorder.

I. Presentation is usually in the fifth to sixth decades.
2. Signs. Blood pressure > 140/90mmHg.
3. Complications
- Ventricular hypertrophy and subsequent failure.
- Increased risk of atherosclerosis resulting in coronary heart disease and stroke, particularly in those with hypertensive retinopathy.
- Renal disease.

4. Treatment options include lifestyle modification (exercise, weight reduction, diminished salt intake and alcohol consumption) and drug therapy (diuretics, beta-blockers, calcium channel blockers, ACE inhibitors, angiotensin II receptor antagonists and alpha-blockers).
5. Ophthalmic features
   a. Common. Retinal arteriolosclerosis and branch retinal vein occlusion.

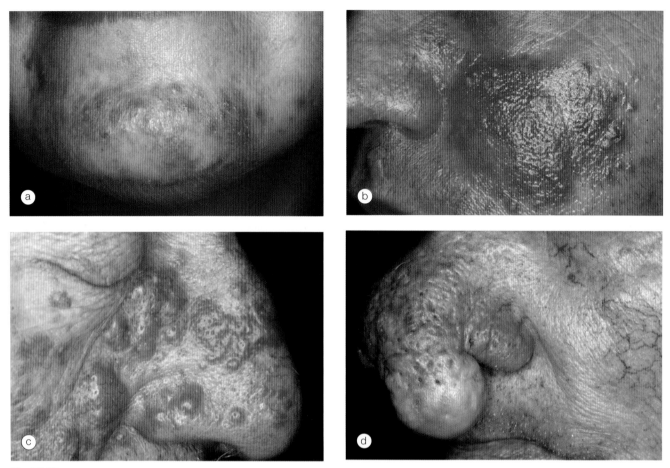

Fig. 24.39
Acne rosacea. **(a)** Erythema and telangiectasia; **(b)** erythema and pustules; **(c)** sebaceous gland hypertrophy; **(d)** rhinophyma

b. Uncommon. Retinopathy, retinal artery occlusion, retinal artery macroaneurysm, anterior ischaemic optic neuropathy, choroidal infarcts and ocular motor nerve palsies.

c. Rare. Exudative retinal detachment in accelerated disease or eclampsia.

Carotid stenosis

Carotid stenosis involves atheromatous narrowing, often associated with ulceration, at the bifurcation of the common carotid artery. The irregularity of the vessel wall may act as a source of cerebral and retinal emboli composed of platelets and fibrin (white emboli) or tiny fragments of atheromatous material (Hollenhorst plaques).

Diagnosis

1. Presentation is in old age with the following:
- Transient retinal ischaemic attacks (amaurosis fugax).
- Retinal artery occlusion.
- Transient cerebral ischaemic attacks (TIA).
- Stroke.

2. Signs

a. Palpation of the cervical carotid arteries should be done gently to avoid dislodging a thrombus. Severe or complete stenosis is associated with a diminished or absent carotid pulse. Other peripheral pulses may also be diminished in generalized atherosclerosis.

b. Auscultation over a partial stenosis gives rise to a bruit, best detected with the bell of the stethoscope. It is important to perform auscultation along the entire length of the artery and to ask the patient to hold his breath. The most ominous bruit is one that is high-pitched and soft because it indicates tight stenosis. When the lumen is narrowed by 90% or more, the bruit disappears.

3. Investigations

a. Duplex scanning is a non-invasive, screening test involving a combination of high-resolution real-time ultrasonography with Doppler flow analysis.

b. Magnetic resonance angiography is non-invasive and accurate.

c. Catheter carotid arteriography is the most accurate method (Fig. 24.40) but carries a significant risk of complications.

Treatment

Treatment is aimed at preventing stroke and permanent visual impairment by the following:

1. **General** measures addressing associated risk factors such as smoking, hypertension, diabetes, obesity, hypercholesterolaemia and cardiac arrhythmias.
2. **Antiplatelet therapy.**
   - Aspirin 75–300mg daily.
   - Combined aspirin and dipyridamole (Persantin) 200mg daily, if aspirin alone is ineffective.
   - Clopidogrel (Plavix) 75mg daily if other measures fail.
3. **Oral anticoagulants** such as warfarin if TIAs continue despite antiplatelet therapy.
4. **Carotid endarterectomy** is indicated in patients with symptomatic stenosis greater than 70%.

Ophthalmic features

1. **Common.** Amaurosis fugax.

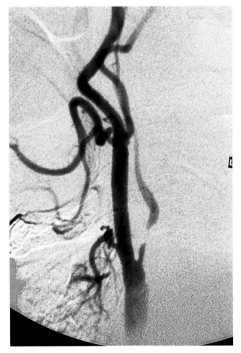

Fig. 24.40
Arteriogram showing severe stenosis of the right internal carotid artery (Courtesy of D Thomas)

2. **Uncommon.** Hollenhorst plaques and retinal artery occlusion.
3. **Rare.** Hypotensive (slow flow) retinopathy and ocular ischaemic syndrome.

METABOLIC DISEASES

Diabetes mellitus

Classification

Diabetes mellitus (DM) is a common disorder characterized by sustained hyperglycaemia of varying severity secondary to lack or diminished efficacy of endogenous insulin. The disease affects about 2% of the population in the UK and can be classified into two types, with some degree of overlap.

1. **Type 1 diabetes** (insulin dependent diabetes mellitus, IDDM, juvenile-onset diabetes) develops most frequently between the ages of 10 and 20 years, with acute polydipsia, polyuria, nocturia and weight loss. There is an association with HLA-DR3 and DR4. Autoimmune destruction of pancreatic islet cells is postulated as instrumental in pathogenesis. Patients are often lean and manifest a total lack of insulin.
2. **Type 2 diabetes** (non-insulin dependent, NIDDM, maturity-onset diabetes) on the other hand, develops most frequently between the ages of 50 and 70 years. Patients are often overweight and manifest relative deficiency of insulin and/or peripheral insulin resistance. Type 2 diabetes is often asymptomatic and discovered by chance. Alternatively, it may present with recurrent infections of the skin, vulva or glans penis or with complications such as vitreous haemorrhage.

Investigations

- Fasting glucose > 6.7mmol/l.
- Random glucose > 10.0mmol/l.
- Glucose tolerance test is performed only if the diagnosis is uncertain.
- Glycosylated haemoglobin (HBA1c) reflects the average level of blood glucose over the preceding 6 weeks. Normally 4–8% of haemoglobin is glycosylated; values in excess of this reflect inadequacy of glycaemic control. It is a better indicator of the efficacy of treatment than a single random glucose level.
- Urine testing for glycosuria is a crude and unsatisfactory means of monitoring diabetic control.

NB Glycosuria per se does not necessarily imply diabetes as it may merely reflect a lowered renal threshold for glucose excretion.

Treatment

Type 1 diabetics require insulin; type 2 diabetics require a regimen involving weight reduction, physical exercise and diet control, often in combination with oral hypoglycaemic agents or insulin. Oral hypoglycaemic agents include sulphonylureas (e.g. gliclazide, glipizide) and biguanides (e.g. metformin). It is also important to aggressively treat any associated problems, particularly hypertension and hyperlipidaemia. Blood pressure should be maintained at or below 140/80mmHg.

Systemic complications

1. **Renal.** Nephropathy is initially characterized by microscopic proteinuria. Severe renal disease may eventually result in renal failure requiring dialysis or transplantation.
2. **Vascular**
   - Accelerated coronary atherosclerosis.
   - Atherosclerosis of lower limb arteries may result in ischaemic ulceration and gangrene of the feet and toes (Fig. 24.41a).

3. **Neurological**
   - Sensory polyneuropathy principally affects the feet in a 'glove and stocking' distribution and may give rise to painless neuropathic perforating ulcers at pressure points in the soles (Fig. 24.41b) and degenerative arthropathy (Charcot joints).
   - Cranial nerve palsies, classically a sixth or a pupil-sparing third, may occur as a result of small vessel involvement.
4. **Cutaneous**
   - Increased susceptibility to bacterial and fungal infections (Fig. 24.41c).
   - Blistering of the feet and toes.
   - Necrobiosis lipoidica characterized by waxy plaques with irregular margins and shiny centres involving the shins (Fig. 24.41d).
   - Lipodystrophy at sites of insulin injection.
   - Granuloma annulare characterized by smooth annular plaques on the extremities is uncommon.

NB Neuropathy in combination with vascular insufficiency and increased susceptibility to infection commonly results in gangrene of the extremities (diabetic foot).

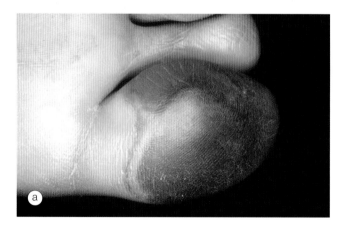
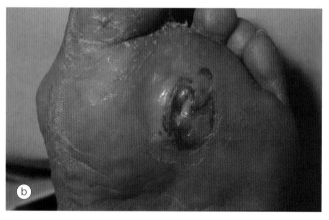
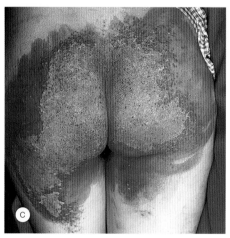
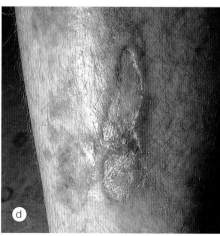

Fig. 24.41
Complications of diabetes mellitus. **(a)** Gangrene; **(b)** neuropathic ulceration; **(c)** severe monilial infection; **(d)** necrobiosis lipoidica

Ophthalmic complications

1. Common
- Retinopathy.
- Iridopathy (increased iris transillumination).
- Unstable refraction.

2. Uncommon
- Recurrent styes.
- Xanthelasmata.
- Accelerated senile cataract.
- Rubeosis iridis which may lead to neovascular glaucoma.
- Ocular motor nerve palsies.
- Reduced corneal sensitivity.

3. Rare
- Papillopathy
- Pupillary light-near dissociation.
- Wolfram syndrome: progressive optic atrophy and multiple neurological and systemic abnormalities.
- Acute-onset cataract.
- Rhino-orbital mucormycosis.

Thyrotoxicosis

Thyrotoxicosis (hyperthyroidism) is caused by excessive secretion of thyroid hormones. Graves disease, the most common subtype of hyperthyroidism, is an autoimmune disorder in which IgG antibodies bind to thyroid stimulating hormone (TSH) receptors in the thyroid gland and stimulate secretion of thyroid hormones. It is commoner in females and may be associated with other autoimmune disorders.

1. Presentation is in the third to fourth decades with weight loss despite good appetite, increased bowel frequency, sweating, heat intolerance, nervousness, irritability, palpitations, weakness and fatigue.

2. Signs
a. External
- Diffuse thyroid enlargement (Fig. 24.42a), fine hand tremor, palmar erythema, and warm and sweaty skin.
- Finger clubbing (thyroid acropachy) (Fig. 24.42b) and onycholysis (Plummer nails).
- Pretibial myxoedema is an infiltrative dermopathy characterized by raised plaques on the anterior aspect of the legs, extending on to the dorsum of the foot (Fig. 24.42c).
- Alopecia and vitiligo.
- Myopathic proximal muscle weakness but brisk tendon reflexes.

b. Cardiovascular
- Sinus tachycardia, atrial fibrillation and premature ventricular beats.
- High output heart failure.

3. Investigations. Abnormal thyroid function – serum T3, T4, TSH, thyroxine-binding globulin (TBG) and thyroid-stimulating immunoglobulin (TSI).

4. Treatment options include carbimazole, propylthiouracil, propranolol, radioactive iodine and partial thyroidectomy.

5. Ophthalmic features
a. Common. Lid retraction, chemosis and proptosis.
b. Uncommon. Superior limbic keratoconjunctivitis, keratoconjunctivitis sicca and diplopia.
c. Rare. Optic neuropathy and choroidal folds.

Homocystinuria

Homocystinuria is caused by deficiency of cystathionine-beta-synthetase leading to accumulation of homocysteine and methionine. The condition is phenotypically similar to Marfan syndrome but carries a thrombotic tendency.

1. Inheritance is AR.

2. Signs
- Blond hair with a malar flush (Fig. 24.43).
- Marfanoid habitus but infrequent arachnodactyly.
- Mental retardation and psychiatric disturbance.

3. Complications
- Osteoporosis and spontaneous crush fractures.
- Thromboses in any vessel and at any age, particularly postoperatively or postpartum.

4. Treatment involves oral pyridoxine to reduce homocysteine and methionine levels.

5. Ophthalmic features
a. Common. Ectopia lentis.
b. Uncommon. Myopia and retinal detachment.

Paget disease

Paget disease is a chronic, progressive bone disease characterized by excessive and disorganized resorption and formation of bone.

1. Signs: enlargement of the skull (Fig. 24.44a) and anterior bowing of the tibias (Fig. 24.44b).

2. Systemic complications include deafness (see Fig. 22.44a), arthropathy, kyphoscoliosis, fractures, compression of spinal and cranial nerves, heart failure and increased risk of osteosarcoma.

3. Ocular features include optic atrophy, proptosis, ocular motor nerve palsies and angioid streaks.

Cushing syndrome

Cushing syndrome is caused by prolonged elevation of free plasma glucocorticoid levels.

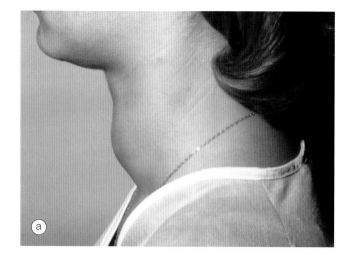

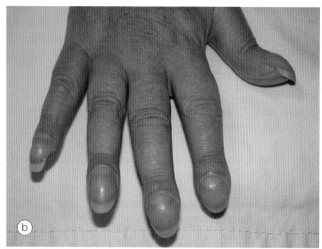

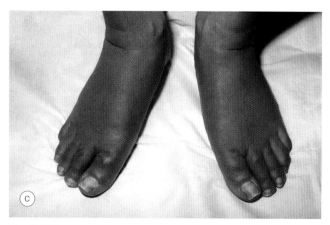

Fig. 24.42
Thyrotoxicosis. **(a)** Diffuse goitre; **(b)** acropachy; **(c)** pretibial myxoedema

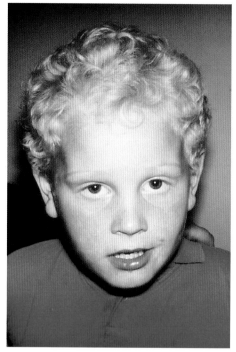

Fig. 24.43
Blond hair and malar flush in homocystinuria

1. **Causes**
   - Iatrogenic due to systemic administration of steroids is the most common.
   - Hypersecretion of glucocorticoids by the adrenal cortex.
   - Hypersecretion of adrenocorticotrophic hormone (ACTH) by a pituitary basophil adenoma (Cushing disease).

2. **Signs**
   a. ***Obesity*** may be generalized or classically involve the trunk, abdomen and neck (buffalo hump).
   b. ***The face*** is swollen (moon face) and the complexion plethoric; females may be hirsute (Fig. 24.45a).
   c. ***The skin*** is thin and susceptible to bruising, and may show purple striae (Fig. 24.45b). Hyperpigmentation may develop with ACTH-dependent Cushing disease (see Fig. 24.45a).
   d. ***Other features*** include depression/psychosis, osteoporosis, poor wound healing and proximal myopathy.

3. **Complications** include hypertension, diabetes, pathological fractures and acute necrosis of the femoral head.

4. **Investigations** are targeted at firstly establishing the presence of elevated cortisol levels and then identifying the underlying cause (unless iatrogenic).

5. **Treatment**
   a. ***Surgical*** removal of pituitary adenoma or adrenal secreting tumour. Ectopic foci of ACTH secretion may also be amenable to excision.

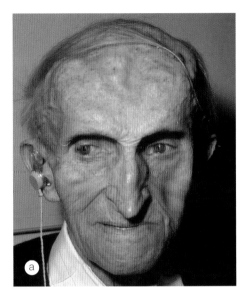
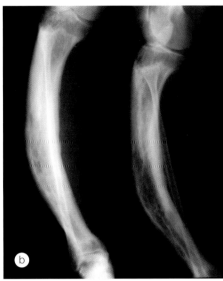

Fig. 24.44
Paget disease. **(a)** Enlargement of the skull and deafness; **(b)** anterior bowing of the tibias

b. Medical suppression of cortisol secretion with metyrapone or aminoglutethimide.
6. **Ophthalmic features**
   a. Common. Steroid-induced cataracts frequently develop in iatrogenic Cushing syndrome but not in Cushing disease.
   b. Uncommon. Bitemporal hemianopia is uncommon with secreting pituitary tumours, which tend to present with systemic features of hypersecretion, as opposed to non-secreting pituitary tumours, which tend to present with chiasmal compression. Glaucoma may develop in susceptible individuals with iatrogenic Cushing syndrome.

Acromegaly

Acromegaly is caused by excessive growth hormone (GH) occurring during adult life, after epiphyseal closure and is almost invariably due to a secreting pituitary acidophil adenoma. (Hypersecretion of growth hormone in childhood, prior to epiphyseal closure, results in gigantism.)

1. **Presentation** is in the fourth to fifth decades.
2. **Signs**
   a. Skin. Hyperhidrosis, seborrhoea, acne and hirsutism in females.
   b. Face.
   – Coarseness of features with thick lips, exaggerated nasolabial folds and prominent supraorbital ridges (Fig. 24.46a).
   – Enlargement of the jaw (prognathism) with dental malocclusion.

   c. Enlargement of the head, hands, feet (Fig. 24.46b), tongue and internal organs.
3. **Complications** include osteoarthritis, carpal tunnel syndrome, cardiomyopathy, hypertension, respiratory disease, diabetes mellitus, gonadal dysfunction and neuropathy.
4. **Investigations.** The diagnosis may be confirmed by noting GH levels in response to an oral glucose tolerance test. Normal individuals manifest suppression of GH levels to below 2mU/L. However, in acromegaly, GH levels do not fall, and may paradoxically rise.
5. **Treatment** options include bromocriptine (a long-acting dopamine agonist), radiotherapy (external beam or by implantation of yttrium rods in the pituitary) and trans-sphenoidal hypophysectomy.
6. **Ophthalmic features**
   a. Common. Bitemporal hemianopia and optic atrophy.
   b. Rare. Angioid streaks and see-saw nystagmus of Maddox.

MYOPATHIES

Myasthenia gravis

Myasthenia gravis is an autoimmune disease in which antibodies mediate damage and destruction of acetylcholine receptors in striated muscle. The resultant impairment of neuromuscular conduction causes weakness and fatigue of skeletal musculature, but not of cardiac and involuntary muscles. The disease affects females twice as commonly as males and may be (a) *ocular*, (b) *bulbar* or (c) *generalized*.

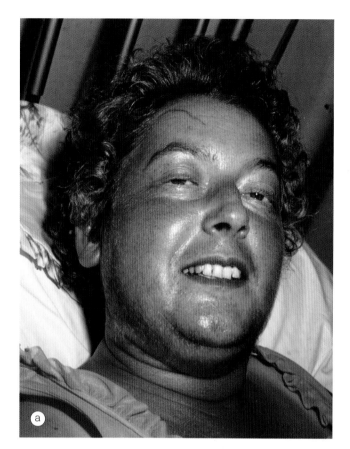

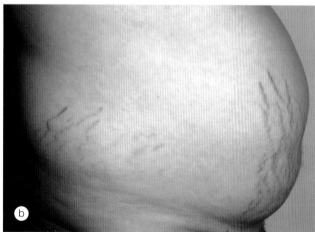

Fig. 24.45
Cushing disease. **(a)** Moon face, hyperpigmentation and hirsutism;
(b) obesity and cutaneous striae

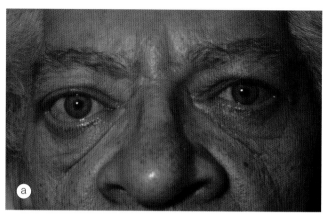

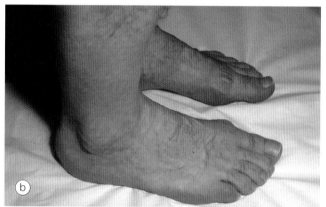

Fig. 24.46
Acromegaly. **(a)** Coarse facial features; **(b)** enlargement of the
feet

Systemic features

I. Presentation is most commonly in the third decade, but
may be at any time after the first year of life, most
frequently with ptosis or diplopia. Patients with generalized involvement then develop fatigue, often brought on
by exercise, which may be worse towards the end of the
day and provoked by infection or stress.

2. **Signs.** The most important feature is excessive fatigue
of muscles, affecting the limbs, facial expression, ocular
movements, mastication and speech.
   a. Peripheral
   – Weakness, particularly of the arms and proximal
     muscles of the legs.
   – Permanent myopathic wasting may occur in long-
     standing cases.
   b. Facial. Lack of expression (myopathic facies) and ptosis.
   c. Bulbar. Difficulties with swallowing (dysphagia),
     speaking (dysarthria) and chewing.
   d. Respiratory. Difficulty with breathing is rare but
     serious.

Investigations

- Positive edrophonium test (see below).
- Raised serum acetylcholine receptor antibody levels.
- Thoracic CT or MR to detect thymoma, which is present
  in 10% of patients. Patients under the age of 40 years
  without thymoma generally have a hyperplastic thymus;
  in older patients the thymus is usually normal (atrophic).

Treatment

Treatment options include anticholinesterase drugs (pyridostigmine, neostigmine), steroids, immunosuppressive drugs (azathioprine, ciclosporin), plasma exchange, intravenous immunoglobulins and thymectomy. Patients with pure ocular myasthenia are usually not helped by thymectomy.

Ocular features

Ocular involvement occurs in 90% of cases and is the presenting feature in 60%. Two-thirds of patients have both ptosis and diplopia. Less than 10% of patients have ptosis alone, and less than 30% have diplopia alone.

1. **Ptosis** is insidious, bilateral and frequently asymmetrical.
   - It is worse at the end of the day and least on awakening.
   - It is worse on prolonged up-gaze due to fatigue.
   - If one eyelid is elevated manually as the patient looks up, the fellow eyelid will show fine oscillatory movements.
   - Cogan twitch sign is a brief up-shoot of the eyelid as the eyes saccade from depression to the primary position.
   - Positive ice test (Fig. 24.47): the degree of ptosis improves after an ice pack is placed on the eyelid for 2 minutes. The test is negative in non-myasthenic ptosis.
2. **Diplopia** is frequently vertical, although any or all of the extraocular muscles may be affected. A pseudo-internuclear ophthalmoplegia may be seen. Patients with stable deviations may benefit from muscle surgery, botulinum toxin injection or a combination of both.
3. **Nystagmoid movements** may be present on extremes of gaze.

   NB Bizarre defects of ocular motility may occur; myasthenia should therefore be considered in the differential diagnosis of any ocular motility disorder that does not fit with a recognized diagnosis.

Edrophonium test

Edrophonium is a short-acting anticholinesterase which increases the amount of acetylcholine available at the neuromuscular junction. In myasthenia this results in transient improvement of symptoms and signs such as weakness, ptosis and diplopia. The estimated sensitivity is 85% in ocular and 95% in systemic myasthenia. Uncommon complications include bradycardia, loss of consciousness and even death. The test should therefore never be performed without an assistant, and a resuscitation trolley should also be close at hand in case of sudden cardiorespiratory arrest. The test is performed as follows (Fig. 24.48):

a. Objective baseline measurements are made of the ptosis or diplopia with a Hess test (see Chapter 20).

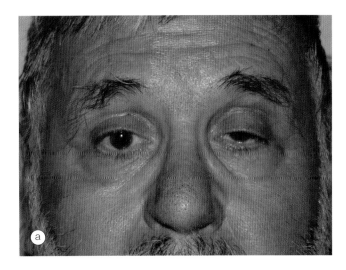

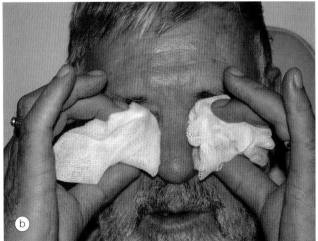

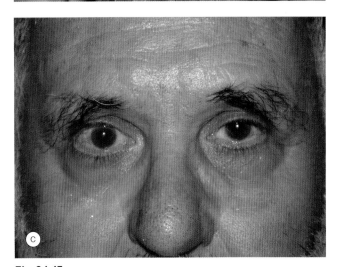

Fig. 24.47
Ice test in myasthenia gravis. **(a)** Asymmetrical ptosis; **(b)** application of ice; **(c)** improvement of ptosis (Courtesy of J Yanguela)

b. Intravenous injection of atropine 0.3mg is given to minimize muscarinic side-effects.

c. Intravenous test dose of 0.2ml (2mg) edrophonium hydrochloride is given. If definite symptomatic improvement is noted the test is terminated forthwith.

d. The remaining 0.8ml (8mg) is given after 60 seconds, provided there is no hypersensitivity.

e. Final measurements are made and the results compared, remembering that the effect lasts only 5 minutes.

Myotonic dystrophy

Myotonic dystrophy (dystrophia myotonica, Steinert disease) is characterized by delayed muscular relaxation after cessation of voluntary effort (myotonia). The gene locus is on 19q13.3.

1. **Inheritance** is AD.
2. **Presentation** is in the third to sixth decades with weakness of the hands and difficulty in walking. Successive generations exhibit progressively earlier onset and greater severity of disease, a phenomenon termed 'anticipation'.
3. **Signs**
   a. *Peripheral.* Difficulty in releasing grip, muscle wasting and weakness.
   b. *Central.* Mournful facial expression (Fig. 24.49) caused by bilateral facial wasting with hollow cheeks and slurred speech from involvement of the tongue and pharyngeal muscles.
   c. *Other.* Frontal baldness in males (Fig. 24.49), hypogonadism, mild endocrine abnormalities, cardiomyopathy, pulmonary disease, intellectual deterioration and bone changes.
4. **Investigations.** Electromyography shows myotonic and myopathic potentials. Serum creatine kinase is elevated.
5. **Treatment** involves exercise and prevention of contractures.
6. **Ophthalmic features**
   a. *Common.* Early-onset cataract and ptosis.
   b. *Uncommon.* External ophthalmoplegia, pupillary light-near dissociation, mild pigmentary retinopathy, bilateral optic atrophy and low intraocular pressure.

Kearns–Sayre syndrome

Kearns–Sayre syndrome is a mitochondrial cytopathy associated with mitochondrial DNA deletions. Histology of extraocular muscles shows ragged red fibres due to intramuscular accumulation of abnormal mitochondria (Fig. 24.50a).

1. **Presentation** is in the first to second decades with an insidious onset of bilateral ptosis and limitation of ocular movements in all directions of gaze (progressive external ophthalmoplegia – Fig. 24.50b, c and d).

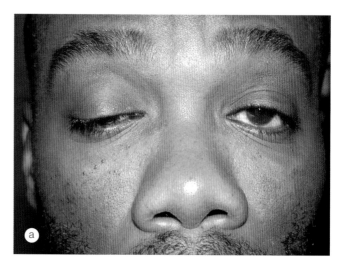
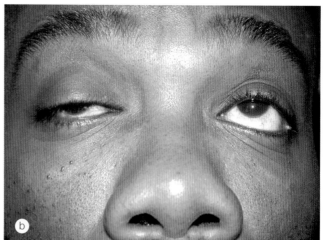
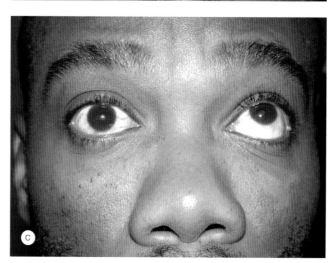

Fig. 24.48
Edrophonium test in myasthenia gravis. **(a)** Severe asymmetrical ptosis in the primary position; **(b)** defective upgaze; **(c)** following injection of edrophonium there is marked improvement of ptosis and modest improvement in upgaze of the left eye

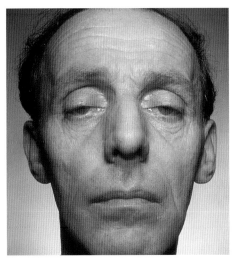

Fig. 24.49
Symmetrical ptosis, frontal baldness and a mournful facial
expression in myotonic dystrophy (Courtesy of M A Mir, from *Atlas
of Clinical Diagnosis*, Mosby, 2003)

2. Signs
- Ataxia and cardiac conduction defects.
- Fatigue and proximal muscle weakness are common.
- Deafness, diabetes, short stature and hypoparathyroidism may be present.
- Pigmentary retinopathy.

3. Diagnostic tests
- Lumbar puncture shows increased CSF protein concentration (> 1g/l).
- ECG demonstrates cardiac conduction defects.

NEUROLOGY

Multiple sclerosis

Multiple sclerosis (MS) is an idiopathic, remitting, demyelinating disease involving white matter within the CNS (Fig. 24.51a, b and c).

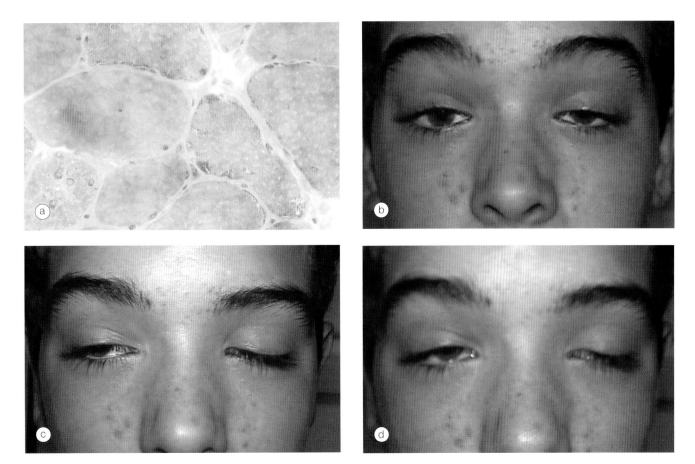

Fig. 24.50
Kearns–Sayre syndrome. **(a)** Histology shows ragged red fibres; **(b)** symmetrical ptosis in the primary position; **(c)** severe restriction of right gaze; **(d)** severe restriction of left gaze (Courtesy of J Harry and G Misson, from *Clinical Ophthalmic Pathology*, Butterworth-Heinemann, 2001 – fig. a; M Parulekar – figs b, c and d)

1. Presentation is in the third to fourth decade in one of two ways:

    a. Relapsing-remitting episodes of demyelination with complete or incomplete recovery is by far the most common. After 10 years about 50% of patients develop continuously progressive disease with occasional remissions.

    b. Progressive disease from the onset, without remissions, affects about 10% of patients and is very difficult to treat.

2. Signs

    a. Spinal cord. Weakness, stiffness, sphincter disturbance and sensory loss with a 'trouser-like' distribution.

    b. Brainstem. Diplopia, nystagmus, dysarthria and dysphagia.

    c. Cerebral hemisphere. Hemiparesis, hemianopia and dysphasia.

    d. Psychological. Intellectual decline, depression, euphoria and dementia.

    e. Transient features include Lhermitte sign (electrical sensation on neck flexion), dysarthria-dysequilibrium-diplopia syndrome and Uhthoff phenomenon (sudden worsening of vision or other symptoms on exercise or increase in body temperature).

3. Investigations

    a. Lumbar puncture shows leucocytosis, IgG level > 15% of total protein and oligoclonal bands on protein electrophoresis.

    b. MR shows ovoid periventricular and corpus callosum plaques with their long axes perpendicular to the ventricular margins (Fig. 24.51d). Acute demyelination plaques may be highlighted with gadolinium on T2-weighted scans.

4. Treatment options in selected cases include systemic steroids and interferon beta-1a.

5. Ophthalmic features

    a. Common. Retrobulbar neuritis, internuclearophthalmoplegia and nystagmus.

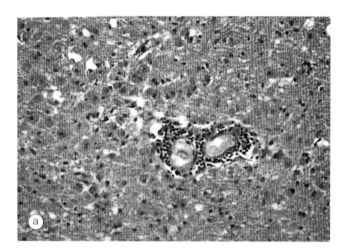

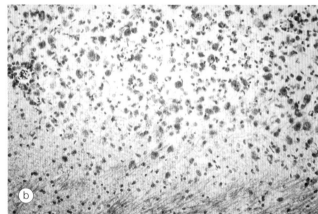

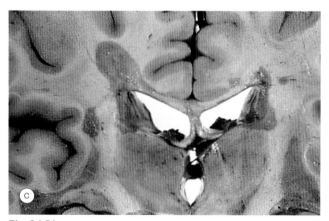

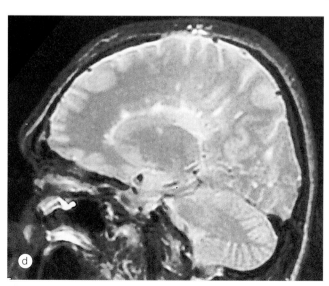

Fig. 24.51
Multiple sclerosis. **(a)** Histology shows a plaque with perivascular cuffing; **(b)** phagocytosis of myelin by macrophages; **(c)** demyelinating plaques in periventricular white matter; **(d)** MR T2-weighted sagittal view shows periventricular plaques (Courtesy of J Harry and G Misson, from *Clinical Ophthalmic Pathology*, Butterworth-Heinemann, 2001 – fig. b)

b. Uncommon. Skew deviation, ocular motor nerve palsies and hemianopia.

c. Rare. Intermediate uveitis and retinal periphlebitis.

Neurofibromatosis type 1

Neurofibromatosis is a disorder that primarily affects cell growth of neural tissues. Inheritance is AD with the gene locus on 17q11 with irregular penetrance and variable expressivity and a high mutation rate. The two main types are: (a) *type 1* (NF-1) and (b) *type 2* (NF-2). Both may show segmental involvement in which the features are confined to one or more body segments. NF-1 (von Recklinghausen disease) is the most common phacomatosis affecting 1:4000 individuals.

Diagnostic criteria

Two or more of the following signs must be present:
- Six or more café-au-lait macules over 5mm in greatest diameter in pre-pubertal children and over 15mm in greatest diameter in post-pubertal individuals.
- Two or more neurofibromas of any type or one plexiform neurofibroma.
- Axillary or inguinal freckling.
- Optic nerve glioma.
- Two or more Lisch spots (iris hamartomas).
- A distinctive osseous lesion such as sphenoid dysplasia or thinning of long bone cortex, with or without pseudoarthrosis.
- A first degree relative (parent, sibling, or offspring) with NF-1 by the above criteria.

Signs

1. **Intracranial tumours,** usually meningiomas and gliomas.
2. **Neurofibromas** may develop anywhere along the course of peripheral or autonomic nerves but do not occur on purely motor nerves. They may also involve internal organs.
   a. Discrete cutaneous neurofibromas are small, soft, violaceous nodules (Fig. 24.52a) or larger pedunculated flabby lesions (Fig. 24.52b).
   b. Nodular plexiform neurofibromas feel like a 'bag of worms' when palpated (Fig. 24.52c). Involvement of the eyelid gives rise to the characteristic S-shaped deformity (Fig. 24.52d).
   c. Diffuse plexiform neurofibromas may infiltrate widely and deeply into surrounding structures. Associated overgrowth of soft tissue and thick redundant folds of skin may result in considerable disfigurement (elephantiasis nervosa – Fig. 24.52e).

2. **Skeletal.** Short stature, mild macrocephaly (enlarged head), facial hemiatrophy, absence of the great wing of the sphenoid bone, scoliosis and thinning of long bone cortex.
3. **Skin**
   - Café-au-lait spots are light-brown macules most commonly found on the trunk (Fig. 24.52f). They appear during the first year of life and increase in size and number throughout childhood; teenagers and adults invariably have more than six.
   - Axillary or inguinal freckles usually become obvious around the age of 10 years and are pathognomonic.
4. **Associations** include malignancies, hypertension and mental handicap.

Ocular features

1. **Orbital** involvement may be caused by one of the following:
   a. Optic nerve glioma develops in about 15% of patients. It may be unilateral or bilateral and may extend posteriorly to involve the chiasm and hypothalamus.
   b. Other neural tumours: neurilemmoma, plexiform neurofibroma and meningioma.
   c. Spheno-orbital encephalocele is caused by absence of the greater wing of the sphenoid bone. It characteristically causes a pulsating proptosis, unassociated with either a bruit or a thrill.
2. **Eyelid neurofibromas,** which may be either nodular or plexiform, tend to develop early in life. When involving the upper lid, they frequently cause a mechanical ptosis.
3. **Iris lesions**
   a. Lisch nodules develop during the second to third decades and are eventually present in 95% of cases.
   b. Congenital ectropion uveae is uncommon and may be associated with glaucoma.
   c. Mammillations are rare.
4. **Prominent corneal nerves** may occur.
5. **Glaucoma** is relatively rare and, when present, is usually unilateral and congenital. About 50% of patients with glaucoma manifest ipsilateral neurofibroma of the upper eyelid and facial hemiatrophy.
6. **Fundus lesions**
   a. Choroidal naevi, which may be multifocal and bilateral, are common and carry an increased risk for the subsequent development of melanoma.
   b. Retinal astrocytomas, identical to those in tuberous sclerosis, are rare.

Neurofibromatosis type 2

Neurofibromatosis 2 (NF-2) is less common than NF-1. Inheritance is AD with the gene locus on 22q12.

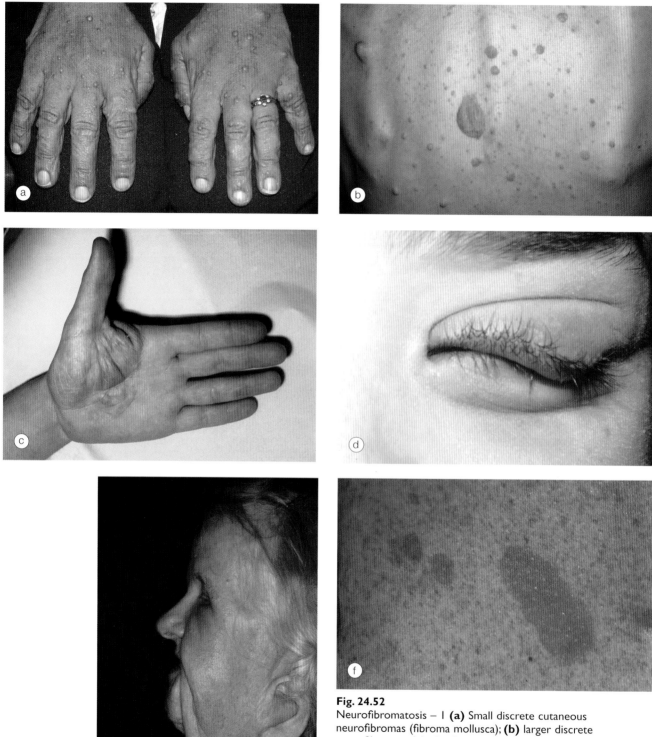

Fig. 24.52

Neurofibromatosis – I **(a)** Small discrete cutaneous neurofibromas (fibroma mollusca); **(b)** larger discrete neurofibromas; **(c)** plexiform neurofibroma; **(d)** plexiform neurofibroma causing an S-shaped eyelid deformity; **(e)** elephantiasis nervosa associated with a diffuse plexiform neurofibroma; **(f)** café-au-lait spots

Diagnostic criteria

1. **Bilateral acoustic neuroma** which usually present in the late teens or early twenties with hearing loss, tinnitus or imbalance (Fig. 24.53). Most acoustic neuromas are schwannomas arising from the vestibular nerve. In young patients tumour growth is invariably fast, whereas in older patients the lesion may be either slow- or fast-growing. Recent advances in microsurgical techniques have significantly improved the results of surgery. The gamma-knife (stereotactic radiotherapy) provides a therapeutic option.
2. **A patient with a first-degree relative with NF-2** who also has either a unilateral acoustic neuroma or two of the following: neurofibroma, meningioma, glioma, schwannoma or early-onset cataract.

Ophthalmic features

The following ocular lesions are often the first signs of the disease and may therefore assist in presymptomatic diagnosis:

1. **Cataract** affects about two-thirds of patients prior to the age of 30 years.
2. **Fundus lesions** consisting of combined hamartomas of the RPE and retina, and perifoveal epiretinal membranes are relatively common.
3. **Ocular motor defects** are present in about 10% of cases.
4. **Less common** findings include optic nerve sheath meningioma, optic nerve glioma, unilateral Lisch nodules and an abnormal electroretinogram.

Tuberous sclerosis

Tuberous sclerosis (Bourneville disease) is an AD phacomatosis characterized by the development of hamartomas in multiple organ systems from all primary germ layers. The classic triad of (a) *epilepsy*, (b) *mental retardation* and (c) *adenoma sebaceum* is only present in a minority of patients, but is diagnostic when present. About 60% of cases are sporadic and 40% are AD.

1. **Cutaneous signs**
   - Adenoma sebaceum, consisting of fibroangiomatous red papules with a butterfly distribution around the nose and cheeks, is universal (Fig. 24.54a).
   - Ash leaf spots are hypopigmented macules on the trunk (Fig. 24.54b), limbs and scalp. In infants with sparse skin pigmentation they are best detected using ultraviolet light, under which they fluoresce (Wood's lamp).
   - Confetti skin lesions.
   - Shagreen patches consist of diffuse thickening over the lumbar region (Fig. 24.54c).
   - Fibrous plaques on the forehead.
   - Skin tags (molluscum fibrosa pendulum).
   - Café-au-lait spots.
   - Subungual hamartomas (Fig. 24.54d).
2. **Neurological features**
   - Intracranial paraventricular (Fig. 24.54e) subependymal astrocytic nodules and giant cell astrocytomas hamartomas.
   - Mental retardation.
   - Seizures.

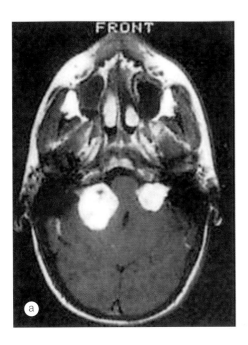
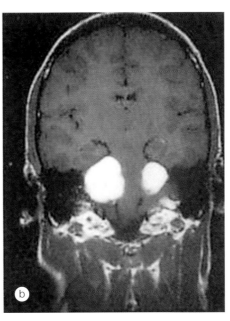

Fig. 24.53
MR with enhancement shows bilateral acoustic neuromas. **(a)** Axial view; **(b)** coronal view

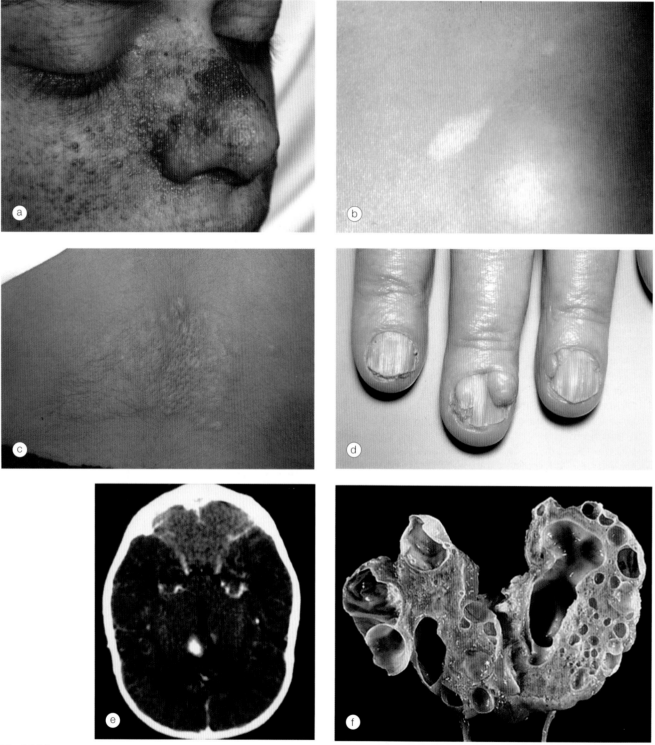

Fig. 24.54
Tuberous sclerosis. **(a)** Adenoma sebaceum; **(b)** ash leaf spots; **(c)** shagreen patch; **(d)** subungual hamartomas; **(e)** axial CT shows a periventricular astrocytic hamartoma at the left foramen of Munro; **(f)** renal cysts (Courtesy of N Rogers – fig. c; M A Mir, from *Atlas of Clinical Diagnosis*, Mosby, 2003 – fig. d; B J Zitelli and H W Davis, from *Atlas of Pediatric Physical Diagnosis*, Mosby, 2002 – fig. f)

3. **Visceral tumours**
   - Renal angiomyolipomas and cysts (Fig. 24.54f).
   - Cardiac rhabdomyomas.
   - Pulmonary lymphangiomatosis.
4. **Ocular features** are fundus astrocytomas, patchy iris hypopigmentation and atypical iris colobomas.

Sturge–Weber syndrome

Sturge–Weber syndrome (encephalotrigeminal angiomatosis) is a congenital, sporadic phacomatosis.

1. **Classification**
   - Trisystem disease involves the face, leptomeninges and eyes.
   - Bisystem disease involves the face and eyes or the face and leptomeninges.
2. **Signs**
   - Facial naevus flammeus (port-wine stain), extending over the area corresponding to the distribution of one or more (Fig. 24.55a) branches of the trigeminal nerve. The lesion is usually unilateral and occasionally bilateral.
   - Ipsilateral parietal or occipital leptomeningeal haemangioma (Fig. 24.55b) may cause contralateral or generalized focal or generalized seizures, hemiparesis or hemianopia.
3. **Ocular features** are ipsilateral glaucoma, episcleral haemangioma, diffuse choroidal haemangioma, and iris heterochromia.

Von-Hippel–Lindau syndrome

V-H-L is caused by a mutation of chromosome 3(3p25-p24). Inheritance is AD.

Clinical features

- CNS haemangioblastoma involving the cerebellum (Fig. 24.56), spinal cord, medulla or pons affects about 25% of patients with retinal tumours.
- Phaeochromocytoma.
- Renal cell carcinoma and pancreatic islet cell carcinoma.
- Cysts of the testes, kidneys, ovaries, lungs, liver and pancreas.
- Polycythaemia, which may be the result of factors released by a cerebellar or renal tumour.

Screening

Screening is vital because it is impossible to predict which patients with retinal haemangiomas will harbour systemic lesions. The ophthalmologist must therefore refer all such patients for systemic and neurological evaluation. Relatives should also be screened because of the dominant inheritance pattern. Apart from physical examination, the following screening protocol should be regularly performed in patients with established V-H-L and relatives at risk.

1. **Annual screening**
   - Physical examination.
   - Ophthalmoscopy from age 5 years, increased to 6-monthly from 10 to 30 years.
   - Renal ultrasonography from age 16 years.
   - 24-hour urine collection for estimation of vanillyl mandelic acid and catecholamine levels from age 10 years to detect phaeochromocytoma.
2. **Screening every 2 years** involves abdominal and brain MR from age 15 years.
3. **Genetic tests** are indicated in all patients with suspected disease and in first- and second-degree relatives. With modern techniques the sensitivity is almost 100%.

LEUKAEMIA

Classification

The leukaemias are malignancies of the haematopoietic stem cells. Acute leukaemias are characterized by replacement of bone marrow with very immature (blast) cells (Fig. 24.57a). Chronic leukaemias are associated, at least initially, with well-differentiated (mature) leucocytes (Fig. 24.57b) and occur almost exclusively in adults. The four major variants of leukaemia are:

1. **Acute lymphocytic** (lymphoblastic) that predominantly affects children; overall, 90% of cases respond to treatment and approximately 70% are cured.
2. **Acute myelocytic** (myeloblastic) is most frequently seen in older adults and is curable in 30% of those under the age of 60 years.
3. **Chronic lymphocytic** has a very chronic course and many patients die from an unrelated cause.
4. **Chronic myelocytic** has a progressive clinical course and a less favourable prognosis.

Systemic features

- Fever, night sweats and weight loss typically occur in chronic leukaemias.
- Anaemia resulting in tiredness, weakness and shortness of breath on exertion.
- Neutropenia may cause recurrent infections.
- Thrombocytopenia may cause purpura, easy bruising or bleeding, especially from the oral mucosa.
- Infiltrative features resulting in lymphadenopathy and hepatosplenomegaly typically occur in chronic leukaemia.

Ocular features

Ocular involvement is more commonly seen in the acute form and may involve virtually any ocular structure.

1. **Primary** or direct leukaemic infiltration may involve the uvea and orbit. Neuro-ophthalmic involvement may

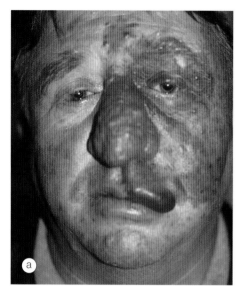

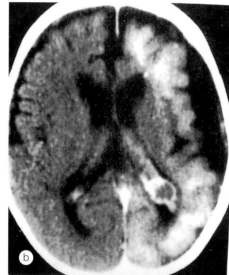

Fig. 24.55
Sturge–Weber syndrome. **(a)** Naevus flammeus; **(b)** axial CT shows an extensive meningeal haemangioma associated with cerebral atrophy (Courtesy of C D Forbes and W F Jackson, from *Color Atlas and Text of Clinical Medicine*, Mosby, 2003 – fig. b)

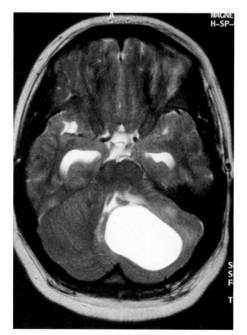

Fig. 24.56
Axial MR shows a cerebellar haemangioblastoma (Courtesy of A Singh)

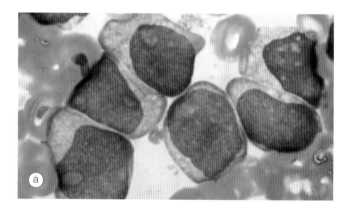

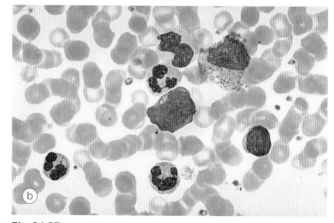

Fig. 24.57
(a) Myeloblasts in bone aspirate shows large nuclei with prominent nucleoli; two of the cells have purple Auer rods in the cytoplasm that are pathognomonic of acute myelocytic leukaemia; **(b)** peripheral blood smear in chronic myelocytic leukaemia shows all stages of maturity of the myeloid series at the same time (Courtesy of N Bienz)

result in optic neuropathy, cranial nerve palsies and papilloedema.

2. **Secondary** or indirect involvement may occur as a result of anaemia, thrombocytopenia and hyperviscosity. These may manifest as intraocular bleeding, infection and vascular occlusion.

Index